D0908568

Levin and O'Neal's

THE
DIABETIC
FOOT

Levin and O'Neal's

THE DIABETIC FOOT

SIXTH EDITION

EDITED BY

JOHN H. BOWKER, MD
Professor, Department of Orthopaedics and
  Rehabilitation
University of Miami School of Medicine
Director, Diabetic Foot and Amputee Services
Jackson Memorial Medical Center
Miami, Florida

MICHAEL A. PFEIFER, MD
Professor and Chief, Section of Endocrinology/
  Metabolism
Director, Diabetes and Obesity Center
Brody School of Medicine
East Carolina University
Greenville, North Carolina

With Forewords By

Paul W. Brand, MD • Gary W. Gibbons, MD • Fred W. Whitehouse, MD

Mosby
A *Harcourt Health Sciences* Company
St. Louis   Philadelphia   London   Sydney   Toronto

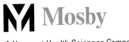

A Harcourt Health Sciences Company

Acquisitions Editor: Kimberley Cox
Production Manager: Donna L. Morrissey

SIXTH EDITION
Copyright © 2001, 1993, 1988, 1983, 1977, 1973 by Mosby, Inc.

Mosby, Inc.
A Harcourt Health Sciences Company
11830 Westline Industrial Drive
St. Louis, Missouri 63146

Printed in the United States of America

Library of Congress Cataloging-in-Publication Data

Levin and O'Neal's The diabetic foot.—6th ed. / edited by John H. Bowker, Michael A. Pfeifer.
   p.   cm.
   Previous editions entered under: The diabetic foot.
   Includes bibliographical references and index.
   ISBN 1–55664–471–X
   1. Foot—Diseases. 2. Diabetes—Complications. 3. Foot—Surgery. I. Bowker, John H.
II. Pfeifer, Michael A. III. Diabetic foot. IV. Title.

RC951.D53 2001
617.5'85—dc21

00-041142

Dedicated to our wives

Alice Bowker and Sonya Pfeifer,
and to our children
Thomas Bowker, and
Katie, Noel, Susan, Ben,
Jake and Zack Pfeifer

with heartfelt gratitude for their support and forbearance
during the long development of this volume

CONTRIBUTORS

JESSIE H. AHRONI, Ph.D., A.R.N.P., C.D.E.
Clinical Faculty, Department of Biobehavioral
Nursing and Health Systems, University of
Washington School of Nursing; Research Nurse
Practitioner and Project Manager, The Seattle
Diabetic Foot Study, Seattle, Washington
Lower Limb Self-Management Education

JAMES E. AIKENS, Ph.D.
Assistant Professor of Clinical Psychiatry,
University of Chicago; Staff Attending
Psychologist, University of Chicago Physician's
Group, Chicago, Illinois
*Psychosocial and Psychological Aspects of
Diabetic Foot Complications*

BRENT T. ALLEN, M.D.,
Vascular Surgeon, Partner, Suburban Surgical
Associates, St. Louis, Missouri
*The Role of Vascular Surgery in the
Diabetic Patient*

JOSEPH C. BENACCI, M.D.
Attending Surgeon, Department of Plastic and
Reconstructive Surgery, Lahey Clinic Medical
Center, Burlington, Massachusetts
*Plastic Surgical Reconstruction of the
Diabetic Foot*

ANDREW J.M. BOULTON, M.D., F.R.C.P.
Professor of Medicine, University of
Manchester; Consultant Physician, Manchester
Royal Infirmary, Manchester, United Kingdom
*Diabetic Foot Problems and their
Management Around the World*

JOHN H. BOWKER, M.D.
Professor, Department of Orthopaedics and
Rehabilitation, University of Miami School of
Medicine; Director, Diabetic Foot and Amputee
Services, Jackson Memorial Medical Center,
Miami, Florida
*Minor and Major Lower Limb Amputation
in Persons with Diabetes Mellitus;*

*Organizing an Education-Based Diabetic
Foot Clinic*

JAMES W. BRODSKY, M.D.
Clinical Professor of Orthopaedic Surgery,
University of Texas Southwestern Medical
School, and Director, Foot and Ankle Surgery
Fellowship Program, Baylor University Medical
Center and University of Texas Southwestern
Medical School, Dallas, Texas
*An Improved Method for Staging and
Classification of Foot Lesions in
Diabetic Patients*

GREGORY M. CAPUTO, M.D.
Professor of Medicine, College of Medicine, The
Pennsylvania State University, University
Park, Pennsylvania; Chief, Division of General
Internal Medicine, Milton S. Hershey Medical
Center, Hershey, Pennsylvania
*The Biomechanics of the Foot in
Diabetes Mellitus*

MOLLY C. CARR, M.D.
Senior Fellow, Department of Medicine,
Division of Metabolism, Endocrinology and
Nutrition, University of Washington, Seattle,
Washington
*Medical Management of Diabetic Patients
During the Perioperative Period*

PETER R. CAVANAGH, Ph.D.
Distinguished Professor of Kinesiology,
Department of Kinesiology, The Pennsylvania
State University, University Park;
Distinguished Professor of Medicine, and
Orthopaedics and Rehabilitation, College of
Medicine, The Pennsylvania State University,
Hershey; Distinguished Professor of
Biobehavioral Health, Department of
Biobehavioral Health, The Pennsylvania State
University, University Park; Director, The
Center for Locomotion Studies, and Director of
Research, Diabetes Foot Clinic, The
Pennsylvania State University, University

Park, Pennsylvania; Director of Research,
Diabetes Foot Clinic, The Pennsylvania State
University, Hershey, Pennsylvania
*The Biomechanics of the Foot in
Diabetes Mellitus*

KARL S. CHIANG, M.D.
Clinical Associate Professor of Radiology,
Section of Vascular and Interventional
Radiology, Brody School of Medicine, East
Carolina University; Eastern Radiologists, Inc.,
Greenville, North Carolina
*Radiologic Intervention in Diabetic
Peripheral Vascular Disease*

PAUL CIANCI, M.D.
Professor of Medicine Emeritus, University of
California, Davis, Davis; Medical Director,
Department of Hyperbaric Medicine, Doctors
Medical Center, San Pablo, John Muir Medical
Center, Walnut Creek, and St. Francis
Memorial Hospital, San Francisco, California
*Adjunctive Hyperbaric Oxygen Therapy in
the Treatment of the Diabetic Foot Wound*

CURTIS R. CLARK, P.T.
Assistant Chief Physical Therapist, Medical/
Surgical Unit, University of Miami/Jackson
Memorial Hospital, Miami, Florida
Rehabilitation of the Diabetic Amputee

WILLIAM C. COLEMAN, D.P.M.
Section Head of Podiatry, Department of
Orthopedics, Ochsner Clinic, New Orleans,
Louisiana
*Footwear for Injury Prevention: Correlation
with Risk Category*

JOHN A. COLWELL, M.D., Ph.D.
Professor of Medicine, and Director, Diabetes
Center, Medical University of South Carolina;
Medical University Hospital, Charleston, South
Carolina
*Atherosclerosis and Thrombosis in Diabetes
Mellitus: New Aspects of Pathogenesis*

KENRICK J. DENNIS, D.P.M.
Volunteer Clinical Faculty, University of Texas
Health Science Center at San Antonio, San
Antonio; Private Practice, Houston, Texas
Role of the Podiatrist

DOROTHY B. DOUGHTY, M.N., R.N., F.N.P.,
C.W.O.C.N.
Director, Wound Ostomy Continence Nursing
Education Center, Emory University, Atlanta,
Georgia
Role of the Wound Care Nurse

NANCY ELFTMAN, C.O., C.Ped.
Guest Lecturer, California State University-
Domingues Hills, Carson, and Rancho Los
Amigos Medical Center, Downey; Certified
Orthotist, Martin Luther King Jr./Drew Medical
Center, Los Angeles, Rancho Los Amigos
Medical Center, Downey, and University of
Southern California University Hospital, Los
Angeles, California
*Alternative Weight Redistribution Methods
in the Treatment of Neuropathic Ulcers*

LOIS S. FINNEY, R.D., M.P.H., C.D.E.
Fairview University Medical Center,
Minneapolis, Minnesota
*Nutritional Issues in the Patient with
Diabetes and Foot Ulcers*

ANDREW J. FISHER, M.D.
Radiologist, Radiology Imaging Associates,
Denver, Colorado
Imaging of the Diabetic Foot

JOHN J. FRANK, J.D.
Professor of Law, (Trial Practice), and Ethics,
St. Louis University School of Law, St. Louis,
Missouri
*Medicolegal Aspects of Care and Treatment
of the Diabetic Foot*

JOSEPH A. FRANK, J.D.
Board of Governors, Missouri Association of
Trial Attorneys, St. Louis, Missouri
*Medicolegal Aspects of Care and Treatment
of the Diabetic Foot*

ROBERT G. FRYKBERG, D.P.M., M.P.H.
Dean for Clinical Affairs, Des Moines
University College of Podiatric Medicine and
Surgery, Des Moines, Iowa
Charcot Neuroarthropathy of the Foot

ROBERT S. GAILEY Jr., Ph.D., P.T.
Assistant Professor, Department of
Orthopaedics and Rehabilitation, Division of
Physical Therapy, University of Miami School
of Medicine, Coral Gables, Florida
Rehabilitation of the Diabetic Amputee

LOUIS A. GILULA, M.D.
Professor of Radiology, Orthopedic Surgery, and
Plastic and Reconstructive Surgery,
Mallinckrodt Institute of Radiology, St. Louis,
Missouri
Imaging of the Diabetic Foot

DOUGLAS A. GREENE, M.D.
Professor, Taubman Health Care Center,
University of Michigan, Ann Arbor, Michigan
*Neuropathic Problems of the Lower
Extremities in Diabetic Patients*

LINDA B. HAAS, Ph.C., R.N., C.D.E.
Assistant Clinical Professor, University of
Washington School of Nursing; Endocrinology
Clinical Nurse Specialist, Veterans Affairs
Puget Sound Health Care System, Seattle,
Washington
Lower Limb Self-Management Education

LAWRENCE B. HARKLESS, D.P.M.
Professor, Department of Orthopaedics, and
Louis T. Bogy Professor of Podiatric Medicine
and Surgery; Director, Podiatry Residency
Training Program, University of Texas Health
Science Center at San Antonio, San Antonio,
Texas
Role of the Podiatrist

FALLS B. HERSHEY, M.D.
Emeritus, St. John's Mercy Medical Center,
Creve Coeur, Missouri
*Noninvasive Vascular Testing: Basis,
Application, and Role in Evaluating
Diabetic Peripheral Arterial Disease*

IRL B. HIRSCH, M.D.
Associate Professor of Medicine and Medical
Director, Diabetes Care Center, University of
Washington, Seattle, Washington
*Medical Management of Diabetic Patients
During the Perioperative Period*

MICHAEL Y. HU, M.D.
Vascular Surgeon, General and Vascular
Surgery Consultants, Abbott Northwestern
Hospital, Minneapolis, Minnesota
*The Role of Vascular Surgery in the
Diabetic Patient*

THOMAS K. HUNT, M.D.
Professor of Surgery, University of California,
San Francisco, San Francisco, California
*Adjunctive Hyperbaric Oxygen Therapy in
the Treatment of the Diabetic Foot Wound*

JOSEPH J. HURLEY, M.D.
Associate Professor, St. Louis University, St.
Louis; Chief, Section of Vascular Surgery, and
Director of Blood Flow Laboratory, St. John's
Mercy Medical Center, Creve Coeur, Missouri
*Noninvasive Vascular Testing: Basis,
Application, and Role in Evaluating
Diabetic Peripheral Arterial Disease*

DENNIS J. JANISSE, C.Ped.
Clinical Assistant Professor, Department of
Physical Medicine and Rehabilitation, Medical
College of Wisconsin; President and Chief
Executive Officer, National Pedorthic Services,
Inc., Milwaukee, Wisconsin
Pedorthic Care of the Diabetic Foot

J.E. JELINEK, M.D.
Clinical Professor of Dermatology, New York
University Medical Center; Attending
Physician, Dermatology, New York Hospital-
Tisch, New York, New York
Cutaneous Aspects of Diabetes Mellitus

JEFFREY E. JOHNSON, M.D.
Associate Professor, Department of Orthopaedic
Surgery, and Chief, Foot and Ankle Service,
Washington University School of Medicine;
Chief, Foot and Ankle Service, Barnes-Jewish
Hospital, St. Louis, Missouri
*Charcot Neuropathy of the Foot:
Surgical Aspects*

RUDOLF J. JOKL, M.D.
Assistant Professor, Endocrinology-Diabetes
Medical Genetics, Medical University of South
Carolina, Charleston, South Carolina
*Atherosclerosis and Thrombosis in Diabetes
Mellitus: New Aspects of Pathogenesis*

MATTHEW JUNG, M.D.
Staff, Vascular and Endovascular Surgeon,
Baptist Hospital East, Louisville, Kentucky
*Noninvasive Vascular Testing: Basis,
Application, and Role in Evaluating
Diabetic Peripheral Arterial Disease*

ALLAN KHOURY, M.D., Ph.D.
Associate Medical Director for Medical
Information and Clinical Innovation, Ohio
Permanente Medical Group, Cleveland; Staff
Internist, Lake Hospital, Willoughby, Ohio
*Improvements in Diabetic Foot Care with
Clinical Information Systems*

RICHARD L. KLEIN, Ph.D.
Assistant Professor, Department of Medicine,
Medical University of South Carolina; Research
Scientist, Veterans Affairs Medical Center,
Charleston, South Carolina
*Atherosclerosis and Thrombosis in Diabetes
Mellitus: New Aspects of Pathogenesis*

DIANE L. KRASNER, Ph.D., R.N., C.E.T.N.,
C.W.S., F.A.A.N.
Adjunct Associate Professor, The Johns Hopkins
University School of Nursing; Clinical Nurse
Specialist for WOCN, Greater Baltimore
Medical Center, Baltimore, Maryland
*Diabetic Foot Ulcer Care: Assessment
and Management*

JANICE F. LALIKOS, M.D.
Assistant Professor of Surgery, Division of
Plastic and Reconstructive Surgery, Brody
School of Medicine, East Carolina University;
Plastic Surgeon, University Health Systems of

Eastern Carolina, Pitt County Memorial
Hospital, Greenville, North Carolina
*Plastic Surgical Reconstruction of the
Diabetic Foot*

PATRICK LANDERS, D.P.M.
Associate Professor of Surgery, Ohio College of
Podiatric Medicine, Cleveland; Staff Podiatrist
and Chief of Section Podiatry for Kaiser
Permanente, SUMMA Health Care Systems,
Akron, and Cleveland Clinic Foundation,
Cleveland, Ohio
*Improvements in Diabetic Food Care with
Clinical Information Systems*

MARVIN E. LEVIN, M.D.
Professor of Clinical Medicine, and Associate
Director of The Diabetes, Endocrinology, and
Metabolism Clinic, Washington University
School of Medicine, St. Louis, Missouri
*Pathogenesis and General Management of
Foot Lesions in the Diabetic Patient*

BENJAMIN A. LIPSKY, M.D., F.A.C.P.,
F.I.D.S.A.
Professor of Medicine, University of Washington
School of Medicine; Director, General Internal
Medicine Clinic, and Head, Infection Control
Program, Veterans Affairs Puget Sound Health
Care System, Seattle, Washington
*Infectious Problems of the Foot in
Diabetic Patients*

MARIA F. LOPES-VIRELLA, M.D., Ph.D.
Professor of Medicine and Pathology,
Department of Medicine, Division of
Endocrinology, Diabetes, and Medical Genetics,
Medical University of South Carolina; Staff
Physician, Veterans Affairs Medical Center,
Charleston, South Carolina
*Atherosclerosis and Thrombosis in Diabetes
Mellitus: New Aspects of Pathogenesis*

PATRICK J. LUSTMAN, Ph.D.
Professor of Medical Psychology, Department of
Psychiatry, Washington University School of
Medicine; Staff Psychologist, Barnes Hospital/
BJC Health System, St. Louis, Missouri
*Psychosocial and Psychological Aspects of
Diabetic Foot Complications*

TIMOTHY J. LYONS, M.D.
Associate Professor of Medicine, Medical
University of South Carolina, Charleston, South
Carolina
*Atherosclerosis and Thrombosis in Diabetes
Mellitus: New Aspects of Pathogenesis*

STEPHEN A. McCLAVE, M.D.
Professor of Medicine, Department of Medicine,
Division of Gastroenterology and Hepatology,

University of Louisville School of Medicine,
Louisville, Kentucky
*Nutritional Issues in the Patient with
Diabetes and Foot Ulcers*

KEVIN W. McENERY, M.D.
Assistant Professor of Radiology, University of
Texas-MD Anderson Cancer Center, Houston,
Texas
Imaging of the Diabetic Foot

DONALD E. McMILLAN, M.D., A.B.
Research Professor of Engineering, Professor
Emeritus of Internal Medicine, and Professor
Emeritus of Physiology, University of South
Florida; Staff Physician, Family Health Center,
Tampa, Florida
Hemorheology: Principles and Concepts

MICHAEL J. MUELLER, Ph.D., P.T.
Associate Professor, Program in Physical
Therapy, Washington University School of
Medicine, St. Louis, Missouri
*Total-Contact Casting in the Treatment of
Neuropathic Ulcers*

LAWRENCE W. O'NEAL, M.D., F.A.C.S.
Emeritus Clinical Professor of Surgery, St.
Louis University School of Medicine, St. Louis,
Missouri
*Surgical Pathology of the Foot and
Clinicopathologic Correlations*

MICHAEL A. PFEIFER, M.D., M.S.
Professor of Medicine, Section of Endocrinology/
Metabolism, and Director, Diabetes Center and
Obesity Center, Brody School of Medicine, East
Carolina University, Greenville, North Carolina
*Neuropathic Problems of the Lower
Extremities in Diabetic Patients*

GAYLE E. REIBER, Ph.D., M.P.H.
Associate Professor, Departments of Health
Services and Epidemiology, University of
Washington; Research Career Scientist,
Veterans Affairs Puget Sound Health Care
System, Seattle, Washington
*Epidemiology of Foot Ulcers and
Amputations in the Diabetic Foot*

MARK ROTH, M.D.
Senior Instructor in Medicine, Case Western
Reserve University College of Medicine; Staff
Internist, Ohio Permanente Medical Group,
Cleveland Clinic Foundation, Cleveland, Ohio
*Improvements in Diabetic Foot Care with
Clinical Information Systems*

RICHARD R. RUBIN, Ph.D.
Assistant Professor in Medicine and Pediatrics,

The Johns Hopkins University School of
Medicine, Baltimore, Maryland
Empowerment in Amputation Prevention

LEE J. SANDERS, D.P.M.
Adjunct Clinical Professor, Temple University
School of Podiatric Medicine, Philadelphia;
Chief, Podiatry Section, Acute Care and
Specialty Service, Department of Veteran's
Affairs Medical Center, Lebanon, Pennsylvania
Charcot Neuroarthropathy of the Foot

THOMAS P. SAN GIOVANNI, M.D.
Institute of Orthopaedic Specialists, Bay Harbor
Islands, Florida
*Minor and Major Lower Limb Amputation
in Persons with Diabetes Mellitus*

V. KATHLEEN SATTERFIELD, D.P.M.
Assistant Professor, Orthopaedics Department,
Director of Academic Affairs, Podiatry
Residency Training Program, and Director of
Research Division, Podiatry Department,
University of Texas Health Science Center at
San Antonio, San Antonio, Texas
Role of the Podiatrist

MARY P. SCHUMER, M.S.
Research Instructor, Brody School of Medicine,
East Carolina University, Greenville, North
Carolina
*Neuropathic Problems of the Lower
Extremities in Diabetic Patients*

R. GARY SIBBALD, M.D., F.R.C.P.C. (Med),
F.R.C.P.C. (Derm)
Associate Professor of Medicine, and Director,
Continuing Medical Education, Department of
Medicine, University of Toronto; Director,
Dermatology Day Care, Sunnybrook Womens
College Healthcare System, Toronto, Ontario
*Diabetic Foot Ulcer Care: Assessment
and Management*

DAVID R. SINACORE, Ph.D., P.T.
Assistant Professor, Program in Physical
Therapy, and Research Instructor, Division of
Geriatrics and Gerontology, Department of
Internal Medicine, Washington University
School of Medicine, St. Louis, Missouri
*Total-Contact Casting in the Treatment of
Neuropathic Ulcers*

JAY S. SKYLER, M.D.
Professor of Medicine, Pediatrics and
Psychology and Director, Division of
Endocrinology, Diabetes and Metabolism,
University of Miami School of Medicine, Miami,
Florida
*Diabetes Mellitus: Old Assumptions and
New Realities*

DAVID L. STEED, M.D.
Professor of Surgery, University of Pittsburgh
School of Medicine, Pittsburgh, Pennsylvania
Modulating Wound Healing in Diabetes

ROBERT J. TANENBERG, M.D., F.A.C.P.
Professor of Medicine, Brody School of
Medicine, East Carolina University, Greenville,
North Carolina
*Neuropathic Problems of the Lower
Extremities in Diabetic Patients*

MICHAEL D. TRIPP, M.D.
Clinical Associate Professor of Radiology,
Section of Vascular and Interventional
Radiology, Brody School of Medicine, East
Carolina University; Eastern Radiologists, Inc.,
Greenville, North Carolina
*Radiologic Intervention in Diabetic
Peripheral Vascular Disease*

JAN S. ULBRECHT, M.D.
Associate Professor of Biobehavioral Health,
College of Health and Human Development,
and Associate Director, General Clinical
Research Center, The Pennsylvania State
University, University Park; Associate Professor
of Clinical Medicine, College of Medicine, The
Pennsylvania State University, Hershey,
Pennsylvania
*The Biomechanics of the Foot in
Diabetes Mellitus*

LORETTA VILEIKYTE, M.D., M.Sc.
Clinical Research Fellow, Departments of
Medicine and Behavioral Sciences, University of
Manchester, and Diabetes Unit, Manchester
Royal Infirmary, Manchester, United Kingdom
*Diabetic Foot Problems and their
Management Around the World*

NANCY P. WADE, B.S.N., M.H.M.
Rehabilitation Clinician, Orthopaedic,
Rehabilitation and Neurology Division, Jackson
Memorial Medical Center, Miami, Florida
*Organizing an Educated-Based Diabetic
Foot Clinic*

WILLIAM J. WISHNER, M.D.
Clinical Professor of Medicine, Division of
Diabetes and Endocrinology, Indiana University
School of Medicine, Indianapolis, Indiana
Empowerment in Amputation Prevention

WILLIAM A. WOODEN, M.D.
Associate Professor of Surgery and Vice
Chairman of Surgery, Division of Plastic and
Reconstructive Surgery, Brody School of

Medicine, East Carolina University; Plastic
Surgeon, University Health Systems of Eastern
Carolina, Pitt County Memorial Hospital,
Greenville, North Carolina
  *Plastic Surgical Reconstruction of the
  Diabetic Foot*

JOHN J. WOODS, Jr., M.D.
Vascular Surgeon, St. John's Mercy Medical
Center, Creve Coeur, Missouri
  *Noninvasive Vascular Testing: Basis,
  Application, and Role in Evaluating
  Diabetic Peripheral Arterial Disease*

FOREWORD

Having been retired from the practice of medicine for 10 years and having been previously in the forefront of the battle to save the diabetic foot from amputation and to emphasize the techniques that were critical in this battle, it is now quite a privilege to be invited to look over the newest edition of the book to which I was once a contributor and to comment on the general direction of change in our profession. It is good to see that the present edition has enlarged beyond the previous one, which in its turn was double the size of the last edition to which I contributed. This means that new ideas continue to arise and need to be recorded and that new areas of specialization have been invoked to take care of the disease itself, the mechanical impact of footwear on the insensitive foot, changes in the vascular supply, and many other areas.

I think that the most important trend I see as we proceed from the old volumes to the new is the increased emphasis on the *team approach.* In this new edition, the team concept has been dignified by having a whole section devoted to it, made up of chapters by contributors from many disciplines. From my own experience I would say that the most important emphasis of all is the recognition that the patient is the most important member of the team. No matter how qualified the other members are, and no matter how ingenious the new techniques, if the patient does not believe they can master the problem and keep their own feet intact for the rest of their life, everything else will be a failure. Thus, each member of the team, in bringing their own particular expertise to bear upon the problems of the diabetic foot, has to remember that their most important contribution is to convince the patient's own mind of the significance of what they advise and to in-volve him or her in the implementation of the program.

Well-designed shoes with pressure-equalizing insoles are useful, but only if they are actually worn every time the patient walks. Diets for the diabetic may be designed with perfection but not only must they be eaten and drunk, the patient must be sufficiently convinced to eat and drink nothing else!

In my own field of biomechanics I used to find it very satisfying to use multiple transducers to record and display graphic images of pressure profiles of the foot in reference to footwear. However, the problem was and is that quite moderate pressures that are acceptable for a few hundred steps may be dangerous after tens of thousands of steps during the day. It is *repetitive* steps and *repetitive* pressure that lowers the threshold for breakdown of the foot. Breakdown is slowly approached through a stage of traumatic inflammation of the tissues that not only increases fragility of the tissue under stress but also concentrates more pressure there because localized swelling is part of inflammation.

Unfortunately, both pressure measurement and the counting of steps per day are beyond the capability of the average patient.

I began to have much better success when I was able to get the patients to look for signs of inflammation at points of stress on their own feet. There is nothing so useful as a skin thermometer to monitor the gradual onset of traumatic inflammation in the foot because it teaches the patient on a daily basis to recognize whether his or her activity that day has been within safe limits.

When my patients understood that on a day-to-day basis the evening temperature of the foot was always an objective statement of what the day's activity had done to them and was a safe guide for future management, then I could relax. Only then did I feel that their feet were safe. Such patients were willing to keep a little thermistor or thermocouple beside their bed. Checking their own temperatures gave my patients a sense of control. That is the secret of success.

In many cases one should include the spouse along with the patient in this type of educational exercise because they are the only other member of the team who is likely to be present every night at the time the shoes are taken off, and it may be easier for them to check the sole of the foot.

I congratulate Drs. Bowker and Pfeifer and their collaborators on the extra emphasis on the team approach. I hope this fine book will continue for many more editions.

Paul W. Brand, M.D.

FOREWORD

The fact that the incidence of diabetes mellitus is increasing and that 15% of diabetics will develop a foot ulcer during their lifetime dramatizes the need for appropriate preventative and management strategies, especially education. Foot ulcer with sequelae such as chronic nonhealing wounds, osteomyelitis, and amputation is a costly complication in both health care expenditures and quality of life. With ever-decreasing health care dollars, health care professionals must educate, prevent, diagnose, and treat problems in the most appropriate, efficient, and cost-effective way. This is best accomplished by practicing evidence-based medicine.

As I have said previously, new knowledge is meaningless unless presented effectively so that it can be understood. The editors of the sixth edition of *The Diabetic Foot* have incorporated the expertise of recognized authorities on all aspects of diabetic lower limb care, assimilating the most current knowledge and concentrating on fundamentals and evidence-based clinical approaches. Today's practice is overwhelming: so many publications on how to do it, new technologies, and new products and concepts, especially dressings and wound care. No wonder there are still wide variations in practice and amputation rates. The sixth edition of *The Diabetic Foot* helps to eliminate anecdotes and misconceptions related to management of the diabetic lower limb. Recognizing a need, the editors added new chapters and authors as well as expanding previous topics to create a multidisciplinary text that has enormous value to all health care professionals interested in caring for diabetic patients with problems of the lower leg and foot. The new edition addresses the patient with a problem (not just focusing on the foot) with input from all over the world.

Although I am a surgeon, and vascular specialist, in my 27 years at our institution, we have practiced as a multidisciplinary team. Clearly recognizing that no one discipline can solve the multidimensional nature of the diabetic patient with a lower limb problem, we all bring strengths to achieve our goal of healing, returning patients to function, well-being, their families and community, and preventing amputation. It has always been our belief that quality of care is the best way to reduce the cost of care.

Gary W. Gibbons, M.D.

FOREWORD

In 1954, my first assignment as a new Fellow at the Joslin Clinic was to organize Foot Rounds. Held on Deaconess Ward 2 every Monday morning, we Fellows presented our "foot cases." Our eight beds were always filled. Attendees included Joslin senior staff led by Dr. Elliott P. Joslin himself, nurses, podiatrists, general surgeons, an orthopedic surgeon, and the Joslin Fellows. We discussed each patient in depth, documenting new decisions and noting progress or lack of progress. No one used the term "multidisciplinary," but what a way to learn how important foot care is to the diabetic patient! And what better way to optimize quality in foot care.

Later, also as a Fellow, I learned the greater importance of *preventing* the foot lesion that would surely lead to Deaconess 2. I understood the importance of properly fitting shoes, the dangers of walking barefoot, the need to avoid applied heat and chemical astringents and unguents, and the reason for regular visits to a foot care specialist, for callus and nail care and, at times, prophylactic surgery. Prior to antibiotics, cellulitis of the foot with lymphangiitis meant amputation. We had the limb-saving measures of early use of antibiotics, early bed rest to decrease local trauma, the aggressive control of hyperglycemia to ensure adequate leukocyte function, and careful local debridement by an experienced surgeon. All measures to "save or salvage a foot."

Great strides in foot care have occurred since those days on Deaconess 2: newer antibiotics that penetrate bone better and overcome resistant organisms, more accurate assessment of polymicrobial infections, and the miracles of better blood supply successfully achieved by vascular surgeons. Their distal grafts seem to tie into smaller and smaller vessels—microsurgery at its best. We and our patients are also grateful to the diagnostic radiologists who more accurately pinpoint the presence of infected bone and chart its progress. Orthopedic and podiatric devices and rehabilitative skills permit earlier ambulation, less loss of job time, and an improved quality of life.

All these approaches and much more have been brought up-to-date in this sixth edition of *The Diabetic Foot.* Drs. Bowker and Pfeifer along with Drs. Levin and O'Neal have mustered an outstanding group of authors to address their areas of expertise, areas that require the touch of the experienced specialist. This book emphasizes the critical need for professional (and patient) education. The professional care team (care of a "diabetic foot" requires a multidisciplinary team as we had in 1954 on Deaconess 2) includes, among others, the primary care physician, the podiatrist, often a nurse care manager, the radiologist and, when required, a vascular surgeon, orthopedist, and a physical medicine expert. At my institution, an infectious disease specialist is another key player. Without identifying the colonizing bacteria and how best to eradicate their influence, we would be no further ahead now than we were prior to World War II.

When a person with diabetes calls me with a foot problem, I say, "One look is worth a thousand words." The patient reports for an examination within 24 hours. The novel Semmes-Weinstein 5.07, 10-gm nylon filament examination, if performed regularly and properly, will identify the patient at high risk for foot ulceration. These people require intensified education in the self-care of the foot as well as a barefoot examination at each

xvii

office visit. Without looking at the feet, no one is prepared to prevent a foot problem. See your patients after they have removed their shoes and stockings.

This text belongs in the office of any provider who sees diabetic people either in a primary care capacity or as a relevant specialist. In particular, the family physician, the internist, the diabetologist, and the nurse care manager must be familiar with much that dwells within this book. Hardly any service to a diabetic patient, simple as it may seem, pays greater dividends than quality foot care. Outcomes of quality care include less grief to the patient, a feeling of achievement for the provider, lower hospital use, and happier fiscal officers, especially those in managed care organizations.

Read *The Diabetic Foot* as an encyclopedic reference, not straight through as a novel, but rather selectively as your patients present or when you are in need of a specific bit of information. Pay heed to the up-to-date chapter references. When a patient visits with a foot problem, read an expert's discussion of it later that day. Notice how often each author offers something new, yet repeats the "tried and true" for emphasis. Though all chapters are pertinent, each reader will identify some of individual interest. For me, Lustman's discussion on psychological aspects of diabetic foot problems, Washington University's contribution on total-contact casting, the biomechanics of the diabetic foot from Penn State, and McMillan's unique information on hemorheology will take top priority in my reading. Foremost, implement what you read. This book contains premier information. When reading *The Diabetic Foot,* you have in your hands a text without peer.

Fred W. Whitehouse, M.D.

PREFACE

With this sixth edition, Marvin Levin and Lawrence O'Neal have passed the responsibility for the continuation of this pioneering work to the present editors. We accepted the challenge with enthusiasm, subject to their willingness to both act in an advisory capacity and to continue as authors. The original intent of Drs. Levin and O'Neal has been maintained; namely, to provide in one text a comprehensive overview of current knowledge regarding both the pathogenesis of diabetic foot lesions and their clinical management. The exponential growth of the pertinent knowledge base has caused the text to expand from a first edition of 10 chapters with 12 contributors and 262 pages to the present text consisting of 38 chapters with 73 contributors and approximately 800 pages.

This edition has been divided into five sections. Section A explores the foundations of diabetic foot management, beginning with Jay Skyler's discussion of "old assumptions and new realities," especially apropos in view of the incontrovertible findings of the Diabetes Control and Complications Trial and the United Kingdom Prospective Diabetes Study. The chapters on epidemiology and foot biomechanics have been expanded with new data. Entirely new chapters on neuropathy and nutrition have been added. The section concludes with an overview of diabetic foot care around the world by Boulton and Vileikyte, a reflection of the spreading pandemic of diabetes mellitus.

Section B deals with nonsurgical management of diabetic foot problems, including evaluation techniques. Of note, Brodsky presents a comprehensive classification of foot lesions that properly weights both depth and level of ischemia, extending the classic work of F.W. Wagner, Jr. There are entirely new chapters on infection, wound repair, wound care materials, weight-relief methods in addition to total-contact casting, and radiologic intervention in peripheral vascular disease.

Section C includes expanded discussion of the surgical aspects of diabetic foot care. New chapters include the perioperative medical management of diabetics, the role of surgery in vascular disease, wound coverage, and Charcot neuroarthropathy of the foot. The chapter on lower limb amputation has been greatly expanded with emphasis on partial foot salvage. This is followed by a comprehensive review of prosthetic rehabilitation of the diabetic amputee.

Section D is devoted to the team approach to diabetic foot care. New chapters deal with the organization of an education-based diabetic foot clinic, patient education in self-management of foot problems, the role of the wound care nurse, psychological aspects, and the impact of modern health management options on foot care.

Section E deals with the medicolegal issues that continue to increase in number as patients and attorneys become more knowledgeable about the results of inappropriate foot care. It is essential that caregivers fully understand their scope of responsibility and that which is assignable to the patient as regards the prevention and management of foot problems in diabetes.

As we enter the new millennium, we hope that the information gathered in this text will help both caregivers and patients, working as a team, to drastically reduce the appalling rate of major lower limb amputation currently associated with the diagnosis of diabetes mellitus.

John H. Bowker, M.D.
Michael A. Pfeifer, M.D.

CONTENTS

Section A ■ THE FOUNDATIONS OF DIABETIC FOOT
MANAGEMENT   1

Chapter 1
Diabetes Mellitus: Old Assumptions and New Realities   3
   JAY S. SKYLER

Chapter 2
Epidemiology of Foot Ulcers and Amputations in the Diabetic Foot   13
   GAYLE E. REIBER

Chapter 3
Neuropathic Problems of the Lower Extremities in Diabetic Patients 33
   ROBERT J. TANENBERG, MARY P. SCHUMER, DOUGLAS A. GREENE,
   and MICHAEL A. PFEIFER

Chapter 4
Atherosclerosis and Thrombosis in Diabetes Mellitus: New Aspects
of Pathogenesis   65
   JOHN A. COLWELL, TIMOTHY J. LYONS, RICHARD L. KLEIN,
   MARIA F. LOPES-VIRELLA, and RUDOLF J. JOKL

Chapter 5
Hemorheology: Principles and Concepts   107
   DONALD E. McMILLAN

Chapter 6
The Biomechanics of the Foot in Diabetes Mellitus   125
   PETER R. CAVANAGH, JAN S. ULBRECHT, and GREGORY M. CAPUTO

Chapter 7
Cutaneous Aspects of Diabetes Mellitus   197
   J.E. JELINEK

Chapter 8
Nutritional Issues in the Patient with Diabetes and Foot Ulcers   212
STEPHEN A. McCLAVE and LOIS S. FINNEY

Chapter 9
Pathogenesis and General Management of Foot Lesions in the
Diabetic Patient   219
MARVIN E. LEVIN

Chapter 10
Diabetic Foot Problems and their Management Around the World   261
ANDREW J.M. BOULTON and LORETTA VILEIKYTE

Section B ■ EVALUATION TECHNIQUES AND NONSURGICAL MANAGEMENT   271

Chapter 11
An Improved Method for Staging and Classification of Foot Lesions
in Diabetic Patients   273
JAMES W. BRODSKY

Chapter 12
Diabetic Foot Ulcer Care: Assessment and Management   283
DIANE L. KRASNER and R. GARY SIBBALD

Chapter 13
Total-Contact Casting in the Treatment of Neuropathic Ulcers   301
DAVID R. SINACORE and MICHAEL J. MUELLER

Chapter 14
Alternative Weight Redistribution Methods in the Treatment of
Neuropathic Ulcers   321
NANCY ELFTMAN

Chapter 15
Imaging of the Diabetic Foot   333
ANDREW J. FISHER, LOUIS A. GILULA, and KEVIN W. McENERY

Chapter 16
Noninvasive Vascular Testing: Basis, Application, and Role in
Evaluating Diabetic Peripheral Arterial Disease   355
JOSEPH J. HURLEY, MATTHEW JUNG, JOHN J. WOODS, Jr.,
and FALLS B. HERSHEY

Chapter 17
Radiologic Intervention in Diabetic Peripheral Vascular Disease   374
KARL S. CHIANG and MICHAEL D. TRIPP

Chapter 18
Modulating Wound Healing in Diabetes   395
    DAVID L. STEED

Chapter 19
Adjunctive Hyperbaric Oxygen Therapy in the Treatment of the
Diabetic Foot Wound   404
    PAUL CIANCI and THOMAS K. HUNT

Chapter 20
Footwear for Injury Prevention: Correlation with Risk Category   422
    WILLIAM C. COLEMAN

Chapter 21
Charcot Neuroarthropathy of the Foot   439
    LEE J. SANDERS and ROBERT G. FRYKBERG

Chapter 22
Infectious Problems of the Foot in Diabetic Patients   467
    BENJAMIN A. LIPSKY

Section C ■ SURGICAL ASPECTS 481

Chapter 23
Surgical Pathology of the Foot and Clinicopathologic Correlations   483
    LAWRENCE W. O'NEAL

Chapter 24
Medical Management of Diabetic Patients During the
Perioperative Period   513
    MOLLY C. CARR and IRL B. HIRSCH

Chapter 25
The Role of Vascular Surgery in the Diabetic Patient   524
    MICHAEL Y. HU and BRENT T. ALLEN

Chapter 26
Plastic Surgical Reconstruction of the Diabetic Foot   565
    JANICE F. LALIKOS, WILLIAM A. WOODEN, and JOSEPH C. BENACCI

Chapter 27
Charcot Neuropathy of the Foot: Surgical Aspects   587
    JEFFREY E. JOHNSON

Chapter 28
Minor and Major Lower Limb Amputation in Persons with
Diabetes Mellitus   607
JOHN H. BOWKER and THOMAS P. SAN GIOVANNI

Chapter 29
Rehabilitation of the Diabetic Amputee   636
ROBERT S. GAILEY, Jr., and CURTIS R. CLARK

Section D ■ TEAM APPROACH   655

Chapter 30
Organizing an Education-Based Diabetic Foot Clinic   657
JOHN H. BOWKER and NANCY P. WADE

Chapter 31
Lower Limb Self-Management Education   665
LINDA B. HAAS and JESSIE H. AHRONI

Chapter 32
Role of the Wound Care Nurse   676
DOROTHY B. DOUGHTY

Chapter 33
Role of the Podiatrist   682
LAWRENCE B. HARKLESS, V. KATHLEEN SATTERFIELD, and KENRICK J. DENNIS

Chapter 34
Pedorthic Care of the Diabetic Foot   700
DENNIS J. JANISSE

Chapter 35
Psychosocial and Psychological Aspects of Diabetic
Foot Complications   727
JAMES E. AIKENS and PATRICK J. LUSTMAN

Chapter 36
Empowerment in Amputation Prevention   737
WILLIAM J. WISHNER and RICHARD R. RUBIN

Chapter 37
Improvements in Diabetic Foot Care with Clinical
Information Systems   749
ALLAN KHOURY, MARK ROTH, and PATRICK LANDERS

Section E ■ MEDICOLEGAL ASPECTS   755

Chapter 38
Medicolegal Aspects of Care and Treatment of the Diabetic Foot   757
JOHN J. FRANK and JOSEPH A. FRANK

Index   766

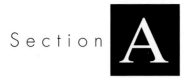

Section **A**

THE FOUNDATIONS OF DIABETIC FOOT MANAGEMENT

Chapter 1

DIABETES MELLITUS: OLD ASSUMPTIONS AND NEW REALITIES

■ Jay S. Skyler

Nearly 16 million Americans suffer from diabetes mellitus, approximately 1 in 16 people.[19] Unfortunately, of these people, 5.4 million are unaware that they have diabetes. Each year, nearly 800,000 Americans develop diabetes. The cost of caring for diabetes now exceeds $137 billion per year, approximately 1 of every 7 health care dollars, including 30% of the Medicare budget. Each year, 182,000 deaths are linked to diabetes, making it the third largest killer in the country, with 57,000 of those deaths directly attributable to diabetes.[8] Yet, the human burden of diabetes is a consequence of the devastating chronic complications of the disease. In the United States, diabetes remains the leading cause of new blindness in adults, with 24,000 individuals becoming legally blind every year due to diabetes. Diabetes now accounts for 40% of patients entering dialysis or transplantation, making it by far the leading cause of end-stage renal disease.[41] Compared to the nondiabetic population, people with diabetes are two- to six-fold more likely to have heart disease and two- to four-fold more likely to have a stroke. Diabetes results in a 15- to 40-fold increased risk of amputations compared to the nondiabetic population, and thus is the nation's leading cause of nontraumatic lower limb amputations.[8] Each year, an estimated 67,000 limbs are lost due to diabetes.

The impact of diabetes is staggering. In the future, this need not be. Future development of blindness, kidney failure, amputation, and heart disease can be markedly lessened by scrupulous attention to therapies and preventive approaches demonstrated to be effective. This includes attainment of meticulous glycemic control, aggressive blood pressure control, careful attention to lipid abnormalities, use of aspirin and other preventive therapies, coupled with appropriate use of proven therapies and technologies (e.g., laser photocoagulation, early introduction of angiotensin converting enzyme inhibitors or angiotensin receptor blockers, routine foot care).

Randomized controlled clinical trials, completed over the last several years, have clearly and unambiguously demonstrated the benefits in diabetic patients of meticulous glycemic control, aggressive blood pressure control, lowering of low-density lipoprotein (LDL) cholesterol, and use of aspirin therapy. There can no longer be any excuse to ignore these important risk factors.

New Diabetes Criteria and Clinical Implications

The American Diabetes Association (ADA) Expert Committee on the Diagnosis and Classification of Diabetes Mellitus released its report in June 1997.[4] This report recommended moving towards an etiopathogenetic classification of diabetes that emphasizes the two principal types. It also recommended that the terminology used in classification of diabetes be changed. The official names for the two principal types become "type 1 diabetes" and "type 2 diabetes" (using arabic numerals "1" and "2") while "IDDM" and "NIDDM" are deleted.

More importantly, the Expert Committee recommended a major shift in the way diabetes is diagnosed. The previous criteria were based on evidence that there is increased retinopathy risk when an oral glucose tolerance test (OGTT) 2-hour value exceeds 200 mg/dL (11.1 mmol/L). The older data implied that retinopathy risk increased when fasting plasma glucose (FPG) exceeded 140 mg/dL (7.8 mmol/L). Newer data suggest that this FPG cutpoint is too high. The Expert Committee also noted that approximately 35 to 40% of people with diabetes in the United States are undiagnosed. One of the reasons they are undiagnosed is that the OGTT is not routinely performed in clinical practice. As a consequence, the default criterion for diagnosis has been an FPG of less than or equal to 140 mg/dL (7.8 mmol/L). The Expert Committee found that by lowering this FPG cutpoint to less than or equal to 126 mg/dL (7.0 mmol/L), two things would happen. First, it would acknowledge that retinopathy risk begins at a lower FPG than now used for diagnosis. Second, most people with undiagnosed diabetes would become recognized, without very much risk of false-positive diagnosis. Thus, 126 mg/dL (7.0 mmol/L) becomes a surrogate for an OGTT 2-hour value of 200 mg/dL (11.1 mmol/L). This change really does not increase the number of people *with* diabetes. Rather, it increases the number of people with *known* diabetes. That is why it is a crucial public health measure.

The old criteria used an FPG of less than 115 mg/dL (6.4 mmol/L) for normal. In contrast, the new ADA criteria use an FPG of less than 110 mg/dL (6.1 mmol/L) for normal. Individuals having FPG levels 110 to 125 mg/dL (6.1 to 6.9 mmol/L), too high to be considered altogether normal, are now defined as having "impaired fasting glucose" (IFG). This group (IFG) is considered to be at increased risk of diabetes, similar to those with impaired glucose tolerance (IGT), who have OGTT 2-hour values of 140 to 199 mg/dL (7.8 to 11.0 mmol/L).

Glycosylated hemoglobin (HbA_{1c}) measurement is not currently recommended for diagnosis of diabetes, although some studies have shown that the frequency distributions for HbA_{1c} have characteristics similar to those of the FPG and the 2-hour plasma glucose. However, both HbA_{1c} and FPG (in type 2 diabetes) have become the measurements of choice in monitoring the treatment of diabetes, and decisions on when and how to implement therapy are often made on the basis of HbA_{1c}. The revised criteria are for diagnosis and are not treatment criteria or goals of therapy. No change was made in the ADA recommendations of FPG below 120 mg/dL (6.7 mmol/L) and HbA_{1c} below 7% as treatment goals.

Screening is important for a variety of reasons. Hyperglycemia is important in the pathogenesis of the specific complications of diabetes mellitus—microangiopathy (retinopathy and nephropathy) and neuropathy. Meticulous glycemic control slows the course of development of diabetic complications. Prolongation of normoglycemia should reduce risk of diabetic complications. Undetected type 2 diabetes is common—it is estimated that 35 to 40% of individuals with type 2 diabetes are unaware that they have the disease and that undiagnosed diabetes exists for 4 to 7 years prior to clinical recognition.[20] Studies suggest that interventions such as diet and exercise may forestall the evolution of type 2 diabetes. Screening for type 2 diabetes is now easy—only a simple FPG is required. The more cumbersome OGTT is no longer the primary screening tool. Screening and early diagnosis of type 2 diabetes should be highly cost effective. All adults over age 45 should be screened every 3 years. All individuals at higher risk (based on obesity, ethnicity, etc.) should be screened annually, starting at an earlier age.

Glycemic Control

The debate over the role of careful glycemic control in the evolution of complications has ended, thanks in particular to the Diabetes

Control and Complications Trial (DCCT), which studied patients with type 1 diabetes, and the United Kingdom Prospective Diabetes Study (UKPDS), which studied patients with type 2 diabetes. Yet, the evidence that hyperglycemia is important had been accumulating from many other epidemiologic studies and small randomized controlled clinical trials, all of which suggested a significant relationship between glycemia and complications.[33]

One of the longest, largest, and most carefully conducted epidemiologic studies is the Wisconsin Epidemiologic Study of Diabetic Retinopathy (WESDR), which although named for retinopathy has examined a whole array of complications.[22–24] The Wisconsin study is a population-based study amongst diabetic patients receiving community care in 11 counties in southern Wisconsin. The sample included a "younger onset cohort" of all diabetic subjects with onset less than age 30 years ($n = 1,210$), presumably mostly with type 1 diabetes; and an "older onset cohort" of a probability sample of those with onset greater than age 30 years ($n = 1,780$ of $5,431$ patients with a confirmed diagnosis of diabetes). For many analyses, the older onset cohort is divided into those not treated with insulin (53.7% of the original sample), presumably with type 2 diabetes; and those treated with insulin (46.3% of the original sample), presumably a mixed group with most having type 2 diabetes. These individuals underwent baseline evaluation in 1980–1982, with follow-up evaluations performed after 4, 10, and 14 years. Evaluations were conducted in a van, and included historical data, blood pressure, visual acuity, seven-field fundus photography, and measurement of HbA_{1c} and urine protein.

Data from the WESDR demonstrate a strong consistent relationship between hyperglycemia and the incidence and/or progression of microvascular (diabetic retinopathy, loss of vision, and nephropathy), neurologic (loss of tactile sensation or temperature sensitivity), and macrovascular (amputation and cardiovascular disease mortality) complications in people with type 1 and type 2 diabetes.

Epidemiologic studies, however, cannot demonstrate a treatment effect. A number of randomized controlled clinical trials have demonstrated that meticulous control of blood glucose dramatically reduces the frequency and progression of diabetic complications.

The DCCT, a randomized, multicenter controlled clinical trial, demonstrated that intensive treatment of type 1 diabetes, with the goal of meticulous glycemic control, reduced the frequency and severity of retinopathy, nephropathy, and neuropathy.[10] The DCCT was conducted in 29 centers across North America (26 in the United States and three in Canada) and included 1,441 subjects with type 1 diabetes. Of the subjects enrolled, 726 were in a "primary prevention cohort," with less than 5 years' duration of diabetes and at baseline both no retinopathy and normal albumin excretion. Another 715 subjects were in a "secondary intervention cohort," with less than 15 years' duration of diabetes and at baseline having "mild to moderate" background retinopathy, and either normal albumin excretion or microalbuminuria. Subjects were randomly assigned either to "intensive therapy" or to "conventional therapy." Intensive therapy consisted of insulin administered either by continuous subcutaneous insulin infusion (CSII) with an external insulin pump or multiple daily insulin injections (MDI) (three or more injections per day); guided by frequent self-monitoring of blood glucose (SMBG) three to four times daily, with additional specified samples including a weekly overnight sample, meticulous attention to diet, and monthly visits to the treating clinic. Conventional therapy consisted of no more than two daily insulin injections, urine glucose monitoring or SMBG no more than twice daily, periodic diet review, and clinic visits every 2 to 3 months.

The intensive group achieved a median HbA_{1c} of 7.2% versus 9.1% in the conventional group ($p < 0.001$). Mean blood glucose was 155 mg/dL in the intensive group and 230 mg/dL in the conventional group. Glycemic separation was maintained for 4 to 9 years, with mean duration of follow-up 6.5 years, for a total of approximately 9,300 patient-years of observation. Of 1,430 subjects alive at the end of the study, 1,422 came for evaluation of outcomes. Risk reductions for microvascular and neurologic end points in the DCCT were dramatic: over 70% for clinically important sustained retinopathy, 56% for laser photocoagulation, 60% for sustained microalbuminuria, 54% for clinical grade nephropathy, and 64% for confirmed clinical neuropathy. Macrovascular end points demonstrated a trend in risk reduction (42% risk reduction), which did not quite reach statistical significance.

In the DCCT, there was a continuous exponential relationship between prevailing glycemia and complications, without evidence of a glycemic threshold.[11]

The beneficial effects and impact of effective glycemic control in type 1 diabetes also has been seen in a number of other smaller studies, which collectively were subjected to a meta-analysis, which was consistent with the findings noted in the DCCT.[42, 43]

The UKPDS, a randomized, multicenter controlled clinical trial, demonstrated that an intensive treatment policy in type 2 diabetes, with the goal of meticulous glycemic control, could decrease clinical diabetic complications.[37, 39] The UKPDS was conducted in 23 centers and included 5,102 subjects with newly diagnosed type 2 diabetes, 25 to 63 years of age at entry (median, 53 years). Subjects were randomly assigned either to "intensive treatment policy" or "conventional treatment policy." Intensive policy aimed at achieving fasting plasma glucose of 108 mg/dL, using various pharmacologic agents. Conventional policy attempted control with diet alone, adding pharmacologic therapy when symptoms developed or FPG exceeded 270 mg/dL.

The intensive policy group achieved a median HbA_{1c} of 7.0% versus 7.9% in the conventional policy group ($p < 0.001$). Although there was a progressive deterioration in glycemia over time, degree of glycemic separation was maintained for 6 to 20 years, with a median duration of follow-up of 11 years. The primary outcome measures in the UKPDS were three aggregate end points— "any diabetes-related endpoint," "diabetes-related death," and "all-cause mortality." Of these, only any diabetes-related end point was significantly impacted—a 12% risk reduction. In addition, risk reductions were seen for other end points. Patients assigned intensive policy had a significant 25% risk reduction in microvascular end points compared with conventional policy—most of which was due to fewer cases of retinal photocoagulation, for which there was a 29% risk reduction. There was also a decreased risk of cataract extraction (24% risk reduction), deterioration in retinopathy (21% risk reduction at 12 years' follow-up), and of microalbuminuria (33% risk reduction at 12 years' follow-up). Reduction in microvascular complications was seen regardless of primary treatment modality for intensive therapy— insulin, sulfonylureas, or metformin. Thus, improved glycemic control is the principal factor. The only macrovascular end point that demonstrated a trend on risk reduction in the main analysis was myocardial infarction (16% risk reduction), which did not quite reach statistical significance.

In the metformin subgroup analysis within UKPDS, however, there were significant risk reductions in diabetes-related deaths (42% risk reduction), any diabetes-related end point (32% risk reduction), and myocardial infarction (39% risk reduction).[37] A combined analysis of all macrovascular end points (myocardial infarction, sudden death, angina, stroke, peripheral vascular disease) showed a risk reduction of 30% over the conventional therapy group.

The beneficial effects and impact of effective glycemic control also was seen in a small study reported from Kumamoto University in Japan that involved 110 nonobese patients with type 2 diabetes.[29] This study contrasted intensive insulin therapy (multiple daily injections—preprandial regular and bedtime intermediate acting insulin) and conventional insulin therapy (once- or twice-daily intermediate acting insulin) in two cohorts, a "primary prevention cohort" and a "secondary intervention cohort." Over 6 years of follow-up, glycemic outcomes and risk reductions were almost identical to those found in the DCCT. The intensive therapy group achieved a mean HbA_{1c} over the 6 years of the study of 7.1% versus a value in the conventional therapy group of 9.4% ($p < 0.001$). Mean fasting blood glucose was 157 mg/dL in the intensive group and 221 mg/dL in the conventional group. Retinopathy progression was reduced by 69%, nephropathy progression by 70%, and motor and sensory nerve conduction velocities and vibration thresholds were better in the intensive group than the conventional group.

Conclusions and Recommendations

Thus, there are consistent and substantial beneficial effects of improved glycemic control in both type 1 and type 2 diabetes, impacting on the entire array of diabetic complications. The current glycemic recommendations of the ADA appear in their Standards of Medical Care for Patients with Diabetes Mellitus.[5] The goal is, ideally, fasting plasma glucose less than 120 mg/dL and HbA$_{1c}$ below 7% (normal range, ~3.0 to 6.0%). The ADA uses the term "action suggested" to define another category, which might also be defined as "unacceptable" glycemic control (i.e., fasting plasma glucose >140 mg/dL and HbA$_{1c}$ >8%).

Contemporary diabetes management is based on the concept of "targeted glycemic control." Therapy, based on glycemic goals, utilizes progressive step-wise additions of whatever treatment modality is necessary to achieve glycemic goals. Medical nutritional therapy and promotion of physical activity are fundamental and needed for all patients, as is basic diabetes education.

Intensive insulin therapy is mandatory in type 1 diabetes. This is accomplished, as in the DCCT, with insulin administered either by CSII with a pump or by MDI; frequent SMBG; and meticulous attention to balancing insulin dose, food intake, and energy expenditure.[21]

In type 2 diabetes, progressive pharmacologic therapy is required, the specific choice based on disease severity and glycemic targets.[14] There are a growing number of classes of pharmacologic agents available to control glycemia. These include insulin secretagogues (i.e., sulfonylureas and repaglinide), which stimulate insulin production; insulin sensitizers (i.e., biguanides and thiazolidinediones), which enhance muscle glucose uptake and decrease hepatic glucose production; α-glucosidase inhibitors, which retard carbohydrate absorption; and replacement of insulin deficiency with insulin or insulin analogues. The availability of agents with differing and complementary mechanisms of action allows them to be used in various combinations, thus increasing the likelihood that satisfactory glycemic control can be achieved in any given patient.

Blood Pressure Control

Several clinical trials have addressed the influence of blood pressure control in diabetes. They have used different outcomes.

The Hypertension in Diabetes Study (HDS) was embedded in the UKPDS by using a factorial design.[38, 40] HDS was conducted in 20 centers amongst 1,148 patients with type 2 diabetes with coexisting hypertension. The design was a randomized controlled trial comparing "tight" control of blood pressure aiming at a blood pressure of less than 150/85 mm Hg with "less tight" control aiming at a blood pressure of less than 180/105 mm Hg. Median follow-up was 8.4 years. The "tight" control group achieved a mean blood pressure of 144/82 mm Hg versus 154/87 mm Hg in the "less tight" control group ($p <$ 0.0001).

Risk reductions in the HDS were substantial. Patients assigned "tight" control had a 24% risk reduction for "any diabetes-related end point" 32% risk reduction for diabetes-related deaths, 56% risk reduction for heart failure, 44% risk reduction for stroke, and a 37% risk reduction for microvascular disease. After 7.5 years of follow-up the group assigned to "tight" control also had a 34% reduction in risk of deterioration of retinopathy and a 47% reduced risk of deterioration in visual acuity.

The Hypertension Optimal Treatment (HOT) Study was a randomized multinational trial involving 18,790 hypertensive patients, aged 50 to 80 years (mean, 61.5 years) with diastolic blood pressure 100 to 115 mm Hg, including 1,501 patients with diabetes at baseline.[18] They were randomly assigned to three different target diastolic blood pressure groups: less than or equal to 90 mm Hg, less than or equal to 85 mm Hg, and less than or equal to 80 mm Hg. Felodipine was given as baseline therapy with the addition of other agents, according to a five-step regimen.

In the patients with diabetes in HOT, with the lowest target blood pressure (≤80 mm Hg), there was a decline in the rate of major cardiovascular events, cardiovascular mortality, and total mortality. In the group randomized to less than or equal to 80 mm Hg the risk of major cardiovascular events was halved in comparison with that of the target group (≤90 mm Hg). This change was attenuated but remained significant when silent myocardial infarctions were included. The approximate halving of the risk was also observed for all myocardial infarction, although it was not significant. Stroke also showed a declining rate with lower target blood pressure groups.

The Systolic Hypertension in Europe (Syst-Eur) Trial included a post hoc analysis of the data in this trial to determine the effects on long-term outcome in diabetic versus nondiabetic patients with hypertension.[36] In Syst-Eur, 4,695 patients (≥60 years of age), including 492 patients (10.5%) with diabetes, with systolic blood pressure of 160 to 219 mm Hg and diastolic pressure below 95 mm Hg, were randomly assigned to receive active treatment or placebo. Active treatment consisted of nitrendipine, with the possible addition or substitution of enalapril or hydrochlorothiazide or both, titrated to reduce the systolic blood pressure by at least 20 mm Hg and to less than 150 mm Hg. In the control group, matching placebo tablets were administered similarly. Amongst the diabetic patients, after a median follow-up of 2 years, the systolic and diastolic blood pressures in the two treatment groups differed by 8.6 and 3.9 mm Hg, respectively. Amongst the diabetic patients, active treatment reduced overall mortality by 55%, mortality from cardiovascular disease by 76%, all cardiovascular events combined by 69%, fatal and nonfatal strokes by 73%, and all cardiac events combined by 63%.

Conclusions and Recommendations

Thus, there are consistent and substantial beneficial effects of improved blood pressure control in diabetic patients, impacting on various diabetic complications. In patients with diabetes, current blood pressure recommendations of the American Diabetes Association appear in their "Standards of Medical Care for Patients with Diabetes Mellitus"[5] and in a consensus statement on "Treatment of Hypertension in Diabetes."[6] Similar recommendations are contained in the "Sixth Report of the Joint National Committee on Detection, Evaluation, and Treatment of High Blood Pressure"[35] and elsewhere.

The primary goal of therapy for (nonpregnant) adults (>18 years of age) with diabetes is to decrease blood pressure to and maintain it at less than 130 mm Hg systolic and less than 85 mm Hg diastolic. In children, blood pressure should be decreased to the corresponding age-adjusted 90th percentile values. It should be noted, however, that in the general population, the risks for end-organ damage appear to be lowest when the systolic blood pressure is less than 120 mm Hg and the diastolic blood pressure is less than 80 mm Hg. For patients with an isolated systolic hypertension of greater than 180 mm Hg, the initial goal of treatment is to reduce the systolic blood pressure to less than 160 mm Hg. For those with systolic blood pressure of 160 to 179, the goal is a reduction of 20 mm Hg. If these goals are achieved and well tolerated, further lowering to less than 140 mm Hg may be appropriate. An approach for achieving such control has recently been reviewed.[27]

Control of Lipids

The Scandinavian Simvastatin Survival Study (4S) was a randomized multinational trial involving 4,444 patients, aged 35 to 70 years (mean, 58.9 years) with known coronary heart disease (CHD) manifested by angina pectoris or previous myocardial infarction, who had serum cholesterol levels of 5.5 to 8.0 mmol/L (213 to 310 mg/dL) while on a lipid-lowering diet.[32] The study included 202 diabetic patients. In 4S, patients were randomly assigned to receive active treatment with simvastatin 20 mg/day (with masked dosage titration up to 40 mg/day, according to cholesterol response during the first 6 to 18 weeks) or placebo. Over the 5.4 years' median follow-up period, simvastatin produced mean changes in total cholesterol, low-density lipoprotein (LDL) cholesterol, and high-density lipoprotein (HDL) cholesterol of −25%, −35%, and +8%, respectively.

The investigators performed a post hoc subgroup analysis comparing the diabetic and nondiabetic patients.[30] Mean changes in serum lipids in diabetic patients were similar to those observed in nondiabetic patients. The results strongly suggest that cholesterol lowering improves prognosis of diabetic patients with CHD. Amongst the diabetic patients, active treatment reduced total mortality by 43%, major cardiovascular events combined by 55%, and any atherosclerotic event by 37%. The corresponding risk reductions in nondiabetic patients were less, such that the investigators asserted that the absolute clinical benefit achieved by cholesterol lowering may be greater in diabetic than in nondiabetic patients with CHD because diabetic patients have a higher absolute risk of recurrent CHD events and other atherosclerotic events.

The Cholesterol and Recurrent Events (CARE) Trial was a randomized multicenter trial involving 4,159 patients with myocardial infarction who had plasma total cholesterol levels below 240 mg/dL (mean, 209) and LDL cholesterol levels of 115 to 174 mg/dL (mean, 139).[31] The study included 586 patients (14.1%) with clinical diagnoses of diabetes, and 342 patients with IFG at entry,[16] as defined by the 1997 American Diabetes Association criteria (i.e., 110 to 125 mg/dL).[4] In CARE, patients were randomly assigned to receive active treatment with pravastatin 40 mg daily or placebo, for 5 years. The primary end point was a fatal coronary event or a nonfatal myocardial infarction. The investigators performed a post hoc subgroup analysis comparing the diabetic and nondiabetic patients.[16] Mean LDL cholesterol reduction was similar (27% and 28%) in the diabetic and nondiabetic groups, respectively. As in 4S, in the placebo group, the diabetic patients suffered more recurrent coronary events (CHD death, nonfatal myocardial infarction, coronary bypass surgery, and coronary angioplasty) than did the nondiabetic patients (37% vs. 25%). Pravastatin treatment reduced the absolute risk of coronary events for the diabetic and nondiabetic patients by 8.1% and 5.2% and the relative risk by 25% and 23%, respectively. In the diabetic patients, the relative risk for revascularization procedures was reduced by 32%. Patients with IFG had a higher rate of recurrent coronary events than those with normal fasting glucose, and in IFG patients recurrence rates for nonfatal MI were reduced by 50%.

Conclusions and Recommendations

Thus, there are consistent and substantial beneficial effects of careful control of lipids—specifically, LDL cholesterol—in diabetic patients, impacting on recurrent coronary disease. Although not directly examined in these studies, it is probably a reasonable assumption that such lipid lowering will reduce the risk from peripheral vascular disease as well.

In patients with diabetes, current lipid treatment recommendations of the American Diabetes Association appear in their "Standards of Medical Care for Patients with Diabetes Mellitus"[5] and in a position statement on "Management of Dyslipidemia in Adults with Diabetes."[3] The primary goal of therapy for adult patients with diabetes is to lower LDL cholesterol to below 100 mg/dL. People with diabetes who have triglyceride levels above 1,000 mg/dL are at risk of pancreatitis and other manifestations of the hyperchylomicronemic syndrome. These individuals need special immediate attention to lower triglyceride levels to below 400 mg/dL. Fur-

ther reduction to a goal of less than 200 mg/dL, as recommended by the National Cholesterol Education Program's Adult Treatment Panel II,[13] may be beneficial. A secondary goal of therapy is to raise HDL cholesterol to above 35 mg/dL in men and above 45 mg/dL in women. An approach for achieving such control has recently been reviewed.[15]

Aspirin and Other Antiplatelet Therapy

The Physicians' Health Study was a randomized trial involving 22,071 healthy U.S. male physicians aged 40 to 84, designed to determine whether low-dose aspirin (325 mg every other day) decreases cardiovascular mortality.[34] The aspirin component was terminated earlier than scheduled after an average follow-up time of 60.2 months, due to the dramatic results. There was a 44% reduction in the risk of occurrence of a first myocardial infarction ($p < 0.00001$) in the aspirin group. Subgroup analyses in the diabetic physicians revealed a reduction in myocardial infarction from 10.1% (placebo) to 4.0% (aspirin), yielding a risk reduction of 61% for the diabetic men on aspirin therapy. This supports use of aspirin therapy for primary prevention in patients with diabetes. In addition, there was a 46% reduction in the risk of peripheral artery surgery in the aspirin group ($p = 0.03$).[17]

The Early Treatment Diabetic Retinopathy Study (ETDRS) was a randomized trial involving 3,711 type 1 and type 2 diabetic men and women, about 48% of whom had a history of cardiovascular disease.[12] The study, therefore, may be viewed as a mixed primary and secondary prevention trial. Patients were randomly assigned to aspirin or placebo (two 325-mg tablets once per day). The risk reduction for myocardial infarction in the first 5 years in those randomized to aspirin therapy was 28%.

In the HOT study mentioned earlier, aspirin reduced major cardiovascular events by 15% and all myocardial infarction by 36%.[18] The effect was seen in both diabetic and nondiabetic patients.

The Veterans Administration Cooperative Study on Antiplatelet Agents in Diabetic Patients After Amputation for Gangrene was a small multicenter randomized trial on the effects of aspirin plus dipyridamole versus placebo on major vascular end points in 231 diabetic men with either a recent amputation for gangrene or active gangrene.[7] Survival curve analyses revealed little difference between groups for major vascular end points, total mortality, all amputations, or myocardial infarctions. However, the overall rate of atherosclerotic deaths was 20.3%, and the overall rate of opposite-side amputations was 22.1%. This suggests that the subjects may have had such advanced disease that precluded an effect of antiplatelet therapy.

An analysis of antiplatelet therapy, particularly with aspirin, has been published.[9] The analysis considered 174 randomized trials involving approximately 100,000 patients. In each of four main high-risk categories (patients with acute myocardial infarction, patients with a past history of myocardial infarction, patients with a past history of stroke or transient ischemic attack, and patients with some other relevant medical history [unstable angina, stable angina, vascular surgery, angioplasty, atrial fibrillation, valvular disease, peripheral vascular disease, etc.]), antiplatelet therapy was definitely protective. Reductions in vascular events were about one quarter in each of these four main categories and were separately statistically significant in middle age and old age, in men and women, in hypertensive and normotensive patients, and in diabetic and nondiabetic patients. Taking all high-risk patients together showed reductions of about one third in nonfatal myocardial infarction, about one third in nonfatal stroke, and about one third in vascular death. It was estimated that 38 ± 12 vascular events per 1,000 diabetic patients would be prevented if they were treated with aspirin as a secondary prevention strategy. The most widely tested regimen was "medium dose" (75 to 325 mg/day) aspirin. Doses throughout this range seemed similarly effective. There was no appreciable evidence that either a higher aspirin dose or any other antiplatelet regimen was more effective than medium-dose aspirin in preventing vascular events. Among low-risk recipients of "primary prevention" a significant reduction of one third in nonfatal myocardial infarction was, however, accompanied by a nonsignificant increase in stroke.

Conclusions and Recommendations

Thus, there are beneficial effects of antiplatelet therapy, particularly with aspirin, in dia-

betic patients, impacting on various diabetic complications. In patients with diabetes, current recommendations of the American Diabetes Association appear in their "Standards of Medical Care for Patients with Diabetes Mellitus"[5] and in a position statement on "Aspirin Therapy in Diabetes."[2] The ADA specifically advocates the use of aspirin therapy as a secondary prevention strategy in diabetic men and women who have evidence of large-vessel disease, including a history of myocardial infarction, vascular bypass procedure, stroke or transient ischemic attack, peripheral vascular disease, claudication, and/or angina. ADA also recommends considering aspirin therapy as a primary prevention strategy in high-risk men and women with type 1 or type 2 diabetes.

Smoking

Although cigarette smoking is a major risk factor for peripheral vascular disease and amputation in nondiabetic people, amongst people with diabetes, the evidence for a relationship between tobacco and ulcers or amputation is variable. In the WESDR mentioned earlier, in type 1 diabetes there was an association between foot ulcers and either being a current smoker or having a 10+ pack-year history of smoking.[26] However, no increased risk was found for smokers with type 2 diabetes in the same population. Most other studies have failed to show an association of cigarette smoking with an increased risk of macrovascular disease, peripheral vascular disease, diabetic foot ulcers, or amputation in diabetic individuals, as recently discussed in an American Diabetes Association "Technical Review on Foot Problems in Diabetes."[28] Only a few studies show a weak relationship between smoking and peripheral vascular disease, ulcers, or amputation risk. On the other hand, in people with diabetes tobacco use has been associated with both microvascular disease (i.e., retinopathy, nephropathy) and cardiovascular disease. As a consequence, smoking cessation should be recommended to all individuals with diabetes, and that recommendation should be continually reenforced.

Concluding Remarks

The American Diabetes Association annually publishes its "Clinical Practice Recommendations,"[1] including its "Standards of Medical Care for Patients with Diabetes Mellitus."[5] These are contained in a supplement to Diabetes Care and are available on the World Wide Web at *www.diabetes.org*. Patients with diabetes mellitus have long suffered from the devastating complications that threaten their lives. The challenge for all health providers caring for diabetic patients is to recognize that there is a growing body of evidence, based on controlled clinical trials, demonstrating that the impact of this dreaded disease can be dramatically lessened. To benefit from recent advances, patients with diabetes must understand the treatment goals and must strive to attain excellent glycemic control, aggressive control of blood pressure, and normalization of lipids. They should avoid cigarette smoking, use prophylactic aspirin therapy, take excellent care of their feet, have regular medical examinations, and avail themselves of appropriate interventions as needed. When this occurs on a regular basis, it should be possible to reduce the risk of complications and lessen the burden of diabetes.

REFERENCES

1. American Diabetes Association: Clinical practice recommendations 1999. Diabetes Care 21(Suppl 1): 1999.
2. American Diabetes Association: Position statement. Aspirin therapy in diabetes. Diabetes Care 21(Suppl 1): S60–S61, 1999.
3. American Diabetes Association: Position statement. Management of dyslipidemia in adults with diabetes. Diabetes Care 22(Suppl 1): S56–S59, 1999.
4. American Diabetes Association: Report of the Expert Committee on the Diagnosis and Classification of Diabetes Mellitus. Diabetes Care 20:1183–1197, 1997.
5. American Diabetes Association: Standards of medical care for patients with diabetes mellitus. Diabetes Care 22(Suppl 1): S32–S41, 1999.
6. American Diabetes Association: Treatment of hypertension in diabetes (consensus statement). Diabetes Care 16:1394–1401, 1993.
7. Antiplatelet Trialists' Collaboration: Collaborative overview of randomised trials of antiplatelet therapy—I: Prevention of death, myocardial infarction, and stroke by prolonged antiplatelet therapy in various categories of patients. BMJ 308:81–106, 1994.
8. Centers for Disease Control and Prevention: The public health of diabetes mellitus in the United States. Atlanta, GA: Department of Health and Human Services, 1997.
9. Colwell JA, Bingham SF, Abraira C, et al: Veterans Administration Cooperative Study on antiplatelet agents in diabetic patients after amputation for gangrene: II. Effects of aspirin and dipyridamole on atherosclerotic vascular disease rates. Diabetes Care 9:140–148, 1986.
10. Diabetes Control and Complications Trial Research Group: The effect of intensive treatment of diabetes on the development and progression of long-term complications in insulin-dependent diabetes mellitus. N Engl J Med 329:683–689, 1993.
11. Diabetes Control and Complications Trial Research Group: The relationship of glycemic exposure (HbA$_{1c}$) to the risk of development and progression of retinopathy in the Diabetes Control and Complications Trial. Diabetes 44:968–993, 1995.
12. ETDRS Investigators: Aspirin effects on mortality and morbidity in patients with diabetes mellitus. Early Treatment Diabetic Retinopathy Study Report 14. JAMA 268:1292–1300, 1992.
13. Expert Panel on Detection, Evaluation, and Treatment of High Blood Cholesterol in Adults: Summary of the second report of the National Cholesterol Education Program (NCEP) Expert Panel on Detection, Evaluation, and Treatment of High Blood Cholesterol in Adults (Adult Treatment Panel II). JAMA 269:3015–3023, 1993.
14. Feinglos MN, Bethel MA: Treatment of type 2 diabetes mellitus. Med Clin North Am 82:757–790, 1998.
15. Garber AJ: Vascular disease and lipids in diabetes. Med Clin North Am 82:931–948, 1998.
16. Goldberg RB, Mellies MJ, Sacks FM, et al, and the Care Investigators: Cardiovascular events and their reduction with pravastatin in diabetic and glucose-intolerant myocardial infarction survivors with average cholesterol levels: Subgroup analyses in the Cholesterol and Recurrent Events (CARE) trial. Circulation 23:2513–2519, 1998.
17. Goldhaber SZ, Manson JE, Stampfer MJ, et al: Low-dose aspirin and subsequent peripheral arterial surgery in the Physicians' Health Study. Lancet 340:143–145, 1992.
18. Hansson L, Zanchetti A, Carruthers SG, et al, and the HOT Study Group: Effects of intensive blood-pressure lowering and low-dose aspirin in patients with hypertension: Principal results of the Hypertension Optimal Treatment (HOT) randomised trial. Lancet 351:1755–1762, 1998.
19. Harris MI, Flegal KM, Cowie CC, et al: Prevalence of diabetes, impaired fasting glucose, and impaired glucose tolerance in U.S. adults. The Third National Health and Nutrition Examination Survey, 1988–1994. Diabetes Care 21:518–524, 1998.
20. Harris MI, Klein R, Welborn TA, Kuiman MW: Onset of NIDDM occurs at least 4–7 yr before clinical diagnosis. Diabetes Care 15:815–819, 1992.
21. Hirsch IB: Intensive treatment of type 1 diabetes. Med Clin North Am 82:689–719, 1998.
22. Klein R: Hyperglycemia and microvascular and macrovascular disease in diabetes. Diabetes Care 18:258–268, 1995.
23. Klein R, Klein BEK, Moss SE: Relation of glycemic control to diabetic microvascular complications in diabetes mellitus. Ann Intern Med 124:90–96, 1996.
24. Klein R, Klein BEK, Moss SE, Cruickshanks KJ: Relationship of hyperglycemia to the long-term incidence and progression of diabetic retinopathy. Arch Intern Med 154:2169–2178, 1994.
25. Klein R, Klein BEK, Moss SE, et al: Glycosylated hemoglobin predicts the incidence and progression of diabetic retinopathy. JAMA 260:2864–2871, 1988.
26. Moss SE, Klein R, Klein BE: The prevalence and incidence of lower extremity amputation in a dia-

betic population. Arch Intern Med 152:610–616, 1992.

27. Marks JB, Raskin P: Nephropathy and hypertension in diabetes. Med Clin North Am 82:877–907, 1998.

28. Mayfield JA, Reiber GE, Sanders LJ, et al: Preventive foot care in people with diabetes (technical review). Diabetes Care 21:2161–2177, 1998.

29. Ohkubo Y, Kishikawa H, Araki E, et al: Intensive insulin therapy prevents the progression of diabetic microvascular complications in Japanese patients with non-insulin-dependent diabetes mellitus: A randomized prospective 6-year study. Diabetes Res Clin Pract 28:103–117, 1995.

30. Pyrälä K, Pedersen TR, Kjekshus J, et al: Cholesterol lowering with simvastatin improves prognosis of diabetic patients with coronary heart disease. A subgroup analysis of the Scandinavian Simvastatin Survival Study (4S). Diabetes Care 20:614–620, 1997.

31. Sacks FM, Pfeffer MA, Moye LA, et al, and the Cholesterol and Recurrent Events Trial Investigators: The effect of pravastatin on coronary events after myocardial infarction in patients with average cholesterol levels. N Engl J Med 335:1001–1009, 1996.

32. Scandinavian Simvastatin Survival Study Group: Randomised trial of cholesterol lowering in 4444 patients with coronary heart disease: The Scandinavian Simvastatin Survival Study (4S). Lancet 344:1383–1389, 1994.

33. Skyler JS: Diabetic complications: Glucose control is important. Endocrinol Metab Clin North Am 25:243–254, 1996.

34. Steering Committee of the Physicians' Health Study Research Group: Final report on the aspirin component of the ongoing Physicians' Health Study. N Engl J Med 321:129–135, 1989.

35. The Sixth Report of the Joint National Committee on Detection, Evaluation, and Treatment of High Blood Pressure. Arch Intern Med 157:2413–2446, 1997.

36. Tuomilehto J, Rastenyte D, Birkenhager WH, et al, for the Systolic Hypertension in Europe Trial Investigators: Effects of calcium-channel blockade in older patients with diabetes and systolic hypertension. N Engl J Med 340:677–684, 1999.

37. UK Prospective Diabetes Study Group: Effect of intensive blood-glucose control with metformin on complications in overweight patients with type 2 diabetes (UKPDS 34). Lancet 352:854–865, 1998.

38. UK Prospective Diabetes Study Group: Efficacy of atenolol and captopril in reducing risk of macrovascular and microvascular complications in type 2 diabetes: UKPDS 39. BMJ 317:713–720, 1998.

39. UK Prospective Diabetes Study Group: Intensive blood-glucose control with sulfonylureas or insulin compared with conventional treatment and risk of complications in patients with type 2 diabetes (UKPDS 33). Lancet 352:837–853, 1998.

40. UK Prospective Diabetes Study Group: Tight blood pressure control and risk of macrovascular and microvascular complications in type 2 diabetes: UKPDS 38. BMJ 317:703–713, 1998.

41. US Renal Data System: USRDS 1997 Annual Data Report. Bethesda, MD: The National Institutes of Health, National Institute of Diabetes and Digestive and Kidney Diseases, 1998.

42. Wang PH, Lau J, Chalmers TC: Meta-analysis of effects of intensive blood glucose control on late complications on type I diabetes. Lancet 341:1306–1309, 1993.

43. Wang PH, Lau J, Chalmers TC: Meta-analysis of effects of intensive glycemic control on late complications on type I diabetes mellitus. Online J Curr Clin Trials 1993; Document No. 60, May 21, 1993.

Chapter 2

EPIDEMIOLOGY OF FOOT ULCERS AND AMPUTATIONS IN THE DIABETIC FOOT

■ Gayle E. Reiber

Half of all lower limb amputations in the United States are performed in persons with diagnosed diabetes even though this group comprises only 4% of the U.S. population.[55] Amputations reduce patient function and quality of life and place a heavy burden on individuals, their families, and their health care systems. This chapter reviews the epidemiology and risk factors for foot ulcers and nontraumatic lower limb amputations in persons with diabetes and describes the associated mortality and economic impact. Data for this chapter were selected from population-based surveys and analytic and experimental studies. The infrequent inclusion of data on nondiabetic individuals is indicated.

Epidemiology of Foot Ulcers

Incidence, Prevalence, and Site of Foot Ulcers

Foot ulcers are cutaneous erosions characterized by a loss of epithelium that extends into

or through the dermis to deeper tissue. Although foot ulcers result from various etiologic factors, they are characterized by an inability to self-repair in a timely and orderly manner.[32] Data from the U.S. National Hospital Discharge Survey indicated that nearly 6% of the hospital discharges between 1983 and 1990 in persons with diabetes were associated with a foot ulcer condition. The average length of hospital stay was 59% longer in these individuals than in diabetic individuals without a foot ulcer.[51]

Considerable variation is reported in incidence (new onset) and prevalence (history) of diabetic foot ulcers. Table 2–1 shows the annual population-based incidence of diabetic foot ulcers ranges from 1.0% to 4.1%, while the prevalence of foot ulcers is reported between 5.3% and 10.5%.[7, 27, 45, 52, 67] The lifetime risk for foot ulcers in persons with diabetes is estimated at 15%.[47]

Population surveillance of new foot ulcer episodes is difficult in out-of-hospital settings and is subject to coding limitations in all settings. Sampled information from the National Ambulatory Medical Care Survey for office visits and the National Hospital

---

All material in this chapter is in the public domain, with the exception of any borrowed figures or tables.

Table 2-1 ■ POPULATION-BASED DIABETIC FOOT ULCER INCIDENCE AND PREVALENCE FROM SELECTED STUDIES

AUTHOR	POPULATION STUDIED	ANNUAL INCIDENCE/100	PREVALENCE/100
Borssen et al.[7]	375 patients Umea County Sweden, age 15–50, type 1 = 298, type 2 = 77	2.0	10.0 Type 1 DM 9.0 Type 2 DM
Kumar et al.[27]	Cross-sectional study of 811 type 2 patients from three U.K. cities	1.0	5.3
Moss et al.[45]	Cohort of 2,990 patients with late and early-onset diabetes	2.4 younger 2.6 older	9.5 younger 10.5 older
Ramsey et al.[52]	Nested case-control study in HMO, 8,905 type 1, type 2	1.9	
Walters et al.[67]	Cross-sectional study of 1,077 type 1, 2 patients in 10 U.K. general medicine practices	4.1	7.4

HMO, health maintenance organization.

Ambulatory Medical Care Survey for outpatient department and emergency room visits was used to identify foot ulcer care in out-of-hospital settings. Excluded were patients served by Veterans Administration (VA) and military hospitals. Table 2–2 shows that the most frequent outpatient ulcer condition in persons with diabetes between 1993 and 1995 was chronic ulcer. When all lower limb conditions in Table 2–2 were combined, the total accounted for only 1% of all office, outpatient, and emergency room visits in persons with diabetes (S. Preston, personal communication, 1997).

The anatomic site of a foot lesion has both etiologic and treatment implications. Table 2–3 presents data from two large prospective studies showing that the most common sites were the toes (dorsal or plantar surface), followed by the plantar metatarsal heads and the dorsum of the foot.[3, 55] The authors caution that ulcer severity is more important than ulcer site in determining the final outcome.[3] While foot ulcers reepithelialized in the majority of patients in these two studies, amputations occurred in 14% of the U.S. and 24% of Swedish patients. A small percentage of patients in each study died; however, their deaths were unrelated to the ulcer and were attributed to other comorbidity.[4, 55]

Risk Factors for Diabetic Foot Ulcers

Demographic characteristics of individuals hospitalized with a foot ulcer condition were identified from the National Hospital Discharge Survey (NHDS), 1983–1990. Figure 2–1 shows the highest percentage of hospital discharges for foot ulcers was in persons ages 45 to 64, while the lowest percentage was in persons younger than 45 years of age. Figure 2–2 displays a higher age-standardized proportion of discharges for lower limb ulcers in males compared to females. This difference was uniform across the 8-year interval. In the analytic studies reported in Table 2–4, male gender was not an independent predictor of foot ulcer.[27, 45, 67] Figure 2–3 shows the year-to-year discharge variation between white and nonwhite individuals.

Recent analytic studies using multivariable modeling techniques to assess independent risk factors for diabetic foot ulcers are presented in Table 2–4. The most consistent independent foot ulcer risk factors were long diabetes duration, select measures of neuropathy and peripheral vascular disease, glycemic control, foot deformity, prior foot ulcer, and prior amputation.

Long duration of diabetes, even after controlling for age, was a statistically significant finding in several studies.[27, 57, 67] In the study

Table 2-2 ■ DISTRIBUTION OF LOWER EXTREMITY CONDITIONS REPORTED IN OFFICE, OUTPATIENT, AND EMERGENCY ROOM SETTINGS IN PERSONS LISTING DIABETES, US, 1993–1995*

CONDITION (ICD CODE)	NUMBER
Abscess (682.6, 682.7)	289,000
Chronic ulcer (707.1, 707.6, 707.7)	675,000
Osteomyelitis (730.×6, 730.×7)	82,000
Open wound foot (892.0–892.9)	166,000
Open toe wound (893.0–893.9)	47,000

* Data from National Ambulatory Medical Care Survey and National Hospital Ambulatory Medical Care Survey; S.D. Preston, personal communication, 1997.

Table 2–3 ■ ANATOMIC SITE AND OUTCOME OF DIABETIC FOOT LESIONS IN TWO PROSPECTIVE STUDIES

	ALL LESIONS (N = 314) APELQVIST et al.[3]*	MOST SEVERE LESION (N = 302) REIBER et al.[55]†
Lesion Site		
Toes (dorsal and plantar surface)	51%	52%
Plantar metatarsal heads, midfoot and heel	28%	37%
Dorsum of foot	14%	11%
Multiple ulcers	7%	NA
Total	100%	100%
Lesion Outcomes		
Reepithelialization/primary healing	63%	81%
Amputation at any level	24%	14%
Death	13%‡	5%
Total	100%	100%

* Apelqvist's study included consecutive patients whose lesions were characterized according to Wagner Criteria from superficial nonnecrotic to major gangrene.
† Reiber's study patients were enrolled with a lesion through the dermis that could extend to deeper tissue.
‡ Includes eight amputees who had not yet met the 6-month healing criterion.

by Rith-Najarian, long duration of diabetes increased the risk of foot ulcers over sixfold comparing persons with a diabetes duration 9 years or less to those with a duration of 20 or more years.[57]

Several semiquantitative and quantitative measures of peripheral neuropathy and neurologic summary scores were used to describe associations between peripheral neuropathy and foot ulcers. In a randomized clinical trial using vibration perception threshold (VPT) greater than or equal to 25 as an entry criterion, Abbott and colleagues identified both baseline VPT and a combined score of re-flexes and muscle strength as significant predictors of incident ulcers.[1] Studies by Boyko and Rith-Najarian identified increased ulcer risk in patients unable to detect the 5.07 monofilament, a semiquantitative measure of light touch.[8, 57]

Parameters of peripheral vascular function appear in the final model in several studies. Low transcutaneous oxygen tension (TcPo$_2$), indicating diminished skin oxygenation, and low ankle-arm index (AAI), suggestive of impaired large-vessel perfusion, were both independent predictors of foot ulcers in the study by Boyko. In this study,

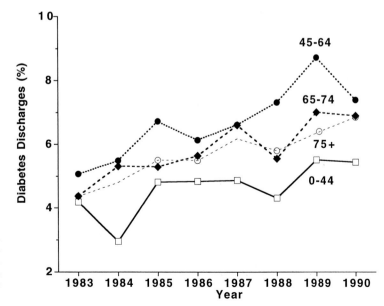

Figure 2–1 ■ Proportion of hospital discharges listing diabetes and lower extremity ulcers by age, United States, 1983–1990. (Data from National Hospital Discharge Survey, CDC.)

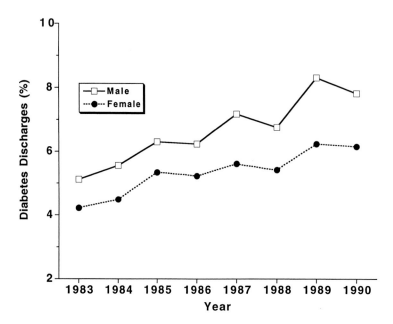

Figure 2–2 ■ Age-standardized proportion of hospital discharges listing diabetes and lower extremity ulcers by gender, United States, 1983–1990. (Data from National Hospital Discharge Survey, CDC.)

laser Doppler flowmetry was not a significant predictor of foot ulcers.[8] Kumar defined peripheral vascular involvement as the absence of two or more foot pulses or a history of previous peripheral revascularization. He reported presence of this variable was a significant predictor of foot ulcer.[27] Walters found that absent dorsalis pedis (DP) pulse was associated with a 6.3-fold increased risk of foot ulcer (95% confidence interval [CI], 5.57 to 7.0).[67]

Elevated levels of glycosylated hemoglobin (HbA_{1c}) or blood glucose have been associated with risk of foot ulcer. The cohort study by Moss identified a statistically significant association between high levels of HbA_{1c} and subsequent foot ulcer with an odds ratio of 1.6 (95% CI, 1.3 to 2.0).[45] Two of the studies reported in Table 3–4 report on the relationship between foot deformity and subsequent foot ulcer. The study by Boyko found an independent association between Charcot deformity and foot ulcer, but other foot deformities were not independent predictors.[8] Foot deformity did not enter the final analytic model in the study by Rith-Najarian.[57]

Smoking was assessed in four of the studies reported in Table 2–4. It was only of borderline significance in the younger population in the Wisconsin study.[45] The risk associated with a prior history of ulcers and amputations was assessed in two of the studies. Boyko reported both a prior history of ulcers and amputation significantly in-

creased the likelihood of a subsequent ulcer, while Kumar only found this relationship between prior amputation and subsequent ulcer.[8, 27] Boyko's cohort study also identified several additional independent predictors of foot ulcer including higher body weight, insulin use, and history of poor vision.[8]

Health care and education variables have been reported as important factors in development of foot ulcers. A randomized trial was conducted by Litzelman in a U.S. population served by a county hospital.[35] Patients were randomized to education, behavioral contracts, and reminders, while their providers received special education and chart prompts. The control population in this study received usual care and education. After 1 year, patients in the intervention group were more likely to report appropriate foot self-care behaviors, including inspection of feet and shoes, washing of feet, and drying between toes. Not all desirable behaviors were adopted. There was no significant difference between patient groups in testing of bath water temperature and reporting of foot problems. Patients in the intervention group developed fewer serious foot lesions including ulcers than did those in the control group.[35]

A study of causal pathways leading to diabetic foot ulcers was performed with U.S. patients from Seattle and U.K. patients from Manchester. Figure 2–4 defines sufficient and component causes.[58, 59] Reiber, Boulton,

Table 2–4 ■ RISK FACTORS FOR FOOT ULCERS IN PATIENTS WITH DIABETES MELLITUS FROM FINAL ANALYSIS MODELS OF SELECT STUDIES

AUTHOR, TYPE OF ANALYSIS	STUDY DESIGN, DIABETES TYPE	LONG DM DURATION	NEUROPATHY (MONOFILAMENT, REFLEX, VIBRATION, OR NEUROLOGIC SUMMARY SCORE)	LOW AAI, TcPo$_2$ OR ABSENT PULSES	HIGH HbA$_{1c}$	DEFORMITY	HISTORY		
							Smoking	Ulcer	Amputation
Abbott et al.[1] Cox regression analysis	RCT, patients with VPT ≥25; (U.S., U.K., Canada) type 1 = 255 type 2 = 780	0	0 Monofilament, + VPT + Reflex	Exclusion criteria			Exclusion criteria	Exclusion criteria	Exclusion criteria
Boyko et al.[8] Cox regression analysis	Cohort, Veterans type 1 = 48 type 2 = 701	0	+ Monofilament	+ AAI + TcPo$_2$	0	+ Charcot	0	+	+
Kumar et al.[27] Logistic regression	Cross-sectional 811 type 2 from U.K. general practices	+	+ NDS	+			0	0	+
Moss et al.[45] Logistic regression	Cohort, 2,990 patients with early- and late-onset diabetes	Borderline older			+		Borderline young		
Rith-Najarian et al.[57] Chi square analysis	Cohort 358 type 2 Chippewa Indians	+	+ Monofilament			0			
Walters et al.[67] Logistic regression	Cohort, 10 U.K. general practices 1,077 type 1, 2	+	+ Absent light touch + Impaired pain, perception, 0 VPT	+ Absent pulses 0 Doppler			0		

AAI, ankle-arm index; DM, diabetes; HbA$_{1c}$, hemoglobin A$_{1c}$; NDS, neuropathy disability score; RCT, randomized controlled trial; TcPo$_2$, transcutaneous oxygen tension; VPT, vibration perception threshold; blank cell, not studied; +, statistically significant finding; 0, no statistically significant finding.

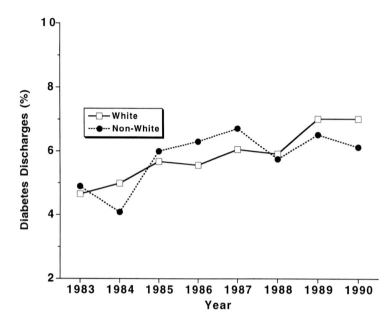

Figure 2–3 ■ Age-standardized proportion of hospital discharges listing diabetes and lower extremity ulcers by race, United States, 1983–1990. (Data from National Hospital Discharge Survey, CDC.)

and colleagues identified a critical triad of neuropathy, deformity, and minor trauma as the most common factors in the pathway to foot ulcer.[53] The temporal relationship of these components is diagrammed in Figure 2–5. Table 2–5 presents the frequency of each component cause that appeared in the multiple pathways leading to diabetic foot ulcers.[53]

Lower limb ulcer recurrences were addressed in a U.K. study by Mantey and colleagues.[37] Diabetic patients with an initial foot ulcer and two ulcer recurrences were compared to diabetic patients who had only one ulcer and no recurrences for at least 2 years. The authors report that increased peripheral sensory neuropathy and poorer diabetes control were higher in the ulcer recurrence group. In addition, the ulcer recurrence group waited longer from observing serious foot problems until reporting them to their clinic provider. The ulcer recurrence group also consumed more alcohol than did the group without ulcer recurrences.[37]

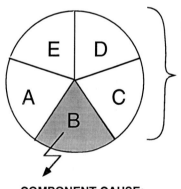

SUFFICIENT CAUSE:

--Inevitably produces an ulcer or amputation

--Restricted to the minimal number of component causes required for a foot ulcer or amputation

COMPONENT CAUSE:

--Not sufficient in itself

--Removal or blocking renders action of other components insufficient

Figure 2–4 ■ Diagram of sufficient and component causes of diabetic foot ulcers. A–E, Causes that are not sufficient in themselves, but are required components of a sufficient cause that will inevitably produce the outcome. (Adapted from Rothman K: Causes. Am J Epidemiol 104:587–592, 1976, with permission.)

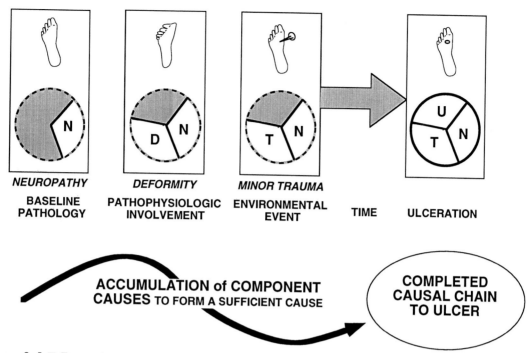

Figure 2–5 ■ Frequent component causes of diabetic foot ulcers. (From Reiber G, Vileikyte L, Boyko E, et al.: Causal pathways for incident lower-extremity ulcers in patients with diabetes from two settings. Diabetes Care 22:157–162, 1999, with permission.)

Epidemiology of Lower Limb Amputation

Incidence, Prevalence, and Amputation Level

Amputation, the removal of the terminal, nonviable part of a limb, is performed with differing frequency in different regions and

Table 2–5 ■ COMPONENT CAUSES PRESENT IN CAUSAL PATHWAYS LEADING TO FOOT ULCERS IN PERSONS WITH DIABETES*

COMPONENT CAUSE	PERCENT PRESENT IN CAUSAL PATHWAYS
Peripheral neuropathy	78
Minor trauma	77
Deformity	63
Edema	37
Peripheral ischemia	35
Callus	30
Infection	1

* From Reiber G, Vileikyte L, Boyko E, et al: Causal pathways for incident lower-extremity ulcers in patients with diabetes from two settings. Diabetes Care 22:157–162, 1999, with permission.

countries. The variation in age-adjusted incidence rates for nontraumatic lower limb amputations is illustrated in Table 2–6. The rates range from 2.1 per 1,000 to 13.7 per 1,000, a sixfold difference.[22, 23, 34, 43, 44, 46, 63, 64, 66] Recent trends in nontraumatic lower limb diabetic amputation in some populations are provocative. Figure 2–6 shows the U.S. 1996 age-adjusted amputation rate in persons with diabetes was 9.8 per 1,000, an increase of 26% from 1990 (L. Geiss, personal communication, 1999). The number of U.S. amputations, excluding VA and military, increased from 36,000 in 1980, to 54,000 in 1990 and to 86,000 in 1996 (L. Geiss, personal communication, 1999).[10] Figure 2–7 shows the hospital length of stay for amputation decreased markedly between 1980 and 1996, largely due to implementation of Diagnostic Related Group (DRG) reimbursement.[11]

Amputation prevalence data are also available from the U.S. National Health Interview survey. Individuals with diabetes had a tenfold higher overall prevalence of amputations than did nondiabetic persons, 2.8% versus 0.29%. In persons with diabetes, the prevalence increased by age from 1.6% in those ages 18 to 44, to 2.4% in those ages

Table 2–6 ■ AGE-ADJUSTED POPULATION-BASED INCIDENCE AMPUTATION RATES* AMONG PATIENTS WITH DIABETES FROM SELECT STUDIES

AUTHOR	POPULATION STUDIED	INCIDENCE RATE/1,000
Humphrey et al.[22]	Nauru	7.6
Humphrey et al.[23]	Rochester, MN, United States	3.8
Letho et al.[34]	East and West Finland	8.0
Morris et al.[43]	Tayside, Scotland	2.5
Moss et al.[44]	Wisconsin, United States	
	Younger onset diabetes	5.1
	Older onset diabetes	7.1
Nelson et al.[46]	Pima Indians, United States	13.7
Siitonen et al.[63]	Incident LEA	3.4 Men
	East Finland	2.4 Women
Trautner et al.[64]	Leverkusen, Germany	2.1
Van Houtum and Lavery[66]	California, United States	4.9
	Netherlands	3.6

* Rates are for any amputation, unless incident amputation specified.

45 to 64, and 3.6% in those age 65 years or older.[54]

The level of amputation differs between people with and without diabetes. The percentage of distal amputations performed in persons with diabetes is higher than in persons without diabetes; conversely, there is a higher percentage of proximal amputations in patients without diabetes. Table 2–7 presents amputation levels from the 1995 U.S. Hospital Discharge Survey and Table 2–8 provides information on amputation levels for diabetic and nondiabetic amputees in 1998 in Department of Veterans Affairs Hospitals. The proportion of diabetic amputations by level is similar for these two settings, with about 41% of amputations performed at the toe level, 11 to 13% of amputations at the transmetatarsal level, 24 to 28% at the transtibial level, and 20 to 21% at the transfemoral level.[11, 38] The overall frequency of amputation in individuals with and without diabetes in the Department of Veterans Affairs decreased as shown in Figure 2–8, yet diabetic amputations, as a proportion of total amputations, increased from 59% to 66% between 1989 and 1998.[38]

Risk Factors for Diabetic Lower Limb Amputations

Demographic characteristics of diabetic individuals with amputations discharged from

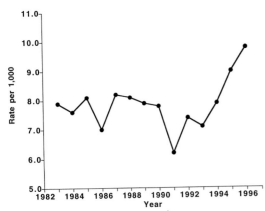

Figure 2–6 ■ Age-standardized hospital discharge rate for nontraumatic lower limb amputations in persons with diabetes, United States, 1983–1996. (Data from National Hospital Discharge Survey, CDC.)

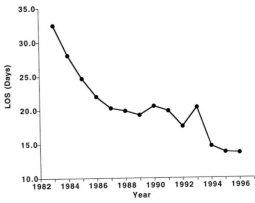

Figure 2–7 ■ Average length of stay for hospital discharges listing diabetes and nontraumatic lower limb amputation, United States, 1983–1996. (Data from National Hospital Discharge Survey, CDC.)

Table 2–7 ■ NUMBER AND PERCENT OF U.S. NATIONAL HOSPITAL DISCHARGE SURVEY
AMPUTATIONS IN PERSONS WITH DIABETES BY AMPUTATION LEVEL, 1995*

AMPUTATION LEVEL	NUMBER	PERCENT
Toe	31,291	40.6
Transmetatarsal	10,386	13.4
Transtibial	18,639	24.2
Knee disarticulation	44	0.1
Transfemoral	16,487	21.4
Hip disarticulation	265	0.3
Total	77,112	100

* Data from National Hospital Discharge Survey 1995.

Table 2–8 ■ NUMBER AND PERCENT OF AMPUTATIONS BY DIABETES STATUS AND HIGHEST
AMPUTATION LEVEL, IN VETERANS HEALTH AFFAIRS HOSPITALS, U.S., 1998*

| HIGHEST LEVEL AMPUTATION (%) | AMPUTATION INDICATION | | |
	DIABETES (N = 3,477)	OTHER INDICATION (N = 1,852)	TOTAL (N = 5,329)
Toe	41.2	25.7	35.8
Transmetatarsal	10.5	5.9	8.9
Transtibial	28.2	26.7	27.7
Transfemoral	20.1	41.7	27.6
Total	100	100	100

* Data from VA patient treatment file, Seattle Rehabilitation Research and Development Center, 1999.

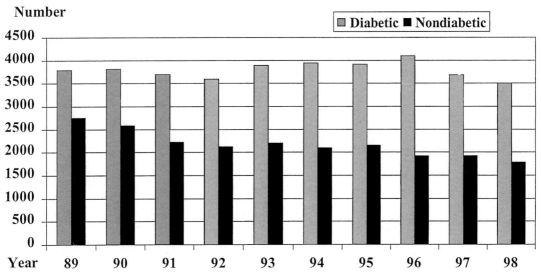

Figure 2–8 ■ Total discharges with lower extremity amputation, VA hospitals, 1989–1998.

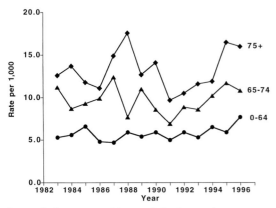

Figure 2–9 ▪ Rate of hospital discharge for nontraumatic lower limb amputation in persons with diabetes, by age, United States, 1983–1996. (Data from National Hospital Discharge Survey, CDC.)

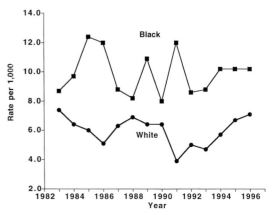

Figure 2–11 ▪ Age-standardized hospital discharge rate for nontraumatic lower limb amputation in persons with diabetes, by race, United States, 1983–1996. (Data from National Hospital Discharge Survey, CDC.)

U.S. NHDS hospitals show the impact of advancing age, male gender, and nonwhite racial status. Figure 2–9 shows that advancing age imparts an increased risk of amputation, with the highest amputation discharge rates occurring in patients ages 75 or older. Figure 2–10 shows age-adjusted amputation rates by gender, with discharge rates consistently higher in males than in females. Black individuals experienced higher hospital amputation discharge rates than did the combined group of whites and Hispanic Americans, although as shown in Figure 2–11 there was considerable year-to-year variation.

Statewide amputation rates show racial disparities in amputation frequency. Wisconsin 1994 hospital discharge rates in persons with diabetes indicated that blacks had 3.1

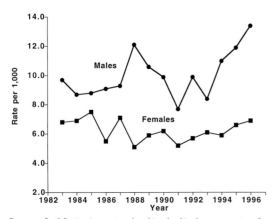

Figure 2–10 ▪ Age-standardized discharge rate for nontraumatic lower limb amputation in persons with diabetes, by gender, United States, 1983–1996. (Data from National Hospital Discharge Survey, CDC.)

times, and American Indians had 4.4 times the amputation rates of whites.[18] Findings from a 1991 California hospital discharge survey indicated the age-adjusted amputation rate was 4.4 per 1,000 in Hispanics, 5.6 per 1,000 in non-Hispanic whites, and 9.5 per 1,000 in African Americans.[30] In California, amputations in African Americans were performed at higher levels than in individuals from other ethnic and racial groups.[31] The importance of access to care and socioeconomic status deserve consideration when assessing racial and ethnic differences and amputations. Findings from a case-control study performed on patients from a large California health maintenance organization and a prospective case-control study in veterans reported no difference in amputation rates by racial and ethnic status. Patients in these health care systems presumably had more consistent access to health care.[56, 61]

Eight analytic studies that reported multivariable analysis of risk factors for amputation in persons with diabetes were selected for this chapter and are presented in Table 2–9. The risk factors identified are long duration of diabetes; select measures of neuropathy and peripheral vascular disease; high levels of HbA_{1c} or fasting plasma glucose; and a history of ulcers, amputations, retinopathy, and patient education.[2, 33, 34, 39, 44, 46, 56, 61] The two protective factors identified were provision of outpatient diabetes education[56] and use of aspirin.[44] Evidence for these risk factors follows.

Diabetes duration was a significant risk factor for amputation in five of the eight stud-

Table 2–9 ■ RISK FACTORS FOR LOWER LIMB AMPUTATIONS IN PERSONS WITH DIABETES IDENTIFIED IN FINAL ANALYSIS MODELS OF SELECT STUDIES

AUTHOR, TYPE OF ANALYSIS	STUDY DESIGN DIABETES TYPE	DURATION	NEUROPATHY (MONOFILAMENT VIBRATION, REFLEX)	PVD, AAI, TcPO₂, PULSES	HBP	HIGH HbA₁c, FPG	HISTORY			
							Smoking	Ulcer	Retinopathy	Pt Ed
Adler et al.[2] Multivariate proportional hazards	Cohort, 776 type 1 and 2 veterans	0	+	+		0	0	+		
Lee et al.[33] Cox regression	Cohort, 875 type 2 Oklahoma Indians	+			+SBP Male +DBP/Female	+ Male	0	0	+	0
Lehto et al.[34] Cox regression	Cohort, 1,044 type 2, Finland	+	+	+	0	+	0		+	
Mayfield et al.[39] Logistic regression	Retrospective case-control, 246 type 2 Pima Indians	+	+	+	0	+	0	+	+	
Moss et al.[44] Logistic regression	Cohort, 2,990 early and late onset, S. WI	0			+DBP	+	+Younger	+	+	
Nelson et al.[46] Stratified	Cohort, 4,399 Pima Indians, AZ, United States	+	+	+	0	+	0		+	
Reiber et al.[56] Logistic regression	Prospective case-control, 316 type 1, 2 veterans	Control variable	+	+	0	+	0		+	+
Selby and Zhang[61] Logistic regression	Nested retrospective case-control, 428 type 1, 2, HMO	+	+		+SBP	+	0		+	

AAI, ankle-arm index; DBP, diastolic blood pressure; HbA₁c, hemoglobin A₁c, HBP, high blood pressure; FPG, fasting plasma glucose; Pt Ed, patient outpatient education; PVD, peripheral vascular disease; SBP, systolic blood pressure; TcPO₂, transcutaneous oxygen tension; blank cell, not studied; +, statistically significant finding; 0, no statistically significant finding.

ies, and in one it was used as a risk adjuster. Risk for amputation increased with increasing duration of diabetes.[33, 34, 39, 46, 61] The exceptions were in the studies by Adler and Moss, which reported no statistically significant association in the multivariable analysis.[2, 44]

The loss of peripheral sensation decreases patients' awareness of foot pressure, discomfort, and even pain and increases the risk of ulceration and amputation.[6] Several measures of peripheral neuropathy were identified as risk factors for amputation. Insensitivity to the 5.07 (10-gm) Semmes-Weinstein monofilament at any of nine sites was found to increase amputation risk in the Seattle study reported by Adler and colleagues. However, this was only in the analysis model using $TcPo_2$.[2] Other measures of peripheral neuropathy associated with amputation risk were absent or diminished bilateral vibration sensation or absent ankle reflexes.[34, 56]

The importance of peripheral vascular function and its relationship to amputation was directly assessed in six studies. Peripheral vascular risk factors included low $TcPo_2$, low AAI, and absent or diminished dorsalis pedis (DP) and posterior tibialis (PT) pulses. Clinicians are increasingly able to distinguish the importance and adequacy of cutaneous circulation measured using $TcPo_2$, and major arterial circulation. Both parameters are important in preventing and healing amputations. Cutaneous perfusion depends not only on the underlying arterial circulation, but may be critically influenced by other factors, including skin integrity, mechanical effects of repetitive pressure, and tissue edema.

Using the cutpoint of less than or equal to 0.80 which is associated with lower limb arterial disease regardless of other symptoms, Adler found AAI was an independent predictor of amputation in one of the final reported models.[2] Absence of peripheral pulses was a risk factor for amputation in three analytic studies[2, 34, 39]; however, in another study absent peripheral pulses were only significant for women in the univariate analysis.[33]

Major symptoms of lower limb arterial disease are intermittent claudication, absent peripheral pulses, and rest pain. Findings on these variables were reported by Palumbo for the Rochester, Minnesota, population. The incidence of lower limb arterial disease was 8% at diabetes diagnosis, 15% at 10 years, and 45% at 29 years.[48] Intermittent claudication, a fairly benign condition, progressed to rest pain or gangrene in only 1.6% and 1.8%

of men and women, respectively, over 10 years.[47] In the Framingham Study, intermittent claudication was 3.8 and 6.5 times more common in diabetic than nondiabetic males and females, respectively.[26]

High blood pressure was an independent predictor of amputation in three analytic studies. In two of these studies there was no direct measure of peripheral vascular function.[44, 61] In the third study, Lee reported that systolic hypertension was significant only in the model for men and diastolic blood pressure was significant only in the model for women. Peripheral vascular function as measured by peripheral pulses was not an independent predictor of amputation in this study population.[33]

Poor glycemic control has been associated with an increased risk of amputation, primarily through the neuropathy pathways. The Diabetes Control and Complications Trial (DCCT) randomized patients with type 1 diabetes to either the intensive blood glucose control group or conventional control. The intensively treated group achieved nearly normal blood glucose levels compared to the control group, whose blood glucose values remained in the conventional range. The intensively treated group had a 69% reduction in subclinical neuropathy, a 57% reduction in clinical neuropathy, and fewer peripheral vascular events than the control group. Elevated HbA_{1c} or plasma glucose was a statistically significant predictor of amputation in seven of the eight analytic studies reported in Table 2–9.[33, 34, 39, 44, 46, 56, 61]

Major alterable risk factors for development of atherosclerosis in nondiabetic persons are cigarette smoking, lipoprotein abnormalities, and high blood pressure. These factors are assumed to be similarly atherogenic in diabetic individuals. Smoking was a risk factor in only one study, and only among persons with younger onset diabetes.[44] There are several possible explanations. Smoking was reported as an infrequent exposure by several authors. Other measures of peripheral arterial disease, more proximal in time to the amputation such as $TcPo_2$, AAI, or peripheral pulses, may better capture this domain in the multivariate analyses. An interesting protective association reported by Moss was the significant protective effect of aspirin on lower limb amputation in younger onset patients and a similar though nonsignificant trend in older onset patients.[44] Aspirin has long been used as a preventive agent for cardiovascular disease.

History of a prior foot ulcer was an independent predictor in three studies.[2, 39, 44] Foot ulcers preceded approximately 85% of nontraumatic lower limb amputations in two clinical epidemiology studies.[29, 49] In studies by Boulton in the United Kingdom and Reiber in the United States 45 to 60% of patients with new-onset ulcers reported a prior history of foot ulcer.[6, 55]

Appropriate footwear for foot ulcer patients and patients with toe or ray amputations has been described in several studies. In a study by Edmonds, a specialized foot care team achieved high rates of ulcer healing and decreased amputations. Therapeutic footwear was provided to ulcer patients who were then monitored for ulcer recurrences for an average of 26 months. The authors reported ulcer recurrences in 26% of persons who wore their special shoes compared to 83% who wore their own footwear.[17] Uccioli randomized patients with a history of prior foot ulcer to therapeutic footwear or their own footwear for a 1-year period. He found a significant decrease in reulceration rates in the group randomized to therapeutic shoes and inserts.[65]

The majority of studies reported that retinopathy was an independent predictor of amputation.[33, 34, 39, 44, 46, 56, 61] Retinopathy may reflect the extent of microvascular disease and may also be a proxy for diabetes severity.

Patient self-management education and self-care behaviors were linked to a decreased amputation risk in two studies. Veterans with high-risk foot conditions were randomized to "usual education" or a 1-hour lecture showing pictures of ulcers and amputations and a one-page instruction sheet. After 1-year follow-up, persons receiving the special educational session had a threefold decrease in ulceration ($p < 0.005$) and amputation rates ($p < 0.0025$).[36] A prospective case-control study, also in veterans, reported a strong protective effect comparing patients who had and had not received prior outpatient education.[56] Several foot care intervention programs reported decreases in amputations, reduced days of hospitalizations, and costs. Their descriptive interventions consisted of patient and professional education and structural changes in organization of foot care services. Given the multidimensional nature of these interventions, there were many components contributing to their reported success.[14, 42, 60]

Although foot examinations take minimal time to complete, patients in national surveys reported that only about 50% of patients with diabetes reported a foot exam from their health care provider within the past 6 months. Foot exam frequency was lowest in type 2 patients on insulin, where only 41% had been examined.[54] The frequency of foot examinations increased when there were chart reminders, clinician prompts, or when the nurse removed the patient's shoes and stockings before the clinician entered the room. However, provider foot exam frequency has not been associated with decreased ulcer amputation rates.

Subsequent Amputations

Subsequent amputations on the same side or contralateral side are common in diabetic amputees. Table 2–10 displays the frequency of subsequent amputations by side, if available, and by year since amputation. State-wide hospital discharge data from California and New Jersey indicated that 1-year following amputation, 9 to 13% of amputees experienced a new same side or contralateral amputation.[41, 68] Denmark has an amputation registry for surveillance purposes that excludes toe amputations. This registry is comprised of 27% of persons who reported diabetes and 73% who did not have a diabetes diagnosis.[16] Danish Registry reports identified that 19% of all patients undergoing a major amputation for arteriosclerosis and gangrene had another same-side amputation within 6 months. This percentage increased to only 23% by 48 months following amputation, suggesting that most same-side amputations above the toe level would be performed within 6 months of the initial amputation.[16]

The study by Braddeley reported 12% of diabetic individuals had a contralateral amputation at 1 year, 23% at 3 years, and 28% at 5 years.[9] According to the descriptive findings available, subsequent contralateral limb amputations occurred in persons with diabetes in 23 to 30% at 3 years and 28 to 51% at 5 years.[9, 28, 62] The notable exception was the study from Newcastle upon Tyne, where the 3-year ipsilateral amputation frequency was 6% and contralateral amputation frquency was 3%. This study did report 3-year mortality rates at 50%.[15] Part of the variation in the frequency of ipsilateral and contralateral amputations reported in these

Table 2-10 ■ PERCENT OF DIABETIC INDIVIDUALS WITH AMPUTATION FROM SELECT STUDIES UNDERGOING SUBSEQUENT IPSILATERAL AND CONTRALATERAL AMPUTATION BY TIME INTERVAL

AUTHOR	POPULATION	1 YEAR			3 YEARS			5 YEARS		
		Ipsilateral	Both	Contralateral	Ipsilateral	Both	Contralateral	Ipsilateral	Both	Contralateral
Braddeley and Fulford[9]				12			23			28
Deerochanawong et al.[15]	Newcastle, United Kingdom				6		3			
Larsson[28]	Lund, Sweden		14			30			49	
Miller et al.[41]	State of New Jersey, United States	9								
Silbert[62]	New York				30		51			
Wright and Kaplan[68]	State of California	13								

studies is related to the age structure of the study population.

Subsequent Mortality

The cause of death among amputees is rarely attributable to amputation, and is usually related to concurrent comorbid conditions such as cardiac or renal disease. Mortality following amputation has been examined by interval; 28 days (perioperative) and 1, 3, and 5 years. Table 2–11 presents amputation mortality data from nine select populations.

U.S. perioperative mortality from the National Hospital Discharge Survey for 1989 and 1992 was 5.8%.[51] Perioperative mortality was 10% in both the Newcastle study and in diabetic amputees in the Department of Veterans Affairs in 1998.[15, 38] Reports indicate the 1-year mortality rates in diabetic amputees range from 13 to 40%, 3-year mortality rates range from 35 to 65%, and the 5-year mortality rates range from 39 to 80%.[9, 15, 16, 29, 33, 38, 46, 50, 54] Amputation mortality varies by racial and ethnic status. In the 1991 Statewide California Hospital Discharge data, the age-adjusted amputation mortality rates were 1.6% among Hispanics, 2.7% among non-Hispanic whites, and 5.7% among African Americans.[30]

Economic Considerations

Economic considerations are an increasing concern for providers and payers. While the exact direct and indirect costs are difficult to ascertain, several studies have addressed direct costs for foot ulcers and amputations. In a study of patients with type 2 diabetes, "chronic skin ulcers" was a subset of all foot ulcers and accounted for $150 million of the $11.6 billion of direct diabetes patient care costs.[24] This study did not report separate costs for peripheral neuropathy, peripheral vascular disease, or amputation.

Most studies assess only direct patient costs (visits, hospitalizations, procedures, pharmaceuticals, dressings, referrals, etc.) and then report only the cost of the incident procedure. There are often recurring costs following ulcers and amputations that will be required over the patient's lifetime. Indirect cost (value of lost income from work, pain, suffering, and family burden, etc.) is difficult to estimate and therefore is seldom provided. The Study Revealing the Costs of Type 2 Diabetes in Europe (CODE-2) is assessing both direct and indirect costs in type 2 patients. The information on foot ulcers and amputations will be available as of late 2000.

Three studies comparing the cost of foot ulcers are presented in Table 2–12. The study by Apelqvist followed 314 patients from ulcer presentation until final resolution.[5] Healing was achieved in 2 months or less in 54% of patients, in 3 to 4 months in 19% of patients, and in 5 months or more in 27% of patients. There were 63% of patients who healed without surgery at an average cost of $6,664. Lower limb amputation was required for 24% of patients at an average cost of $44,790. The 13% of patients who died

Table 2–11 ■ PERCENT MORTALITY IN DIABETIC AMPUTEES FROM SELECT STUDIES BY TIME INTERVAL

AUTHOR	POPULATION	PERIOPERATIVE (28 days)	1 YEAR	3 YEARS	5 YEARS
Braddeley and Fulford[9]	Birmingham, United Kingdom		16%	35%	
Deerochanawong et al.[15]	Newcastle, United Kingdom	10%	40%	50%	
Ebskov and Josephsen[16]	Denmark* excludes toe amputations		32%	55%	72%
Larsson et al.[29]	Lund, Sweden		15%	38%	68%
Lee et al.[33]	Oklahoma Indians, United States			40%	60%
Mayfield et al.[38]	U.S. Veterans	10%	13%	41%	65%
Nelson et al.[46]	Pima Indians				39%
Pohjolainem and Alaranta[50]	S. Finland		38%	65%	80%
Reiber et al.[54]	National Hospital Discharge Survey, United States	5.8%			

* 27% of individuals in Danish Registry have diabetes.

Table 2–12 ■ DIRECT COST FOR DIABETIC FOOT ULCERS IN THREE STUDIES

AUTHOR	NO. OF PATIENTS/STUDY TYPE	OUTCOME	AVERAGE EPISODE COST (U.S. $)	INPATIENT COST	OUTPATIENT COST
Apelqvist et al.[5]	Prospective 314 general internal medicine patients	Primary healing, 63%	$6,664	61%	39%
		Healed after amputation, 24%	$44,790		
Holtzer et al.[21]	Retrospective, administrative records of 3,013 patients, and 3,524 episodes	Primary healing, 52%	$1,929	23%	77%
		Osteomyelitis, 33%	$3,980	23%	77%
		Gangrene/amputation, 14%	$15,792	12%	88%
Ramsey et al.[52]	Nested case-control study in HMO of 8,905 type 1, 2	Primary healing, 84%	$27,987 total attributable cost	18%	82%
		Amputation, 16%			

prior to final ulcer resolution were excluded from this analysis. The proportion of all costs that were related to hospitalization was 39% among ulcer patients and 82% among amputees.[5]

Ramsey conducted a nested case-control study in a large health maintenance organization (HMO) involving 8,905 patients with diabetes. In this group, 514 diabetic individuals developed one or more foot ulcers and 11% of these patients required amputation. Costs were computed for the year prior to the ulcer and the 2 years following the ulcer for both cases and controls. The excess costs attributed to foot ulcers and their sequelae were $27,987 per patient for the 2-year period following ulcer presentation.[52]

Holzer obtained direct cost data on private insurance patients from the MEDSTAT Group, a large U.S. integrated administrative claims system affiliated with private health insurance plans. Study enrollment criteria were ages 18 to 64, employed and not on Medicare, and in this system during 1991 to 1992. Ulcer claims were submitted for 5.1% of diabetic patients. These 3,013 patients had 3,524 ulcer episodes costing an average of $4,595 per episode. When ulcers were categorized by outcome, the costs were $1,929 for ulcers that healed without complications, $3,980 for those complicated with osteomyelitis, and $15,792 for patients whose ulcers were complicated with gangrene and required amputation. In this study, over 70% of total costs were from hospital settings.[21] These direct costs are a conservative estimate, as they exclude amounts paid by the patient, and secondary insurance, episodes of less than 1 week, and individuals who failed to seek treatment.

Frequency and cost of diabetes complications were addressed in two studies. A study by Jacobs on hospitalization for late complications of diabetes in the United States compared 1987 hospital discharge data for diabetic and age- and sex-matched nondiabetic individuals. The authors found the relative risk for skin ulcer/gangrene comparing diabetic to nondiabetic individuals was 21.8 (95% CI, 21.6 to 22.0).[25] A similar study was conducted in Wales by Currie using National Health Service data to examine differences in admissions, length of stay, and costs between diabetic and nondiabetic individuals. The relative risk for a foot ulcer comparing diabetic to nondiabetic individuals was 21.1 (95% CI, 16.6 to 26.9).[13] The authors concluded that only 2% of their population had diabetes, yet they consumed 20% of the inpatient cost.

The costs for treating foot ulcers are not well reimbursed in some settings. For diabetic and nondiabetic patients in the United States hospitalized with select foot conditions, reimbursement for hospital care differed by the patient's payer source. Table 2–13 shows that in fiscal year 1996, under DRG reimbursement code 271 (skin ulcer), private insurance reimbursed hospitals on average $11,199 for an average 12.7-day length of stay, while Medicare reimbursed hospitals an average of $4,855 (43% of the private reimbursement) for an average 7.9-day length of stay.[20, 40] Payment for the health care provider is not included in these figures.

Cost of Lower Limb Amputation

Costs for lower limb amputations vary by amputation level. There are often recurrent direct and indirect health care costs. In 1996, the average reimbursement to private hospitals for DRG 113, a lower limb amputation in persons with and without diabetes, was $26,126 for 14.3 days' hospitalization compared to $13,512 (51.7%) for an average 13.1-day hospital stay for Medicare patients (Table 2–14).[20, 40] Physician, rehabilitation, outpatient, and other follow-up care costs would be added to these figures for a complete estimate of direct care cost.

The rise in U.S. amputation rates reported earlier may be influenced by the disparity in reimbursement between limb salvage and amputation in fee-for-service systems. Hospitals are reimbursed almost twice as much for a lower limb amputation as salvage.[20, 40] Further information on financial impact to health care institutions is provided from the New England Deaconess Hospital. In 100 patients presenting with limb-threatening ischemia between 1984 and 1990, the frequency of diabetic amputation decreased from 44% to 7%, the frequency of popliteal and tibial bypass grafts remained constant, and the frequency of dorsalis pedis bypass grafts increased. The reported length of hospitalization decreased from 1984 levels of 44.1 days for amputees and 34.1 days for bypass grafts recipients to 22 days for both groups in 1990. The average bypass graft cost was $19,808 in 1984 and $15,981 in 1990, while amputation costs were $20,248 in 1984

Table 2–13 ■ ULCER REIMBURSEMENT TO HOSPITALS FOR PATIENTS WITH AND WITHOUT DIABETES, 1996

NO. OF PATIENTS	CONDITION	MEDSTAT (PRIVATE)[40]		MEDICARE[20]	
		LOS	Average Reimbursement	LOS	Average Reimbursement
238	Osteomyelitis	9.6	$10,453	9.3	$6,524
271	Skin ulcers	12.7	$11,199	7.9	$4,855
263	Skin graft/debridement and complications	11.7	$17,395	12.5	$10,837
264	Skin graft/debridement no complications	8.1	$10,168	7.2	$5,220
287	Skin graft/debridement Endocrine	10.7	$16,877	12.2	$10,363

LOS, length of stay (hospital days).

and $18,341 in 1990. Gibbons concluded that even though they were able to improve quality of care, maximize limb salvage, and reduce length of stay and overall cost, their Medicare reimbursement was insufficient and resulted in an average loss of $7,480 per admission.[19]

The discharge status of diabetic amputees has been monitored in several populations. In Colorado, the percentage of patients discharged to home or self-care after amputation gradually declined from 66% for those age 45 years or younger to 23% for those age 75 plus. Conversely, as age increased, an increasing proportion required relocation from home or self-care settings to other acute, skilled, and intermediate care facilities for inpatient care.[12] In Larsson's cohort in Sweden, 93% of patients living independently before their minor index amputation were able to return to living independently compared to 61% after a major amputation.[29] Lavery reported that while 2.3% of amputees in south Texas were admitted from an institutional care facility, over 25% were discharged to one following amputation.[30]

Summary

Lower limb diabetic ulcers and amputations are an important and costly problem for patients and their health care systems. The hospital amputation discharge rates have increased in the United States in recent years, particularly among males who are members of racial and ethnic minority groups. Many of the independent risk factors for ulcers and amputations are identified from population-based, analytic, and experimental studies and are similar. Several have the potential for modification by patients and their health care providers. Specific evidence is available demonstrating the benefit of better blood glucose control, self-care strategies learned through patient education, and use of appropriate footwear to prevent lesions in high-risk patients.

Once an individual has an ulcer, their risk of reulceration is high. Similarly, once an individual has had an amputation, the likelihood of a subsequent amputation reaches 51% at 5 years. Mortality following ampu-

Table 2–14 ■ AMPUTATION REIMBURSEMENT TO HOSPITALS FOR PATIENTS WITH AND WITHOUT DIABETES, 1996

NO. OF PATIENTS		MEDSTAT (PRIVATE)[40]		MEDICARE[20]	
		LOS	Average Reimbursement	LOS	Average Reimbursement
113	Lower limb amputation, except toe	14.3	$26,126	13.1	$13,512
114	Toe and upper limb amputation	7.7	$12,755	8.8	$7,268
285	Endocrine amputation	9.7	$15,496	12.0	$11,345

LOS, length of stay (hospital days).

tation steadily increases to 39 to 80% at 5 years.

The direct economic cost of foot ulcers and amputation is high. Information on indirect costs is not currently available. The majority of the costs are related to hospitalization. The cost for an average uncomplicated ulcer episode ranged from $1,929 to $6,664 in the studies examined. Complicated ulcers that required amputation increased these costs by sevenfold.

U.S. hospital reimbursement for amputations was approximately twice as much to hospitals for patients covered by private insurance compared to those covered by Medicare ($26,126 vs. $13,512). Hospital care of ulcers is reimbursed at less than half of that for amputation. Patient benefit, quality of life, and rehabilitation potential must be carefully assessed before considering economic tradeoffs in decisions regarding limb salvage or amputation.

REFERENCES

1. Abbott C, Vileikyte L, Williamson S, et al: Multicenter study of the incidence of and predictive risk factors for diabetic neuropathic foot ulceration. Diabetes Care 21:1071–1075, 1998.
2. Adler A, Boyko E, Ahroni J, Smith D: Lower extremity amputation in diabetes: The independent effects of peripheral vascular disease, sensory neuropathy and foot ulcers. Diabetes Care 22:1029–1035, 1999.
3. Apelqvist J, Castenfors J, Larsson J: Wound classification is more important than site of ulceration in the outcome of diabetic foot ulcers. Diabet Med 6:526–530, 1989.
4. Apelqvist J, Larsson J, Agard C: Long term prognosis for diabetic patients with foot ulcers. J Intern Med 233:485–491, 1993.
5. Apelqvist J, Ragnarson-Tennvall G, Persson U, Larsson J: Diabetic foot ulcers in a multidisciplinary setting and economic analysis of primary healing and healing with amputation. Intern Med 235:463–471, 1994.
6. Boulton AJM: Diabetic neuropathy. Carnforth, Lancashire, UK, Marius Press, 1997.
7. Borssen B, Bergenheim T, Lithner F: The epidemiology of foot lesions in diabetic patients aged 15–50 years. Diabet Med 7:438–444, 1990.
8. Boyko E, Ahroni JH, Stensel V, et al: A prospective study of risk factors for diabetic foot ulcer: The Seattle Diabetic Foot Study. Diabetes Care 22:1036–1042, 1999.
9. Braddeley R, Fulford J: A trial of conservative amputations for lesions of the feet in diabetes mellitus. Br J Surg 52:38–43, 1965.
10. CDC: Diabetes Surveillance. Atlanta, GA: U.S. Department of Health and Human Services, 1993.
11. CDC: Diabetes Surveillance, 1997: Centers for Disease Control and Prevention, DHHS, 1997.
12. Colorado State Department of Health: Diabetes Prevalence and Morbidity in Colorado Residents, 1980–1991, 1993:119–136.
13. Currie CJ, Morgan C, Peters LI Jr: The epidemiology and cost of inpatient care for peripheral vascular disease, infection, neuropathy, and ulceration in diabetes. Diabetes Care 21:42–48, 1998.
14. Davidson J, Alogna M, Goldsmith M: Assessment of program effectiveness at Grady Memorial Hospital, Atlanta. In Steiner GLP (ed): Educating Diabetic Patients. New York: Springer-Verlag, 1981.
15. Deerochanawong C, Home PD, Alberti KGMM: A survey of lower limb amputation in diabetic patients. Diabet Med 9:942–946, 1992.
16. Ebskov B, Josephsen P: Incidence of reamputation and death after gangrene of the lower extremity. Prosthet Orthot Int 4:77–80, 1980.
17. Edmonds M, Blundell M, Morris M, et al: Improved survival of the diabetic foot. Q J Med 60:763–771, 1986.
18. Ford E, Remington P, Sonnenberg G: The burden of diabetes in Wisconsin: Diabetes-related amputations, 1994. Wisconsin Med J 643, 1996.
19. Gibbons GW, Marcaccio EJ Jr, Burgess AM, et al: Improved quality of diabetic foot care, 1984 vs 1990. Arch Surg 128:576–581, 1993.
20. HCFA: DRG Inpatient Billing Data, 1996: Health Care Finance Administration, Bureau of Data Strategy and Management, 1998.
21. Holzer S, Camerota A, Martens L, et al: Costs and duration of care for lower extremity ulcers in patients with diabetes. Clin Ther 20:169–181, 1998.
22. Humphrey A, Dowse G, Thoma K, Zimmet P: Diabetes and nontraumatic lower extremity amputation: Incidence, risk factors and prevention—a 12 year follow-up study in Nauru. Diabetes Care 19:710–714, 1996.
23. Humphrey L, Palumbo P, Butters M, et al: The contribution of non-insulin dependent diabetes to lower extremity amputation in the community. Arch Intern Med 154:885–892, 1994.
24. Huse DM, Oster G, Killen AR, et al: The economic costs of non-insulin-dependent diabetes mellitus. JAMA 262:2708–2713, 1989.
25. Jacobs J, Sena M, Fox N: The cost of hospitalization for the late complications of diabetes in the United States. Diabet Med 8:S23–S29, 1991.
26. Kannel WB, McGee DL. Diabetes and cardiovascular disease: The Framingham Study. JAMA 241:2035–2038, 1979.
27. Kumar S, Ashe HA, Fernando DJS, et al: The prevalence of foot ulceration and its correlates in type 2 diabetic patients: A population-based study. Diabet Med 11:480–484, 1994.
28. Larsson J: Lower extremity amputation in diabetic patients. Lund University Doctoral Thesis, 1994.
29. Larsson J, Agardh C, Apelqvist J, Stenstrom A: Long term prognosis after healed amputations in patients with diabetes. Clin Orthop 350:149–158, 1998.
30. Lavery LA, Ashry HR, van Houtum W, et al: Variation in the incidence and proportion of diabetes-related amputations in minorities. Diabetes Care 19:48–52, 1996.
31. Lavery LA, van Houtum WH, Armstrong DG, et al: Mortality following lower extremity amputation in minorities with diabetes mellitus. Diabetes Res Clin Pract 37:41–47, 1997.
32. Lazarus GS, Cooper DM, Knighton DR, et al: Definitions and guidelines for assessment of wounds and evaluation of healing. Arch Dermatol 130:489–493, 1994.

33. Lee J, Lu M, Lee V, et al: Lower extremity amputation. Incidence, risk factors, and mortality in the Oklahoma Indian Diabetes Study. Diabetes 42:876–882, 1993.
34. Lehto S, Pyorala K, Ronnemaa T, Laakso M: Risk factors predicting lower extremity amputations in patients with NIDDM. Diabetes Care 19:607–612, 1996.
35. Litzelman DK, Slemenda CW, Langefeld CD, et al: Reduction of lower extremity clinical abnormalities in patients with non-insulin-dependent diabetes mellitus. Ann Intern Med 119:36–41, 1993.
36. Malone JM, Snyder M, Anderson G, et al: Prevention of amputation by diabetic education. Am J Surg 158:520–524, 1989.
37. Mantey I, Foster A, Spencer S, Edmonds M: Why do foot ulcers recur in diabetic patients? Diabet Med 16:245–249, 1999.
38. Mayfield J, Reiber G, Maynard C, et al: Trends in lower extremity amputation in the Veterans Affairs hospitals, 1989–1998. J Rehabil Res Dev 37:23–30, 2000.
39. Mayfield J, Reiber G, Nelson R, Greene T: A foot risk classification system to predict diabetic amputation in Pima indians. Diabetes Care 19:704–709, 1996.
40. MEDSTAT: DRG Guide Descriptions and Normative Values. Ann Arbor, MI, 1998.
41. Miller A, Van Buskirk A, Verhoek W, Miller E: Diabetes related lower extremity amputations in New Jersey, 1979–1981. J Med Society N J 82:723–726, 1985.
42. Miller L: Evaluation of patient education: Los Angeles County Hospital experience: Report of National Commission on Diabetes, Vol 3, 1975: Part V.
43. Morris AD, McAlpine R, Steinke D, et al: Diabetes and lower-limb amputations in the community. Diabetes Care 21:738–743, 1998.
44. Moss S, Klein R, Klein B: The 14-year incidence of lower-extremity amputations in a diabetic population. Diabetes Care 22:951–959, 1999.
45. Moss SE, Klein R, Klein BEK: The prevalence and incidence of lower extremity amputation in a diabetic population. Arch Intern Med 152:610–616, 1992.
46. Nelson R, Gohdes D, Everhart J, et al: Lower-extremity amputations in NIDDM: 12-yr follow-up study in Pima Indians. Diabetes Care 11:8–16, 1988.
47. Palumbo P, Melton L: Peripheral vascular disease and diabetes. In Mi H (ed): Diabetes in America: U.S. Govt. Printing Office, 1985:XV 1–21.
48. Palumbo PJ, Melton LJ III: Peripheral vascular disease and diabetes. Diabetes in America, 1995 (NIH Publication No. 95-1468).
49. Pecoraro RE, Reiber GE, Burgess EM: Pathways to diabetic limb amputation: Basis for prevention. Diabetes Care 13:513–521, 1990.
50. Pohjolainen T, Alaranta H: Ten-year survival of Finnish lower limb amputees. Prosthet Orthot Int 22:10–16, 1998.
51. Preston SD, Reiber GE, Koepsell TD: Lower extremity amputations and inpatient mortality in hospitalized persons with diabetes: National population risk factors and associations. University of Washington Thesis, 1993.
52. Ramsey SD, Newton K, Blough D, et al: Incidence, outcomes, and cost of foot ulcers in patients with diabetes. Diabetes Care 22:382–387, 1999.
53. Reiber G, Vileikyte L, Boyko E, et al: Causal pathways for incident lower-extremity ulcers in patients with diabetes from two settings. Diabetes Care 22:157–162, 1999.
54. Reiber GE, Boyko EJ, Smith DG: Lower extremity foot ulcers and amputations in diabetes. In National Diabetes Data Group (ed): Diabetes in America, 2nd ed. Washington, DC: DHHS, 1995.
55. Reiber G, Lipsky B, Gibbons G: The burden of diabetic foot ulcers. Am J Surg 176:5S–10S, 1998.
56. Reiber GE, Pecoraro RE, Koepsell TD: Risk factors for amputation in patients with diabetes mellitus. Ann Intern Med 117:97–105, 1992.
57. Rith-Najarian SJ, Stolusky T, Gohdes DM: Identifying diabetic patients at high risk for lower-extremity amputation in a primary health care setting. Diabetes Care 15:1386–1389, 1992.
58. Rothman K: Causes. Am J Epidemiol 104:587–592, 1976.
59. Rothman K: Modern Epidemiology. Boston: Little, Brown, 1986.
60. Runyon J: The Memphis diabetes continuing care program. JAMA 3:231–264, 1975.
61. Selby JV, Zhang D: Risk factors for lower extremity amputation in persons with diabetes. Diabetes Care 18:509–516, 1995.
62. Silbert S: Amputation of the lower extremity in diabetes mellitus. Diabetes 1:297–299, 1952.
63. Siitonen O, Niskanen L, Laakso M, et al: Lower extremity amputations in diabetic and nondiabetic patients. Diabetes Care 16:16–20, 1993.
64. Trautner C, Haastert B, Giani G, Berger M: Incidence of lower limb amputations and diabetes. Diabetes Care 19:1006–1009, 1996.
65. Uccioli L, Faglia E, Monticone G, et al: Manufactured shoes in the prevention of diabetic foot ulcers. Diabetes Care 18:1376–1378, 1995.
66. Van Houtum W, Lavery L: Outcomes associated with diabetes-related amputations in the Netherlands and in the state of California. J Intern Med 240:227–231, 1996.
67. Walters DP, Gatling W, Mullee MA, Hill RD: The distribution and severity of diabetic foot disease: A community study with comparison to a non-diabetic group. Diabet Med 9:354–358, 1992.
68. Wright W, Kaplan G: Trends in lower extremity amputations, California, 1983–1987. Sacramento, CA: California Department of Health Services, 1989.

NEUROPATHIC PROBLEMS OF THE LOWER EXTREMITIES IN DIABETIC PATIENTS

■ Robert J. Tanenberg, Mary P. Schumer, Douglas A. Greene, and Michael A. Pfeifer

This chapter reviews the role that neuropathy plays in lower extremity complications. Although diabetic neuropathy is common and is a frequent cause of disability, assessment and management of diabetic neuropathy is often overlooked or forgotten. Physicians and health care providers generally ensure that retinal exams, 24-hour urine collections, blood pressures, cholesterol levels, and glycemic control assessments are done on a routine basis. Neuropathy, on the other hand, is seldom diagnosed until the patient complains of pain or has developed a foot ulcer. It is for this reason that neuropathy is considered, by many health care professionals, to be the "forgotten complication" of diabetes.

Definitions

Diabetic neuropathy is defined as "peripheral, somatic or autonomic nerve damage attributable solely to diabetes mellitus."[70] "Clinical diabetic neuropathy" requires the presence of an abnormal neurologic exam done by a physician skilled in the proper examination technique and that the abnormal neurologic exam be consistent with nerve damage from diabetes. Confirmed clinical neuropathy is defined as clinical neuropathy plus confirmation by abnormal quantitative neurologic function tests (e.g., electrophysiologic tests, quantitative sensory testing, or autonomic function tests) in two or more nerves. "Subclinical diabetic neuropathy" is the presence of abnormal quantitative neurologic function tests with little or no evidence of clinical neuropathy by exam.[25] There are sensory nerves (controlling sensation), motor nerves (controlling the musculature), and autonomic nerves (controlling functions such as sweating, vascular flow, heart rate, gastric emptying, and other visceral organs). Sensory neuropathy can result in abnormal sensations, such as pain, or lack of sensation (numbness). Motor neuropathy can result in muscle atrophy. This may lead to imbalances between muscle groups in the foot. These imbalances can result in foot deformities. A common example is claw toe deformity, which is caused by the constant flexion of the toes. Autonomic neuropathy may lead to decreased sudomotor function and dry feet or abnormal blood flow in the soles of the feet.

Stages

A useful staging method is the one described by the Mayo Clinic.[26] Stage 0 is no evidence of neuropathy. Stage 1 is subclinical neuropathy defined as no signs or symptoms of neuropathic problems but abnormal quantitative neurologic function tests. Stage 2 is clinical neuropathy (i.e., findings of signs and symptoms consistent with diabetic neuropathy). Usually this can be confirmed by evaluating quantitative neurologic function tests. Stage 3 is end-stage, debilitating neuropathy. Typically, people with stage 3 neuropathy have an abnormal gait, can't walk on their heels, or have had a foot ulcer. Table 3–1 summarizes these stages.

Epidemiology

Only a few authors have reported the prevalence of diabetic neuropathy, with varying results. Some of the best information on the prevalence of diabetic neuropathy is from the population-based Rochester Diabetic Neuropathy Study.[27] Between 60 and 65% of either type 1 or type 2 diabetic patients had some (any) neuropathy. Forty to 45% had distal-symmetric polyneuropathy (see definition of this type of diabetic neuropathy below). Approximately 30% had carpal tunnel syndrome. Six percent had autonomic neuropathy. Less than 5% had "other" neuropathies (including plexopathies, mononeuropathies, cranial neuropathies, and radiculopathies). There was no statistically significant difference in the prevalence of neuropathy between the two types of diabetes mellitus.

In a separate study done by Harris, the prevalence of neuropathy in type 1 and type 2 diabetic patients was found to be 35 to 40% compared to the prevalence of neuropathy (10 to 12%) in nondiabetic, matched patients.[40] In addition, the prevalence of neuropathy increased with the duration of diabetes. This confirms previous results published by Pirart, who analyzed the findings of a large population of patients with diabetes over many years.[69] He found an increase in the prevalence of neuropathy with both increased duration of diabetes and worse glycemic control.

Types of Neuropathy

Neuropathy can be divided into several types (Table 3–2). The two major types are focal and diffuse neuropathies. Focal neuropathies can be further divided into ischemic and entrapment neuropathies. Diffuse neuropathy can be divided into distal, symmetric polyneuropathy and autonomic neuropathies.

Focal Neuropathies

Focal ischemic neuropathies are believed to be due to an acute ischemic event to a nerve, a plexus of nerves, or a nerve root. As a result, this type of neuropathy tends to have a sudden onset, to be asymmetric in distribution, and to have a self-limiting course. Examples of acute ischemic focal neuropathies include mononeuropathies, femoral neuropathies, radiculopathies, plexopathies, and cranial neuropathies. Diagnosis is typically via clinical exam and symptoms. Therapy relates to time. Cranial neuropathies (e.g., third-nerve palsy) may improve in days to a few weeks, whereas femoral neuropathies may take months to 1½ years to improve. There is no known therapy that has been proven to shorten the time to recovery.

Table 3–1 ■ STAGES OF DIABETIC NEUROPATHY

STAGE	DESCRIPTION	SIGNS OR SYMPTOMS	ABNORMAL QUANTITATIVE TESTS
0	No neuropathy	No	No
1	Subclinical neuropathy	No	Yes
2	Clinically evident neuropathy	Yes	Yes
3	Debilitating neuropathy	Yes	Yes

Table 3–2 ■ TYPES OF DIABETIC NEUROPATHY

  I. Focal neuropathies
     A. Ischemic neuropathies
        1. Sudden onset
        2. Asymmetric
        3. Ischemic etiology
        4. Self-limited
        5. Examples
           a. Mononeuropathies
           b. Femoral neuropathies
           c. Radiculopathies
           d. Plexopathies
           e. Cranial neuropathies
     B. Entrapment neuropathies
        1. Gradual onset
        2. Usually asymmetric but can be bilateral
        3. Compression etiology
        4. Waxing and waning progressive course
           without spontaneous recovery
        5. Examples
           a. Carpal tunnel syndrome
           b. Ulnar entrapment (tennis elbow)
           c. Lateral cutaneous femoral nerve
              entrapment
           d. Tarsal tunnel syndrome
 II. Diffuse neuropathies
     A. Insidious onset
     B. Symmetric
     C. Abnormalities secondary to vascular,
        metabolic, structural, and autoimmune
        aberrations
     D. Progressive without spontaneous recovery
     E. Examples
        a. Distal-symmetric polyneuropathy
        b. Autonomic neuropathies

Focal entrapment neuropathies occur when a nerve is compressed in a specific body compartment. They tend to have a gradual onset, to occur in an asymmetric distribution (but it can occur bilaterally), and often have a progressive course. Examples include carpal tunnel syndrome, ulnar entrapment, and tarsal tunnel syndrome. Tarsal tunnel syndrome occurs when the tibial nerve becomes entrapped in the tarsal tunnel. The tarsal tunnel is located on the medial surface and just below the medial malleolus. As the tibial nerve traverses into the foot, it splits into two branches, one to the heel and the other to the remainder of the foot. The split of the tibial nerve can occur before or within the tarsal tunnel. Thus, people with tarsal tunnel syndrome may have a variety of symptoms. Symptoms may include paresthesias or numbness in the distal foot with the heel spared, or the heel may be involved as well. Pain from tarsal tunnel entrapment generally worsens throughout the day, as there is increased pain with activity. Thus, the pain is typically worse at the end of the day and improves upon resting the foot. This pain scenario is very different from the pain associated with distal symmetric polyneuropathy.

Signs of tarsal tunnel syndrome include an abnormal two-point discrimination test, abnormal vibratory sensation, and weakness and wasting of foot muscles. Often there is loss of flexibility of the metatarsophalangeal joint (inability to hold a pencil with toes or the inability to grab a handkerchief placed flat on the floor with the toes). A gait disturbance is occasionally observed. Diagnosis is made via appropriate signs and symptoms and confirmed by electrodiagnostic measures above and below the tarsal tunnel. Therapy may include surgery or steroid injections.

Diffuse Neuropathies

Diffuse neuropathies are due to structural, vascular, and metabolic abnormalities (see below). They tend to have an insidious onset. There is a symmetric distribution and progressive course. Examples of diffuse diabetic neuropathies include distal symmetric polyneuropathy and autonomic neuropathy. Distal symmetric polyneuropathy may involve both motor and sensory nerves. Typically, both small nerve fibers, as well as large nerve fibers, are involved. There are, however, cases of diabetic distal symmetric polyneuropathy, limited to the small nerve fibers and cases where the large nerve fibers seem to be almost exclusively involved. These cases of "small fiber neuropathy" or "large fiber neuropathy" are considered variants of distal symmetric polyneuropathy. However, their clinical picture would vary from the more classic variety of distal symmetric neuropathy. For instance, people with small fiber neuropathy may have severe dysesthetic pain but have a relatively normal neurologic exam (see below), since the neurologic exam is, for the most part, an evaluation of large nerve fiber function and integrity. Large fiber neuropathy may not be recognized as different from the more classic form of distal symmetric polyneuropathy unless small fiber tests (see below) are done and found to be disproportionately normal compared to its large fiber counterpart.

Distal symmetric polyneuropathy has a symmetric distribution. There is distal and dying-back (stocking-and-glove) nerve damage (Fig. 3–1). Neuropathy of the motor nerves in the foot may result in muscle wasting, foot deformities, and abnormal pressure points. Sensory neuropathy in the foot may result in pain, in numbness, and/or in decreased position sense, resulting in gait changes.

Clinical neuropathy can be documented by a routine foot exam and confirmed by quantitative nerve testing. Painful diabetic neuropathy, which usually occurs after 8 to 10 years' duration of diabetes, is often brought to the attention of the physician by the patient because the patient is often seeking relief from the pain. In patients with distal symmetric polyneuropathy the pain is usually worse at night (as opposed to the end of the working day), gets worse with rest (rather than better), and is relieved with movement (rather than aggravated). However, the insensate foot is silent and may lead to foot ulcers and

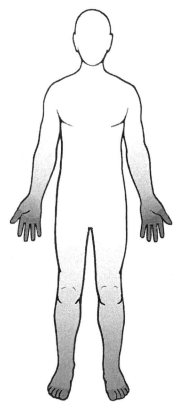

Figure 3–1 ■ Stocking-and-glove distribution of diabetic, distal, symmetric polyneuropathy. Diabetic distal symmetric polyneuropathy involves both sides relatively equally, feet more than hands, is distal rather than proximal, and involves multiple nerves. There is a distal dying of the nerve fiber. This results in a dying-back clinical picture. Thus, the involvement of hands and feet presents as a stocking-and-glove pattern.

amputation if appropriate therapy is not applied.

Autonomic neuropathy can result in a relaxation (opening) of arterial shunts on the plantar surface of the foot. The opening of these shunts because of sympathetic denervation results in a redirection of blood flow away from the nutrient capillaries and the surface of the skin. Figure 3–2 illustrates how opening these shunts will result in a decrease in transcutaneous oxygen and cause arterialization of the venous blood from the foot.[8, 22, 38, 47] The decrease in transcutaneous oxygen level is dependent upon the degree of the neuropathy. Figure 3–3 shows the transcutaneous oxygen levels on the dorsal and plantar surfaces of the feet of diabetic patients with stage 2 and 3 neuropathy. With severe neuropathy (stage 3), there is less transcutaneous oxygen on the plantar surface where the arteriovenous (AV) shunts exist but no difference in trancutaneous oxygen on the dorsum of the foot where no AV shunts exist.

Autonomic neuropathy can also cause a decrease in sudomotor function (loss of sweating). Poor sudomotor function can cause the foot to become dry and cracked. The natural protection and integrity of the skin is lost, and that puts the foot at greater risk for mechanical damage.

There is also loss of subcutaneous fat tissue in the foot. Although the etiology of the loss of this fat tissue is not clearly understood, some investigators believe that it is associated with autonomic neuropathy. The loss of this subcutaneous fat increases the foot pressure points.

Etiologies of Diffuse Neuropathies

Much information as to the etiology of the diffuse neuropathies has been established in the last 25 years. It is unlikely that a single cause is the culprit, but rather a combination of different abnormalities cumulating in a common clinical picture of diabetic neuropathy (Fig. 3–4).

Hyperglycemia

As with most diabetic complications, insulin deficiency and hyperglycemia are considered the initiating factors. Although there are multiple retrospective studies that support

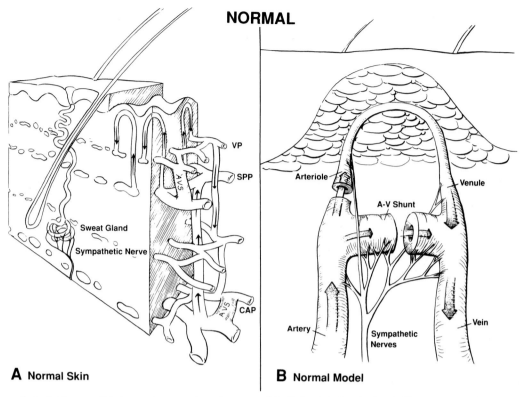

Figure 3–2 ■ Plantar AV shunts in normal and neuropathic diabetic individuals. *A,* The microvasculature of the sole of the foot. Small subcutaneous arteries penetrate the dermis and anastomose in the cutaneous arterial plexus (CAP). Arterioles arise from this plexus and ascend to form the subpapillary plexus (SPP). Arteriovenous anastomoses (AV shunts [AVS]) are richly innervated, are under rigid sympathetic control, and connect small arteries and arterioles to small veins and venules, which form a venous plexus (VP). *B,* A schematic model of the normal artery, arteriole, venule, vein, and sympathetically innervated AV shunt. Under normal circumstances, the AV shunt is closed and blood flow is through the nutrient capillaries.

Illustration continued on following page

this hypothesis, the Diabetes Control and Complications Trial (DCCT)[24] and the United Kingdom Prospective Diabetes Study (UK-PDS)[82, 83] are the strongest evidence supporting this mechanism in both type 1 and type 2 diabetic patients (Table 3–3). Both these trials were prospective and involved randomization to methods to achieve better glucose control or traditional therapy. In both of these trials patients randomized to methods designed to achieve better control had better nerve conduction velocity tests. Furthermore, the DCCT demonstrated better autonomic nervous tests and less "confirmed clinical" neuropathy in patients with better glucose control. Long-term follow-up of the DCCT patients may answer the question of whether as little as 5 years of better glucose control early in the course of diabetes will result in fewer neuropathic foot ulcers and amputations in the future.

Vasa Nervorum

It has been proposed that an abnormal vasa nervorum causing local nerve ischemia will lead to poor nerve function (nerve conduction velocity [NCV], nerve conduction amplitude, quantitative sensory tests [QST], and abnormal autonomic function tests [AFT]) and nerve morphometry. Several studies lend credence to these mechanisms.[6, 11, 49] One study demonstrated that treatment with a prostaglandin I_2 analog (beraprost sodium) resulted in improved nerve function by theoretically inducing relaxation of vascular smooth muscle and reducing nerve ischemia.[43] Furthermore, the angiotensin converting enzyme (ACE) inhibitor, lisinopril, has shown an increase in NCV in diabetic humans and a prevention of the decrease in NCV observed in untreated streptozotocin (STZ)-induced diabetic rats.

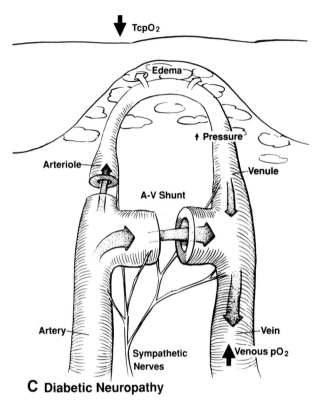

C Diabetic Neuropathy

Figure 3–2 ■ *Continued. C,* Proposed mechanism of AV shunting in diabetic neuropathy. A decrease in sympathetic innervation of the richly innervated AV shunts and less innervated arterioles results in relatively greater dilatation of the AV shunt and only a modest dilatation of the arteriole. This leads to a shunting of blood away from the capillary dermal papillae loops (nutrient capillary), a decrease in transcutaneous oxygen tension at the skin, an increase in foot venous oxygen tension, and low skin temperature.[8, 22, 38, 47]

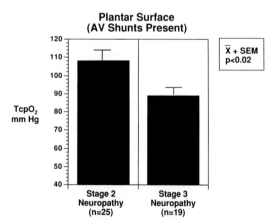

Figure 3–3 ■ Effects of stage of neuropathy on transcutaneous oxygen tension. Diabetic patients with stage 2 (signs and symptoms of neuropathy, confirmed by quantitative tests) and stage 3 (debilitating neuropathy) diabetic neuropathy are compared. Both groups of patients had normal pedal pulses and toe blood pressures. The transcutaneous oxygen tension ($TcpO_2$) on the plantar surface was lower in the patients with the more advanced neuropathy. On the other hand, there was no difference in $TcpO_2$ on the dorsal surface of the feet between the two groups of patients (data not shown). There are AV shunts on the soles of the feet but not the dorsum of the feet. The decrease in $TcpO_2$ may be secondary to lack of innervation of the AV shunts in the stage 3 patients.

The improvement of NCV by lisinopril was hypothesized to be secondary to vasodilatation secondary to increase in nitric oxide.[14, 16, 71] Other work has suggested that the increased aldose reductase activity secondary to hyperglycemia competitively competes with nitric oxide synthetase for NADPH, resulting in decreased nitric oxide. The reduction in nitric oxide reduces nerve blood flow, resulting in nerve ischemia. In this study, NCV did not decrease in STZ-induced diabetic rats if the animals were treated with sorbinil (an aldose reductase inhibitor [ARI]), but nitric oxide synthetase inhibitor could block the effect of sorbinil.[81, 89] This implies that the beneficial effects of ARI seen in diabetic animals and man may be secondary to vascular effects on the nerve. The diacylglycerol (DAG)–protein kinase C (PKC) pathway activation has been proposed to explain some of the complications of diabetes and may help to explain the above findings in a unified hypothesis. Hyperglycemia increases the formation and the metabolism of DAG, which in turn activates PKC.[86] In addition, hyperglycemia activates the polyol pathway, which in turn decreases *myo*-inositol (see below).[35] The altered inositol phospholipid metabolism also

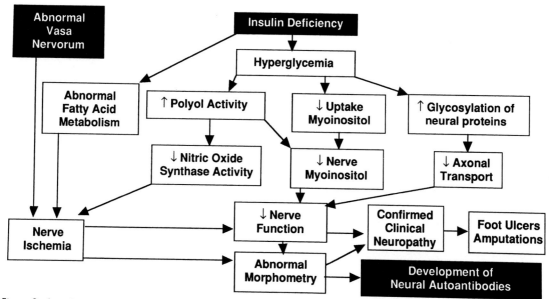

Figure 3–4 ■ Proposed etiologies of diffuse diabetic neuropathy. Abnormal vasa nervorum, insulin deficiency, hyperglycemia, abnormal fatty acid metabolism, increased polyol activity, decrease nerve *myo*-inositol, increased glycosylation of neural proteins, and neural autoantibodies have all been suggested as etiologies of diabetic neuropathy. There appears to be a common end result: confirmed clinical neuropathy. In a single individual one or more of these pathways may be prominent. In another individual other pathways may play a more predominant role. (From Pfeifer MA, Schumer MP: Clinical trials of diabetic neuropathy: Past, present and future. Diabetes 44:1355–1361, 1995, with permission.)

increases PKC activity.[21] PKC mediates a vascular response to hyperglycemia that involves both the endothelium and smooth muscle tissue. PKC regulates vascular permeability, contractility, basement membrane synthesis, and cellular proliferation.[44, 55, 69, 85] Inhibition of the β form of PKC with

LY333531 appears to decrease vascular endothelial growth factor (VEGF) in the retina and transforming growth factor-β (TGF-β) in the kidney.[23, 41] VEGF and TGF-β are believed to play pivotal roles in the development of diabetic retinopathy and nephropathy, respectively.[9, 54] It is anticipated that

Table 3–3 ■ DCCT AND UKPDS LANDMARK CLINICAL TRIALS OF GLUCOSE CONTROL

	DCCT	UKPDS
Type of diabetic patients	1	2
Number of patients	1,441	4,209
Length of study (years)	10	20
Average length of patient follow-up (years)	5	10
Average HbA$_{1c}$ (%)		
Standard therapy	8.9	7.9
Intensive therapy	7.1	7.0
Average glucose level (mg/dL)		
Standard therapy	231	177
Intensive therapy	155	147
Reduction in retinopathy (%)	76	21
Reduction in nephropathy (%)	56	34
Reduction in neuropathy (%)	60	25

DCCT, Diabetes Control and Complications Trial; UKPDS, United Kingdom Prospective Diabetes Study; HbA$_{1c}$, glycosylated hemoglobin.

increased PKC activity may play a role in the development of diabetic neuropathy by changes in the vascular environment.

Abnormal Fatty Acid Metabolism

Linoleic acid is converted to γ-linolenic acid, which is converted to dihomo-γ-linolenic acid. Dihomo-γ-linolenic acid will eventually be converted (through several more steps) to arachidonic acid, which helps dilate blood vessels. In diabetes, the δ-6-desaturation of linoleic acid to γ-linoleic acid (GLA) is impaired. This forces prostaglandin metabolism down an alternate pathway, leading to a decrease in nerve function either directly or indirectly via nerve ischemia as a result of altered prostaglandin metabolism (see above).[10, 13] When patients were given evening primrose oil, which is high in γ-linolenic acid, in a double-blind, placebo-controlled, randomized, multicenter study, both peroneal and median motor NCV and thermal perception threshold improved in the patients randomized to GLA treatment compared to the control patients.[80] However, clinical signs and symptoms were unchanged.

Polyol Pathway

The polyol pathway consists of converting glucose to sorbitol via aldose reductase and then converting sorbitol to fructose via sorbitol dehydrogenase. The pathway is relatively dormant at normal glucose levels and activated during hyperglycemia due to the Km of the aldose reductase enzyme. Besides the competitive consumption of NADPH and the theoretical decrease in nitric oxide synthetase activity, the increased activity of the polyol pathway also decreases nerve *myo*-inositol through mechanisms that are not well understood.[12, 32, 63] Thus, the decrease in nerve *myo*-inositol may also lead to a decrease in nerve function (NCV) and to abnormal morphometry.[76] Clinical studies with ARIs have documented improved morphometry and an improvement in NCV.[68] Only one study using an ARI has attempted to prevent the development of diabetic neuropathy. In this double-blind, randomized, placebo-controlled, multi-center study, results showed an improvement in peroneal motor, median motor and median sensory NCV, but prevention of confirmed clinical neuropathy was not

statistically different between the ARI and the placebo group.[50] However, the statistical power of the study was noted to be inadequate. In a small single-center longitudinal study, long-term treatment with the ARI sorbinil prevented the deterioration of tactile and thermal perception thresholds.[65] In summary, therapy with an ARI is associated with both an improvement of NCV and morphometry, presumably via a restoration of nerve *myo*-inositol concentration and improved nerve blood flow. However, clinical efficacy of this class of medicines has not been established. This may be due to clinical trial design rather than lack of efficacy.

Myo-inositol

Hyperglycemia, per se, competitively inhibits neural uptake of *myo*-inositol (in addition to the polyol pathway decreasing nerve *myo*-inositol). It is hypothesized that Na^+-K^+-ATPase activity is decreased by lower *myo*-inositol concentrations and thus presumably slows NCV.[88] In some studies, patients and animals placed on a high–*myo*-inositol diet showed improvement in NCV, but in other studies the results were contradictory.[36, 52, 53] Improvement in nerve morphometry and autonomic neuropathy has been shown in animals placed on high–*myo*-inositol diets.[15, 20, 77, 87]

Advanced Glycated End Products

Increased levels of glycosylated neural proteins have also been attributed to hyperglycemia. The first step in glycosylation of proteins is bonding of glucose to a free amino group. Subsequent glycosylated neural protein can cross-link, leading to the formation of advanced glycosylated end products (AGEs). Cross-linking changes the three-dimensional configuration of the proteins, and the proteins may become dysfunctional. This may account for the slowing of axonal transport observed in diabetic neuropathy. Aminoguanidine prevents this cross-linking from occurring. Future studies may show that aminoguanidine or similar products may be useful in the prevention of the development of diabetic neuropathy. In addition, aminoguanidine appears to have ARI properties and effect on nitric oxide and vascular flow in animal models of diabetes.[30, 42] However, these latter effects of aminoguanidine have not been confirmed in other studies.

Antibodies to Neural Tissue

Although antibodies to nerve tissue are associated with the presence of neuropathy in both type 1 and type 2 diabetic patients, it is not clear that these antibodies play an initial etiologic role. These antibodies could simply be a response by the immune system to damaged nerves. However, once the autoantibodies have been produced, it is certainly feasible that they may further impair nerve integrity and function.[17, 45, 91] Clinical trials of immune suppression therapy for diabetic neuropathy have not been conducted.

Nerve Growth Factor

Distal dying back of nerves is a common morphometric finding in patients with diabetic neuropathy. Efforts to reverse this process with nerve growth factor and gangliosides have been attempted in clinical trials. Both nerve growth factor and ganglioside treatment result in axonal sprouting and could theoretically improve nerve function, especially in small nerve fibers. To date, results of these trials have been inconsistent and disappointing.[3, 29]

Delineating the Etiologies

It is clear that many etiologies may lead to the common clinical manifestation of diabetic neuropathy. Although all the pathways are feasible and appear to be valid in animal studies, confirmation in human clinical trials is generally lacking. The exception, of course, is hyperglycemia. It is now certain that treatment of hyperglycemia will prevent and/or slow the progression of diabetic neuropathy.

Clinical trials of the chronic complications of diabetes require demonstrating that the progression of development of the complication can be slowed or prevented. This requires adequate time for the control group to develop the complication or demonstrate a worsening of the condition. In diabetic individuals with stage 0 or 1 neuropathy, the rate of progression is very slow. It has been estimated that NCV (one of the most reliable and precise measurements) deteriorates at a rate of 0.5 m/sec/yr. This would imply that the minimum worsening in NCV that would be considered clinically significant (2 to 3 m/sec) in the control group would take 4 to 6 years. This is compounded by the fact that physiologic changes in NCV can be as much as 2 to 3 m/sec. For instance, one study showed that an improvement in serum glucose levels via a 20-minute intravenous insulin infusion can improve NCV 2 m/sec.[51, 78] Furthermore, there appears to be a metabolic component and a structural component to diabetic neuropathy. The metabolic component may be the result of any of the proposed etiologies listed above. Theoretically, this component is reversible if the underlying abnormality is corrected. In fact, many of the clinical trials that test the various hypothesized pathogenic mechanisms demonstrate a small (1 to 2 m/sec) statistical but not clinically meaningful improvement in NCV (Fig. 3–5).[63] Interestingly, the improvement is very consistent among the various trials and methods. This implies that most, if not all, of the proposed mechanisms play a similar contributing role or that they interplay in a single common pathogenic mechanism. The most likely common mechanism may be the vascular component. The structural component does not appear to be reversible and may represent a greater portion of the sum total nerve abnormality and damage over time (Fig. 3–6). Therefore, even small reversibility of late stage 2 or 3 neuropathy is probably not feasible.

Delineation of etiologies also requires clear-cut end points. Clinical trials meeting this requirement have been conducted for retinopathy and nephropathy. However, with the exception of the DCCT, clinical trials of diabetic neuropathy have been too short, underpowered, and conducted in patients with advanced disease, and without clear-cut demonstrable end points. In the future, further delineation of the causes of diabetic neuropathy will be possible only by meeting this requirement.

Documentation of Neuropathy

Neurologic Exam

Quantitative tests are not routinely necessary, as the clinical diagnosis of diabetic distal symmetric polyneuropathy can often

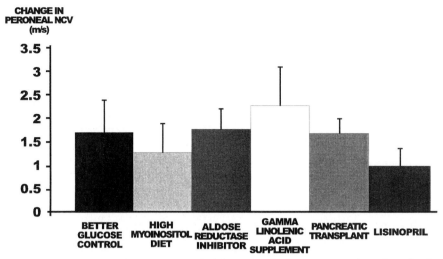

Figure 3–5 ■ Change in peroneal NCV in human diabetic individuals in various clinical trials. Better glucose control, a high–*myo*-inositol diet, use of an aldose reductase inhibitor, γ-linolenic acid oral supplementation, pancreatic transplant, and use of an angiotensin converting enzyme inhibitor (lisinopril) have been evaluated in human clinical trials. Interestingly, the change in peroneal nerve conduction velocity has been very similar (an increase of 1 to 2 m/sec) in all these well-done, controlled clinical trials. Thus, it would not appear that one of the etiologic pathways plays a consistently dominant role. Combined therapies clinical trials have not been done.[18, 19, 34, 50, 71, 80]

be made by a detailed neurologic exam. Occasionally, thermal perception threshold is necessary to confirm the presence of small fiber involvement, and electrophysiologic tests are often needed to confirm tarsal tunnel syndrome.

Distal symmetric polyneuropathy involves both small and large nerve fibers and involves more than one nerve. It is distal (i.e., toes worse than ankles and lower extremity worse than upper extremity), symmetric, and associated with nerve fiber loss with a dying-back presentation. Ideally, the exam would include all these elements. However, small nerve fiber assessment is not easily done in the neurologic exam. Thermal perception threshold or sudomotor function can be performed if the diagnosis is in question after the neurologic exam is complete or if small fiber neuropathy is suspected. Small fiber neuropathy might be suspected if the neurologic exam (which has mostly large fiber elements) is relatively normal or disproportionately less severe than the neuropathic symptoms might suggest. A complete and comprehensive neurologic exam can be quite detailed and exhaustive. However, often a more limited exam as detailed in Table 3–4 is sufficient to enable one to confirm or deny the diagnosis of distal symmetric polyneuropathy in the majority of cases.

In individuals with neuropathy of other etiologies the results of this exam would be markedly different than that detailed in a patient with distal symmetric polyneuropathy. For instance, tarsal tunnel syndrome generally has a unilateral presentation. The hands and the feet are equally involved in the neuropathy from pernicious anemia. Lead poisoning has more proximal than distal nerve involvement. A modified limited neurologic exam should be done on a yearly basis. A suggested modified limited exam would include reflexes, monofilaments, muscle tightness, and muscle strength in the lower extremity. A more complete exam should be done periodically or if there is a significant change in the clinical presentation.

Two-Point Discrimination

Although two-point discrimination may represent lesions in the posterior columns of the spinal cord or lesions in the cerebrum, in diabetic patients without other neuropathies it is used as a rough estimate of nerve fiber density. Although an unwound wire paper clip or a pair of dividers with dull points can be used, it is preferable to use two-point discrimination wheels. These wheels (usually two) consist of pairs of dull, thin rods sepa-

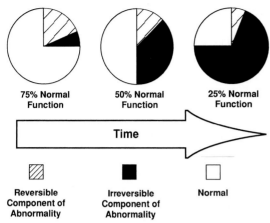

75% Normal
Function

50% Normal
Function

25% Normal
Function

Time

Reversible
Component of
Abnormality

Irreversible
Component of
Abnormality

Normal

Figure 3–6 ■ Reversible and irreversible components of diabetic neuropathy as a function of time. There appears to be both a reversible (metabolic) and irreversible (structural) component to diabetic neuropathy. The reversible component appears to play a greater role earlier in the natural history of diabetic neuropathy. In contrast, the irreversible component appears to play a greater role later. The response of any treatment modality would be limited to the reversible component. Thus, early prevention and consistent treatment of the reversible components appears the only practical approach for the therapy of diabetic neuropathy. It is unlikely that reversibility of advanced neuropathy is any more likely than reversibility of the other chronic complications of diabetes (retinopathy or nephropathy). The DCCT (see text) was able to prevent the development of diabetic neuropathy, in patients without neuropathy at the beginning of the trial, by controlling blood glucose level. However, some patients already had neuropathy at the beginning of the DCCT and there was no difference in the reversibility of neuropathy in these patients with better glucose control compared to the less well-controlled patients.

rated in distance from 1 to 25 mm. One single rod is also placed on one of the wheels. The two points of the pair of rods are placed on the skin simultaneously with equal pressure. The patient is asked if the touch is one or two rods. Randomly one rod is used instead of a pair of rods. The smallest distance of separation of the pair of rods in which the patient can consistently correctly identify is considered the two-point discrimination for that digit. The test is done on both the right and left side and in both the upper (pulp of the index fingers) and lower extremities (pulp of the great toes).[74] The results may be recorded onto a work sheet (Fig. 3–7) for interpretation at a later time. Normal is 2 mm or less in either the index finger or the great toe. Two-point discrimination of greater than 2 mm is consistent with nerve fiber loss. In diabetic distal symmetric polyneuropathy, there should be less nerve fiber

loss in the upper extremity than the lower extremity. The right and left side of the upper extremity and the right and left side of the lower extremity should be similar.

Pinprick

The sense of superficial pain can be tested by pinprick using a sharp pin or the Wartenberg pinwheel. Some examiners prefer a pin with a dull side and a sharp side. The pin is thrown away after each use and thus eliminates the remote chance of contamination. The process of using the pin for evaluating the sharp sense is similar to that of the pinwheel. The pinwheel consists of a wheel with sharp identical pins extending from the center like spokes. The wheel should be slowly rolled across the skin using the weight of the tool as the force pressure (i.e., do not push down on the wheel). The pinprick examination should be done by rolling the pinwheel from the tip of the middle finger to the elbow on the volar surface of both arms. This length is divided into 150 equal segments for scoring purposes (see Fig. 3–7). Similarly, the pinprick examination is done with a pinwheel from the tip of the middle toe to the knee on the anterior surface of both legs. This segment is also divided into 150 equal segments for scoring purposes. Finally the pinprick exam is done with a pinwheel from the tip of the middle toe to the heel on the plantar surface of both feet. In all cases the exam is first done from distal to proximal. Patients are first shown on their face what sharp (one of the spokes) and dull (the handle end) feel like. Patients are not allowed to watch while the tests are being done. Patients are asked if they can feel the wheel at all. If they can then they are asked if the sensation is dull or sharp. Documentation of the level in which the sensation goes from numb to dull or dull to sharp is recorded on the work sheet.

Some patients will start with a sharp feeling at the most distal tip of the toe or finger (normal) and this sensation will not change throughout the testing path. Some patients will start with a dull (muted) feeling, which will either stay dull throughout the entire testing zone or will become sharp somewhere along the path. Some patients will start numb, become dull and then become sharp. Some will start numb and then become dull. Some will stay numb through the entire testing path. These are typical patterns. The sensation should go from abnormal to less abnor-

Table 3–4 ■ LIMITED NEUROLOGIC EXAM

EXAM ELEMENT*	PURPOSE OF EXAM ELEMENT
Two-point discrimination (great toes; index fingers)	Nerve fiber density estimate; upper versus lower
Pinprick (toes to knees; fingers to elbows; soles of feet)	Distal versus proximal; large nerve fibers; sensory nerves; upper versus lower
Deep tendon reflexes (knees and ankles; wrists and arms)	Distal versus proximal; large nerve fibers; motor nerves; upper versus lower
Muscle strength (feet and knees; hands and elbows; flexion and extension)	Distal versus proximal; large nerve fibers; motor nerves; upper versus lower (R versus L)
Position sense (great toes; thumbs)	Large nerve fibers; sensory nerves; upper versus lower
Sense of touch (great toes; index fingers; monofilaments)	Large nerve fibers; sensory nerves; upper versus lower
Vibration sense (base of great toe nails; base of thumb nails; 128-Hz tuning fork)	Large nerve fibers; sensory nerves; upper versus lower
Walk on toes and heels	Large nerve fibers: sensory and motor nerves coordination
Gait	Large nerve fibers; sensory and motor nerves coordination
Muscle tightness (gastrocnemius)	Large nerve fibers; motor nerves
Joint flexibility (toes; hands)†	Limited joint mobility syndrome
Harris foot mat†	Feet pressure points
General exam of feet shape†	Feet deformity

* Exams are done bilaterally to test for symmetry.
† Part of the feet exam but not strictly a neurologic component.

mal as the pinwheel moves from distal to proximal. In diabetic distal symmetric polyneuropathy the upper extremities should be less abnormal than the lower extremities.[56] Furthermore, the pinprick sensation should have a similar pattern bilaterally. Patterns that show more abnormality proximal than distal, asymmetric, or upper extremity equal or worse than lower extremity are not consistent with diabetic distal symmetric polyneuropathy, and other neuropathic etiologies should be sought. Pinprick sensation is a large nerve fiber function.

Deep Tendon Reflexes

The tendon reflex examination is a test of a reflex arc and a number of suprasegmental systems that modify the quality of the reflex. The reflex arc consists of muscle spindles in the tendon, afferent nerves, spinal cord synapses (usually monosynaptic), and efferent nerves from the anterior horn cells of the spinal cord to muscle spindles and motor end plates. Diseases of muscle, afferent nerve, efferent nerve, spinal nerve root, or spinal cord can abolish the tendon reflex. Normality is difficult to assess and therefore the responses are usually classified as present, present with reinforcement, or absent. The following reflexes are frequently done in a limited neurologic exam in the diabetic patient. The patient should be relaxed and the limbs supported. Use a reflex hammer with a soft head and enough weight to be effective (e.g., Traumer hammer). Hold the handle of the reflex hammer between your thumb and index finger. Use your wrist (not your arm) and swing the hammer to strike (i.e., do not poke). Proper action will provide a brisk, direct, striking motion. Reflexes should be tested on both sides and the results recorded for further interpretation.[74] This test provides information of large motor nerves. In distal symmetric polyneuropathy the lower extremity will be more involved than the upper extremity. More distal reflexes should be more involved than proximal reflexes and the reflex responses should be similar bilaterally. If this pattern does not emerge (e.g., upper extremities equal lower extremities, one side more abnormal than the other, proximal reflexes equal or worse than distal reflexes), alternative neuropathic etiologies should be entertained.

ANKLE (ACHILLES)

Have the patient kneel on the edge of a high-back, stable chair with his/her back towards you. Gently apply pressure on the sole of the foot (causing some dorsiflexion and muscle stretching). Strike the Achilles tendon. Observe plantar flexion of the foot via muscle

NAME: _____

DATE: _____

SIU #: _____

RIGHT: LEFT:

A = Becomes or starts to be normal
B = Becomes or starts to be muted
C = Becomes or starts to be numb

	RIGHT	LEFT
DTR		
BRACHIAL:	NL___ ABN___ ABS___	NL___ ABN___ ABS___
EXENSORS:	NL___ ABN___ ABS___	NL___ ABN___ ABS___

TWO POINT DISCRIMINATION
___MM   ___MM

POSITION SENSE
NL___ ABN___ ABS___   NL___ ABN___ ABS___

TUNING FORKS
128: NL___ ABN___ ABS___   128: NL___ ABN___ ABS___
256: NL___ ABN___ ABS___   256: NL___ ABN___ ABS___
FORMAL VIBRATORY TESTING DONE   YES / NO

FORMAL THERMAL TESTING DONE   YES / NO
TEMPERATURE SENSE
NL___ ABN___ ABS___   NL___ ABN___ ABS___

MONOFILAMENTS
_____   _____

INTERPRETATION:
_____   _____

RADIAL PULSE
NL___ ABN___ ABS___   NL___ ABN___ ABS___

A

Figure 3–7 ■ Neurologic exam work sheet. Work sheets such as these are often helpful in performing the limited neurologic exam. The work sheet has places for pinprick exam, tuning fork result (sometimes both 128- and 256-Hz tuning forks are used), monofilaments, two-point discrimination, deep tendon reflexes, and even a place to document whether the quantitative sensory testing was done. These sheets can either be used as the final report or as a work sheet for a formal dictation. The pattern of distal, symmetric, more than one nerve, lower extremities worse than upper extremities, and fiber loss is consistent with distal symmetric polyneuropathy of diabetes. Results not consistent with this pattern would suggest nondiabetic neuropathic etiologies (even if it occurs in an individual who happens to have diabetes). *A*, upper extremities; *B*, lower extremities.

Illustration continued on following page

contraction of the gastrocnemius and soleus muscles.

KNEE (PATELLA)

Have the patient sit with the knee flexed at a right angle and hanging freely. Strike the patellar tendon. Observe the extension of the lower leg and contraction of the quadriceps muscles. Normal responses may vary from a flicker of the quadriceps muscles to a jump of the lower leg.

WRIST (BRACHIORADIALIS)

Flex the patient's arm at the elbow with the hand supported and resting in your hand or in the patient's lap. The hand should be pro-

NAME: _____

DATE: _____

SIU #: _____

RIGHT: LEFT:

A = Becomes or starts to be normal
B = Becomes or starts to be muted
C= Becomes or starts to be numb

	RIGHT	LEFT
DTR		
KNEE:	NL___ ABN___ ABS___	NL___ ABN___ ABS___
ANKLE:	NL___ ABN___ ABS___	NL___ ABN___ ABS___
TWO POINT DISCRIMINATION	___MM	___MM
POSITION SENSE	NL___ ABN___ ABS___	NL___ ABN___ ABS___
TUNING FORKS	128: NL___ ABN___ ABS___	128: NL___ ABN___ ABS___
	256: NL___ ABN___ ABS___	256: NL___ ABN___ ABS___
	FORMAL VIBRATORY TESTING DONE YES / NO	

FORMAL THERMAL TESTING DONE   YES / NO
TEMPERATURE SENSE

NL___ ABN___ ABS___   NL___ ABN___ ABS___

MONOFILAMENTS

_____   _____

INTERPRETATION:

_____   _____

PULSES

POST TIB: NL___ ABN___ ABS___   NL___ ABN___ ABS___
PEDAL: NL___ ABN___ ABS___   NL___ ABN___ ABS___

B

Figure 3–7 ■ *Continued*

nated (palm down). Strike the radius just proximal to the styloid process (about 2 to 3 inches above the wrist on the side of the arm proximal to the thumb). Observe contraction of the brachioradialis muscle and supination of the hand.

ARM (BICEPS)

Rest the patient's arm along your nondominant arm and hand. The patient's arm should be flexed and the palm should be up. Place your thumb on the biceps tendon. In order to slightly stretch the biceps tendon; push slightly into the antecubital fossa. Tap your thumb with the reflex hammer. Observe for contraction of the biceps.

ARM (TRICEPS)

The patient should be supine. Stand on the patient's right to examine the left triceps reflex. Rest the patient's left forearm across his/her abdomen with the elbow at a right angle. Percuss (strike) the triceps tendon just above the olecranon (elbow) process with the reflex hammer. Observe contraction of the triceps muscle.

Muscle Strength

Muscle strength is very difficult to quantitate. Nevertheless, it is important to obtain an overall sense of the muscle strength of the individual. Muscle strength is typically well preserved until the late stages of diabetic neuropathy. These tests assess large nerve fiber function, as well as muscle group action. If the muscle strength appears to be disproportionately abnormal compared to sensory testing (i.e., muscle strength is worse than sensory function), alternative neuropathic etiologies should be considered. The following muscle groups should be tested.[74]

DORSIFLEXION OF THE FOOT (DEEP PERONEAL NERVE)

Patient should be supine and asked to vigorously bend his/her foot towards his/her head against opposition by the examiner's hand. The examiner should apply force toward plantar flexion and eversion.

PLANTAR FLEXION OF THE FOOT (TIBIAL NERVE)

Gastrocnemius: With the patient prone and the knee **extended,** the patient should attempt to flex his/her foot against resistance. *Soleus:* With the patient prone and the knee **flexed,** the patient should attempt to flex his/her foot against resistance.

LEG FLEXION AT THE KNEE (SCIATIC NERVE)

With the patient prone and the knee flexed, the patient attempts to move his/her heel towards the buttock while resisting further flexion.

LEG EXTENSION AT THE KNEE

With the patient prone and the knee flexed, the patient attempts to straighten his/her leg while resisting further flexion.

FLEXION OF THE WRIST (MEDIAN NERVE)

Ask the patient to put the dorsum of his/her hand and forearm on a flat surface and flex his/her wrist against resistance.

EXTENSION OF THE WRIST (RADIAL NERVE)

Place the volar surface of the patient's forearm on a flat surface. Ask the patient to slightly flex his/her fingers. Then ask the patient to forcefully extend his/her hand while resistance is applied to the dorsum of the hand.

FLEXION OF THE FOREARM (RADIAL NERVE)

Place the dorsal aspect of the patient's forearm and hand on a flat surface. Fix the patient's elbow and ask the patient to flex his/her forearm against resistance.

EXTENSION OF THE FOREARM (RADIAL NERVE)

Place the elbow on a flat surface. Ask the patient to flex his/her forearm to 90 degrees. Fix the elbow and ask the patient to straighten his/her arm against resistance.

Position Sense

Position sense (proprioception) is defective in diseases of the posterior spinal roots, posterior spinal columns, and the parietal lobe. Typically, position sense is preserved until the late stages of distal symmetric polyneuropathy of diabetes. If it is abnormal early in the course of the neuropathy of a patient who has diabetes, etiologies other than diabetes should be considered. To test this, with the patient's eyes closed, the great toe is firmly grasped by the examiner's index finger and thumb. The toe is wiggled up and down several times. Finally, the great toe is placed in either the up or the down position. The patient is asked to identify the position of the great toe. This process is repeated several times. This test is repeated on the toe on the opposite foot and in both thumbs. This is considered a large nerve fiber function.

Sense of Touch

Performing monofilament testing on the plantar surface of the great toe and the pulp of the index finger bilaterally can assess the sense of touch. A series of 24 monofilaments that range in size from 2.83 to 6.65 are used. The tip of the monofilament is gently placed perpendicular on the surface until the monofilament buckles. The approach, skin contact, and departure of the monofilament should be approximately 1.5 seconds. Do not allow the filament to slide across the skin or make repetitive contact to the site. Avoid callused areas. The patient should be able to sense the monofilament by the time the monofilament buckles. The thicker (higher the number) the monofilament, the more force is required to cause the buckle. Monofilaments of 4.17 (equivalent of 1 gm of linear pressure) or higher are considered consistent with neuropathy (large fiber modality). Inability to sense a monofilament of 5.07 (equivalent to 10 gm of linear force) is consistent with severe neuropathy and loss of protective sensation. Custom footwear is indicated in diabetic people who cannot feel the 5.07 monofilament.

Vibration Sense

It is difficult to establish a quantitative assessment, so a 128-Hz tuning fork is commonly used. Have the patient close his/her eyes. Demonstrate the feeling to be expected to the patient by touching his/her jaw with the vibrating tuning fork. Make the tuning fork vibrate by hitting it close to the base of the tines with the heel of your hand. Place the tuning fork at the base of the great toenail for at least 10 seconds. The response should be present or absent. The test is repeated in the other foot and at the base of both thumbnails.[74] The inability to feel the tuning fork at the base of the great toenail carries the same significance as the inability to feel a 5.07 monofilament and the patient should be referred for custom footwear. This is considered to be a large nerve fiber function.

Gait

When one walks, the hip flexes (the knee comes away from the floor), the knee flexes (the foot comes away from the floor), and the ankle plantar flexes. All the weight of a person is on the other leg. As the leg comes forward, there is more hip flexion and the beginning of knee extension. The ankle dorsiflexes in preparation for the transfer of weight. As the swing of the leg is progressing and passing the other leg, the contralateral ankle plantar flexes in preparation to push off the floor. The first leg's heel strikes the floor with the ankle dorsiflexed and the weight of the body starts to shift to this foot. As the body comes forward, the first foot flexes and the

knee extends, accepting the full weight of the body as it does so. The second foot then plantar flexes and pushes off the floor and the process continues. The arms reciprocate with the legs.

In order to observe the patient's gait, have the patient walk a straight line, heel to toe. It is important to pay particular attention to the foot and ankle movements. The patient should put his/her right heel immediately in front of the left toes and then the left heel immediately in front of the right toes. The heel should strike before the toes (not at the same time and not slap the floor).[74] Most people with diabetes can walk normally in the examination room. In the advanced stage of distal symmetric polyneuropathy patients may develop defective proprioception (see "Position Sense," above). This may result in an abnormal gait. The patients may walk with a wide gait (feet wide apart), watching the floor and landmarks. Compared to patients with cerebellar ataxia, there is less reeling and lurching. Often the diabetic patients will lift the feet unnecessarily high. There may be an associated foot drop and the patient may slap the floor. Balance is coordinated by the sense of position and feeling in the feet, vision, and the middle ear. Often patients with diabetes have vision problems, which are worse at night, and neuropathy. Thus, two of the three coordination elements of balance may be lacking. This puts the patient at increased risk of falling.

Walk on Heels

Asking the patient to walk on his/her heels is a simple way to find balance problems early, often before the gait becomes very abnormal. These patients have stage 3 diabetic neuropathy and are considered to be disabled by many physicians. Ask the patient to walk forward and backwards on his/her heels.

Muscle Tightness

The gastrocnemius and the foot extensor muscles should be checked carefully for tightness. In patients with muscular pain (see below) these muscles are inappropriately tight for the degree of exercise the muscle groups get on a regular basis.

Joint Flexibility

Limited joint mobility syndrome may occur in people with diabetes. In this syndrome the skin and joint capsules of the feet and hands are stiffened with collagen. The etiology is not well understood but is thought to be related to glycosylation of collagen. The patient is asked to fold his/her hands as if he/she is praying. Normally the palms and fingers of the hand will easily juxtapose and there will be very little space between the hands. In patients with limited joint mobility syndrome, the hands do not become flush with each other. There is a space between the fingers and sometimes the palms of the hands during a prayer pose. This is called the "prayer sign."

Asking the patient to pick up a sock from the floor with his/her toes can assess limited joint mobility syndrome in the feet. Joint flexibility is not a neurologic test but is important to assess and often is easiest to do during the neurologic exam.

Harris Foot Mat

The feet can be evaluated for high pressure points by means of devices that can quantitate the pressure under the foot during walking or standing. These may be important tests but may not be practical in large clinic situations, as they are time consuming and expensive. A relatively inexpensive method to crudely establish the presence or absence of pressure points is the Harris Foot Mat (Fig. 3–8). This is an ink pad with graded depths of grid lines. The patient walks across the pad and pressure points can then be identified by intensity of ink. This, of course, is not strictly part of the neurologic exam but is useful in assessing the diabetic foot.

General Exam of Foot Shape

Examination of the feet for foot deformities, calluses, dryness, fissures, corns, lesions, sores, ulcers, and onychomycoses (nail fungus infection) is important. Although these are not part of the neurologic exam, they impact the care of the foot. Structural deformities such as hammer toes, claw toes, bunions, calluses, and Charcot joint are important to document (see Chapter 2).

Vascular status can be evaluated by palpating the dorsalis pedis pulse, the posterior tibial pulse, foot pallor on elevation, rubor after dependency, and delayed capillary filling (see Chapter 25).

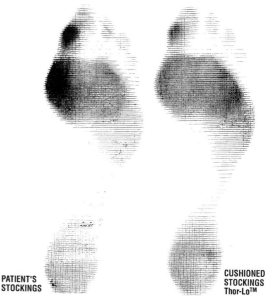

PATIENT'S STOCKINGS

CUSHIONED STOCKINGS Thor-Lo™

Figure 3–8 ■ Harris Foot Mat results before and after wearing a cushioned stocking. The Harris Foot Mat is an inexpensive method to document the presence of increased pressure points in an individual. This person had increased pressure points over the first metatarsal head and great toe on the right foot. Use of a cushioned sock (Thor-Lo) greatly decreased the presence of these pressure points. Harris mat determinations are recommended in all diabetic patients on a routine basis. This serves as both information to the health care provider and as education and motivation for patients.

Quantitative Tests

Large Fiber Tests

Nerve function can be crudely divided into large nerve fiber and small nerve fiber function (Table 3–5). Although there are multiple tests of large nerve fiber function, electrophysiology testing (nerve conduction velocity) and vibratory perception threshold are the two most commonly used. Commercially available equipment makes these tests practical for most clinics. Nerve conduction velocity is mainly a large fiber test. Nerve conduction represents the transmission of electrical impulses through the largest myelinated fibers. The amplitude of the electrical impulse represents large fiber density. Normative data are available for nerve conduction velocity and nerve amplitude. Electrophysiologic tests are fairly reproducible, with a coefficient of variation between 3% and 8%.[1, 56] From a clinical point of view, electrophysiologic tests are seldom needed in making the diagnosis of diabetic distal symmetric poly-

Table 3–5 ■ EXAMPLES OF SMALL AND LARGE
NERVE FIBER FUNCTION

SMALL NERVE FIBER FUNCTIONS	LARGE NERVE FIBER FUNCTIONS
Heat sensation	Vibration
Cold sensation	Pinwheel sensation
Pain sensation	Deep tendon reflexes
Autonomic nervous system functions	Position sense
Sudomotor function	Sense of light touch
Vascular AV shunt control	Motor nerves

AV, arteriovenous.

neuropathy, but these tests are very helpful
in the diagnosis of tarsal tunnel syndrome.

Vibration perception threshold is also a
large fiber test and commercial equipment is
available. Normative data are also available
for vibratory perception threshold and the
coefficient of variation is approximately
15%.[31]

Small Fiber Tests

Small nerve fibers are also affected by diabetic neuropathy. The small nerve fibers are
primarily responsible for heat, cold, and pain
sensation. There are several tests described
in the literature. These tests include heat-
pain threshold, warm thermal perception
threshold, cold thermal perception threshold, and autonomic tests. A common autonomic test used in the foot is sudomotor function. The QSART machine allows for
quantitation of sweating function. Normative data are lacking and the variability of
the test is not well established. Thermal
perception threshold tests can also be done
quite easily with commercially available
devices. Normative data are available, but
the coefficient of variation is unacceptably
high (~50%).[31]

Prevention and Treatment

At present, there is no treatment that will
reverse diabetic distal symmetric polyneuropathy. It is clear that good glucose control
will delay, prevent, and slow the progression
of the development of distal, symmetric polyneuropathy. There are several promising
drugs in development that may also help prevent the development of and/or slow the progression of diabetic neuropathy, but convincing clinical trials are currently lacking.

Currently, therapy of distal symmetric polyneuropathy can be divided into treatment of
risk factors for the development of neuropathy, offering treatment for painful neuropathy in order to achieve a better quality of
life, and avoidance of further complications
from neuropathy.

Risk Factors

There are both modifiable and nonmodifiable
risk factors for the development of diabetic
neuropathy (Table 3–6). Only hyperglycemia
has been proven to be a risk factor via prospective, randomized, multicenter, parallel
design clinical trials. The other factors are
considered to be risk factors via retrospective
or cross-sectional data analysis. Although
other risk factors have been identified, these
risk factors are consistently found in most
analyses. The nonmodifiable risk factors include older age, longer duration of diabetes,
HLA DR 3/4 genotype, and height. Age, duration of diabetes, and the DR 3/4 genotype are
also risk factors for the other two microvascular complications of diabetes, retinopathy
and nephropathy. Many studies have found
that men are at greater risk for neuropathy
than females, but reanalysis of these data
show it to be height rather than gender that
is significant. It is hypothesized that longer
nerves are more prone to nerve damage.[73, 79]

Modifiable risk factors include hyperglycemia, hypertension, elevated cholesterol,
smoking, and heavy alcohol use. The DCCT
and the UKPDS studies have demonstrated
conclusively that better glucose control prevents or slows the progression of diabetic
neuropathy.[25, 82, 83] Hyperglycemia, hypertension, elevated cholesterol, and smoking are

Table 3–6 ■ RISK FACTORS FOR DIABETIC
NEUROPATHY

Nonmodifable risk factors
  Older age
  Longer duration of diabetes
  HLA DR-¾ genotype
  Greater height
Modifable risk factors
  Hyperglycemia
  Hypertension
  Elevated cholesterol levels
  Smoking
  Heavy alcohol use

also risk factors for retinopathy and nephropathy.

Heavy alcohol use can cause neuropathy
in nondiabetic individuals. Therefore, listing
it as an independent risk factor for the development of diabetic neuropathy is problematic.[2, 90] Perhaps the increased incidence of
neuropathy in diabetic patients who are
heavy alcohol users is no more than a combination of two neuropathies occurring in the
same individual. It will be very difficult if
not impossible to ferret out the interaction.

Although only treatment of hyperglycemia
has been proven to help prevent or slow the
progression of diabetic neuropathy, it is prudent to address the other modifiable risk factors as well. Treatment of hypertension has
been shown to prevent or slow the progression of nephropathy and retinopathy in the
UKPDS and other studies.[24, 84] Furthermore,
treatment of elevated cholesterol levels has
also been shown to slow the progression of
nephropathy.[75] There is no reason to believe
that treatment of hypertension and elevated
cholesterol levels would not help neuropathy
as well. Cessation of heavy alcohol use and
smoking should be encouraged in all people.

Pain Management

Pain involves C fibers, which are small-
diameter, unmyelinated slow conduction velocity fibers and A and D fibers, which are
small, myelinated, and have faster conduction than large myelinated fibers. The reason
these nerves begin to fire in a hectic pattern
causing pain is not well understood, but therapy may be initiated in a semiempiric manner. Figure 3–9 details a treatment algorithm for offering an improved quality of life
by decreasing the painful symptoms. It is
important to determine that the painful
symptoms result from diabetic neuropathy.
Pain from other etiologies may respond well
to appropriate therapy once the proper diagnosis is made. In one study, 117 consecutive
diabetic patients who were referred to a ter-
tiary care center for treatment of painful diabetic neuropathy found that only 65% had
distal symmetric polyneuropathy.[66] Other diagnoses included peripheral vascular disease
(11%), femoral neuropathy (7%), tarsal tunnel syndrome (4%), spinal stenosis (4%), reflex sympathetic dystrophy (3%), and other
miscellaneous causes (6%).

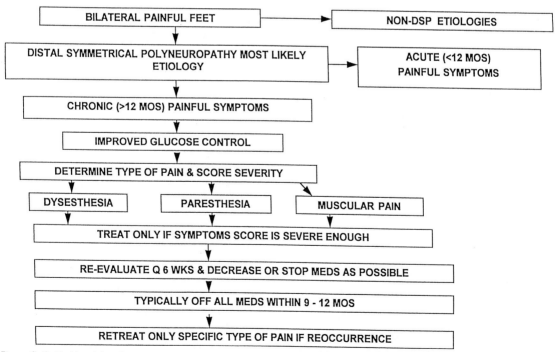

Figure 3–9 ■ Algorithm for the treatment of painful diabetic neuropathy. This algorithm has proven to be successful
in a prospective clinical trial. It requires the health care professional to query the patient as to the type of neuropathic
pain. Therapy is then directed toward the specific type of pain (dysesthesia, paresthesia, muscular pain, or combinations of the three). (From Pfeifer MA, Ross D, Schrage J, et al: A highly successful and novel model for the treatment
of chronic painful diabetic peripheral neuropathy. Diabetes Care 16:1103–1115, 1993, with permission.)

Table 3–7 ■ ACUTE VERSUS CHRONIC PAINFUL DIABETIC NEUROPATHY

FACTOR	ACUTE PAINFUL NEUROPATHY	CHRONIC PAINFUL NEUROPATHY
Duration of diabetes	Short (<3 years)	Intermediate (8 to 12 years)
Onset	Acute	Gradual
Pain duration	Less than 12 months	Greater than 12 months
Etiology	Metabolic > structural	Structural > metabolic
Natural history	Self-limited	May persist for years
Relapses	Rare, if ever	Frequently occur

Once it has been determined that the pain is secondary to distal symmetric polyneuropathy, the pain is divided into acute versus chronic painful neuropathy (Table 3–7). Acute painful neuropathy lasts less than 12 months and is mostly attributable to metabolic abnormalities rather than to structural abnormalities. Proposed etiologies include decreased nerve taurine concentration and endoneurial swelling. The typical scenario is the newly diagnosed diabetic patient just started on insulin. Acute, painful diabetic neuropathy is self-limited. The patient often responds well to analgesic therapy with nonsteroidal anti-inflammatory drugs (NSAIDs).

Chronic, painful diabetic neuropathy typically occurs in patients with intermediate duration (8 to 12 years) of diabetes. It has a gradual and insidious onset and the pain typically lasts more than 12 months. There are structural abnormalities (see below). The pain may persist for years and relapses occur. Treatment of chronic, painful diabetic neuropathy requires a more complex approach but can be greatly or moderately successful in patients who do not have motives for treatment failure (e.g., sympathy-seeking behavior, narcotic-seeking behavior, wishing to gain or maintain disability).

Boulton demonstrated a decrease in painful neuropathic symptoms by intensive glucose control using an insulin pump.[7] However, this finding is not consistent. In fact, pain may worsen in some patients as better glucose control is achieved. Figure 3–10 demonstrates the relationship between nerve function and painful neuropathic symptoms. As nerve function worsens, the pain threshold may be exceeded. Once this occurs the pain continues until the nerve becomes so dysfunctional that pain signals are not easily transmitted to the central nervous system (CNS). Eventually, nerve function worsens to the point that sensation decreases to the point that the foot becomes numb. Some individuals get numb feet without ever breaching the pain threshold. Depending on the location of the patient on the pain curve, an improvement in nerve function could either cause the pain to drop below the pain threshold or increase pain. Glucose control can improve nerve function enough to cause such changes. This would explain the decreased pain in some patients (located on the left side of the curve) and increased pain in other patients (located on the right side of the curve) with better glucose control. Regardless of the change in pain symptoms, glucose control is still desirable and should be initiated in all patients.

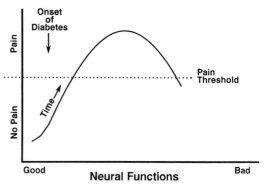

Figure 3–10 ■ The relationship between nerve function and painful symptoms. Nerve function worsens over time (x-axis) and sensation may exceed the putative "pain threshold" (y-axis). If the nerve function worsens to the point that the pain threshold is exceeded, the individual senses pain; but as nerve function worsens (over time) the sensation of pain may completely abate, leaving the patient with numbness. Some individuals become numb without ever breaching the pain threshold. If an individual has pain early in the course of his/her neuropathy, an improvement in nerve function (e.g., better glucose control) may result in the painful symptoms. On the other hand, individuals with the same degree of painful symptoms later in the course of his/her neuropathy may experience worsening pain upon nerve function improvement. (From Pfeifer MA, Greene DA: Diabetic Neuropathy. Kalamazoo, MI: Upjohn Monograph, 1985, with permission.)

Dysesthesia Pain

Three types of pain have been described in patients with painful diabetic neuropathy. According to the pain model developed by David Ross the three categories include dysesthesia, paresthesia, and muscular pain (Fig. 3–11). Dysesthetic pain has been attributed to a cutaneous or subcutaneous distribution and may be attributable to increased firing of damaged or abnormally excitable nociceptive fibers particularly sprouting regenerating fibers. The pain descriptors that a patient may use with this type of pain are "burning sensation," "sunburn-like," "skin tingles," "painful sensation when something touches me" that normally would not hurt, such as bed sheets or stockings (Table 3–8). Suggested therapies for this type of pain are capsaicin or gabapentin. Capsaicin cream comes in 0.25% and 0.075% concentrations. It is a natural substance that occurs in hot peppers. Capsaicin only penetrates to the subdermal layer and, therefore, is considered ideal for treatment of dysesthetic pain. Although direct application of capsaicin to nerves can deplete nerves of substance P, inhibit axonal transport of substance P, and reduce conduction in type C fibers, the action of capsaicin when applied topically is not known. Continued use of topical capsaicin appears to produce desensitization and raise the threshold for mechanical stimulation by blocking the nociceptive afferents. It is applied, thinly, three to four times a day in mapped areas. Fewer applications will not result in an adequate response. At time of initial use, capsaicin briefly stimulates the release of substance P into the dermal area. This may result in a burning sensation. Patients need to be warned about this possibility. Also, the patient should be instructed to use gloves when applying capsaicin or to wash hands thoroughly after applying. The burning sensation usually lasts no more than 3 to 4 days because desensitization occurs with depletion of substance P. Capsaicin does not affect touch, pressure, or vibration sense. Some patients develop topical reactions to capsaicin. Capsaicin is for external use only and contact with eyes should be avoided. Capsaicin decreases the pain 40 to 70% but may take 2 to 3 weeks before significant pain relief is realized.

Gabapentin (Neurontin) is approved by the Food and Drug Administration (FDA) for the treatment of complex partial seizures, but it has also been used successfully in the management of painful diabetic neuropathy.[5] However, large doses (2,400 to 3,600 mg in divided doses per day) may be necessary for gabapentin to achieve pain relief. A common mistake made by physicians is to use too low a dose. Side effects include somnolence, dizziness, ataxia, fatigue, and nystagmus. The mechanism of action is not known. However, it has been hypothesized that gabapentin works through several mechanisms. The known biochemical changes observed after administration of gabapentin, in animal studies, includes increased rate of γ-aminobutyric acid (GABA) synthesis, altered nonsynaptic GABA release, and decreased glutamate synthesis. In addition, it binds with high affinity to the $\alpha_2\delta$ subunit of Ca^{2+} channels in brain membranes.

Paresthesia Pain

Paresthesic pain is thought to occur from several possible etiologies: (1) spontaneous activity and increased mechanosensitivity near the cell body of damaged afferent axons in the dorsal root ganglion; (2) loss of segmental inhibition of large myelinated fibers on small unmyelinated fibers (modified gate control in which pain signals are transmitted from the spinal cord transmission neuron as a result of the input from the unmyelinated, myelinated, and inhibitor cells); (3) ectopic impulses generated from demyelinated patches of myelinated axons; or (4) increased firing caused by physiologic stimulation of endings of nociceptive afferents that innervate the nerve sheaths themselves (nervi nervorum). Morphologic changes in affected nerves include nerve fiber loss, axonal atrophy, nodal swelling, and endoneurial swelling.[28] These abnormalities may lead to other structural changes (e.g., axonal degeneration, myelin wrinkling, and wallerian degeneration). The endoneurial swelling may be secondary to endoneurial sodium accumulation and marked increase in nerve hydration. The pain descriptors used to describe paresthesia include "pins and needles," "electric-like," "numb," "aching feet," "feel as if my feet have been in ice water," "knife-like," "shooting pains," or "lancinating pains." Systemic therapy (as opposed to topical therapy) is often necessary. Several therapies have been tried including tricyclic antidepressants, mexiletine, carbamazepine, phenytoin, α-lipoic acid, and tramadol.[33, 39, 43, 60, 61, 92] Combinations of

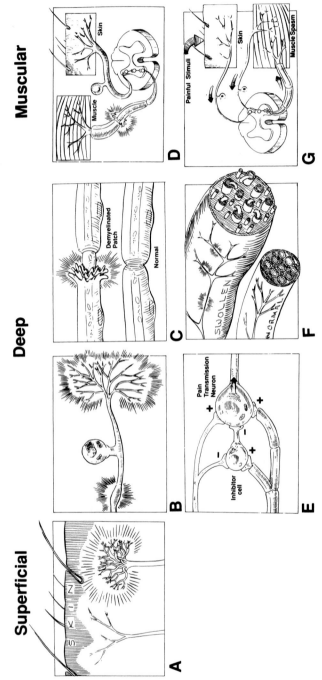

Figure 3–11 ■ The proposed etiologies of the different types of pain. *A*, Dysesthesia pain. Increases firing of damaged or abnormally excited nociceptive fibers, particularly sprouting regenerating fibers in the cutaneous tissue. *B*, Paresthesia pain. Spontaneous activity and increased mechanosensitivity near the cell body of damaged afferents in the dorsal root ganglion. *C*, Paresthesia pain. Ectopic impulses generated from demyelinated patches of myelinated axons. *D*, Muscular pain. Ectopic impulses to the muscle generated from demyelinated patches resulting in muscle spasms and pain. *E*, Paresthesia pain. Loss of large myelinated fibers on the effects of the small unmyelinated fibers (modifed gate control hypothesis). Pain signals are transmitted from the spinal cord pain transmission neuron as a result of the input from the unmyelinated, myelinated, and inhibitor cells. *F*, Paresthesia pain. Increased firing of endings of nociceptive afferents that innervate the nerve sheaths themselves (nervi nervorum). The endoneurial swelling is secondary to endoneurial sodium accumulation and marked nerve hydration. *G*, Muscular pain. Reflex loop (Livingston's vicious cycle) involving a nociceptive input that activates the motor neuron within the spinal cord causing muscle spasms that in turn activate the muscle nociceptors and feeds back to the spinal cord to sustain the spasm. (From Pfeifer MA, Ross D, Schrage J, et al: A highly successful and novel model for the treatment of chronic painful diabetic peripheral neuropathy. Diabetes Care 16:1103–1115, 1993, with permission.)

Table 3–8 ■ PAIN DESCRIPTORS OF DIFFERENT TYPES OF NEUROPATHIC PAIN

DYSESTHESIA	PARESTHESIA	MUSCULAR PAIN
Burning sensation	Pins and needles	Dull ache
Sunburn-like	Electric-like	Night cramps
Skin tingles	Numb but achy	Band-like sensation
Painful sensation when something touches me that normally would not hurt (e.g., bedsheets or stockings)	Like feet in ice water	Drawing sensation
	Knife-like	Deep aches
	Shooting pain	Spasms
	Lancinating pain	Toothache-like

these medicines are often used. Imipramine or amitriptyline are typical tricyclic antidepressants used. The starting dose is 50 mg at bedtime, and may be increased to 150 mg (use smaller doses in the elderly). Side effects include dry mouth, dizziness, somnolence, postural hypotension, and urinary retention in men with prostatic hypertrophy.

Mexiletine is an antiarrhythmic with anesthetic properties. Although it is an antiarrhythmic agent, it can cause ventricular arrhythmias (typically unifocal, benign, premature ventricular contractions) in some people. Therefore, it is dosed in a manner to avoid arrhythmias. An electrocardiogram (ECG) is done before mexiletine is started. Provided there are no arrhythmias, the initial dose is 150 mg after supper for 3 days. A cardiac rhythm strip is then obtained. Provided there is no evidence of arrhythmias, the dose is increased to 300 mg after supper for 3 days. Another cardiac rhythm strip is obtained. Provided there is still no evidence of arrhythmias, the dose is increased to 10 mg/kg of body weight in divided doses after meals for 3 more days. A 24-hour Holter monitor is then obtained. If this is normal, the dosage is continued. The occurrence of ventricular arrhythmias with mexiletine is unusual, but it is important to periodically monitor cardiac rhythm while patients are on this very effective paresthetic pain relief medicine. The most common side effect of mexiletine is nausea, which is greatly ameliorated by taking the medicine on a full stomach at the end of meals.

Carbamazepine (e.g., Tegretol) is an antiseizure medicine. Initial dose is 100 mg twice a day and is increased to a maximum dose of 400 mg three times a day over a 6-week period. Of concern with this medicine is the rare occurrence of aplastic anemia. Therefore, periodic complete blood count (CBC) testing is necessary. Other side effects include nausea and elevated liver function tests. Liver function tests and CBC are usually obtained on a monthly basis for the first 3 months and quarterly thereafter.

Phenytoin (e.g., Dilantin) is another antiseizure medicine. The initial dose is 100 mg three times a day and is increased over 6 weeks to a maximum dose of 200 mg three times a day. It has multiple gastrointestinal and CNS side effects. It can cause a rash and elevated liver function tests. Gingival hyperplasia has been described with long-term use. Liver function tests are done at 6 weeks and quarterly thereafter.

In one randomized, placebo-controlled study, intravenous α-lipoic acid decreased painful symptoms in patients with diabetes.[39] Although this is available in Europe, it is not commercially available in the United States. Clinical trials are now underway to confirm these findings and may be a useful tool for treatment of the pain of neuropathy in the future.

Tramadol (e.g., Ultram) is an analgesic that has shown some efficacy in the treatment of painful diabetic neuropathy.[92] Presumably, it is helpful in paresthetic pain, but therapeutic benefit based on pain descriptors was lacking in the report.

Muscular Pain

The third type of pain is muscular pain. This is believed to be secondary to injury to the motor neurons (e.g., demyelinated patches) or "Livingston's vicious cycle." Ectopic neural impulses to the muscle may be generated from the demyelinated patches in motor nerves. These ectopic impulses would result in muscle spasms and pain. Livingston first described the "vicious cycle" in 1925. It is a reflex loop involving a nociceptive input that activates the motor neuron within the spinal cord causing muscle spasms that in turn activate the muscle nociceptors and feeds back to the spinal cord to sustain the loop and the spasms and pain. Muscular pain descriptors include "dull ache," "night cramps," "band-like sensation," "drawing sensation," "spasms," and "toothache-like." Physical examination often reveals tight, contracted foot extensors and gastrocnemius muscles. Treatment for muscular pain includes lower extremity stretching exercises twice a day, and proper footwear including custom shoes and metatarsal bars where necessary. Patients are encouraged to avoid high heels because they cause undue strain on the gastrocnemius muscles. If the muscular pain continues after 2 weeks of exercise, a muscle relaxant should be considered. Metaxalone, 800 mg three or four times a day for 2 weeks, is generally effective. Alternatively, an NSAID could be used in order to break "Livingston's vicious cycle."

Treatment Algorithm

Initiation of treatment for any of the pain types is based on a pain score deemed severe enough to warrant therapy. A numeric scoring system can be used. A typical scoring system would be from 0 (no pain) to 20 (worst pain imaginable). Using this system, a score of 5 or greater is necessary to initiate therapy for any of the pain types. Patients are reevaluated every 6 weeks during therapy. At each evaluation the pain score is reassessed. Once the pain score drops to less than 5, attempts to decrease or discontinue medicines are initiated. Typically, all medicines are discontinued in 9 to 12 months. Once patients have been able to be relieved of their pain and

have been able to have the medicines discontinued, the pain may reoccur. Unfortunately, these relapses are not uncommon. If a reoccurrence does occur, the medicine that was successful for that specific type of pain can be restarted.

In one case-controlled series of 75 patients, treatment by the above algorithm for the three types of pain was compared to a placebo group. The treatment protocol was highly successful. Not only was there a decrease in pain scores (Fig. 3–12) but there was an improvement of sleeping patterns (Fig. 3–13) and psychosocial distress.

In summary, pain can be divided into three categories (dysesthesia, paresthesia, and muscular pain). The pain model approach to treating distal symmetric polyneuropathy is highly successful (Table 3–9). Future treatments may include topical clonidine, gabapentin cream, pregabalin therapy, and α-lipoic acid.

Avoidance of Future Complications of Diabetic Neuropathy

The ultimate consequences of diabetic neuropathy can be pain or foot ulcers and amputation. Pain was discussed above. In order to avoid ulceration and possible amputation, routine assessment of the foot by health care professionals, proper footwear, and patient education are important. In addition, offering methods and tools to improve the quality of life for patients with diabetic neuropathy is part of good clinical care.

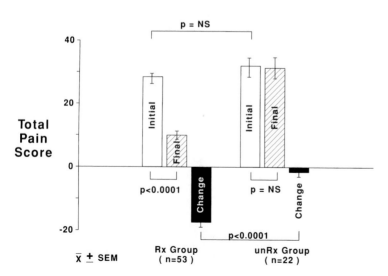

Figure 3–12 ■ Improvement of pain score with therapy. Initial and final treatment pain scores. Before treatment (using the algorithm detailed in Fig. 3–9), no significant difference (p = NS; nonsignificant) was found between the treated (Rx) and untreated (unRx) groups. The treated group, but not the untreated group, demonstrated a significant decrease in the pain score after 3 months. The changes (before vs. after) in the pain score were statistically greater in the treated group. (From Pfeifer MA, Ross D, Schrage J, et al: A highly successful and novel model for the treatment of chronic painful diabetic peripheral neuropathy. Diabetes Care 16:1103–1115, 1993, with permission.)

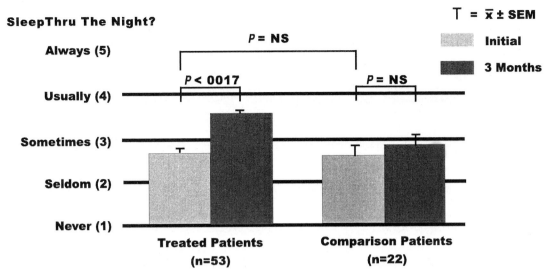

Figure 3–13 ■ Improvement of sleeping pattern with successful treatment of painful diabetic neuropathy. Sleep score (ability to sleep completely through the night) was not different initially between the treated and untreated group, but improved in the treated group with lessening of the painful symptoms. (From Pfeifer MA, Ross D, Schrage J, et al: A highly successful and novel model for the treatment of chronic painful diabetic peripheral neuropathy. Diabetes Care 16:1103–1115, 1993, with permission.)

Routine Assessment by the Health Care Professional

Early identification and appropriate therapy of the patient at increased risk of ulceration and amputation requires routine assessment and examination by the health care professional. The health care provider is responsible for lifelong surveillance, examination of the feet at each office visit, risk stratification, and referral for therapeutic footwear and orthoses when needed. The patient's responsibilities include daily foot inspection and obtaining patient education on self-care practices. The American Diabetes Association (ADA) has estimated that 50% of the limbs with foot ulcers can be saved if both the health care provider and the patient fulfill their respective responsibilities.

ROUTINE OFFICE VISIT EXAM

At each office visit the health care provider should examine the patient's feet. Motor neuropathy can lead to foot deformities from muscle atrophy and imbalance of the muscles. A common deformity is the claw toe deformity (Fig. 3–14). The loss of foot flexor strength allows the foot extensors to contract relatively unopposed. Even at rest the toes are pulled into a claw position. As this occurs the fat pad is pulled off the metatarsal heads. This may lead to high pressure points under the metatarsal heads, the tips of the toes, and the knuckle of the toe. These are common areas for ulceration. Metatarsal bar orthoses help pull the fat pad back into place and straighten the toes. Thus, the metatarsal bar can help prevent ulceration in patients with claw toe deformity.

Other deformities that the health care provider should evaluate include hammer toes, hallux limitus, bunions, Charcot arthropathy, limited joint mobility, abnormal toe position, calluses, and partial foot amputations. Bunions do not allow for proper shoe fitting. Callus formation is secondary to repeated insult from increased pressure. Thus, shoes that fit poorly, shoes that have poor cushioning, going barefoot, and foot deformities may result in heavy callus formation. Although calluses form in order to better protect the foot, calluses are unyielding, fixed tissue that is more prone to injury from shearing and may actually increase the pressure under the callus even more. It is not uncommon to find an ulcer under a callus.[37]

Charcot foot (see Chapter 21) is a progressive destruction of the bones in the foot. The arch of the foot is usually lost. The misshapen foot and bony protrusions lead to increased pressure points in unusual places on the foot.[62] Any foot deformity contributes to increased pressure and shear stress over the bony prominence, putting the foot at in-

Table 3–9 ■ PAIN MODEL APPROACH FOR TREATING DISTAL SYMMETRICAL POLYNEUROPATHY*

Gabapentin
100-mg tablets
   Day 1–3: 1 tablet 2 times a day
   Day 4–6: 2 tablets 2 times a day
300-mg tablets
   Day 7–9: 1 tablet 2 times a day
   Day 10–12: 1 tablet 3 times a day
   Day 13–15: 2 tablets 3 times a day
   Day 16–on: 2 tablets 4 times a day
• Titrate upwards until pain resolves, maximum dose is reached (or) symptoms are too great.
• If symptoms too great, continue for 6 days the last dose tolerated and then try to increase again.
• If unable to tolerate maximum dose continue at last dose tolerated.
Side effects: drowsiness, lethargy, fatigue, depression

Capsaicin
0.025–0.075%
• Use 4 times a day in order to desensitize.
• Warn about increased burning during early part of treatment.

Mexiletine
Day 1:   ECG
Day 1–3:   Mexiletine 150 mg pc supper for 3 days
Day 4:   Rhythm strip (5 mins)
Day 4–6:   Mexiletine 300 mg pc supper for 3 days
Day 7:   Rhythm strip (5 mins)
Days 7–9:   Mexiletine 10 mg/kg divided daily pc meals & snacks for 3 days
Day 10:   Holter (24 hours)
After day 10:   Continue on at last dose
Side effects: nausea, ectopic beats

Tricyclic antidepressants (TCAs)
e.g., Imipramine
50 mg PO qhs, Day 1
Increase to max. dose of 150 mg PO qhs
Side effects: postural hypotension, dry mouth, urinary retention (men), somnolence

Carbamazepine
e.g., Tegretol
100 mg PO bid, Day 1
Increase to max. dose 400 mg PO tid
Side effects: aplastic anemia, nausea, increased LFTs

Phenytoin
e.g., Dilantin
100 mg PO tid, Day 1
Increase to max. dose of 200 mg PO tid
Side effects: multiple, GI, CNS, increased LFT, rhythm disturbance

Skeletal muscle relaxant
e.g., Metaxalone (Skelaxin)
400-mg tablets; 2 PO pc tid–qid
Side effects: lethargy, nausea

* Data from Therapy for Diabetes Mellitus and Related Disorders, 2nd ed., Am. Diabetes Assoc., 1994, Chap 39; Diabetes Care 16:1103–1115, 1993; Diabetes Care 5:386–390, 1982; Clin Pharmacol Ther 22:196–199, 1977; JAMA 251:1727–1730, 1984; Arch Intern Med 151:2225–2229, 1991; and Lancet 2:9–11, 1988.
PC, after meals; qhs, every bedtime; bid, twice daily; tid, three times daily; LFT, liver function tests; GI, gastrointestinal; CNS, central nervous system.

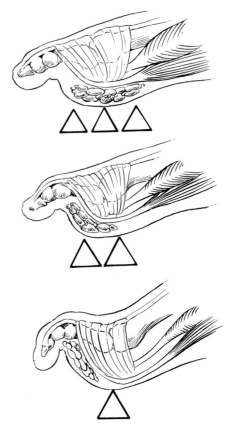

Figure 3–14 ■ Development of claw toe deformity. As the flexor muscles of the foot become weakened disproportionately to the extensor muscles, the toes are pulled into a claw deformity. This action pulls the fat pad off the metatarsal heads of the foot. The pressure is no longer distributed along a wide base but rather a narrow point beneath the metatarsal heads, which no longer have any fat padding. The plantar surface of the metatarsal heads, the cocked-up toe knuckle (more likely to hit the top of the toe box), and the tip of the toe are at increased risk for ulceration with this common deformity.

creased risk of ulceration. Foot deformities should be sought, noted, and evaluated at each office visit. These and other foot deformities are discussed in detail elsewhere in this book.

Sensory neuropathy can easily be evaluated via monofilament testing (see above). Figure 3–15 details the importance of monofilament testing. Individuals who were unable to feel the 5.07 monofilament (insensate) were at greater risk of ulceration at any duration of diabetes.[72] For this reason, diabetic individuals with insensate feet should obtain custom footwear. Lack of vibration sense over the great toenail carries a similar risk. Monofilaments and tuning fork

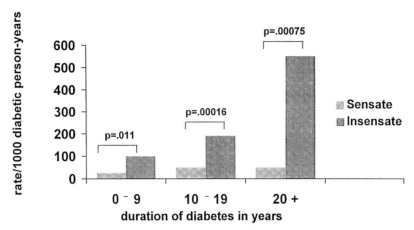

Figure 3–15 ■ Incidence of plantar ulceration by duration of diabetes and sensitivity to 5.07 monofilament; 358 American Indians were screened with the Semmes-Weinstein 5.07 monofilament. The patients were followed prospectively for lower extremity events and changes in sensation. Insensitivity to the 5.07 monofilament occurred in 19% of the patients screened. Among the insensate group the odds ratio of subsequent ulceration was 9.9 (95% CI, 4.8 to 21.0) and amputation was 17.0 (95% CI, 4.5 to 95.0) compared to those individuals who were able to feel the 5.07 monofilament. These relationships were maintained when controlling for the duration of diabetes and vascular indices. (From Rith-Najarian SJ, Stolusky T, Gohdes DM: Identifying diabetic patients at high risk for lower-extremity amputation in a primary health care setting. A prospective evaluation of simple screening criteria. Diabetes Care 15:1386–1389, 1992, with permission.)

evaluation should be determined on an annual basis.

Two common consequences of autonomic neuropathy in the diabetic foot are sudomotor dysfunction and changes in vascular flow within the skin of the sole of the foot. Both of these abnormalities lead to dry feet. Dry, cracked, or fissured skin in the feet is a common problem in people with diabetes. The reason is twofold: (1) lack of skin lubrication, and (2) redirection of blood flow in the microscopic blood vessels in the skin (see Fig. 3–2). Skin lubrication is maintained by oil and sweat secretion by the sebaceous glands. These sweat glands atrophy in the presence of autonomic neuropathy. This natural lubrication is important for maintaining the health of the skin. The other reason for dry feet is because the AV shunts, which are located in the soles (but not the dorsum) of the feet, are inappropriately dilated. Normally, the sympathetic nerves to these channels keep them tightly shut and the blood flows to the skin surface through the nutrient capillaries. These channels (AV shunts) are normally used by the body to help protect an individual from very cold weather. During extreme cold the body allows these channels to open up and redirects the blood away from the surface of the skin back towards the central (core) part of the body. These channels are located in the ear lobes, the fingers, the

tip of the nose, and the soles of the feet. Thus, frostbite occurs in these places first. When the nerves to these channels are damaged from autonomic neuropathy the channels are not kept consistently shut (i.e., the AV shunts dilate). This allows the blood to bypass the surface of the skin. Bypassing of the surface of the skin causes a lack of integrity to the skin and aids in it becoming dry. This is also a common reason for cold feet. The combination of poor natural lubrication and reduction in blood flow in the soles of the feet allow the skin to become dry, crack, form fissures, and become hard. The skin helps protect the feet from injury. If the skin is dry and has lost its integrity, for any reason, the foot is at increased risk for damage, sores, lesions, ulcers, infections, and even amputation. Therefore, keeping the feet well lubricated (not wet) is an important part of foot care.

In choosing an agent to help maintain or replace skin moisture, the health care provider must read the label of the product. Sometimes agents added to creams, ointment, and lotions are not the best for feet. Many of the fragrances used in these products are alcohol based. As alcohols evaporate, they can actually dry the skin further. The patient should be instructed that words ending with "-ol" are often alcohols. If any of the first four items on the label ends with the last two letters "-ol," another product should be chosen. Furthermore, words like "natural," "intensive," "nature's," "diabetic," "diabetes," "pure," "prevention," "dermal," "the best," "formulated," "formula," "secret," "oldest," "doctors," and "physicians," have no bearing on the quality of the product. In addition, petroleum-based products seal the surface of the skin. It keeps what little lubrication is made from evaporating too quickly but it does not penetrate past the surface of the skin. Thus, petroleum-based products do not replace the moisture in the skin. Creams or lotions with substances that are known to help replace the moisture to the skin surface and just below the surface of the skin are better than perfumed lotions or petroleum-based products. Most ointments are petroleum based. Animal oils (e.g., lanolin), urea (a substance commonly found in urine), and fats (e.g., stearates) tend to penetrate deep into the skin and moisturize dry skin well. There are many excellent creams and lotions on the market. One lotion that is commonly used is called Lansinoh. This lotion is a form of lanolin and is often used by nursing mothers in order to avoid cracking of their nipples when breast-feeding. Other commonly used lanolin-based products include Bag Balm and Udder Butter, which were first used to keep cows' udders soft and pliable. These lanolin-based products appear to be safe and work reasonably well. However, Bag Balm and Udder Butter contain an antibiotic that some health care professionals find less than desirable. Urea is found in many lotions and creams.

Urea appears to be fairly efficacious and safe as a moisturizer. Lard is also commonly used by patients to replace moisture in their feet. This appears to be safe and efficacious but somewhat distasteful and foul smelling. To date, no clinical studies have been done to compare the moisturizing effect of these products to a placebo or each other. Nevertheless, moisturizing dry feet is an important part of foot care in people with diabetes and needs to be encouraged.

RISK STRATIFICATION

Several classification schemes for foot risk stratification have been proposed and are discussed elsewhere in this book. Table 3–10 is a convenient, evidence-based classification.[4] In this system, patients are stratified according to the presence or absence of sensa-

Table 3–10 ■ TREATMENT-BASED DIABETIC FOOT INDEX

CATEGORY	PRESENTATION
0	Minimal or no pathology present
1	Insensate foot
2	Insensate foot with deformity
3	Neuropathy with deformity plus history of prior foot ulcer
4	Insensate injury
5	Infected diabetic foot
6	Dysvascular foot

tion, deformity, neuropathic ulceration, infection, and vascular disease. Each category corresponds to a recommended treatment regimen and is discussed in Chapters 11, 18, and 34. Evidence exists that the odds ratio of developing a foot ulcer increases as patients exhibit more of the following characteristics: severe peripheral neuropathy (inability to feel a monofilament of 5.07), advanced peripheral vascular disease (absence of pedal pulses, dependent rubor, pallor on elevation, or history of intermittent claudication or rest pain), foot deformity, history of previous foot ulcer or amputation, presence of plantar callus, and/or limited joint mobility syndrome.[59] Health care professionals need to identify feet at risk for ulceration and seek methods (see below) to prevent the same.

Proper Footwear

Chapter 35 describes appropriate footwear for people with diabetes in detail. Because of the presence of neuropathy, special protective shoes are often necessary.[46] Custom or modified footwear is important for healing (e.g., total contact casting, removable walker, half-shoe) and for prevention (e.g., extra-depth shoe, custom-molded shoes, custom insoles). Metatarsal bars are commonly used in custom insoles and help to correct the claw toe deformity (see above). Rocker-bottom shoes are also commonly used. The rocker-bottom shoe enables the individual to rock or roll the foot from heel to toe without bending the shoe or creating undue pressures on the foot. Custom shoes can decrease the reulceration rate from 60% over 3 years to 20% in over 3 years.[57] The benefit of special shoes and insoles has been recognized and supported by Medicare. The Medicare-supported Therapeutic Shoe Bill allows for payment for special footwear and insoles made for people with diabetes. The ADA states that the objectives of prescription footwear include: (1) to relieve areas of excessive plantar pressure, (2) to reduce shock, (3) to reduce shear stress, (4) to accommodate deformities, (5) to stabilize and support deformities, and (6) to limit motion of joints.

In addition to special shoes, Figure 3–8 demonstrates the advantage of cushioned socks (Thor-Lo). Even in people without neuropathy or foot deformity, well-fitting shoes, especially jogging, tennis, or other cushioned shoes, are essential to avoiding blisters and other foot lesions. Simple habits such as changing the shoes every 4 to 6 hours, breaking in new shoes slowly, and inspecting shoes before wearing each time are also effective preventative measures.

Patient Education

Chapter 31 details the importance and techniques for proper patient education. Table 3–11 summarizes the general principles. Foot soaks; "bathroom surgery"; going bare foot; heating pads; astringents; plastic shoes; and over-the-counter preparations for corns, calluses, and nails should be avoided. It is important for the patient to be actively involved in his or her own care. Proper foot care should be demonstrated by the health care educator and in turn by the patient. The use of a nonbreakable mirror enables the patient to inspect the soles of his or her feet with ease. Specific instructions (such as "don't go barefoot") are often more practical than generalities (such as "avoid hurting your feet"). Liberal use of films, booklets, pamphlets, videos, and handouts is important. The impor-

tance of patient education was well illustrated in one study.[58] This study showed that simple interventions (patient foot care education provided with written information about proper foot care) reduced serious foot problems by 60% in 1 year. Although patient education is important in all people with diabetes, it is especially important to provide patient education to individuals with diabetic neuropathy.

Devices for activities of daily living, including buttoners, zipper assist devices, mirrors, and bath water thermometers, may be helpful to a patient when diabetic neuropathy is advanced.

Summary

In summary, assessment of the "forgotten" complication of diabetes, diabetic neuropathy, is possible, inexpensive, and important. With proper concern and diligence towards the treatment of diabetic neuropathy, the quality of life, treatment modalities, and the lifestyle of diabetic patients can be improved.

REFERENCES

1. Abbruzzese M, Ratto S, Abbruzzese G, Favale E: Electroneurographic correlates of the monosynaptic reflex: Experimental studies and normative data. J Neurol Neurosurg Psychiatry 48:434–444, 1985.
2. Adler AI, Boyko EJ, Ahroni JH, et al: Risk factors for diabetic peripheral sensory neuropathy. Results of the Seattle Prospective Diabetic Foot Study. Diabetes Care 20:1162–1167, 1997.
3. Apfel SC: Neurotrophic factors and diabetic peripheral neuropathy. Eur Neurol 41(Suppl 1):27–34, 1999.
4. Armstrong DG, Lavery LA, Harkless LB: Treatment-based classification system for assessment and care of diabetic feet. J Am Podiatr Med Assoc 86:311–316, 1996.
5. Backonja M, Beydoun A, Edwards KR, et al: Gabapentin for the symptomatic treatment of painful neuropathy in patients with diabetes mellitus. A randomized controlled trial. JAMA 280:1831–1836, 1998.
6. Beggs J, Johnson PC, Olafsen A, Watkins CJ: Innervation of the vasa nervorum: Changes in human diabetics. J Neuropathol Exp Neurol 51:612–629, 1992.
7. Boulton AJ, Drury J, Clarke B, Ward JD: Continuous subcutaneous insulin infusion in the management of painful diabetic neuropathy. Diabetes Care 5:386–390, 1982.
8. Boulton AJM, Scarpello JHB, Ward JD: Venous oxygenation in the diabetic neuropathic foot: Evidence of arteriovenous shunting? Diabetologia 22:6–8, 1982.
9. Bursell SE, Takagi C, Clermont AC, et al: Specific retinal diacylglycerol and protein kinase C beta isoform modulation mimics abnormal retinal hemody-

---

Table 3–11 ■ EDUCATION FOR DIABETIC PATIENTS WITH NEUROPATHY

Appropriate type of exercise	Good communication with health care provider
Wash feet carefully	Dry feet carefully (especially between toes)
Inspect feet every day (especially between toes)	Look for changes in skin color
Feel for increased skin temperature	Avoid extremes in temperature
Trim toe nails straight across	Wear proper footwear
Stop smoking	Avoid minor trauma (i.e., no barefeet)
Good nutrition	Learn (read pamphlet or watch video) about proper foot care

namics in diabetic rats. Invest Ophthalmol Vis Sci 38:2711–2720, 1997.

10. Cameron NE, Cotter MA: Comparison of the effects of ascorbyl μ-linolenic acid and μ-linolenic acid in the correction of neurovascular deficits in diabetic rats. Diabetologia 39:1047–1054, 1996.

11. Cameron NE, Cotter MA: Metabolic and vascular factors in the pathogenesis of diabetic neuropathy. Diabetes 46(Suppl 2):S31–S37, 1997.

12. Cameron NE, Cotter MA, Basso M, Hohman TC: Comparison of the effects of inhibitors of aldose reductase and sorbitol dehydrogenase on neurovascular function, nerve conduction and tissue polyol pathway metabolites in streptozotocin-diabetic rats. Diabetologia 40:271–281, 1997.

13. Cameron NE, Cotter MA, Hohman TC: Interactions between essential fatty acid, prostanoid, polyol pathway and nitric oxide mechanisms in the neurovascular deficit of diabetic rats. Diabetologia 39: 172–182, 1996.

14. Cameron NE, Cotter MA, Robertson S: Angiotensin converting enzyme inhibition prevents development of muscle and nerve dysfunction and stimulates angiogenesis in streptozotocin-diabetic rats. Diabetologia 35:12–18, 1992.

15. Cameron NE, Leonard MB, Ross IS, Whiting PH: The effects of sorbinil on peripheral nerve conduction velocity, polyol concentrations and morphology in the streptozotocin-diabetic rat. Diabetologia 29: 168–174, 1986.

16. Cameron NE, Cotter MA, Robertson S: Rapid reversal of a motor nerve conduction deficit in streptozotocin-diabetic rats by the angiotensin converting enzyme inhibitor lisinopril. Acta Diabetol 30:46–48, 1993.

17. Canal N, Nemni R: Autoimmunity and diabetic neuropathy. Clin Neurosci 4:371–373, 1997.

18. Cardiac Arrhythmia Suppression Trial (CAST) Investigators: Preliminary report: Effect of encainide and flecainide on mortality in a randomized trial of arrhythmia suppression after myocardial infarction. N Engl J Med 321:406–412, 1989.

19. Clemens R: Dietary myoinositol intake and peripheral nerve function in diabetic neuropathy. Metabolism 28(Suppl 1):477–483, 1979.

20. Clements RS Jr, Bell DS: Diabetic neuropathy: Peripheral and autonomic syndromes. Postgrad Med 71:50–52, 55–57, 60–67, 1982.

21. Cole JA, Walker RE, Yordy MR: Hyperglycemia-induced changes in Na+/myo-inositol transport, Na(+)-K(+)-ATPase, and protein kinase C activity in proximal tubule cells. Diabetes 44:446–452, 1995.

22. Corbin DOC, Young RJ, Morrison DC, et al: Blood flow in the foot, polyneuropathy and foot ulceration in diabetes mellitus. Diabetologia 30:468–473, 1987.

23. Danis RP, Bingaman DP, Jirousek M, Yang Y: Inhibition of intraocular neovascularization caused by retinal ischemia in pigs by PKCbeta inhibition with LY333531. Invest Ophthalmol Vis Sci 39:171–179, 1998.

24. DCCT Research Group: The effect of intensive treatment of diabetes on the development and progression of long-term complications in insulin-dependent diabetes mellitus. N Engl J Med 329: 977–986, 1993.

25. DCCT Research Group: The Effect of Intensive Diabetes Therapy on the Development and Progression of Neuropathy. Ann Intern Med 122:561–568, 1995.

26. Dyck PJ: Detection, characterization, and staging of polyneuropathy: Assessed in diabetics. Muscle Nerve 11:21–32, 1988.

27. Dyck PJ, Karnes JL, O'Brien PC, et al: The Rochester Diabetic Neuropathy Study: Reassessment of tests and criteria for diagnosis and staged severity. Neurology 42:1164–1170, 1992.

28. Feldman EL, Stevens MJ, Greene DA: Pathogenesis of diabetic neuropathy. Clin Neurosci 4:365–370, 1997.

29. Freeman R: Human studies of recombinant human nerve growth factor and diabetic peripheral neuropathy. Eur Neurol 41(Suppl 1):20–26, 1999.

30. Friedman EA: Advanced glycosylated end products and hyperglycemia in the pathogenesis of diabetic complications. Diabetes Care 22(Suppl 2):B65–B71, 1999.

31. Gelber DA, Pfeifer MA, Broadstone VL, et al: Components of variance for vibratory and thermal threshold testing in normal and diabetic subjects. J Diabetes Complications 9:170–176, 1995.

32. Goldfarb S, Zihadeh FN, Kern EFO, Simmons DA: Effects of polyol-pathway inhibition and dietary myo-inositol on glomerular hemodynamic function in experimental diabetes mellitus in rats. Diabetes 40:465–471, 1991.

33. Gomez-Perez FJ, Choza R, Rios JM, et al: Nortriptyline-fluphenazine vs. carbamazepine in the symptomatic treatment of diabetic neuropathy. Arch Med Res 27:525–529, 1996.

34. Graf J, Halter JB, Pfeifer MA, et al: Glycemic control and nerve conduction abnormalities in non insulin dependent diabetic subjects. Ann Intern Med 94: 307–311, 1981.

35. Greene DA, Lattimer SA: The polyol pathway in dysfunction of diabetic peripheral nerve. Diabet Med 2:206–210, 1985.

36. Greene DA, Lattimer SA, Carroll PB, et al: A defect in sodium-dependent amino acid uptake in diabetic rabbit peripheral nerve. Correction by an aldose reductase inhibitor or myo-inositol administration. J Clin Invest 85:1657–1665, 1990.

37. Grunfeld C: Diabetic foot ulcers: Etiology, treatment, and prevention. Adv Intern Med 37:103–132, 1992.

38. Guyton AC: Textbook of Medical Physiology, 8th ed. Philadelphia: WB Saunders Company, 1991.

39. Harati Y, Gooch C, Swenson M, et al: Double-blind randomized trial of tramadol for the treatment of the pain of diabetic neuropathy. Neurology 50: 1842–1846, 1998.

40. Harris M, Eastman R, Cowie C: Symptoms of sensory neuropathy in adults with NIDDM in the U.S. population. Diabetes Care 16:1446–1452, 1993.

41. Hata Y, Rook SL, Aiello LP: Basic fibroblast growth factor induces expression of VEGF receptor KDR through a protein kinase C and p44/p42 mitogen-activated protein kinase-dependent pathway. Diabetes 48:1145–1155, 1999.

42. Honing ML, Morrison PJ, Banga JD, et al: Nitric oxide availability in diabetes mellitus. Diabetes Metab Rev 14:241–249, 1998.

43. Hotta N, Koh N, Sakakibara F, et al: Prevention of abnormalities in motor nerve conduction and nerve blood-flow by a prostacyclin analog, beraprost sodium, in streptozotocin-induced diabetic rats. Prostaglandins 49:339–349, 1995.

44. Ishii H, Koya D, King GL: Protein kinase C activation and its role in the development of vascular

complications in diabetes mellitus. J Mol Med 76:21–31, 1998.

45. Jaeger C, Allendorfer J, Hatziagelaki E, et al: Persistent GAD 65 antibodies in longstanding IDDM are not associated with residual beta-cell function, neuropathy or HLA-DR status. Horm Metab Res 29:510–515, 1997.

46. Janisse DJ: Prescription insoles and footwear. Clin Podiatr Med Surg 12:41–61, 1995.

47. Jarret A: The Physiology and Pathophysiology of the Skin, vol 2. New York: Academic Press, 1973.

48. Jarvis B, Coukell AJ: Mexiletine. A review of its therapeutic use in painful diabetic neuropathy. Drugs 56:691–707, 1998.

49. Johnson PC, Beggs JL: Pathology of the autonomic nerve innervating the vasa nervorum in diabetic neuropathy. Diabet Med 10(Suppl 2):S56–S61, 1993.

50. Judzewitsch RG, Jaspan JB, Polonsky KS, et al: Aldose reductase inhibition improves nerve conduction velocity in diabetic patients. N Engl J Med 308:119–125, 1983.

51. Kato N, Makino M, Mizuno K, et al: Serial changes of sensory nerve conduction velocity and minimal F-wave latency in streptozotocin-induced diabetic rats. Neurosci Lett 244:169–172, 1998.

52. Kim J, Kyriazi H, Greene DA: Normalization of Na(+)-K(+)-ATPase activity in isolated membrane fraction from sciatic nerves of streptozocin-induced diabetic rats by dietary myo-inositol supplementation in vivo or protein kinase C agonists in vitro. Diabetes 40:558–567, 1991.

53. Kim J, Rushovich EH, Thomas TP, et al: Diminished specific activity of cytosolic protein kinase C in sciatic nerve of streptozocin-induced diabetic rats and its correction by dietary myo-inositol. Diabetes 40:1545–1554, 1991.

54. Koya D, Jirousek MR, Lin YW, et al: Characterization of protein kinase C beta isoform activation on the gene expression of transforming growth factor-beta, extracellular matrix components, and prostanoids in the glomeruli of diabetic rats. J Clin Invest 100:115–126, 1997.

55. Koya D, King GL: Protein kinase C activation and the development of diabetic complications. Diabetes 47:859–866, 1998.

56. Lang AH, Forsstrom J, Bjorkqvist SE, Kuusela V: Statistical variation of nerve conduction velocity. An analysis in normal subjects and uraemic patients. J Neurol Sci 33:229–241, 1977.

57. Levin M: Diabetic foot wounds: Pathogenesis and management. Adv Wound Care 10:24–30, 1997.

58. Litzelman DK, Slemenda CW, Langefeld CD, et al: Reduction of lower extremity clinical abnormalities in patients with non-insulin-dependent diabetes mellitus. A randomized, controlled trial. Ann Intern Med 119:36–41, 1993.

59. Mayfield JA, Reiber GE, Nelson RG, Greene T: A foot risk classification system to predict diabetic amputation in Pima Indians. Diabetes Care 19:704–709, 1996.

60. McQuay H, Carroll D, Jadad AR, et al: Anticonvulsant drugs for management of pain: A systematic review. BMJ 311:1047–1052, 1995.

61. McQuay HJ, Tramer M, Nye BA, et al: A systematic review of antidepressants in neuropathic pain. Pain 68:217–227, 1996.

62. Murray HJ, Boulton AJ: The pathophysiology of diabetic foot ulceration. Clin Podiatr Med Surg 12:1–17, 1995.

63. Obrosova I, et al: Glycolytic pathway, redox state of NAD (P)-couples and energy metabolism in lens in galactose-fed rats: Effect of an aldose reductase inhibitor. Curr Eye Res 16:34–43, 1997.

64. Park JY, Ha SW, King GL: The role of protein kinase C activation in the pathogenesis of diabetic vascular complications. Perit Dial Int 19(Suppl 2):S222–S227, 1999.

65. Pfeifer MA, Peterson H, Snider H, et al: Long-term open-label sorbinil therapy prevents the progression of diabetic neuropathy. Diabetes 37:45, 1988.

66. Pfeifer MA, Ross D, Schrage J, et al: A highly successful and novel model for the treatment of chronic painful diabetic peripheral neuropathy. Diabetes Care 16:1103–1115, 1993.

67. Pfeifer MA, Schumer MP: Clinical trials of diabetic neuropathy: Past, present and future. Diabetes 44:1355–1361, 1995.

68. Pfeifer MA, Schumer MP, Gelber DA: Aldose reductase inhibitors: The end of an era or the need for different trial designs? Diabetes 46(Suppl)2:S82–S89, 1997.

69. Pirart J: Diabetes mellitus and its degenerative complications: A prospective study of 4,400 patients observed between 1947 and 1973. Diabetes Care 1:168–188, 1978.

70. Proceedings of a consensus development conference on standardized measures in diabetic neuropathy. Diabetes Care 15:1080–1107, 1992.

71. Reja A, Tesfaye S, Harris ND, Ward JD: Is ACE inhibition with lisinopril helpful in diabetic neuropathy? Diabet Med 12:307–309, 1995.

72. Rith-Najarian SJ, Stolusky T, Gohdes DM: Identifying diabetic patients at high risk for lower-extremity amputation in a primary health care setting. A prospective evaluation of simple screening criteria. Diabetes Care 15:1386–1389, 1992.

73. Robinson LR, Stolov WC, Rubner DE, et al: Height is an independent risk factor for neuropathy in diabetic men. Diabetes Res Clin Pract 16:97–102, 1992.

74. Ross RT: How to Examine the Nervous System, 3rd ed. Stamford, CT: Appleton & Lange, 1999.

75. Rossing P: Promotion, prediction and prevention of progression of nephropathy in type 1 diabetes mellitus. Diabet Med 15:900–919, 1998.

76. Sima AA, Greene DA, Brown MB, et al: The Tolerestat Study Group: Effect of hyperglycemia and the aldose reductase inhibitor tolerestat on sural nerve biochemistry and morphometry in advanced diabetic peripheral polyneuropathy. J Diabetes Complications 7:157–169, 1993.

77. Sima AA, Lattimer SA, Yagihashi S, Greene DA: Axo-glial dysjunction. A novel structural lesion that accounts for poorly reversible slowing of nerve conduction in the spontaneously diabetic bio-breeding rat. J Clin Invest 77:474–484, 1986.

78. Singhal A, Cheng C, Sun H, Zochodme DW: Near nerve local insulin prevents conduction slowing in experimental diabetes. Brain Res 763:209–214, 1997.

79. Sosenko JM, Gadia MT, Fournier AM, et al: Body stature as a risk factor for diabetic sensory neuropathy. Am J Med 80:1031–1034, 1986.

80. The γ-Linolenic Acid Multicenter Trial Group: Treatment of diabetic neuropathy with γ-linolenic acid. Diabetes Care 16:8–15, 1993.

81. Tomlinson DR, Dewhurst M, Stevens EJ, et al: Reduced nerve blood flow in diabetic rats: Relationship

to nitric oxide production and inhibition of aldose reductase. Diabet Med 15:579–585, 1998.

82. UK Prospective Diabetes Study Group: Effect of intensive blood glucose control with metformin on complications in patients with type 2 diabetes: UKPDS 34. Lancet 352:854–865, 1998.

83. UK Prospective Diabetes Study Group: Intensive blood glucose control with sulfonylureas or insulin compared with conventional therapy and risk of complications in patients with type 2 diabetes mellitus: UKPDS 33. Lancet 352:837–853, 1998.

84. UK Prospective Diabetes Study Group: Tight blood pressure control and risk of macrovascular and microvascular complications in type 2 diabetes UKPDS 38. BMJ 317:703–713, 1998.

85. Williams B, Gallacher B, Patel H, Orme C: Glucose-induced protein kinase C activation regulates vascular permeability factor mRNA expression and peptide production by human vascular smooth muscle cells in vitro. Diabetes 46:1497–1503, 1997.

86. Xia P, Inoguchi T, Kern TS, et al: Characterization of the mechanism for the chronic activation of diacylglycerol-protein kinase C pathway in diabetes and hypergalactosemia. Diabetes 43:1122–1129, 1994.

87. Yagihashi S, Kamijo M, Ido Y, Mirrlees DJ: Effects of long-term aldose reductase inhibition on development of experimental diabetic neuropathy. Ultra-structural and morphometric studies of sural nerve in streptozocin-induced diabetic rats. Diabetes 39:690–696, 1990.

88. Yorek MA, Wiese TJ, Davidson EP, et al: Reduced motor nerve conduction velocity and Na(+)-K(+)-ATPase activity in rats maintained on L-fucose diet. Reversal by myo-inositol supplementation. Diabetes 42:1401–1406, 1993.

89. Yoshida M, Sugiyama Y, Akaike N, et al: Amelioration of neurovascular deficits in diabetic rats by a novel aldose reductase inhibitor, GP-1447: Minor contribution of nitric oxide. Diabetes Res Clin Pract 40:101–112, 1998.

90. Young RJ, Zhou YQ, Rodriguez E, et al: Variable relationship between peripheral somatic and autonomic neuropathy in patients with different syndromes of diabetic polyneuropathy. Diabetes 35:192–197, 1986.

91. Zanone MM, Burchio S, Quadri R, et al: Autonomic function and autoantibodies to autonomic nervous structures, glutamic acid decarboxylase and islet tyrosine phosphatase in adolescent patients with IDDM. J Neuroimmunol 87:1–10, 1998.

92. Ziegler D, Hanefeld M, Ruhnau KJ, et al: Treatment of symptomatic diabetic peripheral neuropathy with the anti-oxidant alpha-lipoic acid. A 3-week multicentre randomized controlled trial (ALADIN Study). Diabetologia 38:1425–1433, 1995.

ATHEROSCLEROSIS AND THROMBOSIS IN DIABETES MELLITUS: NEW ASPECTS OF PATHOGENESIS

■ John A. Colwell, Timothy J. Lyons, Richard L. Klein, Maria F. Lopes-Virella, and Rudolf J. Jokl

The development of atherosclerosis is accelerated in diabetes mellitus, leading to increased morbidity and mortality and excessive health care costs. Virtually all of the large vessels are involved in this process, and clinical manifestations are apparent as a result of atherosclerotic narrowing and thrombosis of coronary, cerebral, and leg vessels.

These factors have led to a renewed interest in factors present in the diabetic state that may help to explain the acceleration of this process. Work in diabetes has been facilitated by new concepts about the pathophysiology of the process of atherosclerosis in the nondiabetic state.

Review articles, and our previous chapters in this text,[82] have considered atherosclerosis in depth and should be consulted for older references.[79, 81, 82] This chapter provides updated information about the factors associated with the diabetic state that may underlie accelerated atherosclerosis and thrombosis and suggests a pathogenetic scheme that builds on knowledge of these processes in the nondiabetic state. The emphasis is on changes in the endothelium, on qualitative and quantitative changes in lipids and lipoproteins, on glycation and glyco-oxidation, and on altered coagulation in diabetes mellitus.

Historical Perspective

Clinicians have long recognized that peripheral vascular disease is an extremely serious medical complication. Advanced calcification of the aorta was found in a mummy from ancient Egyptian times (approximately 1290 to 1223 BC[243]). It is reported that Hippocrates, in 400 BC, "cut away the mortified parts," presumably in patients with gangrene after trauma or vascular occlusion. The first evidence of an amputation was a picture in the *Field Book of Wound Surgery* in 1517, showing the technique of Hans von Gersdortt. It was clear by the 17th century that amputations were indicated not only after traumatic injury but also for foot ulcers and abscesses. In the mid-1800s, Syme performed his celebrated amputation at the ankle joint, ether anesthesia was introduced, and an association of diabetes with gangrene was described by Marchal. By 1891, Heidenhain had published a thorough review of diabetes and arteriosclerosis of the legs and had recommended levels for amputation if gangrene was found.[97, 238]

Autopsy studies prior to 1930 in diabetic patients showed that 29% of them had gangrene at the time of death, and data from the Joslin Clinic between 1923 and 1969 indicated that amputations accounted for 22 to 40% of major surgical operations in their diabetic patients.[464] In Bell's classic autopsy study of 2,130 diabetic persons who had died from 1911 through 1955, gangrene was found in 21% and was 53 to 71 times more common than in nondiabetic individuals.[20]

As time has progressed, diagnostic techniques have improved. Cross-sectional (prevalence) studies have indicated that about 15 to 30% of a heterogenous group of non–insulin-dependent diabetes mellitus type 2 patients may have evidence of peripheral vascular disease when studied by noninvasive techniques.[19, 79, 111, 187, 294] The disease appears to progress as a function of age, duration of diabetes, or both when extrapolation from cross-sectional data is done. Longitudinal data are limited but suggest that the rate of progression may be about 2.5% per year in newly diagnosed white, type 2 subjects in the United States, whereas it may reach 5 to 7% per year in such type 2 diabetic populations who are followed up after the disease is present.[323] In any case, longitudinal studies agree that macrovascular complications involving both the leg and coronary vessels progress with increasing duration of diabetes. Whether this is related to hyperglycemia or other factors is not clear.

Risk Factors for Peripheral Vascular Disease in Diabetes

Studies of risk factors provide insight into the pathogenesis of peripheral vascular atherosclerosis in diabetes and have been reviewed elsewhere in this volume (see Chapter 9). In addition to the influences of age and duration of diabetes, several studies have indicated that hypertension and cigarette smoking, two classic risk factors for coronary artery disease, are also operative for peripheral vascular disease.[79] These correlations have been seen in populations as geographically diverse as Rochester, Minnesota,[330] Seattle, Washington,[19] Munich, Germany,[187] Kuopio, Finland,[438] and Framingham, Massachusetts.[136] It is not clear whether hyperglycemia is an independent risk factor for peripheral vascular disease. Indeed, in some populations, such as Japan, peripheral vascular disease is rarely seen in type 2 diabetes, despite longstanding hyperglycemia.[79] Studies in the United States and Germany have not established that either fasting glucose or glycosylated hemoglobin (HbA$_{1c}$) values are good predictors of progression of peripheral vascular disease in type 2 diabetes.[19, 28]

Altered lipid and lipoprotein profiles are frequently seen in type 2 diabetic subjects, with or without peripheral vascular disease. Several large-scale studies indicate that certain lipid-lipoprotein changes may be important risk factors for peripheral vascular disease in diabetes mellitus. In a cross-sectional study of 252 individuals with type 2 diabetes, elevated plasma triglyceride levels and decreased high-density lipoprotein (HDL) cholesterol levels emerged as possible risk factors for peripheral vascular disease.[19] In a 5-year prospective study in Finland, claudication was associated with increased plasma cholesterol, very low-density lipoprotein (VLDL) cholesterol, decreased HDL cholesterol, and increased VLDL triglyceride and low-density lipoprotein (LDL) triglyceride levels.[438] Multivariate analysis revealed that high LDL triglyceride and VLDL cholesterol levels had independent associations with claudication. On the other hand, negative correlations with lipids and either prevalence or incidence of peripheral vascular disease has been reported in some studies.[330]

Hyperinsulinemia has been implicated as an independent vascular risk factor in many epidemiologic studies.[104, 120, 347, 460] Generally, prospective studies have used ischemic heart disease and vascular deaths as the vascular end points of interest rather than peripheral vascular disease. In one large cross-sectional study, the greatest risk for coronary heart disease and peripheral vascular disease was seen in diabetic and nondiabetic subjects with the highest plasma C peptide levels.[397] Thus, although data in diabetic subjects with peripheral vascular disease are limited, it is possible that endogenous hyperinsulinemia may interact with other risk factors to accelerate macrovascular disease. There are many reviews of this issue, which should be consulted for details.[83, 414, 415]

Thus there are mixed messages from epidemiologic studies of peripheral vascular disease in diabetes. It is likely that this state of affairs is caused by confounding factors, including: (1) insensitive end points such as claudication and amputation; (2) the likelihood that pathogenesis may differ in type 1 diabetes and in the many stages of impaired glucose tolerance and type 2 diabetes; (3) the probability that multiple risk factors such as hyperglycemia, lipid disturbances, hypertension, and cigarette smoking interact; and (4) the frequent association of diabetic neuropathy with vascular insufficiency in many patients with diabetes. Nevertheless, epidemiologic data suggest that an atherogenic mix of lipids and lipoproteins may, in particular, contribute to peripheral vascular disease and that hypertension, smoking, and perhaps hyperglycemia may interact in many subjects to accelerate the process. Such leads from epidemiologic studies have stimulated research on precise mechanisms that may be involved in the pathogenesis of atherosclerosis in diabetes mellitus.

Pathogenesis of Atherosclerosis

Research in the last two decades suggests that atherosclerosis is a chronic inflammatory process that can be converted into an acute clinical event by plaque rupture.[23] The earliest atherosclerotic lesion is the fatty streak that, although not clinically significant on its own, plays a significant role in the events that lead to plaque progression and rupture. Formation of fatty streaks is induced by the transport of lipoproteins across the endothelium and their retention in the vessel wall. Schwenke et al.[381] have shown that for any given plasma lipoprotein concentration the degree of lipoprotein retention in the artery wall is more important than the rate of transport of the same lipoprotein into the artery wall. Frank et al.[123] demonstrated, using ultrastructural techniques, that LDL can be rapidly transported across an intact endothelium and becomes trapped by the extracellular matrix of the subendothelial space.[316] Once LDL is transported across the artery wall and binds to the extra-

cellular matrix, lipid oxidation is initiated, since microenvironment conditions that exclude plasma-soluble antioxidants are established.[313] With oxidation of LDL, endothelial cells are stimulated to release potent chemoattractants, such as monocyte-chemoattractant protein 1, monocyte-colony stimulating factor,[350] and GRO,[380] and these chemoattractants promote the recruitment of monocytes into the subendothelial space. Recruitment of these cells, due to their enormous oxidative capacity, leads to further oxidation of LDL. The more heavily modified LDL is cytotoxic to endothelial and smooth muscle cells[163, 165] and it is no longer recognized by the LDL receptor. It is taken up by macrophage scavenger receptors, leading to massive accumulation of cholesterol in macrophages and to their transformation into foam cells, the hallmark of the atherosclerotic process.[119, 168] Besides promoting the transformation of macrophages into foam cells, oxidized LDL is a potent inducer of inflammatory molecules and stimulates the immune system, leading to the formation of antibodies and, as a consequence, to the formation of immune complexes. These complexes may play a crucial role in macrophage activation and thus in the rupture of atheromatous plaques, as described later in this chapter.

Diabetes accelerates the sequence of events described above in many ways. Both LDL transport through the endothelium and retention in the subendothelial space are enhanced in diabetes. The rate of transport depends not only on the plasma concentration of LDL but also on its size as well as on the permeability of the endothelium. Small, dense LDL particles permeate more efficiently through the endothelium due to their size. Dense LDL levels are increased both in type 1 and type 2 diabetes, mostly when the patients are in poor glycemic control.[185, 186] Furthermore, increased LDL transport rate due to increased permeability of the endothelium is also observed in diabetes, since increased vascular permeability is one of the earliest abnormalities that occurs in vessels exposed to high glucose concentrations.[45] Besides increased rate of transport, the degree of retention of LDL by the matrix is also markedly increased in diabetes. It has been shown that collagen-linked advanced glycation end-products (AGEs), which are increased in diabetes, can act as reactive "foci" to covalently trap circulating serum proteins including LDL, leading to its increased retention in the subendothelium.[40, 42] AGE products are derived from oxidation of Amadori products, a stable product that results from the nonenzymatic reaction of glucose with primary amino acids. The amount of glycated adducts on amino acids varies directly with the ambient glucose concentration and therefore is increased in diabetes mostly in patients with poor glycemic control. Furthermore, AGE-LDL, like heavily oxidized LDL, is cytotoxic and it is a powerful chemoattractant for monocytes/macrophages thus inducing monocyte recruitment from the circulation across normal endothelium.[112]

AGE-LDL and oxidized LDL may also induce endothelial dysfunction. Kahn et al.[207] showed increased expression of vascular cell adhesion molecule-1 (VCAM-1) in human umbilical vein endothelial cells (HUVECs) and in human aortic endothelial cells (HAECs) exposed to LDL oxidized in vitro and increased expression of intercellular adhesion molecule-1 (ICAM-1) in HAEC but not in HUVEC cells. Interestingly, increased expression of VCAM-1 occurs in HAEC but not in HUVEC cells when exposed to in vitro glycated LDL.[207] AGE-LDL, upon occupancy of macrophage receptors, induces the release of tumor necrosis factor (TNF), interleukin-1 (IL-1), platelet-derived growth factor (PDGF), and immunoglobulin growth factor 1.[102, 448] These mediators, in turn, promote the expression of adhesion molecules and the recruitment of nearby connective tissue cells, inducing their proliferation and activating them to produce extracellular matrix components. AGEs will also lead to the down-regulation of the surface anticoagulant thrombomodulin and to the increase of procoagulant tissue factor.[112] Recently, AGEs were found to chemically inactivate nitric oxide or endothelium-derived relaxing factor.[47]

In addition to the actions described above, both oxidized LDL and AGE-LDL, as previously mentioned, can trigger an immune response, leading to the formation of autoantibodies and subsequently to the formation of immune complexes containing modified LDL. Antibodies to oxidized LDL have been described to occur naturally in humans[371] and to be detectable in a higher proportion of patients with advanced atherosclerosis, mostly in those with inflammatory reaction to the atherosclerotic plaques. Salonen and Cols[370] reported a statistically significant relationship between the tier of

autoantibodies to oxidized LDL and the rate of progression of carotid atherosclerosis. More recently, Maggi et al.[273] described high antibody titers against oxidatively modified LDL but normal susceptibility of LDL to oxidation in patients with severe carotid atherosclerosis.

The presence not only of autoantibodies against LDL but also of immune complexes have been described in patients with coronary artery disease by several independent investigators.[420, 423] Tertov et al.[423] were able to increase the lipid content of cultured human aortic smooth muscle cells by exposure to the sera of patients with coronary heart disease. These authors further demonstrated that when immune complexes were removed from the serum of these patients by precipitation with 2.5% polyethylene glycol, the depleted serum was not able to induce lipid accumulation in the same cells, thus suggesting that the atherogenic potential of the serum was due to the presence of immune complexes.

Thus, in addition to the direct effects of oxidized LDL or AGE-LDL on the endothelium, it could be argued that immune complexes formed as a consequence of the autoimmune response to oxidized and/or AGE-LDL could also have a direct pathogenic effect on endothelial cells. The interaction between immune complexes containing AGE-LDL or oxidized LDL and endothelial cells would be very likely if these cells expressed Fcγ receptors, but this is a point that has been the object of controversy. Some authors claim that Fcγ receptors are only expressed by previously damaged endothelial cells or by endothelial cells infected by latent viruses[69] or bacteria.[22] Thus, it is not clear whether immune complexes can play an initial role in damaging endothelial cells or whether they are solely involved in the evolution of a lesion initiated by some other insult. It is interesting to note that the role of infectious agents in the onset of atherosclerosis has been postulated and has received quite a lot of recent attention.[293] In either case, the binding of immune complexes to endothelial cells can have deleterious consequences by promoting endothelial binding and activation of phagocytic cells. Furthermore, if the endothelial cell-bound immune complexes are able to activate complement and release C5a, this complement fragment can attract and activate neutrophils, further contributing to the recruitment of cells potentially able to damage the endothelium.[30, 428] This mechanism may be particularly relevant to diabetes, since it is well known that immune complexes are present in diabetes in increased levels. It has been proposed that in diabetes the immune system is in a state of polyclonal activation, underlying the production of autoantibodies and the subsequent formation of immune complexes.

Injury to the endothelium may also occur indirectly through activation of macrophages. Macrophage activation leads to the release of biologically active mediators including cytokines such as IL-1 and TNF-α,[312] growth factors such as PDGF-B,[368] proteases,[307] collagenases,[462] oxygen radicals,[310] and other compounds capable of damaging the arterial wall. PDGF is known to play a significant role in the pathogenesis of atherosclerosis by being both chemotactic and mitogenic for intimal smooth muscle cells.[366] It has also been shown that PDGF-β protein can be detected in human and nonhuman primate atherosclerotic lesions, mainly in macrophages.[368] Cytokines have been implicated in the development of atherosclerosis in a variety of ways. They are known to induce adherence of leukocytes to endothelial cells. IL-1 has been shown to activate the expression of several specific cell adhesion molecules (CAMs), which appears to vary according to the stimulus and to the specific stage of cell activation.[259] IL-1 and TNF-α are also known to induce synthesis and cell surface expression of procoagulant activity in endothelial cells,[25] to increase vascular permeability,[280] and to stimulate the synthesis of platelet-activating factor (PAF) by endothelial cells.[35, 487] TNF-α, which can be produced not only by macrophages but also by smooth muscle cells, shares with IL-1 the ability to induce cell surface expression of procoagulant activity[25] and to stimulate the expression of cell adhesion molecules in endothelial cells.[55, 134]

Studies performed in our laboratory have shown[444] that human monocyte-derived macrophages stimulated by LDL-IC release not only superoxide radicals but also increased amounts of TNF-α and IL-1β. The release of these cytokines was not induced by the incubation of macrophages with acetylated LDL, oxidized LDL, and native LDL. These cytokines were released, however, as expected, when macrophages were stimulated with another type of immune complexes,

such as those formed by keyhole limpet hemocyanin (KLH) and the corresponding antibodies (KLH-ICs), although much less efficiently. Therefore, the formation of LDL-IC involving IgG anti-LDL antibodies and LDL has a considerably higher pathogenic potential than the modification of LDL per se, since LDL-ICs not only deliver LDL to a cell in a way that escapes normal metabolic control and leads to foam cell formation, but are also taken up through the Fcγ receptor, whose occupancy delivers an activating signal to the macrophage, leading to the release of cytokines.

Another consequence of the activation of macrophage by immune complexes containing either native or modified LDL is posttranscriptional up-regulation of scavenger receptor expression (unpublished results). Up-regulation of scavenger receptor further contributes to the increased uptake of oxidized LDL by macrophages and, as a consequence, to foam cell formation.[119, 168]

Foam cell formation is believed to be a key event in atherosclerosis and there has been considerable interest in defining mechanisms responsible for the accumulation of cholesteryl esters in macrophages, which eventually leads to the formation of foam cells. Modified lipoproteins have been shown to induce foam cell formation, as previously mentioned.[119, 168] Immune complexes containing native or modified LDL are also able to induce the transformation of macrophages into foam cells. We have demonstrated, using in vitro prepared immune complexes containing native or modified LDL, that these complexes induce a marked accumulation of cholesterol esters (CE) in human monocyte-derived macrophages and the transformation of these cells into foam cells.[140, 147, 176, 248, 251, 256, 296] We also demonstrated that the increased accumulation of CE in human macrophages exposed to LDL-IC was secondary to an increased uptake of the LDL complexed with antibody, followed by altered intracellular metabolism of the particle.[251] In the initial stages the intracellular accumulation of CE reflects the accumulation of intact LDL, in later stages the cell accumulates cholesteryl esters generated by de novo esterification of the free cholesterol released during lysosomal hydrolysis of LDL. Recently, we have shown that, in some instances, immune complexes isolated from type 1 diabetic and control subjects led to increased CE accumulation in human macrophages. We have also demonstrated that the degree of CE accumulation is significantly related to the apolipoprotein B and cholesterol content of the immune complexes.[296]

Subsequent to intimal macrophage accumulation and their transformation into foam cells, smooth muscle cells appear to be attracted from the media into the intima, and many of these cells proliferate, leading to the formation of a fibrofatty lesion. With continuing smooth muscle cell migration and proliferation in the intima, connective tissue is formed by the smooth muscle cells and fibrous plaque formation occurs. The components responsible for the migration and proliferation of smooth muscle cells into the intima are cytokines and growth factors such as IL-1, TNF-α, and PDGF, which are released by activated macrophages, by activated endothelium, by the smooth muscle cells, and perhaps by platelets.

IL-1 and TNF-α are known to affect both endothelial cells and smooth muscle cells. IL-1 can be indirectly responsible for fibroblast and smooth muscle cell proliferation by inducing the production of PDGF-AA by these cells, activating what appears to be an autocrine growth-regulating mechanism.[349] However, since IL-1 induces secretion of prostanoids by smooth muscle cells,[245] and prostanoids are known to have growth-inhibiting properties, the in vivo effect of IL-1 release in the arterial wall is unclear. TNF-α, which can be produced not only by macrophages but also by smooth muscle cells, shares with IL-1 the ability to stimulate IL-1 secretion and indirectly PDGF.

PDGF will derive from at least four sources in the intimal lesion: platelets, macrophages, endothelial cells, and smooth muscle cells. It is known to induce both smooth muscle cell and fibroblast proliferation. The susceptibility of a given cell to respond to PDGF depends on the type of PDGF receptor subunits present in the cell. For instance, it is well known that fibroblasts respond poorly to PDGF-AA but they respond well to PDGF-BB.[373] In contrast, smooth muscle cells respond equally well to both PDGF-AA and PDGF-BB. Both macrophages and endothelial cells can make both chains of PDGF, while smooth muscle cells appear to make only PDGF-AA.[367]

Besides IL-1, TNF, and PDGF, (TGF-β), which is usually formed by macrophages but can also be formed by smooth muscle cells, is also responsible for new connective tissue matrix formation.[367] Furthermore, it seems to be also markedly chemotactic for monocytes and smooth muscle cells. However, TFG-β may also play a role in lesion regression, since it can inhibit cell proliferation. Interferon-γ, which is released by T cells, is also known to inhibit proliferation and thus to contribute to lesion regression.[367] Thus, the balance between growth factors and growth inhibitors may be crucial to the development of the atheromatous lesions.

Platelets are also a source for growth factors. Platelets release numerous growth factors (PDGF, endothelial growth factor/transforming growth factors [EGF/TGF-α, TGF-β] and possibly others) when aggregation and the release reaction occur. Platelet-mediated smooth muscle cell proliferation appears to occur frequently in humans in two particular circumstances: following coronary bypass and after percutaneous transluminal coronary angioplasty. It is also likely that platelets may interact with the vessel wall at particular anatomic sites where exposure of macrophages and connective tissue may occur due to gross endothelial damage. When this occurs, platelet adhesion and aggregation may aggravate the response and further enhance the development of the atheromatous lesion.

Besides contributing to foam cell formation and progression of atherosclerotic plaques, immune complexes containing modified LDL are very likely involved in plaque rupture. Figure 4–1 illustrates some of these newer concepts of the pathogenesis of atherosclerosis.

Whatever the precise pathologic sequence of events, it is clear that advanced atherosclerotic lesions may result from altered function of endothelium, monocytes and macrophages, platelets, smooth muscle cells, lipids, and lipoproteins. Thrombosis may be the final event that leads to vascular occlusion and ischemic injury. This chapter will review recent ideas about the effect of the diabetic state of these variables. It will update and extend observations made in the previous edition of this text. Hopefully, insights into the mechanisms by which diabetes may alter the function of the vascular wall, its various components, as well as the hemorheologic factors involved in vascular thrombosis will emerge. An understanding of these events should lead to improved preventive and ther-

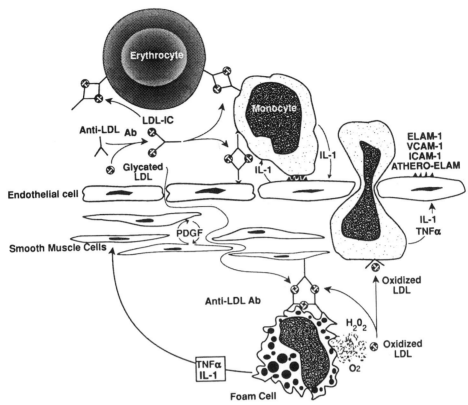

Figure 4–1 ■ New concepts about the pathogenesis of atherosclerosis, with emphasis on the roles of monocyte-derived macrophages, cytokines, immune complexes, glycation and oxidation of LDL, and endothelial adhesion proteins.

apeutic measures for individuals with diabetes.

Endothelium

Vascular endothelial cells participate in a number of important homeostatic and cellular functions such as the coagulation of blood, the activity of leukocytes, the reactivity of platelets, capillary permeability, and regulation of vascular smooth muscle tone. The tonic regulation of vascular smooth muscle cells may be influenced by the endothelium through the release of potent vasorelaxing agents, such as endothelium-derived relaxing factor (EDRF; nitric oxide) and prostacyclin (PGI$_2$), and vasoconstrictors, including thromboxane and endothelin.

Nitric Oxide

The potent vasorelaxation action of EDRF was first demonstrated by Furchgott and Za-

wadzki[132] and the active constituent was later identified to be nitric oxide (NO).[181, 329] NO is synthesized from L-arginine by nitric oxide synthase in endothelial cells and is an antithrombotic product of endothelial cells that has been shown to inhibit the aggregation of platelets,[284, 298] prevent the adhesion of platelets to the endothelium,[298] prolong bleeding time,[169] reduce plasma levels of fibrinogen,[213] and reduce platelet activation.[178] A reduced bioavailability of NO has been suggested to cause thrombotic disorders in humans.[124]

Retinopathy

Studies investigating the role of NO in the development of diabetic complications, or in diabetogenesis per se, have virtually exploded during the last half decade.[73, 90, 286, 334, 409, 410, 430] There is growing evidence from in vitro and in vivo studies that NO-mediated vasodilatation may be impaired in diabetes.[49, 229, 288, 430, 466] Endothelium-derived NO regulates the ocular circulation.[100, 150, 276, 376]

Recently, N^G-monomethyl-L-arginine, an inhibitor of NO-synthase, was administered to ten insulin-dependent diabetic patients. These studies concluded that ocular hemodynamic reactivity to NO-synthase inhibition is reduced in diabetic patients compared to control subjects and further support the hypothesis that NO plays a role in the pathophysiology of diabetic retinopathy.[375]

Neuropathy

A number of metabolic and vascular factors have been implicated in the pathogenesis of diabetic neuropathy and NO may provide the bridge between these two distinct entities.[409, 410] NO-dependent smooth muscle vasodilatation is reduced in type 2 patients with peripheral neuropathy.[337] One metabolic defect that has been implicated in this alteration is disruption of the polyol pathway. NO may be an endogenous regulator of aldose reductase, and consequently the polyol pathway of glucose metabolism.[65] Additional studies in streptozotocin-induced diabetic rats further support the potential for synergistic interactions between the polyol pathway and NO.[51, 62] Elevated glucose levels in diabetic patients may influence vascular tone in cerebral arteries directly via a NO-mediated mechanism.[70] High glucose levels deplete cells of L-arginine, a substrate for NO production and, thus, compromise NO synthesis.[429, 456] It should be noted, however, that not all studies support the role of altered glucose metabolism in NO-mediated changes in vascular tone.[10]

Nephropathy

NO has also been associated with nephropathy in diabetes mellitus.[90] Studies conducted in animal models of diabetes mellitus have utilized the NO precursor L-arginine,[258] N^G-nitro-L-arginine methyl ester (L-NAME)[463] or other inhibitors of NO synthase,[463] or both,[142, 277] to evaluate the role of NO in diabetic nephropathy. One currently favored concept of diabetic nephropathy focuses on increased collagen accumulation in the glomerulus that results from increased collagen synthesis and decreased degradation. Administration of low doses of the NO precursor, arginine, to spontaneously diabetic mice reduced kidney collagen accumulation,[258] supporting a positive role of NO in preventing diabetic nephropathy. Additional studies

in the streptozotocin-induced diabetic rat investigated the contribution of NO to glomerular hyperfiltration in experimental diabetes.[142] These studies concluded that increased NO production may result in a negative contribution to renal hyperfiltration and hyperperfusion in diabetes, but this finding is not universal.[283] Investigations of the contribution of NO to diabetic nephropathy conducted in animal models of diabetes mellitus must be interpreted carefully and cautiously. The results of these studies may be not only species specific, but they may also be specific for the individual type of vascular bed under investigation.[277, 488]

Nitric Oxide and the Pathogenesis of Diabetes

NO has been associated with the pathogenesis of diabetes mellitus type 1.[286] A novel hypothesis has been proposed that implicates NO, a free radical, as the primary effector molecule in cytokine-mediated β-cell dysfunction (decreased insulin secretion) and destruction in vitro.[88, 228, 232, 473] In vivo, each β-cell is located in proximity to at least one capillary islet endothelial cell. Endothelial cells can be activated in vitro to express inducible nitric oxide synthase by the cytokines TNF-γ, interferon-γ, and IL-1β to produce high concentrations of NO.[87] Recent studies using cocultures of rat endothelial cells together with isolated syngeneic islet cells have demonstrated conclusively that activated endothelial cells can function as cytotoxic effector cells and lyse islet cells via nitric oxide.[408] Similar conclusions have resulted from studies employing human islet cells.[348] Studies in vivo have confirmed and extended these in vitro observations.[246, 474] Long-chain fatty acids, like cytokines, upregulate inducible NO synthase and enhance NO generation in islets, and measures to reduce islet triglyceride content may protect against IL-1β–induced NO production and toxicity.[389, 390] NO may also mediate β-cell destruction by an indirect mechanism. Fas is an apoptosis-inducing surface receptor involved in controlling tissue homeostasis and function at multiple sites. NO primes pancreatic β-cells for Fas-mediated destruction in type 1 diabetes.[398] Aminoguanidine, a chemical used extensively in lipoprotein oxidation studies, has been found to be an efficient inhibitor of NO synthase. Studies have been conducted to evaluate its use in preventing insulin-dependent diabetes mellitus but these have met with only marginal success.[398]

Nitric Oxide, Lipoproteins, and Macrovascular Disease

As discussed above, NO plays an important role as the EDRF in the maintenance of normal vascular tone. Recent studies also have demonstrated that a critical relationship between NO and lipoproteins, especially oxidized lipoproteins, exists in the artery wall. The widely accepted "oxidation hypothesis" proposes that lipoprotein oxidation is a causal factor in atherosclerosis.[405] Oxidized lipoproteins can modulate NO activity. Oxidized LDL,[67] oxidized HDL,[67] and oxidized lipoprotein(a)[133] inhibit the biologic activity of NO. Lysophospholipids formed during LDL oxidation seem to be the major mediators of the effect on NO activity.[233] Other studies have demonstrated, paradoxically, that lysophospholipids may increase NO secretion from endothelial cells.[127] Clearly, additional studies are needed to clarify the complex relationship between NO and oxidized lipoproteins in regulating NO availability.

Cells can stimulate LDL oxidation under appropriate conditions.[162, 196, 197] However, if cells are stimulated to express active NO synthase, their oxidative capacity is lost, suggesting that NO, or a product of it, can inhibit lipoprotein oxidation.[195] If conditions in the vascular wall favor the release of superoxide, NO can be converted to peroxynitrite, which is a strong oxidant that can react with proteins.[183] Hypercholesterolemia favors the release of superoxide from arterial tissues. Thus, NO may either protect LDL from oxidation, or it may stimulate the process, depending on the conditions in which it is released. Factors regulating the oxidation of lipoproteins by NO are as complex as those regulating NO availability by oxidized lipoproteins. Additional studies will be required to clarify the relationships between lipoproteins, NO, and atherogenesis in diabetes mellitus.

Prostacyclin

Prostacyclin (PGI$_2$) is synthesized mainly by vascular endothelial cells and is a potent vasodilator and an inhibitor of platelet adhesion and aggregation.[299] Thus, it contributes to the maintenance of vessel wall homeosta-

sis. Previous studies, extensively reviewed in our chapter in the previous edition of this text,[82] have concluded that the synthesis of PGI$_2$ by the vasculature of diabetic patients is reduced.

The decrease in PGI$_2$ concentrations in plasma from diabetic patients may result from a factor originally described in plasma obtained from type 2 diabetic patients.[435] A novel bioactive peptide, prostacyclin stimulating factor (PSF), which produced a stimulation in PGI$_2$ production in vitro, was identified, isolated, and subsequently cloned.[476] High levels of mRNA coding for PSF have been identified in the lungs and kidneys of humans and rats.[322] Subsequent studies identified PSF in human arterial smooth muscle cells by using immunohistochemical techniques.[281] Recently, PSF was localized histochemically in cells from human coronary arteries.[382] Arteries were obtained from four groups of subjects: subjects with or without diabetes, and these two primary groups were subdivided into two additional groups—those with and those without prior myocardial infarction (MI). PSF staining was markedly reduced in coronary artery smooth muscle cells obtained from patients with type 2 diabetes alone or with prior MI, and from nondiabetic subjects with prior MI. The decreased PSF immunostaining in these cells strongly supports the decreased production of PGI$_2$ observed previously in diabetic patients and suggests that the decreased production of PSF may lead to the development of both diabetic macroangiopathy and atherosclerosis. These investigators also determined the effect of high glucose levels on the expression of PSF mRNA and PSF production in cultures of bovine aortic smooth muscle cells. Elevated glucose concentrations in the culture medium decreased both the relative amount of mRNA coding for PSF, and the amount of PSF protein in the cells. Thus, the diabetic milieu, per se, may result in the decreased PSF production and/or secretion observed in diabetic patients. The exact mechanism by which high glucose decreases PSF production remains to be determined, but the effect may be specific for individual arterial beds.[434]

PGI$_2$ is quite active biologically, but it is chemically unstable, and thus its half-life of activity in vivo is quite short. Recently, beraprost sodium, a stable analog of PGI$_2$, has been developed. The development of this stable analog has resulted in a flurry of investigations of its action and efficacy. Beraprost sodium has been shown to be useful for prevention of vascular and neural dysfunction in the retina and peripheral nerves of streptozotocin-induced diabetic rats.[174] In additional studies, beraprost sodium was administered to rats with streptozotocin-induced diabetes, and favorable improvements in diabetic neuropathy,[173, 432] cardiomyopathy,[433] and nephropathy[453] were observed. Studies investigating the effects of this compound in human diabetic patients have begun. Using laser Doppler flowmetry to quantitate changes in skin blood flow, beraprost sodium significantly increased blood flow in both diabetic patients and healthy subjects.[9] The compound has been shown to alleviate autonomic nerve dysfunction in diabetic patients in the absence of severe retinopathy.[320] Beraprost sodium administered to diabetic patients reduced adenosine-stimulated platelet stimulation compared to levels in the same patient before drug administration,[211, 318] suggesting that long-term administration of the drug may favorably influence the occurrence of vascular complications in diabetes mellitus.

Thromboxane

Together with endothelin-1, the endothelium also synthesizes and releases an additional contracting agent, thromboxane A_2 (TXA_2). TXA_2, a product of cyclo-oxygenase, counteracts the vascular effects of NO. TXA_2 and its immediate prostaglandin endoperoxide precursor, prostaglandin H_2, are synthesized by activated platelets as well as by vessel wall tissues. Thus, the increased activation of platelets in diabetes mellitus[75] contributes to both TXA_2 and prostaglandin H_2 in this disease state. Enhanced platelet biosynthesis of TXA_2 has been associated with several cardiovascular risk factors. These include cigarette smoking,[436] diabetes mellitus,[81] type IIa hypercholesterolemia,[94] and homozygous homocystinuria.[101] These studies did not resolve the question, however, of whether persistent platelet activation in these settings results from the consequence of underlying atherosclerotic lesions or whether it reflects the influence of the accompanying metabolic and hemodynamic disturbances on platelet biochemistry and function. To resolve this dilemma, a prospective study of 64 patients was undertaken.[95] Patients with

peripheral arterial disease, as defined by both a history of intermittent claudication localized to the calf with no resting pain and relieved within 10 minutes by rest and by an ankle-arm blood pressure index of less than 0.85 at rest, were selected for having at least one of the following risk factors: cigarette smoking, diabetes mellitus, type IIa hypercholesterolemia, or none of these. TXA_2 biosynthesis was investigated by repeated measurement of the urinary excretion of its major enzymatic metabolite, 11-dehydro-TXA_2, annually for 4 years. Urinary 11-dehydro-TXA_2 levels were significantly higher in patients with peripheral arterial disease than in control subjects. 11-Dehydro-TXA_2 excretion was enhanced only in association with cardiovascular risk factors. Multivariate analysis showed that diabetes, hypercholesterolemia, and hypertension were independently related to 11-dehydro-TXA_2 excretion. During the follow-up period, those patients who experienced major vascular events had significantly higher 11-dehydro-TXA_2 excretion at baseline than did patients who remained event free. These results suggest that the occurrence of large-vessel peripheral arterial disease per se is not a trigger of platelet activation in vivo. Rather, the rate of TXA_2 biosynthesis appears to reflect the influence of coexisting disorders such as diabetes mellitus, hypercholesterolemia, and hypertension on platelet biochemistry and function. Enhanced TXA_2 biosynthesis may represent a common link between these diverse risk factors and the thrombotic complication of peripheral arterial disease.

Endothelin-1

Patients with diabetes often have vascular complications that influence the prognosis of diabetes. Increases in plasma von Willebrand factor and decreases in prostacyclin, plasminogen activator, and fibrinolytic activity, as discussed elsewhere in this chapter, suggest that the endothelium is altered in both humans and in experimental animals with diabetes. Altered endothelial cell metabolism in diabetes may result in altered plasma endothelin concentrations.

Endothelin was first described in 1988,[478, 479] and there has been a virtual explosion of research regarding this potent vasoconstrictor during the ensuing years.[287] Early studies suggested that endothelin-1 concentrations in plasma of type 1 and type 2 diabetic patients were significantly elevated (3.5-fold) compared to levels in nondiabetic subjects[422] and that the elevation could not be explained by secondary changes in blood pressure or renal disease, and did not correlate with the presence of diabetic retinopathy, duration of diabetes, fasting blood glucose, or serum fructosamine in this group of patients. Subsequent studies concluded, however, that elevated plasma endothelin-1 concentrations were associated with retinopathy in diabetic patients[214, 237, 241] and animals,[63, 64, 421] and with nephropathy in diabetic patients[1, 74, 240, 355, 391] and animals.[43, 130, 304, 355] The association between the level of endothelin-1 and the presence of macrovascular disease, however, is controversial.[103, 149] Because of the differences in the conclusions of these studies, subsequent studies have determined plasma endothelin-1 concentrations in well-defined populations of diabetic patients. In a study of 44 type 2 diabetic patients, there were no significant differences in the plasma endothelin-1 concentrations between diabetic patients with and without angiopathy, diabetic patients with different durations of diabetes, and normal subjects.[24]

The plasma concentration of von Willebrand factor has long been considered a marker of endothelial cell damage (see "von Willebrand factor," below). Plasma levels of endothelin-1 and von Willebrand factor were determined in 22 type 2 diabetic patients with and without retinopathy and in normal subjects.[305] Plasma endothelin-1 and von Willebrand factor concentrations were significantly greater in diabetic patients compared to nondiabetic subjects and in diabetic patients with retinopathy compared to patients without retinopathy. Most importantly, there was a strong, positive correlation between the plasma concentration of endothelin-1 and von Willebrand factor. A quantitative immunohistochemical study demonstrated that endothelin-1 and von Willebrand factor immunoreactivity are present in skin biopsies from type 1 diabetic patients and nondiabetic subjects.[344] These studies suggest that endothelin-1 may be a general marker of endothelial cell damage in diabetes mellitus.

Recent studies suggest that simple factors found in the diabetic plasma milieu may influence plasma endothelin-1 concentrations. Circulating endothelin-1 levels increase in lean, type 2 diabetic men,[114, 115] in obese women,[472] and in nondiabetic subjects[339] during euglycemic hyperinsulinemic clamp, suggesting an insulin-endothelin relationship. The role of insulin in the regulation of endothelin production in vivo remains unsettled, however, as an additional study in normal men showed that hyperinsulinemia was not associated with increased plasma endothelin-1 levels.[205, 212] In contrast to studies conducted in vivo, studies in vitro have consistently demonstrated that insulin stimulates the release of endothelin from cultured bovine,[175] porcine,[159] and human[295] endothelial and vascular smooth muscle[7] cells. In addition, the level of glucose in plasma may also contribute to the regulation of plasma endothelin-1 levels.[159, 477]

Disagreement in the conclusions of the studies reported above result, in part, from differences in the diabetic populations studied. However, the type of assay, the difference between commercial assay kits used to quantitate endothelin, and variation between individual laboratories all may influence the determination of endothelin concentration. Until these inconsistencies are resolved, the relationship between diabetes and endothelin will remain uncertain.

Endothelin-1 has been postulated to be a modulator of the erectile dysfunction frequently found in patients with diabetes mellitus.[68, 219] In contrasting studies, concentrations of endothelin-1 were determined in plasma and in the penile cavernous body in ten patients with diabetes mellitus who exhibited erectile dysfunction compared to ten nondiabetic patients.[122] The concentration of endothelin-1 did not differ between the two sites in either population and did not differ between the two populations. Studies in animals that examined the number and density of endothelin-1 receptors in the diabetic penis support the role of endothelin-1 in erectile dysfunction.[369, 417] Clearly, additional studies will be required to resolve the putative role, if any, of endothelin-1 in diabetic erectile dysfunction.

Cell Adhesion Molecules

Endothelial cells elaborate leukocyte-specific adhesion molecules both constitutively and in response to cytokines and other mediators.[54, 98, 431, 481] Circulating monocytes display receptors for these cell adhesion molecules. The adhesion molecules VCAM-1,[93, 327] ICAM-

1,[342, 343] E-selectin,[96, 442] and platelet endothelial cell adhesion molecule (PECAM) (CD31)[96] have been demonstrated to be expressed in atherosclerotic lesions. Recent investigations have documented that soluble forms of these adhesion molecules are present in endothelial cell culture supernatants and human sera.[138, 355, 388] Increased levels of circulating adhesion molecules have been shown in patients suffering from varied disease states including inflammatory diseases, autoimmune disorders, and sepsis.[98] Correlation of the circulating level of adhesion molecules with a disease process would present a useful clinical marker.

L-selectin levels in plasma are increased in patients with recent-onset insulin-dependent diabetes and in subjects at risk for type 1 diabetes.[236] Endothelial cell adhesion molecule-1 (ELAM-1) and VCAM-1 were increased in type 2 diabetic patients; however, ICAM-1 was not.[407] Elevated levels of soluble adhesion molecules may be indicative of the presence of diabetic complications. Diabetic patients with microalbuminuria have increased plasma levels of VCAM-1 compared to diabetic patients without microalbuminuria.[377] There is a positive correlation between the plasma concentration of VCAM-1 and the thickness of the intimal plus medial layer of the carotid arteries in type 2 diabetic patients,[325] suggesting that circulating VCAM-1 levels may be a marker of atherosclerotic lesions in type 2 patients with symptomatic and asymptomatic atherosclerosis. The levels of E-selectin, VCAM-1, and ICAM-1 vary with the extent of retinopathy in type 1 diabetic patients.[321] The concentration of soluble adhesion molecules may be influenced by the level of glycemic control in the diabetic patient.[58, 85, 86, 407] The specificity of the concentrations of the various adhesion molecules with specific diabetic complications remains to be established. Furthermore, the mechanism of the increase in circulating levels of adhesion molecules remains to be determined.

Type 1 diabetes mellitus is caused by a T-cell–mediated destruction of the β-cells in the islets of Langerhans. The interaction between T cells and their antigens or targets is assisted by adhesion molecules on the surfaces of lymphocytes and counterreceptors on antigen-presenting or other cells. As indicated above, soluble forms of these adhesion molecules are increased in diabetic patients. ICAM-1 immunoglobulin fusion proteins have been demonstrated to stop proliferation of T cells in vitro.[362] Similarly, monoclonal antibodies to ICAM-1 reduced the development of hyperglycemia in streptozotocin-induced diabetic rates.[164] The administration of antileukocyte-associated antigen-1 (anti–LFA-1) and anti–ICAM-1 inhibited the development of diabetes in nonobese, diabetic mice.[14, 113, 158] Monoclonal antibodies to the α-4-lymphocyte adhesion molecule administered to nonobese mice also suppressed the development of diabetes in these animals,[482, 483] suggesting that prevention of lymphocyte homing to the pancreatic islets may provide a selective target for prevention/treatment of type 1 diabetics. In order for autoreactive T cells to cause disease, the cells must be able to leave the blood and enter into the target tissue. Thus, the elaboration of adhesion molecules is important in the pathogenesis of insulin-deficient diabetes as well as the vascular disease accompanying this condition.

von Willebrand Factor

The vascular endothelium is intimately involved in the regulation of various metabolic processes (e.g., hemostasis, fibrinolysis, vasomotor control, and vascular permeability), all of which may be relevant to the pathogenesis of diabetic complications. It is very difficult to measure these endothelial functions in vivo; however, it has been suggested that the plasma level of von Willebrand factor (vWF) may serve as a nonspecific marker of endothelial dysfunction.[247] Von Willebrand factor is a complex glycoprotein synthesized by vascular endothelium and megakaryocytes. Diabetic nephropathy and retinopathy are serious complications of diabetes mellitus. Whether dysfunction of the vascular endothelium plays a significant role in the development of these diabetic complications is unknown. To investigate this, recent studies have investigated the relationship between urinary and plasma levels of vWF and diabetic nephropathy and retinopathy.

A prospective, 3-year study of 65 type 1 diabetic patients with and without nephropathy concluded that endothelial dysfunction, as estimated by plasma vWF concentration, precedes and may predict the development of microalbuminuria in type 1 diabetic patients.[402] Similar studies were conducted in patients with non–insulin-dependent diabetes with similar conclusions and further demonstrated that vWF was strongly related to the occurrence of cardiovascular events in these patients.[400] In contrast, a 10-year, prospective study of 209 type 1 patients found no increase in vWF in the patients who developed microalbuminuria.[308] In a larger (2,091 subjects) population-based study of type 1 patients (EURODIAB IDDM Complications Study), there was a statistically significant, positive relationship between the plasma vWF concentration and the albumin excretion rate.[146] The study of Myrup et al.[308] not withstanding, there is an overwhelming consensus that high vWF levels reflect damage to the endothelium or endothelial dysfunction. The measurement of vWF may be considered a noninvasive indicator of the progression of nephropathy in diabetes.

Changes in the level of vWF have also been used to monitor the progress of neuropathy in diabetic patients. In a prospective study of 63 diabetic patients, vWF concentration predicted deteriorating nerve function independently of glycemic control.[338] The Munich General Practitioner Project, a 10-year study of macrovascular and overall mortality in 290 type 2 patients, concluded that vWF was a risk factor for death related to macrovascular disease.[396]

Diabetic retinopathy appears linked to diabetic nephropathy,[333] and, although the nature of this linkage is uncertain, it has been suggested that endothelial dysfunction may represent the pathophysiologic basis for these epidemiologic observations. The relationship between retinal status and plasma vWF concentration was investigated in a cohort of 17 type 1 diabetic patients who were followed prospectively for 42 months.[401] Urinary albumin excretion rates remained normal in all patients throughout the study. Plasma vWF concentrations were similar in patients with or without retinopathy, with the absence of retinopathy defined as less than three microaneurysms observed by an ophthalmologist after dilation of the pupils on two occasions and after fluorescein angiography on a third occasion. Patients in whom plasma vWF concentration increased had higher systolic blood pressure when compared to those in whom the concentration did not increase. This observation suggests that pulse pressure and related shear stress may be determinants of endothelial cell production and secretion of vWF.

Dietary monounsaturated fatty acids have been investigated recently regarding their efficacy in reducing the risk of cardiovascular atherosclerosis, especially as it relates to LDL oxidation. Little information is currently available concerning the effects of monounsaturated fatty acids on vascular endothelial function. One recent study compared the plasma vWF concentration in type 2 diabetic patients before and after consuming a diet high in monounsaturated fatty acids for 3 weeks compared to levels attained while consuming an isocaloric, high-carbohydrate diet. Plasma vWF concentration significantly decreased while consuming the monounsaturated fat diet. In contrast, there were no significant changes observed in plasma vWF concentration when the patients consumed the high-carbohydrate diet.[351, 425] The diet high in monounsaturated fatty acids also reduced blood pressure, suggesting a relationship between vWF, blood pressure, and vascular injury. Of course the beneficial effects of monounsaturated fatty acids in decreasing the susceptibility of LDL to oxidation in vitro and, presumably, in vivo, in view of the many reports of the effects of oxidized LDL on endothelial cell metabolism, cannot be ignored.

Lipids and Lipoproteins

Plasma Levels of Lipoproteins in Diabetes

In poorly controlled diabetic patients, plasma LDL, intermediate-density lipoproteins (IDLs), and VLDL levels are elevated.[205, 235, 253–255, 263, 393] The increase in VLDL levels has been attributed to increased hepatic production or decreased clearance of VLDL[352] and may be more significant in women.[438] High-density lipoprotein levels in diabetes vary with the type of diabetes and, in some groups, with glycemic control. In type 2 diabetic patients, HDL levels are usually low and do not necessarily increase with improved metabolic control.[205, 254, 317] The low HDL levels are thought to be caused by an increased rate of clearance by hepatic triglyceride lipase[210] and may be more significant in men.[437] In type 1 diabetic patients, HDL cholesterol levels are low during poor glycemic control and increase to normal or even above normal concentration when adequate control is achieved.[205, 253, 255, 387] Changes in HDL cholesterol levels with improved glycemic control are less marked in women than in men,[253, 255] and in black women with type 1 diabetes, there seems to be little association between any plasma lipid levels and glycemic control.[387]

Qualitative Lipid Abnormalities

Regardless of the association between lipid levels and atherosclerosis, it is well known that even when lipid levels are similar, the mortality and morbidity from atherosclerotic disease in diabetic patients is higher than in nondiabetic individuals. It is also well known that even normolipemic diabetic subjects are more prone to develop atherosclerosis than nondiabetic individuals. In fact, only a small portion of the increased risk for atherosclerotic disease in diabetes can be explained by consideration of the quantitative abnormalities of plasma lipids.[363] To explain the increased prevalence of atherosclerosis in diabetes, several postulates have been advanced. One of them considers the formation of atherogenic, qualitatively abnormal lipoprotein particles in the diabetic state. Qualitative abnormalities resulting from abnormal lipoprotein glycation, oxidation, and immune-complex formation are considered. Other qualitative abnormalities involve compositional alterations in the particles.

Very Low-Density Lipoprotein

Hypertriglyceridemia is a common lipid abnormality in diabetic patients because of both an increase in VLDL synthesis and an impaired catabolism of triglyceride-rich lipoproteins. Impaired VLDL catabolism, which results from decreased peripheral lipoprotein lipase activity, leads to accumulation of remnant particles and may respond to improved glycemic control.[459] The possible roles of glycation and oxidation in altering VLDL metabolism are considered later on. Compositional abnormalities may also be important. In poorly controlled diabetes, the VLDL remnants are enriched with both free esterified cholesterol and with apolipoprotein B (apo B).[459] The relative proportions of other apoprotein components of triglyceride-rich lipoproteins may also be abnormal. It is known that apolipoprotein E (apo E) facilitates the uptake of triglyceride-rich lipoprotein remnants by the liver, whereas apolipoprotein C-III (apo C-III) inhibits this process.[160, 468] It is also established that apolipoprotein E plays a role in the recognition of VLDL by human macrophages.[454] We found in some groups of diabetic patients that the ratio of apo C/apo E was decreased.[224, 226] This might be expected to enhance hepatic clearance, but any such effect may be overwhelmed by impaired peripheral clearance or unknown effects because of apoprotein glycation or oxidation. Although quantitative abnormalities of VLDL improve with improved glycemic control, at least some of the qualitative abnormalities in this and other lipoproteins persist. In the case of VLDL, these include altered surface rigidity, mediated by an abnormal sphingomyelin/lecithin ratio.[12]

The possibility that abnormal VLDL may contribute to the acceleration of atherosclerosis in diabetes has stimulated a number of studies investigating the metabolism, by cultured cells, of triglyceride-rich lipoproteins isolated from diabetic patients. In the presence of hypertriglyceridemia and diabetes, VLDL and remnant particles are preferentially taken up by murine macrophages, leading to intracellular accumulation of CE or triglycerides.[139, 231] We studied the interaction of VLDL isolated from a group of very well-controlled type 2 diabetic patients with human monocyte macrophages (the precursors of foam cells).[226] No increase in CE synthesis by the cells was observed, though with VLDL from a subset of less well-controlled patients there was a tendency towards increased CE synthesis. VLDL from these type 2 diabetic patients differed from that from controls in having a decreased apo C/apo E ratio, with a tendency toward higher apo E and apo C-I levels, and lower apo C-III levels. In contrast, VLDL from a group of type 1 diabetic patients, who were not so well controlled as the type 2 patients just discussed, did stimulate enhanced CE synthesis in the human macrophages.[224] In this study, VLDL from the diabetic patients was significantly enriched in free cholesterol but otherwise did not differ significantly in composition from that obtained from control patients. Whether the altered VLDL metabolism was the result of altered lipoprotein composition, glycation, or some other undetected alteration (e.g., oxidation) is unknown.

Low-Density Lipoprotein

Qualitative abnormalities of LDL isolated from diabetic patients may alter their cellular recognition. We demonstrated that LDL isolated from type 1 diabetic patients in poor metabolic control was taken up and degraded less efficiently by human fibroblasts than normal LDL or LDL isolated from the same patients after metabolic control was attained.[252] In these studies, in addition to its presumed increased glycation, the LDL isolated from the diabetic patients was triglyceride enriched. Hiramatsu et al.[167] confirmed our studies and demonstrated that triglyceride-enriched LDL isolated from both diabetic and nondiabetic subjects with hypertriglyceridemia was poorly recognized by fibroblasts. Triglyceride enrichment of LDL may therefore, in addition to increased glycation, lead to poor recognition of LDL by the classic LDL receptor in diabetes. Lipoprotein surface lipid composition may also be abnormal even in "normolipemic" type 1 diabetic patients. Bagdade et al.[11] demonstrated altered free cholesterol/lecithin ratios in the combined LDL and VLDL fractions, and these may result in altered lipoprotein metabolism. Similar observations were made in type 2 diabetic patients, and the abnormalities did not respond to improved glycemic control.[12] Recently, the presence of "polydisperse" LDL, that is, LDL particles that are abnormally large and abnormally small, has been described in diabetes.[186] Large quantities of small, dense LDL may enhance the atherogenicity of diabetic plasma and may also simply be higher than expected apolipoprotein B levels for a given LDL cholesterol level.

High-Density Lipoprotein

High-density lipoprotein, because of its role in reverse cholesterol transport, plays an important role in controlling intracellular lipid accumulation.[15, 403] HDL seems to prevent lipid accumulation in macrophages exposed to modified lipoproteins, though the mechanisms for this action are unknown. Recently, the existence of an HDL receptor on human fibroblasts, smooth muscle cells, and aortic endothelial cells has been described; it has been postulated that this receptor may be important in promoting cholesterol efflux.[36, 37]

Although cellular binding of HDL does not seem to be essential for the transport of cholesterol from the cells to HDL, it does appear to facilitate the removal of cholesterol from cells that are overloaded.[36] Whether an identical receptor is present in human macrophages is not known. Foam cells in arterial walls seem, however, to retain large quantities of cholesterol ester even in the presence of a medium containing HDL.[336] The loss of the ability to release accumulated cholesterol ester could be an important difference between foam cells derived from atherosclerotic lesions and those induced in vitro by incubation of abnormal lipoproteins with macrophages.

HDL composition can also be markedly affected by diabetes, and this may impair reverse cholesterol transport. Fielding et al.[116, 117] observed that cholesterol efflux from normal fibroblasts was inhibited when the cells were incubated with plasma from poorly controlled type 2 diabetic patients compared with normal plasma. The defect in cholesterol transport was caused by a spontaneous transfer of free cholesterol from VLDL and LDL to HDL, induced by free cholesterol (and phospholipid) enrichment of both VLDL and LDL present in diabetic plasma. An increase in the triglyceride content of HDL has also been noted in type 2 diabetic patients with hypertriglyceridemia and low levels of HDL cholesterol[12, 27, 28, 437] and cannot be fully corrected by improved glycemic control.[12] The ability of such triglyceride-enriched HDL to remove cholesterol from tissues is not known. Although HDL levels may be normal or increased in type 1 diabetes, the proportion of the less favorable fraction, HDL_3, tends to be increased at the expense of the antiatherogenic HDL_2 fraction.[11] As with VLDL and LDL, the composition of surface lipids in HDL is abnormal in diabetes and, at least in HDL_3, remains so despite improvements in glycemic control.[12]

Alterations in the apoprotein content of HDL in diabetes have been described. Plasma apoprotein A-I levels are increased in diabetic patients,[205] and consequently the HDL cholesterol/apo A-I ratio is reduced,[363] diminishing the particle's antiatherogenic potential. Only some of the abnormalities in apo A-I, apo A-II, and apo E in HDL_2 and HDL_3 could be corrected by improved glycemic control in type 2 diabetes.[12]

Other Factors in Diabetic Plasma That May Alter Lipoprotein Metabolism

Factors other than those inducing alterations of lipoprotein particles may induce a metabolic alteration in cells involved in the arteriosclerotic process. A marked decrease in uptake and intracellular degradation by fibroblasts of LDL isolated from normal and diabetic subjects was observed when the cells were exposed to lipoprotein-deficient serum (LPDS) isolated from poorly controlled diabetic patients.[252] Comparative studies of the composition of LPDS obtained from normal donors and poorly controlled diabetic patient showed an increase in saturated and total unesterified fatty acids, lecithin, apo A-I, and immunoreactive insulin in the LPDS from diabetic patients. Addition of palmitic acid, oleic acid, and lecithin to a pooled LPDS to obtain concentrations similar to those found in the diabetic LPDS led to a decrease in LDL degradation. It is possible that exposure of cells to LPDS obtained from poorly controlled diabetic patients may induce changes in the composition of the fibroblast membrane and alter its fluidity, leading to a decrease in the uptake and degradation of LDL. When diabetic patients are in poor metabolic control, cell membrane changes and modification of LDL composition are likely to act either additively or synergistically to induce an abnormal LDL-cell interaction.

It is therefore apparent that alterations of lipids and lipoproteins are frequently present in diabetes and that insights into mechanisms by which they may accelerate atherosclerosis are emerging. In addition to these critical observations, evidence is accumulating that glycation and glycoxidation of lipoproteins and of other proteins may influence accelerated atherosclerosis in diabetes.

Glycation

In diabetes, increased glycation (nonenzymatic glycosylation) affects any protein exposed to elevated glucose concentrations. Glucose is covalently bound, principally to lysine residues in protein molecules, forming fructose-lysine (FL) (the name of the sugar residue changes because of rearrangement of its double bond in the course of the reaction). Subsequently, especially in long-lived proteins, further ("Maillard") reactions occur, leading to the development of unreactive end-products, many of which are cross-linked, brown, or fluorescent.[239] These end products have been variously termed "browning products," "Maillard reaction products," or "advanced glycation end products" (AGEs). Although numerous, the structures of only a few (e.g., carboxymethyllysine [CML][4] and pentosidine[385]) have been established. Others have been identified in model systems, and by immunologic techniques in vivo: these include pyrraline[161] and "crosslines."[180, 311, 484] Pyrraline has in addition recently been identified in skin collagen in vivo by chromatographic methods[341]: it is a glucose-lysine adduct that may interact with other amino acids in the formation of crosslinks.[309]

Recently, it has been demonstrated that the formation of many of these end products and the accompanying increase in protein fluorescence are mediated by free radical oxidation.[129] Thus, the process involves combined glycation and oxidation reactions, and accordingly the products have been termed "glycoxidation products."[18] In diabetic patients, elevated levels of the initial product of glycation (FL) in skin collagen (a long-lived protein) can be diminished with improved glycemic control, but those of the glycoxidation products, CML and pentosidine, and total protein fluorescence, cannot be reduced.[264] Free radical–mediated oxidation may therefore be regarded as a "fixative" for "glycative" damage: like rust on a car, the oxidative damage cannot be reversed once it has occurred. Theoretically at least, oxidative damage may be enhanced by the process of glycation itself, since glycation may generate free radicals.[471]

More recently, it has been recognized that some so-called advanced glycation end products are actually derived from oxidation of lipids.[128] Oxidation of unsaturated fatty acid side chains (e.g., in triglycerides and cholesteryl esters) yields reactive carbonyl-containing fragments such as glyoxal, 4-hydroxynonenal, and malondialdehyde, any of which may react with and modify amino groups in proteins.[358] Some of the resulting "lipoxidation" products (e.g., CML) are actually identical to "glycoxidation" products derived from carbohydrate sources.[128] This is because the two-carbon intermediate, glyoxal (a reactive dicarbonyl), can be derived by oxidation of either lipids or glucose. Thus, oxidative stress may damage carbohydrates, lipids, or glycated residues already present in proteins, in each case yielding reactive fragments that may further modify proteins. A common feature of these reactions is the generation of carbonyl-containing intermediates, and the term "carbonyl stress" has been used to describe the combined stresses conferred by glucose, lipids, and oxidation. In diabetes, carbonyl stress, and hence protein modification, is increased in several ways: by elevated glucose (always) and hyperlipidemia (often) providing increased substrate, and perhaps by increased oxidative stress, though the latter point is contentious (see below). To make matters more complex, not only proteins may be modified by carbonyl stress but also phospholipids[357] and nucleotides.[346] Furthermore, some reactive carbonyls are generated by nonoxidative processes (e.g., intracellular methylglyoxal formation from glucose-derived triose phosphates is enhanced in diabetes).[426]

The hypothesis that enhanced glycation and carbonyl stress may underlie the development of diabetic complications is attractive. It is consistent with the fact that among individuals as opposed to populations, there is no simple relationship between glycemic control and complication status. Individual variations in antioxidant defenses, perhaps unrelated to the presence of diabetes, may modulate the effects of hyperglycemia, explaining, at least in part, the differing propensities of individuals to develop complications in the face of similar long-term glycemic control. Such variation in antioxidant defenses is likely to be both environmentally (e.g., by diet) and genetically determined. Other related variables influencing complication risk and modulating the effect of hyperglycemia are hyperlipidemia and differences in the composition of fatty acids in lipoproteins and cell membranes: each may influence the flux of lipid-derived oxidation products.

Initial investigations seeking a role for glycation in the development of complications centered around the early stage of the glycation reaction (i.e., FL formation).[215] Later, the roles of glycoxidation, lipoxidation, and AGE-product formation in both atherosclerosis and microvascular complications were investigated.[47, 275, 302, 413] Evidence is presented below that both glycation (particularly in short-lived plasma proteins) and glycoxidation/lipoxidation and carbonyl stress (particularly in long-lived vascular structural proteins)

may be relevant to the accelerated development of atherosclerosis in diabetic patients.

Glycation, Glycoxidation, and Plasma Proteins

Lipoprotein Glycation and its Effect on Lipoprotein Metabolism

It is now established that increased glycation of plasma apolipoproteins occurs from the time of onset of diabetes mellitus,[374] that it correlates with other indices of recent glycemic control,[270] and that for a number of reasons, it may contribute to the acceleration of atherosclerosis. Recognition of glycated LDL (gly-LDL) (whether glycated in vitro[141, 372, 468] or in vivo[252] by the classic LDL receptor) is impaired. This may contribute to hyperlipidemia in poorly controlled diabetes. In contrast, uptake of gly-LDL by human monocytes/macrophages is enhanced, and this may produce foam cells characteristic of the early atherosclerotic plaque.[249, 267]

Recent studies by our group[223] further support the enhanced atherogenicity of glycated LDL in diabetes. Two fractions of *intact* LDL were isolated using boronate affinity chromatography[184] to separate "bound" and "nonbound" (i.e., more and less glycated) LDL. This facilitated concentration of the in vivo–glycated LDL, irrespective of its source (diabetic or control plasma), permitting study of its interactions with cells without the diluting effect of unmodified LDL. The two LDL fractions were isolated from type 1 diabetic patients and nondiabetic control subjects. Glycation of the nonbound fractions was low, and almost identical between control and diabetic samples. Glycation of the bound fractions was increased twofold in control and threefold in diabetic patients, suggesting that, in diabetes, glycation per particle in this fraction is increased.

We studied the metabolic behavior of the fractions using human fibroblasts and monocyte-derived macrophages. Recognition of the nonbound (lightly glycated) LDL by the fibroblasts was normal, whether the particles came from diabetic or nondiabetic subjects. In contrast, recognition of the bound (heavily glycated) LDL by fibroblasts was impaired, again irrespective of the source of the particles, confirming the results of previous studies.[141, 252, 372, 468]

In human monocytes/macrophages, LDL receptor–mediated degradation of both fractions isolated from control subjects was similar, confirming other recent data showing that lesser increases in glycation do not impair LDL recognition by classic receptor in these cells.[226] However, degradation mediated through other receptors was increased twofold for the bound, compared to the nonbound, fraction. LDL receptor–mediated degradation of bound LDL isolated from diabetic patients was mildly impaired, though not to the same extent as was observed in fibroblasts: non–LDL receptor–mediated degradation was significantly increased, as expected. Thus the higher levels of glycation of LDL from diabetic patients both impairs its recognition by the macrophage LDL receptor, and also stimulates its recognition by non–LDL receptor–mediated mechanisms. These data confirm that in humans, while glycated LDL is poorly recognized by the classic LDL receptor on fibroblasts, it is recognized by another high-capacity, low-affinity pathway on monocytes/macrophages, enhancing uptake by these cells and thereby enhancing foam cell formation.

Lipoprotein Glycation and Oxidation

Lipoproteins, containing unsaturated fatty acids in their cores, are particularly vulnerable to oxidative damage, and the role of oxidized lipoproteins in the pathogenesis of atherosclerosis in diabetes has been reviewed.[263, 266] Oxidized LDL is a potent stimulator of foam cell formation, and theoretically at least, glycation may enhance oxidative damage.[306, 471] Despite this, there is little evidence that oxidation of plasma lipoproteins is increased in uncomplicated diabetes, whereas glycation clearly is. Also, no studies have shown a correlation between lipoprotein oxidation and glycemic control in diabetic patients, and there is some evidence that lipid peroxidation, at least in some tissues, is actually reduced in diabetes.[331] A recent study from our group found no evidence of altered susceptibility of plasma LDL from diabetes type 1 patients to (copper ion mediated) in vitro oxidative damage.[191] However, in the vessel wall, glycation enhances covalent binding of lipoproteins to structural proteins, increasing half-life and the likelihood of oxidative damage. Here the processes of glycation, oxidation, and browning may be closely interwoven, causing vicious cycles of vascular injury.

Small AGE peptides in plasma are also thought to modify circulating LDL, increasing its atherogenicity: elevated AGE-modified LDL has been found in patients with macrovascular disease.[413] Retention of these AGE peptides in renal failure may enhance modification of LDL and accelerate atherosclerosis, particularly in diabetes.[118] It has been suggested that AGE peptides of dietary origin may be of significance in promoting atherosclerosis in the presence of renal impairment.[230]

Lipoprotein Glycation and Platelet Function

Increased glycation of LDL may be prothrombotic. In a study by Watanabe et al.,[457] LDL from young diabetes type 1 patients (in good to fair glycemic control) was found to be a more potent stimulator of thromboxane B_2 release and thrombin-induced platelet aggregation than LDL from controls. Glycation of LDL from the diabetic patients was increased, but LDL composition was similar in the two groups. LDL glycated in vitro also caused a marked enhancement in thrombin-, collagen-, and adenosine diphosphate (ADP)-induced platelet aggregation, but this enhancement occurred irrespective of the degree of glycation. Subtle alterations in the composition of platelet membranes, induced by interaction with glycated LDL, were suggested to explain these effects. When bound and unbound (glycated and nonglycated, see above) LDL fractions were isolated from type 1 diabetic patients, platelet aggregation was enhanced to a significantly greater extent by the bound (highly glycated) than by the nonbound (less glycated) fraction.[222]

The effects of modified LDL on the fibrinolytic system have been studied. Jokl et al.[200] showed that LDL isolated from diabetic patients, and also normal LDL oxidized in vitro, failed to stimulate the expected release of the profibrinolytic protein tissue plasminogen activator (t-PA) by cultured human umbilical vein endothelial cells. Furthermore, they found that glycoxidized LDL stimulated the release of plasminogen activator inhibitor 1 (PAI-1), an inhibitor of fibrinolysis, by retinal capillary endothelial cells.[199] All of the above observations suggest that modifications of LDL occurring in diabetes may contribute to an increased tendency towards thrombosis.

Glycation of VLDL, HDL, and Lipoprotein(a)

Increased glycation of VLDL and HDL apoproteins in diabetes has been demonstrated.[92] As with LDL, it is thought to affect cellular interactions, function, and metabolism of the particles. VLDL from normolipemic patients with diabetes types 1 and 2 stimulated increased cholesteryl ester synthesis and accumulation in cultured human monocytes/macrophages,[224, 226] but the effect was less marked than with LDL. Subtle alterations in apoprotein composition are present in VLDL in diabetes,[225] so metabolic differences cannot be attributed to increased glycation with any confidence. Any investigation of the effects of glycation of VLDL is hampered by problems in measuring the separate degrees of modification of its various apoproteins. These degrees of glycation are known to differ because of differing plasma residence times. Use of VLDL glycated in vitro is unsatisfactory because the differential glycation of its several apoproteins occurring in vivo cannot be reproduced. Increased glycation of VLDL apoproteins may therefore have important consequences, but this has not yet been convincingly proven.

Similar problems afflict studies concerning glycation of HDL. Nevertheless, even when mildly glycated in vitro, clearance of HDL from plasma in guinea pigs was accelerated.[468] This effect is opposite to that with glycated LDL, and might partially explain the low plasma levels of HDL in diabetic patients. Duell et al.[105] have demonstrated impaired high-affinity binding of glycated HDL to fibroblasts, with a diminished capacity to remove cholesterol from peripheral cells.[106] Enhanced HDL glycation may therefore contribute to the acceleration of atherosclerotic disease in diabetic patients.

Lipoprotein(a) (Lp[a]) contains an unusual apoprotein, apo(a), which has homology with plasminogen. Lp(a) may contribute to macrovascular disease both by competitively inhibiting the activation of plasminogen, and because it is a cholesterol-rich particle.[192] In the Diabetes Control and Complications Trial (DCCT), Lp(a) levels were lowered with intensive management.[345] There is evidence that plasma Lp(a) is elevated in the presence of diabetic complications.[189, 190] However, a recent study investigating the effects of in vitro glycation of Lp(a) found no evidence that glycation increases its atherogenicity, at least in terms of its interaction with macrophages.[274]

LDL Modification and the Immune System

Modification of LDL may alter its structure sufficiently to provoke an immune response, and the enhanced modifications occurring in diabetes may make this mechanism for vascular disease particularly pertinent in this condition.[21, 91, 248, 250, 261, 469] LDL glycated in vitro in the presence of cyanoborohydride to produce heavily modified particles was found to be strongly immunogenic.[91] However, as detailed above, such LDL contains glucitollysine, a product of "reductive glycation" not present in vivo. FL, which does form in vivo, was not recognized by the antibody raised against reductively glycated LDL. FL itself proved to be a much less potent immunogen, but nevertheless in vitro–glycated LDL, and even control LDL, which always contains some FL, competed for the resulting antibody. The presence of antibodies against "true" glycated LDL had no effect on its rate of clearance from plasma.[470] Nevertheless, the existence of such antibodies even at low levels is probably important, because LDL immune complexes (LDL-ICs) are known to stimulate foam cell formation and to be potently atherogenic.[248, 250, 261] This atherogenicity is thought to be mediated through a variety of interactions between LDL-ICs and vascular cells, in processes involving alterations in cytokine release, coagulant activity, vascular permeability, and vascular growth factors.

In diabetes, the formation of LDL-ICs is likely to be enhanced by the presence of more severely modified ("glycoxidized") lipoproteins sequestered in vessel walls, which may stimulate in situ formation of immune complexes.[42] It is currently unclear whether significant formation of LDL-ICs occurs before, or only after, significant vascular disease has developed. Higher titers of antibodies against oxidized LDL have been demonstrated in patients with diabetes type 2, but it is not clear in this study whether or not the nondiabetic control group had vascular disease.[248] The role of LDL-ICs in the accelerated atherosclerosis of diabetes has been reviewed recently.[248, 250, 261] Recent work from Baynes' group suggests that CML is the dominant epitope for antibody formation against glycoxidation products,[354] and since CML is also a lipoxidation product, it is conceivable that it may also be an important epitope on modified LDL.

Glycation and Antithrombin III Activity

Brownlee et al.[41] have shown that increased glycation of antithrombin III impairs its thrombin-inhibiting activity, and suggested that a resulting defect in inhibition of the coagulation cascade could contribute to the accumulation of fibrin in diabetic tissues. The glycation-induced inhibition of antithrombin III activity is completely reversible by an excess of sodium heparin. Later, Ceriello et al.[59] described an inverse correlation between antithrombin III activity and both HbA_{1c} and plasma glucose, independent of plasma concentrations of antithrombin III. They proposed that antithrombin III activity was probably influenced by glycation. In contrast, in vitro glycation of fibrinogen was not found to influence its function, and therefore does not appear to promote thrombosis.[289]

Glycoxidation/Lipoxidation of Vascular Structural Proteins

Glycation, glycoxidation, and lipoxidation of vascular wall structural proteins may also be important in atherogenesis, not only by altering the characteristics of the vessel wall but also by affecting its interaction with plasma constituents. With age, collagen becomes more insoluble, thermally stable, and resistant to enzymatic attack.[153] Evidence is accumulating that these changes result from glucose-derived crosslinks, formed via the browning or glycoxidation process. These changes are apparently irreversible once they have occurred.[264] This is consistent with the exaggeration of aging changes in collagen in the presence of diabetes. Glycoxidation of vascular connective tissues may contribute to accelerated atherosclerosis in various ways.

Abnormal Vascular Rigidity and Tone

Monnier et al.[302] found an association between skin collagen fluorescence in type 1 diabetic patients and both arterial stiffness (assessed in vivo) and elevated systolic and diastolic blood pressures.[302] Oxlund et al.[326] demonstrated increased aortic stiffness in patients with type 1 diabetes at autopsy, but did not measure glycoxidation products. Decreased elasticity and compliance of arteries and arterioles in diabetes may be due in part to enhanced glucose-mediated crosslinking, and may contribute to the development of hypertension. Arterial stiffness and hypertension combined may result in abnormal shear stresses and endothelial damage, predisposing to injury and atherogenesis. In smaller vessels, similar stresses may contribute to the development of diabetic retinopathy and nephropathy. Collagen glycoxidation products appear to quench the activity of nitric oxide (EDRF) both in vitro and in vivo,[47] potentially causing impairment of endothelium-mediated vasodilation, abnormalities in vascular tone, flow dynamics, perfusion, and blood pressure, all of which may contribute to arterial and arteriolar damage.

Covalent Binding of Plasma Constituents

Endothelial injury causes permeation of plasma constituents into the vessel wall and covalent binding to connective tissue glycoxidation products. Brownlee et al.[40] found increased binding of LDL to glycated versus control collagen, and in diabetic compared to nondiabetic animals, crosslinking of LDL to aortic collagen was increased 2.5-fold. Once trapped in a high-glucose environment in the vessel wall, LDL particles may undergo extensive glycoxidation/lipoxidation, with further increases in atherogenicity. Free radical chain reactions in the trapped LDL may damage its constituent lipids and also neighboring structural proteins and cells. It has been shown, for instance, that products of lipid peroxidation stimulate collagen crosslinking,[166] and recent work from our group suggests they may directly mediate their formation.[359] These interwoven mechanisms may lead to various vicious cycles in the diabetic milieu, leading to damage of arteries and small vessels, and later to in situ formation of lipoprotein-immune complexes, further accelerating foam cell formation. Figure 4–2 illustrates many of these concepts.

The Receptor for Advanced Glycation End Products

Monocytes/macrophages are strongly implicated in the development of atherosclerotic

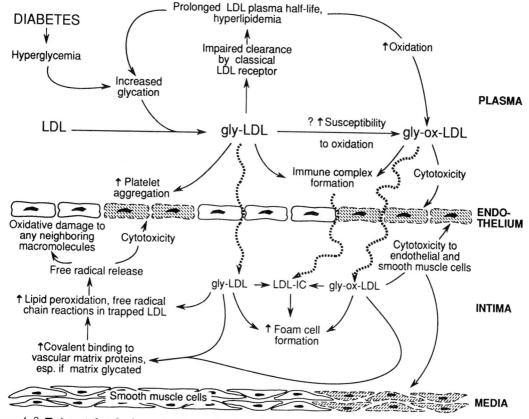

Figure 4–2 ■ A postulated scheme for the mechanism of atherosclerosis in diabetes, which emphasizes the role of glucose in the process.

lesions. AGE products in vessel walls are chemotactic to monocytes, inducing them to migrate through the vascular endothelium.[220] A specific receptor for AGE products on monocytes/macrophages was identified by Vlassara et al. in 1986.[449] Macrophages expressing this receptor may phagocytose proteins and even entire cells expressing glycoxidation products.[446] Consistent with this, AGE products in vessel walls have been localized immunologically to intracellular locations in macrophages, smooth muscle cells, and in foam cells derived from these cells. Two receptors for AGE products (RAGE) on endothelial cells have been characterized in detail, and one was cloned in 1992. Many of the consequences of increased AGE product formation in diabetes may be mediated through various AGE receptors. AGE product/receptor interactions in macrophages may induce release of cytokines, TNF-α and IL-1[448]: these may mediate growth and remodeling and accelerate the atherosclerotic process. They may also induce production of

prothrombotic tissue factor (TF) by macrophages, an action that can be inhibited by antioxidants.[179] In T lymphocytes, AGE product/receptor interactions induce synthesis of interferon-γ, which can enhance immune-mediated mechanisms of tissue injury.[182] In rat renal mesangial cells, AGE products stimulate increased collagen production, an effect probably mediated by TGF-α and by PDGF.[427] Receptor-mediated actions of AGE products have also been implicated in the development of diabetic retinopathy.[66, 412, 475] Infusion of AGE products in rabbits produced a variety of vascular changes. In endothelial cells, these included increased expression of VCAM-1 and ICAM-1, effects seen predominantly in areas affected by atheroma.[450] The induction of VCAM-1 is dependent on AGE product/receptor interactions, and VCAM-1 antigen is elevated in diabetic plasma.[171] Further supporting the significance of these interactions, it has been shown that blockade of RAGE can inhibit AGE product–induced impairment of endothelial barrier function and consequent hyperpermeability. Inhibition of AGE product formation using antioxidants has a similar effect.[458]

Renal Impairment

Accumulation of glycoxidation products in skin collagen is associated with renal impairment in diabetes,[275, 285, 302, 386] suggesting a possible causative role for these products in diabetic nephropathy. Supporting this, infusion of AGE product–modified albumin in rodents induces renal changes (glomerular sclerosis, albuminuria) similar to those occurring in diabetic renal disease.[447] It also induces upregulation of glomerular mRNA for laminin and collagen,[480] proteins that accumulate in glomerulosclerosis. Diabetic nephropathy, and also other forms of renal disease, are characterized by a considerable increase in the expression of RAGE in various renal cell types, many of which do not normally express this receptor.[2] In addition to the kidney-specific effects, if a generalized collagen abnormality is a common underlying mechanism for both microalbuminuria and atheroma, this could partly explain the observation that microalbuminuria is a risk factor for macrovascular disease. The hypertension and lipid abnormalities characteristic of renal impairment may contribute further to the development of atherosclerosis.

Glycoxidation of Collagen and Diabetic Complications: Alternative Hypotheses

The studies discussed demonstrate *associations* between the levels of FL and glycoxidation products in collagen and the presence or severity of several diabetic complications. The data are compatible with, but do not prove, the hypothesis that these products may contribute to complications, including accelerated macrovascular disease. FL, often regarded as a relatively harmless precursor of damaging glycoxidation products, may contribute indirectly, or increased FL and the presence of complications may be related only insofar as both arise from a common origin: either prolonged hyperglycemia itself, or other associated metabolic derangements. In contrast, glycoxidation and lipoxidation products significantly alter the properties of collagen, and so a direct causative role in the development of complications is easier to envisage, yet the case is not proven. Glycoxidation products may simply reflect long-term glycoxidative/lipoxidative stresses: these stresses may cause disease primarily by cumulative effects on substrates other than collagen. Alternatively, complications may arise in association with hyperglycemia but via mechanisms not related to glycoxidation. In this case glycoxidation products in collagen would represent only a record of past events.

Is it Possible to Inhibit the Glycation and Browning of Vascular Structural Proteins?

If carbonyl stress is indeed a significant risk factor in the development of macro- and microvascular complications of diabetes, then reducing this stress would clearly be desirable: it would mitigate recurrent damage to short-lived species, like LDL, and cumulative damage to long-lived species, such as collagen. Possible means to inhibit the glucose-mediated, lipid-mediated, and "oxidative" components of carbonyl stress may be considered separately.

Reducing Glucose-Mediated Stress

Most obviously, glycemic control should be optimized, minimizing FL formation and reducing concentrations of glucose vulnerable to autoxidation. As well as decreasing formation of FL, existing FL levels may be reduced: improved glycemic control has been shown to reduce FL content within a few months even in long-lived proteins.[264] Decreased FL should decrease subsequent formation of glycoxidation products. Optimal glycemic control is an established goal in the management of diabetic patients.

Reducing Lipid-Mediated Stress

Lipoxidative modification of proteins and other molecules may be minimized by decreasing substrate available for oxidative damage, and making it more resistant to oxidation. Thus the plasma lipid profile should be optimized by dietary and pharmacologic means, and by dietary measures to minimize oxidizability of the fatty acid constituents of lipoproteins and cell membranes. Reaven et al. have shown that if monounsaturated fats are substituted for dietary polyunsaturated or saturated fats, LDL is less susceptible to oxidative damage.[353]

Reducing Oxidative Stress

There is little direct evidence concerning the efficacy of any treatment aimed to reduce oxidative damage to proteins and lipids in diabetes. Vitamin C (ascorbate) is thought to be the most important aqueous antioxidant.[125] Plasma vitamin C, and platelet vitamin E, the most important fat-soluble free radical scavenger, tend to be abnormally low in diabetic patients.[193, 209] Dietary supplements of these vitamins may represent a cheap, low-risk intervention. However, under some circumstances, vitamin C may act as a prooxidant,[485] and there are insufficient grounds to recommend its routine use in diabetic patients. In the case of vitamin E (α-tocopherol), there is significant circumstantial but no direct evidence in favor of its use in diabetic patients to reduce oxidative stress and perhaps to slow atherogenesis and the development of microvascular complications. Unfortunately, these same advantages, by leading to widespread use, are likely to impede studies to determine the efficacy of such treatments. Under some circumstances, vitamin E may have pro-oxidant effects.[34] Probucol may be effective in reducing lipid peroxidation,[332] and may have a protective effect in the vessel wall[53, 221, 234]; however, it seems to have few advantages over vitamin E. Butylated hydroxytoluene may also have similar effects[29, 126]; coenzyme Q (ubiquinone), which detoxifies the tocopheroxyl radical (the product of vitamin E oxidation), can also inhibit LDL oxidation. While it may have a role to play, this has not been clearly defined.[424] Other agents inhibiting the toxic consequences of lipid peroxidation, or inhibiting oxidation itself, may be developed as a result of improved understanding of the chemistry involved.[71]

Scavenging Reactive Carbonyls

Aminoguanidine is a scavenger of reactive carbonyl groups, especially of dicarbonyl compounds (e.g., glyoxal formed by oxidative decomposition of fructose-lysine, Schiff base, or fatty acids, or 3-deoxyglucosone formed by decomposition of fructose-lysine), species that may mediate advanced carbonyl reactions. It can prevent the formation of glycoxi-dation and lipoxidation products, and interrupt vicious cycles of oxidative damage. In vitro it may inhibit both collagen crosslinking[39] and lipid peroxidation.[44, 46] In cell culture, recent studies by our group have shown that at concentrations as low as 1 μmol/L, it can significantly inhibit the cytotoxicity that develops in LDL when exposed to glycoxidative stress.[262] The same low concentrations can also inhibit the toxicity of simulated hyperglycemia (25 mmol/L glucose) towards retinal vascular cells (unpublished observations). The results suggest that the observed toxicities may be mediated by oxidation products of LDL and glucose, respectively, and that these products are present at very low concentrations. In vivo, aminoguanidine can inhibit the development[154, 156] and progression[155] of diabetic retinopathy in streptozotocin-diabetic rats, an can also inhibit the development of diabetic nephropathy[110, 394] and neuropathy.[51, 217] Studies are now underway to assess the efficacy of aminoguanidine in diabetic nephropathy in humans, and other similar agents with much greater potency are currently being developed.[26] Another class of experimental agents, the "leumedins" (N-[fluorenyl-9-methoxycarbonyl] amino acids[48]) may also be effective in inhibiting LDL modification.[314]

Possibilities for the Direct Removal of AGE Products from Serum or Dialysis Fluid

AGE products in serum are not effectively removed during hemodialysis. Recent increases in knowledge concerning AGE product receptor recognition have implicated lysozyme, a naturally occurring protein to which AGE products may bind.[244] This has led to experiments using matrix-bound lysozyme as a means of clearing AGE products from serum and dialysis fluid, and initial results are encouraging.[297] Finally, compounds that may cleave existing AGE product–mediated crosslinks in proteins are under investigation.[443]

Eventually, a combination of the measures outlined above may delay the onset and slow the progression of both macro- and microvascular complications of diabetes. They may even be useful in other conditions in the non-diabetic population, including not just atherosclerosis,[404] but also Alzheimer's and other neurodegenerative diseases,[392] other age-related conditions, and even the aging process itself.

Thrombus Formation

Mechanisms

Thrombi may form in atherosclerotic vessels, leading to tissue ischemia, death, or both. Platelets may adhere at areas of endothelial damage or destruction, leading to a local accumulation of platelets at sites of vascular injury. Platelet aggregation occurs with release of intraplatelet materials, and a platelet mass may form that can impede flow and lead to platelet microemboli. This process may be reversible, and its activity and extent depends on the type, size, and configuration of the involved vessels, as well as the local blood flow.

Platelet-fibrin masses are then formed at the next step. It is likely that local fibrinolytic activity is a major determinant of whether the platelet-fibrin masses will break up or will organize further. As thrombi grow, conditions favorable for intravascular coagulation may proceed. Platelets may degenerate, leading to fibrinous transformation. The organizing thrombus may be infiltrated by leukocytes, macrophages, and smooth muscle cells, and thrombin may be incorporated into the vascular wall, contributing to intimal plaque formation.[33]

Recognition of this process has stimulated research into platelet function, the coagulation system, and fibrinolysis in individuals with diabetes mellitus, where thrombosis in large and small vessels often accompanies accelerated atherosclerosis. Atherosclerosis and thrombus formation is a dynamic process that can be reversible and may occur at multiple sites, and it has been difficult to describe the exact sequence of events that may occur in diabetes. Nevertheless, there is evidence that various aspects of platelet function, coagulation, and fibrinolysis are affected by diabetes and that such alterations may help explain thrombotic events in some individuals with diabetes. Furthermore, there is evidence that certain aspects of this process are under metabolic control and that insulin may play a key role in that regulation. For these reasons, a review of platelet function, coagulation, and fibrinolytic activity in diabetes is provided.

Platelets

Many alterations in platelet function are seen in diabetes mellitus.[80, 83, 84] Some of these are summarized in Table 4–1. Studies have shown that platelets from diabetic subjects are more sensitive in vitro to platelet-aggregating agents and that the synthesis of thromboxane is increased. These findings have been reported in type 1 diabetic individuals shortly after the onset of the disease, as well as in diabetic animals, suggesting that altered platelet function may be the consequences of metabolic changes in the diabetic state rather than resulting from the presence of vascular disease. Insulin therapy will decrease platelet thromboxane release in type 1 diabetes, supporting this concept.

On the other hand, there is ample evidence that platelets may be hypersensitive to aggregating agents and may release increased amounts of thromboxane in nondiabetic and diabetic individuals with vascular disease. These observations suggest that platelet damage may occur as a result of diabetic vascular disease, as well as possibly contributing to the development of that process.

Dispersion of platelet aggregates, due to the lysis of the fibrin meshwork, may be the limiting process of thrombus growth when chronic platelet activation and aggregation is present, as in many cases of diabetes. Recently, substantial evidence has accumulated indicating the importance of intraplate-

Table 4–1 ■ ALTERATIONS OF PLATELET FUNCTION IN DIABETES

IN VITRO	IN VIVO
↑ Adhesiveness (vWF?)	↑ Turnover
↑ Aggregability	↓ Survival
↑ Thromboxane release	↑ β-Thromboglobulin
Platelet-plasma interactions	↑ Plasma factor 4
vWF	↑ Platelet-derived growth factor
Fibrinogen	↑ Circulating platelet aggregates
Immune complexes	↑ Platelet-derived urinary TXB$_2$
Glycated LDL	Vessel wall interaction
↑ LDL oxidation	
↓ Phosphoinositide turnover	
↓ Membrane fluidity	

vWF, von Willebrand factor; LDL, low-density lipoprotein; TXB$_2$ thromboxane B$_2$.

let proteins in platelet disaggregation. One of the proteins, PAI-1, is released from activated platelets and bound within the thrombus. The amount of the thrombus-bound PAI-1 determines the resistance to thrombolysis by the activated fibrinolytic system.[416] Recent studies found enhanced platelet PAI-1 expression and release in patients with type 2 diabetes.[198, 201] The platelet PAI-1 concentration was related to plasma insulin concentration. It has been suggested that insulin may modulate intraplatelet protein expression during megakaryocytopoiesis.

Coagulation

Activation of the coagulation system leads to fibrin formation by thrombin. Experimental and clinical data suggest that primary fibrin deposits and mural thrombi lead to the initial endothelial lesion and may contribute to the development of macro- and microvascular disease.[257] In diabetes, there may be a general activation of blood coagulation, and fibrin lesions can be found in several organs of diabetic subjects. Most of the individual factors of both the intrinsic and the extrinsic coagulation pathway, as well as the inhibitors of coagulation, may be altered in diabetes. There are multiple data to support a pathogenetic rather than consequential role of hypercoagulation in the development of vascular disease in diabetes.

Fibrinogen

Attention has been directed at fibrinogen levels and dynamics in diabetes for a variety of reasons. It is now clear that the plasma level of fibrinogen is an independent risk factor for thrombotic events in population-based studies.[208, 291, 465] There have been many studies of fibrinogen levels and dynamics in diabetes mellitus. Generally, plasma fibrinogen levels are found to be elevated in diabetic individuals, particularly in those with previous hyperglycemia.[121, 131, 203, 204, 324] Insulin deficiency results in an increase in fibrinogen synthesis in type 1 diabetes, and an insulin infusion will decrease fibrinogen synthetic rate.[99] Fibrinogen survival has been reported to be decreased in diabetes, and this abnormality is quickly reversed when euglycemia is achieved with insulin.[203, 204] Decreased fibrinogen survival in diabetes is also reversed

by heparin, suggesting that intravascular fibrin formation may be taking place.[204] Fibrinogen is glycated in diabetic subjects, and crosslinking of the α-chains of fibrinogen is impaired.[260] Exercise conditioning will lower plasma fibrinogen levels in type 2 diabetic individuals.[172]

These findings suggest that there may be increased fibrin formation in vivo in individuals with diabetes. Because fibrinogen to fibrin formation may be catalyzed by thrombin, investigations have centered on the regulation of thrombin activity in diabetes and on an in vivo index of thrombin activity, fibrinopeptide A.[202]

Fibrinopeptide A

General activation of blood coagulation in vivo may be assessed by analyzing the final steps of the coagulation cascade (e.g., by fibrinopeptide A [FPA]). FPA is cleaved from the α-chain of fibrinogen by the action of thrombin. This forms the first step in the conversion of fibrinogen to fibrin. FPA levels tend to be elevated in diabetes, especially when control is poor or vascular problems exist.[365] Furthermore, recent studies have indicated that elevated FPA levels may be seen in diabetic individuals before vascular complications are present.[121] A relation between plasma and urinary FPA and hyperglycemia in diabetes has been reported.[202]

Prothrombin Fragment F1+2

Recently, prothrombin activation fragment F1+2 has been identified as a sensitive marker of coagulation activation in vivo.[278] Fragment F1+2 is released from prothrombin when it is converted to thrombin by activated factor X. In type 1 diabetic patients, F1+2 levels have been found lower as compared to the controls.[242] In the same study, microalbuminuria, believed to be a manifestation of generalized angiopathy, was significantly correlated to F1+2 levels.

Antithrombin III

The most important inhibitor of the coagulation system is antithrombin III (AT III). AT III activity may be modulated by glucose both in vitro and in vivo. Hyperglycemia will cause a decrease in AT III activity in nondiabetic subjects, and activity returns to normal after a glucose infusion is stopped.[57] Depressed levels of AT III activity are found in adult type 1 diabetic subjects, and infusion of insulin to produce normoglycemia will return AT III activity to normal.[61] There is an inverse correlation between AT III levels and plasma glucose, as well as the labile component of hemoglobin A_1 in adults with type 1 diabetes.[57]

Activated Protein C

Activated protein C is a vitamin K–dependent plasma protein that is another potent anticoagulant. It acts at the level of factor V and VIII in the intrinsic coagulation scheme. Several investigators have reported decreased protein C antigen and activity levels in type 1 diabetes,[61, 452] and such changes could theoretically promote coagulation. Glucose-induced hyperglycemia will lead to a fall in protein C levels and activity in normal and diabetic individuals. Depressed plasma levels and activity of protein C will rise with insulin-induced normoglycemia in type 1 diabetes.[61]

Fibrinolytic System

The fibrinolytic system controls the patency of the vascular tree by plasmin degradation of fibrin deposits and of thrombi. The generation and activities of plasmin are regulated mainly by the production of two critical proteins by the vascular endothelium, t-PA and the main inhibitor of t-PA, PAI-1. t-PA converts inactive plasminogen into plasmin at the site of fibrin formation. One critical regulator of thrombosis is likely to be the capacity for endogenous fibrinolysis.[419] One hypothesis is that small amounts of fibrin are constantly deposited on the endothelium and that these fibrin deposits are continually dissolved, resulting in a dynamic balance between coagulation and fibrinolysis.

Impaired fibrinolytic activity is characterized by low t-PA activity and high PAI-1 antigen and activity. Studies in man have shown that t-PA antigen concentration (associated with high PAI-1 and low basal or stimulated t-PA activity) may increase as a consequence of preclinical atherosclerosis and may be a

marker of future coronary and cerebrovascular events.[360, 361] Impaired fibrinolysis is an independent risk factor for MI in both nondiabetic and diabetic subjects.[135, 177] Low fibrinolytic activity is a leading determinant of ischemic heart disease in young men.[290] t-PA antigen has been found to have a higher predictive value of mortality in patients with established coronary disease than cholesterol, triglycerides, fibrinogen, blood pressure, diabetes, or smoking.[188]

Conditions favoring enhanced thrombus formation have been frequently documented in type 2 diabetes including decreased t-PA activity, higher basal t-PA antigen, insufficient t-PA release from endothelium under stress, and excess plasma PAI-1 antigen and activity.[77, 201] It has been suggested that normal t-PA and PAI-1 activity levels may be selective factors that influence the survival of diabetic patients.[6] Most studies have been conducted in patients with type 2 diabetes. Decreased fibrinolytic function in type 2 diabetes correlates with the presence and severity of angiopathies.[135, 145] Lower exercise-induced levels of plasma t-PA have been found in early diabetic nephropathy.[194] In patients with type 1 diabetes, higher t-PA antigen levels were associated with the presence of peripheral vascular disease,[418] and increased PAI-1 activity was seen in the presence of microalbuminuria.[148] There appears to be hormonal regulation of PAI-1 gene expression and protein synthesis. Insulin has been shown to induce PAI-1 mRNA expression in hepatocytes, leading to an increased release of this protein by liver cells.[5, 144] Some evidence for this effect of insulin has been shown in in vivo studies[206] but not in others.[440] There is a correlation between PAI-1 and plasma insulin levels in obese individuals.[439, 441] Studies have shown a correlation between PAI-1 and plasma triglyceride levels.[32, 292] Longitudinal studies are needed on the relationships of obesity, plasma glucose, insulin, triglycerides, and PAI-1 in the syndrome of centripetal obesity and insulin resistance.

In vitro studies with cultured endothelial cells have provided some insights into regulation of t-PA and PAI-1 release by lipoproteins. Very low-density lipoproteins harvested from normal individuals will cause release of t-PA and PAI-1 from cultured endothelial cells, whereas VLDLs from hypertriglyceridemic individuals will not.[32] Similar studies showed that endothelial production of PAI-1 is increased by incubation in vitro with VLDL obtained from hyperglycemic patients.[411] Stimulation of endothelial release of t-PA and PAI-1 with desmopressin acetate in type 2 diabetic subjects with hypertriglyceridemia causes a decreased plasma t-PA activity and an elevated PAI-1 response when compared with normal controls.[38] These studies provide some in vivo evidence to support the in vitro reports of increased PAI-1 activity in type 2 diabetes.

The source of physiologically active PAI-1 in plasma is probably the endothelium. Elevated levels may reflect endothelial damage. On the other hand, liver cells and abdominal adipose tissue synthesize and release PAI-1,[5, 144] and studies of PAI-1 in plasma, serum, and platelets have shown that the concentration of PAI-1 antigen in platelets is very high and that platelets account for 93% of PAI-1 antigen in whole blood.[31] Platelet PAI-1 exists primarily in an inactive form.

Discussion

What does all of this mean? Is diabetes characterized by a hypercoagulable state? If so, could this underlie the predisposition toward thrombosis often seen in diabetes? What is the effect of therapy? Can we prevent macrovascular thrombosis?

Clearly, the final answers to all of these questions are not apparent. There is still a lot of work to do. Generalization is dangerous for a number of reasons. First, in clinical studies it is important to differentiate data obtained from type 1 and type 2 diabetic subjects in view of the major differences in pathophysiology between these two syndromes. Second, there is great heterogeneity within type 1 diabetic populations. In some cases, studies are done in prepubertal children; in others, adults of short duration; in others, type 1 diabetic individuals with nephropathy, retinopathy, neuropathy, or macrovascular disease. Third, there is even greater heterogeneity within type 2 diabetic populations. Thus, individuals may be obese or nonobese; have low, normal, or elevated plasma insulin or lipid levels; be free from microvascular of macrovascular disease; be treated with diet, oral agents, or insulin; or have clinically apparent or inapparent microvascular or macrovascular disease. Furthermore, the majority of studies are cross-sectional in nature, and this may give misleading data because of patient selection. Longitudinal data are limited and extremely difficult and costly to pursue.

Nevertheless, from the studies cited in this review and in other sources,[79, 81–84, 324] some trends are apparent. First, even when an abnormal mean value for platelet function or index of coagulation is found and the subjects are well defined (e.g., type 1 diabetes free from clinical vascular disease), there are many patients with normal activity or levels no matter what parameter is measured. On the other hand, there is a certain consistency in reported results in uncomplicated type 1 diabetic subjects with hyperglycemia, and there is increasing evidence that in these individuals, insulin therapy may return altered values to or toward normal. By probing results from a number of different studies in different type 1 diabetic populations, some interesting findings emerge. In all cases, when studied in vivo, insulin administration to hyperglycemic type 1 diabetic subjects has been found to produce changes in platelet function, the intrinsic coagulation system, and in fibrinogen dynamics that could reduce the tendency toward intravascular thrombosis. These findings provide a theoretical basis for intensive insulin therapy in type 1 diabetic subjects. On the other hand, studies in type 2 diabetes are limited, and a role of hyperinsulinism in increasing PAI-1 activity may be postulated. It must be recognized that it will require properly designed, multicenter collaborative trials to definitely answer the question as to whether intensive insulin therapy will alter thrombotic events in type 1 or type 2 diabetic individuals.

In light of current knowledge, however, it is generally accepted that one reasonable approach to the prevention of thrombotic events is the use of agents such as aspirin, which irreversibly acetylates platelet cyclooxygenase and thereby inhibits platelet thromboxane production. Presently, there are more than 200 studies with antiplatelet agents in nondiabetic and in diabetic individuals, in which major vascular events such as strokes, MIs, and vascular death have been monitored before and after antiplatelet therapy. Results have been compared with those obtained in individuals receiving placebo therapy. There is general agreement, as indicated by meta-analyses of published data, that antiplatelet therapy is a safe and effective way to prevent future cardiovascular events in diabetic or nondiabetic individuals who have had one vascular event.[8] Thus, pooled data suggest that vascular morbidity can be lowered about 25%, nonfatal MIs about 30%, and vascular mortality approximately 15% after antiplatelet therapy when it is used as a secondary prevention strategy.[8] It is generally believed that the benefits of antiplatelet therapy outweigh the risks. There is no evidence that aspirin therapy will accentuate diabetic retinopathy or vitreous hemorrhage. Although use of aspirin as a primary prevention strategy is still somewhat controversial, studies in nondiabetic individuals suggest that this may be effective in reducing MI incidence.[399] The American Diabetes Association has published a technical review[76] and a position statement which favor the use of low-dose (81 to 325 mg) enteric-coated aspirin as a primary prevention strategy in high-risk diabetic individuals.[76, 78]

Summary

Is it presumptuous to attempt to define the pathogenesis of atherosclerosis in diabetes mellitus? One could adopt this view because the pathogenesis in nondiabetic individuals is a subject of active research and therefore is open to changing views. Extrapolation from these current postulates to a disease state as complicated and heterogeneous as diabetes mellitus could therefore be dangerous, inaccurate, and misleading. In addition, investigators are limited by a variety of factors in their search to delineate mechanisms involved in the atherosclerotic process in humans. Access to normal arterial tissue for in vitro studies has been limited, and noninvasive techniques for assessing the degree and extent of early lesions of atherosclerosis in vivo are limited. Longitudinal studies are compromised by these limitations in technique and by the slow progression of the process. These factors have led investigators to rely on correlative relationships and studies using cell systems that may not be directly transferable to the atherosclerotic process in humans. The issue is further complicated by the fact that animal models are limited; much of the work has been done in animal species in which atherosclerosis is a difficult lesion to produce. Clinical trials in diabetes that could provide useful indirect information have been sparse and usually have been secondary prevention trials in patients with very advanced vascular disease. Of course, primary prevention of atherosclerosis is of greatest importance.

Nevertheless, the situation is improving. Advances in surgical technique in humans, with close coordination of investigators from various disciplines, have led to the availability of fresh human tissue from coronary bypass patients and other individuals who undergo major surgery. Tissue culture techniques allow investigators to directly study the metabolism and function for critical components of the human arterial tree and to objectively manipulate variables involved in the atherosclerotic process. Noninvasive techniques for assessing the vascular system in humans are undergoing refinement and are becoming more available to clinical investigators. Techniques of molecular biology are opening up new approaches to the genetic influences on atherosclerosis. An explosion of biochemical and physiologic information about prostanoids and their derivatives and about lipids, lipoproteins, and apolipoproteins has occurred in recent years. Improved animal models of atherosclerosis and diabetes mellitus exist, and work using animals such as monkeys and pigs is beginning to appear. Clinical trials are moving in the direction of primary rather than secondary prevention trials and involve lipids, lipoproteins, platelets, and prostanoids, which are postulated to be operative in atherosclerosis associated with diabetes mellitus.

An explosion of information on endothelial function, immune complexes, cytokines, adhesion proteins, glycation, and glycoxidation has occurred and has led to newer concepts. Alterations in the coagulation and fibrinolytic systems may predispose diabetic subjects to vascular thrombosis. As work in these very active areas of research continues, it is likely that improved methods of preventing or forestalling the development of accelerated macrovascular disease in diabetes will emerge.

REFERENCES

1. Abassi AZ, et al: Urinary endothelin: A possible marker of renal damage. Am J Hypertens 6: 1046, 1993.
2. Abel M, et al: Expression of receptors for advanced glycosylated end-products in renal disease. Nephrol Dial Transplant 10:1662–1667, 1995.
3. Ahmed MU, et al: Oxidative degradation of glucose adducts to protein. Formation of 3-(N epsilon-lysino)-lactic acid from model compounds and gly-

cosylated proteins. J Biol Chem 263:8816–8821, 1988.

4. Ahmed MU, Thorpe SR, Baynes JW: Identification of carboxymethyllysine as a degradation product of fructose-lysine in glycosylated protein. J Biol Chem 261:4889–4994, 1986.

5. Alessi MC, et al: Insulin stimulates the synthesis of plasminogen activator inhibitor 1 by hepatocellular cell line Hep G2. Thromb Haemost 60: 491–494, 1988.

6. Almer LO: Fibrinolytic disorders in diabetes mellitus. Diab Metab 14:519–522, 1988.

7. Anfossi G, Cavalot F, Massucco P, et al: Insulin influences immunoreactive endothelin release by human vascular smooth muscle cells. Metabolism 42:1081, 1993.

8. Antiplatelet Trialists' Collaboration: Secondary prevention of vascular disease by prolonged antiplatelet treatment. BMJ 296:320–331, 1988.

9. Aso Y, Inukai T, Takemura Y: Evaluation of microangiopathy of the skin in patients with non-insulin-dependent diabetes mellitus by laser Doppler flowmetry: Microvasodilatory responses to beraprost sodium. Diab Res Clin Pract 36:19, 1997.

10. Avogaro A, et al: Forearm nitric oxide balance, vascular relaxation, and glucose metabolism in NIDDM patients. Diabetes 46:1040, 1997.

11. Bagdade JD, Subbaiah PV: Whole-plasma and high-density lipoprotein subfraction surface lipid composition in IDDM men. Diabetes 38:1226–1230, 1989.

12. Bagdade JD, et al: Persistent abnormalities in lipoprotein composition in noninsulin-dependent diabetes after intensive insulin therapy. Arteriosclerosis 10:232–239, 1990.

13. Bailey AJ, Kent MJC: Non-enzymatic glycosylation of fibrous and basement membrane collagens. In Baynes JW, Monnier VM (eds): The Maillard Reaction in Aging, Diabetes and Nutrition. New York: Alan R Liss, Inc, 1989, pp 109–122.

14. Baron JL, et al: The pathogenesis of adoptive murine autoimmune diabetes requires an interaction between alpha 4-integrins and vascular cell adhesion molecule-1. J Clin Invest 93:1700, 1994.

15. Bates SR, Rothblatt GH: Regulation of cellular sterol flux and synthesis by human serum lipoproteins. Biochim Biophys Acta 360:38, 1974.

16. Baynes JW, et al: Accumulation of Maillard reaction products in skin collagen in diabetes and aging. Diabetologia 34(Suppl 2):A7, 1991.

17. Baynes JW, Monnier VM (eds): The Maillard Reaction in Aging, Diabetes and Nutrition. New York: Alan R Liss, Inc, 1989.

18. Baynes JW: Role of oxidative stress in development of complications in diabetes. Diabetes 40:405–412, 1991.

19. Beach KW, et al: The correlation of arteriosclerosis obliterans with lipoproteins in insulin-dependent and noninsulin-dependent diabetes. Diabetes 28:836–840, 1979.

20. Bell ET: Incidence of gangrene of the extremities in nondiabetic and diabetic persons. Arch Pathol Lab Med 49:469–473, 1960.

21. Bellomo G, et al: Autoantibodies against oxidatively modified low-density lipoproteins in NIDDM. Diabetes 44:60–66, 1995.

22. Bengualid V, et al: *Staphylococcus aureus* infection of human endothelial cells potentiates Fc receptor expression. J Immunol 145:4279, 1990.

23. Berliner JA, et al: Atherosclerosis: Basic mechanisms: oxidation, inflammation and genetics. Circulation 91:2488–2496, 1995.

24. Bertello P, et al: Plasma endothelin in NIDDM patients with and without complications. Diabetes Care 17:574, 1994.

25. Bevilacqua MP, et al: Interleukin-1 induces biosynthesis and cell surface expression of procoagulant activity in human vascular endothelial cells. J Exp Med 160:618–622, 1984.

26. Bhatt L, Terleckyj I, Manjula B: Demonstration of *in vivo* efficacy of aminoguanidine and novel AGE-formation inhibitors: Effects on tissue AGE content and microalbuminuria. Diabetes 45(Suppl 2):130A, 1996.

27. Biesbroeck RC, et al: Abnormal composition of high-density lipoproteins in non-insulin-dependent diabetics. Diabetes 31:126, 1982.

28. Biesbroeck RC, et al: Specific high affinity binding of HDL to cultured human skin fibroblasts and arterial smooth muscle cells. J Clin Invest 71: 525, 1983.

29. Björkhem I, et al: The antioxidant butylated hydroxytoluene protects against atherosclerosis. Arterioscler Thromb 11:15–22, 1991.

30. Boackle R: The complement system. In Virella G, Goust JM, Fudenberg HH (eds): Introduction to Medical Immunology, 2nd ed. New York: Marcel Dekker, 1990, pp 143–168.

31. Booth NA, et al: Plasminogen activator inhibitor (PAI-1) in plasma and platelets. Br J Haematol 70:327–333, 1988.

32. Booyse FM, et al: Normal but not hypertriglyceridemic very low-density lipoprotein induces rapid release of tissue plasminogen activator from cultured human umbilical vein endothelial cells. Semin Thromb Hemost 14:175–179, 1988.

33. Bowie EJ, Owen CA: The hemostatic mechanism. In Kwaan H, Bowie EJ (eds): Thrombosis. Philadelphia: WB Saunders Company, 1982, pp 7–22.

34. Bowry VW, Stocker R: Vitamin E in human low-density lipoprotein: When and how this antioxidant becomes a pro-oxidant. Biochem J 288:341–344, 1992.

35. Breviario F, et al: IL-induced adhesion of polymorphonuclear leukocytes to cultured human endothelial cells. Role of platelet-activating factor. J Immunol 141:3391–3397, 1988.

36. Brinton EA, et al: Binding of HDL to cultured fibroblasts after chemical alteration of apoprotein amino-acid residues. Arteriosclerosis 5:329, 1985.

37. Brinton EA, et al: Binding of HDL to cultured fibroblasts after chemical alteration of apoprotein amino-acid residues. J Biol Chem 261:495, 1986.

38. Brommer EJP, et al: Response of fibrinolytic activity and factor VIII-related antigen to stimulation with desmopressin in hyperlipoproteinemia. J Lab Clin Med 100:105–114, 1982.

39. Brownlee M, et al: Aminoguanidine prevents diabetes-induced arterial wall protein cross-linking. Science 232:1629–1632, 1986.

40. Brownlee M, Vlassara H, Cerami A: Nonenzymatic glycosylation products on collagen covalently trap low-density lipoprotein. Diabetes 34:938–941, 1985.

41. Brownlee M, Vlassara H, Cerami A: Inhibition of heparin-catalyzed antithrombin III activity by non-enzymatic glycosylation: Possible role in fibrin deposition in diabetes. Diabetes 33:532–535, 1984.

42. Brownlee M, Pongor S, Cerami A: Covalent attachment of soluble proteins by non-enzymatically glycosylated collagen: Role in the *in situ* formation of immune complexes. J Exp Med 158:1739–1744, 1983.

43. Bruzzi I, Remuzzi G, Benigni A: Endothelin: A mediator of renal disease progression. J Nephrol 10:179, 1997.

44. Bucala R, Cerami A: Phospholipids react with glucose to initiate advanced glycosylation and fatty acid oxidation: Inhibition of lipid advanced glycosylation and oxidation by aminoguanidine. Diabetes 41(Suppl 1):23A, 1992.

45. Bucala R, Vlassara H: Advanced glycosylation end products in diabetic renal and vascular disease. Am J Kidney Dis 26:875–888, 1995.

46. Bucala R, et al: Inhibition of advanced glycosylation by aminoguanidine reduces plasma LDL levels in diabetes. Clin Res 41:183A, 1993.

47. Bucala R, Tracey KJ, Cerami A: Advanced glycosylation products quench nitric oxide and mediate defective endothelium-dependent vasodilatation in experimental diabetes. J Clin Invest 87:432–438, 1991.

48. Burch RM, et al: *N*-(fluorenyl-9-methoxycarbonyl) amino acids, a class of anti-inflammatory agents with a different mechanism of action. Proc Natl Acad Sci U S A 88:355–359, 1991.

49. Calver A, Collier J, Vallance P: Inhibition and stimulation of nitric oxide synthesis in the human forarm arterial bed of patients with insulin-dependent diabetes. J Clin Invest 90:2548, 1992.

50. Calvo C, et al: Non enzymatic glycation of apolipoprotein A-I. Effects on its self-association and lipid binding properties. Biochem Biophys Res Commun 153:1060–1067, 1988.

51. Cameron NE, et al: Effects of aminoguanidine on peripheral nerve function and polyol pathway metabolites in streptozotocin diabetic rats. Diabetologia 35:946–950, 1992.

52. Cameron NE, Cotter MA, Hohman TC: Interactions between essential fatty acid, prostanoid, polyol pathway and nitric oxide mechanisms in the neurovascular deficit of diabetic rats. Diabetologia 39:172, 1996.

53. Carew TE, Schwenke DC, Steinberg D: Antiatherogenic effect of probucol unrelated to its hypocholesterolemic effect: Evidence that antioxidants in vivo can selectively inhibit low density lipoprotein degradation in macrophage-rich fatty streaks and slow the progression of atherosclerosis in the Watanabe heritable hyperlipidemic rabbit. Proc Natl Acad Sci U S A 84:7725–7729, 1987.

54. Carter AM, Grant PJ: Vascular homeostasis, adhesion molecules, and macrovascular disease in non-insulin-dependent diabetes mellitus. Diabet Med 14:423, 1997.

55. Cavender D, Saegusa Y, Ziff M: Stimulation of endothelial cell binding of lymphocytes by tumor necrosis factor. J Immunol 139:1855–1860, 1987.

56. Cerami A, Vlassara H, Brownlee M: Glucose and aging. Sci Am 256:90–96, 1987.

57. Ceriello A, et al: Induced hyperglycemia alters antithrombin III activity but not its plasma concentration in healthy normal subjects. Diabetes 36:320–323, 1987.

58. Ceriello A, et al: Increased circulating intercellular adhesion molecule-1 levels in type II diabetic patients: The possible role of metabolic control and oxidative stress. Clin Exp Metab 45:498, 1996.

59. Ceriello A, et al: Daily rapid blood glucose variations may condition antithrombin biological activity but not its plasma concentration in insulin dependent diabetes: A possible role for labile non-enzymatic glycation. Diabet Metab 13:16–19, 1987.

60. Ceriello A, et al: Protein C deficiency in insulin-dependent diabetes: A hyperglycemia-related phenomenon. Thromb Haemost 64:104–107, 1990.

61. Ceriello A, et al: Evidence for a hyperglycaemia-dependent decrease of antithrombin III-thrombin complex formation in humans. Diabetologia 33:163–167, 1990.

62. Chakir M, Plante GE: Endothelial dysfunction in diabetes mellitus. Prostaglandins Leukot Essent Fatty Acids 54:45, 1996.

63. Chakrabarti S, Sima AA: Endothelin-1 and endothelin-3-like immunoreactivity in the eyes of diabetic and non-diabetic BB/W rats. Diab Res Clin Pract 37:109, 1997.

64. Chakravarthy U, et al: Endothelin expression in ocular tissues of diabetic and insulin-treated rats. Invest Ophthalmol Vis Sci 38:2144, 1997.

65. Chandra A, et al: Active site modification of aldose reductase by nitric oxide donors. Biochim Biophys Acta 1341:217, 1997.

66. Chibber R, Molinatti PA, Kohner EM: Potential role of glucose-mediated proteins in the pathogenesis of diabetic retinopathy. Diabetes 45(Suppl 2):15A, 1996.

67. Chin JH, Azhar S, Hoffman BB: Inactivation of endothelial-derived relaxing factor by oxidized lipoproteins. J Clin Invest 89:10, 1992.

68. Christ GJ, et al: Endothelin-1 as a putative modulator of erectile dysfunction: I. Characteristics of contraction of isolated corporal tissue strips. J Urol 153:1998, 1995.

69. Cines DB, Lyss AP, Bina M: Fc and C3 receptors induced by herpes simplex virus in cultured human endothelial cells. J Clin Invest 69:123, 1982.

70. Cipolla MJ, Proter JM, Osol G: High glucose concentrations dilate cerebral arteries and diminish myogenic tone through an endothelial mechanism. Stroke 28:405, 1997.

71. Coffey MD, et al: In vitro cell injury by oxidized low density lipoprotein involves lipid hydroperoxide-induced formation of alkoxyl, lipid, and peroxyl radicals. J Clin Invest 96:1866–1873, 1995.

72. Cohen MP, et al: Increased glycosylation of glomerular basement membrane collagen in diabetes. Biochem Biophys Res Commun 95:765–769, 1980.

73. Cohen RA: The role of nitric oxide and other endothelium-derived vasoactive substances in vascular disease. Prog Cardiovasc Dis 38:105, 1995.

74. Collier A, et al: Plasma endothelin like immunoreactivity levels in IDDM patients with microalbuminuria. Diabetes Care 15:1038, 1992.

75. Colwell JA, Jokl R: Clotting disorders in diabetes. *In* Porte D, Sherwin R, Rifkin H (eds): Diabetes Mellitus: Theory and Practive, 5th ed. Norwalk, CT: Appleton & Lange, 1996.

76. Colwell JA: Aspirin therapy in diabetes [technical review]. Diabetes Care 20:1767–1771, 1997.

77. Colwell JA: Vascular thrombosis in type II diabetes mellitus. Diabetes 42:8–11, 1993.

78. Colwell JA: Aspirin therapy in diabetes [position statement]. Diabetes Care 20:1772–1773, 1997.

79. Colwell JA: Peripheral vascular disease in diabetes mellitus. *In* Davidson J (eds): Clinical Diabetes Mellitus. New York: Thieme Medical Publishers, 1986, pp 357–375.

80. Colwell JA: Antiplatelet drugs and prevention of macrovascular disease in diabetes mellitus. Metabolism 41(Suppl 1):7–10, 1992.

81. Colwell JA, Winocour PD, Lopes-Virella MF: Platelet function and platelet interactions in atherosclerosis and diabetes mellitus. *In* Rifkin H, Porte D (eds): Diabetes Mellitus: Theory and Practice. New York: Elsevier, 1989, pp 249–256.

82. Colwell JA, et al: New concepts about the pathogenesis of atherosclerosis in diabetes mellitus. *In* Levin ME, O'Neal LW (eds): The Diabetic Foot, 4th ed. St. Louis: Mosby-Year Book, 1988, pp 51–70.

83. Colwell JA, et al (eds): Workshop on insulin and atherogenesis. Metabolism 12(Suppl 1):1–91, 1985.

84. Colwell JA, Halushka PV: Platelet function in diabetes mellitus. Br J Haematol 44:521–526, 1980.

85. Cominacini L, et al: Elevated levels of soluble E-selectin in patients with IDDM and NIDDM: Relation to metabolic control. Diabetologia 38:1122, 1995.

86. Cominacini L, et al: E-selectin plasma concentration is influenced by glycaemic control in NIDDM patients: Possible role of oxidative stress. Diabetologia 40:584, 1997.

87. Corbett JA, et al: Nitric oxide mediates cytokine-induced inhibition of insulin secretion by human islets of Langerhans. Proc Natl Acad Sci U S A 90:1731, 1993.

88. Corbett JA, McDaniel ML: Does nitric oxide mediate autoimmune destruction of β-cells? Diabetes 41:897, 1992.

89. Cornacoff JB, et al: Primate erythrocyte-immune complex-clearing mechanism. J Clin Invest 71:236–247, 1983.

90. Craven PA, DeRubertis FR, Melhem M: Nitric oxide in diabetic nephropathy. Kidney Int Suppl 60:S46, 1997.

91. Curtiss LK, Witztum JL: A novel method of generating region-specific monoclonal antibodies to modified proteins. Application to the identification of human glucosylated low density lipoproteins. J Clin Invest 72:1427–1438, 1983.

92. Curtiss LK, Witztum JL: Plasma apo-lipoproteins A-I, A-II, B, C-I and E are glucosylated in hyperglycemic diabetic subjects. Diabetes 34:452–461, 1985.

93. Cybulsky M, Gimbrone MA Jr: Endothelial expression of a mononuclear leukocyte adhesion molecule during atherogenesis. Science 251:788, 1991.

94. Davi G, et al: Increased thromboxane biosynthesis in type IIa hypercholesterolemia. Circulation 85:1792, 1992.

95. Davi G, et al: Diabetes mellitus, hypercholesterolemia, and hypertension but not vascular disease per se are associated with persistent platelet activation in vivo. Evidence derived from the study of peripheral arterial disease. Circulation 96:69, 1997.

96. Davies MJ, et al: The expression of the adhesion molecules ICAM-1, VCAM-1, PECAM, and E-selectin in human atherosclerosis. J Pathol 171:223, 1993.

97. Davis NS Jr: Diabetic gangrene. JAMA 31:103–105, 1898.

98. De Meyer GR, Herman AG: Vascular endothelial dysfunction. Prog Cardiovasc Dis 39:325, 1997.

99. De Feo P, Gaisano MG, Haymond MW: Differential effects of insulin deficiency on albumin and fibrinogen synthesis in humans. J Clin Invest 88:833–840, 1991.

100. Deussen A, Sonntag M, Bogel R: L-arginine derived nitrous oxide: A major determinant of uveal blood flow. Exp Eye Res 57:129, 1993.

101. Di Minno G, et al: Abnormally high thromboxane biosynthesis in homozygous homocystinuria: Evidence for platelet involvement and probucol-sensitive mechanism. J Clin Invest 92:1400, 1993.

102. Doi T, et al: Receptor-specific increase in extracellular matrix production in mouse mesangial cells by advanced glycosylation end products is mediated via platelet-derived growth factor. Proc Natl Acad Sci U S A 89:2873–2877, 1992.

103. Donatelli M, et al: Circulating endothelin-1 levels in type 2 diabetic patients with ischaemic heart disease. Acta Diabetol 33:246, 1996.

104. Ducimetier P, et al: Relationship of plasma insulin levels to the incidence of myocardial infarction and coronary heart disease mortality in a middle-aged population. Diabetologia 19:205–210, 1980.

105. Duell PB, Oram JF, Biern EL: Nonenzymatic glycosylation of HDL resulting in inhibition of high-affinity binding to cultured human fibroblasts. Diabetes 39:1257–1263, 1990.

106. Duell PB, Oram JF, Bierman EL: Nonenzymatic glycosylation of HDL and impaired HDL-receptor-mediated cholesterol efflux. Diabetes 40:377–384, 1991.

107. Dunn JA, et al: Age-dependent accumulation of N-(carboxymethyl)lysine and N-(carboxymethyl)hydroxylysine in human skin collagen. Biochemistry 30:1205–1210, 1991.

108. Dunn JA, et al: Reaction of ascorbate with lysine and protein under autoxidizing conditions: Formation of N-(carboxymethyl)lysine by reaction between lysine and products of autoxidation of ascorbate. Biochemistry 29:10964–10970, 1990.

109. Dyer DG, et al: Formation of pentosidine during nonenzymatic browning of proteins by glucose. Identification of glucose and other carbohydrates as possible precursors of pentosidine *in vivo*. J Biol Chem 266:11654–11660, 1991.

110. Edelstein D, Brownlee M: Rapid communication: Aminoguanidine ameliorates albuminuria in diabetic hypertensive rats. Diabetologia 35:96–97, 1992.

111. Epstein FH, et al: Epidemiological studies of cardiovascular diseases in a total community—Tecumseh, Michigan. Ann Intern Med 62:1170–1187, 1965.

112. Esposito C: Endothelial receptor-mediated binding of glucose-modified albumin is associated with increased monolayer permeability and modulation of cell surface coagulant properties. J Exp Med 170:1387–1407, 1989.

113. Fabien N, et al: Lymphocyte function associated antigen-1, integrin alpha 4, and L-selectin mediate T-cell homing to the pancreas in the model of adoptive transfer of diabetes in NOD mice. Diabetes 45:1181, 1996.

114. Ferri C, et al: Circulating endothelin-1 levels increase during euglycemic hyperinsulinemic clamp in lean NIDDM men. Diabetes Care 18:226, 1995.

115. Ferri C, et al: Endogenous insulin modulates circulating endothelin-1 concentrations in humans. Diabetes Care 19:504, 1996.

116. Fielding DF, Reaven GM, Fielding PE: Human noninsulin-dependent diabetes: Identification of a defect in plasma cholesterol transport normalized in vivo by insulin and in vitro by immunoadsorption of apolipoprotein E. Proc Natl Acad Sci U S A 79:6365, 1982.

117. Fielding DF, et al: Increased free cholesterol in plasma low and very low density lipoproteins in noninsulin-dependent diabetes mellitus: Its role in the inhibition of cholesteryl ester transfer. Proc Natl Acad Sci U S A 81:2512, 1984.

118. Fishbane S, et al: Reduction of plasma apolipoprotein-B by effective removal of circulating glycation derivatives in uremia. Kid Int 52:1645–1650, 1997.

119. Fogelman AM, et al: Malondialdehyde alteration of LDL leads to cholesterol ester accumulation in human monocytes/macrophages. Proc Natl Acad Sci U S A 77:2214–2218, 1980.

120. Fontbonne AM, et al: Insulin and cardiovascular disease—Paris prospective study. Diabetes Care 6:461–469, 1991.

121. Ford I, et al: Activation of coagulation in diabetes mellitus in relation to the presence of vascular complications. Diabet Med 8:322–329, 1990.

122. Francavilla S, et al: Endothelin-1 in diabetic and nondiabetic men with erectile dysfunction. J Urol 158:1770, 1997.

123. Frank FS, Fogelman AM: Ultrastructure of the intima in WHHL and cholesterol-fed rabbit aortas prepared by ultra-rapid freezing and freeze-etching. J Lipid Res 30:967–978, 1989.

124. Freedman JE, et al: Decreased platelet inhibition by nitric oxide in two brothers with a history of arterial thrombosis. J Clin Invest 97:979, 1996.

125. Frei B, England L, Ames BN: Ascorbate is an outstanding antioxidant in human plasma. Proc Natl Acad Sci U S A 86:6377–6381, 1989.

126. Freyschuss A, et al: Antioxidant treatment inhibits the development of intimal thickening after balloon injury of the aorta in hypercholesterolemic rabbits. J Clin Invest 91:1282–1288, 1993.

127. Fries ED, et al: Oxidized low-density lipoprotein stimulates nitric oxide release by rabbit aortic endothelial cells. Biochem Biophys Res Commun 207:231, 1995.

128. Fu M-X, et al: The advanced glycation end-product, N-(carboxymethyl)lysine (CML), is a product of both lipid peroxidation and glycoxidation reactions. J Biol Chem 271:9982–9986, 1996.

129. Fu M-X, et al: Role of oxygen in the cross-linking and chemical modification of collagen by glucose. Diabetes 43:676–683, 1994.

130. Fukui M, et al: Gene expression for endothelins and their receptors in glomeruli of diabetic rats. J Lab Clin Med 122:149, 1993.

131. Fuller JH: Haemostatic variables associated with diabetes and its complications. Br Med J 2:964–966, 1979.

132. Furchgott RF, Zawadzki JV: The obligatory role of endothelial cells in the relaxation of arterial smooth muscle by acetylcholine. Nature 299:373, 1980.

133. Galle J, et al: Impairment of endothelium-dependent dilation in rabbit renal arteries by oxidized lipoprotein (a). Role of oxygen-derived radicals. Circulation 92:1582, 1995.

134. Gamble JR, et al: Stimulation of the adherence of neutrophils to umbilical vein endothelium by human recombinant tumor necrosis factor. Proc Natl Acad Sci U S A. 82:8667–8671, 1985.

135. Garcia F, et al: Hypofibrinolysis associated with vasculopathy in non insulin dependent diabetes mellitus. Thromb Res 59:51–59, 1990.

136. Garcia ML, et al: Morbidity and mortality in diabetics in Framingham population: Sixteen year follow-up study. Diabetes 23:105–111, 1974.

137. Garlick RL, Bunn HF, Spiro RG: Non-enzymatic glycosylation of basement membranes from human glomeruli and bovine sources. Diabetes 37:1144–1150, 1988.

138. Gearing AJH, et al: Soluble forms of vascular adhesion molecules, E-selectin, ICAM-1, and VCAM-1: Pathological significance. Ann N Y Acad Sci 667:324, 1992.

139. Gianturco SH, et al: Hypertriglyceridemic very low density lipoproteins induce triglyceride synthesis and accumulation in mouse peritoneal macrophages. J Clin Invest 70:168, 1982.

140. Gisinger C, Virella GT, Lopes-Virella MF: Erythrocyte-bound low density lipoprotein (LDL) immune complexes lead to cholesteryl ester accumulation in human monocyte derived macrophages. Clin Immunol Immunopathol 59:37–52, 1991.

141. Gonen B, et al: Non-enzymatic glycosylation of low-density lipoproteins in vitro. Diabetes 30:875–878, 1981.

142. Goor Y, et al: Nitric oxide in ischaemic acute renal failure of streptozotocin diabetic rats. Diabetologia 39:1036, 1996.

143. Grandhee SK, Monnier VM: Mechanism of formation of the Maillard protein cross-link pentosidine. Glucose, fructose and ascorbate as pentosidine precursors. J Biol Chem 266:11649–11653, 1991.

144. Grant PJ, Ruegg M, Medcalf RL: Basal expression and insulin-mediated induction of PAI-1 mRNA in Hep G2 cells. Fibrinolysis 5:81–86, 1991.

145. Gray RP, Patterson DLH, Yudkin JS: Plasminogen activator inhibitor activity in diabetic and nondiabetic survivors of myocardial infarction. Arteriosclerosis 13:415–420, 1993.

146. Greaves M, et al: Fibrinogen and von Willebrand factor in IDDM: Relationships to lipid vascular risk factors, blood pressure, glycaemic control and urinary albumin excretion rate—the EURODIAB IDDM Complications Study. Diabetologia 40:698, 1997.

147. Griffith RL, et al: LDL metabolism by macrophages activated with LDL immune complexes: A possible mechanism of foam cell formation. J Exp Med 168:1041–1059, 1988.

148. Gruden G, et al: PAI-1 and factor VII activity are higher in IDDM patients with microalbuminuria. Diabetes 43:426–429, 1994.

149. Guvener N, et al: Plasma endothelin-1 levels in non-insulin dependent diabetes mellitus patients with macrovascular disease. Coronary Artery Dis 8:253, 1997.

150. Haefliger IO, Flammer J, Lüscher TF: Nitric oxide and endothelin-1 are important regulators of human ophthalmic artery. Invest Ophthalmol Vis Sci 33:2340, 1992.

151. Hamlin CR, Kohn RR: Determination of human chronological age by study of a collagen sample. Exp Gerontol 7:377–379, 1972.

152. Hamlin CR, Kohn RR, Luschin JH: Apparent accelerated aging of human collagen in diabetes mellitus. Diabetes 24:902–904, 1975.

153. Hamlin CR, Kohn RR: Evidence for progressive, age-related structural changes in post-mature human collagen. Biochim Biophys Acta 236:458–467, 1971.

154. Hammes HP, et al: Aminoguanidine inhibits the development of accelerated diabetic retinopathy in the spontaneous hypertensive rat. Diabetologia 37:32–35, 1994.

155. Hammes HP, et al: Secondary intervention with aminoguanidine retards the progression of diabetic retinopathy in the rat model. Diabetologia 38:656–660, 1995.

156. Hammes HP, et al: Aminoguanidine treatment inhibits the development of experimental diabetic retinopathy. Proc Natl Acad Sci U S A 88:11555–11558, 1991.

157. Harman D: The ageing process. Proc Natl Acad Sci U S A 78:7124–7128, 1981.

158. Hasegawa Y, Yokono K, Taki T, et al: Prevention of autoimmune insulin-dependent diabetes in non-obese diabetic mice by anti-LFA-1 and anti-ICAM-1 mAb. Int Immunol 6:831, 1994.

159. Hattori Y, et al: Effects of glucose and insulin on immunoreactive endothelin-1 release from cultured porcine aortic endothelial cells. Metabolism 40:165, 1991.

160. Havel RJ, et al: Isoprotein specificity in the hepatic uptake of apolipoprotein E and the pathogenesis of familial dysbetalipoproteinemia. Proc Natl Acad Sci U S A 77:4349, 1980.

161. Hayase F, et al: Aging of proteins: Immunological detection of a glucose-derived pyrrole formed during Maillard reaction in vivo. J Biol Chem 263:3758–3764, 1989.

162. Heinecke JW: Mechanisms of oxidative damage of low density lipoprotein in human atherosclerosis. Curr Opin Lipidol 8:268, 1997.

163. Henriksen T, Evensen SA, Carlander B: Injury to human endothelial cells in culture induced by LDL. Scand J Clin Lab Invest 39:361–364, 1979.

164. Herold KC, et al: Prevention of autoimmune diabetes by treatment with anti-LFA-1 and anti-ICAM-1 monoclonal antibodies. Cell Immunol 157:489, 1994.

165. Hessler JR, Robertson AL Jr, Chisolm GM: LDL-induced cytotoxicity and its inhibition by HDL in human vascular smooth muscle and endothelial cells in culture. Atherosclerosis 32:213–218, 1979.

166. Hicks M, et al: Increase in crosslinking of nonenzymatically glycosylated collagen induced by products of lipid peroxidation. Arch Biochem Biophys 268:249–254, 1989.

167. Hiramatsu K, Bierman EL, Chair A: Metabolism of LDL from patients with diabetic hypertriglyceridemia by cultured human skin fibroblasts. Diabetes 34:8, 1985.

168. Hoff HF, et al: Modification of LDL with 4-hydroxynonenal induces uptake by macrophages. Arteriosclerosis 9:538–549, 1989.

169. Högman M, et al: Bleeding time prolongation and NO inhalation. Lancet 341:1664, 1993.

170. Holstad M, Jansson L, Sandler S: Inhibition of nitric oxide formation by aminoguanidine: An attempt to prevent insulin-dependent diabetes mellitus. Gen Pharmacol 29:697, 1997.

171. Hori O, et al: Advanced glycation endproducts interacting with their endothelial receptor induce expression of vascular cell adhesion molecule-1 (VCAM-1) in cultured human endothelial cells and in mice. A potential mechanism for the accelerated vasculopathy of diabetes. J Clin Invest 96:1395–1403, 1995.

172. Hornsby WG, et al: The effect of an exercise program on risk factors for vascular disease in type II diabetes. Diabetes Care 13:87–92, 1990.

173. Hotta N, et al: Prevention of abnormalities in motor nerve conduction and nerve blood-flow by a prostacyclin analog, beraprost sodium, in streptozotocin-induced diabetic rats. Prostaglandins 49:339, 1995.

174. Hotta N, et al: Effects of beraprost sodium and insulin on the electroretinogram, nerve conduction, and nerve blood flow in rats with streptozotocin-induced diabetes. Diabetes 45:361, 1996.

175. Hu R, et al: Insulin stimulates production and secretion of endothelin from bovine endothelial cells. Diabetes 42:351, 1993.

176. Huang Y, Ghosh M, Lopes-Virella MF: Transcriptional and post-transcriptional regulation of LDL receptor gene expression in PMA-treated THP-1 cells by LDL-IC. J Lipid Res 38:110–120, 1997.

177. Huber K, et al: A decrease in plasminogen activator inhibitor-1 activity after successful percutaneous transluminal coronary angioplasty is associated with a significantly reduced risk for coronary restenosis. Thromb Haemost 67:209–213, 1992.

178. Huszka M, et al: The association of reduced endothelium derived relaxing factor-NO production with endothelial damage and increased in vivo platelet activation in patients with diabetes mellitus. Thromb Res 86:173, 1997.

179. Ichikawa K, et al: Advanced glycosylation end products induced tissue factor expression in human monocytes. Diabetes 45(Suppl 2):128A, 1996.

180. Ienaga K, et al: Crosslines, fluorophores in the AGE-related crosslinked proteins. Contrib Nephrol 112:42–51, 1995.

181. Ignarro LJ, et al: Endothelium-derived relaxing factor produced and released from artery and vein is nitric oxide. Proc Natl Acad Sci U S A 84:9265, 1987.

182. Imani F, et al: Advanced glycosylation endproduct-specific receptors on human and rat T-lymphocytes mediate synthesis of interferon gamma: Role in tissue remodeling. J Exp Med 178:2165–2172, 1993.

183. Ischiropoulos H, al Mehdi A: Peroxynitrite-mediated oxidative protein modifications. FEBS Lett 364:279, 1995.

184. Jack CM, et al: Non-enzymatic glycosylation of low-density lipoprotein. Results of an affinity chromatography method. Diabetologia 31:126–128, 1988.

185. James RW, Pometta D: Differences in lipoprotein subfraction composition and distribution between type I diabetic men and control subjects. Diabetes 39:1158–1164, 1990.

186. James RW, Pometta D: The distribution profiles of very low and low density lipoproteins in poorly controlled male, type 2 (non-insulin-dependent) diabetic patients. Diabetologia 34:246–252, 1991.

187. Janka HU, Standl E, Mehnert H: Peripheral vascular disease in diabetes mellitus and its relation to cardiovascular risk factors: Screening with the

Doppler ultrasonic technique. Diabetes Care 3:207–213, 1980.

188. Jansson JH, Olofsson BO, Nilsson TK: Predictive value of tissue plasminogen activator mass concentration on long-term mortality in patients with coronary artery disease. Circulation 88:2030–2034, 1993.

189. Jenkins AJ, et al: Plasma apolipoprotein(a) is increased in type 2 (non-insulin-dependent) patients with microalbuminuria. Diabetologia 35:1055–1059, 1992.

190. Jenkins AJ, et al: Increased plasma apolipoprotein(a) levels in IDDM patients with microalbuminuria. Diabetes 40:787–790, 1991.

191. Jenkins AJ, et al: LDL from patients with well-controlled IDDM is not more susceptible to in vitro oxidation. Diabetes 45:762–767, 1996.

192. Jenkins AJ, Best JD: The role of lipoprotein(a) in the vascular complications of diabetes mellitus. J Int Med 237:359–365, 1995.

193. Jennings PE, et al: Vitamin C metabolites and microangiopathy in diabetes mellitus. Diabetes Res 6:151–154, 1987.

194. Jensen T, et al: Features of endothelial dysfunction in early diabetic nephropathy. Lancet 1:461–463, 1989.

195. Jessup W, Dean RT: Autoinhibition of murine macrophage-mediated oxidation of low-density lipoprotein by nitric oxide synthesis. Atherosclerosis 101:145, 1993.

196. Jessup W, Leake D: Cell-mediated oxidation of lipoproteins. In Rice-Evans C, Bruckdorfer K (eds): Oxidative Stress, Lipoproteins and Cardiovascular Dysfunction. London: Portland Press, 1995, p 99.

197. Jessup W: Oxidized lipoproteins and nitric oxide. Curr Opin Lipidol 7:274, 1996.

198. Jokl R, et al: Release of platelet plasminogen activator inhibitor 1 in whole blood is increased in patients with type II diabetes. Diabetes Care 18:1150–1155, 1995.

199. Jokl R: Glycoxidized LDL modifies PAI-1 release by retinal endothelial cells. Diabetologia 35(Suppl 1):A46, 1992.

200. Jokl R, et al: Low density lipoproteins isolated from diabetic patients alter the release of tissue plasminogen activator (tPA) by cultured human endothelial cells. Diabetes 41(Suppl 1):113A, 1992.

201. Jokl R, et al: Platelet plasminogen activator inhibitor 1 in patients with type II diabetes. Diabetes Care 17:818–823, 1994.

202. Jones RL: Fibrinopeptide-A in diabetes mellitus. Diabetes 34:836–843, 1985.

203. Jones RL, et al: Time course of reversibility of accelerated fibrinogen disappearance in diabetes mellitus: Association with intravascular volume shifts. Blood 63:22–30, 1984.

204. Jones RL, Peterson CM: Reduced fibrinogen survival in diabetes mellitus. J Clin Invest 63:485–493, 1979.

205. Joven J, et al: Concentrations of lipids and apolipoproteins in patients with clinically well-controlled insulin-dependent and non-insulin-dependent diabetes. Clin Chem 35:813–816, 1989.

206. Juhan-Vague L, et al: Effect of 24 hours of normoglycaemia on tissue-type plasminogen activator plasma levels in insulin-dependent diabetes. Thromb Haemost 51:97–98, 1984.

207. Kahn B, et al: Modified LDL and its constituents augment cytokine-activated vascular cell adhesion molecule-1 gene expression in human vascular endothelial cells. J Clin Invest 95:1262–1270, 1995.

208. Kannel WB, et al: Fibrinogen and risk of cardiovascular disease: The Framingham Study. JAMA 258:1183–1186, 1987.

209. Karpen CW, et al: Production of 12 HETE and vitamin E status in platelets from type 1 human diabetic subjects. Diabetes 34:526–531, 1985.

210. Kasim SE, et al: Significance of hepatic triglyceride lipase activity in the regulation of serum high density lipoproteins in type II diabetes mellitus. J Clin Endocrinol Metab 65:183–187, 1987.

211. Kato H, et al: Effect of beraprost sodium, a stable prostaglandin I_2 analogue, on platelet aggregation in diabetes mellitus. Intern J Clin Pharm Res 16:99, 1996.

212. Katsumori K, et al: Lack of acute insulin effect on plasma endothelin-1 levels in humans. Diabet Res Clin Pract 32:187, 1996.

213. Kawabata A: Evidence that endogenous nitric oxide modulates plasma fibrinogen levels in rat. Br J Pharmacol 117:236, 1996.

214. Kawamura M, et al: Increased plasma endothelin in NIDDM patients with retinopathy. Diabetes Care 15:1396, 1992.

215. Kennedy L, Baynes JW: Non-enzymatic glycosylation and the chronic complications of diabetes: An overview. Diabetologia 6:93–98, 1984.

216. Kennedy L, Lyons TJ: Glycation, oxidation, and lipoxidation in the development of diabetic complications. Metabolism 46(Suppl 1):14–21, 1997.

217. Kihara M, et al: Aminoguanidine effects on nerve blood flow, vascular permeability, electrophysiology, and oxygen free radicals. Proc Natl Acad Sci U S A 88:6107–6111, 1991.

218. Kilpatrick JM, Hyman B, Virella G: Human endothelial cell damage induced by interactions between polymorphonuclear leukocytes and immune complex-coated erythrocytes. Clin Immunol Immunopathol 44:335–347, 1987.

219. Kim DC, et al: Endothelin-1-induced modulation of contractile responses elicited by an α_1-adrenergic agonist on human corpus cavernosum smooth muscle. Int J Impot Res 8:17, 1996.

220. Kirstein M, et al: Advanced protein glycosylation induces transendothelial human monocyte chemotaxis and secretion of platelet-derived growth factor: Role in vascular disease of diabetes and aging. Proc Natl Acad Sci U S A 87:9010–9014, 1990.

221. Kita T, Nagano Y, Yokode M, et al: Probucol prevents the progression of atherosclerosis in Watanabe heritable hyperlipidemic rabbit, an animal model for familial hypercholesterolemia. Proc Natl Acad Sci U S A 84:5928–5931, 1987.

222. Klein RL, Lopes-Virella MF, Colwell JA: Enhancement of platelet aggregation by the glycosylated subfraction of low density lipoprotein (LDL) isolated from patients with insulin-dependent diabetes mellitus (IDDM). Diabetes 39(Suppl 1):173a, 1990.

223. Klein RL, Laimins M, Lopes-Virella MF: Isolation, characterization and metabolism of the glycated and nonglycated sub-fractions of low density lipoproteins isolated from type 1 diabetic patients and non-diabetic subjects. Diabetes 44:1093–1098, 1995.

224. Klein RL, et al: Interaction of VLDL isolated from type I diabetic subjects with human monocyte-

derived macrophages. Metabolism 38:1108–1114, 1989.

225. Klein RL, Lopes-Virella MF: Metabolism by human endothelial cells of very low density lipoprotein subfractions isolated from type 1 (insulin-dependent) diabetic patients. Diabetologia 36:258–264, 1993.

226. Klein RL, Lyons TJ, Lopes-Virella MF: Metabolism of very low- and low density lipoproteins isolated from normolipidaemic type 2 (non-insulin-dependent) diabetic patients by human monocyte-derived macrophages. Diabetologia 33:299–305, 1990.

227. Klimov AN, et al: Lipoprotein-antibody immune complexes: Their catabolism and role in foam cell formation. Atherosclerosis 58:1–15, 1985.

228. Kolb H, Kolb-Bachofen V: Type I (insulin-dependent) diabetes mellitus and nitric oxide. Diabetologia 35:796, 1992.

229. Komers R, Allen TJ, Cooper ME: Role of endothelium-derived nitric oxide in the pathogenesis of the renal hemodynamic changes of experimental diabetes. Diabetes 43:1190, 1994.

230. Koschinsky T, et al: Orally absorbed reactive glycation products (glycotoxins): An environmental risk factor in diabetic nephropathy. Proc Natl Acad Sci U S A 94:6474–6479, 1997.

231. Kraemer FB, et al: Effects of noninsulin-dependent diabetes mellitus on the uptake of very low density lipoproteins by thioglycolate-elicited mouse peritoneal macrophages. J Clin Endocrinol Metab 61:335, 1985.

232. Kroncke KD, et al: Cytotoxicity of activated rat macrophages against syngeneic islet cells is arginine-dependent, correlates with citrulline and nitrite concentrations and is identical to lysis by the nitric oxide donor nitroprusside. Diabetologia 36:17, 1993.

233. Kugiyama K, et al: Impairment of endothelium-dependent arterial relaxation by lysolecithin in modified lipoproteins. Nature 344:160, 1990.

234. Kuzuya M, et al: Probucol prevents oxidative injury to endothelial cells. J Lipid Res 32:197–204, 1991.

235. Laakso M, Pyorala K: Lipid and lipoprotein abnormalities in diabetic patients with peripheral vascular disease. Atherosclerosis 74:55–63, 1988.

236. Lampeter ER, et al: Elevated levels of circulating adhesion molecules in IDDM patients and in subjects at risk for IDDM. Diabetes 41:1668, 1992.

237. Laurenti O, et al: Increased levels of plasma endothelin-1 in non-insulin dependent patients with retinopathy but without other diabetes-related organ damage. Exp Clin Endocrinol Diabetes 105(Suppl 2):40, 1997.

238. Lawson RA: Amputations through the ages. Aust N Z J Med 42:221–230, 1973.

239. Ledl F, Schleicher E: New aspects of the Maillard reaction in foods and in the human body. Angew Chem Int Ed 29:565–594, 1990.

240. Lee Y-J, Shin S-J, Tsai J-H: Increased urinary endothelin-1-like immunoreactivity excretion in NIDDM patients with albuminuria. Diabetes Care 17:263, 1994.

241. Letizia C, et al: Circulating endothelin-1 in non-insulin-dependent diabetic patients with retinopathy. Horm Metab Res 29:247, 1997.

242. Leurs, PB, et al: Increased tissue factor pathway inhibitor (TFPI) and coagulation in patients with insulin-dependent diabetes mellitus. Thromb Haemost 77:472–476, 1997.

243. Levin ME, Powers MA: Hypertension and diabetes: Then and now. Diabetes Spectrum 3:274, 1990.

244. Li YM, et al: Opsonization and removal of serum AGEs by coupling to lysozyme. Diabetes 45(Suppl 2):239A, 1996.

245. Libby P, Warner SJC, Friedman GB: IL1: A mitogen for human vascular smooth muscle cells that induces the release of growth inhibitory prostanoids. J Clin Invest 81:487–498, 1988.

246. Lindsay RM, Smith W, Rossiter SP, et al: N^{ω}-nitro-L-arginine methyl ester reduces the incidence of IDDM in BB/E rats. Diabetes 44:365, 1995.

247. Lip GY, Lann A: von Willebrand factor: A marker of endothelial dysfunction in vascular disorders? Cardiovasc Res 34:255, 1997.

248. Lopes-Virella MF, Mironova M, Virella G: LDL-IC and atherosclerosis in diabetes mellitus. Diabetes Rev 5:410–424, 1997.

249. Lopes-Virella MF, et al: Glycosylation of low-density lipoprotein enhances cholesteryl ester synthesis in human monocyte-derived macrophages. Diabetes 37:550–557, 1988.

250. Lopes-Virella MF, Klein RL, Virella G: Modification of lipoproteins in diabetes. Diabetes. Metab Rev 12:69–90, 1996.

251. Lopes-Virella MF, et al: Enhanced uptake and impaired intracellular metabolism of LDL complexed with anti-LDL antibodies. Arterioscler Thromb 11:1356–1367, 1991.

252. Lopes-Virella MF, et al: Surface binding, internalization and degradation by cultured human fibroblasts of low density lipoproteins isolated from type I (insulin-dependent) diabetic patients: Changes with metabolic control. Diabetologia 22:430–436, 1982.

253. Lopes-Virella MF, et al: Plasma lipids and lipoproteins in young insulin-dependent diabetic patients: Relationship with control. Diabetologia 21:216, 1981.

254. Lopes-Virella MF, Stone PG, Colwell JA: Serum high density lipoprotein in diabetes. Diabetologia 13:285, 1977.

255. Lopes-Virella MF, et al: Effect of metabolic control on lipid, lipoprotein and apolipoprotein levels in 55 insulin-dependent diabetic patients: A longitudinal study. Diabetes 32:20, 1983.

256. Lopes-Virella MF, Virella G: Cytokines, modified lipoproteins and arteriosclerosis in diabetes mellitus. Diabetes 45:40–44, 1996.

257. Loscalzo J: The relation between atherosclerosis and thrombosis. Circulation 86(Suppl III):95–98, 1992.

258. Lubec B, Aufricht C, Amann C, et al: Arginine reduces kidney collagen accumulation, cross-linking, lipid peroxidation, glycoxidation, kidney weight and albuminuria in the diabetic kk mouse. Nephron 75:213, 1997.

259. Luscinskas FW, et al: Endothelial-leukocyte adhesion molecule-1-dependent and leukocyte (CD11/CD18)-dependent mechanisms contribute to polymorphonuclear leukocyte adhesion to cytokine-activated human vascular endothelium. J Immunol 142:2257–2263, 1989.

260. Lütjens A, et al: Polymerisation and crosslinking of fibrin monomers in diabetes mellitus. Diabetologia 31:825–830, 1988.

261. Lyons TJ, Lopes-Virella MF: Glycosylation-related mechanisms. *In* Draznin B, Eckel RH (eds): Diabetes and Atherosclerosis—Molecular Basis and Clinical Aspects. New York: Elsevier, 1993, pp 169–189.

262. Lyons TJ, Li W: Aminoguanidine and the cytotoxicity of modified LDL to retinal capillary endothelial cells. Diabetes 43(Suppl 1):112A, 1994.

263. Lyons TJ: Oxidized low density lipoproteins—a role in the pathogenesis of atherosclerosis in diabetes? Diabet Med 8:411–419, 1991.

264. Lyons TJ, et al: Decrease in skin collagen glycosylation with improved glycemic control in patients with insulin-dependent diabetes mellitus. J Clin Invest 87:1910–1915, 1991.

265. Lyons TJ, Jenkins AJ: Lipoprotein glycation and its metabolic consequences. Curr Opin Lipidol 8: 174–180, 1997.

266. Lyons TJ: Glycation and oxidation: A role in the pathogenesis of atherosclerosis. Am J Cardiol 71:26B–31B, 1993.

267. Lyons TJ, et al: Stimulation of cholesteryl ester synthesis in human monocyte-derived macrophages by low-density lipoproteins from type I (insulin-dependent) diabetic patients: The influence of non-enzymatic glycosylation of low-density lipoprotein. Diabetologia 30:916–923, 1987.

268. Lyons TJ, et al: Toxicity of mildly modified low density lipoproteins to cultured retinal capillary endothelial cells and pericytes. Diabetes 43:1090–1095, 1994.

269. Lyons TJ, Kennedy L: Non-enzymatic glycosylation of skin collagen in patients with limited joint mobility. Diabetologia 28:2–5, 1985.

270. Lyons TJ, et al: Glycosylation of low density lipoprotein in patients with type 1 diabetes: Correlations with other parameters of glycaemic control. Diabetologia 29:685–689, 1986.

271. Lyons TJ, Kennedy L: Effect of in vitro non-enzymatic glycosylation of human skin collagen on susceptibility to collagenase digestion. Eur J Clin Invest 15:128–131, 1985.

272. Lyons TJ, Jenkins AJ: Glycation, oxidation and lipoxidation in the development of the complications of diabetes mellitus: A "carbonyl stress" hypothesis. Diabetes Rev 5:365–391, 1997.

273. Maggi E, et al: LDL oxidation in patients with severe carotid atherosclerosis: A study of in vitro and in vivo oxidation markers. Arterioscler Thromb 14:1892–1899, 1994.

274. Makino K, et al: Effect of glycation on the properties of lipoprotein(a). Arterioscler Thromb Vasc Biol 15:385–391, 1995.

275. Makita Z, et al: Advanced glycosylation end products in patients with diabetic nephropathy. N Engl J Med 325:836–842, 1991.

276. Mann RM, et al: Nitric oxide and choroidal blood flow regulation. Invest Ophthalmol Vis Sci 36: 925, 1995.

277. Maree A, et al: Nitric oxide in streptozotocin-induced diabetes mellitus in rats. Clin Sci 90:379, 1996.

278. Marmur JD, et al: Thrombin generation in human coronary arteries after percutaneous transluminal balloon angioplasty. J Am Coll Cardiol 24:1484–1491, 1994.

279. Martin S, Rothe H, Tschoepe D, et al: Decreased expression of adhesion molecules on monocytes in recent onset IDDM. Immunology 73:123, 1991.

280. Martin S, et al: IL-1 and INF-g increase vascular permeability. Immunology 64:301–305, 1988.

281. Masakado M, et al: Immunohistochemical localization of a novel peptide, prostacyclin-stimulating factor (PSF), in human tissues. Thromb Haemost 74:1407, 1995.

282. Mathis KM, Banks RO: Role of nitric oxide and angiotensin II in diabetes mellitus-induced glomerular hyperfiltration. J Am Soc Nephrol 7: 105, 1996.

283. Mattar AL, et al: Renal effects of acute and chronic nitric oxide inhibition in experimental diabetes. Nephron 74:136, 1996.

284. Mazzanti L, Mutus B: Diabetes-induced alterations in platelet metabolism. Clin Biochem 30:509, 1997.

285. McCance DR, et al: Maillard reaction products and their relation to complications in insulin dependent diabetes mellitus. J Clin Invest 91:2470–2478, 1993.

286. McDaniel ML, et al: Cytokines and nitric oxide in islet inflammation and diabetes. Proc Soc Exp Biol Med 211:24, 1996.

287. McMillen MA, Sumpio BE: Endothelins: Polyfunctional cytokines. J Am Coll Surg 180:621, 1995.

288. McVeigh GE, et al: Impaired endothelium-dependent and independent vasodilation in patients with type 2 (non-insulin-dependent) diabetes mellitus. Diabetologia 35:771, 1992.

289. McVerry VA, et al: Non-enzymatic glycosylation of fibrinogen. Haemostasis 10:261–270, 1981.

290. Meade TW, et al: Fibrinolytic activity, clotting factors, and long-term incidence of ischaemic heart disease in the Northwick Park Heart Study. Lancet 342:1076–1079, 1993.

291. Meade TW, et al: Hemostatic function and cardiovascular death: Early results of a prospective study. Lancet 1:1050–1054, 1980.

292. Mehta J, et al: Plasma tissue plasminogen activator inhibitor levels in coronary artery disease; correlation with age and serum triglyceride levels. J Am Coll Cardiol 9:263–268, 1987.

293. Melnick JL, et al: Cytomegalovirus antigen within human arterial smooth muscle cells. Lancet 2:644, 1983.

294. Melton LJ, et al: Incidence and prevalence of clinical peripheral vascular disease in a population-based cohort of 56 diabetic patients. Diabetes Care 3:650–654, 1980.

295. Metsärinne K, et al: Insulin increases the release of endothelin in endothelial cell cultures in vitro but not in vivo. Metabolism 43:878, 1994.

296. Mironova M, et al: Anti-modified LDL antibodies and LDL-IC in IDDM patients and healthy controls. Clin Immunol Immunopathol 85:73–82, 1997.

297. Mitsuhashi T, Li YM, Fishbane S, Vlassara H: Depletion of reactive advanced glycation endproducts (AGEs) from diabetic uremic sera by a lysozyme-linked matrix. Diabetes 45(Suppl 2): 47A, 1996.

298. Moncada S, Palmer R, Higgs E: Nitric oxide: Physiology, pathophysiology, and pharmacology. Pharmacol Rev 43:109, 1991.

299. Moncada S: Biological importance of prostacyclin. Br J Pharmacol 76:3, 1982.

300. Monnier VM, Cerami A: Non-enzymatic browning *in vivo*. Possible process for aging of long-lived proteins. Science 211:491–493, 1981.

301. Monnier VM: Toward a Maillard reaction theory of aging. Prog Clin Biol Res 304:1–22, 1989.

302. Monnier VM, et al: Relations between complications to type I diabetes mellitus and collagen-linked fluorescence. N Engl J Med 314:403–408, 1986.

303. Monnier VM, et al: Collagen browning and cross-linking are increased in chronic experimental hyperglycemia. Relevance to diabetes and aging. Diabetes 37:867–872, 1988.

304. Morabito E, Corsico N, Arrigoni Martelli E: Endothelins urinary excretion is increased in spontaneously diabetic rats: BB/BB. Life Sci 56:PL13, 1995.

305. Morise T, et al: Increased plasma levels of immunoreactive endothelin and von Willebrand factor in NIDDM patients. Diabetes Care 18:87, 1995.

306. Mullarkey CJ, Edelstein D, Brownlee M: Free radical generation by early glycation products: A mechanism for accelerated atherogenesis in diabetes. Biochem Biophys Res Commun 173:932–939, 1990.

307. Musson RA, Shafran H, Henson PM: Intracellular levels and stimulated release of lysosomal enzymes from human peripheral blood monocytes and monocyte-derived macrophages. J Reticuloendothel Soc 28:249–264, 1980.

308. Myrup B, Mathiesen ER, Ronn B, et al: Endothelial function and serum lipids in the course of developing microalbuminuria in insulin-dependent diabetes mellitus. Diabetes Res 26:33, 1994.

309. Nagaraj RH, Portero-Otin M, Monnier VM: Pyrraline ether crosslinks as a basis for protein cross-linking by the advanced Maillard reaction in aging and diabetes. Arch Biochem Biophys 325:152–158, 1996.

310. Nakagawara A, Nathan CF, Cohn ZA: Hydrogen peroxide metabolism in human monocytes during differentiation *in vitro*. J Clin Invest 68:1243–1252, 1981.

311. Nakamura K, et al: Crosslines A and B as candidates for the fluorophores in age- and diabetes-related cross-linked proteins, and their diacetates produced by Maillard reaction of -N-acetyl-L-lysine with D-glucose. J Chem Soc Chem Commun 992–994, 1992.

312. Nathan CF, Murray HW, Cohn ZA: The macrophage as an effector cell. N Engl J Med 303:622–626, 1980.

313. Navab M, et al: Monocyte transmigration induced by modification of low density lipoprotein in cocultures of human aortic wall cells is due to induction of monocyte chemotactic protein 1 synthesis and is abolished by high density lipoprotein. J Clin Invest 88:2039–2046, 1991.

314. Navab M, et al: A new anti-inflammatory compound, Leumedin, inhibits modification of low density lipoprotein and the resulting monocyte transmigration into the subendothelial space of cocultures of human aortic wall cells. J Clin Invest 91:1225–1230, 1993.

315. Nawroth PP, et al: Tumor necrosis factor/cachectin interacts with endothelial cell receptors to induce release of interleukin-1. J Exp Med 165:1363–1375, 1986.

316. Nievelstein PFEM, et al: Lipid accumulation in rabbit aortic intima 2 hours after bolus infusion of LDL: A deep-etch and immunolocalization study of rapidly frozen tissue. Arterioscler Thromb 11:1795–1805, 1991.

317. Nikilla EA: High density lipoproteins in diabetes. Diabetes 30(Suppl 2):82, 1981.

318. Nishimura M, et al: The effect of PGI_2 analogue on vascular endothelial function and platelet aggregation in patients with NIDDM. J Diabetes Complications 9:330, 1995.

319. Njoroge FG, Monnier VM: The chemistry of the Maillard reaction under physiological conditions: A review. Prog Clin Biol Res 304:85–107, 1989.

320. Noda K, Umeda F, Nawata H: Effect of beraprost sodium on response to tests of autonomic control of heart rate in patients with diabetes mellitus. Diabetes Res Clin Pract 31:119, 1996.

321. Olson JA, et al: Soluble leucocyte adhesion molecules in diabetic retinopathy stimulate retinal capillary endothelial cell migration. Diabetologia 40:1166, 1997.

322. Ono Y, et al: Expression of prostacyclin-stimulating factor, a novel protein, in tissues of Wistar rats and in cultured cells. Biochem Biophys Res Commun 202:1490, 1994.

323. Osmundson PJ, et al: Course of peripheral occlusive arterial disease in diabetes. Diabetes Care 2:143–152, 1990.

324. Ostermann H, van de Loo J: Factors of the haemostatic system in diabetic patients: A survey of controlled studies. Haemostasis 16:386–416, 1986.

325. Otsuki M, et al: Circulating vascular cell adhesion molecule-1 (VCAM-1) in atherosclerotic NIDDM patients. Diabetes 46:2096, 1997.

326. Oxlund H, et al: Increased aortic stiffness in patients with type 1 (insulin-dependent) diabetes mellitus. Diabetologia 32:748–752, 1989.

327. O'Brien KD, et al: Vascular cell adhesion molecule-1 is expressed in human coronary atherosclerotic plaques. J Clin Invest 92:945, 1993.

328. Palinski W, et al: Low density lipoprotein undergoes oxidative modification *in vivo*. Proc Natl Acad Sci U S A 86:1372–1376, 1989.

329. Palmer RMJ, Ferrige AF, Moncada S: Nitric oxide release accounts for the biological activity of endothelium-derived relaxing factor. Nature 327:524, 1987.

330. Palumbo PJ, et al: Progression of peripheral occlusive arterial disease in diabetes mellitus—what factors are predictive? Arch Intern Med 151:717–721, 1991.

331. Parinandi NL, Thompson EW, Schmid HH: Diabetic heart and kidney exhibit increased resistance to lipid peroxidation. Biochim Biophys Acta 1047:63–69, 1990.

332. Parthasarathy S, et al: Probucol inhibits oxidative modification of low density lipoprotein. J Clin Invest 77:641–644, 1986.

333. Parving HH, et al: Prevalence of microalbuminuria, arterial hypertension retinopathy and neuropathy in patients with insulin-dependent diabetes mellitus. Br Med J 296:156, 1988.

334. Pierce GN, Maddaford TG, Russell JC: Cardiovascular dysfunction in insulin-dependent and non-insulin-dependent animal models of diabetes mellitus. Can J Physiol Pharmacol 75:343, 1997.

335. Pigott R, et al: Soluble forms of E-selectin, ICAM-1 and VCAM-1 are present in the supernatants of cytokine activated cultured endothelial cells. Biochem Biophys Res Commun 187:584, 1992.

336. Pitas RE, Innerarity TL, Mahley RW: Foam cells in explants of atherosclerotic rabbit aortas have receptors for very low density lipoproteins and

modified low density lipoproteins. Arteriosclerosis 3:1, 1983.

337. Pitei DL, Watkins PJ, Edmonds ME: NO-dependent smooth muscle vasodilatation is reduced in NIDDM patients with peripheral sensory neuropathy. Diabet Med 14:284, 1997.

338. Plater ME, et al: Elevated von Willebrand factor antigen predicts deterioration in diabetic peripheral nerve function. Diabetologist 39:336, 1996.

339. Platti P, et al: Hypertriglyceridemia and hyperinsulinemia are potent inducers of endothelin-1 release in humans. Diabetes 45:316, 1996.

340. Pohlman T, et al: An endothelial cell surface factor(s) induced in vitro by lipopolysaccharide, interleukin-1 and tumor necrosis factor increases neutrophil adherence by a CDw18-dependent mechanism. J Immunol 136:4548–4553, 1986.

341. Portero-Otin M, Nagaraj RH, Monnier VM: Chromatographic evidence for pyrraline formation during protein glycation in vitro and in vivo. Biochim Biophys Acta 1247:74–80, 1995.

342. Poston RN, et al: Expression of intercellular adhesion molecule-1 in atherosclerotic plaques. Am J Pathol 140:665, 1992.

343. Printeseva OY, Peclo MM, Gowen AM: Various cell types in human atherosclerotic lesions express ICAM-1: Further immunocytochemical and immunochemical studies employing monoclonal antibody 10F3. Am J Pathol 140:889, 1992.

344. Properzi G, et al: Early increase precedes a depletion of endothelin-1 but not of von Willebrand factor in cutaneous microvessels of diabetic patients. A quantitative immunohistochemical study. J Pathol 175:243, 1995.

345. Purnell JQ, et al: Levels of lipoprotein (a), apolipoprotein B, and lipoprotein cholesterol distribution in IDDM. Results from follow-up in the Diabetes Control and Complications Trial. Diabetes 44:1218–1226, 1995.

346. Pushkarsky T, et al: Molecular characterization of a mouse genomic element mobilized by advanced glycation endproduct modified-DNA (AGE-DNA). Mol Med 3:740–749, 1997.

347. Pyorala K: Relationship of glucose tolerance and plasma insulin to the incidence of coronary heart disease: Results from two population studies in Finland. Diabetes Care 2:131–141, 1979.

348. Rabinovitch A, et al: Human pancreatic islet β-cell destruction by cytokines involves oxygen free radicals and aldehyde production. J Clin Endocrinol Metab 81:3197, 1996.

349. Raines EW, Dower SK, Ross R: Interleukin-1 mitogenic activity for fibroblasts and smooth muscle cells is due to PDGF-AA. Science 243:393–396, 1989.

350. Rajavashisth TB, et al: Induction of endothelial cell expression of granulocyte and macrophage colony-stimulating factors by modified low density lipoproteins. Nature 344:254–257, 1990.

351. Rasmussen O, et al: Decrease in von Willebrand factor levels after a high-monounsaturated-fat diet in non-insulin-dependent diabetic subjects. Metabolism 43:1406, 1994.

352. Reaven GM, Javorski WC, Reaven EP: Diabetic hypertriglyceridemia. Am J Med Sci 269:382, 1975.

353. Reaven P, et al: Effects of oleate-rich and linoleate-rich diets on the susceptibility of low density lipoprotein to oxidative modification in mildly hyper-cholesterolemic subjects. J Clin Invest 91:668–676, 1993.

354. Reddy S, et al: N epsilon-(carboxymethyl)lysine is a dominant advanced glycation end product (AGE) antigen in tissue proteins. Biochemistry 34:10872–10878, 1995.

355. Remuzzi G, Benigni A: Progression of proteinuric diabetic and nondiabetic renal diseases: A possible role for renal endothelin. Kidney Int Suppl 58:S66, 1997.

356. Requena JR: The main mechanism of action of aminoguanidine. Diabetologia 34(Suppl 2):A162, 1991.

357. Requena JR, et al: N -(carboxymethyl)ethanolamine: A biomarker of phospholipid modification by the Maillard Reaction in vivo. J Biol Chem 272:17473–17479, 1997.

358. Requena JR, et al: Quantitation of malondialdehyde and 4-hydroxynonenal adducts to lysine residues in native and oxidized human LDL. Biochem J 322:317–325, 1997.

359. Requena JR, et al: Lipoxidation products as biomarkers of oxidative damage to proteins during lipid peroxidation reactions. Nephrol Dial Transplant 11(Suppl 5):48–53, 1996.

360. Ridker PM, et al: Prospective study of endogenous tissue plasminogen activator and risk of stroke. Lancet 343:940–943, 1994.

361. Ridker PM, Vaughan DE, Stampfer MJ, et al: Endogenous tissue-type activator and risk of myocardial infarction. Lancet 341:1165–1168, 1993.

362. Roep BO, et al: Soluble forms of intercellular adhesion molecule-1 in insulin-dependent diabetes mellitus. Lancet 343:1590, 1994.

363. Ronnemaa T, et al: Serum lipids, lipoproteins, and apolipoproteins and the excessive occurrence of coronary heart disease in non-insulin-dependent diabetic patients. Am J Epidemiol 130:632–645, 1989.

364. Rosenberg H, et al: Glycosylated collagen. Biochem Biophys Res Commun 91:498–501, 1979.

365. Rosove MH, Frank HJL, Harwing SSL: Plasma beta-thromboglobulin, platelet factor 4, fibrinopeptide A, and other hemostatic functions during improved, short-term glycemic control in diabetes mellitus. Diabetes Care 7:174–179, 1984.

366. Ross R: The pathogenesis of atherosclerosis: A perspective for the 1990s. Nature 362:801–809, 1993.

367. Ross R: Mechanisms of atherosclerosis—a review. Adv Nephrol 19:79–86, 1990.

368. Ross R, et al: Localization of PDGF-B protein in macrophages in all phases of atherogenesis. Science 248:1009–1012, 1990.

369. Saito M, Nishi K, Fukumoto Y, et al: Characterization of endothelin receptors in streptozotocin-induced diabetic rat vas deferens. Biochem Pharmacol 52:1593, 1996.

370. Salonen JT, et al: Autoantibody against oxidized LDL and progression of carotid atherosclerosis. Lancet 339:883–887, 1992.

371. Salonen JT: Is there a continuing need for longitudinal epidemiologic research—the Kuopio ischaemic heart disease risk factor study. Ann Clin Res 20:46–50, 1988.

372. Sasaki J, Cottam GL: Glycosylation of LDL decreases its ability to interact with high-affinity receptors of human fibroblasts in vitro and decreases its clearance from rabbit plasma in vivo. Biochem Biophys Acta 713:199–207, 1982.

373. Scanu AM, Scandiani L: Lipoprotein (a). *In* Stollerman GH (ed): Structure, Biology and Clinical Relevance. St. Louis, Mosby-Year Book, 1991, pp 249–270.

374. Schleicher E, Deufel T, Wieland OH: Nonenzymatic glycosylation of human serum lipoproteins. FEBS Lett 129:1–4, 1981.

375. Schmetterer L, et al: Nitric oxide and ocular blood flow in patients with IDDM. Diabetes 46:653, 1997.

376. Schmetterer L, et al: The effect of systemic nitric oxide-synthase inhibition on ocular fundus pulsations in man. Exp Eye Res 64:305, 1997.

377. Schmidt AM, et al: Elevated plasma levels of vascular cell adhesion molecule-1 (VCAM-1) in diabetic patients with microalbuminuria: A marker of vascular dysfunction and progressive vascular disease. Br J Haematol 92:747, 1996.

378. Schneider SL, Kohn RR: Glycosylation of human collagen in aging and diabetes mellitus. J Clin Invest 66:1179–1181, 1980.

379. Schnider SL, Kohn RR: Effects of age and diabetes mellitus on the solubility and non-enzymatic glucosylation of human skin collagen. J Clin Invest 67:1630–1635, 1981.

380. Schwartz D, et al: The role of a *gro* homolgue in monocyte adhesion to endothelium. J Clin Invest 94:1968–1973, 1994.

381. Schwenke DC, Carew TE: Initiation of atherosclerotic lesions in cholesterol-fed rabbits, II: Selective retention of LDL vs selective increases in LDL permeability in susceptible sites of arteries. Arteriosclerosis 9:908–918, 1989.

382. Sekiguchi N, et al: Immunohistochemical study of prostacyclin-stimulating factor (PSF) in the diabetic and atherosclerotic human coronary artery. Diabetes 46:1627, 1997.

383. Sell DR, Monnier VM: End-stage renal disease and diabetes catalyze the formation of a pentose-derived crosslink from aging human collagen. J Clin Invest 85:380–384, 1990.

384. Sell DR, Lapolla A, Monnier VM: Relationship between pentosidine and the complications of long-standing type 1 diabetes. Diabetes 40:302A, 1991.

385. Sell DR, Monnier VM: Structure elucidation of a senescence cross-link from human extracellular matrix. Implication of pentoses in the aging process. J Biol Chem 264:21597–21602, 1989.

386. Sell DR, et al: Pentosidine formation in skin correlates with severity of complications in individuals with long-standing IDDM. Diabetes 41:1286–1292, 1992.

387. Semenkovich CF, Ostlund RE Jr, Schechtman KB: Plasma lipids in patients with type I diabetes mellitus: Influence of race, gender and plasma glucose control: Lipids do not correlate with glucose control in black women. Arch Intern Med 149:51–56, 1989.

388. Seth R, Raymond FD, Makgoba MW: Circulating ICAM-1 isoforms: Diagnostic prospects for inflammatory and immune disorders. Lancet 338:83, 1991.

389. Shimabukuro M, et al: Role of nitric oxide in obesity-induced β-cell disease. J Clin Invest 100:290, 1997.

390. Shimabukuro M, et al: Leptin- or troglitazone-induced lipopenia protects islets from interleukin-1β cytotoxicity, J Clin Invest 100:1750, 1997.

391. Shin SJ, Lee YJ, Tsai JH: The correlation of plasma and urine endothelin-1 with the severity of nephropathy in Chinese patients with type 2 diabetes. Scand J Clin Lab Invest 56:571, 1996.

392. Smith MA, et al: Advanced Maillard reaction end products, free radicals, and protein oxidation in Alzheimer's disease. Ann N Y Acad Sci 738:447–454, 1994.

393. Sosenko JM, et al: Hyperglycemia and plasma lipid levels: A prospective study of young insulin-dependent diabetic patients. N Engl J Med 302:650, 1980.

394. Soulis-Liparota T, et al: Retardation by aminoguanidine of development of albuminuria, mesangial expansion, and tissue fluorescence in streptozotocin-induced diabetic rat. Diabetes 40:1328–1334, 1991.

395. Stamler J: Epidemiology, established major risk factors, and the primary prevention of coronary heart disease. *In* Parmley W, Chatterjee K (eds): Cardiology. Philadelphia: JB Lippincott Company, 1987, pp 1–41.

396. Standl E, et al: Predictors of 10-year macrovascular and overall mortality in patients with NIDDM: The Munich General Practitioner Project. Diabetologia 39:1540, 1996.

397. Standl E, Janka HV: High serum insulin concentrations in relation to other cardiovascular risk factors in macrovascular disease of type 2 diabetes. Horm Metab Res 17(Suppl):46–51, 1985.

398. Stassi G, et al: Nitric oxide primes pancreatic β-cells for Fas-mediated destruction in insulin-dependent diabetes mellitus. J Exp Med 186:1193, 1997.

399. Steering Committee of the Physician's Health Study Research Group: Final report on the aspirin component of the ongoing physicians' health study. N Engl J Med 321:129–135, 1989.

400. Stehouwer CDA, et al: Urinary albumin excretion, cardiovascular disease, and endothelial dysfunction in non-insulin dependent diabetes mellitus. Lancet 340:319, 1992.

401. Stehouwer CDA, et al: von Willebrand factor and early diabetic retinopathy: No evidence for a relationship in patients with type 1 (insulin-dependent) diabetes mellitus and normal albumin excretion. Diabetologia 35:555, 1992.

402. Stehouwer CDA, et al: Endothelial dysfunction precedes development of microalbuminuria in IDDM. Diabetes 44:561, 1995.

403. Stein Y, et al: The removal of cholesterol from aortic smooth muscle cells in culture and Landschutz ascites cell fractions of human high density apoproteins. Biochem Biophys Acta 380:106, 1975.

404. Steinberg D: Antioxidants and atherosclerosis: A current assessment. Circulation 84:1420–1425, 1991.

405. Steinberg D, et al: Beyond cholesterol. Modifications of low-density lipoprotein that increase its atherogenicity. N Engl J Med 320:915, 1989.

406. Steinbrecher UP, Witztum JL: Glucosylation of low density lipoproteins to an extent comparable to that seen in diabetes slows their catabolism. Diabetes 33:130–134, 1984.

407. Steiner M, et al: Increased levels of soluble adhesion molecules in type 2 (non-insulin-dependent) diabetes mellitus are independent of glycaemic control. Thromb Haemost 72:979, 1994.

408. Steiner L, et al: Endothelial cells as cytotoxic effector cells: Cytokine-activated rat islet endothe-

lial cells lyse syngeneic islet cells via nitric oxide. Diabetologia 40:150, 1997.

409. Stevens MJ, Feldman EL, Greene DA: The etiology of diabetic neuropathy: The combined roles of metabolic and vascular defects. Diabet Med 12:566, 1995.

410. Stevens MJ: Nitric oxide as a potential bridge between the metabolic and vascular hypotheses of diabetic neuropathy. Diabet Med 12:292, 1995.

411. Stiko-Rabrin A, et al: Secretion of plasminogen activator inhibitor l from cultured human umbilical vein endothelial cells is induced by very low density lipoprotein. Arteriosclerosis 10:1067–1073, 1990.

412. Stitt AW, et al: Intracellular advanced glycation endproducts (AGEs) co-localize with AGE-receptors in the retinal vasculature of diabetic and AGE-infused rats. Diabetes 45(Suppl 2):15A, 1996.

413. Stitt AW, et al: Elevated AGE-modified ApoB in sera of euglycemic, normolipidemic patients with atherosclerosis: Relationship to tissue AGEs. Mol Med 3:617–627, 1997.

414. Stolar MW: Atherosclerosis in diabetes: The role of hyperinsulinemia. Metabolism 2(Suppl 1):1–9, 1988.

415. Stout RW: Insulin and atheroma: An update. Lancet 1:1077, 1987.

416. Stringer HAR, et al: Plasminogen activator inhibitor-1 released from activated platelets plays a key role in thrombolysis resistance. Studies with thrombi generated in the Chandler loop. Arterioscler Thromb 14:1452–1458, 1994.

417. Sullivan ME, et al: Alterations in endothelin B receptor sits in cavernosal tissue of diabetic rabbits: Potential relevance to the pathogenesis of erectile dysfunction. J Urol 158:1966, 1997.

418. Suminski R, et al: Plasminogen activator inhibitor-1 (PAI-1) and tissue plasminogen activator-plasminogen activator inhibitor-1 (tPA-PAI-1) in IDDM: Profile by complications. Diabetes 43(Suppl 1):197A, 1994.

419. Swan HJC: Acute myocardial infarction: A failure of timely, spontaneous thrombolysis. J Am Coll Cardiol 13:1435–1437, 1989.

420. Szondy E, et al: Occurrence of anti-low density lipoprotein antibodies and circulating immune complexes in aged subjects. Mech Ageing Dev 29:117–123, 1985.

421. Takagi C, et al: Regulation of retinal hemodynamics in diabetic rats by increased expression and action of endothelin-1. Invest Ophthalmol Vis Sci 37:2504, 1996.

422. Takahashi K, et al: Elevated plasma endothelin in patients with diabetes mellitus. Diabetologia 33:306, 1990.

423. Tertov VV, et al: Low density lipoprotein-containing circulating immune complexes and coronary atherosclerosis. Exp Mol Pathol 52:300–308, 1990.

424. Thomas SR, Neuzil J, Stocker R: Cosupplementation with coenzyme Q prevents the prooxidant effect of α-tocopherol and increases the resistance of LDL to transition metal-dependent oxidation initiation. Arterioscler Thromb Vasc Biol 16:687–696, 1996.

425. Thomsen C, et al: Plasma levels of von Willebrand factor in non-insulin-dependent diabetes mellitus are influenced by dietary monounsaturated fatty acids. Thromb Res 77:347, 1995.

426. Thornalley PJ, et al: Formation of methylglyoxal-modified proteins in vitro and in vivo and their involvement in AGE-related processes. Contrib Nephrol 112:24–31, 1995.

427. Throckmorton DC, Brogden AP, Min B, et al: PDGF and TGF-beta mediate collagen production by mesangial cells exposed to advanced glycosylation end products. Kidney Int 48:111–117, 1995.

428. Tonnensen MG, et al: Adherence of neutrophils to cultured human microvascular endothelial cells. J Clin Invest 83:637, 1989.

429. Trachtman H, Futterweit S, Crimmins DL: High glucose inhibits nitric oxide production in cultured rat mesangial cells. J Am Soc Nephrol 8:1276, 1997.

430. Traub O, Van Bibber R: Role of nitric oxide in insulin-dependent diabetes mellitus-related vascular complications. West J Med 162:439, 1995.

431. Tschoepe D: Adhesion molecules influencing atherosclerosis. Diabetes Res Clin Pract 30(Suppl): 19, 1996.

432. Ueno Y, Koike H, Nakamura Y, et al: Effects of beraprost sodium, a prostacyclin analogue, on diabetic neuropathy in streptozotocin-induced diabetic rats. Jpn J Pharmacol 70:177, 1996.

433. Ueno Y, Koike H, Nishio S: Beneficial effects of beraprost sodium, a stable prostacyclin analogue, in diabetic cardiomyopathy. J Cardiovasc Pharmacol 26:603, 1995.

434. Umeda F, Masakado M, Takei A: Difference in serum-induced prostacyclin production by cultured aortic and capillary endothelial cells. Prostaglandins Leukot Essent Fatty Acids 56:51, 1997.

435. Umeda F, Inoguchi T, Nawata H: Reduced stimulatory activity on prostacyclin production by cultured endothelial cells in serum from aged and diabetic patients. Atherosclerosis 75:61, 1989.

436. Undelhoven WM, et al: Smoking alters thromboxane metabolism in man. Biochem Biophys Acta 108:197, 1991.

437. Uusipupa MIJ, et al: Serum lipids and lipoproteins in newly diagnosed non-insulin-dependent (type II) diabetic patients, with special reference to factors influencing HDL-cholesterol and triglyceride levels. Diabetes Care 9:17–22, 1986.

438. Uusitupa MIJ, et al: 5-year incidence of atherosclerotic vascular disease in relation of general risk factors, insulin level, and abnormalities in lipoprotein composition in non-insulin-dependent diabetic and nondiabetic subjects. Circulation 82:27–36, 1990.

439. Vague P, et al: Correlation between blood fibrinolytic activity, plasminogen activator inhibitor level, plasma insulin level and relative body weight in normal and obese subjects. Metabolism 2:250–253, 1986.

440. Vague P: Insulin and the fibrinolytic system. IDF Bull 36:15–17, 1991.

441. Vague P, et al: Fat distribution and plasminogen activator inhibitor activity in nondiabetic obese women. Metabolism 38:913–915, 1989.

442. van der Wal AC, et al: Adhesion molecules on the endothelium and mononuclear cells in human atherosclerotic lesions. Am J Pathol 141:1427, 1992.

443. Vasan S, et al: Design, synthesis, and pharmacological activity of a novel class of thiazolium-based compounds that cleave established AGE-derived protein crosslinks. Diabetes 45(Suppl 2):28A, 1996.

444. Virella G, et al: Activation of human monocyte-derived macrophages by immune complexes containing low density lipoprotein. Clin Immunol Immunopathol 75:179–189, 1995.

445. Vishwanath V, et al: Glycosylation of skin collagen in type I diabetes mellitus: Correlations with long-term complications. Diabetes 35:916–921, 1986.

446. Vlassara H, et al: Advanced glycosylation end products on erythrocyte cell surface induce receptor-mediated phagocytosis by macrophages. A model for turnover of aging cells. J Exp Med 166:539–549, 1987.

447. Vlassara H, et al: Advanced glycation end products induce glomerular sclerosis and albuminuria in normal rats. Proc Natl Acad Sci U S A 91:11704–11708, 1994.

448. Vlassara H, et al: Cachectin/TNF and IL-1 induced by glucose-modified proteins: Role in normal tissue remodeling. Science 240:1546–1548, 1988.

449. Vlassara H, Brownlee M, Cerami A: Novel macrophage receptor for glucose-modified proteins is distinct from previously described scavenger receptors. J Exp Med 164:1301–1309, 1986.

450. Vlassara H, et al: Advanced glycation endproducts promote adhesion molecule (VCAM-1, ICAM-1) expression and atheroma formation in normal rabbits. Mol Med 1:447–456, 1995.

451. Vogt BW, Schleicher ED, Wieland OH: Episilon-amino-lysine-bound glucose in human tissues obtained at autopsy. Diabetes 31:1123–1127, 1982.

452. Vukovich TC, Schernthaner G: Decreased protein C levels in patients with insulin-dependent type I diabetes mellitus. Diabetes 35:617–619, 1986.

453. Wang LN, et al: Effects of the PGI$_2$ analog beraprost sodium on glomerular prostanoid synthesis in rats with streptozotocin-induced diabetes. Nephron 73:637, 1996.

454. Want-Iverson P, et al: Apo E-mediated uptake and degradation of normal very low density lipoproteins by human monocyte/macrophages: A saturable pathway distinct for the LDL receptor. Biochem Biophys Res Commun 126:578, 1985.

455. Warner SJC, Auger KR, Libby P: Interleukin-1 induces interleukin-1. II. Recombinant human interleukin-1 induces interleukin-1 production by adult human vascular endothelial cells. J Immunol 139:1911–1917, 1987.

456. Wascher TC, et al: Involvement of the l-arginine-nitric oxide pathway in hyperglycaemia-induced coronary artery dysfunction of isolated guinea pig hearts. Eur J Clin Invest 26:707, 1996.

457. Watanabe J, et al: Enhancement of platelet aggregation by low density lipoproteins from IDDM patients. Diabetes 37:1652–1657, 1988.

458. Wautier JL, et al: Receptor-mediated endothelial cell dysfunction in diabetic vasculopathy. Soluble receptor for advanced glycation end products blocks hyperpermeability in diabetic rats. J Clin Invest 97:238–243, 1996.

459. Weisweiler P, Dransner M, Schwandt P: Dietary effects on very low density lipoproteins in type II (non-insulin dependent) diabetes mellitus. Diabetologia 23:101, 1982.

460. Welborne TA, Wearne K: Coronary heart disease incidence and cardiovascular mortality in Busselton with reference to glucose and insulin concentrations. Diabetes Care 2:154–160, 1979.

461. Wells-Knecht MC, et al: Age-dependent increase in orthotyrosine and methionine sulfoxide in human skin collagen is not accelerated in diabetes. Evidence against a generalized increase in oxidative stress in diabetes. J Clin Invest 100:839–846, 1997.

462. Werb Z, Bonda MJ, Jones PA: Degradation of connective tissue matrices by macrophages: I. Proteolysis of elastin, glycoproteins, and collagens by proteinases isolated from macrophages. J Exp Med 152:1340–1357, 1980.

463. Wessels J, et al: Nitric oxide synthase inhibition in a spontaneously hypertensive rat model of diabetic nephropathy. Clin Exp Pharmacol Physiol 24:451, 1997.

464. Wheelock FC, Marble A: Surgery and diabetes. In Marble A, White P, Bradley RF, et al (eds): Joslin's Diabetes Mellitus, 11th ed. Philadelphia: Lea & Febiger, 1971, pp 599–620.

465. Wilhelmsen L, et al: Fibrinogen as a risk factor for stroke and myocardial infarction. N Engl J Med 311:501–505, 1984.

466. Williams SB, et al: Impaired nitric oxide-mediated vasodilation in patients with non-insulin-dependent diabetes mellitus. J Am Coll Cardiol 27:567, 1996.

467. Witztum JL, et al: Nonenzymatic glucosylation of low-density lipoprotein alters its biologic activity. Diabetes 31:283–291, 1982.

468. Witztum JL, et al: Nonenzymatic glucosylation of high-density lipoprotein accelerates its catabolism in guinea pigs. Diabetes 31:1029–1032, 1982.

469. Witztum JL, et al: Autoantibodies to glucosylated proteins in the plasma of patients with diabetes mellitus. Proc Natl Acad Sci U S A 81:3204–3208, 1984.

470. Witztum JL, et al: Nonenzymatic glucosylation of homologous low density lipoprotein and albumin renders them immunogenic in the guinea pig. Proc Natl Acad Sci U S A 80:2757–2761, 1983.

471. Wolff SP, Dean RT: Glucose autoxidation and protein modification: The potential role of "autoxidative glycosylation" in diabetes mellitus. Biochem J 245:243–250, 1987.

472. Wolpert HA, et al: Insulin modulates circulating endothelin-1 levels in humans. Metabolism 42:1027, 1993.

473. Wu G, Flynn NE: The activation of the arginine-citrulline cycle in macrophages from the spontaneously diabetic BB rat. Biochem J 294:113–118, 1993.

474. Wu G: Nitric oxide synthesis and the effect of aminoguanidine and N^G-monomethyl-L-arginine on the onset of diabetes in the spontaneously diabetic BB rat. Diabetes 44:360, 1995.

475. Yamagishi S, et al: Receptor-mediated toxicity to pericytes of advanced glycosylation end products: A possible mechanism of pericyte loss in diabetic microangiopathy. Biochem Biophys Res Commun 213:681–687, 1995.

476. Yamauchi T, et al: Purification and molecular cloning of prostacyclin-stimulating factor from serum-free conditioned medium of human diploid fibroblast cells. Biochem J 303:591, 1994.

477. Yamauchi T, et al: Enhanced secretion of endothelin-1 by elevated glucose levels from cultured bovine aortic endothelial cells. FEBS Lett 267:16, 1990.

478. Yanagisawa M, et al: Primary structure, synthesis, and biological activity of rat endothlin, an endothe-

lium-derived vasoconstrictor. Proc Natl Acad Sci U S A 85:6964, 1988.

479. Yanagisawa M, et al: A novel potent vasoconstrictor peptide produced by vascular endothelial cells. Nature 332:411, 1988.

480. Yang CW, et al: Administration of AGEs in vivo induces genes implicated in diabetic glomerulosclerosis. Kidney Int 49:S55–S58, 1995.

481. Yang XD, et al: The role of cell adhesion molecules in the development of IDDM: Implication for pathogenesis and therapy. Diabetes 45:705, 1996.

482. Yang XD, et al: A predominant role of integrin alpha 4 in the spontaneous development of autoimmune diabetes in nonobese diabetic mice. Proc Natl Acad Sci U S A 91:12604, 1994.

483. Yang XD, et al: Cell adhesion molecules: A selective therapeutic target for alleviation of IDDM. J Autoimmun 7:859, 1994.

484. Yoshimori K, et al: Presence of crosslines, a novel advanced glycosylation end products (AGEs) in diabetics. Diabetes 45(Suppl 2):260A, 1996.

485. Young IS, Torney JJ, Trimble ER: The effect of ascorbate supplementation on oxidative stress in the streptozotocin diabetic rat. Free Rad Biol Med 13:41–46, 1992.

486. Yue DK, et al: The thermal stability of collagen in diabetic rats: Correlation with severity of diabetes and nonenzymatic glycosylation. Diabetologia 24:282–285, 1983.

487. Zimmerman GA, Prescott SM, McIntyre TM: Endothelial cell interactions with granulocytes: Tethering and signaling molecules. Immunol Today 13:93–100, 1992.

488. Zimmermann PA, et al: Increased myogenic tone and diminished responsiveness to ATP-sensitive K⁺ channel openers in cerebral arteries from diabetic rats. Circ Res 81:996, 1997.

Chapter 5

HEMORHEOLOGY: PRINCIPLES AND CONCEPTS

■ Donald E. McMillan

The foot needs blood in order to function. Blood is a fluid that is distributed through the body by the pumping action of the heart. Fluids are a broad class of materials that behave by flowing when acted on by any driving force. Fluids differ from solids because solids resist continuing movement by generating a force through the magnitude of their internal deformation (Fig. 5–1). Fluids continue to move because their resistance to motion is generated by the motion itself. Even solids will flow (or break) when they are placed under sufficient force.

The systematic examination of flow is the scope of the scientific discipline called rheology, taken from *rheos,* the Greek word for a "flow" or "current." The study of blood's flow properties is called hemorheology. Blood has physical flow properties that are unique, and these unique properties are affected by disease states like diabetes. We will review here the features of blood flow and its control that may help in understanding and managing foot problems in diabetes.

The Concept of Blood Flow

Many fluids, including air and water, behave in a very regular way when acted on by force. They are referred to as newtonian because their response is analyzable using Newton's laws. In addition to formulating three basic laws for planetary motion (*Book I. The Motion of Bodies*), Newton experimented with movement of fluids, specifically water (*Book II. The Motion of Bodies in Resisting Mediums*). He found a simple and direct relation between applied force and responsive motion, like that expected from his second law of motion. The ratio of such a fluid's resistive force, σ, to its responsive motion or shear rate, γ, (see section "Blood as a Shear Thinning Fluid," below)

$$\eta = \frac{\sigma}{\dot{\gamma}}$$

where η is the fluid's viscosity, is normally stable at constant temperature. Blood does not respond so simply and hence is said to be nonnewtonian. Nonnewtonian fluids make up a broad class. We have day-to-day contact with many of them, principally as foods, inks, and cosmetics. None of the other nonnewtonian materials behaves exactly like blood.

Blood has unique cellular and plasma components. Its dominant cells are erythrocytes. They typically form 40% of blood's volume. Leukocytes form less than 1% of the volume but become very important in the microcirculation. Electrolytes and glucose are osmoti-

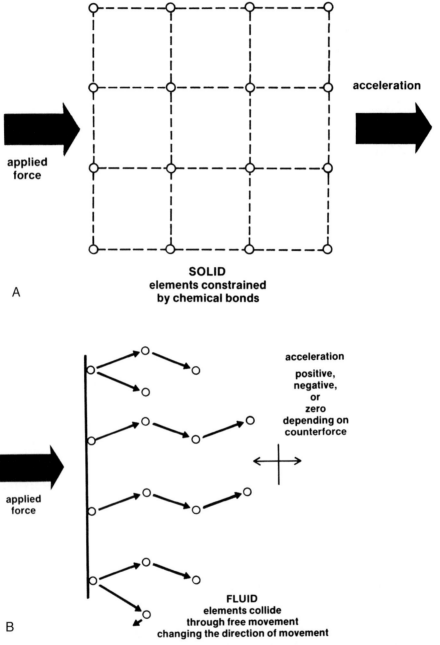

Figure 5–1 ■ Difference between solid (A) and fluid (B) deformation is diagrammed. In solid deformation, the elements of the material are held in place by interactions with their neighbors and resist movement more and more with greater displacement until the solid is disrupted. If no disruption occurs, the solid returns to its original shape by elastic recovery. A fluid resists deformation in proportion to the rate of displacement of its constituents relative to each other as long as there is time for the random motion of the elements relative to each other to dissipate the original momentum.

cally important, affecting red cell size, but they make only a very small direct contribution to blood's flow properties. Proteins in blood have effects on blood flow linked to both their shape and to their concentration. This happens because they interact with red cells based on their shape. The protein–red blood cell mixture in blood generates different flow responses depending on vessel size and flow rate.

Blood is designed to flow and to deliver oxygen to the tissues. But it must also stop flowing when necessary. This happens regularly following trauma, during menstruation, and after parturition. In order to do this, blood contains platelets to plug small defects in the vessel walls, like venipuncture sites and shaving nicks. Larger defects require local blood vessel constriction and the coagulation of the blood. A feature that helps slow local blood flow is the marked rise in blood flow resistance (viscosity; see Fig. 5–5) when flow is slowed. This feature of blood is conferred to it by the plasma proteins, especially fibrinogen. Fibrinogen is also responsible for clot formation. In disease states like diabetes, and in pregnancy, fibrinogen levels rise and blood viscosity at low flow (shear) rates becomes elevated.[62, 70] Fibrinogen and some closely related proteins have been associated cross-sectionally with diabetic complications.[82] Fibrinogen is also now well documented as a risk factor for cardiovascular disease in nondiabetics.[20, 125] Reports show it to have a similarly predictive role in diabetes.[66, 67, 97]

Inertial Versus Viscous Flow

Different blood flow properties are either more or less important in specific flow situations, particularly those seen in blood flow in the leg and foot. A review of both nonnewtonian fluid and circulatory flow concepts can help us understand which blood flow properties are most affected by diabetes. Fluid flow is commonly influenced by inertia, a property linked to mass. Fluids, like all materials in motion, try to continue movement in a straight line.

In the circulation there are very few straight paths so that blood usually cannot maintain straight line flow. It changes direction by using its motion energy and its surrounding vessel walls to generate pressure gradients. These pressure gradients cause blood flow to change in direction. Flow redirecting pressure gradients are seen mainly in large arteries and veins. In capillaries, change in flow direction is controlled by viscous drag generated using the inner wall of the turn.

The relative importance of inertia and viscous drag to the flow of newtonian fluids was systematized by the 19th century work of Sir Osborne Reynolds, who studied liquid flow in straight tubes.[96] He showed that three factors controlled the relative importance of vis-

cosity to inertia in linear flow. They are the velocity of the fluid, u, the diameter of the tube, d, and the kinematic viscosity of the fluid, ν. Kinematic viscosity is the fluid viscosity divided by the fluid's density. The relation is usually represented by an equation as the flow's Reynolds number, Re:

$$Re = \frac{u\ d}{\nu}$$

The ratio of the product of velocity and tube diameter to the kinematic viscosity has no dimension if the units used are the same and the fluid is newtonian. The Reynolds number portrays the relative importance of inertia and viscosity to flow in tubes and in structures roughly similar to tubes, the blood vessels (Table 5–1).

A flow at a Reynolds number that is less than 0.01 is characterized by a nearly uniform shearing motion. Direction change is mediated by the resistive force generated by local differences in rate of shearing. In contrast, flows with a Reynolds number of 100 or more change direction through inertia-generated pressure gradients.

Two important patterns are generated by the contrast between high Reynolds flow (>100) seen in arteries and low Reynolds flow (<0.01) seen in capillaries and small veins. Flow eddies are limited to larger vessels. Eddying has two effects. It causes the flow at the vessel wall to be uneven, increasing the local pressure drop. It also mixes blood locally, an important need in blood's oxygen delivery and other transport functions. In small veins and venules, this mixing

Table 5–1 ■ BLOOD VESSEL
REYNOLDS NUMBERS*

SIZE OF VESSEL	REYNOLDS NUMBER (RANGE)
Intracardiac	400–1,500
Aorta, large arteries	500–5,800
Muscular arteries	100–1,000
Primary arterioles	0.05–1.0
Small arterioles	0.07–0.7
Capillaries	~0.001
Small venules	0.05–0.5
Moderate-sized veins	50–500
Large veins	200–900

* Large Reynolds number flows (>100) are subject to much more inertial influence than lower Reynolds flows, whereas Reynolds number flows < 0.01 are dominated by viscous drag. Reynolds number flows > 2,000 are capable of generating turbulent patterns if tube length is long enough. Reynolds number flows around 1 (0.1 to 10) are mixtures of viscous and inertial behavior.

is absent. The flow is layered, as easily seen in fluorescein studies of the retina. Injected dye returns more rapidly after it passes through shorter and more direct vessel loops. The outer layers of the retinal venules fill with dye first and almost no mixing occurs.[82]

Nonmixing of blood can also be expected in most microvessels in the foot, but capillary flow is a little more complex. Red blood cells pass through capillaries one at a time. They are greater in diameter (8 μm) than true capillaries (usually 4 to 6 μm). The erythrocytes must deform to pass through a capillary. They tend to fill it completely. Their movement disturbs the layered flow of the local plasma. The result is a flow that acts to mix plasma between red cells called bolus flow.[50] This mixing effect enhances oxygen's passage into tissues. By this means, blood is uniquely well designed to defeat the lack of fluid mixing at low Reynolds flow by using red cells to force the needed mixing. This helps to explain why blood can be more viscous than hemoglobin solutions made from it by destroying red cell membranes and still supply oxygen more effectively than oxygen-binding macromolecules in plasma.

Blood flow in arterioles and small veins falls between the two extremes discussed above (see Table 5–1). Both inertial and viscous effects are important. Changes in local flow rate affect mixing efficiency, but slowing always reduces mixing and causes the tangential wall force due to viscous drag to decline.

Arteries to the Leg and Foot

Foot blood flow supplies three major tissue components: skin, muscle and bone. Little is known specifically about blood flow to foot bones; it is often assumed to be modest and stable. On the other hand, muscle flow is closely related to contractile activity, rising strikingly in parallel with oxygen consumption during intrinsic foot muscle contraction. Skin blood flow is determined principally by body core and environmental temperature, rising with the need to dissipate heat. It can change at least as strikingly as the flow associated with intrinsic muscle activity in the foot. A severalfold rise in foot flow is generated by vigorous walking or running.

It is useful to picture the circulation to the foot with both blood flow and blood's flow properties in mind. Blood passes to the foot through the arteries. The aorta gives rise to the common iliac and then the external iliac and femoral arteries. The superficial femoral branch passes medially and posteriorly through the adductor canal to become the popliteal artery. Below the knee, the popliteal gives rise to three arteries (Fig. 5–2). All three supply the foot, but two normally carry most of the flow. The anterior tibial artery changes direction abruptly as it passes forward and then downward with the anterolateral muscles of the leg. It passes then to the front of the ankle where it becomes the dorsalis pedis artery, supplying the dorsal and even plantar foot. The posterior tibial and peroneal arteries arise more directly as medial and lateral branches of the popliteal artery. The posterior tibial artery (medial in Fig. 5–2) is normally considerably larger. It passes behind the ankle's medial malleolus to supply the plantar foot and its muscles. The peroneal artery (lateral in Fig. 5–2) passes behind the lateral malleolus to supply the less muscular lateral foot. The upper leg's arterial anatomy is responsible for some features of arterial pressure around the ankle. The pressure is highest in the large and direct posterior tibial artery. A slightly lower pressure is usually found in the dorsalis pedis artery. Intraluminal pressure is not infrequently low or ultrasonically undetectable in the peroneal arteries at the ankle.

Two leg artery problems develop in diabetes. The more common is atherosclerotic occlusion. It is disproportionately distal in diabetes, affecting the branches of the popliteal more than the iliac and femoral arteries.[58] The development of occlusive disease below the knee enlarges the collateral arteries around the knee. Only infrequently is disease at this low level associated with symptoms of intermittent claudication.[58] Two reasons exist for this absence. First, the low site of occlusion impairs calf flow less than higher blockages. Second, pain appreciation is reduced by diabetic neuropathy and this can hide the symptoms. Clinical problems are commonly associated with ankle artery pressures below 80 mm Hg. At lower arterial perfusion pressure, injury- or infection-mediated gangrene is sometimes the initially recognized event. Several features of diabetic blood flow contribute to the low pressure and to gangrene development. Their detection can justify new treatments effective in reduc-

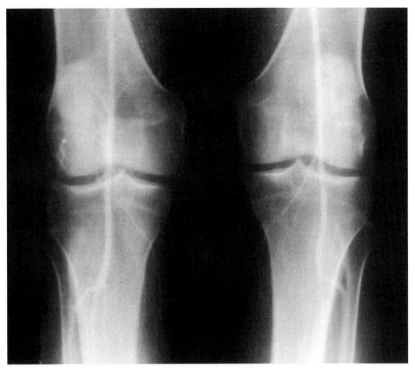

Figure 5–2 ■ Arteriogram of both knee areas shows how the popliteal artery gives rise to three branches after it passes behind the knee. A fork-like configuration on the left deserves the name trifurcation, while on the right the early takeoff of the anterior tibial and size disparity between the smaller posterior tibial and larger peroneal artery destroy the appropriateness of the name, also illustrating the variability of the arterial anatomy.

ing obstruction (see Tables 5–3, 5–4, and 5–5).

The second diabetes-associated problem is arterial wall calcification. This abnormality develops in the middle rather than the inner layer of the vessel wall. It interferes with leg blood pressure evaluation. Leg artery calcification also changes the distal arterial flow pattern and limits maximum blood flow to the foot.[19] Expansion of the artery wall during local systole is prevented so that larger rises in systolic pressure and greater systolic flow are delivered to the microvessels of the foot. Wall expansion is important in preventing atherosclerosis, so that arterial calcification interacts with gravity-mediated rises in intraluminal pressure to set the stage for plaque development at the branches of the popliteal artery.

The plantar forefoot has a deep arterial arch connecting the posterior tibial and dorsalis pedis terminal branches like the one in the palm of the hand that connects radial and ulnar arteries. This arch may be thrombosed by local infection. Blood problems generated by diabetes appear to add to this likelihood. Distal thrombosis can result in digital

artery occlusion and toe gangrene even when proximal foot arteries are completely patent, but leg artery occlusion is a far more common cause of gangrene.

Blood Flow in Leg Veins

Venous return in the leg has some unusual features linked to the dependent position normally occupied by the lower extremities. The saphenous veins have valves, an anatomic feature shared with the superficial forearm veins. The anatomic situation of the deep leg veins below the trifurcation is more unique. They are not only valved but are paired and ensheathed in common with their associated arteries (venae comitantes). This allows the arterial pulse to act to propel deep leg vein blood toward the heart. Arterial stiffening interferes with this mechanism. The result is a rise in intraluminal leg vein pressure. Walking also acts to assist deep vein blood to return to the heart. Loss of muscle due to diabetic neuropathy therefore further reduces blood return. Subcutaneous tissue pressure has been measured and found normally to be less than 3 mm Hg,[121] a value well below the oncotic pressure of the plasma. With a higher venous pressure in the ankle and foot, more fluid passes into the tissues and the efficiency of the lymphatic system is put to the test. This system is also equipped with valves and in health has the ability to contract and pump the lymph.

Effects of Autonomic Neuropathy on Flow

Diabetes is commonly followed by damage to the sympathetic nerves that control blood flow to the feet. The vasoconstrictive response to standing is substantially reduced[115] (Fig. 5–3). When a nondiabetic person stands up, skin blood flow to the feet drops to about 20% of resting supine flow. Reduced auto-

nomic activity in diabetes interferes with this degree of vasoconstriction so that flow to the skin of the feet while standing remains high.[90, 115] This means that leg artery flow in the standing position is unusually high in diabetes at the same time that gravity raises intraluminal leg artery pressure by more than 100 mm Hg. The unusually high intraluminal pressure stretches the arterial wall and reduces its degree of expansion with systole. Persistently high flow acts with reduced wall motion to favor atherosclerotic plaque formation[60] that can develop in leg arteries that would otherwise be protected by reduced flow.

Loss of this reflex may explain why atherosclerotic plaques cause more blockage in the leg than thigh arteries in diabetes and why leg artery atherosclerosis, in contrast with coronary disease, is commonly related in dia-

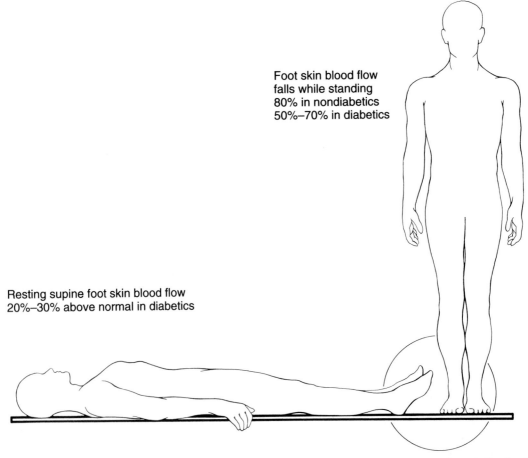

Foot skin blood flow
falls while standing
80% in nondiabetics
50%–70% in diabetics

Resting supine foot skin blood flow
20%–30% above normal in diabetics

Figure 5–3 ■ Figures portray two features of leg and foot blood flow in diabetes that may contribute to the development of leg artery disease in diabetes. Resting (not maximal) skin blood flow is usually high in diabetes, but on standing the normal approximately 80% fall in skin blood flow fails to develop, favoring substantially higher leg artery flow in diabetes when the subject is standing.

betes to disease duration as well as to age.[13] The autonomic neuropathy that allows persistently high foot blood flow in the standing posture[115] is probably also responsible for lowering nutritional flow relative to shunt microvessel flow in the foot in longstanding diabetes.[28]

The Role of Leukocytes in Blood Flow

Leukocytes have unusual importance in the microcirculation. White cells are kept in the main stream by the well-mixed flow present in large arteries and veins. But in smaller vessels, leukocytes tend to make contact with the vessel wall and then roll along if flow is sufficiently rapid. They tend to rest against the wall where flow is slow (in modest-sized venules). The tendency for leukocytes to be near the wall of small vessels is enhanced by high plasma fibrinogen levels,[29] raising the resting leukocyte count in small venules in diabetes.

Adherence of leukocytes to venule walls places them in the path of returning red cells, forcing the small aggregates of erythrocytes that have just passed through capillaries or shunt vessels and are clumped together (Fig. 5–4) to disaggregate again in order to pass the resting leukocytes.[99]

The leukocyte's microcirculatory role as an impeder of movement of red cells as they begin their return to the heart is furthered by fibrinogen. Fibrinogen promotes red cell aggregation. Two other agents that directly influence the leukocyte's role as a microcirculation obstructer are adrenalin and leukocyte-activating peptides. Adrenalin acts to alter microcirculatory flow and pressure. Both injected and endogenous epinephrine dislodge white cells resident in venules, reducing local flow resistance and raising the circulating white blood cell count. Leukocyte activation, by peptides like f-Met*Leu*Phe, that act to signal their increased responsiveness to chemoattractant chemicals and their ability to synthesize strong oxidants, also increases their adherence to vessel walls. Their activation may even result in permanent occlusion of tissue if arterial pressure is insufficient to dislodge them when they become lodged in arterioles and capillaries.[98] This is an attractive mechanism to explain the development of toe gangrene in advanced diabetic occlusive leg artery disease. Both activated monocytes and granulocytes can contribute to capillary nonperfusion in diabetic retinopathy.[101] Pharmacologic agents that can reverse the leukocyte's activation state and thereby improve microvascular flow have a role in management of advanced diabetic leg artery disease by affecting this phenomenon.

Blood As a Shear Thinning Fluid

We have pointed out physical, physiologic, and anatomic components of the diabetic foot's circulation. We now discuss more specific features of blood flow and the effects of diabetes on them. As already mentioned, blood is much more resistant to flow at low than at high shear rates. This property is called shear thinning. Shear is a word used to describe that component of motion within a material that distorts its planes rather than simply changing the relative positions of two points. The rate of distortion of local surfaces during fluid motion is referred to as shear rate. Movement of a small fluid area relative to an adjacent area occurs at one inverse second (the unit of shear rate) if the two areas move relative to each other in both position and rotation the same distance as the distance between them. If a similar amount of motion takes only 10 msec, then the local shear rate is 100 inverse seconds (100 sec^{-1}). For a newtonian fluid, the viscosity or ratio of resistive force generated locally by internal fluid motion is constant. This means that 100 times as much force resisting flow develops at 100 sec^{-1} as at 1 sec^{-1}. Blood is shear thinning (Fig. 5–5) and the flow resistance ratio is only about 20 because its viscosity falls fivefold from 1 sec^{-1} to 100 sec^{-1}. Overall, blood is typically at least 25 times as thick or viscous at very low shear rate (0.01 sec^{-1}) as at high shear rate (500 sec^{-1}).

The basis for blood's shear thinning behavior is the interaction of its red cells during flow. At hematocrits below 10%, blood shows little shear thinning and a 40 to 55% suspension of erythrocytes in saline is also almost newtonian. But as either the concentration of red cells rises to over 60% or plasma globulins are added, red cell suspensions become progressively more shear thinning, their low shear rate viscosity rising higher and higher. The basis for the rise is increasing contact between erythrocytes during flow. In the absence of globulins, each erythrocyte's nega-

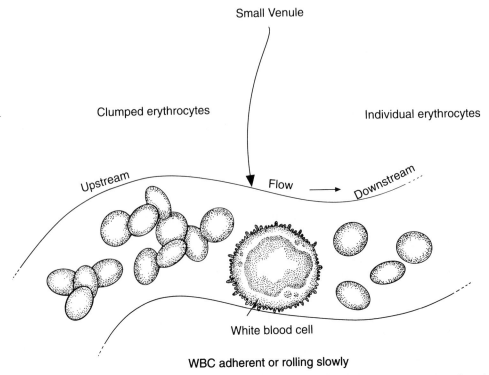

Figure 5–4 ■ Leukocytes tend to stay longest in small venules where they generate small clusters of erythrocytes by slowing their passage. The erythrocytes are forced to disaggregate in order to pass the standing or slowly moving white blood cell.

tive surface charge actively reduces contact with neighbors unless crowding by a hematocrit above 60% forces contact. Plasma globulins overcome the negative red cell charge while albumin has little effect other than to

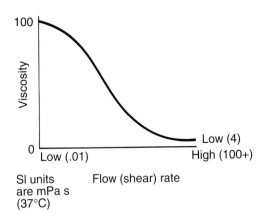

Figure 5–5 ■ Blood's nonnewtonian property of shear thinning is diagrammed. At high flow rates, blood is only five or six times as thick as water, but its flow resistance grows 25-fold as its internal motion slows. This property is useful in blood's need to flow easily and yet stop flowing after injury. A newtonian fluid would produce a horizontal line.

stabilize red cell shape. Other large molecules that similarly enhance red cell contact during flow at low shear rate include dextran (a large carbohydrate molecule) and polyvinylpyrrolidinone (a pyrrole polymer). The plasma globulins share large size and substantial flow eccentricity (molecular elongation) with dextran and polyvinylpyrrolidinone. This physical property also causes increased attractiveness of red cell membranes for each other.

Plasma Proteins and Shear Thinning

Molecular size and elongation affect the protein concentration required to produce red cell aggregation. Fibrinogen is the most potent plasma globulin. Polyvinylpyrrolidinone (360,000 daltons) is ten times as potent as the dextran (150,000 daltons) commonly used in laboratory studies. Fibrinogen and other globulins generate blood's shear thinning properties. Haptoglobin is the most important of the globulins that remain in serum after clotting. In diabetes, all three plasma components favoring increased erythrocyte contact during low shear rate flow—fibrinogen, haptoglobin, and total globulin—are elevated. Total globulin elevation reflects, at least in part, a reduction in plasma albumin. Therefore, diabetic blood typically shows more shear thinning (higher viscosity at low shear rate) than nondiabetic blood,[70] being 25% more viscous at low shear rate. A recent study compared viscosity at a single shear rate (9 sec^{-1}) of blood from diabetic people with and without foot ulcers and showed higher blood viscosity in the former group.[35]

Increased low shear rate blood viscosity alters blood flow by reducing the shearing motion near the center of steady flow. This effect is very modest. Increased shear thinning burdens flow at low to normal rates less than 2%, the burden decreasing as flow rate rises. The pressure rise required to overcome this resistance increase is also less than 2%. This means that variations in plasma protein composition with age, gender, individual genetic predisposition, diabetes, and pregnancy have only this level of direct linkage to blood pressure and do not directly generate measurable changes in cardiac output.

Flow Destabilization

Blood has another continuously present nonnewtonian flow property of interest in addition to shear thinning (Table 5–2). Many nonnewtonian fluids lower fluid drag. Drag is a word used to describe the increased pressure drop generated by newtonian fluids during tube flow at high Reynolds numbers. At Reynolds numbers above 2,000, flow becomes unstable, with local eddies forming and dissipating through the flow. This disturbance causes flow resistance to rise roughly as the 1.4 power of flow velocity.[96] Some substances that make the fluid nonnewtonian also lower this turbulence-related drag when added to the system.[55, 104] Red cells might reduce blood's drag in arteries by damping eddies, but the Reynolds number never achieves a value sufficiently high to make drag clearly important. On the other hand, early destabilization in curving flow (as opposed to straight flow) is seen in many nonnewtonian flows. Fortunately, blood is as stable as newtonian fluids during curvilinear flow, and diabetes has no measurable effect on this flow property.[63]

Time-Based Flow Properties of Blood

Blood also has two time-based flow properties, viscoelasticity and transient resistance (Table 5–2). Both are affected by diabetes. Time-based flow properties are seen only for brief periods when flow conditions change. They are not detectable during steady flow but affect blood flow only when it is pulsatile rather than steady. The pulsatility of blood

---

Table 5–2 ■ TYPES OF NONNEWTONIAN BLOOD FLOW PROPERTIES

A. Time independent (always present during flow)
  1. *Shear thinning* (lower viscosity at higher flow rate)
    Red blood cells interact with plasma globulins to try to aggregate at low flow rates, raising its viscosity. Red blood cells stretch progressively as flow rate rises, becoming more streamlined and continuing to lower blood viscosity.
  2. *Flow destabilization* (favors or opposes kinetically mediated change)
    Fluids fail to flow smoothly at high rates of absolute motion, developing irregular patterns with greater pressure drops. Substances that make the fluid nonnewtonian can affect this property, altering the fluid's ability to flow smoothly in curvilinear vessels, a major feature of artery and vein blood flow.

B. Time dependent (present as flow changes and shortly thereafter)
  1. *Viscoelasticity* (elastic strain energy stored as flow increases)
    Elastic erythrocytes (or stretchable molecules in other fluids) are deformed by the initiation or increase of flow rate. Red cell shape change reduces blood's initial resistance to flow but causes a persistence of internal force as a result of cell motion after the fluid's overall motion has ceased.
  2. *Transient resistance* (increased resistance to flow onset or restoration)
    Nonspherical elements in a fluid (erythrocytes in blood) become oriented to the flow as it is initiated or restored. Red blood cell orientation takes less time but more energy as blood's flow rate increases. Rapid red blood cell relaxation from flow orientation in blood causes its resistance to restarting flow to rise much more rapidly than that of other thixotropic fluids, important in arterial flow.

flow in arteries gives these flow properties special importance in these vessels.

Blood Viscoelasticity

Viscoelasticity is responsible for blood's unusually low initial resistance to flow at low shear rate.[69] Because elastic behavior is characteristically reversible, blood's low initial flow resistance is associated with an essentially symmetric dissipation of resistive force when flow stops. While it is only clearly visible at low shear rate, viscoelastic behavior is a feature of flow initiation at all flow rates. To understand what is happening, we return to the concept of fluid deformation as principally the motion of one fluid area relative to another. Blood contains red cells and plasma, but only plasma can continue to move in this manner. Red cells begin to deform but their solid shape causes them to resist further deformation. They simply achieve a new average shape while flowing. This shape is lost as flow ceases. Erythrocyte shape change is easier to accomplish than plasma deformation at flow onset so that the flow resistance of blood is initially low, but the saving in early resistance shows up when flow stops as a shear stress tail.

While commonly represented as individual red cell deformation, blood's viscoelastic deformation initially involves red cell rouleaux. Red cells normally form rouleaux when flow has stopped. Red cell suspensions that do not form rouleaux show much less viscoelasticity. At low shear rate (<0.5 sec^{-1}) diabetic blood forms rouleaux more vigorously and is more viscoelastic than nondiabetic blood. This difference becomes less evident as shear rate rises. The total elastic strain energy stored at flow initiation rises continuously up to at least 30 sec^{-1}, but less rapidly above 0.5 sec^{-1}.

Blood's Transient Resistance

A number of fluids that have solid components or that gel easily manifest a property called thixotropy,[77] a word coined from Greek to describe fluids and suspensions that fall in flow resistance after they are initially sheared (Fig. 5–6). Good examples are found around the kitchen. Two such materials are mustard and ketchup. When stirred or shaken, both will thin and pour more easily for a few minutes.

Blood was found to be thixotropic a number of years ago, but it does something that no other thixotropic fluid does as well: it recovers its increased flow resistance very quickly, literally between heartbeats. For that reason, this property has been renamed transient flow resistance.[68] Thixotropy has been shown to be caused by the extra work needed to align red cells into the plane of flow as flow begins or restarts. Transient resistance is recovered rapidly because elastic red cells move out of the plane of flow as flow slows or stops as they relax elastically. A large part of blood's transient resistance is mediated by growing contact between red cells as they lose the orientation they maintained during flow.

Transient resistance is the blood flow property most strikingly affected by diabetes. It is elevated about 30%.[72] Its major direct effects are in the arterial system, where flow is clearly burdened more by increased transient resistance than it is benefited by a higher initial drop in flow resistance from increased elasticity in diabetes.[72] But it also has effects whose magnitude have not yet been assessed in local flow situations in which flow velocity suddenly changes at arterial and arteriolar branch sites. In these flow areas, inertial and transient resistance effects are additive. The hemorheologic effects of diabetes should be largest in large artery areas where flow is suddenly accelerated.

Reduced Erythrocyte Deformability in Diabetes

One of the truly unique features of diabetic blood is the reduced ability of diabetic red blood cells to pass through capillary-sized glass tubes[73] and filters.[9, 43, 52, 120] This defect is associated with two other red cell abnormalities. Diabetic red cells also manifest greater flow resistance at low shear rate when resuspended in an artificial medium.[71, 91] Most interesting of all is a slowing and reduced ability to form doublets,[74] the first stage of rouleau formation. This kind of motion is most susceptible to thermodynamic analysis. It indicates that diabetic erythrocyte membranes resist rate of bending about twice normally.[74] This means that diabetic red cells are slow to change shape as they

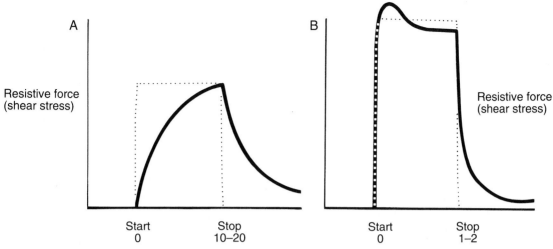

Figure 5–6 ■ Blood's viscoelasticity (A) and transient resistance (B) are diagrammed. The *thicker lines* show blood's behavior and the *thinner dashed lines* a newtonian fluid of similar viscosity to show the normal response. At slow onset of flow (shear rate 0.01 to 0.1 sec^{-1}), red cell bending dominates the fluid's interior motion, reducing its early resistance to deformation. But as flow ceases, the red cells restore their shape and orient more randomly, accounting for the slow decline in internal force seen. At faster onset of flow (shear rate 0.2 to 30 sec^{-1}), red cell bending is dominated by the need to orient the cells to rapidly developing flow. This need is directly linked to the rotation of the cells into line and therefore peaks sharply as shown. The slow red blood cell–based relaxation seen at the end of flow is proportionately smaller but still portrays blood's viscoelastic character.

enter capillaries, explaining the higher pressure at the arteriolar end of the capillaries seen in diabetic extremities even before mural sclerosis has developed.[114]

The basis for the abnormal behavior of diabetic red cells remains unclear. There is evidence that diabetic red cells are more glycated than normal red cells.[64] But rapid reversibility by insulin administration[8, 43, 52] and the uniformity of reduced red cell deformability in 4-μm glass tube flow[73] argue that glycation may not be the basis for the observed reduced deformability. The mechanism has importance because most studies have shown that the erythrocyte deformability problem is reduced when glucose control is better. If a mechanism other than glycation is responsible, then a management strategy other than tight glucose control becomes possible.

Leukocyte Deformability in Diabetes

Diabetic red cell filtration studies were susceptible to leukocyte plugging artifacts, suggesting initially that increased numbers of leukocytes in diabetes might be responsible for slowing filtration of diabetic blood.[111] But changes in technique to deal with this still allowed reduced red cell filterability to be

demonstrated.[22, 48, 112] In the meantime, leukocytes were reported to have slowed passage through capillary-sized (5-μm) filters in diabetes.[26] Chemical activation alters leukocyte behavior,[101] further burdening clinical analysis. Further studies have not made the situation clear. The effect of age is of the same magnitude as the diabetes effect in one study[79] and it eliminated the diabetes effect in another.[57] A recent report confirmed the initial observation but could show no difference when the white cells were divided into polymorphonuclear and mononuclear components.[16] A linkage between the age and activation effects has not been shown yet.

In the microcirculation, leukocytes normally pass through small arteriolovenular shunt vessels rather than true capillaries. Both red and white cells tend to be directed into the shunt vessels by the higher flow that these vessels experience while tissues are at rest. With less arterial pressure from leg artery disease in diabetes, leukocyte shunting loses efficiency, raising leukocyte residency frequency and duration in true capillaries,[98] a phenomenon that can lead to permanent tissue damage.[98] This becomes particularly important in the foot. The cutaneous vessels responsible for heat loss are mainly shunt vessels, while the nutritional vessels are true capillaries.[28] Foot skin nutrition is disproportionately compromised by diabetic leg artery disease.[28] Activation of leukocytes by infection can turn marginal blood flow into toe gangrene. This result illustrates how problems can add to each other to lead to amputation.

Treatment Considerations

As described above, many hemorheologic changes in diabetes have been linked in their severity to poor glucose control. But few randomized tests of the effects of improved glucose control on hemorheologic parameters have been carried out. The cross-sectional and prospective data already cited[20, 97] argue that close control of blood glucose should reduce or prevent rheologically mediated vascular complications of diabetes. But our large study of Diabetes Control and Complications Trial (DCCT) patients failed to show any plasma protein level benefit of intensive treatment in type 1 diabetes.[65]

Exercise (Table 5–3[37, 100, 119, 122]) is reported to lower blood viscosity through plasma protein changes. Both fibrinogen[37, 100, 119] and hap-

toglobin[122] are reported to fall. Haptoglobin's fall is thought to involve the feet; red cells are damaged as they pass through plantar capillaries as the feet hit the ground. Hemoglobin released binds to haptoglobin and both are cleared from the blood stream by the reticuloendothelial system.

Nutritional choices are also thought to affect blood viscosity. Lowering the traditional U.S. dietary fat intake results in less serum triglyceride.[3] Lowering of very low-density lipoprotein (VLDL) triglyceride levels leads in turn to reduced levels of plasminogen activator inhibitor 1 (PAI-1) the major component of plasmin-mediated clot dissolution and fibrinogenolysis. VLDL is a direct stimulator slowing PAI-1 formation by endothelial cells.[108] Adequate protein intake is necessary for normal serum albumin levels.[38, 42] Consumption of high levels of fish[46] or its associated ω-3 unsaturated fatty acids[14, 88, 124] is reported to lower blood viscosity, but effects of the levels of dietary intake achieved by most Americans have not been studied. The fish oil effect appears to be mediated by triglyceride lowering[104] and erythrocyte membrane lipid changes.[44, 86]

A number of parenteral regimens are used to manage serious hemorheologic problems (Table 5–4). Low-molecular-weight dextran, available as 40,000 dalton average Rheomacrodex, has been used in Europe to expand plasma volume as red cells are removed in order to lower the hematocrit and reduce blood's flow resistance. Alternative plasma expanders based on starch and other large molecules have also been examined.[45]

Plasmapheresis is often used to lower the level of a particular plasma protein. Fibrinogen levels remain subnormal for 2 to 3 days while plasma complement and other clotting components are restored in 1 day.[123]

The use of plasmin-activating enzymes to dissolve intravascular clots has become commonplace. Most of these agents also lower blood and plasma viscosity in parallel with their clot-dissolving action, an effect considered to benefit microcirculatory flow.[4] Streptokinase, acting throughout the plasma volume, produces a more striking change than urokinase and tissue plasminogen activator (t-PA; Alteplase) because the latter has a strong tendency to bind to thrombi.[40]

Information about oral pharmacologic agent effects on blood flow properties and fibrinogen levels is shown in Table 5–5. It has been growing steadily, but remains far

---

Table 5–3 ■ NONPHARMACOLOGIC HEMORHEOLOGIC MANAGEMENT

1. *Exercise*
   Generalized hemoconcentration and intravascular hemolysis in the feet occur during activity but fibrinolysis increases as physical condition improves with training[37, 100, 119, 122]
2. *Diet*
   Diabetes control accompanied by an appropriately low fat diet decreases VLDL (triglyceride)[11] and its stimulated endothelial PAI-1 synthesis[108]
3. *Protein intake*
   When adequate and timely, good-quality protein allows a normal albumin synthesis rate when combined with insulin[38, 42]
4. *Garlic / onion oil* (allyl propyl disulfide)
   When consumed in diet acts to lower plasma free fatty acids and increase fibrinolysis[84]
5. *Trans-unsaturated fatty acids*
   Present in margarine and other foods, have been shown to lower plasma fibrinogen levels in rats[84]
6. *Fish oil and supplements*
   Act to lower blood viscosity,[13, 46, 124] fibrinogen,[88] and red cell flow resistance[86] and membrane fluidity[45]
7. *Smoking cessation*
   Fibrinogen and haptoglobin fall slowly after smoking stops in parallel with declining cardiovascular risk[76]
8. *Vitamins and nutrients* (often considered food supplements)
   See Table 7–5

Table 5–4 ■ PARENTERAL AGENT HEMORHEOLOGIC MANAGEMENTS

1. *Hemodilution*

A therapy designed to reduce blood viscosity by lowering hematocrit without decreasing blood volume and oxygen delivery. It is normally accomplished by removal of blood and replacement of plasma by an excess of low-molecular-weight dextran (40,000 daltons) or another oncotically active material. This is done to expand the plasma volume without raising blood viscosity. This management has been used in stroke,[109] peripheral arterial disease,[25, 126] and retinal vein thrombosis[36] with varying degrees of success. Its ultimate methodology and role in disease management are still being explored.[45]

2. *Plasmapheresis*

Undesirable plasma components, usually proteins, are removed by phlebotomy. Red blood cells are separated by centrifugation and returned to the patient during the procedure; the plasma is either processed to remove specific substances and returned to the patient or replaced by salt-poor albumin. Treatment effectiveness depends on the half-life of the material being removed and the benefit derived from the feasible amount of lowering. The technique has been used to remove immune proteins,[102] lipoproteins,[103] and acts to lower plasma fibrinogen,[123] but it is both costly and inconvenient for the patient.

3. *Enzyme administration*

   a. Streptokinase, used in treating early acute myocardial infarction,[39] causes fibrinogen to fall to very low levels, altering blood flow properties.[5, 40]
   b. Urokinase, also used in acute myocardial infarction, has less antibody interference and less drop in fibrinogen[59] and blood viscosity[5] than streptokinase.
   c. Alteplase (tissue plasminogen activator), also used in acute myocardial infarction, has much less effect on fibrinogen and blood flow properties than streptokinase.[40]
   d. Ancrod (Arvin) has been used in treating peripheral artery disease.[53, 54]
   e. Piyavit (enzyme from medicinal leeches), lowers blood viscosity and platelet aggregation.[45]

from complete. I have unpublished data that show that sulfonylurea drugs improve blood viscosity at the same time that they normalize glucose control. Hypoglycemia mediates additional changes in the flow properties of blood that are less desirable. They include increased blood and plasma viscosity, rising von Willebrand factor and t-PA levels, and falling PAI levels without change in fibrinogen level.[32]

Table 5–5 lists aldose reductase inhibitors, used in diabetic neuropathy management in some countries, anabolic steroids, benzoic acid derivatives, and a series of agents used principally in Europe to treat intermittent claudication. They are also commonly employed as vasodilators. A number of antihypertensive drugs used in diabetes have been reported to affect blood flow properties. Some of their therapeutic effect may ultimately be explained by this mechanism, but their major hypotensive effects appear to be from their influence on vascular smooth muscle. The biguanide drugs, recently reintroduced in diabetes management in the United States, have all been shown to lower plasma fibrinogen levels by increasing fibrinolysis.[29, 30, 116] Agents used in controlling hyperlipidemias, also commonly used in diabetes management, make up a large fraction of the table.

The agent in Table 5–5 that is used most frequently in leg and foot disease in diabetes in the United States is pentoxifylline, a xanthine derivative with adenosine agonist effects. It has been shown to improve intermittent claudication.[87] Its effect was initially thought to be generated by improved red cell deformability,[24] but more recent work has suggested that the agent's adenosine action reverses leukocyte activation.[81] Such an inactivation could also help explain its reported ability to lower fibrinogen.[7, 31]

The major feature of Table 5–5 is the effect of many drugs on plasma fibrinogen levels. The mechanism for drug action in lowering or raising plasma fibrinogen is of interest. It is hinted at by an analysis of the cited reports. Fibrinogen is synthesized by the liver and after introduction into the plasma volume has a half-life of 2 to 4 days, a short period for plasma proteins. Valproic acid's effect in lowering fibrinogen is likely to be by direct suppression of hepatic protein synthesis, since it has been reported to disrupt liver metabolism and structure in idiosyncratic hepatotoxic reactions through generation of toxic metabolites.[23]

Cytokines, especially interleukin-6 (IL-6), interact with surface receptors on hepatocytes to increase both fibrinogen and haptoglobin synthesis.[18] Pentoxifylline may act by

Table 5–5 ■ ORAL MEDICATION HEMORHEOLOGIC MANAGEMENT

Aldose reductase inhibitors
  Sorbinil—lowers fibrinogen, improves red cell filterability[93]
  Ponalrestat (statil)—improves red cell suspension viscosity[92]
Anabolic steroids
  Furazabol—activates fibrinolytic system, lowers fibrinogen[1]
  Stanozolol—activates fibrinolytic system, lowers fibrinogen[20]
Anionic amphophiles
  Aspirin—suppresses fibrinogen synthesis,[84] reduces RBC aggregation,[75] enhances RBC flow through glass
    capillaries[89]
  Calcium dobesilate—lowers fibrinogen,[118] blood viscosity[12, 118] reduces red cell aggregation[75]
Anticlaudicants
  Buflomedil—lowers fibrinogen, WBV, WBC activation[17, 117]
  Defibrotide—produces a fall in fibrinogen in claudication patients[20]
  Dipyridamole—improves filterability of processed red cells in vitro[95]
  Pentoxifylline—lowers fibrinogen[7, 31] by a mechanism other than activating fibrinolysis,[84] opposes WBC
    activation[81]
  Suloctidil—lowers fibrinogen, mechanism not clear[94]
  Ticlopidine—lowers fibrinogen in claudication, transient ischemia (TIA) patients[15, 20]
Anticonvulsants
  Valproic acid—acts on liver, probably stops fibrinogen synthesis[113]
Antihypertensives
  β-Blockers
    Celiprolol—lowers fibrinogen in hypertension management[20]
    Propanolol—lowers fibrinogen and increases fibrinolysis together[20]
  Calcium inhibitors
    Diltiazem—reported to lower blood viscosity, basis not clear[27]
    Flunarizine—reported to lower blood viscosity, basis not clear[21]
    Nimodipine—WBV falls without fall in plasma viscosity or fibrinogen[33]
  Central agents
    Clonidine—lowers fibrinogen modestly, basis not clear[84]
Antioxidants
  Idebenone—improves red cell filterability, aggregability, lowers plasma viscosity[80]
  Probucol—lowers fibrinogen and factor VIII in Watanabe rabbits[78]
Biguanides
  Buformin—increases fibrinolysis, decreases fibrinogen[29]
  Metformin—reported to increase fibrinolysis by lowering PAI-1[116]
  Phenformin—reported to increase fibrinolysis, not available in U.S.[30]
Ergot derivatives
  Dehydroergocryptine—decreases RBC flow resistance in acidosis and hyperosmolar states[51]
Fibric acid derived triglyceride-lowering drugs
  Bezafibrate—lowers fibrinogen, more in hypertriglyceridemia[2, 107]
  Ciprofibrate—lowers fibrinogen, more in hypertriglyceridemia[20]
  Clofibrate—lowers fibrinogen, more in hypertriglyceridemia[20, 85]
  Fenofibrate—lowers fibrinogen, more in hypertriglyceridemia[4, 20]
  Gemfibrozil—reported to raise fibrinogen level[110]
HMG-reductase inhibitors
  Lovastatin—raises fibrinogen while improving red cell filterability[10]; lowers plasma viscosity and red cell
    aggregation but does change fibrinogen[48]; has its effect influenced by lipoprotein(a) level[47]
  Pravastatin—lowers fibrinogen, plasma viscosity[41]; produces no change[6]
  Simvastatin—does not change fibrinogen level[60]
Vitamins-nutrients
  Ligustrazine (herb component)—lowers whole blood viscosity, cause not clear[127]
  Niceritrol (nicotinic acid + PETN)—lowers fibrinogen in diabetes[20]
  Nicotinic acid—lowers fibrinogen level in parallel with triglyceride[84, 106]
  Troxerutin—reduces red cell clumping in diabetic retinopathy,[49] reverses WBC wall adhesions in diabetic rats[11]

WBV, whole blood viscosity; WBC, leukocytes; RBC, erythrocytes.

reducing leukocyte-mediated signaling[81] by IL-6 and its resultant fibrinogen and haptoglobin synthesis.

The mechanism of effect of many other drugs listed appears more complex. The relatively short half-life of fibrinogen and associations between hypertriglyceridemia and the coagulation process[105] argue that plasma fibrinogen is lost early in good part because the coagulation process is initiated and/or the enzyme plasmin has been activated. Either mechanism can lead to a fall in plasma fibrinogen level. Plasmin's activation is usually accomplished by t-PA, an enzyme whose two kringles encourage its attachment to coagulated fibrin. This enzyme is efficiently opposed by PAI-1. Both enzymes are principally products of the endothelium that lines the vascular space. Evidence that PAI-1 is directly stimulated from endothelial cells in culture by VLDL[108] creates a potential explanation for the effect of many of the drugs in Table 5-5. But a past report indicting suppression of hepatic synthesis in clofibrate's fibrinogen-lowering action[85] and the ability of gemfibrozil to lower triglyceride while raising fibrinogen[110] suggest that the situation is more complex.

Fibrinogen is a well-documented risk factor predicting future cardiovascular disease[20, 125] that both alters blood's flow properties and accelerates its coagulability. Drug effects on its blood level should receive at least as much attention as drug effects on serum cholesterol. Hemorheologic treatment is currently a decade or more behind management of hyperlipidemia. The interaction of antihyperlipidemic agents with blood fibrinogen levels should assist us in speeding our assimilation of information that will allow us to understand how to restore the health of the feet and other parts of the body through which blood passes in the diabetic patient.

REFERENCES

1. Abiko Y, Kumada T: Enhancement of fibrinolytic and thrombolytic potential in the rat by an anabolic steroid, furazabol. Thromb Res 8:107–114, 1976.
2. Almer LO, Kjellstrom T: The fibrinolytic system and coagulation during bezafibrate treatment of hypertriglyceridemia. Atherosclerosis 61:81–85, 1986.
3. American Diabetes Association: Nutrition recommendations and principles for people with diabetes mellitus. Diabetes Care 20:S15–S20, 1997.
4. Arntz HR, et al: Influence of fenofibrate on blood rheology in type II hyperlipoproteinemia. Clin Hemorheol 10:297–307, 1990.
5. Arntz HR, et al: The effects of different thrombolytic agents on blood rheology in acute myocardial infarction. Clin Hemorheol 11:63–78, 1991.
6. Arntz HR, et al: Influence of pravastatin on blood rheology in type II hypercholesterolemia. Clin Hemorheol 11:785, 1991.
7. Bachet P, Lancrenon S, Chassoux G: Fibrinogen and pentoxifylline. Thromb Res 55:161–163, 1989.
8. Baldini P, et al: Insulin effects on human red blood cells. Mol Cell Endocrinol 46:93–102, 1986.
9. Barnes AJ, et al: Is hyperviscosity a treatable component of diabetic microcirculatory disease? Lancet 2:789–791, 1977.
10. Beigel Y, et al: Lovastatin therapy in heterozygous familial hypercholesterolaemic patients: Effect on blood rheology and fibrinogen levels. J Intern Med 230:23–27, 1991.
11. Berthasult, et al: Hemorheological abnormalities in rats with experimental mild diabetes: Improving effect of troxerutine and α-tocopherol. Clin Hemorheol 14:83–92, 1994.
12. Benarroch IS, et al: Treatment of blood hyperviscosity with calcium dobesilate in patients with diabetic retinopathy. Ophthalmic Res 17:131–138, 1985.
13. Bild DE, et al: Lower-extremity amputation in people with diabetes epidemiology and prevention. Diabetes Care 12:24–31, 1989.
14. Cartwright IJ, et al: The effects of dietary Ω-3 polyunsaturated fatty acids on erythrocyte membrane phospholipids, erythrocyte deformability and blood viscosity in healthy volunteers. Atherosclerosis 55:267–281, 1985.
15. Boisseau MR, et al: Hemorheologically active substances, their profile and clinical impact. Clin Hemorheol 14:171–180, 1994.
16. Caimi G, et al: Rheological and metabolic leucocyte determinants in diabetes mellitus. Clin Hemorheol 15:53–60, 1995.
17. Capecchi PL, et al: Buflomedil prevents ischaemia-dependent changes in blood rheology and neutrophil reactivity. A possible adenosine-mediated mechanism. Clin Hemorheol 15:221–333, 1995.
18. Castell JV, et al: Recombinant human interleukin-6 (IL-6/BSF-2/HSF) regulates the synthesis of acute phase proteins in human hepatocytes. FEBS Lett 232:347–350, 1988.
19. Christensen NJ: Muscle blood flow, measured by xenon-133 and vascular calcifications in diabetics. Acta Med Scand 183:449–454, 1968.
20. Cook NS, Ubben D: Fibrinogen as a major risk factor in cardiovascular disease. Trends Pharmacol Sci 11:444–451, 1990.
21. De Cree J, et al: The rheological effects of cinnarizine and flunarizine in normal and pathologic conditions. Angiology 30:505–515, 1979.
22. Diamantopoulos EJ, Raptis SA, Moulopoulos SD: Red blood cell deformability index in diabetic retinopathy. Horm Metabol Res 19:569–573, 1987.
23. Eadie MJ, Hooper WD, Dickinson RG: Valproate-associated hepatotoxicity and its biochemical mechanisms. Med Toxicol 3:85–106, 1988.
24. Ehrly AM: The effect of pentoxifylline on the deformability of erythrocytes and on the muscular oxygen pressure in patients with chronic arterial disease. J Med 10:331, 1979.
25. Ernst E: Hemodilution for peripheral arterial occlusive disease. Clin Hemorheol 12:35–40, 1992.
26. Ernst E, Matrai A: Altered red and white blood cell rheology in type II diabetes. Diabetes 35:1412–1415, 1986.
27. Ernst E, Matrai A: Diltiazem alters blood rheology. Pharmatherapeutica 5:213–216, 1988.
28. Fagrell B, et al: Vital capillary microscopy for assessment of skin viability and microangiopathy in patients with diabetes mellitus. Acta Med Scand Suppl 687:25–28, 1984.
29. Fahraeus R: The suspension-stability of the blood. Acta Med Scand 55:1–228, 1921.
30. Fearnley GR, Chakrabarti R: Fibrinolytic treatment of rheumatoid arthritis with phenformin plus ethyloestrenol. Lancet 2:757–761, 1966.

31. Ferrari E, et al: Effects of long-term treatment (4 years) with pentoxifylline on haemorheological changes and vascular complications in diabetic patients. Pharmatherapeutica 5:26–39, 1987.

32. Fisher BM, et al: Effects of acute insulin-induced hypoglycemia on haemostasis, fibrinolysis and haemorheology in insulin-dependent diabetic patients and control subjects. Clin Sci 80:525–553, 1990.

33. Forconi S, et al: Effect of treatment with the calcium-entry blocker nimodipine on cerebral blood flow (spect) and blood viscosity of patients affected by cerebral chronic vascular insufficiency. Clin Hemorheol 11:787, 1991.

34. Ghanem MH, Guirgis FK, El-Sawy M: Effect of buformin on fibrinolytic activity in rheumatoid arthritis. Arzneimittelforschung 22:1487–1489, 1972.

35. Giansanti R, et al: Haemorheological profile and retinopathy in patients with diabetic foot ulcer. Clin Hemorheol 15:73–80, 1995.

36. Hansen LL, Wiek J, Wiederholt M: A randomized prospective study of treatment of nonischaemic central vein occlusion by isovolaemic haemodilution. Br J Ophthalmol 73:895–899, 1989.

37. Hornsby G, et al: Exercise conditioning reduces plasma fibrinogen in noninsulin-dependent diabetes mellitus. Diabetes 37(Suppl 1):240a, 1988.

38. Hutson SM, et al: Regulation of albumin synthesis by hormones and amino acids in primary cultures of rat hepatocytes. Am J Physiol 252:E291–E298, 1987.

39. I.S.A.M. Study Group: A prospective trial of intravenous streptokinase in acute myocardial infarction (I.S.A.M.). N Engl J Med 314:1465–1471, 1986.

40. Jan KM, et al: Altered rheological properties of blood following administrations of tissue plasminogen activator and streptokinase in patients with acute myocardial infarction. Circulation 72:417, 1985.

41. Jay RH, Rampling MW, Betteridge, DJ: Abnormalities of blood rheology in familial hypercholesterolaemia: Effects of treatment. Atherosclerosis 85:249–256, 1990.

42. Jeejeebhoy KN, et al: The comparative effects of nutritional and hormonal factors on the synthesis of albumin, fibrinogen and transferrin. Clin Symp 9:217–247, 1973.

43. Juhan I, et al: Effects of insulin on erythrocyte deformability in diabetics-relationship between erythrocyte deformability and platelet aggregation. Scand J Clin Lab Invest 41:159–164, 1981.

44. Kamada T, et al: Dietary sardine oil increases erythrocyte membrane fluidity in diabetic patients. Diabetes 35:604–611, 1986.

45. Kameneva MV, et al: Piyavit—a complex preparation from the medicinal leech improves blood rheology and decreases platelet aggregation. Clin Hemorheol 15:633–640, 1995.

46. Kobayashi S, et al: Epidemiological and clinical studies of the effect of eicosapentaenoic acid (epa c20:5 ω-3) on blood viscosity. Clin Hemorheol 5:493–505, 1985.

47. Koenig W, et al: The effects of lovastatin on blood rheology. Clin Hemorheol 11:785, 1991.

48. Koppensteiner R, Minar E, Ehringer H: Effect of lovastatin on hemorheology in type II hyperlipoproteinemia. Atherosclerosis 83:53–58, 1990.

49. Ledevehat C, Vimeux M, Bondoux G: Hemorheological effects of oral troxerutin treatment versus placebo in venous insufficiency of the lower limbs. Clin Hemorheol 9:543, 1989.

50. Lew HS, Fung YC: The motion of the plasma between the red cells in the bolus flow. Biorheology 6:109–119, 1969.

51. Li A, Sahm U, Artmann GM: Dihydroergocryptine maintains erythrocyte fluidity in acidotic and hyperosmolar buffer solutions modelling hypoxic and ischemic microcirculation. Clin Hemorheol 15:133–146, 1995.

52. Lipovac V, et al: Influence of lactate on the insulin action on red blood cell filterability. Clin Hemorheol 5:421–428, 1985.

53. Lowe GDO: Drugs in cerebral and peripheral arterial disease. BMJ 300:524–528, 1990.

54. Lowe GDO, et al: Subcutaneous Ancrod therapy in peripheral arterial disease: Improvement in blood viscosity and nutritional blood flow. Angiology 30:594–599, 1979.

55. Lumley JL, Kubo I: Turbulent drag reduction by polymer additives: A survey. In Gampert B (ed): The Influence of Polymer Additives on Velocity and Temperature Fields. New York: Springer-Verlag, 1984, pp 3–21.

56. MacRury SM, et al: Evaluation of red cell deformability by a filtration method in type 1 and type 2 diabetes mellitus with and without vascular complications. Diabetes Res 13:61–65, 1990.

57. MacRury SM, et al: Deformability of leukocyte subpopulations in type 1 (insulin-dependent) and type 2 (non-insulin-dependent) diabetic patients. Clin Hemorheol 14:539–544, 1994.

58. Marinelli MR, et al: Noninvasive testing vs clinical evaluation of arterial disease. JAMA 241:2031–2034, 1979.

59. Mathey DG, et al: Intravenous urokinase in acute myocardial infarction. Am J Cardiol 55:878–882, 1985.

60. McDowell IFW, et al: Simvastatin in severe hypercholesterolaemia: A placebo controlled trial. Br J Clin Pharmacol 31:340–343, 1991.

61. McMillan DE: Blood flow and the localization of atherosclerotic plaques. Stroke 16:582–587, 1985.

62. McMillan DE: Hemorheological studies in the Diabetes Control & Complications Trial. Clin Hemorheol 13:147–154, 1993.

63. McMillan DE, et al: Taylor-Couette flow stability of diabetic blood. Clin Hemorheol 9:989–998, 1989.

64. McMillan DE, Brooks SM: Erythrocyte spectrin glycosylation in diabetes. Diabetes 31:64–69, 1982.

65. McMillan DE, Malone JI: Hemorheological effects of intensive diabetes management in the DCCT. Clin Hemorheol 14:481–488, 1994.

66. McMillan DE, Malone JI, Rand LI: Progression of diabetic retinopathy is linked to rheologic plasma proteins in the DCCT. Diabetes 44:54A, 1995.

67. McMillan DE, Malone JI, Steffes MW: Plasma fibrinogen and total globulin are elevated in albuminuria in the DCCT. Diabetes 44:23A, 1995.

68. McMillan DE, Strigberger J, Utterback NG: Rapidly recovered transient flow resistance: A newly discovered property of blood. Am J Physiol 253: H919–H926, 1987.

69. McMillan DE, Utterback NG: Maxwell fluid behavior of blood at low shear rate. Biorheology 17:343–354, 1980.

70. McMillan DE, Utterback NG, Stocki J: Low shear rate blood viscosity in diabetes. Biorheology 17:355–362, 1980.
71. McMillan DE, Utterback NG: Impaired flow properties of diabetic erythrocytes. Clin Hemorheol 1:147–152, 1981.
72. McMillan DE, Utterback NG: Viscoelasticity and thixotropy of diabetic blood measured at low shear rate. Clin Hemorheol 1:361–372, 1981.
73. McMillan DE, Utterback NG, La Puma J: Reduced erythrocyte deformability in diabetes. Diabetes 27:895–901, 1978.
74. McMillan DE, Utterback NG, Mitchell TP: Doublet formation of diabetic erythrocytes as a model of impaired membrane viscous deformation. Microvasc Res 26:205–220, 1983.
75. McMillan DE, Utterback NG, Wujek JJ: Effect of anionic amphophiles on erythrocyte properties. Ann N Y Acad Sci 416:633–641, 1983.
76. Meade TW, Imeson J, Stirling Y: Effects of changes in smoking and other characteristics on clotting factors and the risk of ischaemic heart disease. Lancet 2:986–988, 1987.
77. Mewis J: Thixotropy—a general review. J Non-Newtonian Fluid Mech 6:1–20, 1979.
78. Mori Y, et al: Hypercoagulable state in the Watanabe heritable hyperlipidemic rabbit, an animal model for the progression of atherosclerosis. Thromb Haemost 61:140–143, 1989.
79. Missirlis Y, Kaleridis V: Polymorphonuclear leukocyte deformability in type II diabetes mellitus and in ageing. Clin Hemorheol 14:489–496, 1994.
80. Nagakawa Y, et al: Effect of idebenone on hemorheologic variables in geriatric patients with cerebral infarction. Clin Hemorheol 11:351, 1991.
81. Nash GB, et al: Effects of acute Trental infusion on white blood cell rheology in patients with critical leg ischaemia. Clin Hemorheol 11:309, 1991.
82. Nielsen NV: The normal fundus fluorescein angiogram and the normal fundus photograph. Acta Ophthalmol 64(Suppl 180):1–30, 1986.
83. Ostermann H, Van De Loo J: Factors of the hemostatic system in diabetic patients. Haemostasis 16:386–416, 1986.
84. Pickart L: Fat metabolism the fibrinogen/fibrinolytic system and blood flow: New potentials for the pharmacological treatment of coronary heart disease. Pharmacology 23:271–280, 1981.
85. Pickart L: Suppression of acute-phase synthesis of fibrinogen by a hypolipidemic drug (clofibrate). Int J Tissue React 3:65–72, 1981.
86. Popp-Snijders C, et al: Fatty fish-induced changes in membrane lipid composition and viscosity of human erythrocyte suspensions. Scand J Clin Lab Invest 46:253–258, 1986.
87. Porter JM, et al: Pentoxifylline efficacy in the treatment of intermittent claudication: Multicenter controlled double-blind trial with objective assessment of chronic occlusive arterial disease patients. Am Heart J 104:66–72, 1982.
88. Radack K, Deck C, Huster G: Dietary supplementation with low-dose fish oils lowers fibrinogen levels: A randomized, double-blind controlled study. Ann Intern Med 111:757–758, 1989.
89. Rao PR, et al: Aspirin analogues and flow of erythrocytes through narrow capillaries. Clin Hemorheol 15:877–887, 1995.
90. Rayman G, Hassan A, Tooke JE: Blood flow in the skin of the foot related to posture in diabetes mellitus. Br Med J 292:87–90, 1986.
91. Rillaerts E, et al: Increased low shear rate erythrocyte viscosity in insulin dependent diabetes mellitus. Clin Hemorheol 8:73–80, 1988.
92. Rillaerts EG, Vertommen JJ, De Leeuw IH: Effect of statil (ICI 128436) on erythrocyte viscosity in vitro. Diabetes 37:471–475, 1988.
93. Robey A, et al: Sorbinil partially prevents decreased erythrocyte deformability in experimental diabetes mellitus. Diabetes 36:1010–1013, 1987.
94. Roncucci R, et al: Effects of long-term treatment with suloctidil on blood viscosity, erythrocyte deformability and total fibrinogen plasma levels in diabetic patients. Arzneim-Forsch Drug Res 29:682–684, 1979.
95. Saniabadi AR, Fisher TC, Rimmer AR, et al: A study of the effect of dipyridamole on erythrocyte deformability using an improved filtration technique. Clin Hemorheol 10:263, 1990.
96. Schlichting H: Boundary Layer Theory. New York: McGraw-Hill Book Company, 1979.
97. Schmechel VH, Beikufner P, Panzram G: Langsschnittuntersuchungen zur progrenstischen bedeutung des plasmafibrinogens beim diabetes mellitus. Z Ges Inn Med Jahrg 39:453–457, 1984.
98. Schmid-Schonbein GW: Capillary plugging by granulocytes and the no-reflow phenomenon in the microcirculation. Fed Proc 46:2397–2401, 1987.
99. Schmid-Schonbein GW, et al: The interaction of leukocytes and erythrocytes in capillary and post-capillary vessels. Microvasc Res 19:45–70, 1980.
100. Schneider SH, et al: Impaired fibrinolytic response to exercise in type II diabetes: Effects of exercise and physical training. Metabolism 37:924–929, 1988.
101. Schroder S, Palinski W, Schmid-Schonbein GW: Activated monocytes and granulocytes, capillary nonperfusion, and neovascularization in diabetic retinopathy. Am J Pathol 139:81–100, 1991.
102. Schwab PJ, Okun E, Fahey JL: Reversal of retinopathy in Waldenstrom's macroglobulinemia by plasmapheresis. Arch Ophthalmol 64:515–521, 1960.
103. Seidel D, et al: The HELP-LDL-apheresis multicentre study, an angiographically assessed trial on the role of LDL-apheresis in the secondary prevention of coronary heart disease. Part I. Eur J Clin Invest 21:375–383, 1991.
104. Sellin RHJ, Moses RT: Drag Reduction in Fluid Flows. Chichester: Ellis Horwood, 1989.
105. Simpson HCR, et al: Hypertriglyceridaemia and hypercoagulability. Lancet 1:786–790, 1983.
106. Sirs JA, Boroda C: Variations of blood rheology in diabetic patients on nicofuranose. Clin Hemorheol 11:191, 1991.
107. Specht-Leible N, et al: Fibrinogen and bezafubrate—a pilot study in patients following percutaneous transluminal coronary angioplasty (PTCA). Clin Hemorheol 13:679–685, 1993.
108. Stiko-Rahm A, et al: Secretion of plasminogen activator inhibitor 1 from cultured human umbilical vein endothelial cells is induced by very low density lipoprotein. Arteriosclerosis 10:1067–1073, 1990.
109. Strand T, et al: A randomized controlled trial of hemodilution therapy in acute ischemic stroke. Stroke 15:980–989, 1984.
110. Stringer MD, Rampling MW, Kakkar VV: Rheological effects of gemfibrozil in occlusive arterial disease. Clin Hemorheol 10:339, 1990.
111. Stuart J, et al: Filtration of washed erythrocytes in atherosclerosis and diabetes mellitus. Clin Hemorheol 3:23–30, 1983.

112. Stuart J, Juhan-Vague I: Erythrocyte rheology in diabetes mellitus. Clin Hemorheol 7:239–245, 1987.

113. Sussman NM, McLain LW Jr: A direct hepatotoxic effect of valproic acid. JAMA 242:1173–1177, 1979.

114. Tooke JE: Microvascular dynamics in diabetes mellitus. Diabetes Metab 14:530–534, 1988.

115. Tooke JE, Rayman G, Boolell M: Blood flow abnormalities in the diabetic foot: Diagnostic aid or research tool? *In* Connor H, Boulton AJ (eds): The Foot In Diabetes. New York: John Wiley, 1987, pp 23–31.

116. Vague P, et al: Metformin decreases the high plasminogen activator inhibition capacity, plasma insulin and triglyceride levels in non-diabetic obese subjects. Thromb Haemost 57:326–328, 1987.

117. Van Acker K, Rillaerts E, De Leeuw I: The influence of buflomedil on blood viscosity parameters in insulin-dependent diabetic patients: A preliminary study. Biomed Pharmacother 43:219–222, 1989.

118. Vinazzer H, Hachen HJ: Influence of calcium dobesilate (Doxium) on blood viscosity and coagulation parameters in diabetic retinopathy. Vasa 16:190–192, 1987.

119. Volger E, Pfafferott C: Effects of acute physical effort versus endurance training on blood rheology in coronary heart disease patients. Clin Hemorheol 10:423, 1990.

120. Volger E, Schmid-Schonbein H: Mikrorheologisches verhalten des blutes beim diabetes mellitus. Dtsch Gesellshaft Inner Med 80:963–966, 1974.

121. Wiederhielm CA, Weston BV: Microvascular, lymphatic, and tissue pressures in the unanesthetized mammal. Am J Physiol 225:992–996, 1973.

122. Wolf PL, et al: Changes in serum enzymes, lactate, and haptoglobin following acute physical stress in international-class athletes. Clin Biochem 20:73–77, 1987.

123. Wood L, Jacobs P: The effect of serial therapeutic plasmapheresis on platelet count, coagulation factors, plasma immunoglobulin, and complement levels. J Clin Apheresis 3:124–128, 1986.

124. Woodcock BE, et al: Beneficial effect of fish oil on blood viscosity in peripheral vascular disease. Br Med J 288:592–594, 1984.

125. Yarnell JWG, et al: Fibrinogen, viscosity, and white blood cell count are major risk factors for ischemic heart disease. Circulation 83:836–844, 1991.

126. Yates CJP, et al: Increase in leg blood-flow by normovolaemic haemodilution in intermittent claudication. Lancet 2:166–168, 1979.

127. Zhao C, et al: The hemorheological study of ligustrazine treatment in diabetic subjects. Clin Hemorheol 9:615, 1989.

6

THE BIOMECHANICS OF THE FOOT IN DIABETES MELLITUS

■ Peter R. Cavanagh, Jan S. Ulbrecht, and Gregory M. Caputo

The aim of this chapter is to provide a biomechanical framework on which an understanding of the cause, treatment, and prevention of foot injury in patients with diabetes can be built. Although peripheral vascular disease has long been implicated in lower limb problems in the diabetic patient, it is now well-recognized that the majority of injuries to the foot, principally ulcers, are a consequence of mechanical trauma not recognized by the patient because of neuropathy. Diabetes-related distal symmetric polyneuropathy results in a loss of protective sensation, and subsequently a number of biomechanical risk factors conspire to cause injury. Thus, biomechanics has great relevance to neuropathic injury as has been discussed in a number of articles on the topic in the last decade.[70, 116, 195]

Most of the skin injuries seen on the feet of patients with diabetic neuropathy occur in the forefoot, with approximately equal distribution on the dorsal and plantar surfaces.[107] Those on the plantar surface are frequently at sites of high pressure under the foot.[31, 45, 51, 236, 243, 244, 263] Many of the ulcers on the dorsum are at sites of high pressure

where the patient's footwear creates a lesion,[11] meaning that the majority of foot ulcers have, in large part, a biomechanical etiology. This has been known for some time due mainly to the writing of Brand and his colleagues,[32, 49] who emphasized the role of repetitive stress in foot injury. However, recent developments make this a particularly exciting time for biomechanical studies of the foot in diabetes. The tools are now available to make measurements of pressure under the bare foot during walking and, more importantly, to make measurements inside the shoes of patients who have been prescribed footwear to prevent ulceration or reulceration. There has been rapid growth in the understanding of why people with diabetes have higher pressures under their feet than those without diabetes. The topic of shear stress as a possible mechanism of skin injury is being revisited and the biomechanical consequences of peripheral neuropathy for posture and gait are being explored. Experimental determinations of tissue properties are expanding our knowledge of the effects of diabetes on the mechanical behavior of skin, collagen, and adipose tissue, and objective

125

assessment of footwear designs is providing an understanding of how to best intervene to treat or prevent injury. Evidence dealing with all of these issues (Table 6–1) will be presented in this chapter. It is also extremely important that biomechanical issues be considered when new treatments for wounds on diabetic feet are being evaluated.[62]

In summary, we attempt to describe how the forces that injure the foot are generated, how they may cause injury, and how they might be measured and modified to achieve healing, and better still, to prevent injury. Our concentration is on topics where evidence is available to support our assertions. However, by necessity, we also mention a number of areas in need of further biomechanical study and attempt to provide some hypotheses to guide such study. We also intend to keep this chapter firmly directed at clinical reality, because a frequent and usually valid criticism of biomechanical and bioengineering texts is their inaccessibility to clinicians. After a brief discussion of the mechanics of gait and a review of plantar pressure measurement, we discuss the mechani-

cal factors responsible for the development of foot injuries in diabetes. Following a consideration of the role of unloading in ulcer healing we turn to the mechanics of footwear. Finally we discuss some issues in clinical biomechanics, including "what to look for" in a foot examination, and we discuss the role of surgery in altering the biomechanics of the foot.

Gait: Internal and External Mechanics

Why Study Gait Mechanics?

Most foot injuries occur while the patient is walking and are caused by the forces generated during gait. Thus, a natural place to begin the discussion of injury is with an overview of the mechanics of gait. When we watch a patient ambulate in the clinic, we are attempting to assess certain aspects of the external mechanics of the patient's gait. What we actually see are the limb movements in space, which bear little relationship to the most important quantities in the current con-

Table 6–1 ■ A SUMMARY OF THE EVIDENCE FOR BIOMECHANICAL FACTORS INVOLVED IN THE PROCESS OF ULCERATION, HEALING, AND PREVENTION

PROCESS	REFERENCES
Ulceration	
Elevated peak plantar pressure—a major risk factor	31, 236, 243, 244, 264
Factors affecting peak barefoot plantar pressure	
Thickness of plantar tissue	66
Foot deformity	1, 68
Callus	185, 272
Limited joint mobility	37, 85, 108
Body weight (low correlation)	1, 71
Gait parameters (speed, stride length, etc.)	68
Tissue changes from prior ulceration	185
Threshold normal pressure for injury (estimated at 750 kPa)	13
Pressure-induced dorsal injury is caused by footwear	11
Hallux pressure during turning may be significantly higher than during straight walking	214
Elevated pressure causes tissue ischemia	Studies in progress
Shear stress contributes to neuropathic injury	Studies in progress
Ulcer Healing	
Pressure relief is required	100
The total-contact cast is effective at pressure relief and healing	156, 180, 232
Other pressure relief devices	14
Ideal healing rates can be predicted	134
Ulcer Prevention	
Appropriate footwear reduces plantar pressure	54, 78, 117, 130, 158, 159, 199, 201, 219
Socks reduce plantar pressure	262
Removal of callus reduces plantar pressure by 29%	272
In-shoe pressure facilitates footwear modification	67, 178
Shear stress can be modified by proper footwear fit	Studies in progress
Prophylactic metatarsal head resection causes acute Charcot foot	110

text, the injurious stresses in the tissue, which could be labeled the internal mechanics. Yet it is worth dwelling briefly on the external mechanics of gait, because observation and, preferably, measurement can sometimes provide insight into the reasons for high forces and pressures during gait.

Kinematics

A number of techniques are available to track the spatial position of targets attached to segments of the lower limb during gait.[149, 171] Most commonly, reflective markers are used and tracked by high-speed video (Fig. 6–1A). This allows joint motion in the foot to be quantitatively measured during normal function rather than depending on inferences from a static examination. For example, the pattern of dorsiflexion and plantarflexion of the first metatarsophalangeal (MTP) joint in a diabetic patient during gait is shown in Figure 6–1B. Very few such measurements of foot movement in diabetes have actually been performed to date, although the techniques are widely used in orthopedic biomechanics for the study of conditions such as cerebral palsy[209] and joint replacement.[9]

The example just chosen is quite relevant to the current context, because plantar ulceration of the hallux is a common occurrence in patients with diabetic neuropathy (Fig. 6–1C).[36] Dorsiflexion at the first MTP joint is essential during the toe-off phase of gait. When the ability of that joint to dorsiflex is mechanically limited, very high pressure must be expected under the hallux during toe-off, a common finding in patients who ulcerate in this region. An understanding of the necessary range of dorsiflexion of the first MTP joint during gait, taken together with a static measurement of dorsiflexion at that joint, can provide insight into why high plantar pressure may occur at that particular site.

Forces at the Foot

Although the likelihood of high pressure between a region of the foot and the floor can be inferred from an analysis of movement as described earlier, neither the eye nor the most sophisticated video analysis system can measure these forces and pressures, because it is only the consequences of force that can

actually be "seen." The area of mechanics in which the forces that cause movement are studied is called kinetics, whereas the label kinematics is applied to studies (e.g., those described earlier) when the movement per se is measured. The forces that are most frequently measured and studied are the external forces between the foot and either the floor or the footwear. Less frequently, internal forces in tissues or forces between the articulating surfaces of joints can be measured, estimated, or modeled.

When the foot strikes the ground in gait, Newton's third law tells us that there will be equal forces experienced by both the foot and the floor. Because it is more convenient to measure the force with an instrument mounted on the floor than on the foot, a device called a "force platform" is frequently found in gait laboratories. As demonstrated in Figure 6–2, the force measured by a force platform during a single foot contact is usually expressed in three components: vertical (or normal, to use the engineering term), anteroposterior shear, and mediolateral shear.

Pressure: The Harm Done By Force

The forces shown in Figure 6–2 can be thought of as the mechanical input to the foot, yet their magnitude does not necessarily reflect the risk of injury. As Brand[50] has so aptly said, "Pressure is the critical quantity that determines the harm done by the force." The link between force and pressure is, of course, the area of force application. Much more damage can be done by a force transmitted through a few plantar prominences than by the same force distributed over a larger area of the plantar surface. Consequently, plantar pressure measurement is a topic of critical interest in the field of diabetes-related foot injury and we examine below the way in which this can be achieved.

Average pressure is calculated by dividing the applied force by the area over which it acts. What is widely called "plantar pressure" in the diabetes literature is known in mechanical terms as "normal stress": "stress" because it is the result of force applied to a defined area and "normal" because it is measured at right angles to the supporting surface. Shear stress is calculated in the same manner but using the magnitude of the shear force and its area of application, which

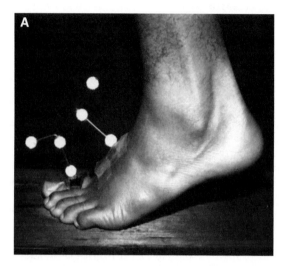

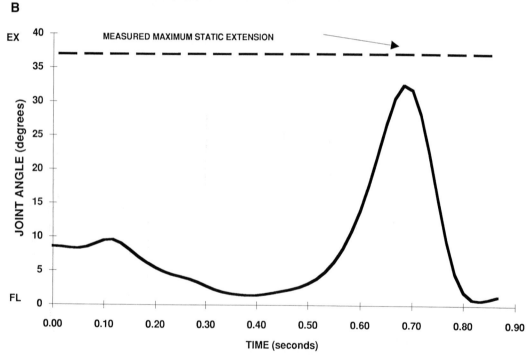

Figure 6–1 ■ *A,* Foot with targets attached for automated video analysis of motion of the first metatarsophalangeal joint. At least three targets must be placed on each segment of interest (or on a base firmly attached to it). If the targets are visible in two or more video cameras, the three-dimensional locations of the targets can be obtained automatically by computer analysis of the resulting images and the unique position of the segment in space determined. *B,* Dynamic flexion-extension pattern of the first metatarsophalangeal joint (MTPJ1) during slow barefoot walking in a patient with diabetic neuropathy and limited joint mobility. Measurements were made using automated analysis of video, as described in *A. Dashed line* represents the maximum extension (37 degrees) measured statically during physical examination. Note that the maximum dynamic value is approximately 90% of the static value.

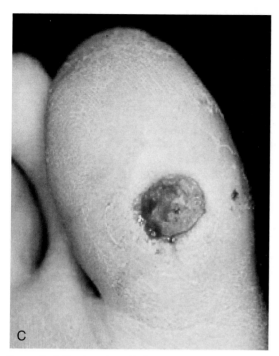

C

Figure 6–1 Continued ■ C, An ulcer under the hallux in a patient with limited joint mobility of MTPJ1.

may be the same as that for the normal stress. For example, consider the effects of the peak ground reaction forces shown in Figure 6–2 on a "rocker bottom foot" with concentrated force application to a midfoot prominence. As shown in Figure 6–3, the calculation leads directly to estimates of large "normal" and "shear" stresses. In practice, however, the areas of application are rarely known, and as we have previously shown,[71] similar calculations of pressures based on body weight or ground reaction forces and total foot area are not valid, because "effective foot area" is much smaller than the area of the footprint. Plantar pressure must therefore be directly measured rather than estimated. Although we measure plantar pressure routinely in all patients in our diabetes foot clinic, we are still frequently surprised by the discrepancies between our preconceptions of how a particular foot functions and the evidence from direct plantar pressure measurement. A clinically apparent plantar bony prominence does not guarantee a high pressure in that region, and more important, the absence of any obvious bony deformity is not a guarantee of low pressure.

Plantar Pressure Measurement

The Devices Used

Methods for the measurement of plantar pressure have been discussed in detail by ourselves and others.[3, 35, 67, 72–74] Many devices for barefoot and in-shoe plantar pressure measurement are currently commercially available,[67] and all require the use of a computer and, usually, proprietary software. Although several different principles of measurement of pressure are used in the manufacture of the sensors that make up the devices,[67] in the majority a matrix of transducers is used. For barefoot measurement, the patient walks onto the platform and continues walking. In this situation, information from a single foot contact is collected. For in-shoe measurement the matrix of transducers is manufactured into a thin pliable "insole," which is placed in the shoe in direct contact with the foot. In this case, information from multiple steps can be obtained.[67]

Two other devices for measuring plantar pressure have been proposed, and both are simple and do not require a computer. The first has a single discrete sensor and a voltage meter.[90] No validation of this approach has yet appeared. The second, called the Podotrack, is in the tradition of the Harris mat[228] and gives a "semiquantitative" estimate of pressure distribution.[255] It consists of a three-layer sandwich on which the patient's foot leaves an impression in different shades of gray. The device was found to be highly specific (>92% for three independent observers) but not very sensitive (32%, 36%, and 69% in three observers). Thus the probability of underestimating pressure was high. In a later study,[253] the same authors found that training of the observers could increase sensitivity to greater than 90%. Vijay et al.[266] have reported on the use of this device in a clinical setting.

When any of these instruments are used, attention must be given to many technical considerations: dynamic range, sampling rate, spatial resolution, frequency response, linearity, hysteresis, temperature sensitivity, reliability, and reproducibility. All of these have been reviewed elsewhere.[72, 73] Of particular importance is an understanding of the relevance of effective sensor size on the pressure measured. Generally speaking, the smaller the sensor, the larger the appar-

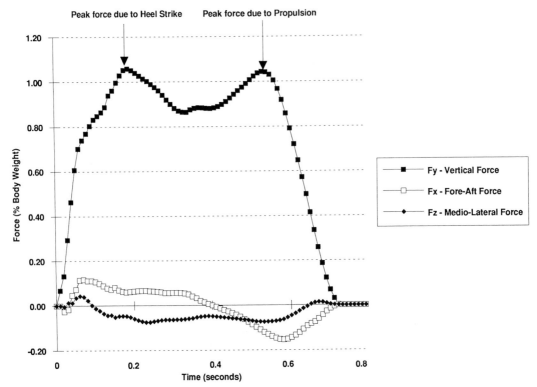

Figure 6–2 ■ Three components of ground reaction force underneath one foot during a single step. The step begins with heelstrike at time 0, and ends with toe-off. The three components of the force are fore-aft shear component (Fx), vertical component (Fy), and mediolateral shear component (Fz). Note that the vertical component is six times larger than the anteroposterior fore-aft shear, and 15 times larger than the mediolateral shear. *Left arrow* marks the peak vertical force after heel strike; *right arrow* marks the peak vertical force during the late part of the step cycle and is used for calculation of pressure in Figure 6–3.

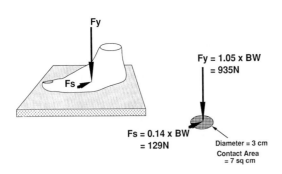

Normal Stress = 935/ (7 x .0001) = 1340 kPa =1.34 MPa
Shear Stress   = 129/ (7 x .0001) =   184 kPa

Figure 6–3 ■ Schematic of a rocker bottom "Charcot" foot in contact with the ground during the late-support phase of gait at the instant shown by the *right arrow* in Figure 6–2. If the contact area is assumed to be circular with a diameter of 3 cm, the normal stress will be 1.34 MPa and the shear stress 184 kPa.

ent pressure recorded in the same region of the same foot.[72–74] Thus, normative data must be developed for each instrument used and cannot be interchanged.

This important point has been investigated theoretically by Lord.[163] Starting with data from an optical pedobarograph (OPBG) with a spatial resolution of approximately 400 pixels/cm², she then created virtual sensors of progressively increasing dimensions to model the effect of transducer size and demonstrated that a sensor with dimensions of 10×10 mm is likely to underestimate the actual plantar pressure (as measured by the OPBG) by 30 to 40%. In a similar study, Davis et al.[98] found that sensors with an effective size of greater than approximately 6×6 would result in significant error in the estimate of pressure compared to a device with 5×5-mm sensors.

This unfortunate situation, where different results are obtained from the same foot under the same conditions, is analogous to that where falsely high blood pressures are obtained with inappropriately small blood pressure cuffs. It is a situation that is unlikely to be resolved in the near future unless manufacturers agree on standard platform characteristics. Unfortunately, a single correction factor to convert estimates from two different systems to a common base will not be appropriate for all regions of the foot. This is because, in systems with large area sensors, a pressure that is applied to a small area, such as a prominent metatarsal head (MTH), will be effectively averaged over a whole large element and will be irreversibly represented as a lower pressure. However, in a region where pressure is more evenly distributed (such as the heel), two devices with different element sizes will provide approximately the same estimates and no correction factor would be required. Perry et al.[199] made region-by-region corrections in order to compare pressures measured during barefoot and shod walking using different devices. Only a few comparisons of different devices have been performed.[174, 274]

Data Collection Issues

Also to be considered are several aspects of the data collection process that will impact the results. These include stride length (natural or mandated), speed of walking (natural or mandated), first step, or midgait.[242] In our daily clinical use, we prefer to make the step as normal as possible for the subject at that point in time. We recognize that step length and speed will affect plantar pressure; however, we believe that, in a clinical setting, measuring the consequences of a normal step for that patient at a given point in time is more meaningful than attempting to make the subject conform to a set of conditions that may be unnatural for him or her. However, speed can be critically important when making comparisons between different types of footwear, since peak pressure is a function of speed.[210] If the patient chooses to walk more slowly during trials with one particular type of shoes, this may lead to the incorrect impression that the footwear is responsible for the observed reduction in plantar pressure.

In their studies of the total-contact cast (TCC), Shaw et al.[226] made sure that speed and step length were maintained between conditions, while Fleischli et al.,[111] Lavery et al.,[156] and Baumhauer et al.[34] allowed the subjects in their studies of different healing devices to choose their own speed for each of the conditions. Both methods are legitimate, but the results of the studies must be interpreted with these conditions in mind. Shaw et al. wanted to understand how a TCC functions and wanted to separate the effects of speed and stride length from those of the cast itself, while the other authors were interested in observing the full clinical effect of the intervention studied.

In our barefoot studies we have chosen to look at the average of five "first steps,"[72] whereas for in-shoe testing we average many (approximately 30) steps during normal gait. The reliability of in-shoe pressure measurements was investigated in symptom-free subjects by Kernozek et al.[146] Subjects walked on a treadmill at three speeds. Reliabilities of greater than 0.9 in the estimates of peak pressure and force-time integral were achieved by the analysis of data from only 8 steps.

Young et al.[271] have shown that plantar callus can significantly increase plantar pressure during walking. It is therefore important that any testing of plantar pressure be preceded by the patient's normal callus care—usually removal by sharp debridement.

Data Analysis

We will now illustrate the collection and analysis of plantar pressure by an example of a patient who has experienced recurrent ulceration under the left first MTP joint. Consider first the measurement of barefoot plantar pressure. The series of images shown in Plate 1 are frames from a movie that can be viewed at *http://www.celos.psu. edu/bowker/movie1.mov*. Note that forefoot pressures are relatively moderate (<400 kPa) at all sites except MTH1, where there is a sustained load applied from before heel-off until the end of stance. This peak reaches a magnitude of greater than 1,275 kPa, which is the limit of measurement of the device. This should be compared to the normal values of 299 kPa (±137 kPa) for MTH1 reported by Rosenbaum et al.[210] for the same device during normal speed walking (see discussion of normal values below).

The Peak Pressure Plot

It is not yet customary to include movies in patient charts (although it is entirely feasible to do so on a CD-ROM and it could become routine once all medical records are computerized) and thus some distillation must be made from the 60 or more images of pressure that are available every second. The peak pressure plot shown in Plate 2 is often chosen for this purpose. This plot was created by simply retaining the largest pressure that every sensor on the platform experienced during the entire contact phase. It can be an extremely useful plot, since the peak loading of every single region can be seen in a single picture.

Regional Analysis Using Masks

A further derivation from Plate 2 is to divide the foot into a number of anatomic regions or masks for a so-called regional analysis. This requires the construction of the masks shown in Figure 6–4. A mask can be as simple as a single square or rectangle that encloses a region of interest on the foot—for example, a hallux, all the metatarsal heads, or the midfoot—where the patient may be experiencing a recurrent ulceration. These masks are created using commercial software supplied by the device manufacturers (in the diagrams in this chapter the software used is NovelWin from Novel Electronics, Inc., St. Paul, MN). Once the mask is created, it can be applied to data from either a single or many foot contacts to generate statistically based estimates of quantities such as peak regional pressures, regional pressure versus time graphs, and force-time impulses (see below).

We suspect that regional analysis may be important because some areas of the foot normally involved in weight bearing may be bet-

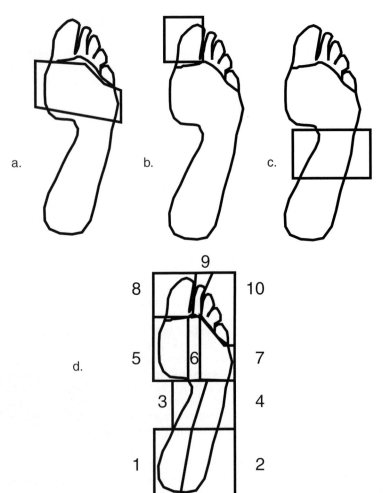

Figure 6–4 ■ Typical masks for regional analysis; *a, b,* and *c* are single masks that examine one anatomic region (metatarsal heads, hallux, and midfoot, respectively). In *d,* ten masks used for regional analysis of plantar pressure are shown (see Fig. 6–5).

ter adapted for this function and may thus tolerate higher pressure before breakdown. Conversely, the pressure threshold for tissue breakdown may be lower in regions of the foot not normally involved in weight bearing. An example of this would be the tip of a very clawed toe or the midfoot exposed to weight bearing because of an underlying Charcot fracture deformity (see Fig. 6–3).

A regional analysis of the data presented in Plates 1 and 2 is shown in Figure 6–5. In this analysis, the ten masks shown in Figure 6–4D were applied to five consecutive steps of the left foot. The resulting peak regional pressure analysis (Fig. 6–5) shows both the mean peak pressures from the five trials and the standard deviation between the five trials. Note that the heel, midfoot, and lesser toe pressures are very consistent in this patient, but the MTH1, lateral MTH, and hallux pressures exhibit high variability. This suggests that the patient does not have a stereotyped loading pattern on successive steps (see discussion of variability below).

Analysis of In-Shoe Plantar Pressure

Because most patients wear shoes and often sustain injury while wearing them, the ability to measure pressures inside the shoe is

an important extension of investigative techniques beyond just barefoot measurement. Bauman and Brand[33] and Brand and Ebner[53] used single in-shoe transducers almost 30 years ago; more recently, similar studies have been performed to investigate principles of footwear management.[88, 142, 164, 178, 191, 199, 201, 202] Although these have been principally research studies, devices suitable for clinical use are now available[70] and it is likely that this approach will revolutionize footwear prescription in the future.

In-shoe peak pressures for the patient whose barefoot data are presented in Plate 2 and Figures 6–4 and 6–5 are shown in Figure 6–6. The patient was wearing a pair of custom molded shoes with rigid rocker outsoles and a dual density PPT and Plastazote #2 insoles (see "Footwear: Theoretical Background," below for more discussion of this type of footwear). Note that the peak pressures are still highest at MTH1 but that they have been reduced from greater than 1,000 kPa in barefoot walking to approximately 150 kPa in the shoes. The patient has remained healed in these shoes.

Loading Analysis Using Impulse

When we change some component of the patient's foot or footwear, an examination of

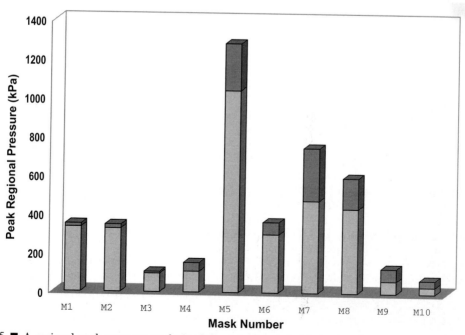

Figure 6–5 ■ A regional peak pressure analysis of the data shown in Plates 1 and 2 using the masks shown in Figure 6–4d. (Standard deviation from five trials shown in darker shading.)

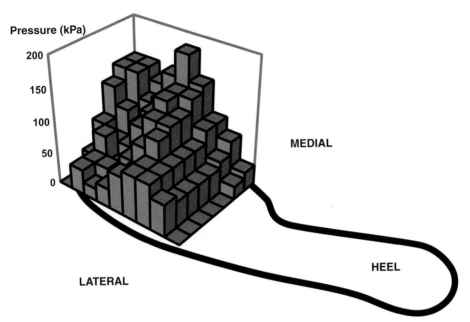

Figure 6–6 ■ In-shoe plantar pressures at a time in the late support phase for the subject whose barefoot data are shown in Plate 2 and Figures 6–4 and 6–5. The highest pressures in the foot are still under MTH1, but the peak pressures are reduced by the footwear to only 180 kPa compared to the mean barefoot value of >1,000 kPa.

the peak pressure response tells us "what" has happened rather than "why" it has happened. Analysis of the distribution of loading throughout the foot contact using an impulse analysis can often provide insight into "why" a change in peak pressure has occurred. Terminology can be confusing here because, in mechanics, an impulse refers to the product of force and time, not pressure and time. But in a system of pressure transducers with the same area (which is always the case in platforms but not in all in-shoe sensors), pressure and force are directly proportional and can be considered interchangeably with just a single multiplicative constant.

More importantly, the terms pressure-time integral and force-time integral are used by software manufacturers to mean quite different approaches to analysis that give totally different results. In the EMED analysis programs (Novel Electronics, Inc., St. Paul, MN), the pressure-time integral gives information from the single sensor in the foot or region on which peak pressure is exerted. However, the force-time integral gives values that represent the summed impulse from every sensor in the entire foot contact area or region (Fig. 6–7).

In either case, the starting point for analysis is the area under the pressure-time curve of a single sensor during the time that the pressure in that sensor was above a predefined threshold value. This threshold is usually the value that distinguishes signal from noise, but some authors have moved the baseline for integration upwards to a value considered to represent a boundary between normal and abnormal values[225] (see below). In the case of the pressure-time integral only the sensor on which peak pressure is exerted is reported in units of kPa-seconds. For the force-time integral, the pressure-time integrals for all sensors in the defined region (entire foot or region) are summed and multiplied by a constant to express the result in units of Newton-seconds (N-s).

Care needs to be taken not only with the selection of the appropriate impulse variables but also with their interpretation. For example, peak pressure and the pressure-time integral can be readily compared between different regions of the foot and different footwear conditions because they both refer to the analysis of a single sensor, but the force-time integral for areas that have the same applied pressure may be quite dif-

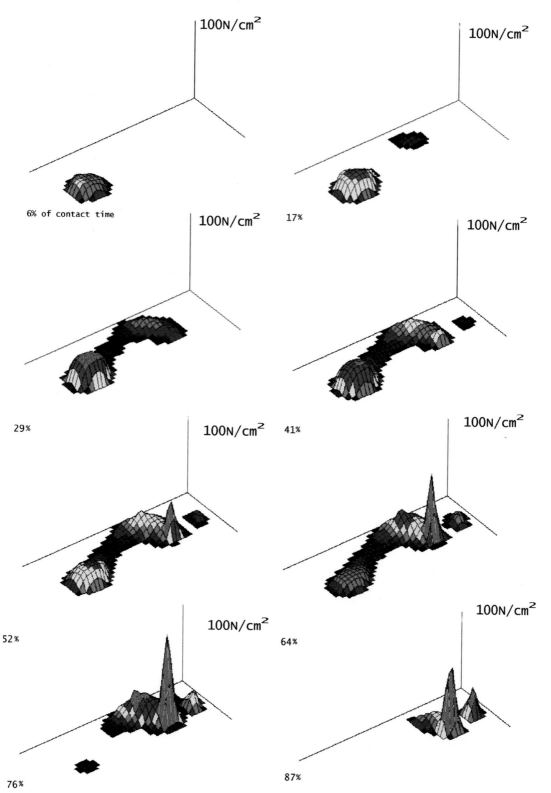

Plate 1 ■ Posteromedial views of individual frames of data from the continuous collection of plantar pressure during barefoot walking in a patient who had experienced recurrent ulcers underneath a prominent first metatarsal head on the left side. See text for details and see movie, which can be viewed at *http://www.celos.psu.edu/bowker/movie1.mov,* for the entire sequence.

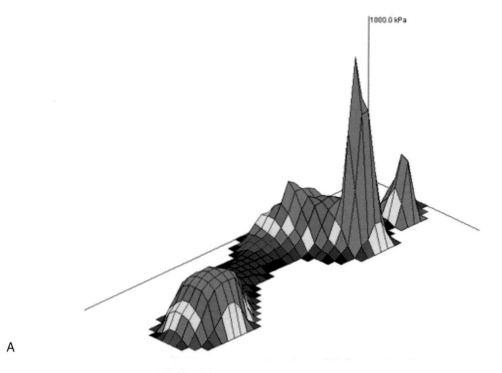

A

1000.0 kPa

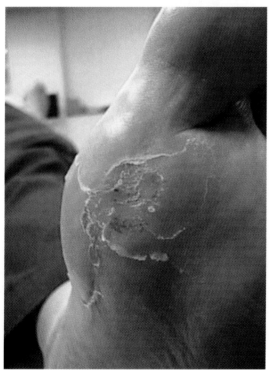

B

Plate 2 ■ Peak pressure plot, which summarizes the data shown in Plate 1. *A,* In this summary plot, the greatest pressure at each location under the foot from any time in the ground contact is shown in the diagram with the same scale and color key used in Plate 1. This display is a useful addition to the patient's chart. *B,* The recently healed ulcer under this patient's left first metatarsal head.

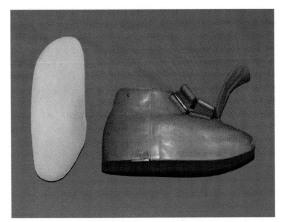

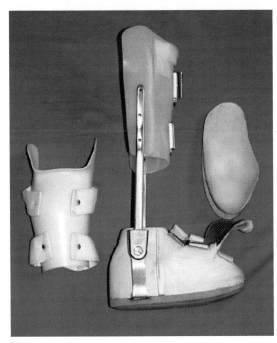

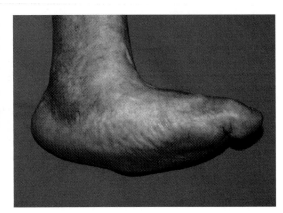

Plate 3 ■ An approach to the determination of ulcer pressure threshold in a patient with a classic midfoot Charcot collapse of the left foot. *A,* Shoe A in which the patient ulcerated. *B,* Shoe B, which did not result in an ulcer when used with the patellar tendon-bearing brace. *C,* The plantar surface of the foot showing the midfoot prominence. *D,* A barefoot peak pressure plot using EMED-SF showing the elevated pressure under the midfoot prominence. It can be seen that the midfoot is the only region of the foot that experiences significant load during the entire contact.

A

B

C

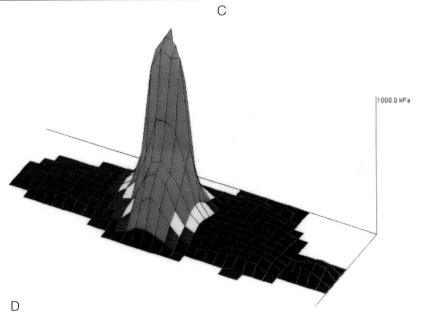

1000.0 kPa

D

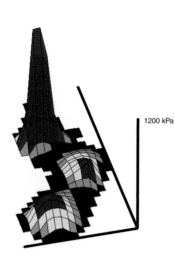

Plate 3 ■ *E*, In-shoe peak pressures in Shoe A, and Shoe B with and without the brace. These tests show that this patient's threshold for ulceration was between 150 and 190 kPa as measured inside the shoe. It is uncertain whether it would be safe to allow the patient to ambulate without the brace, since pressure is marginally reduced by the brace.

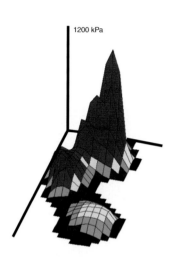

Plate 4 ■ Peak pressures during walking from the feet of patient that had undergone bilateral panmetatarsal amputation. Note the regions of extremely high pressure under the distal metatarsal shafts indicating that pressure relief does not necessarily accompany this procedure.

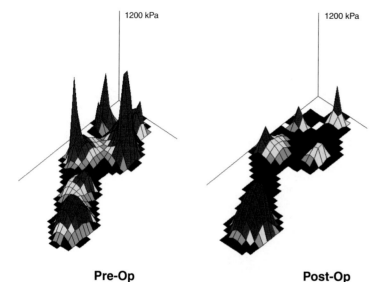

Pre-Op

Post-Op

Plate 5 ■ Pre- and postoperative peak pressures during walking from a patient who underwent a dorsal wedge osteotomy of the first metatarsal, an arthroplasty of MTH2, and a tendo-Achilles lengthening. Note the marked reduction in forefoot peak pressures but the increased heel pressure.

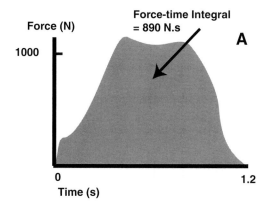

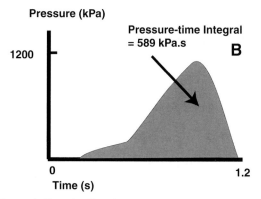

Figure 6–7 ■ *A,* The "force-time integral," which describes the total impulse transmitted to the foot by the ground. *B,* The "pressure-time integral" is simply a summation of the pressure-time curve for the single element that recorded the peak pressure during contact. In this case the element is in the forefoot and thus only begins to experience loading some time after initial foot contact. Both of these data sets are for barefoot walking by the subject whose data are shown in Plates 1 and 2 and Figures 6–5 and 6–6.

ferent depending on the size of the region under consideration. A larger region with the same pressure as a smaller region will yield a larger impulse (consider the heel and hallux, for example). When comparisons between footwear conditions are being made, the force-time integral can be used only if the two regions for which a comparison is being made are identical in area in the two conditions. An example of impulse analysis where in-shoe pressure measurement is used to compare different footwear conditions is given in the section below on the biomechanics of footwear.

Duckworth et al.[104] measured the time during which plantar pressure was above 981 kPa and showed greater times in patients

with an ulcer. Schaff and Cavanagh[223] showed that changes in force-time integral were proportionally much greater than changes in peak pressures in rocker shoes compared to flexible shoes (see "Footwear: Theoretical Background" section, below). Shaw et al.[225] examined the integral of pressure above a threshold value of 490 kPa in patients with and without prior ulceration. They found much greater percentage increases for impulse variables than for peak pressure variables in the ulcer patients. Thus while peak pressure data have received by far the most attention to date in studies of the foot in diabetes, analyses that include time may yet prove to be more useful.

Expected Values for Peak Pressure

The results of a regional analysis of peak pressure for a group of asymptomatic subjects walking at normal speed are shown in Figure 6–8 from the work of Rosenbaum.[210] The mean and the mean plus 2 standard deviations (SD) are shown on the graph. These data (and all the barefoot peak pressure diagrams in this chapter) were collected with an EMED-SF platform (Novel Electronics, Inc., St. Paul, MN) with a sensor area of 0.5 cm². Note that there is considerable between-subject variation in most regions; the coefficients of variation (SD/mean) in the forefoot are approximately 40%.

A number of other workers have reported pressures in various groups of patients with the EMED-SF platform. Armstrong et al.[20] reported peak pressures (regardless of their site of occurrence in the foot) of 627 ± 247 kPa for diabetic patients with no history of ulceration and values of 831 ± 247 kPa for patients who had ulcerated. Both these mean values are outside the range of mean plus 2 SD reported by Rosenbaum et al.[210] Stess et al.[243] reported values of peak pressures in the forefoot of 480 kPa (± 18 kPa SEE) in patients with a history of ulcers, and these values are within the range defined by Rosenbaum et al.[210] Armstrong and Lavery[13] found peak pressures of 1,000 ± 85 kPa in Charcot patients, 900 ± 188 kPa in neuropathic patients with a history of ulceration, 650 ± 256 kPa in patients with neuropathy but no ulceration, and 450 ± 80 kPa in diabetic patients with no neuropathy or history of ulceration. Wolfe et al.[269] reported the results of plantar pressure analysis on nine patients with Charcot feet

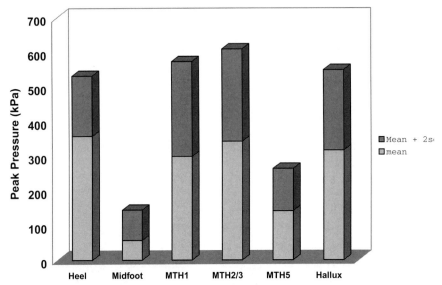

Figure 6-8 ■ Regional analysis of peak pressure (mean and 2 SD) for a group of asymptomatic subjects walking at normal speed (From Rosenbaum D, Hautmann S, Gold M, Claes L: Effects of walking speed on plantar pressure patterns and hindfoot angular motion. Gait Posture 2:191–197, 1994, with permission.)

and found that peak pressure under many of the feet exceeded the 1,275 kPa measurement limit of the EMED-SF platform used.

All four studies described in the previous paragraph used precisely the same measuring device (an EMED-SF platform with a sensor size of 0.5 cm²) and thus the lower values for peak pressure in patients with ulcers found by Stess et al.[243] must be due to either a difference in measuring protocol or a real difference in patient populations. It is quite likely to be the latter, since we have also found pressures of approximately 500 kPa in neuropathic patients who have ulcerated.[135]

Investigators who have used an OPBG have generally reported higher values, as would be expected from the higher spatial resolution of the sensors in the OPBG. Boulton et al.[48] suggested that a value of 1,080 kPa was a threshold for differentiating between normal and abnormal pressures. This group found that 51% of neuropathic feet in their sample had pressures above this value, and all of those with a history of ulceration exceeded this value. In a clinical study[258] and a later prospective study,[264] Veves and his colleagues used a value of 1,207 kPa to distinguish normal from abnormal. They found mean values for peak pres-

sures (regardless of site) of 1,108 kPa in neuropathic patients compared to 795 kPa in nonneuropathic diabetic controls; 39% of the neuropathic patients were above the threshold compared to 15% of controls. In the prospective study, all patients who ulcerated had pressures at baseline of greater than 1,108 kPa.

Frykberg et al.[118] used an F-scan system to record peak pressures from various groups of diabetic patients. They used a value of 600 kPa as their threshold for the definition of "abnormal pressures" and found an association between ulceration and high pressure using this approach. Using a similar device, Pham et al.[200] found a mean peak pressure of 570 ± 30 kPa in a prospective study of a large sample of diabetic patients. This group found pressure measurement to be helpful, but not robust, in predicting ulceration.

Is There a Threshold Pressure for Injury?

Factors That Affect the Threshold

As was discussed above, different authors have used various threshold values to distinguish normal from abnormal pressures. However, this is not the same as defining a threshold for ulceration. As already alluded to, plantar ulceration has been linked to high plantar pressure in several retrospective studies and in one prospective study.[13, 20, 47, 48, 94, 118, 200, 244, 264] However, there is no clear agreement yet on the pressure threshold for ulceration. This may be a consequence of several factors. First, results obtained using one pressure platform cannot be extrapolated to other platforms because of the effect of element size, as discussed above. Second, different regions of the foot may have different pressure thresholds for breakdown. Third, the pressure threshold for tissue breakdown may vary depending on the health of the tissue related to vascular supply, tissue perfusion,[249] amount of glycosylation of the tissues, and scarring. Fourth, shear, although not measured by any of the currently available platforms, may interact with normal forces in ways not yet understood. Fifth, the integral or time-pressure product, currently not often calculated, may be more relevant than simple peak pressure.[72, 73, 225] Sixth, and perhaps most important, barefoot pressures measured during a few steps across a pressure platform do not predict the load that the foot is exposed to. The actual cumulative load during normal daily living depends on activity level and footwear.

The Conventional Approach to Defining Abnormal Values

It is not possible to take the foot pressure distribution of a healthy population and assume that similar values are safe for patients with insensitive feet. Healthy individuals remain ulcer free not necessarily because they have lower plantar pressures, but because they can feel pain. As mentioned earlier, the range of "normal" regional peak pressure values—defined as mean $\pm$ 2 SD—is very wide (see Fig. 6–8), with peak values approaching 600 kPa at several regions. Yet plantar ulcerations can and do occur in the feet of neuropathic patients at sites where peak pressure is as low as 500 kPa, as measured on the EMED-SF platform.[135, 269]

The Evidence for a Threshold Pressure

Although the studies described above that have included patients with a history of ul-

ceration provide some perspective on the issue of a threshold pressure,[13, 48, 104, 118, 200, 225, 264, 269] these studies were not specifically designed to explore the issue of ulceration threshold. Recently, Armstrong et al.[20] have analyzed plantar pressures in patients with a history of ulceration and matched each of them with two control diabetic patients without a history of ulceration. Plantar pressure was measured in cases and controls using an EMED-SF pressure platform. Peak pressures were significantly higher in cases compared to controls (831 $\pm$ 247 kPa vs. 627 $\pm$ 244 kPa) and measures of skewness indicated an opposite pattern of negative skew for cases (more high pressures) and positive skew for controls (more low pressures). The optimal cut-off point that balanced sensitivity and specificity in the data was 700 kPa. However, this value was only 70% sensitive and 65% specific, leaving the authors to conclude that there was no clear value that could be used in screening to predict ulceration. Rather, the higher the pressure, the greater the risk.

These results make great intuitive sense in terms of the skewness described. There will always be patients who ulcerate even at relatively low pressures because of either a traumatic injury or significant walking either barefoot or in very poor footwear on a hard surface. Conversely, there will be patients who, because of low activity and/or very protective footwear, will not ulcerate even with very high barefoot pressure. Thus barefoot pressure can only predict the degree of risk, which is then modified by activity and footwear. It would be unreasonable to expect to find a clear division between ulcer patients and nonulcer patients based on barefoot level gait measurement.

Another related point is that barefoot measurements of pressure do not always predict the highest possible pressure. In general, the faster the gait, the higher the pressure under the foot. At most sites pressure during barefoot walking predicts pressure for more demanding activities. However, during turning, for instance, Rozema et al.[214] have shown that hallux pressure can be very high even in subjects with low hallux pressure during straight level gait. This is consistent with the clinical observation that many hallux ulcers occur despite relatively low pressure measured during straight level gait, and this observation will certainly confound any attempt to define hallux ulcer risk based on level gait pressure measurement.

The work of Shaw and Boulton[225] suggests that a consideration of impulse may also be important in trying to define the ulceration threshold.

Threshold for Injury—the Future

The actual amount of mechanical trauma that is needed for tissue breakdown can be assessed only by documenting the trauma that tissue is exposed to at the time of ulceration. The only practical way to do this is to measure cumulative loading to an ulcer site over a prolonged period while the patient is utilizing footwear that is known from clinical experience to be insufficient to prevent ulceration in that patient. The measurement would then need to be repeated in footwear known to prevent ulceration. The threshold for tissue breakdown would then be found somewhere between the two conditions. Such data would need to be analyzed in many different ways including peak pressure, pressure-time integral, time spent over different pressure values, time spent resting, and the like. As discussed above, barefoot pressure measurement can only ever contribute to estimation of risk, but knowing the true load for tissue breakdown would then, for the first time, allow for more rational footwear prescription: only footwear found by in-shoe load measurement to be safe would be dispensed.

This approach to the determination of ulcer pressure threshold is demonstrated in the case study from the Penn State University Diabetes Foot Clinics shown in Plate 3. The patient's right foot had a classic midfoot Charcot collapse (Plate 3C) with a peak midfoot pressure during barefoot walking (Plate 3D) of 1,019 ± 295 kPa. He ulcerated while wearing a custom molded shoe A (Plate 3A). After healing in a TCC, he was provided with a new custom molded shoe with a redesigned insole and a patellar tendon-bearing brace (Plate 3B). He was able to continue his activities of daily life without ulcerating in this shoe brace combination. Analysis of in-shoe pressure data in these two shoe conditions using a single midfoot mask indicated that peak midfoot pressures in shoe A and B were 190 kPa and 149.5 kPa, respectively (Plate 3F). Thus, it appears possible to identify the threshold for

ulceration in this patient to be somewhere in the 40-kPa range between 149.5 and 190 kPa when measured inside the shoe using a pressure-measuring insole with an average sensor area of approximately 1.5 cm². One additional caveat should be considered. These data were collected during relatively slow, level gait and it is likely that during activities of daily living the plantar surface would actually be exposed to somewhat higher loads than those measured here, even wearing the same shoes. Thus the range of pressure given here as including the ulceration threshold still only represents a window on what is happening. As already discussed, injury must in fact depend not just on some measure of loading, but also on the activity and rest pattern.

Summary of Plantar Pressure Measurement

In summary, the use of plantar pressure measurement is vital from the investigational and clinical standpoints. Potential drawbacks in interpreting the results in the literature are interinstrument variability and gait characteristics such as speed and stride length. From the clinical standpoint, plantar pressure analysis can help refine the assessment of patient risk and give important information for footwear prescription. In daily practice, plantar pressure measurement can identify areas of high pressure unsuspected on clinical examination that will need to be considered in the footwear prescription. Finally, in-shoe measurement represents a major advance and can refine the process of footwear prescription by defining the exact degree of pressure relief at high-risk areas.

Regarding threshold pressure for injury, it is clear that ulceration has been consistently linked to elevated barefoot peak plantar pressure, but there is no agreement regarding the threshold pressure for injury. The studies to date addressing risk of ulceration due to plantar pressure were not designed specifically to address this question. Although a consistent ulcer threshold has not been confirmed, the literature suggests that foci of barefoot pressure measurements above 500 to 700 kPa (as measured on an EMED-SF platform) begin to put the patient at increased risk for ulceration. It is certain, however, that peak plantar pressure as a risk factor does not exist in isolation. Patients with low pressure may ulcerate if they engage in risky behaviors such as barefoot walking and, conversely, patients with high barefoot pressure who are nonambulatory or who consistently use excellent footwear lower their overall risk.

Where Does Ulceration Occur?

Data on the location of ulcers on the feet of patients with diabetes are available from a series of studies by Ctercteko et al.,[94] Birke and Sims[40] (in both Hansen's disease and neuropathic diabetic patients), Calhoun et al.,[60] Edmonds et al.,[107] Apelqvist et al.,[10] and Armstrong et al.[20] Although midfoot ulcers are notably absent from the data presented by Edmonds et al.,[107] their series does allow comparisons of neuropathic with ischemic ulcers and also presents a comprehensive breakdown of ulcers by location on the foot (Fig. 6–9). Of particular interest from a biomechanical perspective is the fact that ulcers on the dorsal and plantar surfaces are approximately evenly distributed. Since dor-

sal ulcers are invariably shoe related, this distribution indicates that approximately half of all neuropathic foot ulcers could be avoided very simply by footwear that is appropriately sized. Preventing plantar ulcers also involves appropriate footwear, and in this case the biomechanical issues are more complex than those affecting dorsal injury prevention (see below).

How Does Foot Injury Occur?

Tissue Ischemia

Although elevated plantar pressure is now accepted as a major factor in the etiopathogenesis of plantar ulcers in diabetics, exactly how tissue damage occurs is not well known. Various mechanisms have been discussed by Brand and Coleman,[52] Delbridge et al.,[101] Pecoraro et al.,[196] and others.[272] It is certain that some regions of the plantar tissue become ischemic when the foot is loaded. A systolic blood pressure of 120 mm Hg is only 15 kPa, and capillary pressure is less than half this value. Reference to Figure 6–8 shows that typical peak plantar pressures in the forefoot during gait are at least 30 times higher, implying that blood flow will be occluded during at least part of the gait cycle. Recovery from this ischemia may be affected by such factors as glycosylation or the state of the microcirculation, which has recently been shown to be abnormal even in early diabetes.[249]

Factors leading to tissue breakdown have been studied much more systematically by those interested in pressure ulcers of the buttocks than by scientists with an interest in the foot. It is believed that pressures as small as 6 to 8 kPa can, when applied for periods of 15 minutes or more, affect the microcirculation, lymph flow, and interstitial transport in the tissues over the ischial tuberosities. Although the loading pattern in this region is fundamentally different from that which occurs in the foot, the protocols used by Bader[27] to examine recovery of tissue transcutaneous oxygen pressure (TcPo$_2$) after repetitive loading would seem to have merit for application to the foot. Delayed recovery of normal tissue oxygenation was found in elderly and neuropathic patients, and this may have been because of the delayed elastic recovery of the aging tissue.

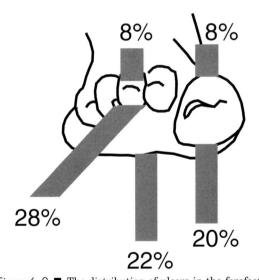

Figure 6–9 ■ The distribution of ulcers in the forefoot from Edmonds et al.[107] The forefoot accounted for 93% of all ulcers in this series. In addition to the locations shown in the figure (plantar and dorsal hallux, plantar, dorsal, and tips of all toes combined), other forefoot ulcers occurred in the following locations: 2% each on the plantar aspect (other than the tip), sides, and between the toes; on the tip and side of the hallux (4% and 1%, respectively); and on the dorsum of the metatarsal head region (1%).

Other Theories of Tissue Damage

It is also likely that unperceived stresses in the plantar soft tissues can be high enough to actually rupture the microanatomic and macroanatomic structures that are usually protected from damage by the exquisite sensitivity of the plantar aspect of a normal foot. Stepping on a sharp object and actually puncturing the skin would be the most severe and the most obvious example. In any case, there can be no doubt that the acute and chronic phases of foot injury deserve more study experimentally than they have received to date.

The classic model of ulceration has been postulated by Delbridge et al.[101] This theory assumes that the initial event in the formation of a typical neuropathic plantar ulcer is the development of plaque (callus) on the surface of the skin. They believe that tissue breakdown then occurs under the callus and that a cavity filled with plasma and blood develops. In their theory, this cavity enlarges until it causes a rupture of the skin surface, forming an ulcer with a small opening but a larger cavity beneath. This view is certainly congruent with the many preulcers that are seen as hemorrhage into callus.

Davis[97] has hypothesized that the irregular interaction of shear and compressive stresses at the skin surface causes tissue damage by a mechanism that he has likened to one region of a carpet slipping under the action of shear while another region remains stationary because of greater frictional forces.

A cellular mechanism for tissue damage has been explored by Landsman and Sage.[151] This group presented data from in vitro studies to show that high rates of tissue deformation cause changes in intracellular concentrations of calcium that do not result if the same magnitude of deformation is applied more slowly. They hypothesize that the altered intracellular environment may lead to cellular death. For this hypothesis to be verified as a causation of foot ulcers, it would be necessary to show that the tissue of patients with foot ulcers is deformed more rapidly than in nondiabetic tissue during typical activities of daily life.

It is interesting to speculate what the different theories might predict about the most appropriate foot-ground interface parameters to measure. For instance, the intermittent ischemia hypothesis would predict that the most important attribute to measure would be time spent above the threshold pressure for vascular occlusion, while the direct tissue-tearing hypothesis might predict that a small number of very-high-pressure events would be sufficient to cause the initial damage.

Causes of High Plantar Pressure and Other Contributors to Ulceration Risk

As noted earlier, pressures generated under apparently healthy feet (Fig. 6–8) can be high enough to cause ulceration in the presence of neuropathy. It is also true that diabetes, and particularly diabetes complicated by neuropathy, is associated with higher than normal plantar pressure.[46, 48] It is generally believed that diabetes mellitus may alter both the musculoskeletal and soft tissue mechanics in a manner that elevates plantar pressure and makes tissue damage more likely. Few of these effects have been observed in prospective studies, and thus evidence rests on retrospective analysis and cross-sectional studies.

Structure and Function Relationships

We have recently examined the relationship between the bony structure of the foot and elevated plantar pressure during controlled speed barefoot walking in 50 symptom-free adults.[68] A variety of angular and linear measurements were taken from standardized anteroposterior and lateral weight-bearing radiographs. A multivariate statistical technique (stepwise multiple regression) was used to identify those structural variables associated with high pressure. Among the strongest predictors of high pressure under the first metatarsal head were soft tissue thickness between the sesamoids and ground, inclination of the metatarsal in a sagittal plane, and frontal plane splay of the first and fifth metatarsals. It is encouraging to find that static structural measurements of the foot are statistically related to dynamic functional characteristics. This suggests that it may be possible in the future to add such measurements as a component of a larger risk-factor profile to predict risk of injury. However, because this approach was only able to predict 38% of the variance in peak plantar pressure at the first metatarsal head, we decided in a second study[176] to add dynamic "functional" variables such as stride parameters, foot motion measures, and electromyographic (EMG) data as possible predictors. With all of these variables in the regression, 50% of the variation in plantar pressure could be predicted and structural variables were still dominant in predicting the metatarsal head pressure, while both structural and functional variables were important at the hallux and heel.

A similar study in neuropathic diabetic patients has recently been reported by Ahroni, Boyko, and Forsberg.[1] These investigators measured in-shoe pressure as the patients walked in their own footwear at a freely chosen speed and foot deformity was assessed subjectively by a nurse practitioner. A wide variety of variables was offered to the subsequent regression models. The inclusion of foot deformity resulted in a significant improvement in the prediction capacity of the model at the metatarsal heads and hallux. However, the maximum amount of explained variance in peak pressure from all variables in the models was only 5.3 to 11.7%. Song et al.[238] used the traditional classification of feet as pes planus and rectus to show that such groups could be distinguished based on functional measurements. They extended this analysis to neuropathic patients and were again able to distinguish between groups based on functional measurements.

Thus it is clear that relationships exist between foot structure and plantar pressure, and we will now examine what is known about how structural and tissue changes in diabetes affect plantar pressure.

Structural Alterations

We have discussed earlier that foot structure is a major determinant of plantar pressure. While some structural factors are independent of diabetes, a number of others that predispose toward elevated pressure appear to be a result of the disease. Obviously, the major collapse of the foot that is seen in Charcot fractures will lead to elevated pressure. However, a number of more subtle changes also appear to contribute. Claw toes are a frequent clinical finding, and this phenomenon has been ascribed to atrophy of the intrinsic muscles that control the position of the proxi-

mal phalanges on the metatarsals.[189] In addition to the fact that claw toes increase the likelihood of dorsal ulceration from footwear, it is hypothesized that the soft tissue "metatarsal cushions"[127] are displaced distally, leaving the condyles of the metatarsal heads exposed. Gooding et al.[122, 123] have investigated tissue thickness under the metatarsal heads using ultrasound, but the results have been inconclusive. Young et al.[273] describe significantly reduced plantar tissue thickness in both neuropathic diabetic patients and those with rheumatoid arthritis and metatarsalgia. They were able to account for almost 70% of the variation in plantar pressure at MTH1 on the basis of soft tissue thickness. Kawchuk and Elliot[145] have provided insight on accuracy and validation of displacements measured using ultrasonic probes. A case study using spiral x-ray computed tomography (CT) in conjunction with plantar pressure measurement to demonstrate the coincidence of bony deformity, lack of underlying soft tissue, and elevated plantar pressure is presented by Mueller et al.[183]

Masson et al.[168] compared plantar pressure distribution in patients with diabetes and with rheumatoid arthritis. Both groups had a similar prevalence of foot deformity and both exhibited similar numbers of patients with plantar pressure above 980 kPa. Thus this study again links deformity and high plantar pressure. Only the diabetic patients experienced plantar ulceration, of course, because of the coexistence of neuropathy.

In a remarkably interesting study, Taylor et al.[246] reported rupture of the plantar fascia in 12 consecutive diabetic patients with clawing of the toes. No such rupture was found in 12 matched control patients with diabetes but without clawing of the toes. If confirmed in a larger study, these observations may reshape our view of the pathogenesis of claw toes and perhaps question the role of intrinsic muscle atrophy as the primary determinant of claw and hammer toes. It should also be noted that Kastenbauer et al.[143] found no differences in peroneal motor nerve conduction velocity (NCV) between groups with and without clawing of the toes. If intrinsic muscle atrophy were to be the cause of the clawing, then a decrease in NCV in the claw toe group would have been expected. Also, the theory of Taylor et al.[246] is supported by observations of Hamel and Sharkey[128] that the plantar fascia is a critical element in the transmission of force through the toes.

Tissue Properties

More direct metabolic consequences of diabetes may also affect plantar soft tissue structure and function. Nonenzymatic glycosylation (NEG) of many proteins in the body has been demonstrated in patients with diabetes,[56] and this process has been shown to affect the mechanical properties of tissue, usually reducing elasticity. The foot is no exception, and Delbridge et al.[102] have shown that keratin in the stratum corneum of the diabetic foot is glycosylated compared with nondiabetic skin. Zilberberg[275] found a higher content of the nonenzymatic crosslink pentosidine in plantar skin samples from the amputated feet of diabetic patients compared to nondiabetic controls. She also found a trend for skin from the diabetic feet to be stiffer as determined by conventional mechanical testing. This may result in a reduced capacity of the skin for the distribution of pressure.

Limited Joint Mobility (LJM)

A further presumed by-product of NEG is the observed limitation of range of movement in many joints of the body in persons with diabetes. Although first demonstrated in the hand,[211] this has now been found in the joints of the foot and ankle.[36, 108] Anecdotally, limitation of motion in the first MTP joint is frequently associated with ulceration of the hallux in neuropathic patients (see earlier discussion and Fig. 6–1C). Birke, Franks, and Foto[37] found that patients with a history of MTH1 ulceration had significantly diminished dorsiflexion range of motion at the first MTPJ. Limited first ray mobility explained almost 50% of the variance in peak MTH1 plantar pressure.

Decreased subtalar joint mobility has been associated with elevated plantar pressure,[108] although there are indications that protective sensation may allow compensation to occur such that pressure may not necessarily be elevated in the setting of subtalar limited joint mobility without neuropathy.[66]

Chantelau et al.[85] reported higher interdigital pressures between the fourth and fifth toes (a common site of ulceration) in patients with limited joint mobility compared to controls and also noted that pressure was higher in shoes with constrained toe caps.

Veves et al.[265] have proposed that diabetic Caucasians may be at greater risk of limited joint mobility compared to diabetic African Americans. The increased range of motion at the subtalar and MTPJ1 joints in African American diabetic patients compared to Caucasian patients was accompanied in their relatively small sample (24 African Americans, 31 Caucasian) by lower plantar pressures.

Although Sabato et al.[215] found an association between high pressure and ulceration in Hansen's disease patients, they reported that a reduced range of motion at the ankle joint was not associated with ulceration. However, others[85, 108] have found that a limited range of motion at several foot and ankle joints in diabetic patients is associated not just with elevated pressure but also with ulceration.

There are some initial indications that pharmacologic interventions may have some impact on LJM. Nargi et al.[190] showed that the use of N-phenacylthiazolium bromide (a substance that cleaves collagen crosslinks) in diabetic rats resulted in increased joint mobility.

Curran et al.[96] were the first to show that a program of physical therapy may be effective in improving joint mobility in diabetic patients with LJM. Armstrong et al.[23] performed an uncontrolled study of ten patients with a history of ulceration and LJM. After a supervised program of passive range-of-motion exercise performed three times per week for 1 month and once daily exercises at home, range of motion at the MTP1 joint increased significantly. There was also a reduction in peak forefoot plantar pressures.

Plantar Callus

It has been suggested that neuropathy predisposes patients to the production of excessive plantar keratoses.[216] Alternately, the formation of callus has been ascribed to elevated shear stress,[127] although experimental evidence for this view is lacking. It is also possible that callus is simply a consequence of elevated vertical pressure, though callus is not found at all sites of high plantar pressure. Whatever the cause of callus may prove to be, recent evidence has shown that the removal of callus from bony prominences in the forefoot reduces plantar pressure by an average of 29%.[272] It appears, therefore, that excessive callus acts to elevate pressure, which may result in positive feedback for the production of further callus. This observation confirms the critical importance of callus care in the patient at risk for neuropathic ulceration.

In a prospective study of 63 neuropathic diabetic patients, Murray et al.[185] found that based on six patients who ulcerated (seven ulcers), relative risk ratios for developing an ulcer were 4.7 for an area of high pressure, 11.0 for patients with areas of plantar callus, and 56.8 for those with a prior ulcer. This points to the importance of callus in the pathogenesis of ulcers, and also suggests that the tissue may be altered after ulceration to make it more susceptible to injury.

Fractures

Several authors have noted a large number of radiographic abnormalities in the feet of neuropathic patients.[95, 120, 129, 161] Cavanagh et al.[79] found a 12% prevalence of fractures (mostly metatarsal shaft) in neuropathic patients, and most of these had not been previously diagnosed. In addition, an 8% prevalence of Charcot joint fractures was found. Fractures can result in alteration of weight bearing and load sharing by regions of the foot not specialized for this purpose. Thus unperceived injury to bone can be a risk factor for elevated plantar pressure and ulceration.

Weakness

Strength loss in the leg as a result of peripheral neuropathy has been well documented by Andersen et al.[8] These authors studied 58 type 1 patients younger than 65 years old, all with a diabetes duration of greater than 20 years. Patients with neuropathy showed a 21% reduction in ankle dorsiflexor and plantar flexor strength, a 16% reduction in knee extensor strength, and a 17% reduction in knee flexor strength as measured with an LIDO isokinetic dynamometer. The most severe strength losses noted in individual patients compared to controls were more than a 50% reduction in the plantar flexors. In a subsequent study using magnetic resonance imaging (MRI), Andersen et al.[7] found a 32%

reduction in the volume of the dorsal and plantar flexors, with more atrophy apparent distally.

It is not yet clear whether strength loss is a factor in altering the load on the plantar surface. Atrophy of the intrinsic foot muscles is widely thought to result in foot deformity, and it may be that loss of more proximal extrinsic muscle mass results in a different interaction of the foot with the ground.

Prior Ulceration

Previous ulceration is a leading risk factor for future ulceration. The initial ulceration represents tangible proof that the patient has the combination of other risk factors that together produce ulceration. In addition, altered mechanical properties of the new tissue generated during the wound repair process may further increase the risk.[55] Although little is known about the mechanical properties of tissue generated during wound repair,[132] clinically one can feel the adhesion between different tissue layers and the lack of mobility of the skin overlying bony prominences. The exact role of adhesion and scar tissue in causing further tissue breakdown is not well known, but certainly stress concentration is a possible explanation. Thus scar tissue may act in much the same way that callus appears to act by transferring large, concentrated loads to the immediately underlying softer tissue. Thus the 56.8 risk ratio conferred by prior ulceration[185] may reflect scar tissue–induced abnormalities as well as other risk factors present at the time of initial ulceration.

Shear Stress

Most of the previous discussion concerning the interaction of the foot with the shoe or ground has centered on the normal (vertical) pressures. But as shown in Figure 6–2, there are also forces during gait, so-called shear forces, that tend to make the foot slip from its relatively fixed position on the ground. These forces generate shear stress in the tissues and in the shoe materials, which are considered on a theoretical basis in the following discussion. Little is known at present about the magnitude and direction of shear stress during everyday activities or its role in causing plantar injury. This is because, until recently, there were only isolated examples in the literature of instrumentation to measure shear stress.[150, 202] Many authorities believe that shear stress is an important pathogenic factor in foot injury,[51, 127, 138] and it should not be ignored simply because there is no satisfactory measurement device at present. Shear stress can probably be modulated by the fit of a shoe (Fig. 6–23), and it may emerge that the minimization of shear stress is an important criterion in defining appropriate fit.

Four new devices to measure plantar shear stress have been described during the last decade. Lord et al.[165] enhanced the magnetoresistive device originally proposed by Tappin et al.[245] by allowing measurement to be made in two orthogonal directions. These authors reported values for shear stress of 20 to 60 kPa, which are approximately 10% of the vertical stress values commonly encountered. Davis and associates[99, 198] have designed and tested a device that is composed of 16 sensors, each 2.54 × 2.54 cm, capable of measuring three components of the applied load. They have derived estimates of 15 to 45 kPa for shear stress under the foot in various conditions. Akhlaghi and Pepper[2] describe preliminary results using thin polyvinylidene fluoride (PVdF) piezoelectric film, which has charge outputs proportional to shear stress in two independent directions. Christ et al.[86] report on a device with 64 elements based on the same capacitance approach as platforms for the measurement of normal stress. All four of these devices are presently being used only in research environments and all have different geometric and physical characteristics. If any or all of them can be shown to be linear and independent of temperature changes, they may offer a new approach to the measurement of foot-floor interaction and the understanding of the etiology of foot injury.

Body Weight: Is It a Factor?

Cavanagh, Sims, and Sanders[71] reported a small but statistically significant association between body mass and peak pressure in diabetic patients. Body weight accounted for only 14% of the variance in peak plantar pressure. Similar results were reported by Ahroni, Boyko, and Forsberg,[1] who were able to explain only 6% of the variance. This some-what counterintuitive finding indicates that foot structure is the dominant factor in determining plantar pressure and that the area over which load is distributed is subject to much more dramatic variations than the load itself. Consider, for example, how a prominent metatarsal head concentrates the forefoot load.

Vela et al.[257] asked young, symptom-free subjects to walk with added weight carried in the pockets of a vest while in-shoe plantar pressure was measured. Not surprisingly, they found that plantar pressure increased as a function of added load. This experiment speaks to a different issue from that described above. Artificially added load to a constant load distribution system (i.e., the individual subject's foot structure) will always increase peak plantar pressure. However, gain in body weight by an individual patient may or may not increase plantar pressure, depending on whether the plantar architecture is altered (e.g., by the deposition of more adipose tissue in the foot). Thus, in any given patient, body weight will be a poor predictor of plantar pressure. A small female weighing 100 lb can easily exhibit higher pressure than a large male weighing 300 lb.

Abnormal Posture and Gait

The standing posture of patients with neuropathy is markedly less stable than the posture of control patients with diabetes of the same duration but with minimal neuropathy.[93, 230, 251] Simoneau et al.[230] have shown that neuropathic patients sway as much with their eyes open and head forward as do non-neuropathic patients in the challenging condition of eyes closed, head back. This may be a factor in the increased number of falls reported by neuropathic patients[64] and may be partly the cause for the increased number of fractures that have been reported in this group.[80, 95, 222]

A number of investigators have explored the effects of diabetic neuropathy on gait and there is considerable speculation that the gait patterns of neuropathic patients may predispose them to injury. Peripheral neuropathy has been shown to be a risk factor for injuries and falls during gait.[65, 205] Courtemanche and colleagues[93] reported that neuropathic patients exhibited conservative gait patterns with increased time spent in double support and lower walking speeds. Increased reaction times to secondary tasks during gait were also found, suggesting that the neuropathic patients had to exert more cognitive control over normal gait compared to controls. Katoulis et al.[144] also found smaller knee joint excursions and lower peaks of vertical and anteroposterior ground reaction forces in neuropathic patients with a history of ulceration compared to nonneuropathic patients. However, these may have been speed effects, since the neuropathic patients walked significantly slower than the control groups. Shaw et al.[227] used matching gait speeds between groups and found slightly higher first peaks in the vertical ground reaction forces of neuropathic patients with a history of ulceration compared to control subjects. Van Schie et al.[252] showed that the peak ground reaction forces in the residual limb of unilateral amputees were lower than those on the unaffected side, but the force-time integral was higher, reflecting the altered gait mechanics necessary for ambulation with only one power input limb.

Different authors have hypothesized that peripheral neuropathy may lead to more variable[70] or less variable[51, 52] gait patterns. It has also been hypothesized that less variable gait might contribute to risk of plantar ulceration. Cavanagh et al.[69] found that neuropathic patients did not exhibit abnormal variability of in-shoe plantar pressure patterns during shod walking, but by studying 10-minute epochs of continuous gait, Dingwell[103] found increased kinematic variability at the ankle joint in neuropathic patients.

Taken together, these studies show that neuropathic gait may be somewhat different from nonneuropathic gait and does exhibit, if anything, slightly more variability compared to normal, thus refuting the hypothesis that less variable plantar loading due to neuropathy at a subconscious level contributes to ulceration. Of course, patients with loss of protective sensation do not vary their gait at a conscious level in response to pain. Neuropathy does cause unstable posture. However, despite the widely agreed upon role of sensory feedback in gait,[213] patients with diabetic neuropathy are able to ambulate in a nonchallenging situation in a manner remarkably similar to their nonneuropathic counterparts. The frequent anecdotal reports from patients that they "do not know where their feet are" and that they "bump their feet

into things" must mean that gait studies to date have failed to successfully characterize the result of proprioceptive deficits. It is likely that the increased number of fractures in neuropathic patients is at least partly the result of these mechanisms.

Footwear

Uccioli et al.[250] conducted a prospective study of patients with previous ulceration. Patients were randomly assigned to wear either their own shoes or an extra-depth shoe with custom molded insoles. After 1 year, reulceration in the two groups was 58.3% and 27.7% for the group wearing their own shoes and the extra-depth shoe group, respectively. Since reimbursement for special footwear was extremely limited in Italy prior to this study, the authors justified their protocol of assigning patients to wear shoes in which they had already ulcerated by the need to influence public health policy. Such a protocol would probably not, and should not, be approved by institutional review boards in the United States, since it is now clear from this and a number of other studies[11] that footwear can play a key role in causing ulceration.

Summary of Causes of High Pressure

In summary, a variety of structural and functional factors in the foot and leg interact to result in elevated plantar pressure or they can cause skin injury directly. Among the most important variables is soft tissue thickness. Other important anatomic and functional factors include the degree of foot deformity, and gait parameters such as speed and instability.

Underlying tissue properties thought to have an effect include inelasticity due to nonenzymatic glycosylation, resulting in limited joint mobility, particularly at the first MTP joint and subtalar joints. Plantar callus is a visible marker for high plantar pressure, perhaps owing its existence to elevated pressure and itself causing an estimated 30% increase in pressure. Scar formation from prior ulceration may result in a focus of elevated pressure. Lastly, body weight has not been found to contribute significantly to elevated peak plantar pressure.

Although vertical pressure is measured in almost every study to date, it is believed that future evaluation of shear forces will further illuminate the pathogenesis of ulceration.

Ulcer Healing: Biomechanical Considerations

The Need for Load Relief

Ulcers develop on neuropathic feet because of trauma not felt by the patient, and it makes sense that they cannot heal if mechanical trauma is ongoing. It is now generally agreed that the terms "chronic ulcer" or "nonhealing ulcer" when applied to feet with adequate vascular supply are misnomers.[75] The evidence for this statement comes from the many studies of the TCC (see section "The Total-Contact Cast," below), which is probably the best and certainly the best studied method of mechanically protecting plantar neuropathic ulcers. De Block et al.[100] found that only 3% of a large group of ulcer patients that they studied actually had "chronic" foot ulcers that were resistant to appropriate treatment. If a typical neuropathic plantar ulcer fails to heal by approximately 8 weeks, it is either being poorly treated or the patient is not being compliant with the treatment. In a recent review, Sinacore[232] summarized 13 studies that describe the efficacy of the TCC in the treatment of 389 neuropathic ulcers. Many of these ulcers had been present for months and even years prior to instituting TCC treatment, yet the reported healing rates were 77 to 100% in 5 to 7 weeks.

By studying uncomplicated patients who have remained in a TCC to complete wound closure, we have been able to define "ideal healing curves" for plantar wounds of different initial sizes.[134] (Uncomplicated patients were those without infection, with good vascular supply, and with continuous healing all the way to closure.) These curves, shown in Figure 6–10A, are derived from the equation:

$$r = b_0 + b_1{}^*r_0 + b_2{}^*t + b_3{}^*r_0{}^*t$$

This equation expresses the equivalent radius (r) of the ulcer at the time (t) in days after presentation. Equivalent radius is the radius of a circle whose area is the same as the (usually noncircular) ulcer. Where r_0 is

the equivalent radius at day 0, and the constants b_0, b_1, b_2, and b_3 were determined to be:

$$b_0 = -0.74$$
$$b_1 = 1.04$$
$$b_2 = -0.10$$
$$b_3 = -0.012$$

Ideal healing curves such as those shown in Figure 6–10 allow healing data for a given patient to be plotted against the ideal. In the clinic, the equivalent radius of a wound can be estimated by measuring the widest (D_w) and narrowest (D_n) diameter and dividing the sum of these measurements by 4.

If the patient's data deviate significantly into the area 1, 2, and 3 standard errors away from the mean (shown as dotted lines on the graph), then the treatment and the patient's compliance and behavior need to be reevaluated. That is not to say that all wounds must or can heal "ideally." Compromises may have to be made in patient care, possibly leading to a healing rate that is less than "ideal," and such an approach may be acceptable to both the patient and the care provider. Nevertheless, having an "ideal" standard is useful even in such a case, since it allows the judgments to be made as to how much of a compromise is actually being made. An example of actual healing data for a large midfoot ulcer (Fig. 6–10B) is shown in Figure 6–10C.

The above equation can be rewritten to predict the time to healing (t_h):

$$t_h = -(b_0 + b_1{}^*r_0) / (b_2 + b_3r_0)$$

and a table of days-to-healing for ulcers of different initial sizes is presented in Table 6–2 and Figure 6–11.

The most common reason for failure to heal a neuropathic ulcer is lack of effective pressure relief at the ulcer site—either due to the failure of the clinician to prescribe the correct measures or to patient nonadherence. The following section will examine ways in which load can be relieved from an active ulcer.

The Total-Contact Cast

The TCC was designed to equalize loading of the plantar surface by equal "total contact"

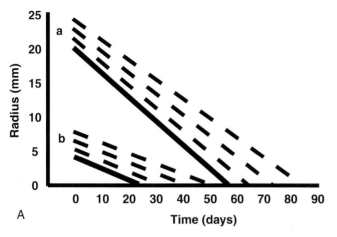

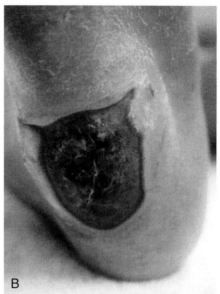

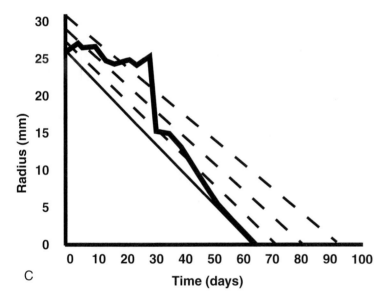

Figure 6–10 ■ A, Ideal healing curves for plantar wounds with initial sizes of 5 mm and 20 mm equivalent radii from Hsi et al.[134] The *dashed lines* associated with each curve are 1, 2, and 3 standard errors from the mean. B, A large midfoot ulcer at the initial visit. C, The ulcer shown in Figure 6–10B was healed in a total-contact cast with the healing curve shown. Note that progress was not along the ideal curve until drainage was controlled at approximately day 30.

Table 6–2 ■ IDEAL HEALING TIMES FOR ULCERS OF DIFFERENT INITIAL SIZES

INITIAL SIZE (EQUIVALENT RADIUS) (MM)	INITIAL AREA (CM²)	TIME TO 50% REDUCTION IN RADIUS (DAYS)	TIME TO COMPLETE HEALING (DAYS)
2.5	0.2	4.7	14.3
5	0.8	12.3	27.9
10	3.1	21.2	43.9
15	7.1	26.3	53.1
20	12.6	29.6	59.0
25	19.6	31.9	63.2
30	28.3	33.6	66.2

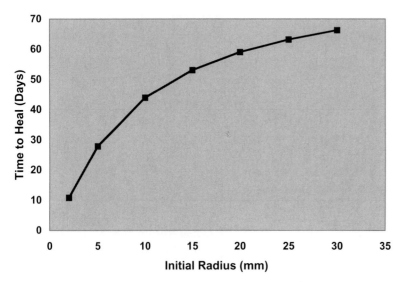

Figure 6–11 ■ Days to healing for ulcers of different initial sizes.

of the plantar skin with the cast material,[89] thereby minimizing pressure at an ulcer site. While the device was not developed by Paul Brand, he and his associates popularized its use, first in India in the treatment of patients with Hansen's disease, and later in the United States in the treatment of the ulcerated diabetic neuropathic foot.[89] In the early publications on the TCC, emphasis was placed on the total contact and it was recommended that the cast be made of plaster, because it is more malleable than fiberglass. Later, outer layers of fiberglass were added for strength. Most centers now make the whole cast from fiberglass[44, 63, 136, 226] without apparent detriment in clinical outcomes. For further information on the use of TCC, see Chapter 13.

The precise mechanism of unloading in the TCC has now been studied by measuring plantar pressure inside the cast. A common design feature of the TCC is to "pad" the ulcer area with a soft foam before putting the cast on.[39, 187] This, in essence, creates a void under the ulcer. In a group of healthy subjects, Shaw et al.[226] demonstrated pressure alteration in the forefoot at an MTH "ulcer site" in a TCC from approximately 350 kPa barefoot to approximately 50 kPa (reduction of 86%). Neither peak pressure nor impulse (total force transmitted during a step) were equalized across the plantar surface in the TCC. While some of the unloading seen in the forefoot was due to transfer of load to other parts of the foot (particularly the heel),

approximately 30% of the unloading was actually due to the leg transferring load directly to the cast walls, and much of the effect was due to the "void" created by the foam under the "ulcer." Midfoot peak pressure was reduced by 28% (92 kPa to 66 kPa, NS), but this cannot be reasonably extrapolated to what might happen in patients with high midfoot pressure due to a Charcot fracture or a similar prominence. Heel pressure was reduced markedly (49%, 354 kPa to 181 kPa), but the overall heel impulse was markedly increased (52%) because of increased time of loading. Shaw et al. did not report any peak pressure-time integrals.

In a very comprehensive study, Lavery et al.[156] found average pressure reductions in a TCC compared to a thin rubber-soled canvas oxford shoe in 25 patients with recently healed forefoot ulcers of 81 to 92% (depending on the site), at the previous ulcer sites. The average pressures in the canvas shoe were 271 kPa at the hallux, 438 kPa at the first MTH, and 506 kPa at the second through fifth MTHs, while the corresponding average pressures at these sites in the TCC with a plastic walking heel were 49, 59, and 39 kPa, respectively. There was a small benefit in terms of pressure relief to the use of a TCC with a plastic walking heel versus a TCC with a canvas cast shoe over it. Armstrong et al.[21] reported on the heel pressures in this cohort. Mean peak pressure of the group was reduced by 33% (approximately 275 kPa to 185 kPa), but the pressure-time integral was not changed (meaning that loading at the point of peak pressure in the TCC was much longer than that in the canvas shoe).

Cogley et al.[87] noted a 91% reduction in forefoot plantar pressure in five subjects in a TCC compared to barefoot walking, and they actually reported an increase in heel pressure, but this was not statistically significant. Baumhauer et al.[34] noted forefoot pressures in a TCC of approximately 85 to 155 kPa. However, their protocol called for casting in 5 to 10 degrees of dorsiflexion at the ankle, which may be responsible for these somewhat higher forefoot pressures than those reported in the other studies. Almost all other descriptions of the TCC procedure call for casting with the ankle in a neutral position.[58, 89] In the Baumhauer study, no data were given for baseline barefoot or similar pressures. Martin et al.[167] reported that a TCC significantly lowered midfoot pressure in Charcot deformity patients.

Three studies have examined whether or not total contact is required to unload an ulcer. Conti et al.[92] reported no difference in pressure reduction between standard short leg orthopedic casts and TCCs both in asymptomatic subjects and in patients with midfoot collapse due to Charcot fracture.[167] Cogley et al.[87] also found no difference in forefoot pressure relief in five subjects making the same comparison (TCC 91% reduction, short leg cast 88% reduction), and similar results had been reported much earlier by Birke et al.[41]

In all of the biomechanical studies just summarized, the emphasis has been on pressure relief, and there can be no doubt that removing injurious forces from the wound is central to healing. However, in all these studies, only peak pressure was measured. Impulse and shear may also be important and may also be reduced in a TCC. Shortened stride length and less walking in general because of the weight and clumsiness of the cast may also be of benefit. Another potential benefit of the TCC that has not been confirmed by clinical studies is reduction of edema. Lastly, an important advantage of the TCC over other measures of pressure relief is ensured patient adherence.

Many studies have been published highlighting the clinical efficacy of the TCC approach, and their summary in 1996 by Sinacore[232] is discussed above. The work of Mueller et al.[180] deserves special mention since, to date, this has been the only randomized controlled trial of TCC therapy published. Forty patients with plantar neuropathic ulcers were randomized to receive either good wound care and a TCC, or just good wound care. Importantly, the patients not casted were instructed to avoid bearing weight on the foot and were given crutches or walkers to that end. They were also given protective footwear in case they should step on the affected foot. The average duration of the ulcers before entry into the study was 155 days in the TCC group and 175 days in the standard care group. Despite the effort to encourage the control group to not bear weight on the ulcer, in the TCC group 19 of 21 ulcers healed in 42 ± 29 days, while in the control group only 6 of 19 ulcers healed in 65 ± 29 days.

Since 1996 several other studies have been published further demonstrating the benefits of the TCC and providing some insights into other factors that affect the healing time. Lavery, Armstrong, and Walker[153] reported on a series that included 25 neuropathic plantar ulcers with a mean surface area of 7.7 ± 4.0 cm² and a duration of 88.5 ± 98.3 days and 22 patients with Charcot fractures and ulcers with a mean surface area of 10.3 ± 4.6 cm² and duration of 17.7 ± 12.9 days. All of the ulcers healed in a TCC in 38.8 ± 21.3 days, while all of the Charcot-related ulcers healed in a TCC in 28.4 ± 13.0 days. Short duration, small size, and association with a Charcot fracture all predicted a shorter healing time. A related study[17] reported that among the 25 noninfected ulcers, higher plantar pressures at the ulcer site predicted a longer duration of casting until healing. Sinacore[233] reported on a series of patients with various fixed deformities of the foot. He found a gradient of healing times for ulcers in the forefoot (35 ± 12 days), 73 ± 23 days in the midfoot, and 90 ± 12 days in the rearfoot, with the overall average being 67 ± 29 days. The extent of the fixed deformity was also correlated with healing time. Caravaggi et al.[63] followed 50 patients with neuropathic foot ulcers to healing in a fiberglass TCC. All the ulcers healed in 58.5 ± 38.0 days, and size predicted time to healing. Patients preferred fiberglass casts to plaster casts. Finally, Lin et al.[160] reported that a group of 21 patients with neuropathic foot ulcers randomly selected from those that healed using a TCC in their clinic did so on average in 43.5 days. Importantly, they found that the sole cause of nonhealing of a forefoot plantar ulcer in their series was inability to dorsiflex at the ankle (dorsiflexion range of motion in nonhealers was −20 to − 5 degrees; in those who healed it was −5 to +10 degrees). Fourteen of the 15 ulcers that had failed to heal initially did so in an average 39.3 days after a tendo Achilles lengthening (TAL) procedure (and ongoing TCC). It is perhaps relevant that Lin et al.[160] applied the TCC with 5 degrees of dorsiflexion at the ankle, while others describe TCCs applied with the ankle neutral.[58, 89]

Exact and consistent data on the complications of the TCC are hard to come by. Reported rates of complications vary from 6 to 43%,[232] and this variability depends on what is reported as a complication. Minor abrasions are common and heal in the next TCC. Major abrasions are rare and the devastating complication of a major unrecognized infection is very rare, as are falls that lead to fractures.

To summarize the pressure and clinical data on the TCC, it is reasonable to conclude that the TCC is very effective at reducing forefoot and probably midfoot plantar pressure and at healing plantar ulcers. The data are less clear with respect to heel ulcers. It may be that to accomplish efficient healing of a heel ulcer in a TCC a significant foam cover creating a "void" under the ulcer (as is done routinely in many but not all centers) may be particularly useful since, while heel pressure is reported to be decreased in a TCC in at least two studies, one found increased impulse and the other no improvement in the pressure-time integral in a TCC intimately molded at the heel. Many centers report that their results are as good with all fiberglass TCCs as with plaster TCCs. Both the clinical data of Lin et al.[160] and the pressure data of Baumhauer et al.[34] suggest that the efficacy of the TCC in healing forefoot ulcers may depend critically on the angle at which the ankle is fixed with respect to the available range of dorsiflexion. In both studies the TCC was applied with dorsiflexion at the ankle. Lin et al.[160] found unusually poor healing compared to other studies, and Baumhauer et al.[34] found relatively high forefoot pressures in a TCC compared to other studies. Based on the available data, there seems to be no reason to cast with the ankle in dorsiflexion and the possibility that a few degrees of

plantar flexion may be additionally helpful should be explored. The pressure studies of Birke et al.,[41] Conti et al.,[92, 167] and Cogley et al.[87] with standard short leg casts, as well as the study of Shaw et al.[226] suggest that the "total-contact" concept may not be as critical to healing casts as had been previously thought.

The total-contact cast can be bivalved by making a saw cut on the medial and lateral midlines, in effect making a "clamshell" type of front section that is held in place by Velcro straps. This approach has both advantages (ease of removal for bathing or sleeping) and disadvantages (easy for noncompliant patients to remove at inappropriate times). A loosely applied bivalved cast probably does not unload the plantar surface as well as a full TCC (see above discussion of Shaw et al.[226]). To date, no quantitative comparison of pressure relief in the two devices has been performed. Another version of a bivalved cast, in which the front shell is not replaced, is called a walking or "Carville" splint.[38, 234] In a small study, Foster et al.[112] found that five of seven ulcers with a duration of 32 ± 31 weeks healed in a splint in 11 ± 8 weeks, while four of seven ulcers with a duration of 29 ± 16 weeks healed in a TCC in 7 ± 16 weeks.

Other forms of casts are also used, particularly a cast boot that does not extend above the ankle.[57, 139, 140, 234] The mechanism of action of the cast boot is different from the TCC, since no load can be shared by the leg. Usually a large cut-out around the ulcer site is made in the thick foam padding lining the boot and this probably serves to mechanically isolate the wound. Plantar pressure was measured in a small study of five volunteers in a cast boot, and pressure reduction in the forefoot compared to barefoot was only approximately 50% of the barefoot value—which is unlikely to be enough to promote good healing.[87] However, in one clinical study of a cast boot,[57] 35 of 40 patients healed in a mean of 3 months (range, 1 to 8 months), and in another study ulcers that healed did so by 130 days despite mean ulcer duration prior to entry into the study of 912 days.[172]

Another unloading method that uses casting is the MABAL shoe proposed by Hissink et al.[131] These authors describe a removable fiberglass "combicast" that is applied to the ulcerated foot over a thick felted foam dressing. A rocker outsole is attached and the cast ends below the level of the malleoli. Velcro straps are used to stabilize the shoe to the foot. Better than 90% healing with mean healing times of 34 days (range, 7 to 75 days) are reported for a group of 23 ulcers with a mean area of 2 cm^2.

All of the removable devices can be used with infected wounds, since they allow for frequent dressing changes and wound inspection. Once infection is under control and the patient is clearly improving on antibiotics, it is a matter of clinical judgment as to whether a full TCC with frequent changes should be employed for optimal wound protection.

Other Approaches to Unloading

The absence of information on pressure thresholds for healing complicates the interpretation of studies of the various unloading devices. Strict non–weight bearing should be completely efficacious, of course, but in a clinical setting it is never as good as a TCC.[180] This may be because the TCC has other benefits over non–weight bearing, but more likely it is a function of some steps taken by the insensate patient despite his or her best efforts. Clinical experience suggests that when non–weight bearing is to be part of the protocol, very specific and explicit instructions need to be given to the patient about how to accomplish non–weight bearing in each situation they may encounter at home, at work, at night, and so forth. It is a matter of clinical experience that patients who bear weight even a few steps per day do not heal particularly well. It should also be recalled that balance is compromised in neuropathy and therefore any intervention that requires the patient to balance on one leg may be dangerous.

A number of approaches to unloading the foot are discussed by Knowles[18, 148] and by Armstrong and Lavery.[14] Many footwear interventions for healing can benefit by the added use of a walking aid such as crutches or the use of a wheelchair. A novel approach to unloading has been suggested by Roberts and Carnes,[207] who designed an "orthopedic scooter." This device consists of a metal frame attached to a trolley with four small wheels and an adjustable-height padded channel on which the patient can rest their lower leg and foot while propelling themselves with the contralateral foot. A similar device has been used by others,[109] and the design has also been refined with the addition of a brake (Roll-A-Bout Corp., Boca Raton, FL).

Chantelau et al.[82] describe the use of "half shoes" in the healing of forefoot plantar ulcers. These shoes offer support only under the rear and midfoot, leaving the forefoot "suspended." Despite the risk of blunt trauma to the forefoot and of the additional load added to the midfoot, these shoes appear to be successful in healing forefoot ulcers. In the study by Chantelau et al.,[82] 96% of patients healed with a mean time to ulcer closure of 70 days. Because of the inherent instability of this approach, Chantelau et al. insisted that patients also use crutches. Needleman[192] presents a retrospective case series of 33 patients who had been treated with a "half shoe" (IPOS, Niagara Falls, NY); 77% of patients healed in an average of 8 weeks. Among the complications from wearing the IPOS shoe were balance problems or falls (8 of the 33 patients reviewed), new ulcers or preulcers (4 of 33 patients), and bone pain (2 of 33 patients). Needleman also presented a comparison of charges for a course of treatment. The figures he proposed (as of 1997) were $82 plus the cost of daily wound care for the IPOS shoe, $800 to $1,400 plus four to seven episodes of wound care for the TCC, and approximately $1,000 plus daily wound care for the bivalved cast. He also estimated the cost of hospital bed rest at $390 per day plus daily wound care and a one-time charge for crutches plus daily wound care. This figure is already a significant underestimate of actual costs in many hospitals. A full cost-benefit analysis is not possible because of the lack of comparative data for wound healing by these different methods.

An important point to make about "half shoes" is that they are not all created equal. In the studies of Chantelau et al.[82] and Needleman,[192] the shoes used had no support surface for the forefoot (true half shoes). Fleischli et al.[111] studied unloading in terms of plantar pressure in the Darco half shoe. This version of the half shoe has a forefoot support and it is in reality a negative heel shoe with a large rocker (see "Footwear Theoretical Background," below). Pressure reduction in this type of shoe as reported by Fleischli et al. was only 64 to 66% compared to a canvas shoe. The published healing data were on true half shoes.[82, 192]

A number of braces and orthosis-like devices have also been explored as alternatives to TCCs. Most of these have a rigid rocker or roller sole, some method of attachment of vertical members up the sides or back of the leg, and a soft insole. Among the devices that have been most studied are the AirCast brace,[34, 111, 157] the CAM walker,[157] the DH Walker,[111, 157] and the Easy Step Walker.[16]

The AirCast brace has four inflatable chambers that are designed to provide an enhanced fit to the leg, though there are no published data to support this feature as additionally helpful in plantar pressure relief. No data on clinical efficacy of this device have been published either. However, Lavery et al.[157] noted a 60 to 73% reduction of plantar pressure at forefoot ulcer sites among 25 subjects with recently healed ulcers, and an approximately 26% reduction in the heel peak pressure without a change in the pressure-time integral[21] compared to a canvas Oxford with a thin rubber sole. The absolute forefoot peak pressures in the device were 111 to 150 kPa, significantly higher than TCC pressures in the same subjects (53 to 83 kPa). The heel peak pressures were approximately 200 kPa in the Air-Cast brace, 275 kPa in the canvas shoe, and 185 kPa in the TCC. In a similar study, Baumhauer et al.[34] found similar forefoot pressures (approximately 65 to 155 kPa) in the brace in ten healthy volunteers, and these values were not significantly different from TCC pressures (but see earlier discussion of the TCC technique used in this study).

The insole of the DH Walker consists of small hexagonal foam columns that can be removed to provide pressure relief for an ulcer. While this has been shown to be effective when brand new in normal subjects in terms of pressure relief, care is needed when the device is used clinically to ensure that columns surrounding the ulcer site do not collapse into the void, resulting in a significant loading of the ulcer site. Again, no published clinical data are available. However, forefoot pressure relief in the DH Walker as demonstrated by Lavery et al.[157] was in the range of 77 to 84%, with absolute pressures of 64 to 83 kPa. Similarly, Fleischli et al.[111] noted pressure reductions of 76 to 85% in 26 patients with recently healed ulcers, with absolute peak pressures of 49 to 77 kPa at the ulcer sites in the device. Both studies used a simple canvas shoe for comparison.

Armstrong and Stacpoole-Shea[21] reported that heel pressures in the DH Walker were 195 kPa compared to a shoe baseline of 275 kPa.

Saltzman et al.[217] reported reduced pressures under a Charcot midfoot prominence when using a patellar tendon-bearing brace, and Guse and Alvine[125] have also recommended such a brace to unload plantar ulcers. Further studies need to be conducted to determine the optimal design characteristics of such devices for unloading the foot, since a poorly designed or fitted device may result in little unloading. In fact, Salzman et al.[217] noted that the longer a device had been used, the looser the cuff and the less well the brace functioned to unload the foot. Landsman and Sage[152] have presented some successful case studies in which an ankle-foot orthosis was used during the healing of plantar ulcers in patients with Charcot fractures. Their pressure measurements showed that the brace offered considerable relief at the ulcer site compared to a shoe alone.

Morgan et al.[177] described a device called the Charcot Restraint Orthotic Walker (CROW), which has some similarity to a bivalved TCC. It is constructed from a bivalved polypropylene shell but, in contrast to the TCC or Carville splint, there is a layer of deep padding under the footbed. The outsole is rockered. These authors and others[175] described the successful use of the CROW as a follow-up to TCCs in patients with Charcot fractures. It has been speculated that the CROW could be used to treat ulcers, but such use is not supported by any published data. A similar device was used by Boninger and Leonard[43] to treat Charcot fractures and ulcers. Healing of 12 ulcers was very slow in this small study (eight ulcers healed in an average of 10 months).

Various types of felt and foam dressings are used at a number of centers for healing plantar ulcers.[126, 186] This approach consists of adhering a bilayer of felt and foam to the patient's foot (foam layer next to the skin). A region of pressure relief is created by removing the foam and felt material from the area of the ulcer and thus transferring load to the surrounding tissue. A surgical shoe is then worn to accommodate the bulk of the dressing. While no large controlled study of this method exists, a number of anecdotal reports suggest that it can be effective for patients who insist on remaining ambulatory during ulcer healing. Without providing specific data, Ritz et al.[206] state that more than 90% of neuropathic plantar ulcers can be healed in an average of 8 weeks using the felted foam approach. In a study comparing ten patients with plantar ulcers due to Hansen's disease treated with traditional care plus felt dressings to seven patients treated without felt, Kiewied[147] noted that, at 4 weeks, five of ten patients had healed with felt dressings, while no patients of seven healed with traditional care only. Off-loading of between 34 and 48% in terms of forefoot peak pressure at previous ulcer sites was noted by Fleischli et al.[111] when felt dressings were compared to walking in simple canvas shoes. This therapy is also said to be helpful for healing nonplantar wounds. However, some have expressed concern about the possible edge effects of such dressings, particularly when used on the plantar surface of the foot.[12, 19]

Connelley[90] has suggested from anecdotal observations that a pressure of 55 kPa (8 psi) measured inside footwear during walking will allow plantar ulcers to heal. This value is similar to those presented above for unloading in the TCC, AirCast brace, and DH Walker (although different devices were used by these two investigators to measure the pressure—see earlier discussion on this issue). For a discussion of the implementation of alternatives to the TCC see Chapter 14.

Most of the methods for off-loading the plantar ulcer described in this section have the advantage over the TCC that they can be easily removed and that they can therefore be used in the setting of infected ulcers, where frequent wound inspection and dressing changes are important.

Unloading the Plantar Ulcer—a Summary

Neuropathic ulcers should heal easily if given proper mechanical protection. The best studied and best established method for protecting the plantar neuropathic wound is the TCC.[62] Extensive data on normal healing in a TCC have been presented here and some of the design features of the TCC have also been discussed. Interestingly, equalization of pressure across the plantar surface is probably not an important feature of the cast and total contact may not be key. The TCC is labor intensive and therefore expensive, and it can lead to serious complications such as

unrecognized infection and iatrogenic lesions.

Only a few of the other methods discussed above for protecting the plantar surface are supported by clinical data, and even then, only small numbers of patients had been studied. The half shoe for healing plantar forefoot ulcers has been evaluated the most, but, as discussed above, not all brands/types of half shoes are likely to be equally efficacious. Several other commercial devices (in particular the AirCast brace and DH Walker) appear promising in terms of peak pressure relief, but that is not the same as clinical efficacy (particularly if peak pressure turns out not to be the key variable that determines tissue breakdown). Many experts support the use of felt and foam dressings.

As discussed earlier, patients with neuropathy fall more often, have more injuries, and sway more during standing than do persons without neuropathy. All of the devices intended to unload a neuropathic ulcer would seem intuitively to be likely to increase the risk of falling just because of their clumsiness, and this hypothesis is supported for the TCC with a plastic heel by Lavery et al.,[154] who demonstrated approximately 20% more sway during standing in a TCC with a plastic heel compared to standing in a simple canvas sports shoe. Interestingly, a TCC with a cast shoe, a CAM-type cast walker, and a Darco half shoe had little effect on postural sway. It still seems prudent to pay attention to the risk of falling and injury in all patients being treated for neuropathic plantar ulcers. However, casting with a cast shoe may be preferable in patients at very high risk for falling compared to casting with a plastic heel (but it should be recalled that a TCC with a cast shoe does not reduce pressure as well as a TCC with a plastic heel).[156]

Patients who have ulcerated often continue to wear footwear that had been prescribed to prevent ulceration. It is the common clinical experience that patients do not heal in shoes, even though the shoes may be good enough to prevent recurrence. It is worthwhile to consider this point in terms of what is known about pressure relief that can be achieved in a TCC compared to "therapeutic" shoes. The data just reviewed for pressure relief in a TCC show that 80 to 90% of the peak plantar pressure can be removed in a cast, while in sport shoes that figure is around 30% and may be no more than 50% in therapeutic shoes.

Footwear: Theoretical Background

That footwear is thought to be so central to injury prevention in diabetes is emphasized by the fact that other chapters in this book deal with the various aspects of footwear design and prescription (see Chapters 20 and 34). Footwear can "cushion" the plantar surface from the injurious high pressures that we discussed above, and through proper or improper fit, can both prevent and cause dorsal injury. Footwear can thus be critical in preventing the first injury in patients with newly diagnosed neuropathy and becomes an issue of lifetime concern for a patient who has experienced a neuropathic ulcer. Given the emphasis on the practical aspects of footwear in other chapters, in this section we describe some of the principles behind the action of footwear and explore ways in which some science may be applied to this area, which has been widely described as "an art."

Cushioning: Static and Dynamic

If asked to choose a single word to describe the objective of footwear for the neuropathic foot, many workers in the field would probably choose the term cushioning. Yet the definition of cushioning in a footwear context is elusive: it has no units, it is not easily measured, and it is often misinterpreted. Webster's dictionary[268] offers the definition "to protect against force or shock," and goes on to define a cushion as "an elastic body for reducing shock." This definition might be paraphrased in more mechanical terms as "controlling the energy of a collision." To understand the inadequacy of this definition and to seek a better one, it is helpful to divide the contact of the shoe and the floor into two

distinct phases: a dynamic phase, which starts at heel strike and ends at foot flat; and a quasistatic phase, which includes the remainder of ground contact. It may come as a surprise that late support and toe-off are considered quasistatic, but compared with the high impact forces of landing[204] the rather slowly changing forces of the second part of support have minimal dynamic components.

The major difference between these two phases is that the net or total force acting on the foot through the shoe can be reduced by the cushioning effect of footwear during the dynamic phase, but the net force during the quasistatic phase cannot be changed. However, during both phases, the net force can be distributed so that local pressures on the foot are reduced. By net force, we mean the total, at any instant in time, of all the forces acting on each part of the foot. For example, if there were forces of 300 N and 200 N on the forefoot and hindfoot, respectively, at 0.3 second after footstrike, a net force of 500 N would be acting, and this could be recorded by a force platform as shown in Figure 6–2.

To appreciate the difference between the dynamic and static phases, consider the two situations shown in Figure 6–12. In Figure 6–12A, an egg is dropped from the same height onto surfaces of successively softer characteristics. On the hard surface, it breaks, but on the foams the impact is "cushioned" and breakage does not occur. The appropriate models are of a mass with velocity V and acceleration g, contacting first a rigid link and then springs of stiffness $k1$ and $k2$ (where $k1 > k2$). Hypothetical force-time curves show that the peak force at impact would be reduced and the time to peak force increased. Both of these effects are forms of cushioning that can occur in a dynamic situation.

Figure 6–12 ■ Schematic illustrations on the effects of different types of "cushioning" during the dynamic phase and quasi-static phases of contact. *A*, Dynamic phase. Egg falling from the same height onto surfaces of successively softer characteristics. The appropriate models are of a mass with velocity v and acceleration g, contacting first a rigid link, then springs of stiffness k1 and k2 (k1 > k2). Hypothetical force-time curves show that the peak impact force would be reduced and the time to peak force increased by the softer material; however, the area under each curve (which represents the change in momentum of the egg) is the same in each case. Thus, in the dynamic phase (as occurs during gait primarily only at foot strike) soft materials can change the peak force acting on the foot. *B*, Static phase. Flat plate standing on materials of progressively increasing softness: rigid; stiffness, k1; stiffness k2 (k1 > k2). Note that despite the fact that the plate sinks more deeply into the softer material, the net (total) force acting on the plate is the same in each case and is equal to its weight. Therefore, in the static phase of foot contact with the ground (as occurs in the later phases of support) soft materials cannot change the total force acting on the foot, but can affect the distribution of the force (see also Fig. 6–13).

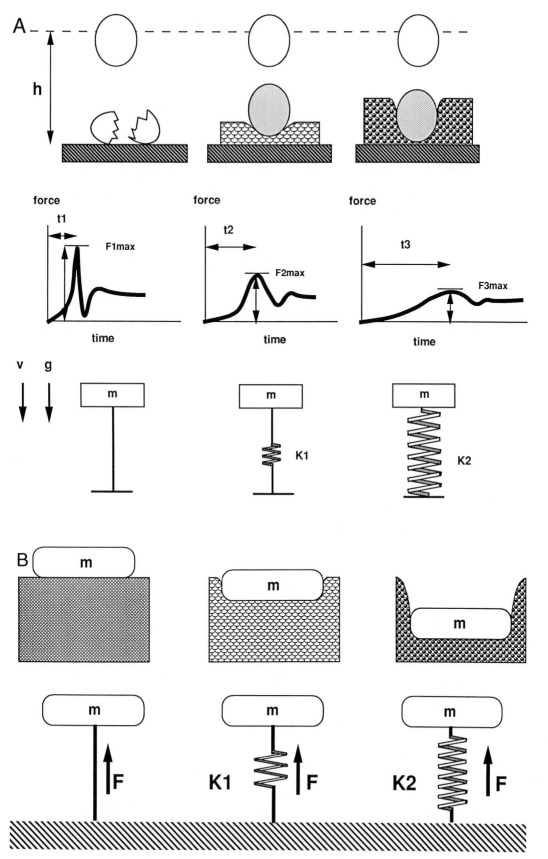

Figure 6-12 ■ *See legend on opposite page*

In the static situation, a flat plate is shown standing on the same materials (see Fig. 6–12B). Despite the fact that the plate sinks more deeply into the softer foams, the net (or total) force acting on the plate is the same in each case and is equal to its weight.

In the case of a collision, as occurs at heel strike, Webster's definition of cushioning is appropriate, because we are concerned with managing the energy of the collision to reduce the force on the foot. Certainly therapeutic shoes can be cushioned in this way, but we know that neuropathic ulceration rarely occurs in the heel regions except for ulcers caused by continuous application of pressure (similar to decubitus ulcers in the bedridden patient), which have a different etiology. Thus collision energy is not really what causes ulcers. Because the static example (Fig. 6–12B) shows that net force cannot be reduced during the midsupport phase when forefoot plantar pressures are largest (Plate 2), we must search elsewhere to find a definition of cushioning that is relevant to the prevention of neuropathic foot injury.

Footwear as a Distributor of Force

This search leads to a definition of cushioning that is based on "distribution" of force (and accompanying reduction of pressure) rather than attenuation of net force. As mentioned earlier, the term "net" is key to understanding the action of footwear because, although the net or total force acting on the forefoot at any instant in time may remain the same, the local forces acting on individual anatomic structures, which, when totaled, must equal the net force, can be altered dramatically by footwear.

A further model of cushioning in the context of forefoot deformity is proposed in Figure 6–13. If a bony prominence such as the head of a plantarflexed metatarsal contacts a rigid surface, most of the ground reaction force will be applied to the small area of the bony prominence, with resultant large local pressures (Fig. 6–13A). Patients are always encouraged to avoid walking barefoot for precisely this reason. The model of this foot in a conventional (nontherapeutic) shoe is shown in Figure 6–13B. The uniform stiffness of the midsole material (i.e., its spring constant k) is so large that even though the shoe does deform slightly, the amount of deformation is not enough to engage the adja-

cent spring elements with the foot so that the load can be shared. Thus no pressure reduction occurs.

When a compliant material is placed in the shoe, the situation becomes much more favorable for the soft tissue. The appropriate model now consists of a series of springs with lower spring constants than before, arranged in parallel with each other (Fig. 6–13C). Because the spring constant is smaller, more deformation will occur, allowing adjacent spring elements to begin to share the load as the material under the bony prominence is compressed. This action results in the so-called accommodative behavior of shoes for the neuropathic foot. The total force from all the spring elements at any instant will be the same as the force in Figure 6–13A but the local pressure (force in each spring element divided by its area of application) will be reduced.

This situation in Figure 6–13C clearly is not perfect, because the greater compression of the spring element under the prominence will still result in greater local pressure. The available options are to increase the length of the adjacent springs (Fig. 6–13D) or to reduce both the stiffness and the length of the spring under the prominence (see Fig. 6–13E). In practice, the first of these options is easier to achieve, because the deformation range over which a less stiff spring could work is limited by the room in the shoe. Molding of the insole to the shape of foot is the practical embodiment of this theory. This process brings the insole up to meet those parts of the plantar aspect that would otherwise not share in the load-bearing process. A firm molded insole should in theory equalize loading. However, relative movement between foot and footbed would bring prominent parts of the foot into contact with raised parts of the rigid insole, leading to tissue damage. Thus we depend on soft materials that modify their contour and keep the load shared between adjacent regions even when shearing movements occur. The "softness" of various insole materials is compared in Figure 6–14A.[219]

It has recently been shown that socks must be considered in this equation,[261, 262] because special thick socks alone can reduce barefoot peak pressures by approximately 30%. One can conceptualize the way they achieve this in the same manner as insoles have their effect, by providing a large number of short springs that can bring new, albeit small, re-

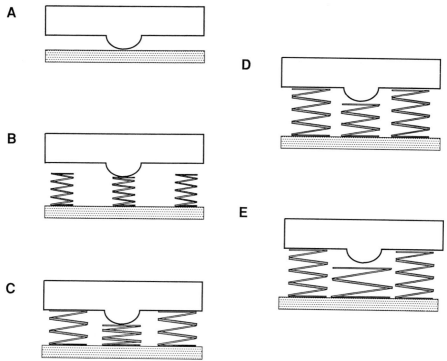

Figure 6–13 ■ Role of footwear during the quasi-static phase of ground contact in "cushioning" by distribution of load. *A,* Schematic cross-section of a foot with a plantar prominence resting on a flat rigid surface. *B,* Conceptual model of the foot in contact with a rigid shoe. Spring elements are all the same, and extremely stiff. Even though slight deformation occurs under the prominence, this does not cause enough deflection to bring other regions of the foot-shoe interface into the load-bearing process. Thus the pressure under the prominence is as high as in *A,* because the total force still is transmitted through this region. *C,* When a more compliant material is placed in the shoe the appropriate model now consists of springs with lower spring stiffness than before in parallel with each other. Because the spring stiffness is smaller, more deformation will occur, and as the material under the bony prominence is compressed, adjacent spring elements begin to share the load. This action results in the "accommodative" behavior of shoes for the neuropathic foot. The force transmitted through the prominence now will be less. *D,* Alternative solution (shown for the almost unloaded foot) is to reduce the length of the spring under the prominence and/or increase the length of the springs away from this region, so that all springs will engage immediately on loading. This occurs with a molded insole, where load sharing begins as soon as the foot is loaded and peak pressures are reduced. *E,* Better solution still is to make the spring under the prominence both shorter and less stiff. This reduces the loading on the prominence and increases loading on other structures. This occurs with a composite insole with different material under the bony prominence.

gions of the foot surrounding bony prominences into a weight-bearing role.

Even with a well-molded insole (e.g., Plastazote backed with PPT), there will still be elevated pressures under bony prominences compared with the adjacent regions. This is because the molding results in a thin, compressed layer of material under the prominence, which probably acts as a stiffer spring and will give greater force for a given compression than the uncompressed material in surrounding areas. There are presently no data in the literature on the mechanical characteristics of moldable materials after they have been reduced in thickness.

From the point of view of equalizing the pressure in different areas of the foot, the ideal foot-shoe interface would be a hydrostatic cushion (a fluid-filled bag) that could adapt to local curvatures and apply equal loads to all regions of the foot. This principle has been implemented in the area of pressure ulcers of the buttocks[26] and there are reports of investigations into fluid-filled insoles.[229] However, fluid has no ability to resist movement of the foot in the anteroposterior or mediolateral directions, providing a very unstable platform for the foot. The depth would also have to be great enough to prevent bottoming out. These problems do not appear to be insurmountable, however, with an appropriate restraint applied through the upper and with the kind of depth that is already incorporated into a rocker shoe. The problem

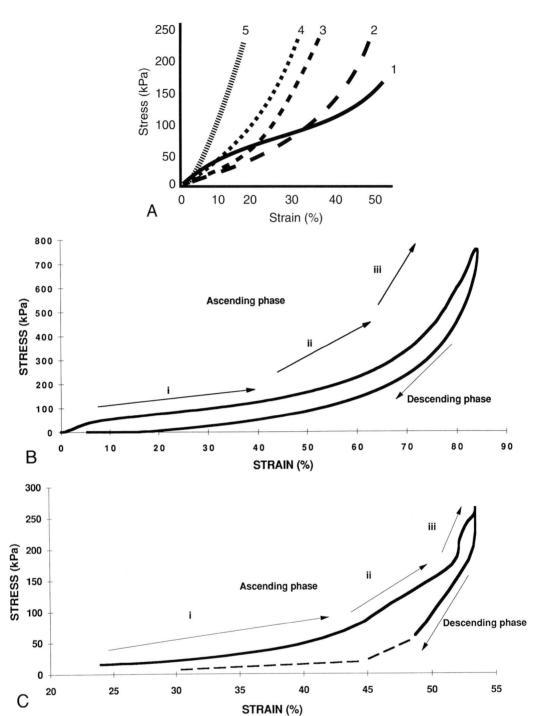

Figure 6–14 ■ Results of compression tests for *A*, several insole materials, *B*, a material used in insole construction (Plastazote 1), *C*, the human heel pad, and *D*, a perfect spring. The variation in mechanical properties of typically used insole materials is apparent from *A*. The materials shown are: *1*, Poron (PPT); *2*, Spenco; *3*, Plastazote #1; *4*, Plastazote #2; and *5*, Soft Pelite. (From Sanders JE, Greve JM, Mitchell SB, Zachariah SG: Material properties of commonly-used interface materials and their static coefficients of friction with skin and socks. J Rehabil Res Dev 35:161–176, 1998, with permission.) Graphs for materials (*B* and *C*) have a standard form: stress is plotted on the *y*-axis and strain on the *x*-axis. No single value can be used to characterize the slopes of the curves for the Plastazote material and the human heel pad, because these curves get steeper in three phases (i.e., the materials become stiffer) as more compression occurs. Stiffness (or modulus) can be calculated for each of these phases. Both insole material and the heel show hysteresis, meaning that loading and unloading follow different paths. Note that the idealized spring (*D*) is linear and follows the same path during the ascending (loading) and descending (unloading) phases but that a "bottoming-out" point is reached where force increases sharply with minor change in compression. Gradient of the graph (change in force divided by change in deformation) in its linear portion is known as spring "stiffness." *Illustration continued on opposite page*

158

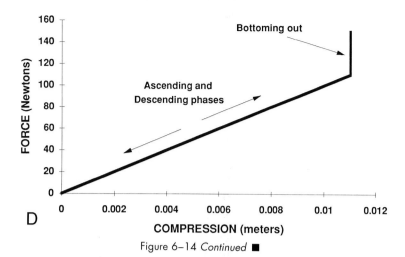

Figure 6–14 Continued ■

of excessive weight in fluid-filled insoles may prove more difficult to resolve.

Properties in the Plane of the Ground

The example of lack of control in the "fluid bag" brings us to the last additions to the conceptual model of the shoe-foot interface, and these are damping and spring stiffness in the anteroposterior and mediolateral directions. We note from the stress-strain experiments on both a shoe material and the heel shown in Figure 6–14B and C that these structures exhibit hysteresis, showing that energy-absorbing (damping) elements are present. Hysteresis is said to occur when the behavior of a material is different during loading and unloading. Perfect springs store all of the available energy when they deform and return that energy during the rebound phase. If no damping were present in the earlier example of the falling egg (Fig. 6–12), the egg would rebound from the foam cushions up to its initial height.

Whereas springs store energy, dampers redirect it. The first law of thermodynamics tells us that energy cannot be created or destroyed; it can only be transformed. Energy used to deform a damper is converted to heat and thus cannot be usefully recovered as mechanical energy. When a viscous element is cyclically loaded, stress and strain are not in phase, and a characteristic loop is developed (Fig. 6–14B). The area enclosed by the loop is a measure of how much energy has been lost. Practically speaking, the damping elements control the rate of compression of

the spring and its tendency to oscillate or bounce. They are usually represented as "dashpots" (Fig. 6–15), which in our model would be in parallel with the spring. Thus each spring element in our cushioning models of Figures 6–12 and 6–13 should be replaced with the combined element shown in Figure 6–15A.

Finally, we turn to the issue of stiffness and damping in shear directions. The potential role of shear stress in causing foot injury has been discussed earlier, and we consider here how footwear may affect shear stress. As long as there is sufficient friction between the insole and the foot or sock, points on the foot will tend to remain in contact with the same points on the surface of the insole when shear forces are applied, causing the insole material to experience shear strain. When there is not enough friction, the foot will, of course, slip. Exactly how much strain occurs for a given shear stress will be determined by the stiffness of the material in shear, and this can be added conceptually to our unit element by a spring in the horizontal plane as shown in Figure 6–15B. In the examples discussed previously, the spring constant of the horizontal components would be extremely small in the hydrostatic cushion, extremely large on a rigid surface, and intermediate in value in traditional insole materials. The provision of a material that allows an appropriate amount of shear strain to occur is a critically important factor in the specification of an insole. There will also be a damping action in the horizontal plane, and this is shown by the added horizontal dashpot in Figure 6–15C, which represents the final

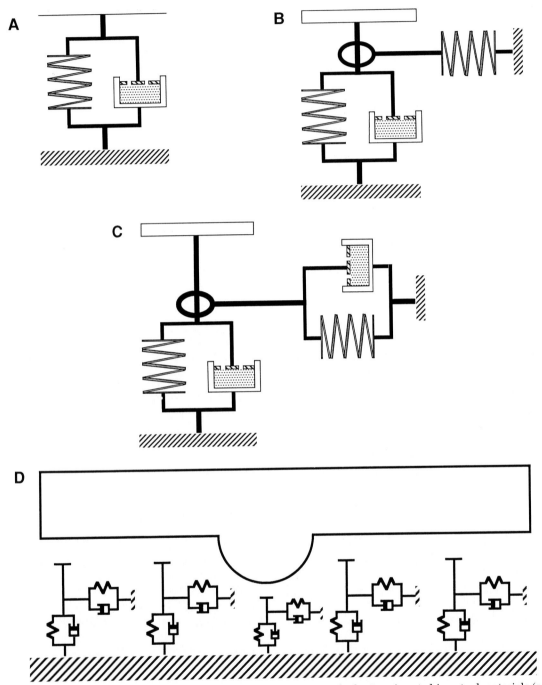

Figure 6–15 ■ Single-spring models cannot describe shear stress or the hysteresis noted in actual materials (see Fig. 6–14). However, refinements to such simple models are possible. *A,* Damping element is added in parallel with the spring. This controls the rate at which the spring compresses and controls the rebound. It also can model hysteresis in the materials. *B,* Stiffness of the material in shear is modeled by a spring rounded at one end and attached to the vertical element at the other. Stiffness of the spring can be measured as the shear stiffness (or modulus) in actual shoe materials. *C,* Model element with both compliance and damping in both vertical and horizontal directions (see text for further details.) *D,* Refined large conceptual model of the foot in cross-section. Load sharing will begin as soon as the foot is loaded in both horizontal and vertical directions. Damping is incorporated into each element, and the spring constants of the materials under the prominence are smaller than those elsewhere.

configuration of a conceptual model that is appropriate for the consideration of cushioning in the shoe. The complete conceptual model, which incorporates different spring constants under the bony prominence, as well as compliance and damping in both vertical and horizontal directions, is shown in Figure 6–15D.

Although the concepts of individual springs and dampers are useful for discrete conceptual models, when the materials are continuous, the compression modulus and shear modulus are better quantities for the characterization of the vertical and horizontal spring stiffness. Values for these quantities are not common knowledge at the present time although, as will be discussed below, information on the material properties of insoles is now available[61, 114, 219] and it is expected that they will become the basis for a more quantitative approach to footwear design and manufacture in the near future.

Tissue and Material Properties

Many of the presumed reasons for elevated plantar pressure in diabetes have to do with changes in the plantar soft tissues, whereas footwear is prescribed to redistribute plantar forces and thereby lower plantar pressure. Thus, a deeper understanding of the properties of footwear materials and the plantar tissues, in particular, how they respond to force, is key in providing further insight into why high pressure may occur and how it may be dealt with. The excellent chapter by Thompson[247] in the fourth edition of this book is recommended as a good primer on tissue mechanics, as is the more mathematical treatment presented by Sharkey.[224]

When a force is applied to an object, some deformation always occurs. If the material is very hard (e.g., bone), the deformation may not be visible to the naked eye, but if the material is soft (e.g., the heel pad), deformation is obvious. Because both the area over which the force is applied and the initial length of the material will affect the outcome of a given interaction, engineers have chosen to standardize the approach to these kinds of problems using the quantities stress and strain. As discussed earlier, stress is synonymous with pressure and is calculated by dividing force by the area over which it acts. Strain is simply fractional deformation, calculated by dividing the change in length by

the original length. Thus, stress causes strain; it is important that these terms not be used interchangeably.

The field of solid mechanics examines the relationship between stress and strain in materials. In a biologic context, it is most developed in the area of tensile (elongation) testing of hard tissues; for example, both experimental and theoretical determination of the effects of stress on bone are well documented.[224] In contrast, soft tissues have received less attention, particularly in compression, and little is known about the mechanical properties of the tissues of the plantar surface of the foot. The same is true for the mechanical properties of the materials that are typically put in contact with the foot, such as polyethylene foam (e.g., Plastazote) and urethane foam (e.g., PPT). Both soft tissues and these materials are complex because they exhibit large deformation, nonlinearity, and viscoelastic behavior —all properties that make theoretical approaches difficult.

Figure 6–16 shows theoretical examples of deformation (strain) under the action of stress. A normal (vertical) stress causes both compression in the direction of the stress and expansion at right angles to the stress (Fig. 6–16B). When a shear stress is applied (Fig. 6–16C), the entire material "rotates"; that is, it experiences the most absolute deflection at the free surface and possibly zero deflection at the opposite surface. In general, tissues in the foot will experience both shear and normal stress (Fig. 6–16D), with resultant compression along the line of normal stress, expansion at right angles to the stress, and "rotation" simultaneously. The same will be true of insole materials.

The mechanical properties of materials can be characterized by performing controlled tests on uniformly shaped samples such that the strain resulting from a known stress can be measured. In the present application, compression and shear tests are most relevant, although these are less frequently conducted than tension tests. Tests can be done either in vitro or, in some cases, in vivo.

Examples of the results of compression tests for a perfect spring, an insole material (Plastazote I closed-cell polyethylene foam), and the human heel pad and a perfect spring are shown in Figure 6–14B–D. Note that the graphs for materials have a standard form. Stress is plotted on the y-axis (in units of force divided by area, kilopascals in the SI

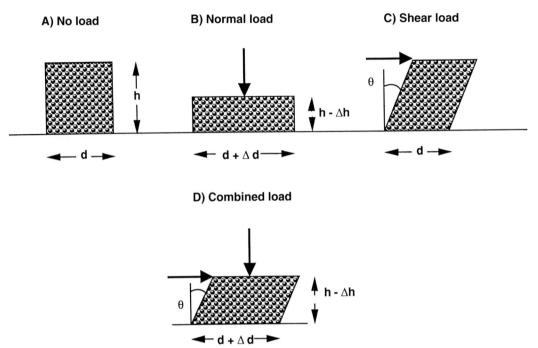

Figure 6–16 ■ Tissue deformation (strain) under the action of stress. From the unloaded position (*A*), normal stress applied to the top of the cube (*B*), causes compression in the direction of the stress by an amount d. When a shear stress is applied (*C*) the entire material "rotates" and the deflection is measured by the angular change θ. In the general case (*D*), tissue in the foot will express all consequences of stress; compression along the line of normal stress, expansion at right angles to the stress, and rotation will occur simultaneously.

system), and strain on the *x*-axis in dimensionless form (change in thickness divided by initial thickness).

The relationship between stress and strain in the working range of a perfect spring is linear (Fig. 6–14*D*), and this curve can therefore be described by a single constant equal to the gradient of the curve, the so-called spring constant. Notice, however, that in this idealized spring a point is reached when further application of force causes no further change in thickness and the spring is said to be "bottomed out."

In almost all biologic tissues and in most insole applications, the materials are nonlinear in compression. The particular form of nonlinearity most often seen is the stiffening of materials as strain increases (Fig. 6–14*B* and *C*). When stress is high enough to cause materials to reach that part of their range where they become extremely stiff (Fig. 6–14*C*), this is the equivalent of the spring bottoming out. Although an objective in insole design is to avoid bottoming out, prolonged use causes degradation of material, which

may bring it closer to the bottoming out regions.[54, 61, 114]

The curve for Plastazote I shown in Figure 6–14*B* is clearly nonlinear and thus cannot be described by a single "spring constant." As shown in this figure, a variety of slopes (equivalent to spring constants) can be used to characterize these curves, and their values describe the stiffness of the materials over different regions of their operating ranges. If we compare Plastazote I with another insole material (Pelite), we find that Pelite is three times stiffer than Plastazote I in the middle part of the range. Similar tests can be performed with the materials being subjected to shear stress.

There are several points of interest about the heel pad data (Fig. 6–14*C*). Note that the early part of the curve (phase 1) is quite flat. This indicates that very little stress is required to produce significant strain. The tissue then seems to "stiffen" first along one line (phase 2) and then along another steeper line (phase 3). The anatomic correlates of this behavior remain to be identified. A comparison of the heel pad data with the insole material is also of interest. Note that the initial stiffness of the heel pad is less than that of the insole material, the phase 2 slope is about equal, and the phase 3 slope is stiffer.

Another major departure from perfect spring behavior is that both the insole material and the heel pad follow different paths during loading and unloading. This feature, which is discussed later, is known as "hysteresis" and results in energy loss during repeated loading and unloading.

Although some data describing the mechanical properties of commonly used shoe materials are available[54, 61, 114] most prescribers and fabricators follow an empiric approach to insole and shoe manufacture at the present time. However, reference to such data will become vital as more quantitative methods of footwear design become possible. Similarly, investigation of the mechanical properties of the plantar soft tissues will be helpful in ascertaining the presumed role of soft tissue change in the increase in plantar pressure associated with diabetes. With better understanding of the relationship between these relatively simple material characteristics and cushioning, it should be possible to pick the correct material for a given situation.

Computer Models of Foot and Shoe Biomechanics

The models presented earlier are useful to help understand the concepts behind therapeutic footwear interventions in the diabetic patient. They do not, however, allow direct predictions of the efficacy of different approaches to be made, because they lack the quantitative detail and sufficient complexity to approximate the real situation. The two most accessible methods presently available to assess different types of footwear are (1) to use different materials in experiments with patients and measure plantar pressure at the interface of the foot with the inside of the shoe, and (2) to try to predict plantar pressure from known forces, material properties, and tissue architecture by modeling. Most previous models have attempted to explore the effects of major structural or surgical changes, but little has been done on the modeling of events leading to tissue breakdown in the normal foot with relatively normal gross structure but with important changes in the plantar adipose tissue, for example.

Although calculations of the effects of stress on uniform rigid solids (e.g., beams and plates) are routinely performed in engineering, the effects of stress on multiple layers of soft, irregular, nonlinear, viscoelastic tissues is more problematic. We have explored a technique known as finite element analysis,[159] and some of the preliminary results from this technique are shown in Figure 6–17. The basic approach is to divide the problem into small geometric elements (in either two or three dimensions) that can be mathematically characterized one at a time by a sophisticated computer program. The geometry and mechanical properties of each element are first defined; the boundary conditions and external loads are then added, and the program is set in motion. The model allows the combined effects of all these factors to be used in the prediction of the resulting deformations and stresses at any point in the model.

The particular benefit of this approach is that any of the input parameters can be varied at will and a set of new predictions obtained. In the examples shown (Fig. 6–17A and B), a two-dimensional model of a single weight-bearing metatarsal head has been formulated. Bone, muscle, tendon, adipose tissue, and skin all have been included, and the three different weight-bearing surfaces (a rigid floor, a stiff shoe, and a compliant shoe) have been modeled. Also, the effects of changes in the thickness of the adipose tissue layer have been explored.

The results provide considerable insight into mechanical conditions under the foot that could lead to tissue damage. The model correctly predicts the higher pressures that are found under a foot with inadequate plantar cushioning and also shows the effect of different thicknesses of soft insole material under the foot (see the following section, "Biomechanical Studies of Footwear," for more discussion of these results). We expect that further development of the modeling approach in three dimensions will yield significant insight into the etiology of elevated plantar pressures (Fig. 6–17C).

Thompson et al.[248] also used finite element modeling to explore the effects of changes in the mechanical properties of skin and other soft tissues as a result of diabetes. They predicted an approximately 25% increase in

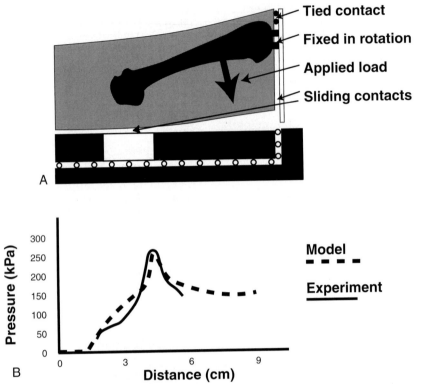

Figure 6–17 ■ Examples of a modeling approach to the calculation of plantar pressures. *A,* A conceptual model used to develop a two-dimensional finite element model of an isolated second metatarsal segment, the surrounding soft tissue, and footwear that may include a different density plug. *B,* Experimental and model results for plantar pressure distribution under the model shown in Figure 6–17A. Note remarkably close correspondence between the two approaches. *C,* Part of a mesh used for a three-dimensional finite element model of the second metatarsal and surrounding soft tissue. (From Saucerman J: Finite element analysis of plantar pressure distribution of the forefoot. Undergraduate Honors Thesis. Penn State University [in preparation]).

Illustration continued on opposite page

stresses at the skin/adipose tissue interface in the subcalcaneal tissue for diabetic patients with stiffer skin and more compliant adipose tissue. Finite element analysis was also employed by Patil, Braak, and Huson,[194] who chose to concentrate on stresses in the tarsal bones with various simulated muscle actions. This approach has some potential for understanding damage to the bones of neuropathic feet.

Biomechanical Studies of Footwear

The previous section reviewed in mostly theoretical terms the principles that might be employed in the design of the foot-shoe interface. We will now review what is known about the biomechanical effects of frequently employed footwear modifications. The foot-shoe interface, outsole modifications, and modifications of the upper will be discussed.

Chapters 20 and 34 emphasize the clinical perspective of footwear prescription.

Insoles

The mechanical properties of commonly used insole materials have been studied by several authors. The classic approach to mechanical testing of materials is to subject them to progressively increasing stress and to measure the amount of strain that results. When this is done for typical insole materials, a characteristic sigmoid curve is generated (see Fig. 6–14A). The material is initially relatively stiff to small stresses; it then has a period of being less stiff in response to midrange stresses; and finally, as compaction of the material occurs, it becomes very stiff (showing little strain) in response to further increases in stress. Thus insole materials have a nonlinear response to loading and this is

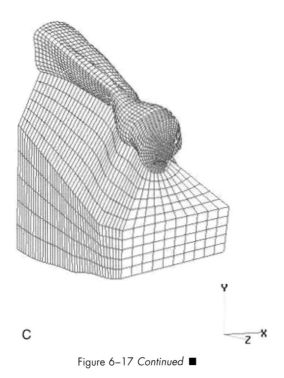

C

Y

Z X

Figure 6–17 Continued ■

perhaps why the responses have not been used by insole designers—because a single number cannot characterize the entire stress-strain behavior. The "operating range" of different insole materials is not yet clear in terms of compression, but it is almost certain that many soft materials (particularly those in thin insoles) are used beyond 50% compression, which will move them to the stiff region of the curves (Fig. 6–14A).

Campbell et al.[61] were the first to attempt to define insole materials in a rigorous engineering manner. They subjected 31 foamed rubber and plastic materials to accelerated aging, including heat, sustained compression, and cyclic loading using both novel tests and formal protocols such as ASTM D395.[25] Materials were placed into four groups based on the magnitude of changes that occurred with the various duty cycle tests. Reduction in thickness following sustained compression ranged from barely measurable change (Poron 20125, also known as PPT) to approximately 50% (Aliplast, Cetite, Ethafoam, Evasote, Neoprene, and Pelite). The reduction in thickness following cyclic compression tests varied from almost zero (PPT) to more than 80% (Pelite, Evasote, Ensolite, Aliplast).

Leber and Evanski[158] examined the pressure reduction properties of seven commonly used insole materials using a Harris and

Beath mat in patients with metatarsalgia. They attempted to quantify the results using the calibration procedures proposed by Silvino, Evanski, and Waugh.[228] The range of pressure reduction measured was between 28 and 53%. The most effective materials identified were PPT, Spenco, and Plastazote.

Another significant effort to characterize a number of materials used for insoles was conducted by Sanders et al.[219] These authors examined 11-mm diameter × 4-mm-thick specimens of eight commonly used materials in a 1-Hz cyclic loading protocol up to pressures of 220 kPa for 60-minute periods. Coefficients of friction between the material and skin, material and sock, and skin-sock interface were also determined. Recovery from compression set was assessed 1 hour and 168 hours after the 60-minute compression test. The shapes and stiffness of the curves varied considerably. There was appreciable deformation in some of the materials after the 60-minute tests but most materials recovered well in 168 hours (although several recovered poorly in 1 hour). Sanders et al.[219] include in their article a comprehensive description of the chemical composition of the various materials.

Brodsky et al.[54] examined the response of five commonly used insole materials to repeated compression and repeated shear and compression combined. They proposed that the ideal material would exhibit a combination of durability and moldability. After 10,000 cycles, loss of thickness ranged from zero (for PPT) to 55% (Plastazote #1). These results have important implications for the replacement of insoles at regular intervals, since it is clear that many regularly used insole materials lose their effectiveness rapidly with use.

Foto and Birke[113] conducted a survey of health professionals who treat diabetic patients to determine the most commonly used multidensity materials (such as a layered combination of Plastazote #2 and Poron). They then devised a testing method[114] to measure how the materials behaved when new and when aged in terms of their mechanical properties. The authors presented stress-strain curves for the various materials after 40 cycles, 10,000 cycles, and 100,000 cycles and examined each material against their criterion that the material should be capable of maintaining a dynamic strain of 50% or less at a stress of 350 kPa. The key findings

Table 6–3 ■ PERCENT LOSS IN PERFORMANCE DURING DYNAMIC COMPRESSION OF DUAL-DENSITY INSOLE MATERIALS ON REPEATED CYCLES.*

NUMBER OF CYCLES	MATERIALS				
	a	b	c	d	e
1,000	7%	13%	8%	4%	22%
10,000	12%	22%	27%	36%	50%
100,000	26%	25%	36%	49%	61%

* From Foto JG, Birke JA: Who's using what? An orthotic materials survey. Biomechanics 3:63–68, 1996, with permission.
a, Poron + Plastazote #2; b, Spenco + Microcell Puff light; c, Plastazote #1 + Poron; d, Plastazote #1 + Poron + Microcell Puff; e, Plastazote #1 + Plastazote #2.

of the study are summarized in Table 6–3 and Figure 6–18. The authors concluded that the Poron/Plastazote #2 and Spenco/Microcel Puf Lite combinations exhibited the best dynamic material deformation and compression set properties of all the materials tested and these materials were the preferred choice for insoles to be used in insoles for diabetic patients from those examined. Lavery et al.[156] have also described a methodology for the evaluation of the change in material properties over time.

The practitioner will often choose materials based on whether or not they are capable of being molded to match a positive cast of the foot. These thermoplastic properties are fundamental to the formulation of the polymers used but few data are readily available regarding ease of molding, temperature requirements, and the like; nor has the efficacy of molded insoles been well studied. Hewitt[130] examined the peak pressures under the feet of neuropathic patients as they walked in insoles molded in the heel and arch area and in flat insoles of approximately the same thickness. He found mixed results, with metatarsal head pressures being relieved in some patients by the molded insole while other patients showed increases in peak pressure. Pitei et al.[201] found that peak pressure was decreased by ethyl vinyl acetate (EVA) insoles as compared to the patients' conventional street shoes by 31% when new and by 50% as they became molded to the foot during "break-in."

The basic philosophy of most molded insole approaches is to increase the load in "safe regions" in order to decrease the load over "at-risk" regions. A simply molded insole offers, at least in theory, the same support to all points under the foot (although the compression of each region of the insole will differ depending on the load immediately above it and the thickness). However, molding can also be "exaggerated" or "customized"; in other words, areas of the foot that are considered "safe" can be loaded preferentially. This can be accomplished with extra support in a "safe" area (e.g., metatarsal pads, bars, or more individualized insole build up), or with an extra relief under the at risk area (i.e., "plugs" of a "softer" material or simply thinning of the material to provide less contact between the foot and insole).

The most popular class of "extra loading" devices is the metatarsal pad that is placed under the metatarsal shafts to unload the MTHs. The traditional metatarsal pad can be quite effective in relieving metatarsal head pressure if it is correctly placed and can be tolerated by the patient. Edington[106] examined metatarsal head peak pressures as patients walked barefoot across a pressure platform with metatarsal pads of various dimensions directly attached to their feet. He found significant and substantial reductions in peak pressure at the metatarsal heads (53 kPa for ³⁄₁₆-inch and 80 kPa for ⁵⁄₁₆-inch pads) for pads that were placed ³⁄₁₆ to

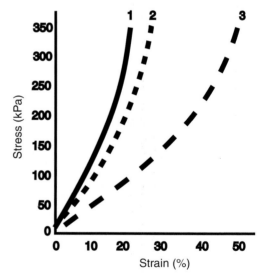

Figure 6–18 ■ The results of simulated wear tests on insole materials. Stress-strain curves for a sample of dual density material (Plastazote #1 and Plastazote #2) after cycling under a 350-kPa stress for (1) 40 cycles, (2) 10,000 cycles, and (3) 100,000 cycles. Note the increase in stiffness of the material as cycling increases shown by the steeper curves. (From Foto JG, Birke JA: Who's using what? An orthotic materials survey. Biomechanics 3:63–68, 1996, with permission.)

¼ inch behind the palpated third metatarsal head. Holmes and Timmerman[133] found reductions between 12 and 60% in metatarsal head peak pressures using a protocol similar to that of Edington. They also reported that three of their ten subjects showed either no change or an increase in MTH pressure and speculated that this was because of incorrect positioning of the pad. Chang et al.,[81] using an in-shoe protocol, found only minor reductions in plantar pressures with metatarsal pads. This may have been due to positioning of either the pad or the small discrete sensors used, which had a metal disk backing. Metatarsal bars, thick straight support wedges just proximal to the MTHs and tapering proximally, and custom pads designed to relieve just one or two metatarsal heads are also used but no experimental studies have been performed on such devices. Frykberg[117] has presented preliminary data to suggest that a rockered insole may be effective in reducing plantar pressure under the forefoot, and this device could be considered to be a prefabricated metatarsal bar. Lord and Hosein[164] have provided insight into the redistribution of plantar pressure that can occur with customized insoles.

As discussed above, the effective thickness of an insole can be increased under an area of particular concern by using a firmer, less compressible material under areas of the foot judged to be able to take greater loads and using softer materials under the area of concern. For instance, a two-layer composite insole could have a firm material as its base, a thin layer of soft material over the whole surface, and a soft material all the way through to the base layer at the area of concern. Such a relief or "plug" can be extended into the midsole of the shoe and take any shape needed. A small circular plug might be used under an MTH, while a large plug involving a third of the insole could be used for a foot badly deformed by a Charcot fracture (Fig. 6–19). Little is known about the ideal geometry and material properties required for such plugs, and there is concern that a ring of high stress can be created at the edges of the plug.[162]

The thickness of insoles is usually limited by the space available in the shoe, but this can be substantial (up to half an inch) in a super-extra-depth shoe. No study has systematically examined the effects of insole thickness on pressure relief in a large group of patients with different characteristics.

Our own data, which were used to validate the FEM models described above, suggest that the effect will be different depending on the foot deformity and baseline pressure of the patient. Lemmon et al.[159] used PPT insoles of various thicknesses in two individuals with markedly different MTH2 plantar pressures. Their results indicated a steeper gradient of pressure versus insole thickness in a patient with reduced submetatarsal tissue and higher baseline plantar pressure compared to an individual with more plantar tissue. A reduction of approximately 6 kPa/mm versus 2 kPa/mm was obtained in the two individuals.

As expected on a theoretical basis, the thicker the insole, the less the incremental improvement in pressure reduction per millimeter of added thickness. For the subject with lower barefoot peak pressure, adding thickness beyond 12.5 mm (0.5 inch) led to little incremental improvement in pressure. However, for the individual with higher barefoot peak pressure, the curve was still reasonably steep even around 12.5 mm (0.5 inch), indicating continuing benefit from increasing thickness. While this work is preliminary, it underscores the importance of insole thickness, which was predicted theoretically (see "Footwear as a Distributor of Force," above). In our own clinics, we do not use insoles that are less than 6.25 mm (0.25 inch) thick for any at-risk patient and we try to approach the 12.5-mm (0.5 inch) thickness for all high-risk patients. In the individual with higher baseline pressure in the Lemmon et al. study,[159] the overall pressure reduction (from the moderate value of only 279 kPa) by the 12.5-mm insole was 25%. This could be expected to be even higher for an individual with still higher baseline pressures, since the pattern of greater plantar pressure relief by the same intervention for feet with higher baseline pressure has been found in other studies.[197]

Conti[91] has pointed out that there are many unanswered questions regarding appropriate insole prescription, and Janisse[137] has described a number of practical implementations of the theories discussed above. He also provides recommendations for the manufacture of a variety of therapeutic footwear devices. Some of these approaches (including metatarsal pads) were used by Ashry et al.,[24] who examined four different insole designs in a group of 11 patients with great toe amputation. Surprisingly, they found no

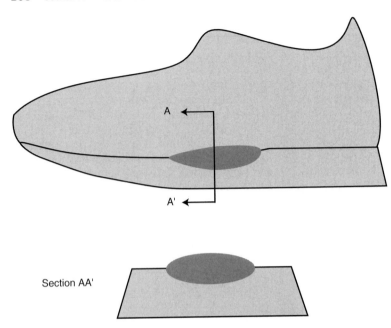

Section AA'

Figure 6–19 ■ A compliant insole "plug" under a prominent area in the midfoot of the patient whose plantar pressures were shown in Plate 3. A schematic cross-section of the shoe is also shown.

significant differences in peak plantar pressures with their various interventions. This may be due to the poor performance characteristics of the device they used for in-shoe pressure measurement,[270] but their conclusion that insole modification is unwarranted would seem to be premature.

It is noteworthy that simple athletic shoes have been observed to reduce the incidence of callus,[240] and in three studies have been found to reduce pressures by 25 to 30% on average compared to leather-soled shoes or subjects' own over-the-counter shoes.[142, 197, 201] In addition, Perry et al.[197] found that the peak pressure reduction in the forefoot as a result of cushioned running shoes compared to leather Oxfords (expressed as percentage reduction) was much greater in individuals with high initial peak pressure. For example, those with peak MTH1 pressures of 200 kPa in the Oxfords typically experienced little change in running shoes, but those with peak pressures of 600 kPa in the Oxfords experienced approximately 50% reduction in running shoes. Thus the combination of insole and midsole in these shoes can often be effective, particularly in patients with higher baseline pressure, in reducing pressure below the level of injury threshold.

Fluid-filled insoles have been described,[229] but no data are available on their performance in diabetic patients. There is also a complete class of commercial "over-the-counter" devices that purport to combine

molding, relief, load transfer, and support, but the efficacy of these devices has not been tested in published studies of either pressure reduction or clinical efficacy.

Our own studies[59] suggest that customized insoles of appropriate design can play a significant role in pressure and impulse reduction at the metatarsal heads if load can be transferred to the arch and other regions of the foot. Loading at the heel also seems particularly amenable to reduction by insoles that provide a "cupping" of the heel. A case study demonstrating redistribution of load away from the first metatarsal head in a patient with recurrent ulceration and elevated pressure at this location is presented in Figure 6–20A–C. The customized insole in this case incorporated molding, a metatarsal pad, pressure relief under the metatarsal heads, and a substantial build-up in the medial arch area. A Novel PEDAR system was used to measure in-shoe pressure.

During barefoot walking, this patient's MTH1 plantar pressure was 1,058 kPa. Even with a ¼-inch PPT insole, the peak pressure at this location was 552 kPa, much higher than in-shoe pressures usually observed in this region. Figure 6–20B shows a comparison between the regional plantar pressures in the ¼-inch PPT flat insole and in the customized insole during normal walking in the same shoe. The largest changes that occurred were in the medial midfoot, where increased load was being taken by the built-up arch in

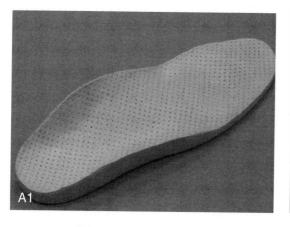
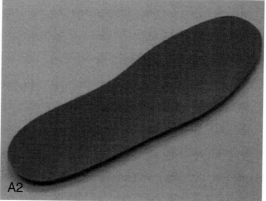

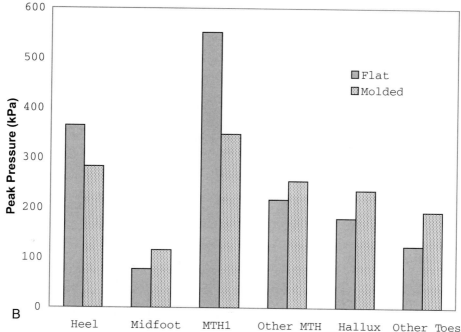

Figure 6–20 ■ A case study showing redistribution of load away from a high-risk region. The graphs show a comparison of plantar pressure in the same shoe with a molded insole (A1) and a flat insole (A2) in a patient who had previously ulcerated at the first metatarsal head. *B,* Peak pressure at MTH1 was markedly reduced in the molded insole but increased at other sites.

Illustration continued on following page

the customized insole. The peak pressure in this region increased by 61.2% (from 72 to 115 kPa). While this change is substantial, it is small in comparison to the change in force-time integral, which increased by 1,041% (from 3.9 to 44.5 N-s). This and other features in the insole resulted in a decrease of peak pressure in the patient's region of concern, MTH1, by 37% (from 552 kPa to 348 kPa). The MTH1 force-time integral showed a somewhat lower (24%) percentage reduction (from 100.2 N-s to 76.6 N-s). A useful insight is gained by expressing the re-

gional force-time integrals in the MTH1 and medial arch as a percentage of the total force-time integrals in all regions. In the flat insole this approach indicates that the MTH1 and midfoot were responsible for 17% and 4%, respectively, of the force-time integrals in the flat insole. In the molded insole these values change to 13% and 12%, respectively, reflecting the unloading of MTH1 and the transfer of load to the medial arch. In many respects, the prescription of insoles can be characterized as a process of experimental load transfer until enough load relief to prevent injury

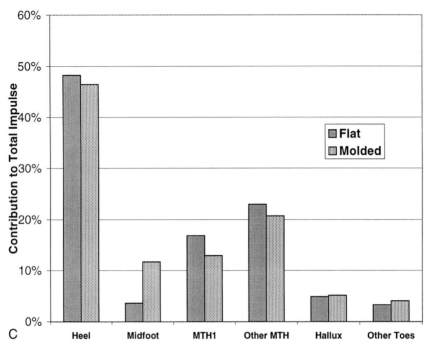

Figure 6–20 ■ *Continued C,* The contribution of each region to the total force-time integral or impulse shows that the midfoot increased its load-sharing role in the molded insole while other regions were reduced or unchanged.

has occurred. As was discussed earlier, we can now document changes caused by footwear in peak pressure, pressure-time integral, force-time integrals, time over a certain pressure, and the like. However, the relative importance of each quantity and the absolute relief required to prevent injury is not yet clear.

In summary, when prescribing an insole for an individual at risk for neuropathic ulceration, one must consider the material or combination of materials, thickness, molding, supports (e.g., metatarsal pads), and reliefs (e.g., plugs). This is a useful and important checklist to consider when a prescription is being written. While we know something about the individual effects of these various insole attributes, as was just reviewed, there are very few data on how they should be most efficaciously combined. In the absence of such data, it is reasonable to take cost into consideration. Flat insoles are relatively inexpensive, even when thick, while the more customized an insole is, the more expensive it generally is.

Another point worthy of emphasis is that in the entire discussion of insoles only reduction of the loading forces to areas of the plantar surface at risk was considered. Insoles or in-shoe orthoses are often made in settings other than the neuropathic foot to "correct" or "control" the motions of the foot. Such corrections load one part of the foot more than another and thereby increase pressure in areas that, in a neuropathic foot, may not necessarily be able to tolerate higher pressures. Thus any such correction or control must be performed with extreme caution and only with very good reason in the neuropathic foot.

Socks

Socks should be considered as part of the cushioning system. Veves and colleagues[259, 260, 262] have shown in patients with both diabetes and rheumatoid arthritis that special padded socks can significantly reduce plantar pressures. In their initial studies, ten neuropathic subjects with plantar pressures greater than 980 kPa wore specially padded socks for 6 months. Reductions of 31.3% in peak forefoot plantar pressure were found when the socks were new. After 3 and 6 months of wear the socks had lost some of their efficacy and offered reductions in peak pressure of only 15.5% and 17.6%, respectively. Patient acceptance of the socks was good and no patient developed an ulcer during the study. The authors also experimented with the use of over-the-counter padded sport socks designed for tennis and running and found that if the socks had high-density padding, a reduction of 17% could be achieved when the socks were new. In studies of patients with rheumatoid arthritis,[259] peak forefoot pressures and perceived pain were both significantly reduced in padded socks. In all of these studies, the patients' own socks (usually thin) had no significant effect on plantar pressure.

Stacpoole-Shea et al.[241] measured pressure distribution during a benchtop simulation of compression of seamless and seamed sock material between two flat plates. They reported a tenfold concentration of pressure at the seams and recommended that seamless socks should be used by neuropathic patients.

It is obviously important that shoes with enough room in the toe box should be used by patients to whom padded socks are prescribed. Otherwise, significant injury to the dorsum of the toes can result.

Outsole Modifications

The discussion of footwear so far has concentrated principally on the interface between the foot and shoe, and there is no doubt that this is the most important aspect of footwear for the neuropathic foot. However, a number of investigators have shown either clinically or through direct measurement of plantar pressure that outsole modifications can also have an important effect on preventing injury.[84, 88, 191, 223, 231, 254] The commonest of these is the rigid rocker bottom shoe, or a variant thereof, called a "roller," which has been advocated by Dr. Paul Brand[52] for many years. The rocker has a break in the contour of the outsole, while the roller has a smooth curve (Fig. 6–21). The general principle behind these designs is that they allow the patient to walk with minimum motion of the joints of the foot. In particular, no extension of the MTP joints is required during the phase of forefoot weight bearing, and this appears to reduce forefoot pressures by up to 50% compared to walking in flexible shoes.[191, 223, 231, 254]

However, it is not known whether the lack of motion in the foot joints is important or if other factors predominate. It is frequently said that the rigid sole, usually accompanied by a molded insole, loads the entire foot throughout the support phase. While this is certainly not true, pressure measurements have confirmed that the duration of loading in all areas but the forefoot is increased in a rocker shoe.[223] These increases in loading time are marked in the hindfoot and midfoot but only small in the toes. The hindfoot and midfoot force-time integrals are also dramatically increased, indicating the change in load-sharing that is taking place, while the force-time integral at the forefoot is markedly decreased. Thus the actual changes in loading that occur with rocker shoes have been determined.

However, functional effects of several important design variables remain to be fully explored. These include the location of the rocker or roller axis along the anteroposterior axis (APA) of the shoe, the angle of the rocker or roller axis with respect to the APA, the amount of toe spring (see below), the height of the outsole at the rocker or roller axis (and thereby the angle of the rocker or the anteroposterior curvature of the roller), and the height differential of the sole between heel and the rocker and roller axis. In addition, it has been shown that a given shoe can actually increase the load under some parts of the foot while reducing it elsewhere.[223] Another extremely important issue is that individual variability in response to rigid shoes is significant. Thus the process of prescribing shoes for a given individual is complex.[254]

The characteristics of roller placement and geometry have been addressed systematically by Coleman[88] and Nawoczenski[191] (see Table 6–4). Both studies examined the effects of these shoe design variables in young healthy male volunteers using the same brand of footwear. Coleman controlled cadence (80 steps per minute), but not speed or stride length, while Nawoczenski et al. did not mention gait parameters. Plantar pressures were measured in both studies using discrete transducers. Coleman placed the roller axis "just behind the 5th MTH" (probably approximately 60% of shoe length), while Nawoczenski et al. explored take-off points of 50 and 60%.

As is apparent from Table 6–4, there were remarkable differences between the results of Nawoczenski et al.[191] and those of Coleman[88] for the same type of footwear modifications (compare, for instance, lines 2 and 3

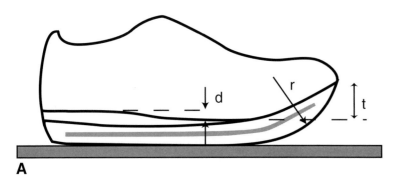

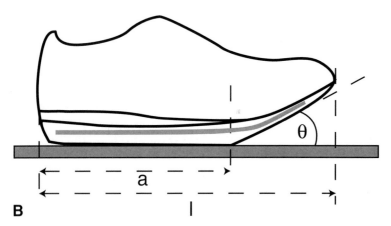

Figure 6–21 ■ Design parameters for rigid shoes. *A,* A roller shoe with a constant curvature outsole, radius **r,** in the forefoot region. The heel-forefoot height differential is **d,** and the "toe spring," **t,** is defined as the height of the anterior tip of the shoe sole above the plane of the ball of the foot. *B,* A rocker shoe with a rocker angle θ beginning at a ratio of (**a/l**) of shoe length. The rigid roller or rocker effect should be achieved by minimizing toe-spring, since this high toe spring probably increases toe pressures.

in Table 6–4). The effect demonstrated by Nawoczenski was always much less than that shown by Coleman. While there may have been differences in speed, cadence, and stride length between the two studies, the most striking difference may have been design of the toe spring, defined as the height of the anterior tip of the shoe sole above the plane of the ball of the foot (see Fig. 6–21). It appears that Coleman maintained the

Table 6–4 ■ EFFECTS OF ROLLER SHOES ON PLANTAR PRESSURE REDUCTION

| AUTHOR | TAKE-OFF (% OF SHOE LENGTH FROM HEEL) | RADIUS (% OF SHOE LENGTH) | PRESSURE REDUCTION EXPRESSED AS % FROM CONTROL | | | | | |
			Hallux	MTH1	MTH2	MTH3	MTH4	MTH5
C	60%†	60%‡	−21%		−31%		−34%	
N*	60%	75%	−5%	−7%		−12%		−10%
C	60%†	77%‡	−15%		−24%		−25%	
N*	60%	125%	−3%	−2%		−8%		−6%
N*	50%	75%	−11%	−9%		−26%		−13%
N*	50%	60%	−8%	−4%		−28%		−12%

* Percent effects estimated from a figure in the paper.
† Estimated based on data from van Schie et al.[252]
‡ Estimated based on assumed shoe size #10 measuring 30 cm.
N, Nawoczenski et al.[191]; C, Coleman.[88]

"normal" toe spring of the shoes used in his study, while Nawoczenski et al. manufactured their shoes with 20 degrees of toe spring. Based on the photograph in the Nawoczenski et al. paper,[191] this was probably more toe spring than that initially built into the shoes. Since Coleman's results showed more pressure relief, it would appear that rigid shoes should be built with minimal toe spring. This is supported by the observations of Bauman et al.,[33] who found only a 6 to 14% reduction in forefoot pressure by a wooden rigid rollered sandal with significant toe spring, while they found pressure reductions of 29 to 41% in wooden flat shoes with a roller. Concerning take-off and radius parameters, it appears from these two studies that with the 60% take-off the shortest radius tested was best (60%), but that the 50% take-off may be better than 60%.

Another important parameter of rocker and roller shoe design that is somewhat related to toe spring is the differential in height between the heel and forefoot of the insole/midsole/outsole combination (see Fig. 6–21). In most commercially manufactured shoes, the rear part of the foot is at least ⅜ to ¼ inch above the forefoot and the upper is made to fit this design. Patients do not like shoes that appear high, and one way to make rollered and rockered shoes appear less high is to even out this difference by making the heel no higher than the forefoot. The efficacy of this has never been addressed experimentally.

In the studies mentioned above, Coleman[88] examined three rocker shoe designs and Nawoczenski et al.[191] examined one. A modular shoe has been proposed for the investigation of the effects of different outsole configurations without altering the foot-shoe interface.[78] Using this device, van Schie[254] systematically explored the pressure distributions inside nine different rigid rocker shoe designs and compared them with the control condition of a flexible, nonrockered extra-depth shoe with the same flat insole. Speed of walking between trials in this study was kept constant. Peak pressure was reduced by rocker shoes compared to control at most forefoot locations, but increased in the midfoot and heel. Axis location was found to have an important effect, particularly on hallux pressures. There was a mean trend towards optimal reduction of pressure in one of the rocker shoe conditions at each anatomic location, but the axis position for this optimal

placement was variable across subjects and anatomic locations. While most configurations of the rocker shoe were superior to the control shoe, no single configuration was optimal for all subjects at all sites or even at the same site. This suggested that some form of in-shoe plantar pressure measurement is ideal to ensure a rigid rocker bottom shoe design that is optimized. On average, the best axis location for reducing MTH pressure was in the region of 55 to 60% of shoe length, while for the toes it was 65%. Van Schie et al.[254] proposed a conceptual model linking the various rocker design parameters and their effects (Fig. 6–22).

The results of the studies that have explored effects of rocker shoe design on pressure relief are presented in Table 6–5. For reasons that have not been fully explained, hallux pressure reduction in the study of van Schie[254] was much less than in the other studies. The summary data as presented in the table neither add to nor detract from the conclusion of van Schie that hallux pressure is best relieved by the 65% take-off rocker. While none of the other studies systematically explored the effect of the take-off position on plantar pressure, the results of all the studies are similar with respect to pressure reduction at the MTHs, and in general these

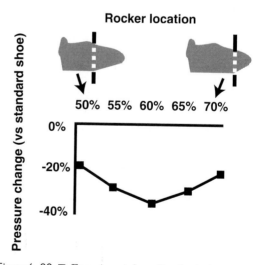

Figure 6–22 ■ Experimental results of a study to examine the effects of variation in the placement of a rocker shoe axis. Peak pressure at the first metatarsal head is shown as a function of rocker axis location. Note that all peak pressures in this region were reduced by at least 20% but there was an optimal location for the axis where pressure relief was maximized.

Table 6–5 ■ EFFECTS OF ROLLER SHOES ON PLANTAR PRESSURE REDUCTION

AUTHOR	TAKE-OFF (% OF SHOE LENGTH FROM HEEL)	ROCKER ANGLE (DEG)	PRESSURE REDUCTION EXPRESSED AS % FROM CONTROL					
			Halllux	MTH1	MTH2	MTH3	MTH4	MTH5
v	70%	20	−4%	−19%	−38%	−38%		
v	70%	30	−12%	−23%	−40%	−41%		
Average			†	**−21%**	**−39%**	**−40%**		
v	65%	20	−1%	−26%	−43%	−44%		
S	67%	24	−32%	−29%		−33%		12%
v	65%	26	−19%	−31%	−48%	−49%		
N	65%*	30	−32%	−16%		−25%		−6%
Average			†	**−25%**	**−45%**	**−38%**		**3%**
C	60%*	15	−16%		−36%		−35%	
C	60%*	20	−23%		−45%		−45%	
v	60%	20	4%	−29%	−46%	−48%		
v	60%	22	−2%	−35%	−52%	−56%		
C	60%*	30	−37%		−51%		−49%	
Average			†	**−32%**	**−46%**	**−46%**		
v	55%	20	8%	−28%	−47%	−50%		
v	55%	21	6%	−30%	−51%	−56%		
Average			†	**−29%**	**−49%**	**−53%**		
v	50%	20	23%	−19%	−39%	−45%		

* Estimated based on data from van Schie et al. (in preparation).
† Averages are not calculated for the hallux data because of the unexplained differences among the studies.
N, Nawoczenski et al.[191]; C, Coleman[88]; v, van Schie[252] (reported results for lateral MTHs rather than 3, 4, and 5 individually; S, Schaff and Cavanagh[223] (reported results for medial, middle, and lateral forefoot).

summary data confirm that best pressure reduction at the MTHs occurs with the 55 to 60% take-off point. The 65% take-off rocker may be acceptable at MTHs 1 to 4, but perhaps not MTH5. Whether MTH5 would be better relieved by a more proximal rocker has not been extensively addressed, though Sims and Birke[231] noted, in apparent agreement with van Schie et al.[254] that "progressive decrease in pressure was noted as the rocker apex was moved posteriorly. . . . the 3^d MTH showed a decrease at all positions," but "rocker placement had minimal effect on . . . pressure at 5th MTH." The expected result, that the higher the rocker (and therefore the greater the rocker angle) the better the pressure relief, is a clear trend.

Van Schie et al.[254] also observed that pressure reduction depends on gait style. The preferred use of the rocker shoe is to dwell on the flat portion of the sole until the last stages of swing. This should then be followed by a rapid rocking forward on the "knife edge" of the rocker and then toe-off of the support foot. However, some patients appear to rock forward and spend considerable time bearing load on the anterior flattened portion of the outsole. This is believed to be associated with an increase in pressure under the forefoot and highlights the importance of training the patient to use a rocker shoe correctly. Short strides are probably the key to successful use of a rocker shoe, since it is more likely that the patient will use the rocker appropriately (without maintaining the flat area of the front part of the shoe in contact with the ground). These same observations and comments were also made much earlier by Bauman et al.[32]

We have recently observed a patient with remarkable "out-toeing" and a first MTH ulcer. A standard rocker was not successful at keeping this patient healed, and observation revealed that design modifications to the shoe were required. With the standard rocker axis orientation (with respect to the APA), this patient rolled right over the first MTH. We changed the axis of the rocker to be perpendicular to the foot position at toe-off (approximately 25 degrees to the APA). In-shoe plantar pressure at that site was markedly reduced and the patient has remained healed in the modified shoe while continuing his "out-toed" gait.

Only in the studies of Coleman[88] and Nawoczenski et al.[191] were the effects of rockers and rollers compared using the same methodology. In the three comparisons shown in Table 6–6, rockers were generally but not always somewhat better than rollers at reducing pressure. The mean difference in pressure reduction was −9% at the hallux

Table 6-6 ■ COMPARISON OF ROCKER AND ROLLER SHOES OF THE SAME HEIGHT

AUTHOR		PRESSURE REDUCTION EXPRESSED AS % FROM CONTROL					
		Hallux	MTH1	MTH2	MTH3	MTH4	MTH5
C (0.75 in height)	15-degree rocker	−16%		−36%		−35%	
(60% take-off)*	77% R Roller†	−15%		−24%		−25%	
Difference		−1%		−12%		−10%	
C (1.25 in height)	20-degree rocker	−23%		−45%		−45%	
(60% take-off)*	60% R Roller†	−21%		−31%		−34%	
Difference		−2%		−14%		−11%	
N‡ (0.75 in)	30-degree rocker 65% take-off	−32%	−16%		−25%		−6%
	60% R roller 50% take-off	−8%	−4%		−28%		−12%
Difference		−24%	−12%		3%		6%

* Estimated based on data from van Schie et al. (in preparation).
† Estimated based on assumed shoe size #10 measuring 30 cm.
‡ Percentage effects estimated from a figure in the paper.
N, Nawoczenski et al.[191]; C, Coleman[88] lower and higher shoes; R, radius.

and −7% at the MTHs, or about −8% overall, favoring rockers.

A careful reader will notice that many footwear modifications can reduce plantar pressure significantly and may speculate that simply adding these reductions can lead to pressures below zero. Obviously, that is not reasonable. In the absence of data on combinations of modifications, it may be reasonable to assume that each added modification reduces pressure further by its own percentage effect from the baseline of the previous modification. The basis for this hypothesis is the study by Perry et al. already mentioned,[199] in which the lower the initial pressure, the lower were both the absolute and the percentage pressure reductions.

Fit

Shoe fit is a critical issue in the prevention of both dorsal and plantar ulcers. Despite its importance, it is usually left to the subjective opinion of the fitter and the wearer. When the fitter is inexperienced and the wearer has limited sensation, it is clear that this approach can lead to a less than perfect outcome. A shoe with ideal fit would control the motion of the foot relative to the weight-bearing surface without applying any pressure whatsoever to the dorsum of the foot. This is not possible in practice, however, and thus a working definition of shoe fit might be "a covering for the dorsum of the foot that minimizes the application of pressures to the dorsum while controlling mediolateral and anteroposterior foot movement." The only study that has examined nonplantar pressure in diabetic patients is that mentioned above by Chantelau, Schroer, and Tanudjaja.[85] Jordan[141] has measured dorsal pressure in relation to comfort in nondiabetic subjects, and her methodology could be readily applied to the issue of dorsal ulceration. It is desirable and expected that such measurements will become routine in footwear prescription for high-risk patients in the near future.

In the absence of experimental data on shoe fit, the following represents a working hypothesis of the role of fit of the upper in providing a safe shoe. Although relief of pressure over bony prominences is an obvious need, a less frequently expressed role of the upper may be to limit the amount of shear strain that the tissue on the plantar aspect of the foot experiences. As shown in Figure 6–23, in the presence of shear forces, the upper acts on the dorsum of the foot to generate opposing forces. This has the effect of reducing the forward movement of the foot on the shoe compared with what would occur with the shoe platform alone, consequently reducing the amount of shear strain in the plantar tissues. An insole that allows shear strain will facilitate this forward movement of the foot relative to the shoe and allow the upper to "engage" the dorsum at a lower value of shear strain. Because excessive shear strain in the tissue is likely to be damaging, the combination of an appropriate in-

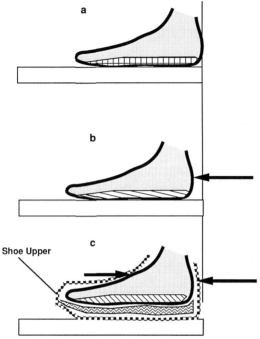

Figure 6–23 ▪ Hypothesis for the role of the shoe upper and a soft insole in reducing the shear strain of the plantar tissues. Soft tissues on the plantar surface of the foot are shown with schematic shading to indicate the amount of shear stress experienced. From the resting position on a flat surface with minimum shear stress in the tissues (*a*), an anteriorly directed shear force applied to a foot with no upper (*b*) causes forward movement of the foot about the fixed plantar surface, which will lead to high shear stress in the tissues. If the same force is applied to a foot in a shoe with an upper and a compliant insole (*c*) the resulting shear stress is reduced because the upper applies a restraining force to the foot once the insole has allowed forward movement. Note that there would be no reduction in the shear of the plantar tissue without the restraint of the shoe upper. Thus the shoe and the insole together reduce the amount of shear stress in the plantar tissues, and possibly the risk of injury. This hypothesis can be investigated experimentally.

sole and a well-fitting upper has the potential to reduce plantar injury based on the principles described here rather than from a simple cushioning approach. If the upper does not fit correctly or the insole does not permit shear strain, this role can be lost; if the upper fits too tightly, direct injury can result.

In practice, the shoe fitter attempts by palpation to establish that any bony prominences will be given adequate pressure relief and to locate the position of the most distal toe. Once this latter position has been determined, there must be some attempt to determine how much relative movement between foot and shoe will occur with the given combination of insole materials, upper, gait, and physical characteristics of the patient. There are, at present, almost no quantitative tools available to assist with this extremely complex process.

Modifications to the upper that are intended to accommodate dorsal deformities include depth shoes, stretching of the upper, soft leather "windows," and custom molding, are discussed in Chapter 34.

Plantar Pressure Measurement in Footwear Prescription

In-shoe plantar pressure measurement, as reported in the scientific literature, has been applied most frequently to the evaluation of off-loading devices that are designed to heal ulcers (see "Ulcer Healing: Biomechanical Considerations," above) and to the elucidation of the general effects of various footwear design features (see earlier part of this section). Such efforts to evaluate prescription footwear quantitatively date back almost 40 years to the work of Bauman, Girling, and Brand.[32] However, there have been only a few reports[178, 220] of the use of this methodology in the prescription of shoes for individual patients, perhaps because this does not fit the randomized controlled trial approach that dominates many scientific journals. This is unfortunate because, while the definition of general principles from experimental studies is important, we believe that the care of individual patients could be greatly enhanced by in-shoe pressure measurement. In the Penn State Diabetes Foot Clinics we use in-shoe pressure measurement for patients who have proven extremely difficult to keep from reulcerating. Although we rarely know the threshold for ulceration (but see case study in the section above on ulcer threshold), we invariably have a shoe in which the patient has already ulcerated. Thus the goal for the design of new footwear is to provide "substantial" pressure relief compared to that shoe. An example of this approach is shown in Plate 3.

Acceptance of Footwear

Compliance with the wearing of prescription footwear is obviously a key to successful treatment. Chantelau and Haage[83] reported that patients who were compliant in the use of prescribed therapeutic footwear (reported use for >60% of the day) experienced significantly fewer ulcer recurrences than noncompliant patients.

No studies of psychological factors involved in the acceptance of prescription footwear are available, but obviously the most sophisticated biomechanical approach to footwear design will fail if the shoes are not worn. It is true that many of the styles of footwear that are currently prescribed to diabetic patients in the United States are not aesthetically pleasing. Several European manufacturers of extra-depth shoes are providing much more attractive styles that may promote better patient compliance. McLoughlin et al.[173] reported a remarkable gender difference in compliance with therapeutic footwear in the United Kingdom. In an audit performed 2 years after an initial footwear prescription, records indicated that while 71% of men received new shoes, only 35% of women obtained a repeat prescription; 65% of women failed to attend a foot review clinic, while male attendance was described as "much better."

Summary of Footwear Biomechanics

In summary, from the biomechanical perspective the primary goal of footwear is to redistribute force over a large area (i.e., reduce pressure), thereby "cushioning" foci of elevated pressure. Ideally this would involve redistributing the pressure throughout the surface of the foot by using an insole that conformed to all curvatures of the foot. This hydrostatic insole model has the drawback of not resisting shear stress, however. The spring and damper concepts help in the understanding of foot-shoe interface material design, but progress is also being made rapidly in the area of computer modeling for footwear design.

Many basic principles of footwear design for the neuropathic foot remain to be elucidated. The uncertainty over the positioning of the rocker axis is a good example of why more objective research is needed in this field before footwear can be designed according to established principles rather than simply being based on designs from clinical experience. Many of the ideas outlined in this section on footwear need to be confirmed by further experimental investigations. The entire field of therapeutic footwear biomechanics is

still in a primitive stage, where trial and error is the principal modus operandi. This is not a satisfactory situation for either patient or provider, and it frequently results in a long and frustrating search for a solution that will keep the patient healed. One can only hope that the continued application of technologies such as biomechanical modeling, pressure measurement, materials testing, and foot shape measurement will result in a more complete understanding of the principles of different approaches and faster convergence toward appropriate interventions.

Clinical Biomechanics: What to Look for and What to Do About It

So far we have discussed the biomechanics of gait, of the soft tissues of the foot, of various devices for healing neuropathic plantar ulcers, and of footwear, all in the context of understanding the cause and options for treatment and prevention of diabetic foot injury. At each point we have tried to offer clinical implications. The goal of the next section of this chapter is to pull together the information provided so far into a coherent, usable clinical strategy. The reader may also wish to consult a recent monograph by Warren and Nade,[267] which offers much practical advice on the treatment of neuropathic limbs.

The key permissive factor in diabetic foot injury is loss of protective sensation because of the distal symmetric peripheral neuropathy that can result from diabetes (see Chapter 3). The degree of nerve damage can be assessed in many ways, and it has been proposed that to fully define the degree of neuropathy an objective assessment of symptoms, function, and electrophysiologic tests should be performed.[6] However, in the context of defining the level of sensory loss that is permissive of unperceived injury, simple functional sensory tests appear to provide the best discrimination.[40, 48, 72, 235, 239] Loss of protective sensation has been defined in terms of touch-pressure sensation using the Semmes-Weinstein monofilaments[40, 239] and in terms of vibration perception threshold using the Biosthesiometer[42, 48] and the Vibratron.[239] A calibrated tuning fork is in use in Switzerland.

We use primarily the Semmes-Weinstein monofilaments and believe that, in clinical practice, this simple tool provides the quickest and best method of confirming and measuring loss of protective sensation. In several studies using a "method of limits" rather than a "forced choice" protocol,[40, 72] the 10-gm monofilament was found to be discriminatory. We believe that this extremely simple and inexpensive tool should be in the office of all physicians who care for patients with diabetes. Just as an annual examination of the retina is viewed as essential to good diabetes care,[4] an annual assessment of sensory level in the feet should be seen as critical. If the patient can perceive the 10-gm monofilament at multiple sites in the feet, he or she can be considered to require little or no additional special foot care. An exception to this would be a patient with good sensation but very ischemic feet, for whom even a simple cut or blister, even though it would be painful, might lead to gangrene and amputation. Regardless of an ability to feel pain and recognize injury, that patient needs to be educated about sensible foot care. Likewise, a patient with good sensation who wears shoes that are inappropriate even for a healthy person, such as those with high heels and a cramped toe box, should also receive education about healthy foot care habits and reasonable footwear styles, as an "investment" for the future.

A number of clinical recommendations for the patient with loss of protective sensation, which are based on biomechanical principles, are contained in two important documents that have emerged from the activities of the American Diabetes Council on Foot Care.[5, 169] The earliest of these[169] is concerned with preventive foot care and identifies several biomechanical risk factors that the clinician should be aware of. The components of an adequate foot examination are also discussed. The second[5] is the result of a Consensus Conference on Ulcer Healing, and many of the recommendations on unweighting parallel the remarks made in the ulcer healing section of this chapter. In a recent publication, we describe what the practicing physician should know about foot biomechanics[77] and how an examination should be conducted. Once the loss of protective sensation is identified, a detailed evaluation of foot structure and function and of gait and footwear is essential. From sources described at the start of this paragraph and on the evidence described in this chapter, the following sections have been compiled in order to help

the clinician determine what to look for. Many of the clinical recommendations are components of a brief examination that we have called "The 2-Minute Foot Exam," which is presented in Table 6–7.

Plantar Pressure

Based on the many studies linking high barefoot pressure to ulceration, it makes sense to measure barefoot plantar pressure in all patients with loss of protective sensation if equipment is available. The best study that defines risk is that of Armstrong et al.[20] They suggest that a pressure of 750 kPa provides the best level of discrimination between low-risk and high-risk patients (as measured using an EMED-SF system). They do point out, however, that the higher the pressure, the higher the risk, and that there is no clearly safe pressure. We have utilized barefoot pressure assessment routinely in all patients with loss of protective sensation at the Penn State Diabetes Foot Clinics for several years, and we tend to think of pressure greater than 500 kPa as conferring some risk at forefoot or midfoot sites. At the hallux clearly high pressures confer risk but low pressures do not exclude risk, since the hallux behaves differently during activities of daily living than during level walking.[214] The recommendation to perform barefoot plantar pressure measurement on all patients with loss of protective sensation must be tempered somewhat by the fact that there is no prospective study showing better patient outcomes due to plantar pressure testing.

If plantar pressure measurement is not available, a clinical assessment of all the factors that contribute to high pressure and therefore to ulceration, as reviewed in the section on causes of high pressure, above, is needed. This includes clinical assessment of deformity, the soft tissue plantar cushion, range of motion of key joints, callus and pre-ulcers and, of course, ulcers and scar tissue. Even when plantar pressure measurement is available, assessment is needed of strength, balance, and the intended activity level, including special activities such as golfing, horse riding, and the like. In each of the following subsections we first offer what the clinician needs to assess, followed by some intervention options. Therapeutic footwear is of course an option that can be utilized to deal with all of the abnormalities that cause

Table 6–7 ■ A "2-MINUTE FOOT EXAM" TO CHECK FOR BIOMECHANICAL AND OTHER RISK FACTORS ONCE A PATIENT HAS BEEN JUDGED TO BE AT RISK BECAUSE OF SIGNIFICANT NEUROPATHY OR VASCULAR DISEASE*

EVALUATION COMPONENT	DETAILS	ACTION
1. Examine all surfaces	Feel for: 　Pulse in posterior tibial artery behind medial malleolus 　Pulse in dorsalis pedis artery on the dorsum of the foot Look for: 　Ulcer 　Callus 　Hemorrhage into callus 　Blister 　Maceration between toes 　Other breaks in the skin 　Skin infection 　Edema, erythema, elevated temperature	Prescribe unweighting device to heal ulcer Remove callus (sharp débridement and/or dremmel or emery board) Treat skin infection or injury Refer if Charcot fracture suspected
2. Examine the nails	Look for: 　Fungal infections 　Ingrown toe nails 　Evidence of injury from nail self-care	Consider treating fungal infections Advise against self-care of nails Suggest chiropody care
3. Identify foot deformity	Look for: 　Prominent metatarsal heads 　Claw or hammer toes 　Rocker bottom foot deformity 　Hallux valgus and bunions 　Prior amputation	The presence of foot deformity will dictate footwear specifications (see text and Table 6–8)
4. Examine the shoes Have the patient put their shoes and socks on as the last component of the examination. This will show the patient's ability to examine their own feet.	Look for: 　Drainage into socks 　Worn out (flattened) insoles 　Shoes that are leaning badly to one side 　Poorly fitting shoes (too tight, too loose, too short, not enough room for the toes) 　Gait pattern	Prescribe appropriate footwear if necessary (see text and Table 6–8) Suggest replacement shoes if necessary
5. Establish need for education	Ask: 　Why do you think I am concerned about your feet? 　Do you walk without shoes at home? 　Who takes care of your nails?	Schedule patient for education visit with diabetes educator/nurse if understanding is lacking or if behaviors are unacceptable.

* From Boulton AJM, Connor H, Cavanagh PR (eds): Biomechanics for the Practicing Physician. *In* The Foot in Diabetes, 3rd ed. Chichester: John Wiley & Sons, 2000, with permission.

high pressure; footwear is dealt with separately in its own subsection. Many of the deformities can also be treated by surgery, which has its own section.

Foot Deformity

High pressure on both the dorsal and plantar surfaces is the immediate cause of most skin injury. The key foot deformities that must be identified as potential risk factors for foot injury are shown in Table 6–7. On the dorsal aspect of the foot, skin breakdown is usually the result of deformity. The most common deformity is clawing of toes. On occasion the toes will actually become dorsally dislocated, and standard off-the-shelf shoe fit is usually not possible in that situation. At the very least, extra-depth shoes must be utilized. Although uncommon, bony prominences on the dorsal aspect of the midfoot are very troublesome because this region of the foot is likely to be particularly involved in the transfer of propulsive forces from the foot through footwear to the floor during gait. Such dorsal prominences are sometimes seen in patients with Charcot fractures. Bunions, secondary to hallux valgus, are important deformities, particularly when associated with a wide forefoot. They are usually covered by very little soft tissue, making shoe fitting difficult.

Another important deformity is that of forefoot supination or pronation (rotation of the plane of the metatarsal heads so that they are no longer in the same plane as the hindfoot).[208] When the forefoot is in supination, the fifth metatarsal head tends to hit the ground first during gait so that higher plantar pressure in this region would be predicted. Similarly, when the forefoot is in pronation, one could predict higher plantar pressure under the first metatarsal head. However, this is a good example of how very difficult it is to predict plantar pressure from just an examination of the foot. The pressures just implied will, in fact, depend on whether the supination or pronation is fixed or flexible; in other words, on how difficult it is to bring all the metatarsal heads onto the ground during stance and gait. Plantarflexed metatarsals (particularly the first) can also result in focal areas of pressure if the deformity is relatively rigid.

Unusual deformities or prominences frequently imply underlying fractures that are often not noted by the patient,[79] and radiographs of a patient with a major deformity are mandatory. Unusual prominences of the midfoot are of particular relevance because they are usually an indication of an underlying Charcot fracture. In the acute stages of a Charcot process, the foot is also erythematous, hot, and swollen, but in the "healed" stage of a Charcot fracture these findings are absent (see Chapter 21).

Soft Tissue Changes

Bones can appear to be prominent either because of deformity or because of changes in the soft tissues overlying the bones. The plantar surface is normally well "padded" with soft tissue so that some attempt at an examination of the soft tissues there is important. Because most ulcers occur under the hallux and metatarsal heads, these are the regions that should be inspected most carefully.

Because there is an association between soft tissue thickness under a metatarsal head and peak plantar pressure in that re-

gion,[68, 176, 273] an assessment of the quantity of the soft tissues under the metatarsal heads is relevant. In a healthy young foot, the metatarsal heads are not visible through the plantar skin or palpable to a light stroking movement by the examiner's finger across them. As the toes become clawed as a consequence of intrinsic muscle atrophy and/or tearing of the plantar fascia, the plantar fat pad slides forward away from the metatarsal heads so that the tissue between the skin and the metatarsal heads becomes thinner. In an extreme case the metatarsal heads will be directly palpable, seeming to be covered by skin only. On average, pressure under a metatarsal head covered by skin only will be much greater than when there is a good amount of healthy plantar tissue between the metatarsal head and the floor. As discussed earlier, the quantity and quality of the plantar soft tissues may also be affected by glycosylation. Tissue "quality" may be an important factor but there are no ways to measure this at present. Scarring and adhesions of the soft tissues of the plantar surface can also be detected clinically; because of their possible consequences to plantar soft tissue function and thus to ulceration, we teach our patients to try to mobilize scar tissue by massage. Scarring implies, of course, that an ulcer had been present, identifying that patient as almost certainly still having all the characteristics necessary for further ulceration.

An intriguing anecdotal approach to the alleviation of soft tissue deficits using injected liquid silicon has been reported for a number of years by Balkin.[28–30] Recently a controlled study of this approach reported that patients who had been injected with silicon had lower MTH pressures up to 12 months after the treatment.[256] If this procedure can be shown to be medically safe it would appear to offer a useful way to reduce plantar pressure at metatarsal head prominences.

Obviously, if an ulcer is currently present, the treatments described in the section on ulcer healing must be employed to off-load the ulcerated region.

Callus

Even though the etiology of callus is not clear, the fact that callus contributes to high plantar pressure is clear.[185] Furthermore, in the study of Murray et al.[185] the presence of callus in a patient with loss of protective sensation conferred a very high risk ratio for ulceration. It is therefore strongly recommended that callus be looked for and that appropriate measures be taken to prevent, limit, and remove it. Appropriate footwear prevents callus,[240] and one measure of how efficacious footwear is, short of preventing ulceration, is prevention of callus. One can feel very confident that a patient is doing well if callus is being prevented. Patients can contribute to limiting callus by daily self-care—filing the callus with an emery board or pumice stone. Removal of callus is also a very important part of professional foot care.

An extremely important sign in the evaluation of the neuropathic foot is hemorrhage into a callus, also called a preulcer. Although this may be quite subtle at times, it implies that enough trauma has occurred to cause tissue damage. Therefore, hematoma in a callus must be taken as seriously as an ulcer: it is an ulcer "but for a few more steps." Health care providers must share their concern about such a lesion with their patients as part of patient education, teaching them how to recognize this lesion and report it immediately.

Limited Joint Mobility

Limited joint mobility is statistically associated with higher plantar pressure.[36, 37, 108] The possible mechanisms for this association have been discussed. Although direct prediction of plantar pressure from measurement of the range of motion of a joint is not possible, there is nevertheless one measurement that is probably worthwhile: the measurement of hallux dorsiflexion. Normal range of hallux dorsiflexion is approximately 50 degrees when measured with a simple goniometer in relation to the floor.[115] Marked reductions of hallux dorsiflexion are associated with high hallux pressure.[36] One would similarly predict that a reduction in ankle dorsiflexion would tend to increase forefoot plantar pressure. In general, however, this is not convincing on a patient-by-patient basis, probably because many other factors contribute to forefoot pressure. On the other hand, if a patient is having ongoing problems with recurrent forefoot ulceration, the discovery of a very limited range of dorsiflexion at the ankle might lead to a recommendation for TAL (see the section "Surgery to Alter Biomechanics," below). For completeness, both ankle dorsiflexion, with the knee flexed and extended, and subtalar range of motion should be assessed. Since accuracy and interrater reliability are controversial topics in such measurements,[212] those made by a single examiner are preferable. Certain measurements (e.g., subtalar neutral position) may be almost worthless because of lack of appropriate landmarks.

There is now preliminary evidence that passive range of motion and other exercises may be effective in increasing the range of motion at the joints of the foot and perhaps also in reducing plantar pressure during walking.[23, 96]

Weakness and Balance

Although much emphasis in the evaluation and treatment of the diabetic patient is placed on sensory neuropathy, patients with a significant motor component to their neuropathy can also display major functional problems with the feet. A quick evaluation of the patient's ability to rise repeatedly on the toes from a neutral standing position is a worthwhile component of the clinical examination to reveal triceps surae weakness. Loss of strength of the ankle dorsiflexors will be apparent in gait, during which foot drop, a steppage gait, or both will be seen. Patients with foot drop can injure their toes by dragging them on the floor; this can be prevented if good shoes are always worn. Falling because of the toes catching on the floor can be prevented using an ankle-foot orthosis.

Sensory neuropathy also affects the afferent nerves relevant to balance, as was reviewed earlier, and neuropathic patients fall more often than those without neuropathy. Patients should therefore be asked whether or not they have fallen recently. The traditional Romberg test with the eyes open and closed can also be revealing. A detailed monofilament test using multiple monofilaments of different thicknesses that can establish the threshold for touch sensation (rather than just the presence or absence of protective sensation) can be reasonably predictive of postural stability.[230] However, in the clinic it is worth remembering that a patient who cannot feel the 10-gm monofilament can be expected to sway while trying to stand still as much as a nonneuropathic patient would sway with their eyes closed and head back.[230]

If there does appear to be risk for falling, the provision of an assistive device such as a cane or a walker would seem intuitively reasonable. Patients often report that they feel more stable when their shoes are rockered rather than rollered, but we have no quantitative data to support this observation. Patients with short amputations, such as a transmetatarsal amputation (TMA), also report less of a balance problem with an ankle-foot orthosis (AFO) of some type. Mueller and Strube[184] found that an AFO led to the best biomechanical function in such patients. Although there are no papers in the literature on strength or balance training in patients with diabetes, there are many studies showing the benefits of both these interventions in elderly individuals.[170] It is reasonable to assume that diabetic patients with strength and balance problems would benefit from such a program.

Activity and Gait

An important question to ask patients is how much they use their feet and in what activities. It is important to ask about both the amount and type of use because, for example, running leads to much greater forces being transmitted through the plantar tissues than walking.[214] A patient who is bed- or chair-bound will not need sophisticated footwear to protect the feet, whereas a very athletic patient who has significant foot problems may have to consider altering his or her behavior as well as footwear. We have, at times, made rigid roller bottom modified golf shoes with molded insoles as well as English style riding boots to allow patients to continue as normal a life style as possible while minimizing the risk to their feet. Chair- or bed-bound patients have their own particular problems. Heel decubitus ulcers are well known, but decubitus ulcers can also develop over the malleoli in patients who have a preference for lying on one side or the other. These ulcers will not heal until pressure from lying in bed or on a recliner chair is relieved.

Watching the patient walk, before prescribing footwear or any other intervention, is obviously highly relevant and useful, since most foot injuries occur during gait. While much can be inferred about foot function from the static examination described so far, weakness, balance problems and any un-usual gait due to hip or knee problems become apparent only while walking.

Shoes and Footwear Prescription

The topic of footwear prescription is dealt with more comprehensively in Chapters 20 and 34. We will discuss here some recommendations that flow from the biomechanical studies mentioned above. It is through shoes that the forces of gait that can potentially damage the foot are transmitted from the ground, and it is therefore in shoes that most injuries occur. Shoes can protect from injury, but they can also cause injury directly. A thorough examination of footwear must be considered an essential component of the clinical biomechanical examination of the patient at risk for neuropathic injury.

Concepts of fit must be applied to the clinical situation, with particular attention to dorsal deformities, clawed toes, and forefoot width. Construction of the insole will depend on what the clinical situation demands, but an insole already used must be examined for excessive wear (bottoming out). This can provide insight into the location of high plantar pressure and will also suggest that a particular type of insole is not sufficient (e.g., if it bottoms out very quickly) or is simply too old.

Evaluation of the wear of both the outsoles and uppers of the shoes worn by a patient can also be helpful. Excessive wear of the outsole is probably a consequence of relative movement ("scuffing") during the early and late phases of foot contact and is probably not helpful in predicting where high plantar pressure occurs. Deformations of the upper, however, are often extremely useful because they are evidence of shear forces tending to move the foot off the platform of the shoe. Significant uncompensated supination and pronation deformities of the forefoot can usually be inferred from deformations in the shoe upper.

The approach to footwear prescription should be graded. The simplest intervention for a patient who is at risk for ulceration would be a well-fitting and well-cushioned pair of athletic shoes. A number of studies have shown that athletic shoes can reduce plantar pressure[142, 199, 201] and lead to fewer calluses.[240] Thus athletic shoes can be the first line of defense if the patient's foot fits well in the upper. The next step is to provide extra-depth shoes, which typically add from

¼ inch to ½ inch of space to the toe box, thus allowing for accommodation of significant dorsal deformity or thicker insoles. It is generally advisable to replace the insoles that are supplied with these shoes with a thick foam insole. The next level of complexity in footwear is to make a custom molded and/or a customized insole (see section on footwear, above). A patient who is still not adequately protected will need the outsoles of their depth shoes made rigid and either rockered or rollered (see below). Finally, feet with significant deformity, or feet in need of a very thick insole, will need custom molded shoes. As is apparent from the foregoing, a large majority of patients can be accommodated using footwear that is available over-the-counter from a therapeutic shoe supplier. The manufacture of molded and customized insoles, however, requires specialist care. This fact is implied in the "footwear pyramid" presented in Figure 6–24.

We believe that the factors that drive a decision regarding which of the above types of footwear to prescribe are a combination of the patient's activity level and their plantar pressure (see Table 6–8). If barefoot plantar pressure measurement is not available, then deformity can be used as a surrogate measure for elevated pressure. The more active the patient and the higher the plantar pressure (or the greater the deformity) the more sophistication is needed in the footwear. As is apparent from the table, the process of footwear prescription is not an exact science. The table represents the consensus of several clinicians, but there are few data to support

it, and because of this the table allows much "latitude." Only when the ulceration threshold has been defined in terms of some measure of loading in a shoe (see section on threshold) will it be possible to prescribe footwear with precision. In the meantime, the proof of the shoe is its wearing. In other words, whether a shoe is efficacious or not can be judged only by whether an ulcer, or preferably callus, blister, redness, or preulcer, can be prevented.

The literature regarding rocker and roller outsole shoes was presented earlier. There is conclusive evidence that shoes with rigid soles and a curved or rockered outsole are effective in relieving plantar pressure, and clinical experience suggests that such footwear can help keep patients from experiencing recurrent ulceration.[84, 88, 191, 223, 231, 254]

In summary, taking all of the studies of rocker and roller shoes together, we currently recommend the following in the design of rigid footwear:

1. *Minimize toe spring.* Pending definitive investigation of this variable, this recommendation is suggested by comparing the studies of Coleman[88] and Nawoczenski et al.[191]
2. *Maintain heel/forefoot height difference of the original shoe, but pick a shoe with minimal initial difference to avoid ending up with very high shoes.* This recommendation is made empirically, since no published evidence is available; there is concern that altering the heel/forefoot height difference might cause problems with the upper, since this difference was inherent in the original shoe design.
3. *Consider adjusting the axis of the rocker/roller with respect to the long axis of the shoe to accommodate for significant toe-out.* This particularly makes sense if the area of concern is MTH1, but again, no published evidence is available to support this recommendation at present.
4. *Teach patients who use rocker shoes not to dwell on the forward flat part of the rocker for support.* This recommendation is suggested by Van Schie et al.[254] and much earlier by Bauman et al.[33] Shortening the stride will promote this goal.
5. *Rockers are preferred over rollers.* Rocker shoes of the same height probably reduce pressure more than rollers (perhaps by an additional 8% from baseline; see

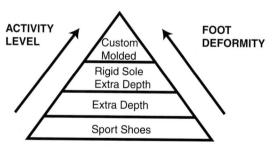

Figure 6–24 ■ The "footwear pyramid." The width of the base of each segment is proportional to the number of patients who can be accommodated in the type of footwear indicated. Thus, custom molded shoes are reserved for only a small group of patients who cannot be accommodated by any of the other designs, which increase in complexity from the base upwards. Activity level and foot deformity (which is a surrogate measure for plantar pressure) are used to define the appropriate footwear for a given patient.

Table 6–8 ■ THE INTERACTION OF PLANTAR PRESSURE (OR DEFORMITY) AND ACTIVITY LEVEL IN THE SELECTION OF APPROPRIATE FOOTWEAR*†

DEFORMITY	ACTIVITY‡		
	Low (Household/Minimal Ambulator)	Moderate (Community Ambulator)	High (Active Ambulator)
None No deformity	• Standard shoe w/soft insole (usually an athletic shoe)	• Standard shoe w/soft insole (usually an athletic shoe) • Standard shoe w/added flat insole • Standard shoe w/added molded insole	• Standard shoe w/added flat insole • Standard shoe w/added molded insole • Extra-depth shoe w/flat insole • Extra-depth shoe w/ molded insole

Moderate
  Limited hallux motion
  Prominent metatarsal heads
  Severe claw or hammer toes
  Callus
  Single lesser ray amputation
  Plantar bony prominences
  Hallux valgus
  Dystrophic nails
  Dorsal exostoses
	• Standard shoe w/soft insole (usually an athletic shoe)
	• Standard shoe w/added flat insole
	• Standard shoe w/added molded insole
	• Extra-depth shoe w/ flat insole
		• Standard shoe w/added flat insole
		• Standard shoe w/added molded insole
		• Extra-depth shoe w/flat insole
		• Extra-depth shoe w/ molded insole
		• Custom molded shoe w/ custom molded insole
		Additional features (+/−)
		• Compliant plugs
		• Roller soles
			• Standard shoe w/added molded insole
			• Extra-depth shoe w/flat insole
			• Extra-depth shoe w/ molded insole
			• Custom molded shoe w/ custom molded insole
			Additional features (+/−)
			• Compliant plugs
			• Differential insoles
			• Roller soles
			Lifestyle modifications

Severe Charcot ≥ Ray amputation ≥ First ray/multiple	• Extra-depth shoe w/ flat insole • Extra-depth shoe w/ molded insole • Custom molded shoe w/custom molded insole • Unweighting orthosis (e.g., PTB)	• Extra-depth shoe w/ molded insole • Custom molded shoe w/ custom molded insole • Unweighting orthosis (e.g., a PTB) Additional features (+/−) • Compliant plugs • Differential insoles • Roller soles • Rocker soles	• Custom molded shoe/w custom molded insole • Unweighting orthosis (e.g., PTB) Additional features (+/−) • Compliant plugs • Differential insoles • Roller soles • Rocker soles *Refer to specialist for management* *Requires lifestyle and/or job modification*

* From Brill LR, Cavanagh PR, Doucette MM, Ulbrecht JS: Treatment of chronic wounds: Prevention, protection and recurrence reduction of diabetic neuropathic foot ulcers. East Setauket, NY: Curative Technologies, Inc, 1994, p 9, with permission.
† Patient history of previous plantar ulcers may require a more aggressive approach to protection than the prescription footwear options suggested in this table.
‡ Footwear and footbed options.

Table 6–6) and rockers are less labor intensive to make.

6. *Consider flaring out the outsole of rollers and rockers for added stability.*

7. *Consider in-shoe pressure measurement in difficult cases and certainly if a shoe "failed."* This recommendation is suggested because of the individual variability in response to rocker and roller shoes as demonstrated, for instance, by Van Schie et al.[254]

8. *Try the suggested rocker and roller designs in Table 6–9.* Most patients will not recognize Shoe 1 as "abnormal." While the take-off point in Shoe 2 favors the toes and hallux, relief at MTHs should be reasonable (see Table 6–5), and using the take-off point of 65% allows the shoe to have a very reasonable height. Shoes 3 to 5 all have the same height, but the different shoes are biased towards different clinical situations. Finally, Shoe 6 is

Table 6–9 ▪ RECOMMENDATIONS FOR THE DESIGN OF RIGID SHOES WITH ROCKER AND ROLLER OUTSOLES

SHOE DESCRIPTION	HEIGHT* AT FULCRUM (APPROX, CM)	CLINICAL INDICATIONS
Roller, 60% take-off, 75% radius	2.25	Low level of concern; cosmetically almost not noticeable
Rocker, 65% take-off, 20 degrees	2.75	"Standard" rocker
Roller, 60% take-off, 60% radius	3.25	High risk, but will not accept rocker over roller
Rocker, 60% take-off, 20 degrees	3.25	High risk, MTHs greater concern than hallux
Rocker, 65% take-off, 22.5 degrees	3.25	High risk, hallux and toes greater concern than MTHs
Rocker, 65% take-off, 25 degrees	3.75	Extremely high risk; use boot or AFO for stability

* Height at fulcrum is for a size #10 male shoe 30 cm in length; it will be less for smaller shoes. Degree indications are for rockers, % radii for rollers.

very high and cosmetically troublesome for many patients, but can be considered in extreme cases, perhaps with a brace and/or an assistive device that will prevent ankle sprains and falls.

Patients with partial amputations of the foot need special footwear attention, but little quantitative work has been done to explore optimal design characteristics for this group of patients. Mueller, Strube, and Allen[184] examined a number of "functional measures" in patients with TMA while they were wearing six different shoes (short and full length with different inserts to take up the residual space in the shoe). They reported that appropriate footwear could significantly improve the function of patients with TMA. The best overall performance and patient acceptance was with a full-length shoe with a total-contact insert and a rigid rocker bottom sole. Footwear with an AFO proved to be most effective in reducing pressures on the residual foot, but patients did not like the reduced range of ankle motion. Similarly, although a short shoe was biomechanically effective, patients complained of the cosmetics of short shoes—they preferred a full-length shoe with toe filler. The very high complication rate after foot-shortening surgery[179] suggests that pressure measurement could be extremely useful in the management of such patients. Some of the more unusual amputations (e.g., Chopart's and Syme's amputations) present special biomechanical challenges in footwear management, and it is often because of the difficulties faced in providing adequate footwear that these procedures are not performed more frequently. Based principally on the work of Mueller, Strube, and Allen,[184] our clinical recommendations for patients with short feet secondary

to TMA surgery are shown in Table 6–10. Unfortunately, these still contain many principles in need of further study.

As was discussed and illustrated in the section above on plantar pressure measurement, in-shoe pressure measurement can be invaluable to guide footwear prescription in patients who reulcerate in newly provided footwear.

It is extremely important to realize that insoles degrade, sometimes rapidly, with normal use. An insole that is protective when prescribed may become dangerous after a few months or sometimes even weeks. The clinician should be vigilant for signs of bottoming out of the insole to the point where it appears to provide little cushioning and distribution of load. At present, Medicare provisions allow each patient one pair of extra-depth shoes and three pairs of insoles per calendar year. It is not known at present whether this is sufficient for a typical patient.

It is worth noting in closing that just because shoes are "special" does not make them right. Unfortunately, many specialist clinics still see patients with recurrent ulceration wearing "special" (and often expensive) shoes that are simply inappropriate for the situation.

Surgery to Alter Biomechanics

Since both dorsal and plantar ulceration often occur over bony prominences, it is not surprising that "prophylactic" bone surgery in patients with neuropathy and deformity has been proposed. It is difficult to quantify the absolute risk of a first ulcer occurring, and the surgical benefit (of a bunion procedure, for instance) in terms of ulcer prevention as well as the risk of bone altering proce-

Table 6–10 ■ FOOTWEAR RECOMMENDATIONS FOR PATIENTS WITH SHORT FEET SECONDARY TO TRANSMETATARSAL AMPUTATION

	SHOE DESCRIPTION	CLINICAL INDICATIONS
1	Flexible full-length depth sports shoe, simple insole†	Reasonably long TMA; patient not very active; dorsal fit not a concern; stability not a concern
2	Full-length shoe, upper based on fit needs, appropriate insole,† rigid rocker with outsole height at rocker fulcrum such that a 20-degree rocker would result if take-off was at 60%. Place rocker axis just proximal to TMA line	"Standard" shoe; however, this shoe should be strongly discouraged if rocker axis would be at < 50% of shoe
3	Same as 2, but with AFO built-in to shoe	Offer to patient for better stability
4	Less than full-length custom molded shoe; upper based on fit needs; appropriate insole†; 20-degree rigid rocker with take-off just proximal to TMA line, such that this is 65% of shoe length‡	A compromise between a full-length shoe and a short shoe for patients with short TMA
5	Same as 4, but with AFO built-in to shoe	Offer to patient for better stability
6	Short custom molded shoe; upper based on fit needs; appropriate insole; 20-degree rigid rocker with take-off at 75%	For use with short TMAs
7	Same as 6, but with AFO built-in to shoe	Offer to patient for better stability

* Data from Mueller MJ, Strube MJ, Allen BT: Therapeutic footwear can reduce plantar pressures in patients with diabetes and transmetatarsal amputation. Diabetes Care 20:637–641, 1997.
† Based on needs to reduce plantar pressure.
‡ Example—TMA foot 16 cm long; axis of rocker at 15 cm; 15 cm = 65% therefore, full length of shoe is 15 × 100/65 = 23 cm.

dures have not been clearly established. There are concerns, however, about surgery in the neuropathic foot causing Charcot fractures (see below). It seems prudent to advise against truly prophylactic surgery, although this recommendation may change as more data become available. However, at some point after an ulcer develops, it may be appropriate to consider surgery to alter the biomechanics of the foot to cure an ulcer and/or prevent recurrence. Obviously, the more likely the ulcer is to recur and the more safe and beneficial the procedure is, the more likely it is that surgery will lead to a better outcome. Unfortunately, just as is the case for footwear prescription, this type of decision is a matter of experience and judgment rather than a matter of precise "rules."

What do we know about the risks and benefits of various surgical procedures? Of considerable concern is a report by Fleischli et al.[110] describing a case series of 22 dorsiflexion metatarsal osteotomies for treatment of chronic persistent or recurrent forefoot ulcers. The authors reported a 68% complication rate, with the most prevalent complication being a Charcot fracture "with rapid destruction of the midfoot." Presumably, many of these Charcot fractures were induced by the surgical and/or rehabilitation procedure. Since the majority of the ulcers were Wagner grade I or II (that is, superficial

or deep to tendon, capsule, or bone without osteomyelitis or deep abscess), the evidence cited elsewhere in this chapter would suggest that at least 90% of these ulcers should have healed in 6 to 8 weeks with a standard total-contact cast regimen, unless complicated by noncompliance, significant vascular disease, or significant infection. The probability that they would have remained healed cannot be estimated, but healing should certainly have been possible. This report from Fleischli et al. further confirms the position against truly prophylactic surgery on the neuropathic foot.

Actual removal of some or all metatarsal heads has been recommended by some for patients with recurrent forefoot ulcers. Patel and Weiman[193] used an EMED-SF platform to show that peak pressures at the site of single MTH resections were significantly reduced without any significant increase in pressure at adjacent sites, and Giurini et al.[121] have reported a successful series of patients on whom this procedure was performed. In contrast, we have presented case studies of patients with panmetatarsal head resection where the peak pressures were markedly elevated at several sites under the metatarsal head remnants (Plate 4), with subsequent almost intractable recurrent ulceration.[76] Our suspicion is that this procedure is very technique dependent, but further study is required to confirm this.

A surgical approach to the treatment of midfoot Charcot fractures has become much more commonplace in the last decade. Using a cadaver model, Marks et al.[166] have shown that a plantar third tubular midfoot plate provides a better stabilization for midfoot instability than screw fixation, and they have applied this approach to Charcot patients. Myerson et al.[188] describe a series of 68 patients who were treated by open reduction and arthrodesis, TCC, or amputation. These authors state that surgical salvage of feet with Charcot fractures, once bony coalescence has begun, is reasonable and appropriate. Sammarco and Conti[218] also reported a series of 27 feet in which surgical repair was performed. A complication rate of approximately 30% was described. Early and Hansen[105] reported on an average 28-month follow-up (range, 6 to 84 months) of 21 feet with midfoot collapse on which reconstruction with reduction, fusion, and internal fixation was performed. Seventy percent of the patients with midfoot ulcers healed without incident and there were no recurrent midfoot ulcers in the follow-up period. There is, as yet, no published study in which pre- and postsurgical biomechanical assessment has been performed in a group of Charcot patients who have been surgically reconstructed. Such a study is certainly needed to provide information on the kind of plantar pressure reduction that is required to create a plantar surface that is viable for weight bearing. So far, the clinical results are very encouraging. For further discussion of this issue see Chapter 27.

Tendo Achilles lengthening has often been mentioned anecdotally as a means of relieving forefoot pressure in patients with a history of chronic ulceration, but few authors have reported on outcome and/or plantar pressure measurement after TAL. Lin et al.[160] performed percutaneous TAL and follow-up TCC on 15 patients with forefoot ulcers who initially failed to heal in a TCC. All but one of the ulcers progressed to healing in a mean of 39 days. There was no ulcer recurrence in this group of patients at a mean follow-up time of 17.3 months. Armstrong et al.[22] reported on ten similar patients with recurrent forefoot ulceration. Forefoot plantar pressure was reduced by 230 kPa following percutaneous TAL, and mean range of dorsiflexion was increased by approximately 9 degrees. Although "calcaneal gait" has been mentioned as a complication of TAL,[237] none of these groups reported such a complication. However, we have had a patient develop intractable heel ulceration after a TAL procedure that led to a transtibial amputation. TAL has also been recommended for patients with Charcot neuroarthropathy,[124] but this approach remains to be explored quantitatively.

All the procedures mentioned above fit more or less into the category of attempting to reconstruct anatomy. Not mentioned so far are procedures to straighten clawed or hammered toes to prevent recurrent ulcers of the toe tips. We find these procedures very helpful, but there are no supporting data for them. Ablative procedures, usually due to infection, ischemia, or both, are often necessary. What is known about the biomechanical consequences of amputation procedures and what are the principles that should govern amputation site selection and method? More often than not, the choice of a site for amputation is governed by a bias for preserving tissue at all cost, without regard to subsequent function. This often leaves the patient and the orthotist with the impossible task of living with and dealing with a foot that cannot be maintained in a healed condition. A good example would be a foot with rays 3, 4, and 5 amputated. Ideally, only defined amputations with well-described surgical methods, defined biomechanical consequences, and well-established footwear approaches should be utilized, but too little is currently known about amputation consequences (other than extreme examples such as that just described) to make clear recommendations.

Even minor amputation surgery of the forefoot is associated with significant secondary deformity. Quebedeaux et al.[203] and Lavery et al.[155] reported more deformities of the second and third toes and the lesser MTP joints, and more elevated pressures under the metatarsal heads and toes in feet with hallux amputations, compared to the intact contralateral sides. They also found that ulcers were much more common on the amputated side. Similarly, Armstrong and Lavery[15] reported that a history of surgical procedures within the foot (digital or ray amputation distal to the tarsometatarsal joint) was associated with an odds ratio of 9.8 for limited joint mobility or rigid deformity compared to controls who had never had a foot amputation. Peak pressures were also higher in the feet with amputation. However, this study was not designed to establish a cause-and-effect relationship. Similarly, Lavery et al.[155] reported elevated pressure under the metatarsal heads and toes in feet with a hallux amputation compared to the contralateral side.

It is not surprising that the mechanics of feet that have undergone partial midfoot amputation are also altered. Garbalosa et al.[119] reported elevated forefoot pressure in patients with unilateral TMA compared to their intact side. These investigators also found reduced functional dorsiflexion during gait in the TMA feet. Both these findings suggested that careful footwear management after TMA surgery is essential, but it is also possible that better surgical technique (e.g., incorporation of TAL or tendon transfers as has been suggested) might improve outcomes. Mueller et al.[181] also reported that patients with TMA showed reduced ranges of motion, and reduced joint moments and power during gait compared to control patients although, again, speeds were not controlled. Mueller and Sinacore[182] presented a biomechanical rationale for problems during rehabilitation and shoe prescription of patients with TMA.

As implied above, it is logical to assume that surgical correction of deformity should be useful in prevention of neuropathic ulceration and reulceration. However, much remains to be learned before specific recommendations can be made. Several case studies from our own clinical practice of plantar pressure measurements with patients who have undergone surgery are presented in Plate 5.

Concluding Remarks

It is our hope that the techniques and principles presented here will make the biomechanical aspects of etiology and prevention of foot injury in the setting of diabetic neuropathy more understandable, and hence more accessible to those involved in the treatment of diabetic foot problems. The growth in this field in the last 5 years has been remarkable, reflecting the important role of biomechanics in the understanding and management of diabetic foot problems. Much remains to be learned. Some of the immediate challenges for the future include the quantification of tissue properties, the definition of objective algorithms for footwear prescription, the reduction of high ulcer recurrence rates, and the introduction of simple in-shoe pressure measurement into a clinical environment.

Present economic forces that require clinicians to spend less time with patients will also mean that careful justification will need to be made for additional measurements performed in the clinic. However, it is anticipated that the acceptance of quantitative approaches to what was formerly seen frequently as a subjective field will eventually benefit patients.

ACKNOWLEDGMENTS

We are grateful to the many patients from whom we have learned and to staff of the Penn State Diabetes Foot Clinics past and present for their devotion to quality patient care. Mary Becker, R.N., M.S., has greatly facilitated our experimental efforts. We thank our colleagues Dr. David Lemmon and Dr. Paul Juliano for their contributions. The contributions of the graduate students and staff of the Center for Locomotion Studies at Pennsylvania State University are also gratefully acknowledged. In particular, Mrs. Esther Y. Boone and Mrs. Diane Plummer have provided superb and dedicated editorial assistance without which the production of this chapter would not have been possible.

Our research has been supported by the American Diabetes Association, the National Institutes of Health, and ConvaTec Inc.

REFERENCES

1. Ahroni JH, Boyko EJ, Forsberg RC: Clinical correlates of plantar pressure among diabetic veterans. Diabetes Care 22:965–972, 1999.
2. Akhlaghi F, Pepper MG: In-shoe biaxial shear force measurement: The Kent shear system. Med Biol Eng Comput 34:315–317, 1996.
3. Alexander IJ, Chao EYS, Johnson KA: The assessment of dynamic foot-to-ground contact forces and plantar pressure distribution: A review of the evolution of current techniques and clinical applications. Foot Ankle 11:152–167, 1990.
4. American College of Physicians, American Diabetes Association, American Academy of Opthalmology: Screening for diabetic retinopathy [position statement]. Diabetes Care 15:16–18, 1992.
5. American Diabetes Association: Consensus development conference on diabetic foot wound care. Diabetes Care 22:1354–1360, 1999.
6. American Diabetes Association/American Academy of Neurology: Consensus Statement. Report and recommendations of the 1988 San Antonio Conference on Diabetic Neuropathy (AK Asbury and D Porte, Jr, Co-chairmen). Diabetes Care 11:592–597, 1988.
7. Andersen H, Gadeberg PC, Brock B, Jakobsen J: Muscular atrophy in diabetic neuropathy: A stereological magnetic resonance imaging study. Diabetologia 40:1062–1069, 1997.
8. Andersen H, Poulsen PL, Mogensen CE, Jakobsen J: Isokinetic muscle strength in long-term IDDM

patients in relation to diabetic complications. Diabetes 45:440–445, 1996.

9. Andriacchi TP, Yoder D, Conley A, et al: Patellofemoral design influences function following total knee arthroplasty. J Arthroplasty 12:243–249, 1997.

10. Apelqvist J, Castenfors J, Larsson J, et al: Wound classification is more important than site of ulceration in the outcome of diabetic foot ulcers. Diabet Med 6:526–530, 1989.

11. Apelqvist J, Larsson J, Agardh C-D: The influence of external precipitating factors and peripheral neuropathy on the development and outcome of diabetic foot ulcers. J Diabetes Complications 4:21–25, 1990.

12. Armstrong DG, Athanasiou KA: The edge effect: How and why wounds grow in size and depth. Clin Podiatr Med Surg 15:105–108, 1998.

13. Armstrong DG, Lavery LA: Elevated peak plantar pressures in patients who have Charcot arthropathy. J Bone Joint Surg 80-A:365–369, 1998.

14. Armstrong DG, Lavery LA: Evidence-based options for off-loading diabetic wounds. Clin Podiatr Med Surg 15:95–104, 1998.

15. Armstrong DG, Lavery LA: Plantar pressures are higher in diabetic patients following partial foot amputation. Ostomy/Wound Management 44:30–39, 1998.

16. Armstrong DG, Lavery LA: Shoes and the diabetic foot. Practical Diabetol 17:23–26, 1998.

17. Armstrong DG, Lavery LA, Bushman TR: Peak foot pressures influence the healing time of diabetic foot ulcers treated with total contact casts. J Rehabil Res Dev 35:1–5, 1998.

18. Armstrong DG, Lavery LA, Harkless LB: Healing the diabetic wound with pressure off-loading. Biomechanics 4:67–74, 1997.

19. Armstrong DG, Liswood PJ, Todd WF: Potential risks of accommodative padding in the treatment of neuropathic ulcerations. Ostomy/Wound Management 41:44–48, 1995.

20. Armstrong DG, Peters EJG, Athanasiou KA, Lavery LA: Is there a critical level of plantar foot pressure to identify patients at risk for neuropathic foot ulceration? J Foot Ankle Surg 37:303–307, 1998.

21. Armstrong DG, Stacpoole-Shea S: Total contact casts and removable cast walkers. Mitigation of plantar heel pressure. J Am Podiatr Med Assoc 89:50–53, 1999.

22. Armstrong DG, Stacpoole-Shea S, Nguyen H, Harkless LB: Lengthening of the Achilles tendon in diabetic patients who are at high risk for ulceration of the foot. J Bone Joint Surg 81-A:535–538, 1999.

23. Armstrong DG, Steinberg JS, Stacpoole-Shea S, et al: The potential benefit of passive range of motion exercises to reduce peak plantar foot pressure in the diabetic foot. Proceedings of the 3rd International Symposium on the Diabetic Foot 1999, p 76.

24. Ashry HR, Lavery LA, Murdoch DP, et al: Effectiveness of diabetic insoles to reduce foot pressures. J Foot Ankle Surg 36:268–271, 1997.

25. ASTM Designation: D-395-68. Standard methods of test for compression set of vulcanized rubber. American National Standards Institute 1971, pp 195–201.

26. Bader DL: Effects of compressive loading regimens on tissue viability. *In* Bader DL (ed): Pressure Sores—Clinical Practice and Scientific Approach. New York: Macmillan, 1990.

27. Bader DL: The recovery characteristics of soft tissues following repeated loading. J Rehabil Res Dev 27:141–150, 1990.

28. Balkin SW: Plantar keratoses: Treatment by injectable liquid silicone—a report of an 8-year experience. Clin Orthop 87:235–247, 1972.

29. Balkin SW: Fluid silicone implantation in the diabetic foot. A twenty-one year study. Unpublished Handout Material at the XII Congress of The International Diabetes Federation, 1985.

30. Balkin SW, Kaplan L: Injectable silicone and the diabetic foot: A 25-year report. Foot 1:83–88, 1991.

31. Barrett JP, Mooney V: Neuropathy and diabetic pressure lesions. Orthop Clin North Am 4:43–47, 1973.

32. Bauman J, Girling E, Brand PW: Plantar pressures and trophic ulceration. An evaluation of footwear. J Bone Joint Surg 45-B:652–673, 1963.

33. Bauman JH, Brand PW: Measurement of pressure between foot and shoe. Lancet 1:629–632, 1963.

34. Baumhauer JF, Wervey R, McWilliams J, et al: A comparison study of plantar foot pressure in a standardized shoe, total contact cast, and prefabricated pneumatic walking brace. Foot Ankle Int 18:26–33, 1997.

35. Betts RP, Franks CI, Duckworth T: Foot pressure studies: Normal and pathologic gait analyses. *In* Jahss MH (ed): Disorders of the Foot and Ankle, 2nd ed, vol 1. Philadelphia: WB Saunders Company, 1991, pp 434–519.

36. Birke JA, Cornwall MA, Jackson M: Relationship between hallux limitus and ulceration of the great toe. J Orthop Sports Phys Ther 10:172–176, 1988.

37. Birke JA, Franks BD, Foto JG: First ray joint limitations, pressure, and ulceration of the first metatarsal head in diabetes mellitus. Foot Ankle Int 16:277–284, 1995.

38. Birke JA, Novick A, Graham SL, et al: Methods of treating plantar ulcers. Phys Ther 71:116–122, 1991.

39. Birke JA, Novick A, Hawkins ES, Patout CJ: A review of causes of foot ulceration in patients with diabetes mellitus. J Prosthet Orthot 3:13–22, 1991.

40. Birke JA, Sims DS: Plantar sensory threshold in the ulcerative foot. Lepr Rev 57:261–267, 1986.

41. Birke JA, Sims DS J, Buford WL: Walking casts: Effect on plantar foot pressures. J Rehabil Res Dev 22:18–22, 1985.

42. Bloom S, Till S, Sonksen P, Smith S: Use of a biothesiometer to measure individual vibration perception thresholds and their variation in 519 non-diabetic subjects. Br Med J 288:1793–1795, 1984.

43. Boninger ML, Leonard JA J: Use of bivalved ankle-foot orthosis in neuropathic foot and ankle lesions. J Rehabil Res Dev 33:16–22, 1996.

44. Borssen B, Lithner F: Plaster casts in the management of advanced ischaemic and neuropathic diabetic foot lesions. Diabet Med 6:720–723, 1989.

45. Boulton AJM: The pathogenesis of diabetic foot problems: An overview. Diabet Med 13(Suppl 1):S12–S16, 1996.

46. Boulton AJM, Betts RP, Franks CI, et al: Abnormalities of foot pressure in early diabetic neuropathy. Diabet Med 4:225–228, 1987.

47. Boulton AJM, Betts RP, Franks CI, et al: The natural history of foot pressure abnormalities in neuropathic diabetic subjects. Diabetes Res 5:73–77, 1987.

48. Boulton AJM, Hardisty CA, Betts RP, et al. Dynamic foot pressure and other studies as diagnostic and management aids in diabetic neuropathy. Diabetes Care 6:26–33, 1983.

49. Brand PW: Insensitive Feet. A Practical Handbook on Foot Problems in Leprosy. London: Leprosy Mission, 1981.

50. Brand PW: The diabetic foot. In Davidson JK (ed): Clinical Diabetes Mellitus: A Problem Oriented Approach. New York: Thieme Medical Publishers, 1986, pp 376–382.

51. Brand PW: Repetitive stress in the development of diabetic foot ulcers. In Levin ME, O'Neal LW (eds): The Diabetic Foot, 4th ed. St. Louis: CV Mosby, 1988, pp 83–90.

52. Brand PW, Coleman WC: The diabetic foot. In Rifkin H, Porte DJ (eds): Ellenberg and Rifkin's Diabetes Mellitus: Theory and Practice, 4th ed. New York: Elsevier Science, 1990, pp. 792–811.

53. Brand PW, Ebner JD: Pressure sensitive devices for denervated hands and feet. J Bone Joint Surg 51–A:109–116, 1969.

54. Brodsky JW, Kourosh S, Stills M, Mooney V: Objective evaluation of insert material for diabetic and athletic footwear. Foot Ankle 9:111–116, 1938.

55. Brown GL, Curtsinger LJ, White M, et al: Acceleration of tensile strength of incisions treated with EGF and TGF-B. Ann Surg 208:788–794, 1988.

56. Brownlee M: Lilly Lecture. Glycation and diabetic complications. Diabetes Care 43:836–841, 1994.

57. Burden AC, Jones GR, Jones R, Blandford RL: Use of the "Scotchcast boot" in treating diabetic foot ulcers. Br Med J 286:1555–1557, 1983.

58. Burnett O: Total contact cast. In Harkless LB, Dennis KJ (eds): Clinics in Podiatric Medicine and Surgery: The Diabetic Foot, vol 4.2. Philadelphia: WB Saunders Company, 1987, pp 471–479.

59. Bus S, Cavanagh PR: Redistribution of plantar load with molded insoles (in preparation).

60. Calhoun JH, Cantrell J, Cobos J, et al: Treatment of diabetic foot infections: Wagner classification, therapy, and outcome. Foot Ankle 9:101–106, 1988.

61. Campbell GJ, McLure M, Newell EN: Compressive behavior after simulated service conditions of some foamed materials intended as orthotic shoe insoles. J Rehabil Res Dev 21:57–65, 1984.

62. Caputo GM, Ulbrecht JS, Cavanagh PR: The total contact cast: A method for treating neuropathic diabetic ulcers. Am Fam Physician 55:605–611, 1997.

63. Caravaggi C, Faglia E, Sacchi G, et al: Effectiveness and tolerability of fiberglass total contact cast in the treatment of neuropathic foot ulcer. Diabetes 47(Suppl 1):A169, 1998.

64. Cavanagh PR, Derr JA, Ulbrecht JS, et al: Problems with gait and posture in neuropathic patients with insulin-dependent diabetes mellitus. Diabet Med 9:469–474, 1992.

65. Cavanagh PR, Derr JA, Ulbrecht JS, Orchard TJ: Problems during gait and posture in patients with insulin dependent diabetes mellitus [abstract]. Presented to the Fall Meeting (September 6–7) of The British Diabetic Association, Newcastle Upon Tyne, 1990.

66. Cavanagh PR, Fernando DJS, Masson EA, et al: Limited joint mobility (LJM) and loss of vibration sensation are predictors of elevated plantar pressure in diabetes [abstract 2119]. Diabetes 40(Suppl 1):531A, 1991.

67. Cavanagh PR, Hewitt FG J, Perry JE: In-shoe plantar pressure measurement: A review. Foot 2:185–194, 1992.

68. Cavanagh PR, Morag E, Boulton AJM, et al: The relationship of static foot structure to dynamic foot function. J Biomech 30:243–250, 1997.

69. Cavanagh PR, Perry JE, Ulbrecht JS, et al: Neuropathic diabetic patients do not have reduced variability of plantar loading during gait. Gait Posture 7:191–199, 1998.

70. Cavanagh PR, Simoneau GG, Ulbrecht JS: Ulceration, unsteadiness, and uncertainty: The biomechanical consequences of diabetes mellitus. J Biomech 26(Suppl 1):23–40, 1993.

71. Cavanagh PR, Sims DS, Sanders LJ: Body mass is a poor predictor of peak plantar pressure in diabetic men. Diabetes Care 14:750–755, 1991.

72. Cavanagh PR, Ulbrecht JS: Biomechanics of the diabetic foot: A quantitative approach to the assessment of neuropathy, deformity, and plantar pressure. In Jahss MH (ed). Disorders of the Foot and Ankle, 2nd ed. Philadelphia: WB Saunders Company, 1991, pp 1864–1907.

73. Cavanagh PR, Ulbrecht JS. Plantar pressure in the diabetic foot. In Sammarco GJ (ed): The Diabetic Foot. Philadelphia: Lea & Febiger, 1991, pp 54–70.

74. Cavanagh PR, Ulbrecht JS: Clinical plantar pressure measurement in diabetes: Rationale and methodology. Foot 4:123–135, 1994.

75. Cavanagh PR, Ulbrecht JS, Caputo GM: The nonhealing diabetic foot wound: Fact or fiction? Ostomy/Wound Management 44(Suppl 3A):S6–S13, 1998.

76. Cavanagh PR, Ulbrecht JS, Caputo GM. Elevated plantar pressure and ulceration in diabetic patients after pan-metatarsal head resection: Two case reports. Foot Ankle Int 20:521–526, 1999.

77. Cavanagh PR, Ulbrecht JS, Caputo GM. What the practicing physician should know about foot biomechanics. In Boulton AJM, Connor H, Cavanagh PR (eds): The Foot in Diabetes, 3rd ed. Chichester, UK: John Wiley & Sons, 2000.

78. Cavanagh PR, Ulbrecht JS, Zanine W, et al: A method for the investigation of the effects of outsole modifications in therapeutic footwear. Foot Ankle Int 17:706–708, 1996.

79. Cavanagh PR, Young MJ, Adams JE, et al: Bony abnormalities in the feet of neuropathic diabetic patients [abstract 5]. In The Diabetic Foot. Proceedings of the First International Symposium and Workshop, May 3–4, Noordwijkerhout, The Netherlands, 1991.

80. Cavanagh PR, Young MJ, Adams JE, et al: Radiographic abnormalities in the feet of patients with diabetic neuropathy. Diabetes Care 17:201–209, 1994.

81. Chang AH, Abu-Faraj ZU, Harris GF, et al: Multistep measurement of plantar pressure alterations using metatarsal pads. Foot Ankle Int 15:654–660, 1994.

82. Chantelau E, Breuer U, Leisch AC, et al: Outpatient treatment of unilateral diabetic foot ulcers with "half shoes." Diabet Med 10:267–270, 1993.

83. Chantelau E, Haage P: An audit of cushioned diabetic footwear: Relation to patient compliance. Diabet Med 11:114–116, 1994.

84. Chantelau E, Kushner T, Spraul M: How effective is cushioned therapeutic footwear in protecting diabetic feet? A clinical study. Diabet Med 7:355–359, 1990.

85. Chantelau E, Schroer O, Tanudjaja T: Between-toe pressure in patients with limited joint mobility (LJM): The effect of footwear [abstract 1003]. Diabetologia 39(Suppl 1):A264, 1996.

86. Christ P, Gender M, Seitz P: A 3-D pressure distribution measuring platform with 8 × 8 sensors for simultaneous measurement of vertical and horizontal forces. Proceedings of the VI EMED Scientific Meeting, 1998.

87. Cogley D, Laing P, Crerand S, Klenerman L: Foot-cast interface vertical force measurements in casts used for healing neuropathic ulcers [abstract 58]. In The Diabetic Foot. Proceedings of the First International Symposium and Workshop, May 3–4, Noordwijkerhout, The Netherlands, 1991.

88. Coleman WC: The relief of forefoot pressures using outer shoe sole modifications. In Patil KM, Srinivasa H (eds): Proceedings of the International Conference on Biomechanics and Clinical Kinesiology of Hand and Foot. Madras, India: Indian Institute of Technology, 1985, pp 29–31.

89. Coleman WC, Brand PW, Birke JA: The total contact cast: A therapy for plantar ulceration on insensitive feet. J Am Podiatr Assoc 74:548–552, 1984.

90. Connelley LKJ: Verifying successful off-loading of neuropathic pressure ulcers [letter]. J. Am Podiatr Med Assoc 89:147–149, 1999.

91. Conti SF: In-shoe plantar pressure measurement and diabetic inlays: A series of questions and a few answers. Biomechanics 3:47–8, 74–5, 1996.

92. Conti SF, Martin RL, Chaytor ER, et al: Plantar pressure measurements during ambulation in weightbearing conventional short leg casts and total contact casts. Foot Ankle Int 17:464–469, 1996.

93. Courtemanche R, Teasdale N, Boucher P, et al: Gait problems in diabetic neuropathic patients. Arch Phys Med Rehabil 77:849–855, 1996.

94. Ctercteko GC, Dhanendran M, Hutton WC, Le Quesne LP: Vertical forces acting on the feet of diabetic patients with neuropathic ulceration. Br J Surg 68:608–614, 1981.

95. Cundy TF, Edmonds ME, Watkins PJ: Osteopenia and metatarsal fractures in diabetic neuropathy. Diabet Med 2:461–464, 1985.

96. Curran F, Nikookam K, Garrett M, et al: Physiotherapy: A novel intervention in diabetic pre-ulceration. Proceedings of the 2nd International Symposium on the Diabetic Foot, 1995.

97. Davis BL: Foot ulceration: Hypotheses concerning shear and vertical forces acting on adjacent regions of skin. Med Hypotheses 40:44–47, 1993.

98. Davis BL, Cothren RM, Quesada P, et al: Frequency content of normal and diabetic plantar pressure profiles: Implications for the selection of transducer sizes. J Biomech 29:979–983, 1996.

99. Davis BL, Perry JE: Development of a device to measure plantar pressure and shear [abstract]. In Hakkinen K, Keskinen KL, Komi PV, Mero A (eds): Book of Abstracts, 15th Congress of the ISB. Jyvaskyla, Finland, 1995.

100. de Block C, van Acker K, de Leeuw I: Chronic diabetic foot ulcers: What is in a name? [abstract 0651]. Diabetes 47(Suppl 1):A168, 1993.

101. Delbridge L, Ctercteko G, Fowler C, et al: The aetiology of diabetic neuropathic ulceration of the foot. Br J Surg 72:1–6, 1985.

102. Delbridge L, Ellis CS, Robertson K: Nonenzymatic glycosylation of keratin from the stratum corneum of the diabetic foot. Br J Dermatol 112:547–554, 1985.

103. Dingwell JB: Variability and nonlinear dynamics of continuous locomotion. Applications to treadmill walking and diabetic peripheral neuropathy. Doctoral Dissertation. University Park, PA: The Pennsylvania State University, 1998.

104. Duckworth T, Boulton AJM, Betts RP, et al: Plantar pressure measurements and the prevention of ulceration in the diabetic foot. J Bone Joint Surg 67-B:79–85, 1985.

105. Early KJS, Hansen ST: Surgical reconstruction of the diabetic foot: A salvage approach for midfoot collapse. Foot Ankle Int 17:325–330, 1996.

106. Edington CJ: The effect of metatarsal pads on the plantar pressure distribution of the foot. Master's Thesis. University Park, PA: The Pennsylvania State University, 1990.

107. Edmonds ME, Blundell MP, Morris ME, et al: Improved survival of the diabetic foot: The role of a specialised foot clinic. Q J Med 60:763–771, 1986.

108. Fernando DJS, Masson EA, Veves A, Boulton AJM: Relationship of limited joint mobility to abnormal foot pressures and diabetic foot ulceration. Diabetes Care 14:8–11, 1991.

109. Fisher A: Neuropathic plantar ulcers: Relief of weight bearing using an orthopaedic knee scooter [abstract 59]. In The Diabetic Foot. Proceedings of the First International Symposium and Workshop, May 3–4, Noordwijkerhout, The Netherlands, 1991.

110. Fleischli JE, Anderson RB, Davis WH: Dorsiflexion metatarsal osteotomy for treatment of recalcitrant diabetic neuropathic ulcers. Foot Ankle Int 20:80–85, 1999.

111. Fleischli JG, Lavery LA, Vela SA, et al: Comparison of strategies for reducing pressure at the site of neuropathic ulcers. J Am Podiatr Med Assoc 87:466–472, 1997.

112. Foster A, Eaton C, Gibby D, Edmonds ME: The posterior splinted cast: A new treatment for long-standing neuropathic ulcers [abstract]. Diabet Med 7(Suppl 1):35A, 1990.

113. Foto JG, Birke JA: Who's using what? An orthotic materials survey. Biomechanics 3:63–68, 1996.

114. Foto JG, Birke JA: Evaluation of multidensity orthotic materials used in footwear for patients with diabetes. Foot Ankle Int 19:836–841, 1998.

115. Fromherz WA: Examination, physical therapy of the foot and ankle. In Hunt GC (ed): Clinics in Physical Therapy, vol 15. New York: Churchill Livingstone, 1988.

116. Frykberg RG: Biomechanical considerations of the diabetic foot. Lower Extremity 2:207–214, 1995.

117. Frykberg RG: Offloading properties of a new rocker insole [abstract 0650]. Diabetes 47(Suppl 1):A168, 1998.

118. Frykberg RG, Lavery LA, Pham H, et al: Role of neuropathy and high foot pressures in diabetic foot ulceration. Diabetes Care 21:1714–1719, 1998.

119. Garbalosa JC, Cavanagh PR, Wu G, et al: Foot function in diabetic patients after partial amputation. Foot Ankle Int 17:43–48, 1996.

120. Geoffroy J, Hoeffel JC, Pointel JP, et al: The feet in diabetes. Roentgenologic observations in 1501 cases. Diagn Imag 48:286–293, 1979.

121. Giurini JM, Basile P, Chrzan JS, et al: Panmetatarsal head resection. A viable alternative to the transmetatarsal amputation. J Am Podiatr Med Assoc 83:101–107, 1993.

122. Gooding GAW, Stess RM, Graf PM: Sonography of the sole of the foot: Evidence for loss of foot pad thickness in diabetes and its relationship to ulceration of the foot. Invest Radiol 21:45–48, 1986.

123. Gooding GAW, Stess RM, Graf PM, Grunfeld C: Heel pad thickness: Determination by high-resolution ultrasonography. J Ultrasound Med 4:173–174, 1985.

124. Grant WP, Sullivan R, Sonenshine DE, et al: Treatment of Charcot neuroarthropathy with Achilles tendon lengthening [abstract 1772]. Diabetes 48(Suppl 1):A401, 1999.

125. Guse ST, Alvine FG: Treatment of diabetic foot ulcers and Charcot neuroarthropathy using the patellar tendon-bearing brace. Foot Ankle Int 18:675–677, 1997.

126. Guzman B, Fisher G, Palladino SJ, Stavosky JW: Pressure-removing strategies in neuropathic ulcer therapy. An alternative to total contact casting. Clin Podiatr Med Surg 11:339–253, 1994.

127. Habershaw G, Donovan JC: Biomechanical considerations of the diabetic foot. In Kozak GP, Hoar CS, Rowbotham JL (eds): Management of Diabetic Foot Problems. Philadelphia: WB Saunders Company, 1984, pp 32–44.

128. Hamel AJ, Sharkey NA: Proper force transmission through the toes and forefoot is dependent on the plantar fascia. Proceedings of the American Society of Biomechanics, 1999.

129. Heath H III, Melton LJ III, Chu C-P: Diabetes mellitus and risk of skeletal fracture. N Engl J Med 303:567–570, 1980.

130. Hewitt FG Jr: The effect of molded insoles on in-shoe plantar pressures in rockered footwear. Master's Thesis. University Park, PA: The Pennsylvania State University, 1993.

131. Hissink RJ, Manning HA, van Baal JG: The mabal shoe, an alternative method in contact casting for the treatment of neuropathic diabetic foot ulcers. Foot Ankle Int 21:320–323, 2000.

132. Holm-Pederson P, Viidik A: Tensile properties of and morphology of healing wounds in young and old rats. Scand J Plast Reconstr Surg 6:24–35, 1972.

133. Holmes GB, Timmerman L: A quantitative assessment of the effect of metatarsal pads on plantar pressures. Foot Ankle 11:141–145, 1990.

134. Hsi WL, Ulbrecht J, Caputo G, et al: Normal healing rates for diabetic neuropathic foot ulcers [abstract 0639]. Diabetes 47(Suppl 1):A165, 1998.

135. Hsi WL, Ulbrecht JS, Perry JE, et al: Plantar pressure threshold for ulceration risk using the EMED SF platform [abstract 324]. Diabetes 42(Suppl 1):103A, 1993.

136. Huband MS, Carr JB: A simplified method of total contact casting for diabetic foot ulcers. Contemp Orthop 26:143–147, 1993.

137. Janisse DJ: Prescription insoles and footwear. Clin Podiatr Med Surg 12:41–61, 1995.

138. Jenkin WM, Palladino SJ: Environmental stress and tissue breakdown. In Frykberg RG (ed): The High Risk Foot in Diabetes Mellitus. New York: Churchill Livingstone, 1991, pp 103–123.

139. Jones GR: Walking casts: Effective treatment for foot ulcers? Practical Diabetes 8:131–132, 1991.

140. Jones R, Beshyah SA, Curryer GJ, Burden AC: Modification of the "Leicester (Scotch Cast) boot." Practical Diabetes 6:118–119, 1994.

141. Jordan C: The relationship between plantar and dorsal pressure distribution and perception of comfort in casual footwear. Gait Posture 2:251, 1994.

142. Kastenbauer T, Sokol G, Auinger M, Irsigler K: Running shoes for relief of plantar pressure in diabetic patients. Diabet Med 15:518–522, 1998.

143. Kastenbauer T, Sokol G, Stary S, Irsigler K: Motor neuropathy does not increase plantar pressure in NIDDM patients [abstract]. Program of the 5th EMED User Meeting, 1996.

144. Katoulis EC, Ebdon-Parry M, Lanshammar H, et al: Gait abnormalities in diabetic neuropathy. Diabetes Care 20:1904–1907, 1997.

145. Kawchuk GN, Elliott PD: Validation of displacement measurements obtained from ultrasonic images during indentation testing. Ultrasound Med Biol 24:105–111, 1998.

146. Kernozek TW, LaMott EE, Dancisak MJ: Reliability of an in-shoe pressure measurement system during treadmill walking. Foot Ankle Int 17:204–209, 1996.

147. Kiewied J: Felt therapy for leprosy patients with an ulcer in a pressure area [letter]. Lepr Rev 68:378–381, 1997.

148. Knowles A: The role of pressure relief in diabetic foot problems. Diabetic Foot 1:55–56, 58–60, 62–63, 1998.

149. Krag MH: Quantitative techniques for analysis of gait. Automedica 6:85–97, 1985.

150. Laing P, Cogley D, Crerand S, Klenerman L: The Liverpool shear transducer [abstract]. In The Diabetic Foot. Proceedings of the First International Symposium and Workshop, May 3–4, Noordwijkerhout, The Netherlands, 1991.

151. Landsman A, Sage R: High strain rate tissue deformation and its role in formation and treatment of foot ulcerations in patients with diabetes [abstract 255]. Diabetes 45(Suppl 2):71A, 1996.

152. Landsman A, Sage R: Off-loading neuropathic wounds associated with diabetes using an ankle-foot orthosis. J Am Podiatr Med Assoc 87:349–357, 1997.

153. Lavery LA, Armstrong DG, Walker SC: Healing rates of diabetic foot ulcers associated with midfoot fracture due to Charcot's arthropathy. Diabet Med 14:46–49, 1997.

154. Lavery LA, Fleishli JG, Laughlin TJ, et al: Is postural instability exacerbated by off-loading devices in high risk diabetics with foot ulcers? Ostomy/Wound Management 44:26–34, 1998.

155. Lavery LA, Lavery DC, Quebedeax-Farnham TL: Increased foot pressures after great toe amputation in diabetes. Diabetes Care 18:1460–1462, 1995.

156. Lavery LA, Vela SA, Fleischli JG, et al: Reducing plantar pressure in the neuropathic foot. A comparison of footwear. Diabetes Care 20:1706–1710, 1997.

157. Lavery LA, Vela SA, Lavery DC, Quebedeaux TL: Reducing dynamic foot pressures in high-risk diabetic subjects with foot ulcerations. Diabetes Care 19:818–821, 1996.

158. Leber C, Evanski PM: A comparison of shoe insole materials in plantar pressure relief. Prosthet Orthot Int 10:135–138, 1986.

159. Lemmon D, Shiang TY, Hashmi A, et al: The effect of insoles in therapeutic footwear: A finite element approach. J Biomech 30:615–620, 1997.

160. Lin SS, Lee TH, Wapner KL: Plantar forefoot ulceration with equinus deformity of the ankle in diabetic patients: The effect of tendo-Achilles lengthening and total contact casting. Orthopedics 19:465–475, 1996.

161. Lithner F, Hietala S-O: Skeletal lesions of the feet in diabetics and their relationship to cutaneous erythema with or without necrosis on the feet. Acta Med Scand 200:155–161, 1976.

162. Loppnow BW: The effect of plugs on reducing pressure under the second metatarsal head. Master's Thesis. University Park, PA: The Pennsylvania State University, 1998.

163. Lord M: Spatial resolution in plantar pressure measurement. Med Eng Phys 19:140–144, 1997.

164. Lord M, Hosein R: Pressure redistribution by molded inserts in diabetic footwear: A pilot study. J Rehabil Res Dev 31:214–221, 1994.

165. Lord M, Hosein R, Williams RB: Method for in-shoe shear stress measurement. J Biomed Eng 14:181–186, 1992.

166. Marks RM, Parks BG, Schon LC: Midfoot fusion technique for neuroarthropathic feet: Biomechanical analysis and rationale. Foot Ankle Int 19:507–510, 1998.

167. Martin RL, Conti SF: Plantar pressure analysis of diabetic rockerbottom deformity total contact casts. Foot Ankle Int 17:470–472, 1996.

168. Masson EA, Hay EM, Stockley I, et al: Abnormal foot pressure alone may not cause foot ulceration. Diabet Med 6:426–428, 1989.

169. Mayfield JA, Reiber GE, Sanders LJ, et al: Preventive foot care in people with diabetes [technical review]. Diabetes Care 21:2161–2177, 1998.

170. Mazzeo RS, Cavanagh PR, Evans WJ, et al: Exercise and physical activity for older adults [position stand]. Med Sci Sports Exerc 30:992–1008, 1998.

171. McBride ID, Wyss UP, Cooke TDV, et al: First metatarsophalangeal joint reaction forces during high-heel gait. Foot Ankle 11:282–288, 1991.

172. McGill M, Collins P, Bolton T, Yue DK: Management of neuropathic ulceration. J Wound Care 5:252–254, 1996.

173. McLoughlin C, Southern S, Lomax G, Jones GR: These shoes are made for walking [abstract 10]. In 6th Malvern Diabetic Foot Conference, 1996.

174. McPoil TG, Cornwall MW, Yamada W: A comparison of two in-shoe plantar pressure measurement systems. Lower Extremity 2:95–103, 1995.

175. Mehta JA, Brown C, Sargeant N: Charcot restraint orthotic walker. Foot Ankle Int 19:619–623, 1998.

176. Morag E, Cavanagh PR: Structural and functional predictors of regional peak pressures under the foot during walking (ISB Keynote Paper 1997). J Biomech 32:359–370, 1999.

177. Morgan JM, Biehl WC III, Wagner FW Jr: Management of neuropathic arthropathy with the Charcot restraint orthotic walker. Clin Orthop 296:58–63, 1993.

178. Mueller MJ: Therapeutic footwear helps protect the diabetic foot. J Am Podiat Med Assoc 87:360–364, 1997.

179. Mueller MJ, Allen BT, Sinacore DR: Incidence of skin breakdown and higher amputation after transmetatarsal amputation: Implications for rehabilitation. Arch Phys Med Rehabil 76:50–54, 1995.

180. Mueller MJ, Diamond JE, Sinacore DR, et al: Total contact casting in treatment of diabetic plantar ulcers: Controlled clinical trial. Diabetes Care 12:384–388, 1989.

181. Mueller MJ, Salsich GB, Bastian AJ: Differences in the gait characteristics of people with diabetes and transmetatarsal amputation compared with age-matched controls. Gait Posture 7:200–206, 1998.

182. Mueller MJ, Sinacore DR: Rehabilitation factors following transmetatarsal amputation. Phys Ther 74:1027–1033, 1998.

183. Mueller MJ, Smith KE, Commean PK, et al: Use of computed tomography and plantar pressure measurement for management of neuropathic ulcers in patients with diabetes. Phys Ther 79:296–307, 1999.

184. Mueller MJ, Strube MJ, Allen BT: Therapeutic footwear can reduce plantar pressures in patients with diabetes and transmetatarsal amputation. Diabetes Care 20:637–641, 1997.

185. Murray HJ, Young MJ, Hollis S, Boulton AJM: The association between callus formation, high pressures and neuropathy in diabetic foot ulceration. Diabet Med 13:979–982, 1996.

186. Myerly SM, Stavosky JW: An alternative method for reducing plantar pressures in neuropathic ulcers. Adv Wound Care 10:26–29, 1997.

187. Myerson M, Wilson K: Management of neuropathic ulceration with total contact cast. In Sammarco GJ (ed): The Foot in Diabetes. Philadelphia: Lea & Febiger, 1991, pp 145–152.

188. Myerson MS, Henderson MR, Saxby T, Short KW: Management of midfoot diabetic neuroarthropathy. Foot Ankle Int 15:233–241, 1994.

189. Myerson MS, Shereff MJ: The pathological anatomy of claw and hammer toes. J Bone Joint Surg 71–A:45–49, 1989.

190. Nargi SE, Colen LB, Liuzzi FJ, et al: PTB treatment restores joint mobility in a new model of diabetic cheiroarthropathy [abstract 0072]. Diabetes 48(Suppl 1):A17, 1999.

191. Nawoczenski DA, Birke JA, Coleman WC: Effect of rocker sole designs on plantar forefoot pressures. J Am Podiatr Med Assoc 78:455–460, 1988.

192. Needleman RL: Successes and pitfalls in the healing of neuropathic forefoot ulcerations with the IPOS postoperative shoe. Foot Ankle Int 18:412–417, 1997.

193. Patel VG, Weiman TJ: Effect of metatarsal head resection for diabetic foot ulcers on the dynamic plantar pressure distribution. Am J Surg 167:297–301, 1994.

194. Patil KM, Braak LH, Huson A: Analysis of stresses in two-dimensional models of normal and neuropathic feet. Med Biol Eng Comput 34:280–284, 1996.

195. Payne CB: Biomechanics of the foot in diabetes mellitus. Some theoretical considerations. J Am Podiatr Med Assoc 88:285–289, 1998.

196. Pecoraro RE, Reiber GE, Burgess EM: Pathways to diabetic limb amputation: Basis for prevention. Diabetes Care 13:513–521, 1990.

197. Perry JE, Cavanagh PR, Ulbrecht JS: The use of conventional footwear to relieve plantar pressures in the diabetic foot [abstract]. *In* Proceedings of the May 5–8, 1992 8th Annual East Coast Clinical Gait Laboratories Conference, Rochester, MN, 1993, pp 121–122.
198. Perry JE, Davis BL, Hall JO: Profiles of shear loading in the diabetic foot [abstract]. *In* Hakkinen K, Keskinen KL, Komi PV, Mero A (eds): Book of Abstracts, 15th Congress of the ISB, Jyvaskyla, Finland, 1995, pp 722–723.
199. Perry JE, Ulbrecht JS, Derr JA, Cavanagh PR: The use of running shoes to reduce plantar pressures in patients who have diabetes. J Bone Joint Surg 77-A:1819–1828, 1995.
200. Pham H, Lavery LA, Harvey C, Rosenblum BI, et al: Risk factors of foot ulceration in a large diabetic population: Two year prospective follow-up [abstract 284]. Diabetologia 41(Suppl 1):A73, 1998.
201. Pitei DL, Watkins PJ, Foster AVM, Edmonds ME: Do new EVA moulded insoles or trainers efficiently reduce the high foot pressures in the diabetic foot? [abstract 87]. Diabetes 45(Suppl 2):25A, 1996.
202. Pollard JP, Le Quesne LP, Tappin JW: Forces under the foot. J Biomed Eng 5:37–40, 1983.
203. Quebedeaux TL, Lavery LA, Lavery DC: The development of foot deformities and ulcers after great toe amputation in diabetes. Diabetes Care 19:165–167, 1996.
204. Radin EL, Yang KH, Riegger C, et al: Relationship between lower limb dynamics and knee joint pain. J Orthop Res 9:398–405, 1991.
205. Richardson JK, Hurvitz EA: Peripheral neuropathy: A true risk factor for falls. J Gerontol Med Sci 50A:M211–M215, 1995.
206. Ritz G, Kushner D, Friedman S: A successful technique for the treatment of diabetic neurotrophic ulcers. J Am Podiatr Med Assoc 82:479–481, 1992.
207. Roberts P, Carnes S: The orthopaedic scooter. An energy-saving aid for assisted ambulation. J Bone Joint Surg 72-B:620–621, 1990.
208. Rose GK: Pes planus. *In* Jahss MH (ed): Disorders of the Foot Ankle, Medical and Surgical Management, 2nd ed. Philadelphia: WB Saunders Company, 1991.
209. Rose SA, DeLuca PA, Davis RB III, et al: Kinematic and kinetic evaluation of the ankle after lengthening of the gastrocnemius fascia in children with cerebral palsy. J Pediatr Orthop 13:727–732, 1993.
210. Rosenbaum D, Hautmann S, Gold M, Claes L: Effects of walking speed on plantar pressure patterns and hindfoot angular motion. Gait Posture 2:191–197, 1994.
211. Rosenbloom AL, Silverstein JH, Lezotte DC, et al: Limited joint mobility in childhood diabetes mellitus indicates increased risk for microvascular disease. N Engl J Med 305:191–194, 1981.
212. Rothstein JM, Miller PJ, Roettger RF: Goniometric reliability in a clinical setting: Elbow and knee measurements. Phys Ther 63:1611, 1983.
213. Rothwell JC, Traub MM, Day BL, et al: Manual motor performance in a deafferented man. Brain 105:515–542, 1982.
214. Rozema A, Ulbrecht JS, Pammer SE, Cavanagh PR: In-shoe plantar pressures during activities of daily living: Implications for therapeutic footwear design. Foot Ankle Int 17:325–359, 1996.
215. Sabato S, Yosipovitch Z, Simkin A, Sheskin J: Plantar trophic ulcers in patients with leprosy: A correlative study of sensation, pressure and mobility. Int Orthop 6:203–208, 1982.
216. Sage RA: Diabetic ulcers: Evaluation and management. *In* Harkless LB, Dennis KJ (eds): Clinics in Podiatric Medicine and Surgery: The Diabetic Foot, vol 4.2. Philadelphia: WB Saunders Company, 1987, pp 383–393.
217. Saltzman CL, Johnson KA, Goldstein RH, Donnelly RE: The patellar tendon-bearing brace as treatment for neurotrophic arthropathy: A dynamic force monitoring study. Foot Ankle 13:14–21, 1992.
218. Sammarco GJ, Conti SF: Surgical treatment of neuroarthropathic foot deformity. Foot Ankle Int 19:102–109, 1998.
219. Sanders JE, Greve JM, Mitchell SB, Zachariah SG: Material properties of commonly-used interface materials and their static coefficients of friction with skin and socks. J Rehabil Res Dev 35:161–176, 1998.
220. Sarnow MR, Veves A, Giurini JM, et al: In-shoe foot pressure measurements in diabetic patients with at-risk feet and in healthy subjects. Diabetes Care 17:1002–1006, 1994.
221. Saucerman J: Finite element analysis of plantar pressure distribution in the forefoot. Undergraduate Honors Thesis. Penn State University (in preparation).
222. Schaff P, Wetter O, Haslbeck M: Changes in foot loading and pressure patterns during standing of patients with diabetic neuropathy. *In* Hotta N, Greene DA, Ward JD, et al (eds): Diabetic Neuropathy: New Concepts and Insights. New York; Elsevier Science BV, 1995, pp 279–284.
223. Schaff PS, Cavanagh PR: Shoes for the insensitive foot: The effect of a "rocker bottom" shoe modification on plantar pressure distribution. Foot Ankle 11:129–140, 1990.
224. Sharkey NA: Skeletal Tissue Mechanics. New York: Springer-Verlag, 1998.
225. Shaw JE, Boulton AJM: Pressure time integrals may be more important than peak pressures in diabetic foot ulceration [abstract A21]. Diabet Med 13(Suppl 7):S22, 1996.
226. Shaw JE, Hsi WL, Ulbrecht JS, et al: The mechanism of plantar unloading in total contact casts: Implications for design and clinical use. Foot Ankle Int 18:809–817, 1997.
227. Shaw JE, van Schie CHM, Carrington AL, et al: An analysis of dynamic forces transmitted through the foot in diabetic neuropathy. Diabetes Care 21:1955–1959, 1998.
228. Silvino N, Evanski PM, Waugh TR: The Harris and Beath footprinting mat: Diagnostic validity and clinical use. Clin Orthop 151:265–269, 1980.
229. Simon SR, Berme N, Sawyer F: Measurement of plantar foot soft tissue properties of patients with diabetic neuropathy for prediction of plantar foot pressures and assessment of plantar ulceration risk. Rehabil Res Dev Progr Rep 34:318–319, 1996.
230. Simoneau GG, Ulbrecht JS, Derr JA, et al: Postural instability in patients with diabetic sensory neuropathy. Diabetes Care 17:1411–1421, 1994.
231. Sims DS, Birke JA: Effect of rocker sole placement on plantar pressures [abstract]. *In* Proceedings of the 20th Annual Meeting of the USPHS Professional Association. Atlanta, GA: 1985, p 53.
232. Sinacore DR: Total contact casting for diabetic neuropathic ulcers. Phys Ther 76:296–301, 1996.

233. Sinacore DR: Healing times of diabetic ulcers in the presence of fixed deformities of the foot using total contact casting. Foot Ankle Int 19:613–618, 1998.

234. Sinacore DR, Mueller MJ: Total-contact casting in the treatment of neuropathic ulcers. In Levin ME, O'Neal LW, Bowker JH (eds): The Diabetic Foot, 5th ed. St. Louis: Mosby Year Book, 1993, pp 283–304.

235. Smieja M, Hunt DL, Edelman D, et al: Clinical examination for the detection of protective sensation in the feet of diabetic patients. J Gen Intern Med 14:418–424, 1999.

236. Smith L, Plehwe W, McGill M, et al: Foot bearing pressure in patients with unilateral diabetic foot ulcers. Diabet Med 6:573–575, 1989.

237. Sobel E, Glockenberg A: Calcaneal gait: Etiology and clinical presentation. J Am Podiatr Med Assoc 89:39–49, 1999.

238. Song J, Hillstrom HJ, Secord D, Levitt J: Foot type biomechanics. Comparison of planus and rectus foot types. J Am Podiatr Med Assoc 86:16–23, 1996.

239. Sosenko JM, Kato M, Soto R, Bild DE: Comparison of quantitative sensory-threshold measures for their association with foot ulceration in diabetic patients. Diabetes Care 13:1057–1061, 1990.

240. Soulier SM: The use of running shoes in the prevention of plantar diabetic ulcers. J Am Podiatr Med Assoc 76:395–400, 1986.

241. Stacpoole-Shea SJ, Walden JG, Gitter A, et al: Could seamed socks impart unduly high pressure to the diabetic foot? [abstract 0776]. Diabetes 48(Suppl 1):A179, 1999.

242. Stehr M, Dietz HG, Morlock MM: Clinical application of pressure distribution measurements during full gait [abstract]. Program of the 2nd EMED User Meeting, 1991.

243. Stess RM, Jensen SR, Mirmiran R: The role of dynamic plantar pressures in diabetic foot ulcers. Diabetes Care 20:855–858, 1997.

244. Stokes IAF, Faris IB, Hutton WC: The neuropathic ulcer and loads on the foot in diabetic patients. Acta Orthop Scand 46:839–847, 1975.

245. Tappin JW, Pollard J, Beckett EA: Method of measuring "shearing" forces on the sole of the foot. Clin Phys Physiol Measurements 1:83–85, 1980.

246. Taylor R, Stainsby GD, Richardson DL: Rupture of the plantar fascia in the diabetic foot leads to toe dorsiflexion deformity [abstract 1071]. Diabetologia 41(Suppl 1):A277, 1998.

247. Thompson DE: The effects of mechanical stress on soft tissue. In Levin ME, O'Neal LW (eds): The Diabetic Foot, 4th ed. St. Louis: Mosby-Year Book, 1988.

248. Thompson DL, Cao D, Davis BL: Effects of diabetic-induced soft tissue changes on stress distribution in the calcaneal soft tissue. Proceedings of XVII International Society of Biomechanics Congress, 1999, p 12.

249. Tooke JE, Brash PD: Microvascular aspects of diabetic foot disease. Review. Diabet Med 13(Suppl 1):S26–S29, 1996.

250. Uccioli L, Faglia E, Monticone G, et al: Manufactured shoes in the prevention of diabetic foot ulcers. Diabetes Care 18:1376–1377, 1995.

251. Uccioli L, Giacomini P, Monticone G, et al: Body sway in diabetic neuropathy. Diabetes Care 18:339–344, 1995.

252. van Schie CHM, Abbott CA, Vileikyte L, et al: Gait analysis in diabetic unilateral lower limb amputees [abstract 1886]. Diabetologia 40(Suppl 1):A–480, 1997.

253. van Schie CHM, Abbott CA, Vileikyte L, et al: A comparative study of the Podotrack, a simple semi-quantitative plantar pressure measuring device, and the optical pedobarograph in the assessment of pressures under the diabetic foot. Diabet Med 16:154–159, 1999.

254. van Schie CHM, Becker MB, Ulbrecht JS, et al: Optimal axis location in rocker bottom shoes [abstract]. Presented to The Diabetic Foot: Second International Symposium, May 1995, Amsterdam 1995.

255. van Schie CHM, Vileikyte L, Abbott CA, et al: Comparing a new simple plantar pressure measuring device with pedobarographically measured pressures [abstract 1005]. Diabetologia 39(Suppl 1):A264, 1996.

256. van Schie CHM, Whalley A, Vileikyte L, et al: The efficacy of injected liquid silicone in the reduction of foot pressures and callus formation in the diabetic foot [abstract 1074]. Diabetologia 41(Suppl 1):A278, 1998.

257. Vela SA, Lavery LA, Armstrong DG, Anaim AA: The effect of increased weight on peak pressures: Implications for obesity and diabetic foot pathology. J Foot Ankle Surg 37:416–420, 1998.

258. Veves A, Fernando DJS, Walewski P, Boulton AJM: A study of plantar pressures in a diabetic clinic population. Foot 2:89–92, 1991.

259. Veves A, Hay EM, Boulton AJM: The use of specially padded hosiery in the painful rheumatoid foot. Foot 1:1–3, 1991.

260. Veves A, Masson EA, Fernando DJ, Boulton AJM: Studies of experimental hosiery in diabetic neuropathic patients with high foot pressures. Diabet Med 7:324–736, 1990.

261. Veves A, Masson EA, Fernando DJS, Boulton AJM: Sustained pressure relief under the diabetic foot with experimental hosiery, and comparison of different padding densities [abstract]. Diabet Med 6(Suppl 2):3A, 1989.

262. Veves A, Masson EA, Fernando DJS, Boulton AJM: Use of experimental padded hosiery to reduce abnormal foot pressures in diabetic neuropathy. Diabetes Care 12:653–655, 1989.

263. Veves A, Murray H, Young MJ, Boulton AJM: Do high foot pressures lead to foot ulcerations? A prospective study [abstract]. Diabetologia 34(Suppl 2):A40, 1991.

264. Veves A, Murray HJ, Young MJ, Boulton AJM: The risk of foot ulceration in diabetic patients with high foot pressure: A prospective study. Diabetologia 35:660–663, 1992.

265. Veves A, Sarnow MR, Giurini JM, et al: Differences in joint mobility and foot pressures between black and white diabetic patients. Diabet Med 12:585–599, 1995.

266. Vijay V, Seena R, Lalitha S, et al: A simple device for foot pressure measurement. Evaluation in South Indian NIDDM subjects [letter]. Diabetes Care 21:1205–1206, 1998.

267. Warren G, Nade S: The Care of Neuropathic Limbs. Pearl River, NY: Parthenon, 1999.

268. Webster: Webster's Collegiate Dictionary, 9th ed. Springfield, MA: Merriam-Webster, 1986.

269. Wolfe L, Stess RM, Graf PM: Dynamic pressure analysis of the diabetic Charcot foot. J Am Podiatr Med Assoc 81:281–287, 1991.

270. Xia B, Garbalosa JC, Cavanagh PR: Error analysis of two systems to measure in-shoe pressures [abstract]. *In* Proceedings of the American Society of Biomechanics, 1994, pp 219–220.

271. Young MJ, Cavanagh PR, Thomas G, et al: Callus and elevated dynamic plantar pressures—does chiropody help? [abstract]. Diabet Med 8(Suppl 1):45A, 1991.

272. Young MJ, Cavanagh PR, Thomas G, et al: The effect of callus removal on dynamic plantar foot pressures in diabetic patients. Diabet Med 9:55–57, 1992.

273. Young MJ, Coffey J, Taylor PM, Boulton AJM: Weight bearing ultrasound in diabetic and rheumatoid arthritis patients. Foot 5:76–79, 1995.

274. Young MJ, Murray HJ, Veves A, Boulton AJM: A comparison of the Musgrave and optical pedobarograph systems for measuring foot pressures in diabetic patients. Foot 3:62–64, 1993.

275. Zilberberg J: Fluorescence and pentosidine content of diabetic foot skin. Master's Thesis. University Park, PA: The Pennsylvania State University, 1998.

7

CUTANEOUS ASPECTS OF DIABETES MELLITUS

■ J. E. Jelinek

Diabetes mellitus affects every organ system of the body. Thus it is not surprising that the skin, the largest organ, participates with numerous manifestations related to this disease.

Although there is uncertainty about the pathogenesis of many of the skin conditions affecting diabetic patients, in no small part because of our imperfect understanding of the metabolic abnormalities of diabetes itself, many cutaneous signs are easily recognizable so as to make them diabetic markers and a few (diabetic bullae, limited joint mobility and waxy skin, and diabetes dermopathy), when strict clinical criteria are observed, are virtually diagnostic of diabetes.

Some cutaneous conditions appear to be caused by the primary abnormalities of diabetes or by its major complications, vasculopathy and neuropathy. Others are linked to altered immunologic causes and to changes in collagen, and some are a consequence of treatment. Several dermatoses, not generally thought to be linked to abnormal glucose metabolism, appear with greater than expected frequency in diabetics. The numerous skin problems of the diabetic have recently been addressed in a text specifically devoted to that subject.[60]

Dermatologic disorders generally appear after diabetes has developed, but they may signal or appear coincidentally with its onset or even precede the disease by many years. Interestingly, many cutaneous signs and complications often occur on the lower parts of the legs and on the feet. It is the purpose of this chapter to review the major dermatologic manifestations of diabetes with particular emphasis to that region of the body.

Cutaneous Signs Associated with Vascular Changes in Diabetes

Atherosclerosis

Atherosclerosis occurs both frequently and earlier in diabetics. On the skin of the legs the condition is associated with atrophy, coldness of the toes, loss of hair, and dystrophy of the nails.[55] A waxy pallor of the feet when the legs are raised, with a delayed return of color and in the filling of the superficial veins, is a reliable sign of occlusive arterial disease.

Periungual Telangiectasia

Periungual telangiectasia, seen often in connective tissue diseases, has been found more frequently in diabetics.[68] Although more apparent at the proximal nail folds of finger-nails, they may be found affecting the toes as well. Detection of early morphologic changes in nail fold capillaries has also been reported in diabetic children.[131] The vascular dilatations appear to be not only a diabetic marker but also an indicator of functional microangiopathy and a measure of long-term control of glucose metabolism.[52]

One study claims that morphologic differ-ences differentiate the dilated vessels in these areas caused by diabetes from those caused by connective tissue diseases.[39] A re-cent report found nail fold capillary abnor-malities in 17 of 43 non–insulin-dependent patients, but these correlated only with ne-phropathic findings.[93]

The value of this sign is challenged by Trapp et al.,[129] who found no statistical differ-ence in capillaries of the nail folds of insulin-dependent diabetics and limited joint mobil-ity, and by Trevisan et al.,[130] who found no connection between single modification of capillary loops and the levels of glucose in sera and urine in diabetic children or com-plex changes in nail fold capillaries in well-controlled patients.

Erythema of the Feet

Lithner and Hietala[80] describe a cutaneous sign of vascular insufficiency in diabetics. This erythema without necrosis appears to be a sign of incipient gangrene in the diabetic foot. The well-demarcated redness correlates with underlying bone destruction, which can be confirmed by x-ray film. The erythema can involve the lower leg, as well as the foot. It is differentiated from erysipelas by the normal temperature of the patient and by the ab-sence of a polymorphonuclear leukocytosis. Small vessel involvement appears to be im-portant, although cardiac decompensation is the most common precipitating factor. The same author[76] noted the frequent nonpalpa-ble purpura evident in both erythematous and nonerythematous areas on the legs of elderly diabetics.

Diabetic Markers in Skin

Necrobiosis Lipoidica Diabeticorum

Necrobiosis lipoidica diabeticorum (NLD) was first described in 1929 by Oppenheim[95]

and received its current name from Urbach[132] 3 years later. The disease, which is quite dis-tinct clinically and unusual but diagnostic histologically, has, however, no clearly ex-plainable pathogenesis, and its very name poses difficulties. The word "necrobiosis" lit-erally means a state of life and death, better discussed in a religious or philosophic trea-tise than a medical textbook. "Lipoidica" re-fers to deposits of extracellular fat that is neither a primary histologic event nor even a constant finding. Finally, "diabeticorum" could strictly be left out of the title in as many as one third of newly diagnosed cases.

The name, nevertheless, is here to stay, and NLD remains the best-known cutaneous marker of diabetes. This is despite its rela-tive rarity, even in diabetics, where it is reported to occur in between 0.3% and 1.2%.[88, 118] It is much less common in nondia-betics. At the time of diagnosis, two thirds of patients will have overt diabetes. Of the rest, all but 10% will either develop diabetes within 5 years, have abnormal glucose toler-ance (some shown by cortisone challenge), or a history of the disease in at least one par-ent.[88] Although diabetes is usually the first of the two to be diagnosed, in as many as one third, necrobiosis lipoidica diabeticorum precedes diabetes, sometimes by several years.[2] Where the two conditions coexist, the diabetes is often more severe. There is a mean delay of 10 years of necrobiosis lipoi-dica diabeticorum developing in those having diabetes first.[118]

Necrobiosis lipoidica diabeticorum is four times more common in women; the sexual preferment is even more obvious in patients who are nondiabetic.[46] The condition may ap-pear at any age from infancy to septuagenari-ans but generally favors young adults. It is curiously selective of whites, although a few cases have been mentioned in the Japa-nese literature.[116]

The characteristic lesion of necrobiosis li-poidica diabeticorum is a slowly enlarging, irregularly contoured plaque. The border is often slightly elevated and has a reddish blue periphery. The central portion, at first ery-thematous, becomes yellow or sclerotic and resembles glazed porcelain (Fig. 7–1). The plaque often atrophies further and may soften and become entirely brown. In the later stages of development, visible telangi-ectasias on the surface are common (Plate 6). Lesions vary in size from a few millimeters to several centimeters. Although initially sin-

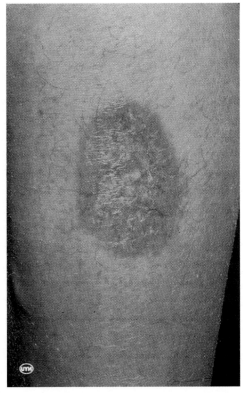

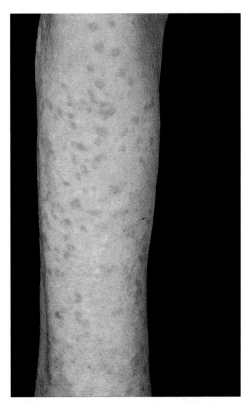

Plate 6 ■ Necrobiosis lipoidica diabeticorum. Plaque on leg, with a yellow, atrophic, and telangiectatic center and an elevated red border. (From Jelinek JE (ed): The Skin in Diabetes. Philadelphia: Lea & Febiger, 1986, with permission.)

Plate 7 ■ Granuloma annulare. Multiple papules of the disseminated form. (From Jelinek JE (ed): The Skin in Diabetes. Philadelphia: Lea & Febiger, 1986, with permission.)

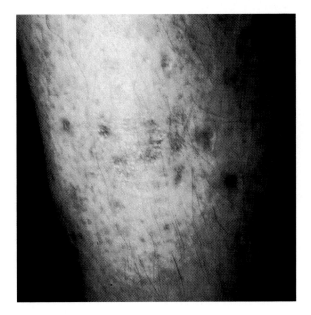

Plate 8 ■ Diabetic dermopathy. Multiple brown, atrophic lesions on the anterior and lower portions of the legs. (From Jelinek JE (ed): The Skin in Diabetes. Philadelphia: Lea & Febiger, 1986, with permission.)

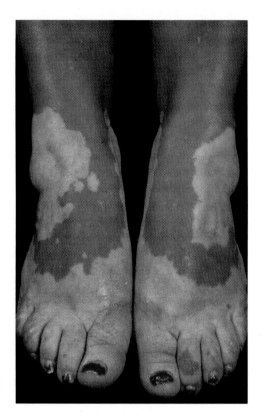

Plate 9 ■ Vitiligo. Loss of pigment on the lower legs and feet. (From Jelinek JE (ed): The Skin in Diabetes. Philadelphia: Lea & Febiger, 1986, with permission.)

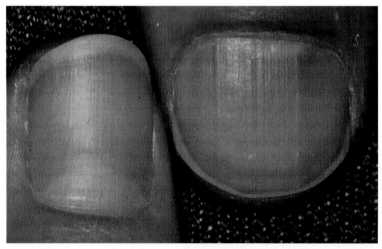

Plate 10 ■ Yellow nail. Discoloration of the nails often is independent of dermatophytosis or vascular disease. (Courtesy of Arthur C. Huntley, M.D.)

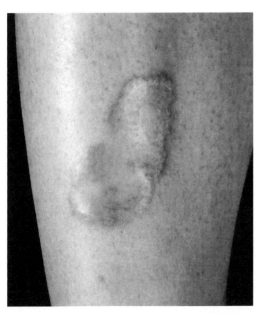

Figure 7–1 ■ Necrobiosis lipoidica diabeticorum. Plaque with an atrophic center and an active and geographic border. (From Jelinek JE [ed]: The Skin in Diabetes. Philadelphia: Lea & Febiger, 1986, with permission.)

Among proposed causative factors are microangiopathy,[65] obliterative endarteritis,[47] immune-mediated vasculitis,[103] other immune factors,[16] delayed hypersensitivity,[121] nonenzymatic glycosylation and other defects in collagen,[10] trauma,[71] platelet aggregation,[127] defective mobility of neutrophils,[35] and vascular insufficiency.[12] It is uncertain whether any of these are primary or secondary, what relationship they bear to one another, and whether any are central, significant, or even relevant to the etiologic explanation of the disease.[58]

Necrobiosis lipoidica diabeticorum can usually be diagnosed by a dermatologist on clinical appearance alone. If the diagnosis is not certain, a biopsy should reveal characteristic changes. These are degeneration of collagen throughout the dermis, particularly in the lower two thirds, histocytes in a palisaded arrangement around the degenerated collagen, and obliterative granulomatous vasculitis. It should be stressed, however, that it is preferable to avoid, whenever possible, surgical procedures on the lower legs of

gle lesions herald the condition, most patients develop multiple plaques, usually more than four.[88] Eighty-five percent are in pretibial and medial malleolar locations (Fig. 7–2), generally bilateral but not in perfect symmetry. Lesions of necrobiosis lipoidica may, however, appear elsewhere on the body, including the thighs, feet, arms, face and scalp, and even the penis, but in diabetics they almost always involve the classic area of the lower legs in addition to those less usual areas. Lesions may have decreased or absent sensation to pinprick and fine touch.[81] One third of lesions ulcerate, sometimes spontaneously, sometimes as a result of trauma (Fig. 7–3).[71] This may be because of local destruction of cutaneous nerves by inflammation.[10] Other findings are partial alopecia and significant hypohidrosis, within the lesions, a finding that may serve as a differential point of diagnosis in cases of granuloma annulare.[45] The sensory and sweating deficits may well be secondary to destruction of the nerves and sweat glands by the disease rather than pathogenic.

Even though ulceration is fairly common and often longstanding, squamous cell carcinoma as a complication is, happily, very rare. Only six such cases have been reported up to 1991, one half of these in diabetics.[102]

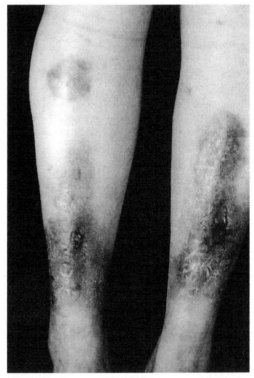

Figure 7–2 ■ Necrobiosis lipoidica diabeticorum. Multiple bilateral plaques on the pretibial region. (From Jelinek JE [ed]: The Skin in Diabetes. Philadelphia: Lea & Febiger, 1986, with permission.)

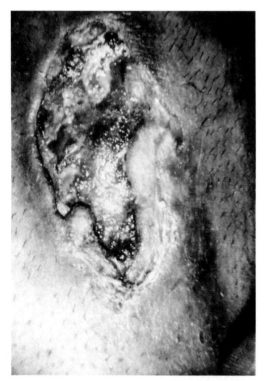

Figure 7–3 ■ Necrobiosis lipoidica diabeticorum. Ulceration, which indicates need for active treatment. (From Jelinek JE [ed]: The Skin in Diabetes. Philadelphia: Lea & Febiger, 1986, with permission.)

these patients, particularly those who are diabetic.

The variety of suggested treatment for necrobiosis lipoidica diabeticorum betrays the efficacy of a single one. Where there is no ulceration and, as is most common, little in the way of subjective symptoms, the approach should be conservative. Protection from injury is important and patients should avoid crowds, wear shin pads if likely to be traumatized, and, if getting out of bed at night, put on the light to avoid collision with furniture. Topical corticosteroids, sometimes under occlusive dressings, may be helpful. Intralesional triamcinolone acetonide for both ulcerated and nonulcerated lesions has its advocates,[122] but this treatment is best reserved for the borders or just beyond the borders of either ulcerated, or symptomatic, or advancing lesions. The demonstration of inflammation extending beyond the clinical borders would suggest this therapy may be useful in these areas in these circumstances.[10]

Aspirin and dipyridamole modify aggregation of platelets and have been used, either alone or in combination, with reported success,[23, 48, 104] but others have found this treatment disappointing.[5] The efficacy of this treatment in preventing new lesions or stemming progression of old ones is still unproved. Pentoxifylline, which decreases the viscosity of blood by increasing fibrinolysis, in addition to inhibiting aggregation of platelets, has been reported as useful in the healing of ulcers.[92]

Several patients have recently been successfully treated with short-term oral steroids. This approach appears to work better in the early, nonulcerated phase.[100] It would seem a reasonable approach in nondiabetic subjects. In those patients who are diabetic, where this approach is elected, a close watch, together with an endocrinologist to monitor glucose levels, would be mandatory.

Active treatment is always called for when ulceration occurs. In addition to the previously mentioned approaches, attention should be given to the prevention and treatment of secondary infection by compresses and local and systemic antibiotics.[56] Topical administration of benzoyl peroxide has been found useful.[43] The new hydrocolloid occlusive dressings may prove helpful in treating noninfected ulcers. When conservative treatment fails, radical excision of the muscularis fascia, ligation of perforating vessels, and split-thickness grafting is a therapeutic option.[30]

Granuloma Annulare

Granuloma annulare has several forms that are identical on histology. The classic and commonest type manifests as one or more localized annular or arciform lesions with flesh-colored papular borders and flat centers. These are seen most often on the dorsal and lateral aspects of the hands and feet of children and young adults (Fig. 7–4). Granuloma annulare is a benign, usually asymptomatic, and generally self-limiting dermatosis.

Less common varieties include generalized, multiple, perforating, and subcutaneous forms. The generalized form may consist of multiple classic lesions or a type in which numerous, disseminated, flesh-colored papules are symmetrically distributed on the arms, neck, and upper half of the trunk and less often on the legs (Plate 7). The cause of granuloma annulare is not known. Treat-

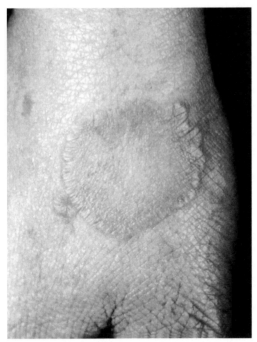

Figure 7-4 ■ Granuloma annulare. Flesh-colored plaque with papular border. (From Jelinek JE [ed]: The Skin in Diabetes. Philadelphia: Lea & Febiger, 1986, with permission.)

ment is similar to the nonulcerated forms of necrobiosis lipoidica diabeticorum and meets with about equal success.

All forms of granuloma annulare share common histologic features, namely, focal degeneration of collagen in the upper and middermis, with histiocytic palisaded arrangement around collagen bundles, and abundant mucin.[72] These features, although distinguishable from necrobiosis lipoidica diabeticorum, bear enough resemblance to that disease to invite the question of the relationship of granuloma annulare to diabetes mellitus. (Rheumatoid nodules and necrobiosis lipoidica diabeticorum also show histologic similarities, yet no association of diabetes and rheumatoid arthritis exists.) Although there is considerable similarity under the microscope, the two conditions of granuloma annulare and necrobiosis lipoidica diabeticorum have only been reported to occur together in the same patient seven times.[1, 22]

Approximately 120 patients have indeed been reported to have coexistent diabetes and granuloma annulare in reported series of some 1,100 patients.[58, 87] In most of these, no distinction was made as to the type of diabetes. Despite a natural bias in such re-ports and the usually transient course of granuloma annulare, there appears to be a greater than expected incidence of abnormal carbohydrate metabolism in these patients, particularly in the disseminated and perforating forms.[59, 120] Evidence for a link of diabetes and granuloma annulare in the localized and generalized forms is much less firm, but it is appropriate to obtain glucose measurements on all patients with the dermatosis and to be particularly watchful for diabetes in adults with disseminated or generalized forms of the condition.

Diabetic Dermopathy

In 1964, Melin[83] noted that his chief, Nils Tornblom, pointed out characteristic, atrophic, circumscribed brown patches on the front and sides of the lower portions of the legs in diabetic subjects. It is probable that Kramer[66] described the same condition 30 years earlier. Binkley[9] coined the name "diabetic dermopathy" for the condition, and it is this term that is now generally used.[9] Others have written of this condition as "the spotted leg syndrome,"[89] shin spots,[24] and pigmented pretibial patches.[4] Despite the name "dermopathy," there is little evidence of angiopathy or a kinship to other diabetic angiopathies. It appears that microangiopathy, when present, reflects the underlying diabetes rather than the cutaneous problem itself.

The lesions are at first small, dull red, scaly papules and small plaques. They eventuate to the characteristic, multiple, bilateral, circumscribed, round or oval, shallow pigmented scars on the pretibial areas (Plate 8). Diabetic dermopathy is the commonest cutaneous sign of diabetes. Its relatively late recognition is explained by the absence of symptoms. The condition has been seen in nondiabetics,[24] but the majority of patients are adult diabetics. The incidence correlates with the duration and severity of diabetes and with the three major microvascular complications,[119] although it may precede that condition.[3] A recent report indicates that most patients with diabetic dermopathy have an increase in glycosylated hemoglobin levels and a long history of diabetes.[125] It is twice as common in men.

The predilection for the pretibial area invites speculation on the relationship of diabetic dermopathy to necrobiosis lipoidica diabeticorum; the matter is easily settled under the microscope. Necrobiosis lipoidica diabeticorum has diagnostic histologic features, whereas diabetic dermopathy is nonspecific. The second question, the role of trauma, is less easily answered. Although the history of repeated physical insults is usually not forthcoming, and attempts to produce the lesions by repeatedly striking the areas of the leg with a rubber hammer failed,[83] experimental thermal injuries[75] and reports linking the dermatosis to peripheral neuropathy[89] suggest that trauma may be a modifying factor.

Other pigmented lesions of the legs are differentiated from diabetic dermopathy by their localization, associated peripheral vascular disease, and the presence of purpura. Diabetic dermopathy, being asymptomatic, requires no treatment except for protection from trauma.

Diabetic Bullae

Although not common, the sudden appearance of one or more tense blisters, generally on the acral portions of the body, is a clinically distinct diabetic marker. Referred to in 1930 by Kramer,[66] the recognition of it as a separate entity was made by Rocca and Pereyra in 1963.[106] The name "bullosis diabeticorum" was coined in 1967.[15] Fewer than 100 cases have been reported up to 1991.[96]

The characteristic history is spontaneous blisters appearing suddenly, most commonly on the dorsa or sides of the hands and feet (Fig. 7–5), forearms, and lower legs. The bul-

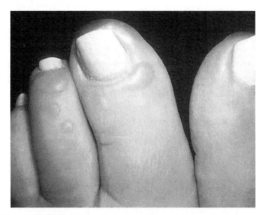

Figure 7–5 ■ Diabetic bullae. Spontaneous lesions appeared on the hands as well as the feet. (From Jelinek JE [ed]: The Skin in Diabetes. Philadelphia: Lea & Febiger, 1986, with permission.)

lae range from 0.5 to several cm, are often bilateral, and contain generally clear fluid, which is invariably sterile. There is no surrounding erythema. The lesions are usually asymptomatic and heal by themselves in a few weeks, usually without scarring. They may recur.

The patients are always adults, more often men, and their diabetes is often, though not invariably, severe and longstanding. The abnormalities of carbohydrate metabolism are not proportionate to the clinical manifestation. Outside of preventing secondary infection, no treatment is necessary.

Diabetic bullae are usually intraepidermal (explaining the lack of scarring), though a subepidermal location has also been reported. Heterogeneity of histologic appearance may be explained by different pathogenesis or by obtaining biopsy specimens at different stages of development. Although insulin-dependent diabetics appear to have a reduced threshold to blister formation,[8] the appearance at the same time of the bullae at widely separated sites argues against trauma as a pathogenic factor.

Diabetic bullae resemble those seen in patients in coma from overdosing on barbiturates or from poisoning with carbon monoxide, but the clinical picture is easily differentiated.

Limited Joint Mobility and Waxy Skin Syndrome

A new clinical syndrome, originally described in insulin-dependent adolescent diabetics in 1974 by Rosenbloom and Frias,[111] consists of two major components: limitation of mobility, primarily of the small joints of the hands, and thickening and stiffness of the skin, most marked on the dorsa of the fingers. Apart from functional limitations of mobility, the condition is asymptomatic, and the lack of pain probably explains why it has only recently been delineated in spite of being evidently common. It appears to be the earliest clinically detectable complication of childhood and adolescent diabetics.[110]

The stiffness usually begins in the metacarpophalangeal and proximal interphalangeal joints, generally of the fifth digit, and then progresses to involve one or more other adjoining fingers.[108] It is bilateral, symmetric, and painless. The limitations of movement initially in active, and later even in

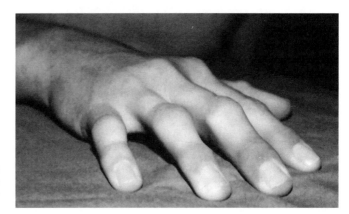

Figure 7–6 ■ Limited joint mobility. The patient could not flatten the hand on a table top. (From Hempstead RW: J Assoc Mil Dermatol 9[2]:30, 1983, with permission.)

passive, extension may less frequently involve larger joints of the wrist, elbow, and even the spine.[40] Flexion limitation occurs much later, if at all.

Recently, the syndrome of limited joint mobility has become recognized as an important contributor to abnormal mechanics in the diabetic foot. Campbell et al.[13] first mentioned limitation of motion of the ankle, and subsequently Deldridge et al.[26] confirmed the presence of the entity in diabetics and commented on its relation to neuropathic ulceration. Similar findings were reported by Mueller et al.[86] Fernando et al.[31] pointed out the relationship of limitation of joint mobility to abnormal pressures in the feet in patients with diabetic neuropathy. In their group two thirds of the patients developed foot ulcers. Patients who had limited joint mobility without neuropathy also had abnormal foot pressures but did not develop ulcers.

Limited joint mobility of the hand can be demonstrated by the inability to flatten the affected hand on a table top (Fig. 7–6) and by failure to approximate the two palms with the fingers fanned and the wrists maximally flexed (the prayer sign). The most accurate sign, however, is limitation of extension with the examiner passively testing the interphalangeal and metacarpophalangeal joints (Fig. 7–7).[110] Skin thickening is assessed by palpation and can also be demonstrated by ultrasound-A scanning.[20]

Although in early reports the condition appeared to be found only in juvenile insulin-dependent diabetics, it is now apparent that it can also affect adult non–insulin-dependent diabetic patients.[32, 69, 114] Although clearly related to and much commoner in diabetics, both components of the syndrome have been described in nondiabetic controls.[69, 97] More than 4,500 diabetic patients have been assessed for this condition from 1974 to 1985. The incidence of the syndrome has ranged from 8% to 50%, with variation probably explainable by the age of the popu-

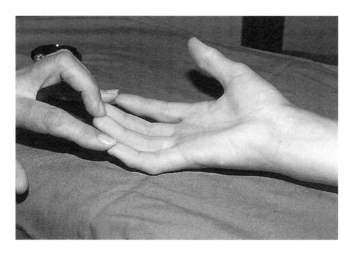

Figure 7–7 ■ Limited joint mobility. Resistance to passive extension. (From Hempstead RW: J Assoc Mil Dermatol 9[2]:30, 1983, with permission.)

lation studied, duration of diabetes, and different examination techniques.[110]

Although contractures of the joints seem related to duration of hyperglycemia, particularly in those with insulin dependence,[124] it is probable that if a patient will develop this complication he or she will do so by the end of the first decade of disease.[17] There is less agreement as to the relationship of the syndrome to diabetic control. No such association was found in several studies,[113, 123] but a strong inverse correlation was reported in another.[14] The importance of strict control is certainly implied in a report of diminished thickness of the skin following careful control of levels of glucose by using an insulin infusion pump.[73] Recently, Lyons et al.[80] also showed decrease in skin collagen glycation with improved glycemic control in insulin-dependent diabetes. Maintaining this control could potentially, therefore, limit subsequent long-term damage.

The abnormal waxiness and thickening of the skin appears in about one third of patients with limited joint mobility, more predictably in the more severe cases,[112] although at times evident without joint involvement.[117] Clinically the taut, shiny skin bears similarity to scleroderma, but that condition is excluded by the absence of Raynaud's phenomenon, ulceration, tapering and calcinosis of the fingers, and the lack of visceral involvement. Histologic appearance of waxy skin is marked by thickening of the dermal collagen and especially by a paucity of elastic fibers.[29]

The pathogenesis of the thickened skin and limitation of mobility of the joints seem interrelated. Despite the name, the joints themselves are not directly involved. The fault apparently is in the collagen of the periarticular tissues. The abnormal collagen of both components may be a reflection of nonenzymatic glycosylation of protein, an accompaniment of persistent hyperglycemia, although tissue glycosylation is not greater in diabetics with the syndrome than in those without it.[79] Because the condition occurs primarily in young patients, it appears not to be vascular in origin.[109]

The suggestion has been made that the syndrome is a harbinger of retinopathy with a threefold to fourfold increased chance of developing this complication in later years,[13, 63, 112, 124] especially in poorly controlled and younger patients.

In older patients, especially those with non–insulin-dependent diabetes, the association of limited joint mobility and microvascular disease is less marked.[69] Others, however, have questioned the syndrome as an indicator of future problems in all patients.[134]

Scleredema Diabeticorum

Scleredema is a rare disorder of diffuse, symmetric induration, and thickening of the skin favoring the posterior side of the neck and upper half of the back. It has two forms. The classic type is known as "scleredema adultorum of Buschke," which, despite its name, more commonly affects children, is usually heralded by an acute infection (frequently streptococcal), followed a few weeks later by a progressive induration of the posterolateral portion of the neck, upper half of the back, and shoulders. The diagnosis is clinically evident by palpation, which demonstrates a hardened, nonpitted skin, often shiny, and with absent superficial markings, that can be neither wrinkled nor pressed together into folds. On rare occasions, the cutaneous involvement is much more widespread, and internal organs may be affected. The condition is painless, and symptoms, if any, are caused by limitation of movement. This type generally resolves spontaneously in about 18 months.

Histologically, the enlarged collagen bundles are separated by an accumulation of hyaluronic acid and glycosaminoglycans.[115]

Scleredema is also seen in diabetics and, although sharing certain characteristics with the "adultorum" type, has distinct differences. Like the classic type, the disease initially affects the upper half of the back and the neck but subsequently tends to involve a much greater part of the body, especially the trunk and sometimes the arms and legs.[107]

Demarcation from the normal skin may be obvious or imperceptible. Not infrequently there is diminished response to pain and light touch in affected areas.[19] There usually is no prodromal infection.

Some 140 patients with scleredema diabeticorum have now been described in the world's literature,[57, 128] about one half as many as of the classic type. The diabetic patients are normally middle-aged men, almost invariably obese, and although their diabetic state varies from mild to severe, most are in need of insulin and many have associated microvascular complications.[19] The cutaneous problem is not only generally more widespread than in the classic type but also has little tendency to resolution. The histology is identical in both types, and both also share a lack of effective treatment.

Although regarded as a rare disease, in a prospective study of 484 diabetics, scleredema had an incidence of 2.5%.[19] Collier et al.[21] found that patients who had diabetes for more than 10 years had thicker skin on their arms than either patients with a shorter duration of diabetes or nondiabetic controls. This thickening was found in another recent study and differentiated by both conventional and electron microscopic appearance from scleroderma.[44] Huntley and Walter[53] have shown thickness of the skin in diabetics not only of the hands but also of the feet. They considered this thickness independent of the syndromes of limited joint mobility and scleredema and found no correlation with retinopathy. The thickening that diabetics have on their extremities may be unapparent clinically but is measurable. In this study it was demonstrated with ultrasonography.[53]

Recently, encouraging therapeutic responses in scleredema have been reported, both in the nondiabetic type with cyclosporine[82] and in the nondiabetic form using high doses of penicillin[67] and in both types following bath psoralen plus ultraviolet A (PUVA) treatments.[41]

Dermatoses Reported to be More Frequent in Diabetics

Perforating Dermatoses

There are several acquired cutaneous disorders having as a common histologic denominator the transepidermal elimination of degenerative material, chiefly collagen and elastic fibers. Although these dermatoses have been reported independently of associated internal problems, many are in patients with chronic renal failure, particularly those on either hemodialysis or peritoneal dialysis, where the incidence has been as high as 11%, and the majority have been diabetic.[85]

Attempts to separate the perforating dermatoses, chief of which are Kyrle's disease, perforating folliculitis, and reactive perforating collagenosis, have been made on both clinical and histologic grounds. Their similarities, however, outweigh their differences,

and the term "acquired perforating dermatoses" seems appropriate.[105]

Clinically, patients have multiple umbilicated keratotic papules, sometimes with a tendency to linear formation (Fig. 7–8). They favor the extensor surface of the trunk and extremities. They are often very itchy, with little tendency to spontaneous resolution. Most patients are middle aged, and often black. Slightly more males than females are affected.

Improvement has been achieved with topical retinoic acid[7] and with protection from scratching, combined with diabetic control,[18] and ultraviolet therapy.[133]

Often, unfortunately, treatment is not too effective. The phenomenon of transepidermal elimination is probably multifactorial. Changes in epidermal keratinization, immunologic and inflammatory factors, alteration of the underlying glycosylation, and contributions from lysosomal enzymes released from leukocytes all have been suggested as being responsible.[27, 99, 136]

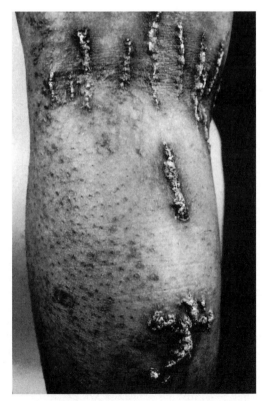

Figure 7–8 ■ Perforating disease, Kyrle's disease. Keratotic lesions showing the isomorphic (Koebner's) phenomenon. (From Jelinek JE [ed]: The Skin in Diabetes. Philadelphia: Lea & Febiger, 1986, with permission.)

Vitiligo

Vitiligo is a disease in which diminished or absent function of melanocytes results in macular depigmentation, most often seen periorificially and on the extensor aspects of the extremities (Plate 9). It is asymptomatic but emotionally stressful, particularly in people with darker skin. It is regarded as an autoimmune disorder. The higher than expected incidence of vitiligo in diabetics seems further evidence for an immunologic basis. Vitiligo, however, has been reported in maturity-onset diabetics,[25] as well as in insulin-dependent ones,[38] making it more difficult to advance autoimmune and genetic factors as the only explanation for their coexistence. The frequency of diabetes in patients with vitiligo, however, seems no higher than would be expected.[59]

A recent report from Japan[64] claims that vitiligo can be divided into types that are confined to a dermatome and others that are generalized and usually progressive. The latter form seems to be associated with conditions that have an allergic or immune basis.

Lichen Planus

Lichen planus, a disease of unknown cause, has a distinctive morphologic and histologic appearance. Clinically, it is characterized by itchy, flat-topped, violaceous papules, most often on the flexor aspects of the forearms and wrists, lower portions of the legs, and the lower back. Mucous membranes, including the mouth and genitalia, are involved in two thirds of cases. In the buccal mucosa, lichen planus forms a white lacework pattern that can become erosive.

An increased incidence of diabetes and abnormalities of insulin response to glucose challenge have been claimed in patients with lichen planus.[91] This is particularly true of adults and more so in those with the erosive oral form.[78]

Whether there is a relationship of diabetes to lichen planus, a usually transient condition, remains speculative. In one report, an increase of A28-HLA antigen among nondiabetic patients with lichen planus but not those with diabetes suggests that there may be two forms of this disease.[42] This concept of two types of lichen planus, one of an immunologic, the other of a metabolic defect linked to diabetes, is supported by the studies of Lisi and Giommoni.[74]

Carotenoderma, Yellow Skin, and Yellow Nails

Carotenes are lipid-soluble pigments. All green vegetables, some fruits, and dairy products contain carotene, but the red and yellow vegetables have the richest content. Carotene contributes a yellow component to normal skin, and in excessive amounts imparts a deep yellow-orange tint, especially on the palms, soles, and the nasolabial folds, where there is either thicker keratin or an abundance of sebaceous or sweat glands. Carotenemia does not alter the color of the sclerae or that of urine. The normal value of carotene is 1 mg/mL in the serum, and levels have to be about 25 times that amount to give clinical evidence of carotenoderma.[70] Carotenoderma, which is asymptomatic, may appear in response to a variety of mechanisms, including excessive intake of foods rich in carotenes, defective conversion of carotene to vitamin A, and in hyperlipidemic conditions.[84] The most common cause is dietary. In preinsulin days, this probably accounted for the reported high incidence of this phenomenon in diabetics. Although diabetics frequently have a yellowish color,[51] there appears in most cases to be no correlation to elevations of carotene levels in the serum.[49] A possible explanation of the yellow color may lie in the consequences of nonenzymatic glycosylation and storage temperatures of the stratum corneum.[126] One of the advanced glycosylatious products that has been identified, 2-(2-furoyl)-4(5)-(2-furanyl)-1H-imadozole, has a distinctly yellow hue.[101]

As many as 50% of diabetics have been reported to have yellow nails, best seen on the distal hallux (Plate 10). One study of fingernails showed diabetics have high levels of fructose-lysine, another marker of nonenzymatic glycosylation.[94] Yellow nails are seen in association with onychomycosis and psoriasis and in the elderly but seem to be a common diabetic marker unassociated with these causes. The early sign is a yellow or brown color of the distal part of the hallux nail plate. Later a canary yellow color can affect nails on both toe and fingernails.

Eruptive Xanthomas

Eruptive xanthomas may appear when serum triglycerides rise to high levels. The majority of patients with this condition are diabetics in poor control. The eruption is of multiple, firm pink-yellow papules and nodules appearing in crops (Fig. 7–9). There is often an erythematous halo surrounding individual papules. The favored sites are the extensor aspects of the extremities and trunk. The oral mucosa may be involved on occasion. The condition is pruritic. With the correction of the hyperlipidemia and control of diabetes, the lesions involute.

The mechanism of the formation of xanthomas is not known. There is some evidence that eruptive xanthomas in diabetes result from macrophages incorporating circulating plasma lipoproteins, forming foamy or xanthoma cells.[98]

Kaposi's Sarcoma

Multiple idiopathic hemorrhagic sarcoma, first described by Kaposi in 1872,[62] is a neoplasm that usually begins on the lower parts of the legs, most often in elderly Jewish and Italian men. The lesions, usually multiple, are purple macules, nodules, or plaques. Later, other areas of the skin, mucous membranes, and internal organs may be involved. Edema of the legs is frequent and may even be a prodrome. The classic form of the disease is uncommon, generally indolent, and usually not aggressive. Histologic examination shows an accumulation of spindle cells forming vascular slits containing erythrocytes.

Diabetes mellitus has been reported with greater than expected frequency in Kaposi's sarcoma,[28, 33] but confirmation is still needed because others have not found a statistically significant association.[11] In a recent study from Sweden that found a 27% incidence of diabetes in 63 patients with Kaposi's sarcoma, the authors[6] related the pathogenesis to cardiac failure with edema in the elderly as the more important factor.

Glucagonoma

Tumors of the α-cell, glucagon-secreting portion of the pancreas have a cutaneous component that may precede other evidence of its existence, sometimes by several years. The distinct skin eruption is necrolytic migratory erythema and is characterized by eczematous patches in annular and gyrate forms that eventuate in plaques, erosions, and crusts. Although preferring the lower abdomen, buttocks, and periorificial areas, the dermatosis may be found not infrequently on the lower portions of the legs (Fig. 7–10). The condition fluctuates but is chronic and persistent. The histology resembles that found in pustular psoriasis with features of intracellular edema in the upper epidermis, acanthosis, subcorneal pustules, and dyskeratosis.[50]

Systemic accompaniments include weight loss, weakness, diarrhea, and, frequently, diabetes. Glossitis and paronychial candidiasis are frequent.

Diagnosis is confirmed by elevated plasma glucagon levels. Hypoaminoacidemia is often an associated finding. Several medications have been reported to ameliorate the cutaneous part of the syndrome, but in the majority of patients the cause is a pancreatic neoplasm, and its surgical removal is the definitive treatment.

Werner's Syndrome

Werner's syndrome is a rare autosomal recessive disease remarkable for premature and accelerated aging. Approximately half of the patients have nonketotic, relatively insulin-resistant, mild diabetes. The skin becomes taut and thin, with loss of subcutane-

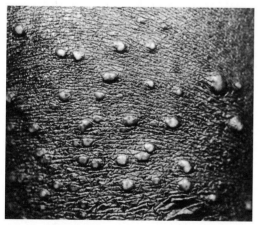

Figure 7–9 ■ Eruptive xanthoma. The condition resolves when metabolic control is established. (From Jelinek JE [ed]: The Skin in Diabetes. Philadelphia: Lea & Febiger, 1986, with permission.)

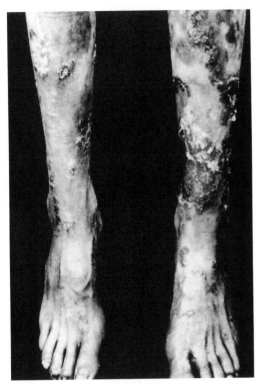

Figure 7-10 ▪ Glucagonoma. Necrolytic migratory erythema. Serpigenous erosions with crusts, vesicles, and pustules at the periphery. (From Shupack JL, Berczeller PH, Stevens DM: J Dermatol Surg Oncol 4:242–247, 1978, with permission.)

ous tissue and diminished sweat glands. This is most evident on the lower parts of the legs, where ulcers often supervene, and on the face, resulting in a bird-like appearance. Poikiloderma marked by both hypopigmentation and hyperpigmentation and telangiectasia, alopecia, hyperkeratoses, and skin cancers are common.[37, 135]

Patients with Werner's syndrome showed a reduction in the growth of skin fibroblasts when compared with subjects with diabetes and those with normal aging, and even more so in normal controls.[36]

Pruritus

It is a commonly held belief that generalized itching is a symptom of diabetes mellitus. This relationship is highly questionable. In recent studies[61, 90] there was no statistical basis for this belief. Localized anogenital pruritus (particularly pruritus vulva associated with moniliasis) is, however, more common in diabetics.[90]

Itching on the legs in elderly diabetics is not a feature of hyperglycemia but a manifestation of xerosis. Simple lubricants or low-potency corticosteroid creams usually suffice to control this symptom.

REFERENCES

1. Abraham Z, et al: Psoriasis, necrobiosis lipoidica, granuloma annulare, vitiligo and skin infection in the same diabetic patient. J Dermatol 17:440–447, 1990.
2. Abramova EA, Polyanskaya NP: Relationship between lipoid necrobiosis and diabetes mellitus. Vestn Dermatol Venerol 2:36–38, 1985.
3. Bauer M, Levan NE: Diabetic dermangiopathy: A spectrum including pretibial patches and necrobiosis lipoidica diabeticorum. Br J Dermatol 83:528–535, 1970.
4. Bauer ME, et al: Pigmented pretibial patches: A cutaneous manifestation of diabetes mellitus. Arch Dermatol 93:282–286, 1966.
5. Beck HI, Bjerring P: Skin blood flow in necrobiosis lipoidica during treatment with low-dose acetylsalicylic acid. Acta Derm Venereol (Stockh) 68:364–365, 1988.
6. Bendsoe N, et al: Increased incidence of Kaposi sarcoma in Sweden before the AIDS epidemic. Eur J Cancer 26:699–702, 1990.
7. Berger RS: Reactive perforating collagenosis of renal failure—diabetes responsive to topical retinoic acid. Cutis 43:540–542, 1989.
8. Bernstein JE, et al: Reduced threshold to suction-induced blister formation in insulin-dependent diabetics. J Am Acad Dermatol 8:790–791, 1983.
9. Binkley GW: Dermopathy in the diabetic syndrome. Am Dermatol 92:625–634, 1965.
10. Boulton AJM, et al: Necrobiosis lipoidica diabeticorum: A clinicopathologic study. J Am Acad Dermatol 18:530–537, 1988.
11. Brambilla L, et al: Sarcoma di Kaposi mediterraneo patologie associate in una casistica di 100 pazienti. G Ital Dermatol Venereol 123:477–480, 1988.
12. Brungger A: Transkutane Sauerstoff—und Kohlendioxiddruck-messung bei Necrobiosis Lipoidica. Hautarzt 40:231–232, 1989.
13. Campbell RR, et al: Limited joint mobility in diabetes mellitus. Ann Rheumatol Dis 44:93–97, 1985.
14. Canfield WK, Chase HP, Hambidge KM: Limited joint mobility (LJM) in insulin dependent diabetes mellitus (IDDM): Relationship to glucose control and zinc nutriture. Pediatr Res 16(Suppl):135A, 1982.
15. Cantwell AR, Martz W: Idiopathic bullae in diabetics: Bullosis diabeticorum. Arch Dermatol 96:42–44, 1967.
16. Chambers B, Milligan A, Fletcher A: Epidermal dendritic S100 positive cells in necrobiosis lipoidica and granuloma annulare. Br J Dermatol 123:765–768, 1990.
17. Chapple M, et al: Joint contracture and diabetic retinopathy. Postgrad Med J 59:291–294, 1983.
18. Cohen RW, Auerbach R: Acquired reactive perforating collagenosis. J Am Acad Dermatol 20:287–289, 1989.
19. Cole GW, Headley J, Skowsky R: Scleredema diabeticorum: A common and distinct cutaneous man-

ifestation of diabetes mellitus. Diabetes Care 6:189–192, 1983.

20. Collier A, et al: Change in skin thickness associated with cheiroarthropathy in insulin dependent diabetes mellitus. Br Med J 292:936, 1986.

21. Collier A, et al: Relationship of skin thickness to duration of diabetes, glycemic control, and diabetic complications in male IDDM patients. Diabetes Care 12:309–312, 1989.

22. Crosby DL, Woodley DT, Leonard DP: Concomitant granuloma annulare and necrobiosis lipoidica: Report of a case and review of the literature. Dermatologica 183:225–229, 1991.

23. Csaszar A, et al: Necrobiosis lipoidica without diabetes mellitus (diagnostic and therapeutic possibilities). Orv Hetil 130:2141–2145, 1989.

24. Danowski TS, et al: Skin spots and diabetes mellitus. Am J Med Sci 251:570–575, 1966.

25. Dawber RPR: Vitiligo in mature onset diabetes mellitus. Br J Dermatol 80:275–278, 1968.

26. Deldridge L, et al: Limited joint mobility in the diabetic foot: Relationship to neuropathic ulceration. Diabetic Med 5:333–337, 1988.

27. Detmar M, et al: Kyrle disease in juvenile diabetes and chronic renal failure. Z Hautkr 65:53–61, 1990.

28. Digiovanna JJ, Safai B: Kaposi's sarcoma: Retrospective study of 90 cases with particular emphasis on the familial occurrence, ethnic background and prevalence of other disease. Am J Med 71:779–783, 1981.

29. Dowd PM, et al: Diabetic sclerodactyly. Br J Dermatol 115:21, 1986.

30. Dubin BJ, Kaplan EN: The surgical treatment of necrobiosis lipoidica diabeticorum. Plast Reconstr Surg 60:421–427, 1977.

31. Fernando DJS, et al: Relationship of limited joint mobility to abnormal foot pressures and diabetic foot ulceration. Diabetes Care 14:8–11, 1991.

32. Fitzcharles MA, et al: Limitation of joint mobility (cheiroarthropathy) in adult non-insulin dependent diabetic patients. Ann Rheum Dis 43:251–257, 1984.

33. Friedman-Birnbaum R, Weltfriend S, Katz I: Kaposi's sarcoma: Retrospective study of 67 cases with the classical form. Dermatologica 180:13–17, 1990.

34. Gannon TF, Lynch PJ: Absence of carbohydrate intolerance in granuloma annulare. J Am Acad Dermatol 30:662–663, 1994.

35. Grange RW, Black MM, Carrington P: Defective neutrophil migration in granuloma annulare, necrobiosis lipoidica and sarcoidosis. Arch Dermatol 155:32–35, 1979.

36. Goldstein S: Studies on age-related diseases in cultured skin fibroblasts. J Invest Dermatol 73:19–23, 1979.

37. Goto M, et al: Family analysis of Werner's syndrome: A survey of 42 Japanese families with a review of the literature. Clin Genet 19:8–15, 1981.

38. Gould IM, et al: Vitiligo in diabetes mellitus. Br J Dermatol 113:153–155, 1985.

39. Grassi W, Gasparini M, Cervini C: Nail fold computed videomicroscopy in morphofunctional assessment of diabetic microangiopathy. Acta Diabetol Lat 22:213–228, 1985.

40. Grgic A, et al: Joint contracture in childhood diabetes. N Engl J Med 292:372, 1975.

41. Hager CM, et al: Bath-PUVA therapy in three patients with scleredema adultorum. J Am Dermatol 38:240–292, 1998.

42. Halevy S, et al: HLA system in relation to carbohydrate metabolism in lichen planus. Br J Dermatol 100:683–686, 1979.

43. Hanke CW, Bergfeld WF: Treatment with benzoyl peroxide of ulcers on legs within lesions of necrobiosis lipoidica diabeticorum. J Dermatol Surg Oncol 4:701–704, 1978.

44. Hanna W, et al: Pathologic features of diabetic thick skin. J Am Acad Dermatol 16:546–553, 1987.

45. Hatzis J, et al: Sweat gland disturbances in granuloma annulare and necrobiosis lipoidica. Br J Dermatol 108:705–709, 1983.

46. Heite HJ, Scharwenka HX: Erythema elevatum diutinum Granuloma annulare, Nekrobiosis lipoidica und Granulomatosis disciformis Gottron-Miescher. Arch Klin Exp Dermatol 208:260–290, 1959.

47. Heng MCY, et al: Focal endothelial cell degeneration and proliferative endarteritis in trauma-induced early lesions of necrobiosis lipoidica diabeticorum. Am J Dermatopathol 13:108–114, 1991.

48. Heng MCY, Song MK, Heng MK: Healing of necrobiotic ulcers with antiplatelet therapy correlation with plasma thromboxane levels. Int J Dermatol 28:195–197, 1989.

49. Hoerer D, Dreyfuss F, Herzberg M: Carotenemia, skin colour and diabetes mellitus. Acta Diabetol Lat 12:202–207, 1975.

50. Hunt SJ, Narus VT, Abell E: Necrolytic migratory erythema: Dyskeratotic dermatitis, a clue to early diagnosis. J Am Acad Dermatol 24:473–477, 1991.

51. Huntley AC: Diabetes mellitus and miscellaneous metabolic conditions affecting the skin. In Jelinek JE (ed): The Skin and Diabetes. Philadelphia: Lea & Febiger, 1986, pp 136–137.

52. Huntley AC: Cutaneous manifestations of diabetes mellitus. In Sammarco GJ (ed): The Foot in Diabetes. Philadelphia: Lea & Febiger, 1991, pp 124–125.

53. Huntley AC, Walter RM Jr: Quantitative determination of skin thickness in diabetes mellitus: Relationship to disease parameters. J Med 21:257–264, 1990.

54. Husz S, et al: Disseminated atypical granuloma annulare. J Dermatol 14:67–69, 1987.

55. Jelinek JE: The skin in diabetes mellitus: Cutaneous manifestations, complications and associations. In Yearbook of Dermatology. Chicago: Mosby-Year Book, 1970, pp 5–35.

56. Jelinek JE: Necrobiosis lipoidica diabeticorum. In Maddin S (ed): Current Dermatologic Therapy. Philadelphia: WB Saunders Company, 1982, p 325.

57. Jelinek JE: Collagen disorders in which skin changes and cutaneous features co-exist. In The Skin in Diabetes. Philadelphia: Lea & Febiger, 1986, pp 155–173.

58. Jelinek JE: Cutaneous markers of diabetes mellitus and the role of microangiopathy. In The Skin in Diabetes. Philadelphia: Lea & Febiger, 1986, pp 31–72.

59. Jelinek JE: Dermatoses reported to be more frequent in diabetes. The Skin in Diabetes. Philadelphia: Lea & Febiger, 1986, pp 175–202.

60. Jelinek JE: The Skin in Diabetes. Philadelphia: Lea & Febiger, 1986.

61. Kantor GA, Lookingbill DP: Generalized pruritus and systemic disease. J Am Acad Dermatol 9:375–382, 1983.

62. Kaposi M: Idiopathisches multiples Pigmentsarkom der Haut. Arch Dermatol Syphilol 4:265–273, 1872.

63. Kennedy L, et al: Limited joint mobility in type I diabetes mellitus. Postgrad Med J 58:481–484, 1982.

64. Koga M, Tango T: Clinical features and course of type A and type B vitiligo. Br J Dermatol 118:223–228, 1988.

65. Koh MS, et al: Increased plasma fibronectin in diabetes mellitus, necrobiosis lipoidica and widespread granuloma annulare. Clin Exp Dermatol 9:293–297, 1984.

66. Kramer DW: Early or warning signs of impending gangrene in diabetes. Med J Rec 132:338–342, 1930.

67. Krasagakis K, et al: Persistent scleredema of Buschke in a diabetic: Improvement with high-dose penicillin. Br J Dermatol 132:597–598, 1996.

68. Landau J, Davis E: The small blood vessels of the conjunctive and nail bed in diabetes mellitus. Lancet 2:731–734, 1960.

69. Larkin JG, Frier BM: Limited joint mobility and Dupuytren's contracture in diabetic hypertensive and normal populations. Br Med J 292:1494, 1986.

70. Lascari AD: Carotenemia: A review. Clin Pediatr 20:25–29, 1981.

71. Laukkanen A, et al: Necrobiosis lipoidica: Clinical and immunofluorescent study. Dermatologica 172:89–92, 1986.

72. Lever WF, Schaumberg-Lever G: Histopathology of the Skin, 6th ed. Philadelphia: JB Lippincott, 1983, pp 234–236.

73. Lieberman LS, et al: Reduced skin thickness with pump administration of insulin. N Engl J Med 303:940–941, 1980.

74. Lisi P, Giommoni V: A study on the carbohydrate metabolism in lichen planus patients in time. Ann Ital Dermatol Clin Sper 37:29–33, 1983.

75. Lithner F: Cutaneous reactions of the extremities of diabetics to local thermal trauma. Acta Med Scand 198:319–325, 1975.

76. Lithner F, Hallmans G, Hietala S-O: Cutaneous hemorrhages and gangrenes localized to the lower limbs in patients with collagen diseases and in diabetes. Upsala J Med Sci 83:141–151, 1978.

77. Lithner F, Hietala S-O: Skeletal lesions of the feet in diabetes and their relationship to cutaneous erythema with or without necrosis of the feet. Acta Med Scand 200:155–161, 1976.

78. Lundström IM: Incidence of diabetes mellitus in patients with oral lichen planus. Int J Oral Surg 12:147–152, 1983.

79. Lyons TJ, Kennedy L: Non-enzymatic glycosylation of skin collagen in patients with type I (insulin-dependent) diabetes mellitus and limited joint mobility. Diabetologia 28:2–5, 1985.

80. Lyons TJ, et al: Decrease in skin collagen glycation with improved glycemic control in patients with insulin-dependent diabetes mellitus. J Clin Invest 87:1910–1915, 1991.

81. Mann RJ, Harman RRM: Cutaneous anaesthesia in necrobiosis lipoidica. Br J Dermatol 110:323–325, 1984.

82. Mattheou-Vakali G, et al: Cyclosporine in scleredema. J Am Acad Dermatol 35:990–991, 1996.

83. Melin H: An atrophic circumscribed skin lesion in the lower extremities of diabetics. Acta Med Scand 176(Suppl 423):9–75, 1964.

84. Monk B: Carotenemia. Int J Dermatol 22:376–377, 1983.

85. Morton CA, et al: Acquired perforating dermatosis in a British dialysis population. Br J Dermatol 135:671–677, 1996.

86. Mueller MJ, et al: Insensitivity, limited joint mobility and plantar ulcers in patients with diabetes mellitus. Phys Ther 69:453–462, 1989.

87. Muhlemann MF, Williams DRR: Localized granuloma annulare is associated with insulin-dependent diabetes mellitus. Br J Dermatol 111:325–329, 1984.

88. Muller SA, Winkelmann RK: Necrobiosis lipoidica diabeticorum, a clinical and pathological investigation of 171 cases. Arch Dermatol 93:272–281, 1966.

89. Murphy R: Skin lesions in diabetic patients: The "spotted leg" syndrome. Lahey Clin Found Bull 14:10–14, 1965.

90. Neilly JB, et al: Pruritus in diabetes mellitus: Investigation of prevalence and correlation with diabetes control. Diabetes Care 9:273–275, 1986.

91. Nigam PK, Singh G, Agrawal JK: Plasma insulin response to oral glycemic stimulus in lichen planus. Br J Dermatol 19:128–129, 1988.

92. Noz KC, Korstanje MJ, Vermeer BJ: Ulcerating necrobiosis lipoidica effectively treated with pentoxifylline. Clin Exp Dermatol 18:78–79, 1993.

93. Ohtsuka T, et al: Nailfold capillary abnormality and microangiopathy in patients with diabetes mellitus. Eur J Dermatol 6:101–105, 1996.

94. Oimomi M, et al: Glycosylation levels of nail proteins in diabetic patients with retinopathy and neuropathy. Kobe J Med Sci 31:183–188, 1985.

95. Oppenheim M: Eigentümliche disseminerte Degeneration des Bindegewebes der Haut bei einem Diabetiker. Zentralbl Haut Geschlechtskr 32:179, 1930.

96. Oursler JR, Goldblum OM: Blistering eruption in a diabetic. Arch Dermatol 127:247, 1991.

97. Pal B, et al: Limitation of joint mobility and shoulder capsulitis in insulin and non-insulin dependent diabetes mellitus. Br J Rheumatol 25:147–151, 1986.

98. Parker F, et al: Evidence for the chylomicron origin of lipids accumulating in diabetic eruptive xanthomas: A correlative lipid biochemical, histochemical and electron microscope study. J Clin Invest 49:2172–2187, 1970.

99. Patterson JW: The perforating disorders. J Am Acad Dermatol 10:561–581, 1984.

100. Petzelbauer P, Wolff F, Tappeiner G: Necrobiosis lipoidica: Treatment with systemic corticosteroids. Br J Dermatol 126:542–545, 1992.

101. Pongor S, et al: Aging of proteins and identification of a fluorescent chromophore from the reactions of polypeptides with glucose. Proc Natl Acad Sci U S A 81:2684–2688, 1984.

102. Porneuf M, et al: Carcinoma cuniculatum arising in necrobiosis lipoidica. Ann Dermatol Venereol 118:461–464, 1991.

103. Quimby SR, Muller SA, Schroeter AL: The cutaneous immunopathology of necrobiosis lipoidica diabeticorum. Arch Dermatol 124:1364–1371, 1988.

104. Quimby SR, et al: Necrobiosis lipoidica diabeticorum: Platelet survival and response to platelet inhibitors. Cutis 43:213–216, 1989.

105. Rapini RP, Hebert AA, Drucker CR: Acquired perforating dermatosis. Arch Dermatol 125:1074–1078, 1989.
106. Rocca FF, Pereyra E: Phlyctenar lesions in the feet of diabetic patients. Diabetes 12:220–223, 1963.
107. Roenigk HH Jr, Taylor JS, Binkley GW: Scleredema adultorum of Buschke (case in society transactions). Arch Dermatol 99:124–125, 1969.
108. Rosenbloom AL: Skeletal and joint manifestations of childhood diabetes. Pediatr Clin North Am 31:569–589, 1984.
109. Rosenbloom AL: Diabetic thick skin and stiff joints [letter]. Diabetologia 32:74–75, 1989.
110. Rosenbloom AL: Limited joint mobility in insulin dependent childhood diabetes. Eur J Pediatr 149:380–388, 1990.
111. Rosenbloom AL, Frias JL: Diabetes, short stature and joint stiffness—a new syndrome. Clin Res 22:92A, 1974.
112. Rosenbloom AL, et al: Limited joint mobility in childhood diabetic mellitus indicated increased risk for microvascular disease. N Engl J Med 305:191–194, 1981.
113. Rosenbloom AL, et al: Limited joint mobility in diabetes mellitus of childhood: Natural history and relationship to growth impairment. J Pediatr 101:874–878, 1982.
114. Rosenbloom AL, et al: Limited joint mobility in childhood diabetes: Family studies. Diabetes Care 6:370–373, 1983.
115. Roupe G, et al: Biochemical characterization and tissue distribution of the scleredema in a case of Buschke's disease. Acta Derm Venereol (Stockh) 67:193–198, 1987.
116. Sawada Y: Successful treatment of ulcerated necrobiosis lipoidica diabeticorum with prostaglandin E and skin flap transfer: A case report. J Dermatol 12:449–454, 1985.
117. Seibold J: Digital sclerosis in children with insulin dependent diabetes mellitus. Arthritis Rheum 25:1357–1361, 1982.
118. Shall L, et al: Necrobiosis lipoidica: "The foot-print not the footstep." Br J Dermatol 123(Suppl 37): 47, 1990.
119. Shemer A, et al: Diabetic dermopathy and internal complications in diabetes mellitus. Int J Dermatol 37:113–115, 1998.
120. Shimizu H, et al: Perforating granuloma annulare. Int J Dermatol 24:581–583, 1985.
121. Smolle J: T-zone histiocytes in granulomatous skin disorders. Dermatologica 171:316–320, 1985.
122. Sparrow G, Abell E: Granuloma annulare and necrobiosis lipoidica treated by jet injector. Br J Dermatol 93:85–89, 1975.
123. Starkman H, Brink S: Limited joint mobility of the hands in type I diabetes mellitus. Diabetes Care 5:534–536, 1982.
124. Starkman HS, et al: Limited joint mobility (LJM) of the hand in patients with diabetes mellitus: Relation to chronic complications. Ann Rheum Dis 45:130–135, 1986.
125. Sueki H, Fujisawa R: Pigmented pretibial patches with special references to the clinical classification and the correlation to HbA1 which serves as an index of diabetic control. Jpn J Dermatol 96:157–163, 1986.
126. Sueki H, et al: Effects of non-enzymatic glycosylation and heating on browning of human stratum corneum and nail. Dermatologica 183:197–202, 1991.
127. Tkach JR: Platelet-inhibition therapy of ulcerated necrobiosis lipoidica diabeticorum. Dermatol Allergy 5:9–12, 1982.
128. Toyota T, et al: Diabetic scleredema. Tohoku J Exp Med 141:457–461, 1983.
129. Trapp RG, Soler NG, Spencer-Green G: Nail fold capillaroscopy in type I diabetics with vasculopathy and limited joint mobility. J Rheumatol 13:917–920, 1986.
130. Trevisan G, Rizzi MG, Tonini G: Capillaroscopia del vallo ungueale e diabete insulino-dipendente osservazioni in ambiente pediatrico. Giornale Ital Dermatol Venereol 122:621–624, 1987.
131. Tubiana-Rufi N, et al: Detection by nail fold capillary microscopy of early morphologic capillary changes in children with insulin dependent diabetes mellitus. Diabet Metab 15:118–122, 1989.
132. Urbach E: Beitrage zu einer physiologischen und pathologischen Chemie der Haut. Eine neue diabetische Stoff wechseldermatose: Nekrobiosis lipoidica diabeticorum. Arch Derm Syph 166:273–285, 1932.
133. Vion B, Frenk E: Erworbene reaktive kollagenose des Erwachsenen: Erfolgreiche behandlung durch UV-B Licht. Hautarzt 40:448–450, 1989.
134. Weber B: Pathophysiology of diabetes mellitus. In Brook CGD (ed): Clinical Paediatric Endocrinology. Cambridge, MA: Blackwell Scientific Publications, 1989, pp 579–581.
135. Zalla JA: Werner's syndrome. Cutis 25:275–278, 1980.
136. Zelger B, et al: Acquired perforating dermatosis: Transepidermal elimination of DNA material and possible role of leukocytes in pathogenesis. Arch Dermatol 127:695–700, 1991.

NUTRITIONAL ISSUES IN THE PATIENT WITH DIABETES AND FOOT ULCERS

■ Stephen A. McClave and Lois S. Finney

Very little information exists in the literature regarding the nutritional status or the incidence of nutritional deficiencies in the patient with diabetes who develops a foot ulcer. Clinicians should closely scrutinize the nutritional status of these patients, especially those with persistent nonhealing lesions that cannot be explained by inappropriate weight-bearing on the ulcer site, inadequate blood flow, excessive weight gain, or persistent infection. Unfortunately, no prospective randomized clinical trials currently exist to guide the clinician in the nutritional management of these patients. Certainly, basic principles of nutritional management of the patient with diabetes mellitus regarding control of serum glucose, hyperlipidemia, and hypertension have been defined[1, 3] and should be applied to the patient who has developed angiopathic or neuropathic foot ulcers. Theoretically, a patient's baseline nutritional status and certain pre-existing nutritional deficiencies might affect outcome and prognosis, not only due to increased susceptibility to the development of foot ulcers but also due to increased time

needed for wound healing and increased likelihood for recurrence. Whether aggressive nutritional support and correction of any nutritional deficiencies can speed the healing of foot ulcers or reduce the need for amputation is unclear from the literature. We will raise a number of issues related to nutrition that should be addressed by the clinician, and we will outline considerations for the nutritional management of the patient challenged with both diabetes and foot ulcers.

Background

In patients without diabetes, a state of malnutrition has a well-documented deleterious effect on patient outcome, ranging from decreased tensile strength and delayed healing of a surgical wound, to increased infection and overall postoperative complications.[12] Adequate nutritional and metabolic status is an essential part of wound healing. Certainly, most patients with diabetes and foot ulcers are outpatients on oral diet, with no defined nutritional deficiency. Vitamin or trace mineral supplementation has not been shown to speed the healing of lesions in patients having no nutritional deficiencies.[9] Therefore, clinicians must focus on risk factors that promote development of nutrient deficiencies, on diagnostic tests that identify deficiencies, and on the management required for correcting the deficiencies, not just augmenting nutrition in patients who are already adequately nourished. Consequently, to determine risk factors, this chapter discusses a standard nutrition assessment and its components (evaluation of macro- and micronutrient intakes, comorbidities, use of pharmacologic agents, and an evaluation of overall medical nutritional status), biochemical nutritional assessment, medical nutrition intervention, and surgical nutrition guidelines.

Nutrition Assessment

The comprehensive evaluation of the patient with diabetes and a foot ulcer should include a standard nutritional assessment that looks at macro- and micronutrient intake. In addition, a careful review of diabetic comorbidities (which may affect ingestion or assimilation of nutrients), use of pharmacologic agents that may affect wound healing or control of glucose levels, and an evaluation of overall medical nutritional status must be completed.

Standard Nutritional Assessment

To ascertain adequacy of oral intake, a standard nutritional assessment should be completed by a registered dietitian using either a patient recall of intake over a usual 24-hour period of time or a review of a patient's record of food intake over a specified period of time, preferably 3 days. Because the healing process can be delayed by poor appetite or poor nutritional status, a close evaluation of overall caloric requirement versus actual intake must take place, paying particular attention to intakes of protein, key vitamins (A, B_6, B_{12}, C, D, E, and K) and folacin, and key minerals (zinc, iron, copper, magnesium, chromium, and phosphorus), whether the sources of these nutrients are actual foods or supplements.

Calories and Weight Loss

The caloric requirements for a patient with diabetes and foot ulcers differs minimally from the requirements of stressed patients with no diabetes. Energy requirements are a function of metabolically active tissue, especially lean body mass, and can vary tremendously among patients. Although energy expenditure may be difficult to determine using only predictive equations, the most commonly used formula for determining resting energy expenditure (REE) is the Harris-Benedict equation (Table 8–1).[5]

A simplified empiric formula of 22 to 25 kcal/kg actual body weight per day correlates to the measured resting energy expenditure in a fashion similar to more sophisticated equations. Accurately measuring energy expenditure is particularly important to the patient who requires aggressive nutritional support (through total parenteral nutrition or enteral tube feedings) or a surgical procedure.

Weight as a percentage of ideal body weight or as a percentage of weight loss compared to the patient's usual weight is still one of the easiest markers to identify patients who have preexisting compromised nutritional status. Weight loss as a percentage of the patient's usual weight is considered mild if 10% or less, moderate if 10 to 20%, and severe when 20% or greater.[13] Significant marasmus is suggested by an actual weight less than 85% of ideal body weight. Of the two parameters, weight loss as a percentage of the patient's usual weight is a more sensitive marker of preexisting deterioration of nutritional status than weight as a percentage of the ideal body weight. Unfortunately, the major limiting factor is that individuals are often aware of their "usual" weight.

Regarding weight loss, mild to moderate weight loss of 10 to 20 lb may improve diabetes control even if desired weight is not reached.[1] However, since these individuals are often instructed to not put weight on their feet, it is very difficult to achieve weight loss.

Table 8–1 ■ HARRIS-BENEDICT EQUATION

Men: 66.473 + 13.752W + 5.003H − 6.755A
Women: 66.096 + 9.563W + 1.85H − 4.676A

where W is weight in kilograms; H is standing height in centimeters; and A is age in years

In fact, it may be necessary to avoid weight reduction until the wound is healed, unless the degree of obesity is directly contributing to the formation or continuation of a foot ulcer.[9]

Macronutrients (Protein, Carbohydrates, and Fat)

The macronutrients—protein, carbohydrate, and fat—have been shown to have a dramatic effect on wound healing and may be a factor in the outcome of individuals with diabetes and foot ulcers. Protein provision is required to stimulate fibrin and collagen deposition, to blunt catabolism, to enhance immunity, and to improve overall wound healing. Protein depletion suppresses the immune response, inhibits angiogenesis, decreases fibroblast generation and remodeling of collagen, and impairs overall wound healing.[12] Obtaining positive nitrogen balance is important to counter the effects of nitrogen losses and maximize the retention of nitrogen. The protein intake goal is to provide 1.2 to 1.7 gm protein per kilogram actual dry body weight.[4] If the individual has nephropathy, a range of 1.0 to 1.5 gm protein per kilogram actual dry body weight is recommended. (To achieve that goal all sources of protein need to be calculated, whether from plant or animal sources.) Of interest, a recent study demonstrated that two amino acids, arginine and glutamine, selectively improve wound healing and blunt protein catabolism to a greater extent than other amino acids.[12]

Carbohydrate and fat intake may also affect the healing process, although usually to a lesser extent than protein intake. Since tissue granulation is an obligate glucose consumer, it can be postulated that adherence to a high-carbohydrate, low-fat diet, as is recommended for all individuals with diabetes, may accelerate wound healing. Essential fatty acid deficiency, which can develop within 4 weeks in an adult on total parenteral nutrition, has been shown to adversely affect wound healing.[12]

Micronutrients (Vitamins and Minerals)

A number of specific vitamins play a key role in wound healing. Vitamin A moderates cell differentiation and reverses the inhibitory effects on growth and wound healing by corticosteroids. Vitamin A deficiency may decrease epithelialization, collagen synthesis, production of macrophages, and overall resistance to infection.[9] Vitamins B_6 and B_{12} are important stimulants for wound healing, and a deficiency of either may result in decreased protein synthesis.[7] Vitamin C affects the speed and strength of wound healing, and deficiencies promote collagen instability, decreased collagen formation, and decreased tensile strength of the wound. Profound deficiencies of vitamin C may promote capillary fragility.[9] Theoretically, extensive wounds can exhaust vitamin C stores. Vitamin D is required for repair of bone fractures and/or healing after amputation. Vitamin E acts as an antioxidant and may serve to enhance immunity and reduce overall inflammatory response. Vitamin K, important in blood clotting, may be necessary in supplement form if long-term anticoagulant therapy or prolonged antibiotics are used. Folate deficiency may play a role in decreasing protein synthesis.

To assess intake of the key vitamins, special attention should be paid to intake of fruits and vegetables, especially those rich in vitamins A and C and folacin, which are usually the dark green and deep yellow fruits and vegetables. Meat, poultry, and seafood are main contributors of vitamins B_6, B_{12}, and K. Vitamin E is present in oils and vitamin D in milk products.

Deficiencies of certain minerals have been documented as having an effect on healing. Zinc plays a key role in protein synthesis and tissue repair. Its deficiency reduces collagen synthesis and tensile strength of the wound and leads to abnormalities in neutrophil and lymphocyte function, the end result being an increase in overall infection and delayed wound healing.[13] Iron deficiency interferes with wound healing as a result of tissue hypoxemia, and if prolonged, anemia may develop, further aggravating the healing process.[13] Copper is required for maintenance and repair of bones. Low serum levels of either magnesium or chromium can play a key role in carbohydrate intolerance and resistance to insulin,[1] although magnesium or chromium deficiency is rare. Zinc, iron, and copper are found primarily in meats and to a lesser extent in whole grains, while magnesium and chromium are principally found in whole grains and copper is readily available in organ meats, nuts, and seeds.

Unfortunately, the incidence of specific vitamin and mineral deficiencies in the patient with diabetes and foot ulcers is not known.

However, there is clear evidence in other disease processes that the identification and correction of certain nutrient deficiencies improves management and accelerates wound healing. Zinc supplementation has been shown to accelerate wound healing in patients following surgery and severe burns, but probably only in the presence of zinc deficiency.[12] Vitamin E supplementation has been shown in clinical studies to accelerate the healing of chronic stasis ulcers. Copper supplementation has been shown to potentially increase the rate of healing from bone fractures.[12] However, the likelihood of a deficiency of one of these vitamins or minerals (from dietary deficiency alone) is extremely low in clinic patients with diabetes and foot ulcers.

Evaluation of the Comorbidities of Diabetes Which Can Lead to Micronutrient Deficiencies

The comorbidities of diabetes, which may affect absorption of micronutrients or accelerate their losses, include diabetic enteropathy with bacterial overgrowth, short bowel syndrome, previous gastric surgery, large gaping wounds, or prolonged used of total parenteral nutrition.[9] The detection of inadequate micronutrient levels and the diagnosis of classic vitamin or mineral deficiencies can be difficult and frustrating for the clinician. Determination of serum levels of vitamins and minerals is often expensive, inaccurate, and may not adequately reflect tissue stores of micronutrients. The routine use of serum vitamin or trace element levels in nutritional assessment is discouraged. Clinicians are better served by efforts that either identify factors potentially promoting losses of micronutrients or look for certain clinical signs of severe nutrient deficiencies. The patient with enteropathy complicated by bacterial overgrowth is at risk for vitamin B_{12} and folate deficiencies due to the inability of the small bowel bacteria to incorporate these vitamins. Gastric bypass surgery for obesity or a partial gastrectomy with a Billroth II anastomosis for peptic ulcer disease increases risk of deficiencies of vitamin B_{12}, calcium, and iron. Short bowel syndrome with resection of any portion of the terminal ileum increases the likelihood of deficiency of any of the fat-soluble vitamins (A, D, E, or K). Large, chronic, poorly healing surgical wounds can be a source of loss of vitamin C and zinc, thus leading to deficiency of these nutrients over time. Overall, though, by far the most common clinical factor increasing a patient's risk of any vitamin or mineral deficiencies is prolonged use of total parenteral nutrition, where deficiencies of especially magnesium and chromium may become evident.[1]

Evaluation of Pharmacotherapy

Patient medication should be reviewed for pharmacologic agents that may affect wound healing or control of glucose levels.[12] Corticosteroids often inhibit wound healing by adversely affecting connective tissue formation, collagen synthesis, and wound contraction. Use of nonsteroidal anti-inflammatory drugs improves wound strength but may adversely increase the rate of wound reinfection. Antiemetics such as prochlorperazine may delay gastric emptying and contribute to nausea and vomiting. Agents such as cyclosporine, sympathomimetics, and corticosteroids may be key factors in worsening glycemic control. Review of patient medication should include bringing *all* pharmacologic agents and any over-the-counter supplements, since patients often forget key medications that may have profound side effects with other medicines.

Evaluation of Overall Medical Nutritional Status

An extremely important part of the comprehensive nutritional assessment is a medical diabetes evaluation as it relates to dietary practices. This assessment should include evaluation of relevant clinical data, including glycosylated hemoglobin levels, blood pressure readings, lipid levels, blood urea nitrogen (BUN) levels, and serum creatinine. A patient's dietary prescription, specific restrictions, and a sense of dietary compliance should be obtained. The dietitian working with the patient and medical team must determine the patient's method of food procurement and preparation, financial constraints that may impact food procurement, current living conditions, support system, and any educational gaps that would impede dissemination of information. Cultural, ethnic, and financial considerations are all factors that affect the ability of patients to adhere to particular dietary programs. If possible, it is advisable to assess clients in their homes. One of the main advantages of completing home assessments is being able to obtain visual data regarding how food is prepared, how the family interacts regarding diabetes and food, and the cultural background of the family. For example, it may be noted that only a hot plate is used for cooking or that many snack foods high in salt and fat are available. This latter observation would severely limit the ability to follow a meal plan for a patient who is both hyperlipidemic and hypertensive.

Biochemical Nutrition Assessment

Visceral Protein Levels

Biochemical components of a nutritional assessment are an initial evaluation of visceral protein levels, including albumin, prealbumin, and transferrin levels. The serum albumin level is a valid prognosticator, with decreasing levels accurately predicting increases in morbidity and mortality.[12] Surprisingly, hypoalbuminemia is an excellent marker for the stress response, but a poor marker for overall nutritional status.[8] A recent study reviewed the association between serum albumin levels and the stress response in patients with and without diabetes and patients with and without foot ulcers. The study found that those patients with diabetes and foot ulcers had significantly higher levels of C-reactive protein and fibrinogen, and lower albumin levels when compared to two groups of control patients, those with diabetes but no foot ulcers and those with neither diabetes nor foot ulcers. These results further demonstrate that patients with diabetes and foot ulcers undergo a reaction that significantly increases acute-phase proteins and diminishes serum albumin levels. The decrease in albumin level shown in this research is theorized to result from a reprioritization of hepatic protein synthesis.[8] This reprioritization results in decreased production of homeostatic proteins and increased production of both acute-phase protein and vascular permeability. Vascular permeability often results in extravasation of the proteins from the vascular space.

A common mistake made by clinicians in treating patients with diabetes and foot ulcers is to interpret hypoalbuminemia as a sign of malnutrition.[4] If malnutrition is suspected, calorie prescription is often increased significantly, leading to hyperglycemia and weight gain, both of which further complicate healing of the ulcer.[10] Fluid shifts, duration of the stress response, and poor response to nutritional therapy limit the value of serial visceral protein levels. Therefore, the use of any visceral protein levels after an initial evaluation is discouraged.

Medical Nutrition Intervention

One of the basic premises of the medical/nutritional therapy of the patient with diabetes and foot ulcer is to maintain serum glucose levels as close to normal as possible while minimizing extremes of hyper- and hypoglycemia.[7] Table 8–2 lists factors to consider when planning perioperative nutrition therapy.

Poorly controlled hyperglycemia has wide-ranging deleterious effects on patient outcome, including neural, skeletal, and smooth muscle dysfunction. Immune abnormalities associated with hyperglycemia (which may actually improve with aggressive glycemic control) include abnormalities of chemotaxis, phagocytosis, and production of superoxide anions by diabetic neutrophils and macrophages.[7] Combined with abnormalities of complement function, the overall impact of poorly controlled hyperglycemia is increased rate of infection. In the stressed patient with diabetes and foot ulcers requiring hospital-

---

Table 8–2 ■ PARAMETERS TO CONSIDER WHEN PLANNING PERIOPERATIVE NUTRITION THERAPY*

Type of surgery and ramifications to gastrointestinal tract
Medications
Degree of diabetic gastroparesis
History of ketoacidosis or nonketotic hyperosmolar coma
Weight loss despite normal or increased intake (>10% usual body weight is significant)
Recent polydipsia, polyuria, polyphagia
Dietary adherence
Serial glycated hemoglobin values
Glycosuria/ketonuria
Serial blood glucose values
Intraoperative or postoperative complications

---

* From Gaare-Porcari J, O'Sullivan-Maillet J: Care for persons with diabetes during surgery. *In* Powers M (ed): Handbook of Diabetes Medical Nutrition Therapy. Gaithersburg, MD: Aspen Publishers, 1996, pp 602–617, with permission.

ization, maintaining glucose levels between 100 and 200 mg/dL may be reasonable, while the more stable outpatient should be controlled between 100 and 150 mg/dL.[7] Any risk factors that might promote hyperglycemia should be identified and corrected (i.e., infection, overfeeding, volume depletion, medications, and insufficient insulin therapy). Also, the clinician needs to pay attention to factors that may precipitate hypoglycemia (i.e., gastroparesis, hepatitis, sepsis associated with nephropathy, discontinuation of nutritional support, resolution of the stress response, or weaning from steroid therapy).

Controlling hyperglycemia is particularly important in the patient with diabetes and foot ulcers who requires aggressive nutritional support and/or surgical intervention. The rate of catheter-related infection is five times higher in the patient with diabetes receiving total parenteral nutrition (TPN) than in the nondiabetic on TPN.[7] Hyperglycemia occurring within 3 days of diagnosing candidemia has been identified as the major risk factor in the development of systemic fungal infections. Poor control of postoperative hyperglycemia in a recent study predicted the likelihood of serious infection. Patients with poor control of glucose ($\geq$220 mg/dL) on the first day following surgery had a 24.6% incidence of serious infection, compared with 4.2% in those patients in whom glucose control was less than 220 mg/dL.[8] In a number of prospective, randomized, controlled trials comparing routes of nutritional support (enteral tube feeding vs. TPN), the groups receiving TPN had significantly higher mean glucose levels and required more insulin to sustain euglycemia.[6]

For any patient with diabetes, whether or not a foot ulcer is present, nutritional management should consist of following an individualized meal plan based on the nutrition recommendations set forth by the American Diabetes Association.[1] Individuals should be encouraged to eat at consistent times throughout the day, synchronized with the peak action of their insulin or oral diabetes medication, and focus on improvement in overall food choices. The clinician and patient should determine a reasonable goal weight (often not the same as the ideal body weight), but a weight that is achievable and maintainable by the patient.

Reduction in total fat intake (especially saturated fats) is important. Approximately 10 to 20% of calories should be from protein sources and less than 30% of the calories as fat (with less than 10% of the calories coming from saturated fat). While the remaining calories should be made up of carbohydrates, little science supports the concept that "simple" sugars should be replaced by complex carbohydrates.[1] The total amount of carbohydrate is more important than the actual source of carbohydrate. Ethanol intake should be restricted, substituting alcohol calories for fat exchanges and limiting those patients on insulin to less than two alcoholic beverages per day.

Diagnosis of a micronutrient deficiency should prompt the use of a general multivitamin/mineral supplement and possible repletion of a specific nutrient determined to be deficient. Dietary plans should be designed according to what the patient is able or willing to do, taking into account the likelihood of adhering to the dietary prescription and any cultural, ethnic, or financial considerations that may affect compliance.[11] Tailoring the diet to the patient's individual needs, providing frequent follow-up and feedback (thereby empowering the patient), and keeping a food diary (helping the patient be aware of what is consumed), often improve glycemic control and will promote adherence to the dietary plan.

Surgical Nutrition Guidelines

The patient with diabetes undergoing an uncomplicated surgical procedure should be able to resume adequate oral intake within several days. Clear liquid diets may be unavoidable in the preparation for surgery or diagnostic tests, but the emphasis should be on provision of obligatory glucose (approximately 150 gm/day) in these situations. Unsupplemented clear liquid diets will not meet the patient's nutrient needs. Although advancement to solid foods as quickly as possible should be encouraged by the clinician, there is often significant appetite suppression following surgery. Patients often try to resume solid food intake too quickly, resulting in severe nausea. Therefore, until the appetite returns, use of one of the numerous oral supplements may be necessary. Since erratic oral intake disrupts blood glucose control when oral hypoglycemic agents or intermediate/long-acting insulin is used, steady caloric intake should be a primary goal. A notation of any uneaten carbohydrate should be made and replacement carbohydrates should be provided, particularly for the patient with type 1 diabetes. In these patients a minimum of 150 gm carbohydrate per 24 hours is needed to prevent ketosis.[6]

Rarely, the patient with diabetes and a foot ulcer may require aggressive nutritional support by enteral tube feeding or TPN. Over the short-term, indications for nutritional support and daily estimates of calorie, protein, and lipid requirements are similar in the hospitalized patient with diabetes compared to the patient with comparable medical problems, but no diabetes.

Surgical intervention with amputation for the patient with foot ulcer is not a reason by itself for TPN. Enteral tube feedings are the superior route of nutritional support, with a lower incidence of nosocomial infections, organ failure, and problems with hyperglycemia when compared to the parenteral route.[7] As a first step, clinicians should use short-acting insulin in case there is a sudden discontinuation of feed. Feeds should be slowly advanced toward the goal, keeping the glucose level below 200 mg/dL.[7] Although formulas with selected soluble fiber may be capable of delaying glucose absorption from the small bowel, the overall effect on glycemic control is probably insignificant. In patients with renal insufficiency and creatinine levels greater than 2.0 mg/dL, cycling the nutritional support with sudden discontinuation may precipitate severe hypoglycemia.

Avoidance of overfeeding an enteric formula is probably of greater importance than the use of a specific formula. Twice-daily intermediate-acting with regular or Humalog may be effective for the patient with diabetes on continuous enteral feeding. For the patient on cycling nocturnal feeds, use of an intermediate-acting insulin prior to initiation of the infusion should adequately control glucose levels.

Conclusion

The optimal management of the diabetes and foot ulcers includes adequate control of glucose, lipids, and blood pressure. A comprehensive nutrition assessment should evaluate macro- and micronutrient intake, comorbidities, pharmacologic therapy, and overall medical nutrition status. Careful nutrition counseling and patient education should be utilized to encourage adherence to basic diabetes dietary recommendations, keeping in mind that weight loss in the obese patient with diabetes may need to be deferred pending the healing of the foot ulcer. Nutritional support by the enteral/parenteral route should be reserved only for those patients who cannot maintain adequate oral intake. In conclusion, more research, especially controlled clinical trials, is needed on the possible role of vitamin or mineral supplements for these individuals, keeping in mind that adhering to overall nutrition principles is of utmost importance.

REFERENCES

1. American Diabetes Association: Nutrition recommendations and principles for people with diabetes mellitus: Diabetes Care 18:S16–S19, 1995.
2. Barbul A, Lazarou S, Efron D, et al: Arginine enhances wound healing and lymphocyte immune responses in humans. Surgery 108:331–337, 1990.
3. Franz M, Horton E, Bantle J, et al: Nutrition principles for the management of diabetes and related complications. Diabetes Care 17:490–518, 1994.
4. Gaare-Porcari J, O'Sullivan-Maillet J: Care for persons with diabetes during surgery. In Powers M (ed): Handbook of Diabetes Medical Nutrition Therapy. Gaithersburg, MD: Aspen Publishers, 1996, pp 602–617.
5. Harris J, Benedict T: Biometric Studies of Basal Metabolism in Man. Washington, DC: Carnegie Institute of Washington, 1919, publication No. 279.
6. McClave S, Snider H, Spain D: Preoperative issues in clinical nutrition. Chest 115:S64–S70, 1999.
7. McMahon M, Rizza R: Nutrition support in hospitalized patients with diabetes mellitus. Mayo Clin Proc 71:587–594, 1996.
8. Pomposelli J, Baxter T, et al: Early postoperative glucose control predicts nosocomial infection rate in diabetic patients. J Parenter Enter Nutr 22:77–81, 1998.
9. Silane M, Oot-Giromini B: Systemic and other factors that affect wound healing. In Eaglstein H (ed): New Directions in Wound Healing. Princeton, NJ: Squib and Sons, Inc, 1990, pp 40–44.
10. Solomon S, Kirby P: The refunding syndrome: A review. J Parenter Enter Nutr 14:90–97, 1990.
11. Snetselaar L (ed): Nutrition Counseling Skills, 2nd ed. Rockville, MD: Aspen Publishers, 1989, pp 315–317.
12. Telfer N, Moy R: Drug and nutrient aspects of wound healing. Dermatol Clin 11:729–737, 1993.
13. Trace Elements. In Recommended Dietary Allowances. Washington, DC: National Academy Press, 1989, pp 195–246.
14. Upchurch G, Keagy B, Johnson G: An acute phase reaction in diabetic patients with foot ulcers. Cardiovasc Surg 5:32–36, 1997.

PATHOGENESIS AND GENERAL MANAGEMENT OF FOOT LESIONS IN THE DIABETIC PATIENT

■ Marvin E. Levin

Diabetes is one of the oldest diseases known to mankind. The Ebers Papyrus of 1500 BC mentions its symptoms and suggests treatment. Moreover, the history of gangrene of the foot was known in biblical times, when the first case, perhaps due to diabetes, was described:

In the 39th year of his reign, King Asa became affected with gangrene of his feet; he did not seek guidance from the Lord but resorted to physicians. He rested with his forefathers in the 41st year of his reign
(Chronicles XVI: 12–14)

Whether King Asa had diabetic gangrene is a moot point. Certainly, in biblical times there was not much one could do for a foot lesion but pray. By the 1500s healing continued to depend on prayer alone. The famous surgeon Ambroise Pare (1510–1590) said, "I dressed him and God healed him." Today the skills of multiple medical disciplines are significantly reducing amputation rates. With increased awareness of diabetic foot problems and improved treatment, amputation rates will continue to decrease.

The human foot is a mechanical marvel. It consists of 26 bones, 29 joints, 42 muscles, and a multitude of tendons and ligaments. In a lifetime this phenomenal machine with its multiple moving parts walks between 75,000 and 100,000 miles, a distance equivalent to three to four times around the world, and is exposed to significant pressures with each step. In the diabetic patient, particularly those with ulceration, the foot is exposed to significantly elevated pressures (see Chapter 6).

Foot problems are common in the population at large. However, the diabetic patient is especially vulnerable because of the complications of peripheral neuropathy (PN), peripheral arterial disease (PAD), and infection. The combination of this triad leads to the final cataclysmic events, gangrene and amputation.

Recent reviews have stressed the magnitude and importance of aggressive management in the prevention of amputation.[17, 77, 79] A very common cause for hospitalization of individuals with diabetes is foot ulceration.[77] Six percent (162,500) of the diabetic population in the United States are hospitalized annually because of foot ulceration.[123] Martin and colleagues found leg and/or foot ulcers to be present in 14% of the Hispanic patients, 9% of the blacks, and 7% of the whites.[94] Smith et al.[137] found that in a 2-year period, foot problems were responsible for 23% of the hospital days. At the India Institute of Diabetes in Bombay, more than 10% of the patients with diabetes are admitted for foot management. More than 70% of these patients required surgical intervention and 40% of these interventions consisted of either toe or limb amputations.[129] In the United Kingdom more than 50% of the bed occupancy of persons with diabetes is due to foot problems.[151] A large survey in the United Kingdom found that of 6,000 patients attending diabetes clinics, more than 2% had an active foot ulcer and 2.5% were amputees.[88] In the United States 50% of all nontraumatic amputations occur in diabetic persons. Reiber et al. reported the location of the amputations as toes (24%), midfoot (5.8%), below the knee (BK) (38.8%), and above the knee (AK) (21.4%). The remaining 10% included hip, pelvis, knee, and sites not listed.[123] The finding that almost twice as many amputations are BK rather than AK is explained by the fact that most PAD in people with diabetes occurs below the knee.

The loss of a single toe may seem insignificant. However, Quebedeux et al. have shown that amputation of a great toe can contribute to development of deformities of the second and third toes and lead to ulceration of this foot as well as the contralateral foot.[119]

The average length of hospitalization for a patient undergoing amputation as reported by Reiber et al. was 20.3 days for patients with private insurance and 12.4 days for patients on Medicare. Similar differences occurred for persons with diabetes who were hospitalized for foot ulcers. Those with private insurance averaged a stay of 17.8 days; those on Medicare, 12 days.[123]

The exact cost of an amputation is difficult to ascertain because of the differences in payment by Medicare and other third-party carriers. Reiber et al. found that reimbursement for patients with private insurance averaged $26,000. The charges for Medicare patients averaged $23,976 but reimbursement averaged $10,969.[123] Eckman et al.[36] reported the average cost of hospitalization for amputation of a toe to be $22,026; a transmetatarsal, $22,373; and BK, $22,419. The cost of a toe

amputation was essentially the same as for a BK.[36] For the patient who had amputation but died during the hospitalization, the costs were astronomical: $59,017 for a toe, $59,365 for a metatarsal, and $59,410 for a BK.[36]

Multiple epidemiologic factors are associated with diabetic foot problems and amputation (see Chapter 2). The diabetic patient most likely to develop a foot lesion is older than 40 years. Today, 90% of diabetic patients in the United States are in this age group.[32] Most of these ulcers are the result of peripheral neuropathy leading to an insensate foot, which is then vulnerable to painless trauma and ulceration. Peripheral neuropathy is extremely common in type 1 diabetes, with the incidence gradually increasing with age and duration. After 20 years' duration of diabetes, 42% of patients have clinical evidence of peripheral neuropathy.[107]

Peripheral arterial disease is present at diagnosis in 8% of diabetic patients, in 15% after 10 years, and in 42% after 20 years.[111]

The long- and short-term prognosis for the diabetic undergoing amputation has always been poor. In the preantibiotic era, the principal cause of in-hospital mortality in patients with diabetic gangrene was infection and toxemia.[91] With the availability of antibiotics and newer management techniques, a mortality rate of 50% in the 1930s[74] is now in the range of 1.5 to 3%.[10] McDermott and Rogers[96] stated that curing all cancers would add just 2 years to the life expectancy for Americans, but the introduction of antibiotics has added 10 years.

Postoperative morbidity is a frequent occurrence in these patients. Fearon et al.[42] found local complication rates of 18% and systemic complication rates of 36%, including gastrointestinal hemorrhage, myocardial infarction, congestive heart failure, and cerebral vascular accident. In the diabetic the major postoperative concern is not the operative site but control of blood glucose and management of medical problems, such as cardiac and renal complications. These require the constant attention of trained medical personnel. It is my opinion that any diabetic patient undergoing surgery should be followed closely by the medical team for systemic and metabolic postoperative care.

The long-term outlook for the diabetic amputee has not improved significantly since Silbert's report in 1952.[135] In a follow-up of 294 cases he found a 65% survival rate for 3 years but only a 41% rate at the end of 5 years. Eighteen years later, Ecker and Jacobs[35] found data similar to those of Silbert. In their series of 103 patients they found a survival rate of only 61% 3 years after the first amputation. Because of the high mortality in this group of diabetic patients, primarily from heart attack or stroke, many do not live long enough to undergo an amputation of the contralateral leg. For those who do, the long-term outlook for the remaining leg is poor. This poor prognosis is not new. Marchel de Calvi[92] in 1864 stated that "often the opposite leg is affected, gangrene sets in and soon the patient succumbs to horrible suffering. Having relieved him only of his local affliction [by amputation], I have done nothing but mutilate him." This problem still exists. On average, 40% of these patients will have amputation of the remaining leg in 1 to 3 years, and 55% in 3 to 5 years.

Risk Factors for Amputation

Risk factors for amputation and ulceration vary from report to report. Selby and Zhang[131] found that blood glucose level, duration of diabetes, and systolic blood pressure were independent risk factors. The microvascular complications of retinopathy, neuropathy, and nephropathy were found in patients who had an amputation. A history of stroke was independently predictive; myocardial infarction was not.[131] Other studies[72, 102, 105, 124] also confirmed the role of neuropathy, retinopathy, and hyperglycemia and included male sex in predicting the probability of lower extremity amputation. One study showed that elevation of the serum cholesterol was a risk factor in women but not in men.[72] In a study in the United States of whites, it was found that in the younger onset persons with diabetes, cigarette smoking was predictive of amputation; it was not predictive in the older onset individual with diabetes.[102] Being black has been reported as a risk factor for amputation.[99, 103] Peripheral neuropathy is a major contributing factor, leading to the development of 90% of all foot ulcers.[11] Patients with diabetes and PN have a sevenfold increased risk of ulceration.[158] Humphrey et al.[56] demonstrated the importance of good blood sugar control in preventing amputation. They found that patients whose fasting blood glucose levels were below 140 mg/dL did not have amputation.

In my opinion, the major risk factors leading to amputation are age, duration of diabetes, sex, race, poor glycemic control, PAD and PN, with loss of protective sensation of the feet, foot deformities, ulceration, failure and/or delay to aggressively treat ulceration, and failure to educate the patient in appropriate foot care.

The Pathogenesis of Diabetic Foot Ulcers

The pathogenesis of diabetic foot ulcers leading to amputation stems from a variety of pathways (Fig. 9–1).[75] The combination of PN, PAD, and infection are the major factors leading to gangrene and amputation. However, both PN and PAD can be independent risk factors for the development of foot ulcers. McNeely et al.[98] found three areas to be significant and independent predictors of foot ulceration. These included the absence of the Achilles tendon reflex, a foot insensate to the 5.07 Semmes-Weinstein monofilament, and a transcutaneous oxygen tension (TcPo$_2$) less than 30 mm Hg with impaired cutaneous oxygenation being the most significant risk factor. They found that ankle-arm pressure index (AAI) was not a significant independent risk factor. However, it should be kept in mind that low ankle-brachial indexes (ABI) and the absence of pulses are indications for a vascular consultation, possible angiography, and, if indicated, peripheral vascular bypass surgery. McNeely and colleagues[98] also stressed that in a clinical setting insensitivity to the 5.07 monofilament was probably the most practical method of risk assessment. Therefore, PN with insensitivity, and PAD are significant risk factors, acting independently and/or in combination. A third and extremely important factor leading to ulceration is increased plantar pressure (see Chapter 6).

Peripheral Arterial Disease

The content of the atherosclerotic plaque—cholesterol, lipids, smooth muscle cells, monocytes, phagocytes, and calcium—is the same for individuals with or without diabetes. However, there are significant differences (Table 9–1). Atherosclerosis in a person with diabetes occurs at a younger age and advances more rapidly than in a person without

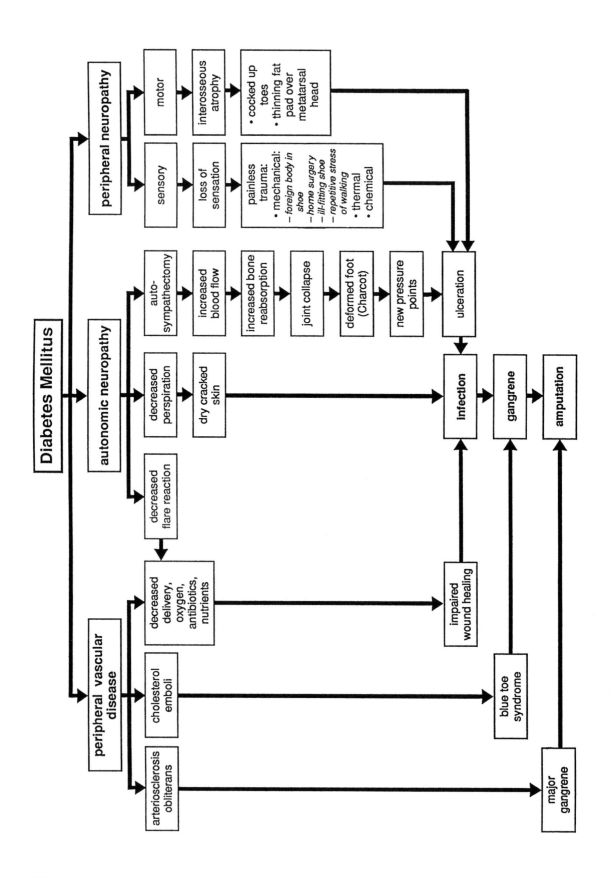

222

Table 9–1 ■ DIFFERENCES IN DIABETIC AND NONDIABETIC ARTERIAL VASCULAR DISEASE

	DIABETIC	NONDIABETIC
Clinical	More common	Less common
	Younger patient	Older patient
	More rapid	Less rapid
Male/female	M = F	M > F
Occlusion	Multisegmental	Single segment
Vessels adjacent to occlusion	Involved	Not involved
Collateral vessels	Involved	Usually normal
Lower extremities	Both	Unilateral
Vessels Involved	Tibial Peroneal	Aortic Iliac Femoral

diabetes. Nondiabetic men have more PAD than nondiabetic women. However, men and women who are diabetic are equally affected. In the Framingham Study, women with diabetes had a greater annual risk of cardiac disease and intermittent claudicaton than did women without diabetes.[154] A significant difference in PAD between the individual with diabetes and one without diabetes is the vessels involved. In the person with diabetes the vessels involved in the lower extremity are usually below the trifurcation, the tibials and the peroneal, whereas the person without diabetes tends to have involvement of the more proximal vessels, the femoral, iliac, and the aorta.

Further evidence of which vessels are involved is demonstrated by the type of vascular surgery that is performed in these patients. Although vascular surgery of all types is more common in the diabetic than in the nondiabetic, the procedure most frequently performed in the diabetic is tibioperoneal bypass surgery, involving the vessels below the knee.[80] Large and smaller vessel disease does not progress at the same rate. It is not uncommon for the small vessels in the toes to have evidence of ischemia, even though the dorsalis pedis or posterior tibial pulses may be present and adequate. Figure 9–2 illustrates a significant decrease in toe pressure

in a patient with normal ankle pressure. It is also common in the diabetic to have very high ankle Doppler pressure compared with brachial pressure. This occurs in about 15% of diabetics, because of deposits of calcium in the arteries, making them noncompressible.

Microangiopathy is not a significant factor in the pathogenesis of diabetic foot lesions. Although there may be capillary basement membrane thickening, there is no evidence that this contributes to the foot ischemia. This has been well documented by LoGerfo and Coffman.[86] They stressed that in many instances there are enough patent vessels at the ankle to allow vascular surgery, usually a tibioperoneal bypass procedure, from the femoral arteries in the thigh to the tibial vessels at the ankle, and that microangiopathy is not a contraindication to vascular bypass surgery (see Chapter 25).

The risk factors for the development of PAD include genetic predisposition, age, duration of diabetes, smoking, hypertension (systolic or diastolic), hypercholesterolemia, hypertriglyceridemia, hyperglycemia truncal obesity, hyperinsulinemia, proteinuria, dialysis, and drugs (e.g., inotropic agents or β-blockers). Age, duration of diabetes, diabetes itself, and genetic factors may be the most important factors, but these cannot be corrected; other risk factors can be treated.

Of the correctable risk factors, smoking tops the list. King James I of England (1566–1625) noted the evils of smoking many years ago:

A custom loathsome to the eye, hateful to the nose, harmful to the braine, dangerous to the lungs and the black stinking fume therefore, nearest resembling the horrible stigian smoke of the pit that is bottomless.

An excellent review on the consequences of smoking has been written by Couch.[25] Pollin[118] has estimated that cigarette smoking causes an estimated 325,000 to 355,000 deaths annually in the United States. This is more than all other drug and alcohol abuse deaths combined, seven times more than all automobile fatalities per year, more than 11 times all reported deaths caused by acquired immune deficiency syndrome (AIDS), and

Figure 9–1 ■ Pathogenesis of diabetic foot lesions leading to amputation. (From Levin ME: Diabetic foot lesions: Pathogenesis and management. *In* Kerstein MD, White JW [eds]: Alternatives to Open Vascular Surgery. Philadelphia: JB Lippincott Company, 1995, with permission.)

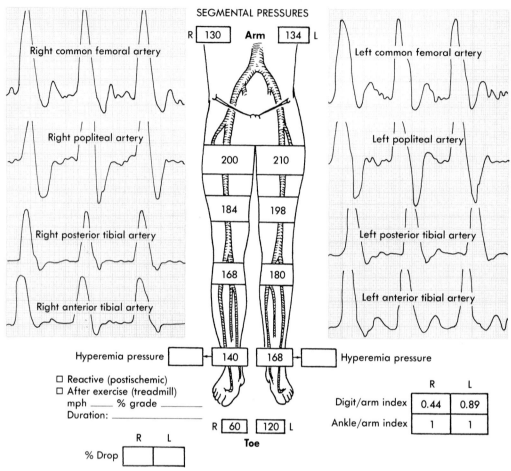

Figure 9–2 ■ Doppler waveforms in lower extremity of 62-year-old woman with type 2 diabetes who had ischemic changes in right great toe. Low toe pressure and normal ankle pressure confirm small-vessel disease of the great toe.

more than all American military fatalities in World War I, World War II, and Viet Nam combined. A clinical series from New Zealand found that cigarette smoking was noted two and one half times more frequently in diabetic patients with ischemia and gangrene as in a control series of persons without diabetes.[28] Kannel,[63] in a 26-year follow-up of the Framingham Study of 5,209 subjects, found that cigarette smoking together with impaired glucose tolerance and hypertension were powerful predisposing factors for PAD. The series of Beach and Strandness[8] on arteriosclerosis obliterans and associated risk factors in diabetics showed a high correlation between smoking and atherosclerosis. They found this to be one of the most important risk factors and presented evidence to show that the cessation of smoking was associated with a decrease in the progression of atherosclerosis. Cigarette smoking approximately

doubled the risk in both sexes. The impact was discernible into advanced age and was dose-related.[8] Smoking is atherogenic, decreases blood flow through vasospasm, and increases blood viscosity and clotting factors (Table 9–2).

Atherosclerotic involvement of the larger proximal vessels, the aorta and the iliac and femoral arteries, is accelerated by smoking. For example, we saw a 27-year-old patient with type 1 diabetes since age 5 years who had been a heavy smoker since age 13 years. At age 27 years severe intermittent claudication developed in his right leg. Vascular laboratory studies demonstrated a right superficial femoral artery obstruction (Fig 9–3). It was believed that his prolonged heavy smoking contributed significantly to the proximal artery atherosclerotic process. He required vascular surgery, which was successful. Despite warnings to stop smoking, he contin-

Table 9–2 ■ VASCULAR COMPLICATIONS OF SMOKING

Atherosclerosis	
↑	Carboxyhemoglobin
↑	Carbon monoxide
↑	Cholesterol
↑	Triglycerides
↑	Very low-density lipoproteins
↓	High-density lipoproteins
↓	Prostacyclin
↑	Truncal obesity
↑	Hypertension
↑	Albuminuria
Decreased blood flow	
↑	Vasospasm
↑	Hypercoagulability
↑	Viscosity
↓	Red blood cell deformability
Increased clotting	
↑	Thrombus formation
↑	Platelet aggregation
↑	Fibrinogen
↑	von Willebrand factor
↓	Plasminogen
↓	Plasminogen activator

ued. Two years later severe PAD developed in the left lower extremity. This time vascular surgery was unsuccessful, and the left leg was amputated. He continued to smoke. Angina developed, and the patient died of a massive myocardial infarction 2 years later at age 31 years. This young patient's inability to stop smoking is not unique. Ardron et al.[2] found conventional antismoking strategies to be completely ineffective in young diabetic subjects.

A final comment on smoking comes from the cigar-smoking Mark Twain's Aunt Mary, who said to him, "I beg you. I beseech you. I implore you, crush out that fatal habit."

Hypertension is a well-known risk factor for atherosclerosis. Approximately 2.5 million Americans have both diabetes and hypertension.[157] Hypertension, both systolic and diastolic, is a risk factor for PAD. The initial treatment of hypertension is a low-salt diet, weight reduction, and exercise. When these approaches are unsatisfactory, pharmacologic treatment is indicated. The older antihypertensive drugs, β-blockers, and diuretics, especially thiazides, may have an adverse effect on atherosclerosis. β-Blockers increase fasting blood glucose levels, hemoglobin A_{1c} (HbA$_{1c}$) levels, insulin levels, very low-density lipoprotein (VLDL) levels, triglyceride levels, and lower high-density lipo-

protein (HDL) levels. Thiazides, in high doses, increase blood glucose, cholesterol, LDL cholesterol, and triglyeride levels and insulin resistance. A report by Warram et al.[149] showed that the use of diuretics was associated with a higher degree of mortality than in patients receiving no antihypertensive treatment or antihypertensive drugs other than diuretics. Diuretics were associated with a fourfold risk for cardiovascular mortality in patients without proteinuria and a tenfold risk in those with proteinuria. Multivariate analysis revealed that diuretic therapy alone as treatment of hypertension was associated with increased risk for cardiovascular mortality in both the proteinuric and nonproteinuric groups, and especially those with proteinuria. Thiazides sometimes are indicated as an adjunct in the treatment of hypertension, but in these cases the dose should be low, not exceeding 12.5 to 25 mg/day. There is some evidence that thiazide therapy in low doses may be more effective in black patients. The antihypertensive drugs of choice for diabetics are angiotension converting enzyme (ACE) inhibitors.

There is no question that a strong correlation exists between hypercholesterolemia and cardiovascular disease. However, not all authorities have found a correlation between PAD and hypercholesterolemia.[58, 105] In most of these studies, triglyceride, LDL, and HDL levels were not reported. Laakso and Pyorala[67] have confirmed a strong relationship between total cholesterol and lipid abnormalities and PAD, as demonstrated by intermittent claudication in both type 1 and type 2 diabetes. They found that the total LDL cholesterol, VLDL, and triglyceride levels tended to be higher and HDL and HDL2 cholesterol levels to be lower in those patients with claudication. Therefore, control of cholesterol and lipid abnormalities should be as vigorous in patients with PAD as in those with coronary artery disease.

Hyperglycemia has been correlated with macrovascular disease.[105] Jensen-Urstad et al. reported that improved glucose control was related to slower development of atherosclerosis in people with diabetes.[59] The Diabetes Control and Complications Trial (DCCT) also showed a trend of macrovascular disease to be correlated with hyperglycemia.[145]

Hyperinsulinemia itself may be atherogenic by contributing to hypertension and

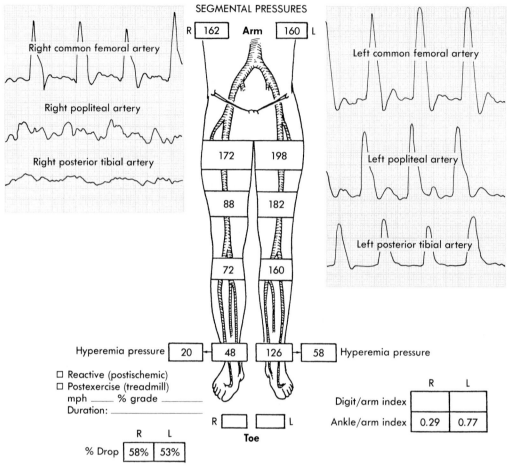

Figure 9–3 ▪ Severe PVD in 27-year-old man. Doppler pressures reveal evidence of right superficial femoral artery obstruction. Note blunted waveforms is right popliteal and right posterior tibial arteries, with ankle-arm index of only 0.29. Patient had been diabetic since age 5 years, and a heavy smoker since his early teens. He required right femoropopliteal Gore-Tex bypass graft. (Courtsey of Dr. Charles B. Anderson, St. Louis.)

dyslipidemia and by indirectly causing atherosclerotic changes in the arteries.

Adiposity, especially the fat distribution, is also a vascular risk factor. Distribution of body fat has been found to be an independent predictor of metabolic aberrations, including cardiovascular morbidity and mortality.[69] Abdominal or truncal obesity has been associated with hyperinsulinemia, hypertriglyceridemia, hypertension, and decreased HDL levels.[53] An excellent review of the reasons why abdominal fat may relate to insulin resistance has been reported by Bjorntorp.[9] Peiris et al.[115] measured intra-abdominal fat using computed tomography (CT). They found that intra-abdominal fat deposition constitutes greater cardiovascular risk than obesity alone. They also reached the conclusion that hyperinsulinemia is associated with abdominal obesity and is an important component of increased vascular risk associated with abdominal obesity. Kaplan[64] has aptly termed the deadly quartet as upper body obesity, glucose intolerance, hypertriglyceridemia, and hypertension.

A cluster of variables—resistance to insulin-stimulated glucose uptake, glucose intolerance, hyperinsulinemia, increased VLDL triglyceride levels, decreased HDL, cholesterol levels, and hypertension—have been termed syndrome X by Reaven.[122] These factors may be of enormous importance in the pathogenesis of macrovascular disease. Proteinuria is also an established macrovascular risk factor.

Another serious risk associated with diabetes and vascular disease is a tendency for increased coagulability and thrombosis.

McGill et al.[97] have shown a threefold increase in tissue plasminogen activator (t-PA) inhibitor type 1 in obese and diabetic subjects compared with lean control subjects. Hyperinsulinemia is common in obesity and type 2 diabetes and may be an important factor in increasing t-PA inhibitor in type 1.

Gangrene of the Toes

Gangrene of the toes can result from atherosclerosis with thrombosis, and microthrombi formation resulting from infection. Microthrombi secondary to infection can convert the small vessels in the toes to end-arteries with resultant gangrene (see Chapter 23). Cholesterol emboli and drugs that decrease blood flow can also result in gangrene. The classic blue toe syndrome[21, 109, 112] is caused by cholesterol emboli that break off from ulcerated atheromatous plaques in the proximal larger vessels. The toe takes on a deep purplish color, and gangrene can develop. Cholesterol emboli to the foot result in painful petechiae, a livedo reticularis pattern of the skin due to embolization of the arterioles in the skin. The atheromatous plaques may be present in the aorta, iliac artery, or more distant vessels. The syndrome is characterized by the sudden onset of pain in the toe or foot. Leg and thigh myalgia may be present if muscular arteries are involved. When digital artery blood flow becomes sluggish, the toe becomes bluish purple. A sharp demarcation frequently occurs between normally perfused skin and ischemic areas. Some patients who develop the blue toe syndrome have received anticoagulation therapy with warfarin.[100] Thrombolytic therapy with streptokinase[120] and t-PA[132] can also result in the blue toe syndrome. Therefore, it is extremely important to check the toes and feet of patients receiving anticoagulants or thrombolytic therapy.

Repeated attacks of acute ischemic changes in the toes occurring bilaterally suggest that the ulcerated atherosclerotic plaque is in the aorta. The development of painful cyanotic toes, myalgias, painful petechia, and a livedo reticularis pattern of skin strongly suggests microemboli. Plate 11 shows purplish discoloration of the right fifth toe and a livedo reticularis pattern on the sole of the foot in a 60-year-old man with a painful, cyanotic fifth toe on his right foot and painful petechial lesions on both feet. These did not blanch on compression. He also complained of myalgias of the lower extremities. An arteriogram (Fig. 9–4) showed a large atheromatous plaque in the left lateral wall of the infrarenal portion of the aorta with ulceration; the ulcerated plaque was removed successfully. The treatment in such cases is vascular surgery with removal of the plaque, thereby preventing further embolization.

Certain drugs can cause gangrenous changes in the toes. Vasopressors frequently are used to treat shock. Because of the norepinephrine-like and vasoconstriction effects of these agents, ischemic gangrene can develop in the toes and feet. Pressure agents should be used with caution, in as low a dose as possible. If a patient is in shock, the risk/benefit ratio will dictate the use of this family of drugs despite the peripheral vascular risks. However, the feet of these patients must be observed daily. Plate 12 shows gangrene of the toes and forefoot of a 40-year-old patient who developed shock secondary to sepsis. He required pressor agents and unfortunately developed gangrene of all of his toes and fingers.

Peripheral circulation can also be impaired by β-blockers, which are commonly used for treatment of angina and hypertension and after myocardial infraction. Zacharias et al.[160] found peripheral vascular complications to be a side effect in 22 of 305 patients given a β-blocker. This mechanism appears to result from unopposed α-vasoconstriction subsequent to β-blockade.

Signs and Symptoms of PAD

The signs and symptoms of PAD are listed in Table 9–3.

Intermittent claudication is a common symptom of PAD. It was originally described by veterinary surgeons as a disease of horses. The first case of intermittent claudication in humans was described by Charcot in 1858.[19] The word "claudication" comes from the Latin word *claudicatio,* meaning to limp, but patients with claudication do not limp; they stop to rest. The pain associated with intermittent claudication is characterized by cramping or aching, most often in the calf. It occurs with walking, and is relieved when the person stops walking, without the need to sit down. The ischemic pain of intermittent claudication must be differentiated from similar pain that may also be induced by walking

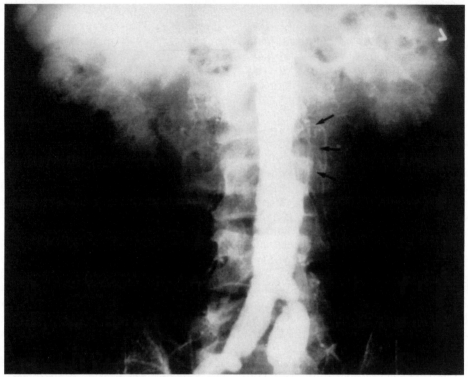

Figure 9–4 ■ Arteriogram shows large filling defect caused by an atheroscleromatous plaque of the aorta just inferior to the renal artery in a patient with evidence of cholesterol emboli to the foot (see Plate 11). (Courtesy of Georgio Sicard, M.D., St. Louis.)

but is caused by arthritis, muscle pain, radicular pain, spinal cord compression, thrombophlebitis, anemia, and/or myxedema. This is referred to as pseudoclaudication. Patients with diabetes may have significant PAD without symptoms of claudication because peripheral neuropathy has led to loss of pain sensation.

Table 9–3 ■ SIGNS AND SYMPTOMS OF PAD

Intermittent claudication
Cold feet
Nocturnal pain
Rest pain
Nocturnal and rest pain relieved with dependency
Absent pulses
Blanching on elevation
Delayed venous filling after elevation
Dependent rubor
Atrophy of subcutaneous fatty tissues
Shiny appearance of skin
Loss of hair on foot and toes
Thickened nails, often with fungal infection
Gangrene
Miscellaneous: blue toe syndrome, acute vascular occlusion

Pseudoclaudication can also be relieved by rest. However, pain associated with pseudoclaudication usually takes longer to disappear. To obtain relief, these patients usually need to sit down and/or change position. Thus, nonischemic causes of intermittent claudication must be considered in the differential diagnosis of leg pain associated with walking. Intermittent claudication most commonly occurs as calf pain, but higher vascular obstruction (e.g., in the aorta) will cause pain in the buttocks and upper thighs and frequently is accompanied by impotence. This is known as Leriche's syndrome. Obstruction of the iliac arteries will cause pain in the lower thigh.

The symptoms of intermittent claudication depend on ischemia in the muscle. Thus, despite extensive involvement of the small vessels in the diabetic foot, symptoms of claudication in the foot may be infrequent because of the small muscle mass. Some investigators believe that claudication does not occur in the foot. Pain occurs after a shorter distance if a person is walking uphill, walking on a hard surface, or walking fast. Persons with progressive intermittent claudication note that over time they are able to walk a shorter distance before the discomfort develops.

Examination of the patient with intermittent claudication involving the calf muscle may reveal both femoral and pedal pulses but no popliteal pulse. The pedal pulses are present because of the collateral arteries. After the patient takes a brisk walk the foot will become pale and pulseless because the blood bypasses the skin of the foot and flows to the skeletal muscles of the calf instead. Intermittent claudication usually results from a single arterial block. However, because of multiple-vessel involvement in the diabetic, several blocks may be present.

Among the several approaches to the treatment of intermittent claudication, the most important is cessation of smoking; the next is walking. Jonason et al.[61] demonstrated the beneficial effects of a supervised training and exercise program in patients with intermittent claudication. Patients with angina were limited in their ability to participate in the program. A minimum of 3 months of training was required to achieve maximum improvement.

Exercise is the cornerstone of conservative management. A regular walking program will improve distance in 80% of the patients. Although leg exercises may be helpful, walking is the best exercise. Bicycling is probably less beneficial, because it exercises the thigh muscles more than the calf muscles. A good walking program consists of a definite daily walking routine over and above normal activities. The exercise can be divided to suit the patient's daily schedule, but a physician should supervise the program.

Surgery is rarely indicated as therapy for intermittent claudication, and then only if the patient is severely disabled. The strongest indication would be for persons whose livelihood depends on walking (e.g., mail carriers). The long-term outlook for the extremity with intermittent claudication is good and in most patients the condition will stay the same or actually improve. However, the long-term outlook for the patient with intermittent claudication is not good because atherosclerosis in the lower extremity is strongly correlated with coronary artery disease and stroke.

Barzilay et al. found lower extremity arterial disease to be an independent risk factor for mortality among all the diabetic patients who had coronary artery disease.[14] There-fore, any patient with lower extremity artery disease must be carefully examined for the presence of coronary, carotid, or aortic vascular disease.

Cold feet are a common complaint in patients with peripheral vascular insufficiency, prompting them to use hot water bottles, heating pads, and hot water soaks. These practices can result in severe burns to a foot that has become insensitive to heat because of peripheral neuropathy. Rest pain usually indicates at least two hemodynamically significant arterial blocks in a series. Rest pain is persistent pain caused by nerve ischemia. It has peaks of intensity, is worse at night, and may require the use of narcotics for relief. Rest pain decreases with dependency of the lower extremities and is aggravated by heat, elevation, and exercise. Nocturnal ischemic pain is a form of ischemic neuritis that usually precedes rest pain. It occurs at night because during sleep the circulation is essentially of the core variety, with decreased perfusion of the lower extremity. The resulting ischemic neuritis becomes intense and disrupts sleep. The patient invariably gains relief by standing up or dangling the feet over the edge of the bed, and on occasion by walking a few steps. This increases cardiac output, leading to improved perfusion of the lower extremities and relief of ischemic neuritis. If the lesions that produce nocturnal and rest pain are not corrected by vascular surgery, tissue necrosis and gangrene are likely to develop, necessitating amputation. Rest pain and nocturnal pain therefore are indications for vascular surgery to relieve arterial occlusions. In the diabetic, rest and nocturnal pain may be absent despite severe ischemia because diabetic neuropathy has destroyed the sensory perception of pain.

Diabetic neuropathy or vascular insufficiency may cause severe pain in the legs at night. To differentiate the two, keep in mind that the diabetic with vascular disease gets relief by sitting up and dangling the legs. Walking more than a few feet makes the pain worse. The patient with neuropathic pain tends to get relief by walking.

If the popliteal area is obstructed, there may be a difference in skin temperature in the two patellar areas. The skin around the knee on the ischemic side often is warmer, due to collateral vessels that form around the obstructed popliteal artery.[27]

Pallor of the foot on elevation and delayed venous capillary filling is indicative of isch-

Table 9–4 ■ CAPILLARY FILLING TIME ON DEPENDENCY

Normal: 10–15 sec
Moderate ischemia: 15–25 sec
Severe ischemia: 25–40 sec
Very severe ischemia: ≥40 sec

emia. With the patient in the supine position, the feet are elevated to a 45-degree angle and held in this position until one or both feet blanch. The patient is then instructed to sit upright with the feet in a dependent position. Normally the venous and capillary filling time is less than 15 seconds; it can be prolonged to minutes in the severely ischemic extremity. A capillary venous filling time of more than 40 seconds indicates very severe ischemia (Table 9–4).

The extremity with severe PAD will develop rubor after dependency. Patients with varicose veins also may have dependent rubor because of venous stasis. Pallor on elevation, prolonged filling time, and dependent rubor are the hallmarks of significant lower extremity vascular insufficiency.

Ischemic skin changes are characterized by shiny atrophic cool skin, loss of hair on the dorsum of the foot and toes, thickening of the nails, and frequently fungal infections. The nails tend to grow more slowly when the blood supply is decreased. As further ischemia develops, the subcutaneous tissue atrophies. The skin appears shiny and tightly drawn over the foot. Ulceration in these vulnerable feet may occur from minor trauma (Fig. 9–5).

Peripheral arterial disease contributes to amputation by impeding the delivery of oxygen, nutrients (necessary for wound healing), and antibiotics to fight infection. Taylor and Porter[144] reported that aggressive therapy with debridement, antibiotic therapy and, when indicated, revascularization resulted in long-term salvage of 73% of threatened limbs even in high-risk patients. Eradication of infection and wound healing is unlikely if the ABI is less than 0.45 or the $TcPo_2$ is less than 30 mm Hg. If $TcPo_2$ is less than 20 mm Hg, healing is very unlikely.

Acute Occlusion

In the diabetic patient most ischemic changes occur slowly, although sudden occlu-

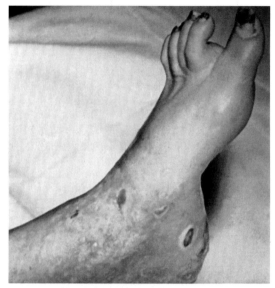

Figure 9–5 ■ Classic diabetic foot with ischemic skin changes: atrophy of subcutaneous tissues, hair loss on dorsum of foot, thickening of nails, atrophy of interosseus muscles resulting in cocked-up toes, and commonly seen superficial ulcerations. (Courtsey of John F. Flarbaim II, M.D., Rochestar, MN, and The Upjohn Company, Kalamazoo, MI.)

sion from emboli or acute complete thrombosis can occur. Most emboli (>70%) originate in the heart. The most common underlying cardiac pathologic condition is atrial fibrillation. Myocardial infarction with mural thrombi is the second most common cause. Acute thrombosis has atherosclerosis as the underlying cause. The signs and symptoms of acute arterial occlusion usually are referred to as the "five Ps" (Table 9–5). The leg becomes pale and may appear waxy. Paresthesias and numbness are common. The patient may have sudden weakness in the leg, and on physical examination, pallor, paralysis, and pulselessness below the block are noted. Most sudden occlusions are the result of emboli. The extent of ischemia and final outcome depend on collateral circulation, size, clot location, and the time between on-

Table 9–5 ■ "FIVE Ps" OF ACUTE ARTERIAL OCCLUSION IN LOWER EXTREMITY

Pain: sudden onset
Pallor: waxy
Paresthesias: numbness
Pulselessness: no pulse below block
Paralysis: sudden weakness

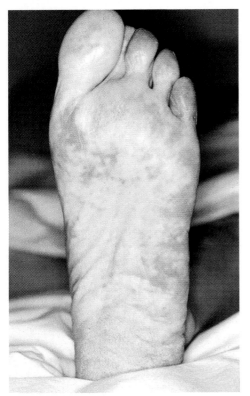

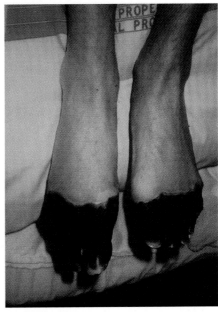

Plate 12 ■ Gangrene in forefoot secondary to use of a pressor agent in a 40-year-old patient who was in shock secondary to sepsis.

Plate 11 ■ Cyanotic changes in the fifth toe and livedo reticularis pattern on the foot secondary to cholesterol emboli from atheroscleromatous plaque (see Fig. 2–4). (Courtesy of Gregorio Sicard, M.D., St. Louis.)

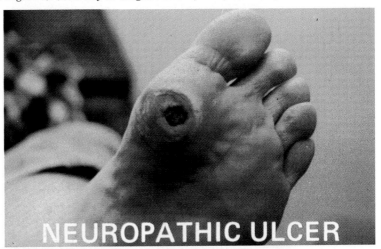

Plate 13 ■ Classic neuropathic diabetic foot ulcer. Note ulceration in callus is well-circumscribed. Lesion is painless. (From the Michigan Diabetes Research and Training Center, University of Michigan, Ann Arbor, 1983, with permission.)

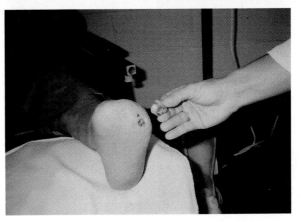

Plate 14 ■ A plantar ulcer resulting from a patient with severe peripheral neuropathy who wore his hearing aid in his shoe. (Courtesy of Susan Graddy, R.N., B.S.N.)

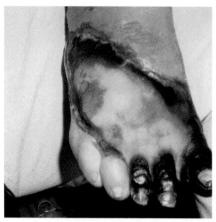

Plate 15 ■ Diabetic patient with peripheral neuropathy and an insensate foot. Cold packs were applied to her foot for treatment of a sprain. She developed frostbite and required a transmetatarsal amputation.

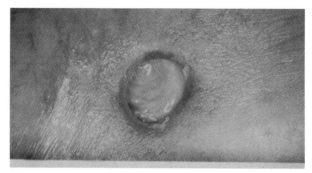

Plate 16 ■ Ischemic ulcer. Note the punched-out appearance. An ischemic ulcer occurs at the tip of the toes or, as in this case, around the ankle, and is very painful.

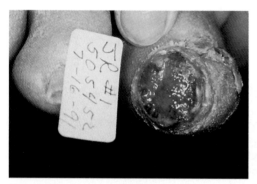

Plate 17 ■ Amelanotic ulcer at the tip of a toe (Courtesy J. Jeffrey Ruegemer, M.D., Edina, MN.)

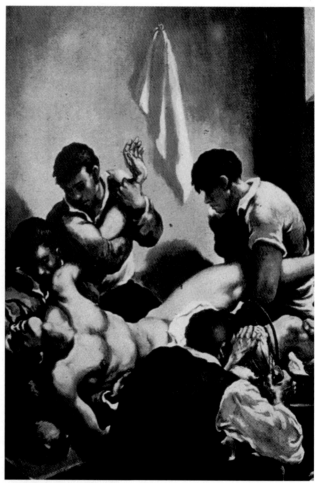

Plate 19 ■ Painting depicts agonies of patient undergoing amputation in ancient times. Amputations were performed with only alcohol as anesthetic. Many patients died during this guillotine operation; some even died of shock and terror before the operation began! Teamwork today should be geared to saving, not removing, the leg. *(Painting by Italian Count Gregorio Calvi de Bergolo in 1953. From the International Museum of Surgical Sciences and Hall of Fame, International College of Surgeons, Chicago.)*

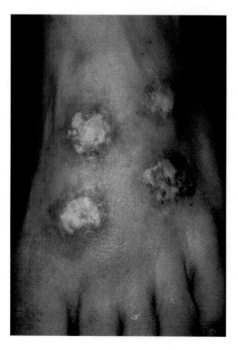

Plate 18 ■ Factitial ulcers. (Courtesy of Arthur Z. Eisen, M.D., St. Louis, MO.)

set of acute occlusion and treatment. These occlusions must be treated as soon as possible because peripheral nerve and skeletal muscles have less resistance to ischemia than does skin and bone. Irreversible changes of skeletal muscle and peripheral nerves may occur after 4 to 6 hours of severe ischemia. The skin may tolerate severe ischemia for 10 hours. Pallor is usually more severe with embolism than with thrombosis. With embolism the effected extremity is waxlike and lemon yellow. With thrombosis the extremity appears less cadaverous and tends to be somewhat cyanotic. Paresthesias are caused by peripheral nerve ischemia. Treatment of sudden arterial occlusion requires surgical intervention or thrombolytic therapy.

A detailed discussion of the pathogenesis of atherosclerosis can be found in Chapter 4.

Peripheral Neuropathy

The first description of the manifestations of diabetic neuropathy was made by Marchel de Calvi[92] in 1864. More than 130 years later, despite much research and many publications, the exact cause of diabetic neuropathy remains unexplained. The pathogenesis is multifactorial. Decreased blood flow in the vasonervorum caused by vascular narrowing of the vessel or increased blood viscosity is a factor. Another possible factor under investigation is the trapping of immunoglobulins on peripheral nerve myelin.[16] This does not occur in the brain, and may account for the fact that rarely is there central nervous system (CNS) neuropathy.[16] Metabolic change probably is the most significant factor.[114] A detailed discussion of the pathogenesis and treatment of diabetic neuropathy is found in Chapter 3.

The most important and most common complication leading to ulceration, and ultimately to amputation, is the loss of protective sensation resulting from PN.

Amputation is the result of either a single factor or a combination of factors. Pecoraro and colleagues[114] found that 81% of the amputations were the result of faulty wound healing, 84% were from ulceration, 55% were from gangrene, and 81% were from initial minor trauma. In 36% of the cases, ill-fitting shoes were a precipitating factor leading to cutaneous ulceration, infection and, ultimately, amputation.

A number of syndromes affecting the foot and leg are associated with diabetic neuropathy. The most common of these involving the foot are distal symmetric sensorimotor polyneuropathies, resulting in pain, paresthesias, muscle atrophy, and loss of sensation. Autonomic neuropathy leads to dry, scaly feet. Radiculopathy due to thrombosis of the vasonervorum leads to unilateral leg pain and weakness. Entrapment syndromes are common in the diabetic. An important entrapment syndrome affecting the foot is the tarsal tunnel syndrome. This syndrome results from compression of the posterior tibial nerve at the tarsal tunnel, causing sensory impairment in the sole of the foot and weakness of the intrinsic pedal musculature. Tarsal tunnel syndrome usually occurs unilaterally, which differentiates it from metabolic bilateral symmetric polyneuropathy. Symptoms include burning pain and paresthesias at the ankle and plantar surface of the foot.[1]

Peripheral neuropathy in diabetic patients is not always due to the diabetes; other causes include alcoholism, herniated nucleus pulposus, heavy metals, vitamin deficiencies, collagen disease, pernicious anemia, malignancy, pressure neuropathy, uremia, porphyria, Hansen's disease (leprosy), and drugs. Malignancies may cause peripheral neuropathy by humoral effect or by nerve compression. Recently we saw a woman with diabetes and peripheral neuropathy. The neuropathy was unilateral, which is atypical. Since diabetic PN is primarily due to abnormal metabolism in the nerve, it is therefore bilateral. Further evaluation revealed a meningioma of the spinal cord. Treatment for diabetic PN in this patient would have resulted in a missed diagnosis.

As noted in Figure 9–1, neuropathy ultimately can result in amputation through various pathways including loss of autonomic, sensory, or motor nerve function. Autonomic involvement results in decreased perspiration. This leads to dryness, cracking, and fissures of the skin, which can be portals of entry for bacteria. Autonomic dysfunction also can lead to loss of the flare reaction.[110] Any noxious stimuli to the skin results in increased blood flow. In the diabetic this effect can be blunted, thereby impeding blood flow to the wound or infected area.

Painless mechanical trauma can occur from a variety of causes. The most common is walking. The repetitive stress of walking results in callus buildup and hot spots. Be-

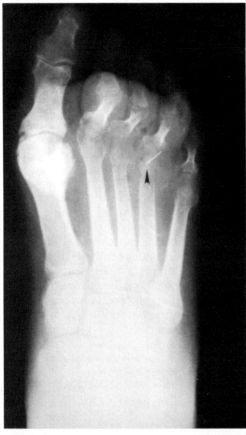

Figure 9-6 ■ Carpenter's nail present for approximately 1 month in tissues of foot of an insulin-requiring diabetic patient. He had no knowledge of having stepped on this nail, nor did he have any pain or discomfort. (Courtesy of Dr. J. Joseph Marr, President and Chief Executive Officer of ImmuLogic Pharmaceutical Corporation, Waltham, MA.)

cause there is no pain, the patient continues to walk. Callus builds up, and ischemic pressure necrosis and ulceration result (Plate 13). Abnormally high pressures, especially on the plantar surface of the forefoot, have been found in these ulcerated feet.[12]

Trauma from painless puncture wounds is not rare. Figure 9-6 shows a carpenter's nail deep in the tissues of the foot of a 45-year-old who had required insulin for 10 years. He had a small, painless draining area on his foot for approximately 1 month, and sought medical attention only because the area had failed to heal. The dorsalis pedis and posterior tibial pulses were of good quality; however, vibratory sensation to pain and touch was markedly diminished. Radiographs of the foot revealed the carpenter's nail, which must have been present for at least a month without any discomfort to the patient. The area involved had caused severe osteomyelitis, and the foot ultimately was amputated.

I agree with Dr. Paul Brand, who stated that the diabetic who claims his/her shoes are killing him/her may well be right. Painless ulceration from ill-fitting shoes may become infected; gangrene may follow, and amputation may be necessary. Ulcers caused by ill-fitting shoes occur most often on the side of the foot (Fig. 9-7). The number of foreign objects found in patients' shoes that they have walked on without pain or awareness is legend, and includes pebbles, coins, and large objects such as doll chairs (Fig. 9-8) and shoehorns (Fig 9-9). Plate 14 shows an ulcer of a foot, resulting from the patient walking on a hearing aid that had found its

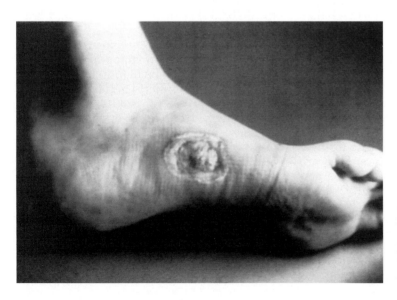

Figure 9-7 ■ Ulceration on the side of the foot, suggestive of ill-fitting shoe. (From Levin ME: Diabetic foot lesions. In Young JR, Graor RA, Olin JW, et al [eds]: Peripheral Vascular Diseases. St. Louis: Mosby–Year Book, 1991, with permission.)

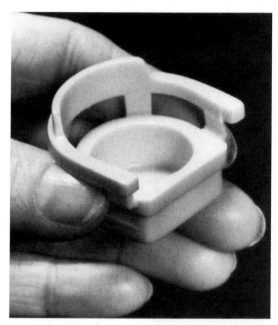

Figure 9–8 ■ Doll's chair measuring 2.5 × 3.8 cm found in patient's shoe. He had worn the shoe all day without being aware of the chair's presence because of almost total absence of sensory perception produced by severe diabetic neuropathy.

way into his shoe. He was totally unaware of its presence.

Another extreme example of painless trauma is noted in Figure 9–10A, which shows ulceration over the Achilles tendon of a patient who kept the back of his heel against a chair while on jury duty. Blisters developed, which ulcerated and penetrated to the Achilles tendon. The patient's physician advised using a bandage and returning to work. Fortunately, the patient sought a second opinion. A skin graft flap procedure was done (Fig. 9–10B) and the ulceration

healed (Fig. 9–10C). This type of surgery affirms the benefit of having a plastic surgeon as a team member caring for patients with diabetes.

A common cause of painless injury results from home surgery. Because persons with diabetic neuropathy feel no pain, they frequently cut their calluses too deep and their nails too short, resulting in ulceration and infection. Figure 9–11 shows an infected and gangrenous great toe that resulted when a patient practiced home surgery. Even though she was partially blind, she attempted to cut the nail, and in doing so, cut into the tissue. This resulted in infection and gangrene, which necessitated amputation of her great toe.

Chemical trauma results from the use of callus and corn removers, and also has occurred from soaking the feet in chemical solutions and strong antiseptics.

Thermal injuries are common in the insensitive diabetic foot. Figure 9–12 shows gangrene of the toes of a diabetic who had soaked his cold foot in a bucket of hot water. The patient had good dorsalis pedis and posterior tibial pulses, and transmetatarsal amputation was successful. Severe burns have occurred in patients with insensitive feet who have walked on hot sandy beaches or other hot surfaces. We have seen a number of these patients ultimately require amputation of the feet. Diabetic patients going to the beach or to swimming pools should wear protective footwear. Not uncommonly, patients who have placed their feet in front of the fireplace to warm them have sustained severe burns. Perhaps the most dramatic case of painless thermal injury that I have seen was in a diabetic patient who had had a previous

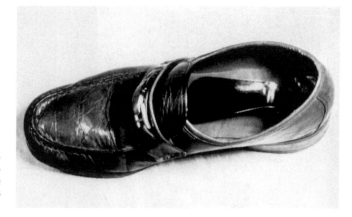

Figure 9–9 ■ Shoehorn in shoe worn by patient who, because of insensitive foot resulting from diabetic neuropathy, was unaware of its presence until removing the shoe at end of day.

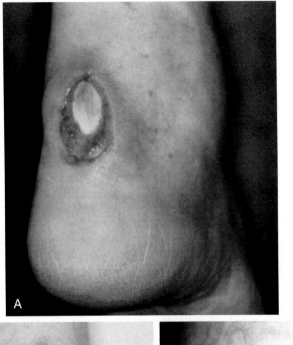

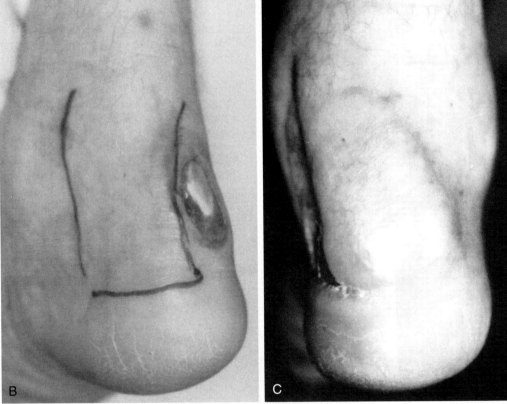

Figure 9–10 ■ *A,* Ulceration resulting from breakdown of painless blisters that penetrated to the Achilles tendon. *B,* Outline of skin flap for treatment of ulceration. *C,* Healed skin flap graft. (Courtesy of Leroy Young, M.D., St. Louis.)

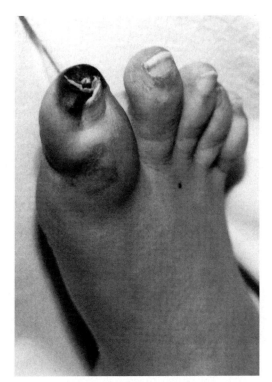

Figure 9–11 ■ Gangrenous toe resulting from patient's attempt at home surgery. Toenail was cut too short and became infected, and gangrene developed.

below-knee amputation. He had purchased a riding lawn mower, and in positioning the good leg, inadvertently placed it on the manifold, which became extremely hot. Only when he smelled something burning did he look down to discover that his shoe and foot were on fire. Subsequent amputation of his remaining foot was necessary.

Plate 15 shows a gangrenous foot lesion in a 58-year-old diabetic woman with longstanding type 2 diabetes, peripheral neuropathy, and loss of protective sensation who, because of a sprained foot, had cold packs applied to her foot and ankle. This figure shows gangrenous changes in the toes and forefoot, the result of application of the ice pack with subsequent frostbite. This woman required a midfoot amputation. Thus, it is important to avoid extremes of temperature, both hot and cold, in people with diabetes, peripheral neuropathy, and loss of protective sensation.

When examining diabetic patients, it is very important to observe the patient's gait. Gait abnormalities are common due to peripheral neuropathy. An abnormal gait can cause falling, foot injury, and abnormal pressure on the foot.[65] Physicians frequently do not notice the patient's gait because the patient is usually seated in the examination room when the physician arrives and departs

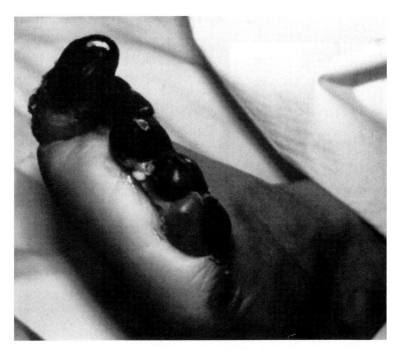

Figure 9–12 ■ Gangrene in toes of patient who had soaked his cold foot in hot water.

before the patient leaves the room. Evidence of an abnormal gait can sometimes be detected by checking the patient's shoes for unusual wearing patterns.

The least expensive and easiest method of testing for PN and loss of protective sensation is with the monofilament (Fig. 9–13). A 5.07 monofilament is applied to various areas of the foot. The examiner applies pressure on the monofilament until it buckles. This pressure equals 10 gm of linear strength. A patient's inability to feel the monofilament on buckling indicates loss of protective sensation. The monofiliment should not be applied to a callus.

Foot Deformities

Muscle atrophy caused by involvement of the motor nerves leads to an imbalance of the interosseous muscles in the foot. This frequently leads to cocked-up toes. Ulceration may occur on the tips and tops of the toes. I refer to this as tip-top-toe ulcer syndrome. Because of thinning or shifting of the fat pads underneath the metatarsophalangeal joints, ulceration may occur in these areas as well (Fig. 9–14). Prevention of ulceration in these areas requires straightening of these cocked-up, claw, or hammer toes at a time when circulation is good. However, if this cannot be done, it is important to make sure the toe box of the

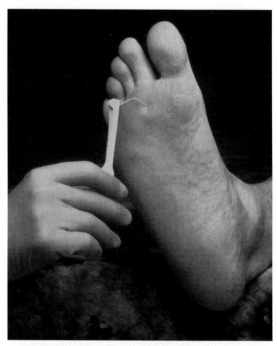

Figure 9–13 ■ The Semmes-Weinstein monofilament. The 5.07 monfilament is pressed against the skin until it buckles. This equals 10 gm of linear pressure. If the patient cannot feel this buckled monofilament, he or she has lost protective sensation. (Courtesy Curative Health Services, Hauppauge, NY.)

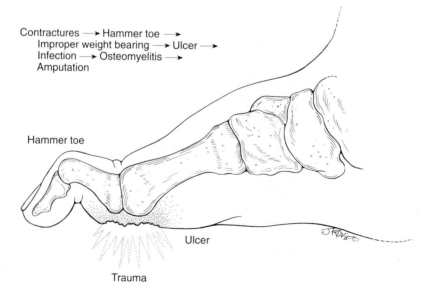

Figure 9–14 ■ Progression of contractures leading to hammer toes, improper weight bearing, ulceration, infection, and osteomyelitis. Because ulcerations can occur at tip and on top of toe, I refer to this as tip-top-toe ulcer syndrome. (From the Michigan Diabetes Research and Training Center, University of Michigan, Ann Arbor, 1983, with permission.)

shoe is large enough to accommodate the top of these deformed toes. Cushioned insoles should be worn to protect the planter tips of the toes and the metatarsophalangeal areas.

The most extreme example of diabetic foot deformity is the Charcot foot, or neuroarthropathy. Classically, the Charcot foot at its onset is hot, erythematous, and swollen, with bounding pulses and prominent veins. Despite what has been written in some textbooks, patients with Charcot foot frequently have moderate pain and discomfort. The patient frequently gives a history of mild trauma to the foot having occurred in the preceding week. It may be difficult to differentiate the warm, red Charcot foot from cellulitis. However, the patient with Charcot foot is afebrile and the white blood cell (WBC) count normal. The sedimentation rate may be slightly elevated. With cellulitis, there is usually a portal of entry for bacteria. A neuropathic component of the Charcot foot probably stems from involvement of the autonomic nervous system. The result is the equivalent of sympathectomy to the arteries in the foot. The arteries dilate, and arteriovenous (AV) shunts have been demonstrated in these feet.[13] X-ray examination in the acute stage usually reveals no bony abnormality (Fig. 9–15A). If the patient continues to walk, there can be gradual dissolution and fragmentation of the distal ends of the metatarsals (Fig. 9–15B) and the ankle bones. The distal ends of the meta-

tarsals become pointed, the peppermint stick sign, as if the ends of the bones were licked away. X-ray films also show the absence of calcification in the interosseous arteries, further evidence that, as a rule, there is no significant vascular insufficiency. It is believed that the increased circulation causes resorption of the bone. Evidence that increased circulation contributes to Charcot foot has been suggested by the report of Edelman et al.[38] These authors reported three cases of deformed Charcot foot that developed after successful peripheral vascular surgery. These cases demonstrate the important role of increased blood flow in the absorption of calcium from the bones in the foot, their collapse, and the development of the deformed Charcot foot. Because there is relative insensitivity in these feet, patients continue to walk, subsequently developing stress fractures and further bone destruction. Treatment in the acute stage is non–weight bearing, frequently with the aid of a contact cast or other non–weight-bearing devices. If the process is allowed to progress, fractures develop and the arch collapses, and the foot becomes inverted and shortened and takes on a clubfoot shape. The arch is lost and the foot takes on a rocker bottom configuration (Fig. 9–16A). Maximum pressure now occurs at the plantar surface of the arch. This area breaks down and becomes ulcerated (Fig. 9–16B). The plantar surface of the arch is the classic site of ulceration in Charcot's foot.

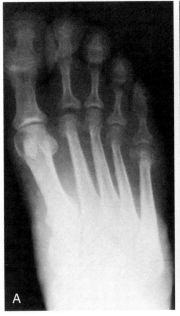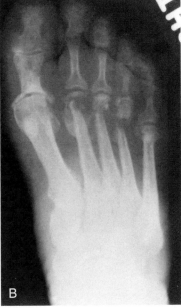

Figure 9–15 ■ A, Radiograph of the foot of a 60-year-old with known diabetes of 4 years' duration who presented with acute Charcot foot. B, Same foot 3 months later shows classic osteolytic bone changes of diabetic-osteoneuropathy involving the distal segment of the metatarsals and the ankle. (Courtesy of Robert Karsh, M.D., St. Louis.)

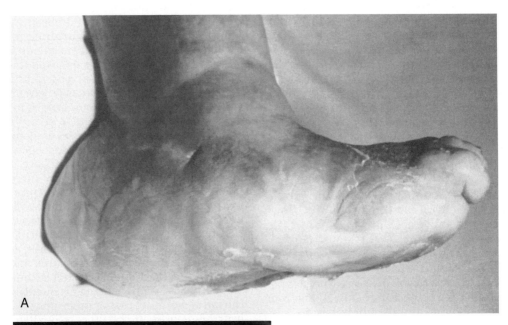

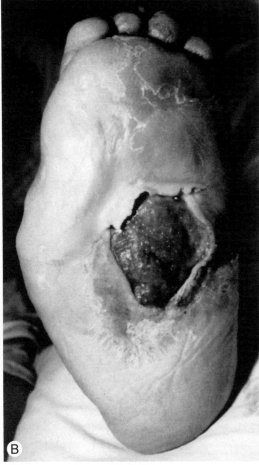

Figure 9–16 ■ Charcot foot. *A,* Note clubfoot appearance, with collapse of tarsal
metatarsal joints. *B,* Massive ulcer on plantar surface of arch. (From Levin ME: Pathophysiology of diabetic foot lesions. *In* Davidson J [ed]: Clinical Diabetes Mellitus: A
Problem-Oriented Approach. New York:
Thieme Medical Publishers, 1986, with permission.)

The treatment for Charcot foot is primarily non–weight bearing and supportive. However, a report by Selby et al. has shown that diphosphonate, pamidronate, can decrease the inflammation.[130]

Immobilization of the Charcot foot is usually needed for a minimum of 8 to 12 weeks.[39, 153] However, a longer period of time is not uncommon. If conservative methods fail and fractures and deformities develop, surgery can be another approach.[60]

Infection

Infection is the third major factor in the pathogenesis of diabetic foot lesions and, when associated with ischemia, frequently leads to amputation. Infections can lead to loss of a patient or a larger part of him.[133] If sepsis develops, the patient may require immediate amputation and/or death may result.

Breaks in the skin, which may be almost imperceptible (e.g., cracks, fissures in calluses), and major wounds such as neurotrophic foot ulcers, puncture wounds, or skin abrasion from trauma provide portals of entry for bacteria. A variety of factors contribute to the diabetic's difficulty in handling infection. In the nondiabetic, infection leads to increased blood flow. In the diabetic, however, infection frequently leads to microthrombi formation in the small arterioles, which further impairs circulation. When this occurs in the small arteries of the toes, the vessels can convert to end-arteries, resulting in gangrene of the toes (see Chapter 23). Vascular disease impairs the delivery of antibiotics and oxygen to the infected areas. Leukocyte function necessary to fight infection is frequently impaired, with defective adherence, diapedesis, chemotaxis, phagocytosis, and microbicidal activity, particularly in patients with uncontrolled diabetes and ketosis.

Puncture wounds of the foot are common in diabetics. Laverly et al. showed that puncture wounds in diabetics were polymicrobial and that resulting osteomyelitis was also polymicrobial. The puncture wounds of diabetics frequently have delayed treatment, probably because there is decreased sensation and the patient does not immediately seek care.[70]

Infection results in increased blood flow locally. This is called a flare reaction. However, the vasodilatory microcirculation in type 1 and type 2 diabetics can be impaired as evidenced by blunted dilatory response to heat and/or injury to the foot.[121, 147]

Successful treatment of infection requires debridement, removing all necrotic material, anaerobic and aerobic cultures and sensitivities, appropriate antibiotics, recognition of osteomyelitis, appropriate treatment, and when indicated consultation with an infectious disease expert (see Chapter 22).

Osteomyelitis can be very difficult to diagnose. Newman et al. found that the diagnosis of proven osteomyelitis was missed in two thirds of bone culture–proven osteomyelitis.[106] Furthermore, primary care physicians rely too heavily on plain x-rays.[37] Grayson et al. have shown, in a high percentage of cases, that simply probing to bone can make the diagnosis of osteomyelitis in 85% of the cases.[51] Scanning techniques for osteomyelitis are not always successful. The triple-phase scan with technetium lacks specificity.[84] Magnetic resonance imaging (MRI) is proving to be a helpful technique[33] (see Chapter 15). Conservative surgery for osteomyelitis contributes to an increased healing rate of foot ulcers with osteomyelitis compared with medical treatment alone.[54] Conservative surgery was defined as a limited resection of the infected part of phalanx or metatarsal bone under the wound.[54]

A new addition to the armamentarium for fighting infection has been suggested by Gough et al. They used granulocyte colony-stimulating factor (G-CSF) to increase the WBC count. The patients in the G-CSF group did better than the placebo group in resolution of cellulitis.[50]

Special Diabetic Foot Problems in the Heel

The heel of the diabetic foot is particularly vulnerable to trauma. The heel is exposed to a great deal of pressure, resulting in callus buildup. As the callus becomes thicker it tends to crack, and becomes a site of infection. When the heel is infected, the infection tends to penetrate deeply. The skin of the heel is tightly bound by numerous vertical septa extending through the subcutaneous tissue to the surface of the calcaneous. These septa result in formation of small cylinders packed with fatty tissue. These small fat-containing tubes act like shock absorbers on heel impact. With ischemic changes there is atrophy of the subcutaneous fatty tissue, thus decreasing the effectiveness of the shock absorber effect. When the skin covering the heel is destroyed, much of the subcutaneous fat colliquates and the septa are disrupted. If healing does occur, a tight scar will result, which makes the heel susceptible to further trauma and infection.

When the diabetic patient requires bed rest for any length of time, as when hospitalized, particular attention must be paid to the heel. Because of loss of sensation the patient with diabetes tends to keep the heels in the same position, which results in pressure necrosis (Figs. 9–17 and 9–18). The skin breaks down, and infection and gangrene can develop. The heels of these patients should be inspected at least once, and preferably twice, daily. If erythema develops, aggressive protective intervention must be instituted at once. Erythema is indicative of rapid tissue breakdown. Stotts et al. found that new heel pressure ulcers occurred in 45% of patients confined to bed because of hip fracture.[142] Therefore, special attention must be paid to the heels of all patients confined to bed, particularly those with diabetes and peripheral neuropathy. The heels must be inspected daily and prophylactic pressure-reducing devices instituted at the time of bed confinement.

Prevention is critically important. Turning the patient and use of heel protectors or foam rubber or egg crate-type sponge rubber mattresses is essential. The heel protectors may

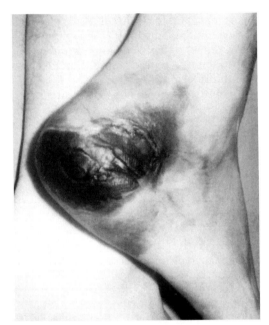

Figure 9–18 ■ Gangrene of heel of bedridden diabetic patient caused by weight of immobile neuropathic foot on mattress.

not stay in place; therefore, daily checks of the heel are necessary.

Examination of Diabetic Foot

One of the most important aspects of the office or clinic visit is examination of the diabetic patient's foot and leg. Despite the problems associated with the diabetic foot, it is frequently the most neglected part of the examination. The low rate of foot inspection in a clinic setting has been documented by Cohen.[22] He found that only 19 to 25% of the patients who entered the examining room had their feet inspected. Bailey and colleagues[94] reported that only 12.3% of the diabetic patients' feet were examined. In one health maintenance organization (HMO) setting, foot examinations were mentioned, at least annually, for 60% of the patients, which meant that 40% probably did not have a foot examination.[94] In another HMO, Peters et al. noted that no documentation of foot examination was made in 94% of the patients.[116]

The foot and lower extremity of the diabetic patient should be examined at every office visit, at least three or four times each year, and more often when indicated. This examination should include the removal of shoes and stockings and trousers or pantyhose as

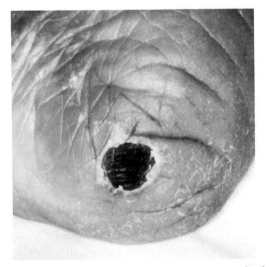

Figure 9–17 ■ Small painless gangrenous area on heel of the foot caused by pressure necrosis in a diabetic neuropathic foot.

well. Only then can the lower extremity be properly examined. Patients are reluctant to remove their shoes and stockings because they seldom feel pain or discomfort and therefore assume that all is well. Patients are also embarrassed to remove their shoes and stockings. However, if the feet are not examined on a routine basis, lesions will be missed and treatment delayed. Amputation may result. Examination of the foot and lower extremity should include inspection, palpation, and neurologic and vascular examination.

Inspection

Simply inspecting the legs and feet will give many clues to the vascular status. Evidence of significant ischemia in the foot includes loss of hair on the dorsum of the foot and toes, and skin that is shiny and atrophic and appears to be drawn tightly around the foot because of loss of the subcutaneous fat layers and dependent rubor (Fig. 9–5). Absent pulses are the hallmarks of significant lower extremity vascular insufficiency.

Inspection between the toes is of the utmost importance. Figure 9–19 shows an example of a painless interdigital ulcer in an elderly woman. When this patient came into the office and was asked to remove her shoes and socks, she refused, saying that her feet felt fine and that she had no problems with them. After much insistence she removed her shoes and stockings, and the ulcer was identified. When asked how long the ulcer had been present, the patient looked down and with great surprise stated that she did not

know that she had an ulcer because she had felt no pain.

Palpation

Touching the skin is a simple and important part of the examination. The experienced hand and eye are extremely important in the evaluation of PAD. Palpation consists of evaluating the femoral, popliteal, dorsalis pedis, and posterior tibial pulses. Auscultation for bruits will help identify the presence of atheromatous plaques and narrowing of the arterial lumen. One of the most important aspects of palpation is detecting whether the skin is warm or cool. Sophisticated instruments are available for quantitative measurements of skin temperature. However, palpation with the hand is sufficient. The use of Doppler and other laboratory techniques for evaluating PAD are discussed in Chapter 16.

Sensory Examination

Although a variety of sophisticated techniques are available for measurement of vibratory sense (large nerve fibers), such as the Biothesiometer, a simple tuning fork with a 128 cycle is sufficient. This examination should include vibratory sense, not only at the ankle but also at the tips of the toes. Once the patient can no longer feel the vibration the examiner can apply the tuning fork to the same area of his or her own foot to see whether further vibrations can be detected.

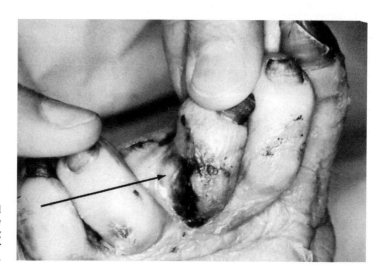

Figure 9–19 ■ Nonpainful interdigital ulcer in elderly diabetic woman. *Arrow* points to exposed tendon, indicating depth of ulceration. The painless ulcer was found on routine foot examination.

The examination to assess the ability to perceive temperature, a small nerve fiber modality, also can be carried out. Guy et al.[52] found the lateral aspect of the foot to be the most sensitive location for the measurement of thermal sensation. These authors noted loss of thermal sensation in all feet with neuropathic ulceration and in feet with Charcot joint. When thermal sensitivity was compared with vibratory perception threshold, it was found that thermal sensitivity sometimes was selectively affected, especially in those patients with painful neuropathy, suggesting that the small fibers are more vulnerable in the diabetic.[52]

In the past, sensory evaluation to perceive protective sensation was frequently carried out by using a pin. This is an inadequate and outdated method of evaluating protective sensation because it varies with each investigator, depending on how forcefully the pin is used. Today's state-of-the art evaluation of the ability to perceive protective sensation is done using the Semmes-Weinstein monofilaments. These filaments come in three thicknesses, 4.17, 5.07, and 6.10. The monofilament is placed against the skin and pressure applied until the filament buckles (Fig. 9–13). When the monofilament is applied to the bottom of the foot at different areas, the patient should be able to identify the area being touched and should also be able to detect the presence of the monofilament at the time it buckles. A thickness of 5.07 is equal to 10 gm of linear pressure and is the limit used to determine protective sensations. McNeely

Table 9–6 ■ ANCIENT TREATMENT OF WOUNDS*

Wine
Dung
Mud
Cow's urine
Beer/hot water
Honey (Egyptian)
Boiling oil
Bread mold (Chinese)
Phenol tar (Gypsies)
Hot vinegar
To make flesh grow combine:
Bitter root (onion)
Goat grease
Swine grease
Oil
Frankincense
Zinc oxide

* Data from Majno (1975) and Brown (1992).

Table 9–7 ■ MANAGEMENT OF DIABETIC FOOT ULCERS

1. Evaluation
   a. Location
   b. Appearance
   c. Depth of penetration
   d. X-rays to detect:
      1. Foreign body
      2. Osteomyelitis
      3. Subcutaneous gas
   e. Biopsy
   f. Vascular examination
2. Debridement, radical
3. Bacterial cultures (aerobic and anaerobic)
4. Metabolic control
5. Antibiotics
   a. Oral
   b. Parenteral
6. Do not soak feet
7. Do not use whirlpool
8. Decrease edema
9. Non–weight bearing
10. Improvement of circulation (vascular surgery)

et al.[98] also stressed that in a clinical setting, the insensitivity to the 5.07 monofilament was the single most practical measurement of risk assessment. Thus, PN with loss of protective sensation and PAD are the most important risk factors, acting independently and in combination, leading to amputation. Both of these factors must be assessed when evaluating the foot of the diabetic.

Treatment of Diabetic Foot Ulcers

The treatment of foot ulcers goes back to ancient times, when every imaginable topical substance was applied (Table 9–6).[15, 89]

Table 9–7 outlines the essential components for assessing and managing the diabetic foot ulcer. Evaluation of the ulcer consists of identifying its location, appearance, presence or absence of pain, and depth of the ulcer. Plate 13 is of the typical neuropathic ulcer, which occurs over the metatarsal heads or on the plantar surface of the hallux. It is painless. Plate 16 is of an ischemic ulcer. It is small, punched out in appearance and typically occurs at the tip of the toes, or around the ankle. It is very painful. Figure 9–7 is of an ulcer on the side of the foot. This is an ischemic pressure ulcer due to ill-fitting shoes. A factitial ulcer (Plate 17) is atypical in appearance. These ulcers occur in malingerers or neurotic patients.

Any foot with an ulcer should be x-rayed. X-rays are necessary to rule out osteomyelitis, gas formation, and the presence of a foreign body.

A retained foreign body is frequently missed because the treating physician fails to take the appropriate x-rays. Kasier et al. reviewed a series of 32 patients who had filed claims involving foreign bodies in their feet. Glass was the most frequently retained foreign body, constituting 53% of the claims. X-rays were ordered for only 35% of these patients.[62] These findings confirmed those of Montano et al., who found glass embedded in 7% of the wounds. The highest prevalence of retained glass was found in puncture wounds, caused by stepping on glass.[101]

Biopsy should be considered when an ulcer appears in an atypical location (e.g., not over the metatarsal heads or plantar surface of the hallux) when it cannot be explained by trauma and is unresponsive to aggressive therapy. On numerous occasions biopsy of an atypical ulcer has revealed malignancy. Plate 18 is an ulceration of the tip of the toe of a 58-year-old type 2 diabetic who had no history of trauma to the toes. He had palpable pulses and severe PN. He had had a variety of local treatments and antibiotics in the past 6 months, without improvement. He ultimately had biopsy of the area, which revealed an amelanotic melanoma.

What may appear to be a superficial ulcer may in fact be just the "tip of the iceberg." There may be deep penetration into the tissues. Figure 9–20A shows what appears to be a relatively small ulcer on the plantar surface of the foot in a 60-year-old woman. She had been diabetic for 20 years and had severe peripheral neuropathy with an insensate foot. While walking barefoot she stepped on a nail and developed a painless ulcer on the plantar surface in the area of the instep. She had treated this with a variety of home remedies. When the wound failed to heal after several weeks, she sought medical attention. The wound appeared to be a small superficial ulcer with minimal infection. However, extensive debridement in the operating room revealed the infection to have penetrated deep into the interfascial space (Fig. 9–20B). Because her circulation was good she responded to parenteral antibiotic therapy, and a skin graft was successful (Fig. 9–20C).

Multiple lessons can be learned from this case. Patients should not go barefoot. A physician should not assume that what appears

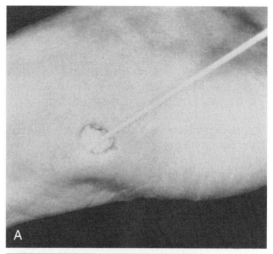

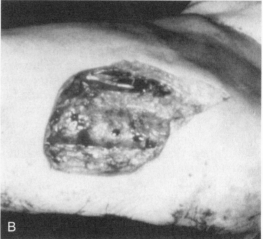

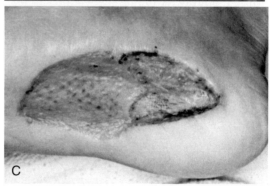

Figure 9–20 ■ A, Ulcer appears to be small and superficial on plantar surface of foot. B, Exploration of ulcer reveals infection to penetrated tissues and interfascial plane. C, Successful skin graft of lesion. (Courtesy of Dr. Dravid Caplan, St. Louis.)

to be a superficial ulceration is simply that and treat it only with topical agents. Vigorous sharp debridement of the ulcer must be done to establish the degree of penetration and to remove all necrotic material. Debridement should be taken down to healthy, bleeding tissue. The ulcer following debridement will in all probability be larger than it was before debridement. When the foot is insensitive, minor debridement can be carried out at the bedside. However, frequently patients must be taken to the operating room for adequate debridement under anesthesia.

Eschars should be completely removed. It is not uncommon to find significant infection under the eschar. However, if there is poor circulation, removing the eschar will not facilitate healing. In such cases consideration should be given to vascular reconstruction.

Steed et al. have shown that sharp wound debridement down to healthy bleeding tissue is a vital adjunct to the care of chronic diabetic foot ulcers. They also suggested that debridement may be of additional benefit because it removes senescent cells from the wound. These cells may have lost to some degree their ability to produce cytokines. The granulation tissue that forms following debridement may perpetuate the wound healing cascade.[140]

Superficial wounds may not be infected. However, when there is suspicion of infection, cultures of the wound should be obtained. Simply swabbing the wound can lead to erroneous results. Cultures should be taken aerobically and anaerobically following debridement and should be obtained from tissue deep in the wound, usually by curettage or aspiration.

Antibiotic therapy should be instituted with a broad-spectrum antibiotic immediately after obtaining the cultures. It can be changed depending upon the organisms identified and the sensitivities. The selection of an oral or parenteral antibiotic for the treatment of a diabetic foot infection depends on medical judgment. Many diabetic foot infections contain gram-negative organisms. Therefore, the oral antibiotic chosen should be effective for gram-positive and gram-negative organisms (see Chapter 22).

Infection in the diabetic foot can deteriorate within 24 to 48 hours. If an oral antibiotic is selected in an outpatient setting, I believe the patient should be seen every 2 to 3 days until the infection is under control. The patient must be carefully instructed to notify the phy-

sician at once should there be increased redness, drainage, pain, or evidence of lymphangitis (Table 9–8). In patients who have insensate feet, the development of pain is indicative of deep infection and requires immediate attention. The development of odor indicates worsening infection and frequently the presence of anaerobes. It is important that patients with infection monitor their blood glucose levels closely. A rising blood glucose level strongly suggests worsening infection. The instructions given to the patient should be documented in the patient's chart. The patients must be informed to notify the health care provider at once should any of the signs and symptoms of worsening infection develop.

When infection does not respond to aggressive debridement and antibiotic therapy, the wound should be debrided again and recultured because the flora may have changed. Chronic recurrent or resistant infection suggests the presence of osteomyelitis. Vascular status should be evaluated carefully and vascular surgery considered when indicated. The worst combination leading to amputation is infection and PAD.

The criteria for hospitalizing a patient for treatment of infection with parenteral antibiotics includes sepsis, temperature elevation, leukocytosis, significant PAD, and uncontrolled diabetes. It must be kept in mind that diabetics may have severe infection and not have temperature elevation or leukocytosis. Leichter et al.[73] have reviewed the laboratory results in a series of 55 patients with diabetes and serious pedal infections. In this series, the sedimentation rates were significantly elevated, with a mean of 58.6 mm Hg. Surprisingly, the mean WBC count was only 9,700. Gibbons and Eliopoulos[49] have also doc-

Table 9–8 ■ INDICATIONS OF WORSENING INFECTION

1. Signs and symptoms
   a. ↑ Drainage
   b. ↑ Erythema
   c. ↑ Pain
   d. ↑ Temperature
   e. Foul odor
   f. Lymphangitis
   g. Lymphadenopathy
   h. Gangrene
2. Laboratory results
   a. ↑ Blood glucose level
   b. ↑ WBC level
   c. ↑ Sedimentation rate

umented that temperature elevation, chills, and leukocytosis may be absent in two thirds of the patients with limb-threatening infections.

If a patient has what appears to be a minor infection on the plantar surface of the foot and develops erythema, edema, or blistering on the dorsum of that foot, he or she should be hospitalized. Even though the patient is not septic, there is a high probability that the infection has penetrated deep into the tissues and has spread to the dorsum of the foot. These patients require parenteral antibiotics and, frequently, incision and drainage and usually hospitalization. Parenteral antibiotics achieve a higher concentration in the peripheral tissues than antibiotics given orally. The antibiotic of choice frequently can only be given parenterally.

Soaking the feet has no benefit, although it has been a traditional approach.[81] Soaking can lead to maceration and further infection. Because of the insensitivity of the foot, the patient may soak it in water that is too hot, resulting in severe burns (Fig. 9–12). Chemical soaks can also result in burns.

Edema is frequently present. Elevation of the feet, no more than the thickness of one pillow, can be beneficial. Higher elevation may impede circulation. In selected cases careful compression can be employed.

In some centers, putting an ulcerated foot into a whirlpool has been an accepted and routine form of therapy. However, this traditional technique is no longer acceptable and may actually be detrimental. The whirlpool can only accomplish superficial debridement and does not improve circulation. Prolonged use can cause maceration and infection. Dangling the lower extremity in a whirlpool can increase edema. Furthermore, a whirlpool can harbor bacteria, especially *Pseudomonas,* a hydrophilic organism. A whirlpool used at home or without supervision can contain water that is too hot, and because of loss of protective sensation the patient does not realize this and can suffer severe thermal injury. The use of a whirlpool delays aggressive sharp debridement and can delay wound healing.

The prolonged use of chemical antiseptics such as povidone-iodine (Betadine), acetic acid, hydrogen peroxide, or Dakin's solution has also become outdated. These antiseptics can injure granulation tissue and impede wound healing.[82, 125]

Non–weight bearing is essential. Because the feet are insensitive and the ulcer does not hurt, patients continue to walk. The result is increased pressure necrosis, forcing bacteria deeper into the tissues, and failure to heal. The use of crutches and wheelchairs is seldom successful in achieving total and consistent non–weight bearing. Many patients with neuropathy have ataxia, making the use of crutches potentially dangerous. One of the best techniques to insure non–weight bearing in appropriately selected patients is the use of a contact cast.[3, 104, 136] This cast allows the patient to be ambulatory by redistributing the weight, thereby decreasing the pressure on the ulcer area. The use of the cast guarantees non–weight bearing all of the time as opposed to devices that can be taken off (see Chapter 13). Other techniques for non–weight bearing can be found in Chapter 14.

Many types of dressings have been advocated to cover and aid in wound healing. These are discussed in detail in Chapter 12. Because there is no universal agreement on the proper dressing, Fisken has suggested that the best policy is to use the safest, simplest, and least expensive dressing.[44] In our institution wet to moist, not wet to dry, saline dressings are used most often.

When an ulcer does not heal despite good metabolic control, adequate debridement, parenteral antibiotic therapy, and non–weight bearing, underlying osteomyelitis, changes in bacterial flora, and an inadequate blood supply should be considered. ABIs of less than 0.45 or $TcPo_2$ less than 30 mm Hg, and certainly less than 20 mm Hg, are highly predictive that the infection will not resolve and that the ulcer will not heal. For example, Pecoraro et al.[113] found a 39-fold increased risk of early wound failure if the average periwound $TcPo_2$ was less than 22 mm Hg.

Figure 9–21A shows ulceration on the plantar surface of the left heel. The patient was hospitalized, and aggressive therapy was carried out. Debridement was carried down to the periosteum of the calcaneus, but after 4 weeks there had been no healing. A vascular consultation was obtained. Arteriograms revealed a previously transplanted kidney in the left iliac fossa, and normal aorta and iliac vessels (Fig. 9–21B); and slight atherosclerosis in both superficial femoral arteries but occlusion of both left an right tibial and peroneal vessels at their ori-

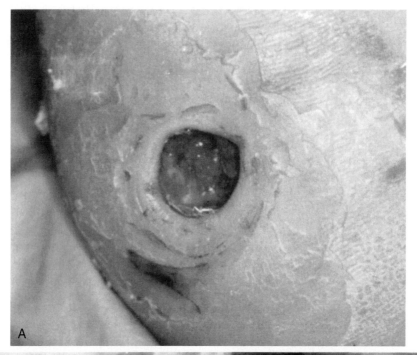

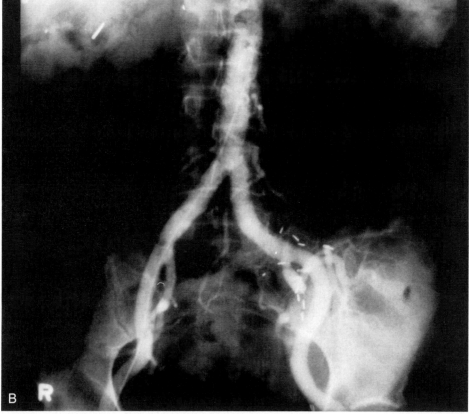

Figure 9–21 ■ *A,* Ulceration of plantar surface of heel, which was debrided to the periosteum of the calcaneus. *B,* Arteriogram revealed normal aorta and iliac arteries. Previously transplanted kidney is noted on left side of the pelvis. *C,* Arteriogram shows occlusion of both left and right tibial and peroneal vessels at their origin. *D,* Extent of surgery for popliteal posterior tibial bypass. *E,* Healed ulcer 3 weeks after vascular surgery. (Courtesy of Dr. Gregorio Sicard, St. Louis.)

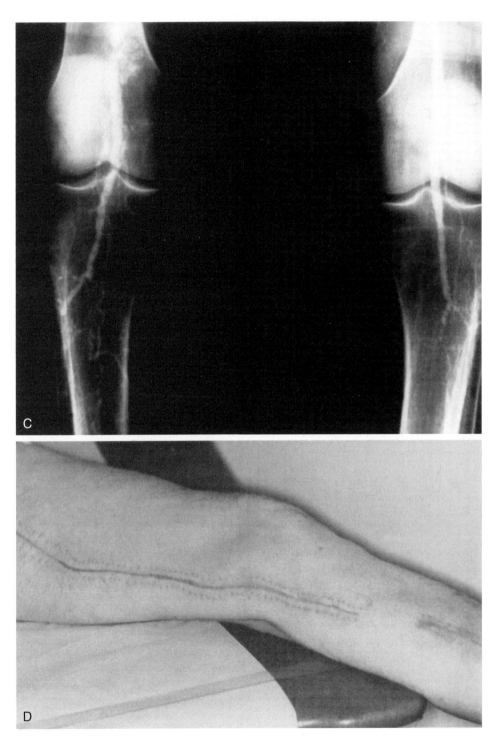

Figure 9–21 *Continued*

Illustration continued on following page

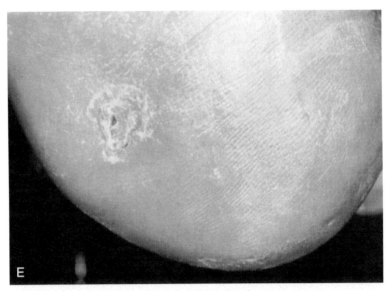

Figure 9–21 *Continued*

gins (Fig. 9–21*C*). The patient underwent a left posterior tibial in situ bypass (Fig. 9–21*D*). The initial left ankle Doppler index of 0.66 preoperatively, probably an erroneously high reading because of noncompressible vessels, had now risen to 0.95. Within 3 weeks, the plantar ulcer had completely healed (Fig. 9–21*E*). The degree of ischemia, not necessarily the size of the ulcer, is the most significant factor in predicting the potential outcome of treatment (See Chapter 26).

He is a good surgeon who can amputate.
He is a better surgeon who can save a limb.
Sir Astley Paston Cooper 1768–1841

Perhaps the "eleventh commandment" should be "Thou shalt not amputate." Loss of limb and a bad outcome does not necessarily mean bad care. Unfortunately, we cannot save all diabetic limbs, but aggressive approaches can save many more limbs and significantly decrease the number of amputations currently being done in the United States.

Impediments to Wound Healing

Wound healing can be impaired by a variety of factors (Table 9–9). Poor circulation due to atherosclerosis inhibits the delivery of oxygen, nutrients, and antibiotics necessary to promote wound healing and to fight infection. A painless ulcer, due to PN, can give the patient a false sense of security. This can result in poor compliance and neglect of the wound. The end result is delayed care of the

---

Table 9-9 ■ IMPEDIMENTS TO WOUND HEALING

1. Vascular
   a. Atherosclerosis
   b. Increased viscosity
2. Neurologic
   a. Insensate foot
   b. Foot deformities
3. Infection
   a. Inadequate debridement
   b. Poor blood supply
   c. Microthrombi
   d. Hyperglycemia
   e. Decreased polymorphonuclear neutrophil function
   f. Polymicrobial infection
   g. Changing bacterial flora
   h. Osteomyelitis
4. Mechanical
   a. Edema
   b. Weight bearing
5. Poor nutrition
   a. Low serum albumin level
6. Immunosuppression
7. Foreign bodies
8. Malignancies
9. Factitial
10. Decreased growth factors
11. Poor patient compliance
12. Poor physician compliance
13. Managed care

---

wound and poor wound healing. Infection if not aggressively attacked will not only impair wound healing but can lead to gangrene and amputation.

While good nutrition is very important, it is difficult to achieve in patients who frequently have a poor appetite and are in a catabolic state. Adequate nutrients are necessary for wound healing. Iron, vitamin B_{12}, and folic acid enable red cells to carry oxygen to healing tissue.[126] Iron is also a cofactor in collagen synthesis. Vitamin C and zinc are vital to tissue repair.[134, 143] Zinc also functions in the immune response.[127] While these vitamins and micronutrients are important, an adequate diet, good metabolic balance, and glucose control are the most important nutritional factors. Protein is essential to wound healing. A serum albumin less than 3 gm/dL significantly impairs wound healing. Leukocyte production is decreased when protein is inadequate.[126] A serum albumin level of less than 3 gm/dL or a lymphocyte count of less than 1,500/mm^3 is evidence of preexisting malnutrition.[30]

An increasing number of hospitalized patients are in a catabolic state, with resultant increased caloric and protein needs. Patients can enter the hospital malnourished or develop malnutrition while in the hospital. Today's shorter length of hospitalization limits the time available for patient assessment and improved nutrition.

The healing of a foot ulcer in the immunosuppressed patient with diabetes is markedly impaired, and these patients also have a higher amputation rate.[45] Immunosuppression is common because of increasing frequency of kidney and pancreas transplants. In kidney transplant patients, limb amputation is required for at least 15% of the kidney recipients who are short term, and 33% of the 10-year survivors.[46] Patients with renal failure are at high risk for amputation. Renal failure compromises the wound healing ability. Wounds in these patients take three times longer to heal than in the nondiabetic.[5] Of the patients with renal failure who present with an infected or gangrenous foot, 25 to 40% underwent immediate amputation without any salvage attempt.[5]

Today, a major impediment to wound healing in some areas is managed care.[78] Managed care can limit the time allotted to see a patient. Adequate care of the diabetic, glucose regulation, education, dietary instruction, and wound care cannot be accomplished in the allotted 15 to 20 minutes allowed for each patient in a managed care setting. Furthermore, limiting consultation and delays in hospitalization can result in delays in wound healing and can lead to amputation.

Adjunctive Therapy for Wound Healing

Despite following the instructions for management of foot ulcers listed in Table 9–7, some chronic diabetic foot wounds heal slowly or not at all.

The healing of a wound is a complex process requiring the collaborative efforts of many different tissues, cell lineages, and growth factors. The contribution of each of these cell types during the phases of proliferation, migration, matrix synthesis, and contraction, as well as the growth factors and matrix signals present at a wound site, are now roughly understood. Details of how these signals control wound cell activities are beginning to emerge, and studies of healing in embryos have begun to show how the normal adult repair process might be readjusted to resemble regeneration rather than "patching up."[93]

Investigations have shown that autologous platelet-derived growth factor formula (PDGF) can be an important adjunct to healing wounds that have shown resistance to comprehensive approaches.[66, 141] Steed has shown that recombinant PDGF significantly achieved complete healing in diabetic foot wounds when compared to standards of care alone.[139] Recombinant PDGF in a gel becaplermin (Regranex, Ortho-McNeil Pharmaceuticals, Inc., Raritan, NJ), is applied once a day to the wound and covered with moist gauze dressing. A dressing change without Regranex is applied approximately 12 hours later. Regranex should not be used when there is extensive necrosis, active infection, and/or ischemia.

The use of living tissue equivalent is another new technique for accelerating wound healing of diabetic foot ulcers. Dermagraft (Advanced Tissue Science, La Jolla, CA) is derived from cultured human dermis. It is derived from foreskin tissue cultures. Dermagraft consists of neonatal dermal fibroblasts cultured in vitro onto a bioabsorbable mesh. This produces living metabolically active tissue containing normal growth factors and cytokines.[48]

In a prospective double-blind study of ulcers treated with Dermagraft, one piece applied weekly for 8 weeks, the ulcers healed significantly more often than those treated with standard wound care alone. Fifty percent of those treated with Dermagraft and 8% of the control ulcers healed completely in 12 weeks.[48]

Hyperbaric oxygen (HBO) is gaining favor as treatment for diabetic foot wounds.[146] Oriani et al. found that amputation rates in 62 diabetics who were treated for foot ulcers with HBO was only 4% compared to 49% of the control group who were unable or unwilling to undergo therapy with HBO.[108] In another study of 30 diabetics with foot lesions, fewer patients in the HBO group required above the ankle amputation.[31] In a recent study by Faglia et al. of 70 patients with diabetes and foot ulcers treated with HBO, only 8.6% underwent major amputation. In the untreated group 33.3% underwent major amputation.[41]

Systemic hyperbaric oxygen greatly increases tissue oxygen levels. Oxygen tension values remain elevated for several hours after exposure. It must be kept in mind that HBO is a supplemental treatment to standard wound care. It is ineffective in patients with severe peripheral vascular disease. Hyperbaric oxygen delivered by a hyperbaric boot is of no value. It must be delivered by putting the patient into single or multiple person chambers (see Chapter 19).

Electrical stimulation is another form of therapy for wound healing. William Gilbert proposed the use of electrical stimulation for wound healing as far back as 1600. This was followed by a number of contributions over the years.[47] Wood and colleagues found that pulse lower intensity direct current represented a useful approach for the treatment of stage II and III chronic decubitus ulcers.[155]

Recently, Baker et al.[7] found that electrical stimulation given daily with short pulsed asymmetric biphasic waveform was effective for enhancement of healing rates for patients with diabetes and open wounds. Using this technique they found a significant increase in the healing rate by nearly 60% in patients treated with electrical stimulation compared to controls. Patients treated with asymmetric biphasic square wave pulse did not show increased wound healing.[7] Lundeberg et al.[87] have also reported improved healing of diabetic ulcers using electrical nerve stimulation.

Ultrasound has also been suggested as a treatment for healing diabetic wounds. Ultrasound refers to high-frequency, mechanical vibrations that are produced when electrical energy is converted to sound waves. Ultrasound gets its name because the sound is beyond the range of human hearing.[95] Ultrasound may be helpful because of its stimulatory effects in fibroblasts and macrophages,[34] and on angiogenesis.[159] Ultrasound can cause dire consequences when applied in an improper manner, and this may result in tissue destruction.[95]

Again, it must be kept in mind that wound healing using electrical stimulation or ultrasound is still experimental and further control studies will be necessary to prove conclusively their efficacy in the treatment of diabetic foot wounds.

Management of Healed Foot Ulcers

Management of the healed ulcer is very important in order to prevent recurrence of the ulcer. The underlying etiologies responsible for the ulcer—PN, PAD, foot deformities, calluses, and increased pressure—must be addressed. Scar tissue from previously healed ulcers is not strong and is vulnerable to the shearing forces of walking. Special measures are therefore necessary to protect the vulnerable sites of previous ulceration. These include education of the patient in walking; for example, taking shorter steps and decreasing overall walking. Patients whose jobs require standing or walking, such as waiters or waitresses or letter carriers, may need to change jobs. The patient with a healed ulcer must carefully inspect their feet every day and report at once any skin changes. Therapeutic shoes play a very important role in preventing recurrence of these ulcers.

Therapeutic Shoes

The use of special therapeutic shoes is very important in preventing ulceration or recurrence of ulcers. Patients who have cocked-up toes require a shoe with a bigger toe box. An extra-depth shoe with a molded plastic-like insole is frequently required to redistribute the weight away from the previous ulcer site and prevent recurrence of ulceration. This was clearly demonstrated in a study at King's

College in London, which showed an 83% recurrence of ulcers when patients returned to wearing regular shoes. However, with the use of special shoes, there was only a 17% recurrence of ulceration.[40] The importance of therapeutic shoes and proper fitting is being recognized with increasing frequency. A study by Ucclolli et al. reported that manufactured shoes specially designed for individuals with diabetes were effective in preventing relapses in patients with previous ulceration.[148]

Patients with a markedly deformed foot, such as a Charcot, require a specially molded shoe. An unusual foot deformity requiring a specially molded shoe was that of a patient with eight toes and eight metatarsal bones of both feet (Fig. 9–22). This person's major problem was finding a shoe that fit. He obviously required very special shoes (see Chapters 20 and 34).

As previously noted, abnormally high pressures contribute to callus buildup and ulceration. A cushioned running style shoe can decrease pressure by 45% (see Chapter 6). Wearing running shoes can decrease ulceration and callus build-up and help to prevent recurrent ulceration.[138]

A recent demonstration study that supplied therapeutic shoes to people with diabetes and selected foot problems showed no increase in cost to Medicare.[156] As a result, Medicare now provides partial payment of therapeutic shoes for the person with diabetes and PAD, peripheral vascular disease, peripheral neuropathy, foot deformity, preulcerative callus, previous ulceration, and amputation or partial amputation of the foot or contralateral foot. Proper fitting of therapeutic shoes and insoles requires the skill of podiatrists and certified pedorthists.[57]

Teamwork

The team needed for the care of the diabetic is not the one depicted in Plate 19. It is a team that will save the foot, not amputate it.

It is obvious that the management of the diabetic foot requires many medical disciplines (see Table 9–10). The primary physician's most important role is examining the foot at every visit and educating the patient in foot care and maintaining good blood sugar control. The physician who does not carry out these tasks loses the advantage of the old adage, "an ounce of prevention is worth a pound of cure." The nurse educator is probably the most important member of the team other than the patient. The educator who carefully and repeatedly teaches foot care accomplishes this while examining the feet,

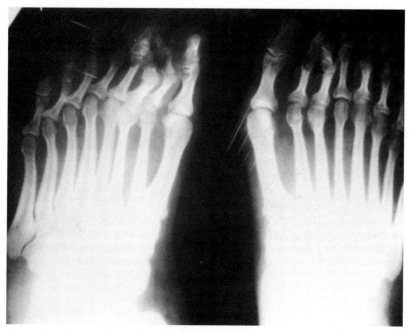

Figure 9–22 ■ This patient has difficulty finding shoes that fit because he had eight toes and eight metatarsal bones on each foot. (Courtesy of Cheryl Strickland Allen, P.T., Oklahoma City.)

Table 9–10 ▪ THE DIABETIC FOOT CARE TEAM

Primary care physician
Internist
Endocrinologist
Diabetologist
Podiatrist
Nurses:
  Educator
  Enterostomal
  Practitioner
  Assistant
Dietitian
Surgeons:
  General
  Vascular
  Plastic
  Orthopedic
Wound care specialist
Infectious disease specialist
Radiologist
Physiatrist
Physical therapist
Occupational therapist
Orthotist
Pedorthist
Dermatologist
Pharmacist
Psychologist
Psychiatrist
Social worker
Home care nurse
Sex therapist

and helps prevent foot problems. Many enterostomal nurses have developed an expertise in wound management and have assumed a significant role in diabetic foot care, including debridement and dressing wounds. The vascular surgeon has saved many patients from amputation. Unfortunately, this surgeon frequently is not called in early enough (see Chapter 25).

The podiatrist is frequently the first health care professional to detect a diabetic foot lesion and occasionally the first to diagnose the patient's diabetes. The podiatrist can surgically correct foot problems such as cocked-up toes and bunions and can treat chronic nail problems. The podiatrist's role in patient education in foot care is paramount. Ronnemaa et al. have shown that education by the podiatrist in foot care and preventive measures results in a significant decrease in foot problems.[128] Neuropathic syndromes are common, and determining a differential diagnosis may require the expertise of a neurologist. The orthopedist frequently sees the patient because of foot deformities. The expertise of the orthopedist

in prophylactic or other corrective surgery is of the utmost importance. Other important members of the team managing diabetic foot deformities are the certified pedorthist and the orthotist. These specialists play an important role in fitting therapeutic shoes and braces. The physical therapist may have two roles. In medical centers where contact casting is practiced, it is frequently the physical therapist that is trained to apply these casts. When amputation occurs, the physiatrist's skills, as well as the physical therapist and the prosthetist, are required for rehabilitation. Treatment of diabetic foot lesions can be prolonged, and because hospital stays today are shortened, many patients require home nursing care services. The home care nurse may be needed to carry out prolonged parenteral antibiotic therapy, change dressings, debride, and observe the patient's clinical course.

Financial problems resulting from loss of a job can be monumental. The social worker becomes an important team member in these cases. Psychiatrists and psychologists are also important team members. Carrington et al. found there was poor pyschosocial adjustment in people with diabetic foot ulcers and/or amputation. They found that patients with diabetic foot ulcers were significantly depressed. This study confirmed the need for psychological and psychiatric care for diabetic patients with foot ulcers and/or amputation.[18]

The management of diabetic foot problems is complicated. Success in saving the foot is achieved only with the expertise of multiple disciplines.

Exercise for Persons with Diabetes and Foot Problems

Exercise is an important modality in the management of diabetes. However, in patients with PAD, PN, previous healed ulceration, or deformed feet, weight-bearing exercises, jogging, prolonged walking, treadmill, and step exercises should be avoided. The presence of an active foot ulcer is an absolute contraindication for weight-bearing exercise. The patients with PN and insensate foot can do a variety of non–weight-bearing exercises such as swimming, bicycling, rowing, chair, and upper body exercises (Tables 9–11, 9–12, and 9–13).[76] Patients, particularly those with

Table 9–11 ■ DIABETIC FOOT CONDITIONS LIMITING EXERCISE

Insensate foot
Deformed foot
  Cocked-up toes
  Charcot foot
Foot ulcer
Previous ulcer

PAD, PN, and a previously healed ulceration, should have specific detailed instructions in foot care and techniques for decreasing foot pressure before undertaking an exercise program.

Exercise for the amputee wearing a prosthesis represents a major problem. Walking speed is significantly impaired. Pinzur[117] has shown that a normal walking speed is 50 m/min or about 2 mph, but in a BK amputee with a prosthesis it is reduced to 40 m/min or about 1.6 mph. The energy cost of ambulating is also markedly increased.[43, 150] Therefore, exercise for the diabetic amputee can be extremely limited. In addition, exercise in the amputee may subject the patient to ulceration of the stump. Many amputees also have coronary artery disease, which can be aggravated by exercise. Therefore, physical therapists and personnel in exercise centers, before recommending an exercise program to the patient with diabetes, should discuss with the referring physician the type of exercise suitable for this particular patient.

Patient Education

Of all the approaches to saving the diabetic foot, the most important is patient education. Despite our current knowledge and good diabetic control, physicians cannot totally prevent PAD and PN. However, patients can be educated in proper foot care, teaching them how to prevent injury and detect foot lesions as early as possible. At the time of the office visit and while the shoes and socks are off, the nurse or physician should review the do's and dont's of foot care with the patient. This cannot be adequately accomplished by simply handing the patient a list of instructions. The instructions should be explained and questions encouraged and answered. If this is done, the patient will have a better understanding of the importance of foot care. The patient should be instructed to not only look at the feet but to also inspect the areas between the toes. Patients with impaired vision, extreme obesity, or arthritis who cannot inspect their feet adequately can have this performed by a family member. If a family member is not available to do this, the patient can place a mirror on the floor, allowing him or her to inspect the bottom of the foot. The feet should be kept clean, and the patient should be cautioned to dry them carefully, making sure that the areas between the toes are dried thoroughly. Moisture left in these areas can lead to maceration and infection.

Because autonomic neuropathy leads to the inability of the foot to perspire, the skin becomes dry, flaky, and cracked. The application of a very thin coat of lubricating material to the foot after bathing helps to seal in the moisture. It is moisture rather than the oil alone that keeps the skin pliable and decreases the dryness. Any type of cream can be used. Each practitioner has his or her favorite. Even vegetable oils can be used. It is important that lubricants not be placed between the toes, because this can cause moisture to accumulate and lead to maceration and infection.

Extremes of temperature should be avoided. Many patients with cold-insensitive feet because of PN and PAD have incurred severe burns by using a heating pad or hot water bottle or by soaking them in water that is too hot. The temperature of the water should be tested before bathing. This should be done with the elbow or a thermometer, not with the hand, which may also be insensitive because of PN. Hot cement around swimming pools and hot sandy beaches are potentially disastrous for the diabetic foot. Many diabetic patients with insensitive feet have suffered severe burns secondary to walking on these surfaces. Patients should be advised to wear protective footwear at the beach and around the pool.

Chemical burns can occur from agents used to remove corns and calluses. The use

Table 9–12 ■ CONTRAINDICATED EXERCISES FOR PATIENTS WITH DIABETIC FOOT PROBLEMS

Treadmill
Prolonged walking
Jogging
Stairmaster

Table 9–13 ■ EXERCISES FOR DIABETIC PATIENTS WITH FOOT PROBLEMS

Non–weight bearing
Swimming
Chair
Cycling
Rowing

of these substances should be avoided. The diabetic should inspect the inside of the shoes daily for foreign objects, nail points, and torn linings.

A very important part of the diabetic's educational program is instruction in proper footwear. The shoes should be comfortable at the time of purchase, and the patient should not depend on them to stretch out. Shoes should be purchased late in the day when the feet are at their largest. Shoes that feel comfortable at the time of purchase may actually be too small, because the patient with an insensitive foot cannot detect discomfort. New shoes should be worn only a few hours each day. The shoes should be made of leather, not man-made materials. However, walking or running shoes may reduce the rate of callus buildup.[138] Patients with foot deformities should wear special therapeutic or molded shoes. The patient should be instructed not to wear thongs. Figure 9–23 shows ulceration between the first and second toes of a patient who had worn thong sandals.

The patient should be taught the proper method of cutting nails straight across or following the curve of the nails but never to cut deep into the corners. Improper trimming can result in an ingrown toenail. Recurring ingrown toenails can be treated conservatively but are always a potential source of infection and should receive definitive therapy. Patients must be instructed repeatedly not to do home surgery. Serious complications can result when the patient operates on insensitive feet.

Calluses should be planed down with pumice stones, and emery boards. Patients with insensitive feet should be cautioned on the use of the callus file, because there is a tendency to file too deeply. If the callus is particularly thick, it should be trimmed by a physician, surgeon, or podiatrist. Patients should be reminded to inform any physician working with their feet that they are diabetic

so that the necessary precautions can be taken. See Table 9–14 for a list of patient instructions for foot care.

Malone et al. have documented the importance of patient education in foot care.[90] Unfortunately, some patients have inadequate functional health literacy. This poses a major barrier to educating patients with a chronic disease such as diabetes.[152] Barriers to foot care also include poor vision, fatigue, lack of motivation, and age.[71] Many patients do not avail themselves of diabetes self-management training programs.[24]

The effectiveness of education and total foot care programs in reducing amputation has been noted in many instances. The amputation rate has been reduced by 50% or more in such programs.[4, 26, 85] Lippman[83] has reduced the amputation rate of 8 to 15 cases a year to zero with a special foot care program in nursing homes.

Legal Issues

This chapter would not be complete without mentioning litigation, which frequently follows amputation in people with diabetes. A diabetic foot problem resulting in amputation is a time bomb waiting to go off.[68] Lane has enumerated various problems that can be encountered in treatment of the diabetic

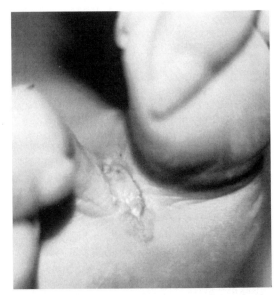

Figure 9–23 ■ Ulceration between toes from wearing thong sandals.

Table 9–14 ■ PATIENT INSTRUCTIONS FOR THE CARE OF THE DIABETIC FOOT

1. Do not smoke.
2. Inspect the feet daily for blisters, cuts, and scratches. The use of a mirror can aid in seeing the bottom of the feet. Always check between the toes.
3. Wash feet daily. Dry carefully, especially between the toes.
4. Avoid extremes of temperatures. Test water with hand, elbow, or thermometer before bathing.
5. If feet feel cold at night, wear socks. Do not apply hot water bottles or heating pads. Do not use an electric blanket. Do not soak feet in hot water.
6. Do not walk on hot surfaces such as sandy beaches or cement around swimming pools.
7. Do not walk barefoot.
8. Do not use chemical agents for removal of corns and calluses, corn plasters, or strong antiseptic solutions.
9. Do not use adhesive tape on the feet.
10. Inspect the inside of shoes daily for foreign objects, nail points, torn linings, and rough areas.
11. If your vision is impaired, have a family member inspect feet daily, trim nails, and buff calluses.
12. Do not soak feet.
13. For dry feet, use a very thin coat of a lubricating oil or cream. Apply this after bathing and drying the feet. Do not put the oil or cream between the toes. Consult your physician for detailed instructions.
14. Wear properly fitting stockings. Do not wear mended stockings or stockings with seams. Change stockings daily.
15. Do not wear garters.
16. Shoes should be comfortable at time of purchase. Do not depend on them to stretch out. Shoes should be made of leather. Purchase shoes late in the afternoon when feet are the largest. Running or special walking shoes may be worn after checking with your physician. Purchase shoes from shoe salesman who understands diabetic foot problems.
17. Do not wear shoes without stockings.
18. Do not wear sandals with thongs between the toes.
19. In winter time, take special precautions. Wear wool socks and protective foot gear such as fleece-lined boots.
20. Nails should be cut following the shape of the nail.
21. Do not cut corns and calluses: follow instructions from your physician or podiatrist.
22. See your physician regularly and be sure that your feet are examined at each visit.
23. Notify your physician or podiatrist at once should you develop a blister or sore on your feet.
24. Be sure to inform your podiatrist that you are diabetic.

foot, which may result in litigation.[68] Insurance companies have reported a high incidence of malpractice claims resulting from diabetic foot problems and amputation. A survey in Indiana found relatively few diabetes-related malpractice cases. However, a number were related to amputation.[20] Hyams et al. have outlined how practice guidelines are used in litigation.[55] I have reviewed a number of these cases. Some of the most common complaints leading to litigation are: failure to educate the patient in proper foot care, delay or failure to obtain consultation, failure to obtain cultures of the wound and to culture for anaerobes and aerobes, failure to do neurologic and/or vascular examination, failure to recognize worsening infection, failure to control blood glucose, failure to improve blood supply with vascular surgery, and failure to instruct the patient in the signs and symptoms of worsening infection. A bad outcome does not necessarily mean a deviation from the standards of care. However, when the standards of care are not met and amputation results, the likelihood of a successful defense is markedly impaired (see Chapter 38).

Rehabilitation After Lower Limb Amputation in the Diabetic

Unfortunately, not all amputations can be prevented. Therefore, rehabilitation becomes an important facet in the overall management of the diabetic amputee. If we achieve our goal of reducing the amputation rate by 50%, we will still have more than 25,000 to 30,000 amputations each year. A significant number of these patients can benefit from a prosthetic rehabilitation program (see Chapter 29).

Summary

The pathogenesis of diabetic foot lesions is multifactorial. Physicians involved in the management of the diabetic foot must understand the pathogenesis and risk factors involved so that whenever possible the development of foot problems can be prevented.

Foot lesions, especially ulceration, are common in persons with diabetes. If treatment is delayed or inappropriate, the ulceration can become infected and gangrene and amputation can develop. Physicians, clinics, hospitals, and wound care centers who repeatedly educate the patient in foot care, prescribe therapeutic shoes, aggressively treat foot ulcers, and utilize the team approach have significantly reduced the amputation rate and length of hospitalization in diabetic patients. The U.S. Department of Health's goal for the year 2000 is a 40% reduction in the amputation rate in patients with diabetes.[29] This should be the goal of everyone who cares for the patient with diabetes.

REFERENCES

1. Aguayo AJ: Neuropathy due to compression and entrapment. *In* Dyck PJ, Thomas PK, Lambert EH (eds): Peripheral Neuropathy. Philadelphia: WB Saunders Company, 1975.
2. Ardron M, MacFarlane IA, Robinson C, et al: Antismoking advice for young diabetic smokers: Is it a waste of breath? Diabet Med 5:677, 1988.
3. Armstrong DG, Lavery LA, Bushman TR: Peak foot pressures influence the healing time of diabetic foot ulcers treated with total contact casts. J Rehab Res Dev 35:1–5, 1998.
4. Assal JP, Muhlhauser I, Pernat A, et al: Patient education as the basis for diabetes care in clinical practices. Diabetologia 28:602, 1985.
5. Attinger CE: Re-examining limb salvage in diabetic patients with renal failure. Biomechanics 3:67–70, 1996.
6. Bailey TS, Yu HM, Rayfield EJ: Patterns of foot inspection in a diabetes clinic. Am J Med 78: 371, 1985.
7. Baker LL, Chambers R, DeMuth SK, et al: Effects of electrical stimulation on wound healing in patients with diabetic ulcers. Diabetes Care 20:405–412, 1997.
8. Beach KW, Strandness DE Jr: arteriosclerosis obliterans and associated risk factors in insulin dependent diabetes. Diabetes 29:882, 1980.
9. Bjorntorp P: Abdominal obesity and the development of noninsulin-dependent diabetes mellitus. Diabetes Metab Rev 4:615, 1988.
10. Bodily KC, Burgess EM: Contralateral limb and patient survival after leg amputation. Am J Surg 146:280, 1983.
11. Boulton AJM: The diabetic foot: Of neuropathic aetiology? Diabetes Care 17:557–560, 1994.
12. Boulton AJM, Hardisty CA, Betts RP, et al: Dynamic foot pressure and other studies as diagnostic and management aids in diabetic neuropathy. Diabetes Care 6:26, 1983.
13. Boulton AJM, Scarpello JHB, Ward JD: Venous oxygenation in the diabetic neuropathic foot: Evidence of arterial venous shunting. Diabetologia 22:6, 1981.
14. Brazilay JI, Kronmal RA, Bittner V, et al: Coronary artery disease in diabetic patients with lower-extremity arterial disease: Disease characteristics and survival. Diabetes Care 20:1381–1387, 1997.
15. Brown H: Wound healing research through the ages. *In* Cohen IK, Diegelmann RF, Lindblad WJ (eds): Wound Healing Biochemical and Clinical Aspects. Philadelphia: WB Saunders Company, 1992.
16. Brownlee M, Vlassara H, Cerami A: Trapped immunoglobulins on peripheral nerve myelin from patients with diabetes mellitus. Diabetes 35:999, 1986.
17. Caputo GM, Cavanagh PR, Ulbrecht US, et al: Current concepts: Assessment and management of foot disease in patients with diabetes. N Engl J Med 331:854–860, 1994.
18. Carrington AL, Mawdsley SKV, Morely M, et al: Psychological status of diabetic people with or without lower limb disability. Diabetes Res Clin Pract 32:19–25, 1996.
19. Charcot JM: Sur la claudication intermittente, observee dans un cas d'obliteration complete de l'une des arteres iliaque primitive. C R Soc Biol 10:225, 1858.
20. Clark CM, Kinney ED: The potential role of diabetes guidelines in the reduction of medical injury and malpractice claims involving diabetes. Diabetes Care 17:155–162, 1994.
21. Coffman JD: Atheromatous embolism. Vasc Med 1:267–273, 1996.
22. Cohen SJ: Potential barriers to diabetes care. Diabetes Care 6:499, 1983.
23. Consensus Development Conference on Diabetic Foot Wound Care: Diabetes Care 22:1354–1360, 1999.
24. Coonrod BA, Betschart J, Harris MI: Frequency and determinants of diabetes patient education among adults in the U.S. population. Diabetes Care 17:852–858, 1994.
25. Couch NP: On the arterial consequences of smoking. J Vasc Surg 3:807, 1986.
26. Davidson JK, Alogna M, Goldsmith M, et al: Assessment of program effectiveness at Grady Memorial Hospital—Atlanta. *In* Steiner G, Lawrence PA (eds): Educating Diabetic Patients. New York: Springer-Verlag, 1981.
27. DeLaurentis DA: Do you know the treatment of choice in peripheral arterial occlusive disease? Geriatrics 34:33, 1979.
28. Delbridge L, Appleburg M, Reeve TS: Factors associated with the development of foot lesions in the diabetic. Surgery 93:78, 1983.
29. Department of Health and Human Services: Healthy People 2000: National Health Promotion and Disease Prevention Objectives. Washington, DC: U.S. Government Printing Office, Department of Health and Human Services Publ No. 91-50213, 1991.
30. Dickhaut SC, Delee JC, Page CP: Nutritional status: Importance in predicting wound-healing after amputation. J Bone Joint Surg 66:71, 1984.
31. Doctor N, Pandya S, Supe A: Hyperbaric oxygen therapy in diabetic foot. J Postgrad Med 38:112–114, 1992.
32. Drury TF, Danchik KM, Harris MI: Sociodemographic characteristics of adult diabetes. *In* Harris MI, Hammer RF (eds): Diabetes in America. Bethesda, MD: National Institutes of Health Publ No. 85-1468, 1985.
33. Durham JR: The role of magnetic resonance imaging in the management of foot abscess in the diabetic patient. *In* Yao JST, Pearce WH (eds): The

Ischemic Extremity: Advances in Treatment. East Norwalk, CT: Appleton & Lange, 1995.

34. Dyson ML: Mechanisms involved in therapeutic ultrasound. Physiotherapy 73:116–120, 1987.

35. Ecker LM, Jacobs BS: Lower extremity amputation in diabetic patients. Diabetes 19:189, 1970.

36. Eckman MH, Greenfield S, Mackey WC, et al: Foot infections in diabetic patients: Decision and cost-effective analyses. JAMA 273:712–720, 1995.

37. Edelman D, Matchar DB: Clinical and radiographic findings that lead to intervention in diabetic patients with foot ulcers: A nationwide survey of primary care physicians. Diabetes Care 19:755–757, 1996.

38. Edelman SV, Kosofsky EM, Paul RA, et al: Neuro-osteoarthropathy (Charcot's joint) in diabetes mellitus following revascularization surgery: Three case reports and a review of the literature. Arch Intern Med 147:1504, 1987.

39. Edmonds ME: The diabetic foot: Pathophysiology and treatment. Clin Endocrinol Metab 15:889–916, 1991.

40. Edmonds ME, Blundell MP, Morris ME, et al: Improved survival of the diabetic foot: The role of a specialized foot clinic. Q J Med 60:763, 1986.

41. Faglia E, Faveles F, Aldeghi A, et al: Adjunctive systemic hyperbaric oxygen therapy in treatment of severe prevalently ischemic diabetic foot ulcer: A randomized study. Diabetes Care 19:1338–1343, 1996.

42. Fearon J, Campbell DR, Hoar CS Jr, et al: Improved results with diabetic below-knee amputations. Arch Surg 120:777, 1985.

43. Fisher SV, Gullickson G: Energy cost of ambulation in health and disability: A literature review. Arch Phys Med Rehabil 59:124–133, 1978.

44. Fisken RA, Digby M: Which dressing for diabetic foot ulcers? Pract Diab Int 13:107–109, 1996.

45. Fletcher F, Ain M, Jacobs R: Healing of foot ulcers in immunosuppressed renal transplant patients. Clin Orthop 296:37–42, 1993.

46. Friedman EA: Diabetic renal disease. In Rifkin H, Porter D (eds): Ellenberg & Rifkin's Diabetes Mellitus, 4th ed. New York: Elsevier, 1990.

47. Gentzkow GD: Electrical stimulation to heal dermal wounds. J Dermatol Surg Oncol 19:753–758, 1993.

48. Gentzkow GD, Iwasaki SD, Hershon KS, et al: Use of Dermagraft, a cultured human dermis, to treat diabetic foot ulcers. Diabetes Care 19:350–354, 1996.

49. Gibbons GW, Elipoulos GM: Infection of the diabetic foot. In Kozak GP, Hoar CS Jr, Rowbotham L, et al (eds): Management of Diabetic Foot Problems: Joslin Clinic and New England Deaconess Hospital. Philadelphia: WB Saunders Company, 1984.

50. Gough A, Clapperton M, Rolando N, et al: Randomised placebo-controlled trial of granulocute-colony stimulating factor in diabetic foot infection. Lancet 350:855–859, 1997.

51. Grayson ML, Gibbons GW, Balogh K, et al: Probing to bone in infected pedal ulcers: A clinical sign of underlying osteomyelitis in diabetic patients. JAMA 273:721–728, 1995.

52. Guy RJC, Clark CA, Malcolm PN, et al: Evaluation of thermal and vibration sensation in diabetic neuropathy. Diabetologia 28:131, 1995.

53. Haffner SM, Fong D, Hazuda HP, et al: Hyperinsulinemia, upper body adiposity and cardiovascular risk factors in non-diabetics. Metabolism 37:333, 1988.

54. Ha Van G, Siney H, Danan JP, et al: Treatment of osteomyelitis in the diabetic foot: Contribution of conservative surgery. Diabetes Care 19:1257–1260, 1997.

55. Hyams AL, Brandenburg BA, Lipsitz SR, et al: Practice guidelines and malpractice litigation: A two-way street. Ann Intern Med 122:450–455, 1995.

56. Humphrey ARG, Dowse GK, Thoma K, et al: Diabetes and non-traumatic lower extremity amputations: Incidence, risk factors and prevention: A 12 year follow-up study in Nauru. Diabetes Care 19:710–714, 1996.

57. Janisse DJ: A scientific approach to insole design for the diabetic foot. Foot 3:105–108, 1993.

58. Janka HU, Standl E, Mehnert H: Peripheral vascular disease in diabetes mellitus and its relation to cardiovascular risk factors: Screening with Doppler ultrasonic technique. Diabetes Care 3:207, 1980.

59. Jensen-Urstad KJ, Reichard PG, Rosfors JS, et al: Early atherosclerosis is retarded by improved long-term blood glucose control in patients with IDDM. Diabetes 45:1253–1258, 1996.

60. Johnson JE: Charcot surgery offers alternative when other methods fail. Biomechanics 4:61–69, 1997.

61. Jonason T, Jonzon B, Ringyvist I, et al: Effect of physical training on different categories of patients with intermittent claudication. Acta Med Scand 206:253, 1979.

62. Kaiser CW, Slowick T, Pfeifer-Spurling K, et al: Retained foreign bodies. J Trauma Injury Infect Crit Care 43:107–111, 1997.

63. Kannel WB: Cigarette smoking and peripheral arterial disease. Prim Cardiovasc 12:13, 1986.

64. Kaplan NM: The deadly quartet: Upper body obesity, glucose intolerance, hypertriglyceridemia and hypertension. Arch Intern Med 149:1514, 1989.

65. Katoulis EC, Ebdon-Parry M, Lansshammar H, et al: Gait abnormalities in diabetic neuropathy. Diabetes Care 20:1904–1907, 1997.

66. Knighton DR, Fiegel VD: Growth factors and repair of diabetic wounds. In Levin ME, O'Neal LW, Bowker JH (eds): The Diabetic Foot, 5th ed. St. Louis: Mosby Year Book, 1993.

67. Laakso M, Pyorala K: Lipid and lipoprotein abnormalities in diabetic patients with peripheral vascular disease. Atherosclerosis 74:55, 1988.

68. Lane SM: Minimize your risk of a malpractice suit. Biomechanics 4:59–60, 70–72, 1997.

69. Lapidus L, Bengtsson C, Larsso B, et al: Distribution of adipose tissue and risk of cardiovascular disease and death: A 12 year follow-up of participants in the population study of women in Gothenburg, Sweden. Br Med J (Clin Res) 289:1257, 1984.

70. Lavery LA, Walker SC, Harkless LB, et al: Infected puncture wounds in diabetic and nondiabetic adults. Diabetes Care 18:1588–1599, 1995.

71. Ledda MA, Walker EA, Basch CE: Development and formative evaluation of a foot self-care program for African Americans with diabetes. Diabetes Ed 23:48–51, 1997.

72. Lee JS, Lu M, Lee VS, et al: Lower-extremity amputations: Incidence, risk factors, and mortality in the Oklahoma Indian Diabetes Study. Diabetes 42:876–882, 1993.

73. Leichter SB, Allweiss P, Harley J, et al: Clinical characteristics of diabetic patients with serious pedal infections. Metabolism 37:22–24, 1998.
74. Levin CM, Dealy FN: The surgical diabetic, a five year survey. Ann Surg 102:1029, 1935.
75. Levin ME: Diabetic foot lesions: Pathogenesis and management. *In* Kerstein MD, White JV (eds): Alternatives to Open Vascular Surgery. Philadelphia: JP Lippincott Company, 1995.
76. Levin ME: Exercise in patients with diabetic complications: The diabetic foot. *In* Ruderman N, Devlin JT (eds): The Health Professional's Guide to Diabetes and Exercise. Alexandria, VA: American Diabetes Association, 1995.
77. Levin ME: Preventing amputation in the patient with diabetes. Diabetes Care 18:1383–1394, 1995.
78. Levin ME: Managed care and diabetes: The best of times or the worst of times? Biomechanics 4:67–70, 1997.
79. Levin ME: Prevention and treatment of diabetic foot wounds. J WOCN 25:129–146, 1998.
80. Levin ME, Sicard GA: Evaluating and treating diabetic peripheral vascular disease: Part I. Clin Diabetes 5:62, 1987.
81. Levin ME, Spratt IL: To soak or not to soak. Clin Diabetes 4:44, 1986.
82. Lineweaver W, Howard R, Sorecy D, et al: Topical antimicrobial toxicity. Arch Surg 120:267–270, 1985.
83. Lippmann HI: Must loss of limb be a consequence of diabetes mellitus? Diabetes Care 2:432, 1979.
84. Littenberg B, Mushlin AI: The diagnostic technology assessment consortium: Technetium bone scanning in the diagnosis of osteomyelitis: A meta-analysis of test performance. J Gen Intern Med 7:158–163, 1992.
85. Litzelman DK, Slemenda CW, Langefeld CD, et al: Reduction of lower extremity clinical abnormalities in patients with non-insulin dependent diabetes mellitus. Ann Intern Med 119:36–42, 1993.
86. LoGerfo FW, Coffman JD: Vascular and microvascular disease of the foot in diabetes. N Engl J Med 311:1516, 1984.
87. Lundeberg TCM, Eriksson SV, Malm M: Electrical nerve stimulation improves healing of diabetic ulcers. Ann Plast Surg 29:328–331, 1992.
88. MacLeod AF, Williams DRR, Sonksen PH, et al: Risk factors for foot ulceration in hospital clinic attenders [abstract]. Diabetologia 34(Suppl 2):A39, 1991.
89. Majno G: The Healing Hand. Man and Wound in the Ancient World. Cambridge, MA: Harvard University Press 1:571, 1975.
90. Malone JM, Snyder M, Anderson G, et al: Prevention of amputation by diabetic education. Am J Surg 158:520, 1989.
91. Mandelberg A, Scheinfeld W: Diabetic amputations: Amputation of lower extremity in diabetes, analysis of one hundred twenty-eight cases. Am J Surg 71:70, 1944.
92. Marchel de Calvi CJ: Recherches sur les accidents diabetiques. Paris: Asselin, 1864.
93. Martin P: Wound healing: Aiming for perfect skin regeneration. Science 276:75–81, 1997.
94. Martin TL, Selby JV, Zhang D: Physician and patient prevention practices in NIDDM in a large urban managed-care organization. Diabetes Care 28:1124–1132, 1995.
95. McCulloch J: Physical modalities in wound management: Ultrasound vasopneumatic devices and hydrotherapy. Ostomy Wound Management 42:30–37, 1995.
96. McDermott W, Rogers DE: Social ramifications of control of microbial disease. Johns Hopkins Med J 151:302, 1982.
97. McGill JB, Schneider DJ, Arfken CL, et al: Factors responsible for impaired fibrinolysis in obese subjects and NIDDM patients. Diabetes 43:104–109, 1994.
98. McNeely MJ, Boyko EJ, Ahroni JH, et al: The independent contributions of diabetic neuropathy and vasculopathy in foot ulceration: How great are the risks? Diabetes Care 18:216–219, 1995.
99. Miller AD, Van Busirk AH, Verhoek-Oftedahl W, et al: Diabetes related lower extremity amputations in New Jersey, 1979–1981. J Med Soc N J 82:723–726, 1985.
100. Moldveen-Geromimus M, Merriam JC Jr: Cholesterol embolization, from pathologic curiosity to clinical entity. Circulation 35:946, 1967.
101. Montano JB, Steele MT, Watson WA: Foreign body retention in glass-caused wounds. Ann Emerg Med 21:1360–1363, 1992.
102. Moss SE, Klein R, Klein BEK: The prevalence and incidence of lower extremity amputation in a diabetic population. Arch Intern Med 152:610–616, 1992.
103. Most RS, Sinnock P: The epidemiology of lower extremity amputations in diabetic individuals. Diabetes Care 6:87–91, 1983.
104. Myerson MS, Henderson MR, Saxby T, et al: Management of midfoot diabetic neuroarthropathy. Foot Ankle Int 15:233–241, 1994.
105. Nelson RC, Gohdes DM, Everhart JE, et al: Lower extremity amputation in NIDDM: 12 year follow-up study in Pima Indians. Diabetes Care 11:8, 1988.
106. Newman LG, Walker J, Palestro CJ: Unsuspected osteomyelitis in diabetic foot ulcers. JAMA 266:1246–1251, 1991.
107. O'Brien IAD, Corrall RJM: Epidemiology of diabetes and its complications. N Engl J Med 318:1619, 1988.
108. Oriani G, Meazza D, Favales F, et al: Hyperbaric oxygen therapy in diabetic gangrene. J Hyperbaric Med 5:171–175, 1990.
109. O'Keefe ST, Woods BB, Reslin DJ: Blue toe syndrome causes and management. Arch Intern Med 152:2197–2202, 1992.
110. Parkhouse N, LeQuesne PM: Impaired neurogenic vascular response in patients with diabetes and neurogenic foot lesions. N Engl J Med 318:1306, 1988.
111. Palumbo PJ, Melton LJ III: Peripheral vascular disease and diabetes. *In* Diabetes in America, Diabetes Data Compiled in 1984. National Institutes of Health Publ No. 85-1468, Washington, DC: U.S. Government Printing Office, 1985.
112. Pearce WH, Wiet SP: Noninvasive evaluation of atherosclerotic emboli. *In* Yao JST, Pearce WH (eds): The Ischemic Extremity: Advances in Treatment. East Norwalk, CT: Appleton & Lange, 1995.
113. Pecoraro RE, Ahroni JH, Boyko EJ, et al: Chronology and determinants of tissue repair in diabetic lower-extremity ulcers. Diabetes 40:1305–1313, 1991.

114. Pecoraro RE, Reiber GE, Burgess EM: Pathways to diabetic limb amputation: Basis for prevention. Diabetes Care 16:1187–1189, 1993.
115. Peiris AN, Sothmann MS, Hoffman RG, et al: adiposity, fat distribution, and cardiovascular risk. Ann Intern Med 110:867, 1989.
116. Peters AL, Legorreta AP, Ossorio RC, et al: Quality of out-patient care provided to diabetic patients. Diabetes Care 19:601–606, 1996.
117. Pinzur MS: Amputation level selection in the diabetic foot. Clin Orthop 296:68–70, 1993.
118. Pollin W: The role of the addictive process as a key step in causation of all tobacco-related diseases. JAMA 252:2874, 1984.
119. Quebedeaux TL, Lavery LA, Lavery DC: The development of foot deformities and ulcers after great toe amputation in diabetes. Diabetes Care 19:165–167, 1996.
120. Queen M, Biem HJ, Moe GW, et al: Development of cholesterol embolization syndrome after intravenous streptokinase for acute myocardial infarction. Am J Cardiol 6:1042–1043, 1990.
121. Rayman G, Williams SA, Spencer PD, et al: Impaired microvascular hyperaemic response to minor skin trauma in type 1 diabetes. Br Med J 292:1295–1298, 1986.
122. Reaven GM: Banting lecture 1988: Role of insulin resistance in human disease. Diabetes 37:1595, 1988.
123. Reiber GE, Boyko EJ, Smith DG: Lower extremity foot ulcers and amputation in individuals with diabetes. In Harris MI, Cowie CC, Stern MP, et al (eds): Diabetes in America, 2nd ed. Washington, DC: U.S. Government Printing Office, Department of Health and Human Services Publ No. 95-1468, 1995.
124. Reiber GE, Pecoraro RE, Koepsell TD: Risk factors for amputation in patients with diabetes mellitus. Ann Intern Med 117:97–105, 1992.
125. Rodeheaver G: Controversies in topical wound management. Ostomy Wound Management 20:58–68, 1988.
126. Rodeheaver G, Baharestani MM, Brabec ME, et al: Wound healing and wound management: Focus on debridement: An interdisciplinary round table, September 18, 1992, Jackson Hole, WY. Adv Wound Care 7:22–36, 1994.
127. Ronaghy HA: The role of zinc in human nutrition. World Rev Nutr Diet 54:237–254, 1987.
128. Ronnemaa T, Hamalainen H, Toikka T, et al: Evaluation of the impact of podiatrist care in the primary prevention of foot problems in diabetic subjects. Diabetes Care 20:1833–1837, 1997.
129. Sathe SR: Managing the diabetic foot in developing countries. IDF Bull 38:16–18, 1993.
130. Selby PL, Young MJ, Boulton AJM: Biphosphonates: A new treatment for diabetic Charcot neuroarthropathy? Diabetes Med 11:28–31, 1996.
131. Selby JV, Zhang D: Risk factors for lower extremity amputation in persons with diabetes. Diabetes Care 18:509–516, 1995.
132. Shapiro LS: Cholesterol embolization after treatment with tissue plasminogen activators [letter]. N Engl J Med 321:1270, 1989.
133. Shaw RS, Baue AE: Management of sepsis complicating arterial reconstructive surgery. Surgery 53:75–86, 1962.
134. Sieggreen M: Healing of physical wounds. Nurs Clin North Am 22:439–447, 1987.
135. Silbert S: Amputation of the lower extremity in diabetes mellitus: A follow-up study of 294 cases. Diabetes 1:297, 1952.
136. Sinacore DR: Total contact casting for diabetic neuropathic ulcers. Phys Ther 76:296–301, 1996.
137. Smith DM, Weinberger M, Katz BP: A controlled trial to increase office visits and reduce hospitalizations of diabetic patients. J Gen Intern Med 2:232–238, 1987.
138. Soulier SM: The use of running shoes in the prevention of plantar diabetic ulcers. J Am Podiatr Med Assoc 76:395, 1986.
139. Steed DL, and The Diabetic Ulcer Study Group: Clinical evaluation of recombinant human platelet-derived growth factor for the treatment of lower extremity diabetic ulcers. J Vasc Surg 21:71–81, 1995.
140. Steed DL, Donohoe D, Webster MW, Lindsley L, and the Diabetic Ulcer Study Group: Effect of extensive debridement and treatment on the healing of diabetic foot ulcers. J Am Coll Surg 183:61–64, 1996.
141. Steed DL, Goslen JB, Holloway GA, et al: Randomized prospective double-blind trial in healing chronic diabetic foot ulcers: CT-102 activated platelet supernatant, topical versus placebo. Diabetes Care 15:1598–1604, 1992.
142. Stotts NA, Deosaransingh K, Roll FJ, et al: Underutilization of pressure ulcer risk assessment in hip fracture patients. Adv Wound Care 11:32–38, 1998.
143. Stotts NA, Washington DC: Nutrition: A critical component of wound healing. AACN Clin Issues 1:585–594, 1990.
144. Taylor LMP Jr, Porter JM: The clinical course of diabetics who require emergent foot surgery because of infection or ischemia. J Vasc Surg 6:454, 1987.
145. The Diabetes Control and Complications Trial Research Group: The effect of intensive treatment of diabetes on the development and progression of long term complications in insulin-dependent diabetes mellitus. N Engl J Med 329:977–986, 1993.
146. Tibbles PM, Edelsberg JS: Hyperbaric-oxygen therapy. N Engl J Med 334:1642–1648, 1996.
147. Tribe RM, Poston L: Oxidative stress and lipids in diabetes: A role in endothelium vasodilator dysfunction? Vasc Med 1:195–206, 1996.
148. Uccioli L, Faglia E, Monticone G, et al: Manufactured shoes in the prevention of diabetic foot ulcers. Diabetes Care 18:1376–1382, 1995.
149. Warram JH, Laffel LMB, Valsania P, et al: Excess mortality associated with diuretic therapy in diabetes mellitus. Arch Intern Med 151:1350, 1991.
150. Waters RL, Perry J, Antonelli D, et al: Energy cost of walking of amputees: The influence of level of amputation [abstract]. J Bone Joint Surg 58A:42–46, 1976.
151. Waugh NR: Amputations in diabetic patients: A review of rates, relative risks, and resource use. Comm Med 10:279–288, 1988.
152. Williams MV, Baker DW, Parker RM, et al: Relationship of functional health literacy to patients' knowledge of their chronic disease: A study of patients with hypertension and diabetes. Arch Intern Med 158:166–172, 1998.
153. Wilson M: Charcot foot osteoarthropathy in diabetes mellitus. Mil Med 156:563–569, 1991.

154. Wilson PWF, Kannel WB: Epidemiology of hyper-glycemia and atherosclerosis. *In* Ruderman N, Williamson J, Brownlee M (eds): Hyperglycemia, Diabetes and Vascular Disease. New York: Oxford University Press, 1992.
155. Wood JM, Evans PE, Schallreuter KU, et al: A multicenter study on the use of pulsed low-intensity direct current for healing chronic stage I and stage II decubitus ulcers. Arch Dermatol 129:999–1009, 1993.
156. Wooldridge J, Moreno L: Evaluation of the costs to Medicare of covering therapeutic shoes for diabetic patients. Diabetes Care 17:541–547, 1994.
157. Working group on hypertension in diabetes: Statement on hypertenison in diabetes mellitus, final report. Arch Intern Med 147:830, 1987.
158. Young MJ, Breddy J, Veves A, et al: The prediction of diabetic neuropathic foot ulceration using vibration perception thresholds. Diabetes Care 19:710–714, 1996.
159. Young SR, Dyson M: The effect of therapeutic ultrasound on angiogenesis. Ultrasound Med Biol 16:261–269, 1990.
160. Zacharias FJ, Cowen KJ, Prestt J, et al: Propranolol in hypertension: A study of long-term therapy. 1964–1970. Am Heart J 83:755, 1972.

10

DIABETIC FOOT PROBLEMS AND THEIR MANAGEMENT AROUND THE WORLD

■ Andrew J. M. Boulton and Loretta Vileikyte

One day everything will be well, that is our hope. Everything is fine today—that is our illusion.
Voltaire

The words of Voltaire summarize the global situation with regard to the diagnosis and management of diabetic foot problems. In recent years there has been an increasing interest in research and into improvements of service provision in this area. This has partly been driven by the realization of the vast economic consequences of the lower limb diabetic complications. In a recent study, Holzer et al.[50] studied a database of 7 million U.S. patients for health insurance: in 2 years, the total expenditure for treated diabetic foot ulcers was $16 million, an average of $4,595 per ulcer episode.

In the United Kingdom, diabetic patients are four times more likely to be admitted to hospital, and this figure rises to 16 for those with peripheral neuropathy.[27] The data from Sweden are more depressing[5]: in a careful study of the economics of healing of foot ulcers, the cost of healing with hospitalization and surgery was $57,300 per case, compared with $8,500 per case for primary healing alone (1990 prices). However, as pointed out by Johnson and Williams,[34] many of these economic analyses failed to take account of the indirect costs, such as absence from work, disability benefits, costs of home alterations, and so on.

Reassuringly, however, it has not only been health care economics that have re-sulted in an increase of the awareness of foot problems: there has been a steady rise in the volume of research and presentations in this area that has been observed worldwide. The American Diabetes Association (ADA) has an active foot council with a large membership, and the European Association for the Study of Diabetes has regular presentations on foot problems at its annual meetings and also established a Diabetic Foot Study Group in 1998. Symposia on the diabetic foot were recently held at annual meetings in South Africa, South America, and Australia, and one of the main sessions at the 1998 Alfadiem (World French Speaking Diabetes Group) in Marrakesh, Morocco, was on *"le pied diabetique."*

A library of all publications on the diabetic foot is kept at Penn State University,[17] and continues to record increasing numbers of publications on these topics. Moreover, groups are now established with multinational representation to gather data and institute multinational studies and guidelines. Examples include the Lower Extremity Amputation (LEA) group, which has a study in progress designed to compare the incidence of LEA over time within and between communities across the world.[37] The International Consensus Group on the Diabetic Foot was established in 1997 and guidelines on diagnosis and management issues were published in 1999. Similar guidelines on diabetic neuropathy were published in 1998.[11]

Finally, strong evidence of increasing activity in the diabetic foot clinical and research areas is provided by the large number of national and multinational meetings that are being held solely on this topic. The Third International Meeting on the Diabetic Foot was held in the Netherlands in 1999, and the Eighth National UK Meeting (held in alternate years) will be held in Malvern, UK, in 2000.

Regular national meetings are also held in Scandinavia, Belgium, the United States, Canada, Italy, and many other countries. Thus, reverting to Voltaire's words, it appears that whereas the illusion of good global footcare remains, we have reason to be hopeful that improvements will continue.

When approaching the vast topic of this chapter, it soon became apparent that no expert could possibly be all inclusive on global foot care. Whereas the risks and prevalence of foot problems vary according to geographic location, there is no diabetic population that is immune from neuropathy, vascular disease, or ulceration/amputation. However, published data on the epidemiologic aspects of foot problems are of variable quality, and in Table 10–1 we have attempted to provide a global overview of the problem, with references taken from published articles or presentations at national meetings.

As the only authors in this volume not working in North America, we have attempted to collect data from countries representing all the remaining continents, but again, the sources of data vary from regional experts to papers in peer-reviewed journals. In our defense, we felt it important to include data from as many countries as possible, even if published data were unavailable.

Europe

With the exception of North America, among the remaining continents, most information on research and clinical management of diabetic foot problems is available from Europe. The St. Vincent Declaration of the European Divisions of the World Health Organization (WHO) and the International Diabetes Federation[2] was signed by most European countries: amongst its many aims was to strive

to achieve a 50% reduction in amputations in diabetic patients within a 5-year period. Several national diabetes associations established St. Vincent Taskforces to try and monitor success in achieving the set targets, and these will be referred to under individual countries.

There have been collaborative ventures between European countries in the area of the diabetic foot. In one example, no major differences were observed when comparing risk factors for foot ulceration between large clinics in four countries, two in northern and two in southern Europe.[60] Thus it was concluded that similar strategies for the prevention of foot problems should be equally successful in different European countries.

United Kingdom

Many reports and publications on the diabetic foot have been produced from the United Kingdom over the years. It was Pryce, a surgeon working in Nottingham, who realized the importance of peripheral neuropathy in the pathogenesis of diabetic foot ulcers,[46] and it was almost 60 years ago that the first successful wedge or ray excision was performed by McKeown in London.[39] More recently, the first detailed reports on the potential success of the team approach and the combined diabetic foot clinic were reported.[22, 56] Despite this, "Everything is fine today—that is our illusion" is sadly true.

In the National Health Service, every resident is entitled to free health care, and all have access to a general practitioner (GP) at the primary care level. Many type 2 diabetic patients are cared for in primary care by the GP, often with a practice nurse. Some, but certainly not all, practices can provide podiatry care. Onward referral to hospital diabetes clinics may occur, especially if there are complications. However, there are probably no more than 20 specialist multidisciplinary diabetic foot clinics in the United Kingdom (population approximately 55 million). Diabetes care is provided with the annual review[10] being the cornerstone of management. Detailed guidelines have been published as part of the St. Vincent initiative.[23] Disturbing evidence, for example, as to the lack of chiropody (podiatry) care in certain districts of the United Kingdom is highlighted in this report.

The difficulties of achieving the St. Vincent target for reducing amputations in a rural

Table 10–1 ■ EPIDEMIOLOGIC DATA ON DIABETIC FOOT PROBLEMS WORLDWIDE, INDICATING THE PREVALENCE AND INCIDENCE OF FOOT ULCERS AND AMPUTATIONS IN DIABETIC POPULATIONS

STUDY AND COUNTRY	N	PREVALENCE (%)		INCIDENCE (%)		RISK FACTORS FOR ULCERS (%)	NOTE
		Ulcers	Amp	Ulcers	Amp		
Population-Based Studies							
Borssen et al., 1990 (Sweden)[8]	395	0.75	—	—	—	—	Age 15–50 only
Bouter et al., 1993 (Netherlands)[12]	300,000	—	—	0.8	0.4	—	
Carrington et al., 1996 (UK)[16]	9,710	4.8	1.4	—	—	67	
Humphrey et al., 1996 (Nauru, Pacific Region)[31]	1,564	—	—	—	0.76	—	From estimate 7.6/1,000 person-yr
Kumar et al., 1994 (UK)[35]	811	1.4	—	—	—	41.6	Type 2 diabetes only
Moss et al., 1992 (USA)[40]	2,900	—	3.6	10.1	2.1	—	Incidence figures over 4 yr
Siitonen et al., 1993 (Finland)[51]	477	—	—	—	0.5	—	
Vozar et al., 1997 (Slovakia)[61]	1,205	2.5	0.9	0.6	0.2	—	
Clinic-Based Studies							
Belhadj, 1998 (Algeria)[7]	865	11.9	6.7	—	—	58.4	
Pendsey, 1994 (India)[42]	11,300	3.6	—	—	—	—	
Urbancic-Rovan et al., 1998 (Slovenia)[58]	701	7.1	—	—	—	86.3	
van Rensberg & Kalk 1995 (South Africa)[59]	125	11.2	—	—	—	68.0	

N, total diabetic population; Amp, amputation.

UK health district were highlighted in a recent audit article.[3] Instead of a reduction, an increase in amputations was observed. Faults were discovered at almost all levels of management, and it is clear that if we are to reduce lower limb complications, as well as guidelines, there must be a clear strategy for their implication and regular audit to monitor progress.

France

There is increasing interest in diabetic foot problems in France, but most diabetic patients with type 2 diabetes are cared for by GPs as in the UK. Moreover, there are no podiatrists in France, although local nail care is provided for by pedicures. For a country of approximately 60 million population, it is estimated that there are only around 10 multidisciplinary diabetic foot clinics.

However, with increasing realization of the problem, there have been recent efforts to improve the knowledge of diabetic foot problems among health care professionals.[48] Studies from Grenoble have also attempted to estimate cost of diabetic foot care in one center.[15] The average direct cost of a hospital admission for a foot ulcer was Fr103,718, (US $17,000) which included direct and indirect costs. The costs varied from Fr55,500 (US $8,770) for a Wagner grade 1 lesion up to Fr175,700 (US $28,800) for a gangrenous grade 4 foot.[15] The establishment of a team approach in a Paris clinic has recently been shown to be beneficial with 33% reduction in hospital inpatients' stay and significance with regard to the St. Vincent Initiative, a 50% reduction of major amputations.[28]

Germany

As in other European countries, diabetes care is mainly based upon a GP primary care model, especially for type 2 diabetes. Because of current funding difficulties, referral from primary care to hospital clinics is restricted and poses financial difficulties. For the largest country in Europe (population approximately 80 million), there are about 50 multidisciplinary diabetic foot clinics, but these are nearly all hospital based. As in France, there is no formal podiatry: chiropodists are available but have little training in the diabetic foot. In contrast, there are well-trained orthopedic shoemakers and reimbursement is available for bespoke shoes.

The German Diabetes Association has established a working party on the provision of foot care across the country, and some progress is being made with the St. Vincent Initiative. However, as in the United Kingdom, Stiegler et al. have reported difficulties in achieving a reduction in amputations.[54]

Italy

There are a number of major centers with a particular interest and excellence in diabetic foot care in Italy, but as in other countries, large rural areas have no specific foot services. Podiatry services are not routinely available, but there are a number of good footwear suppliers. Indeed, one of the first randomized studies to demonstrate the efficacy of therapeutic footwear in reducing recurrent ulcers was performed in Rome.[57]

Benelux Countries

The Netherlands, unlike many other European countries, have a well-developed network of podiatrists, all of whom undergo a 3-year training degree course. Bakker et al. have reviewed the role of podiatrists and diabetic foot care and found, in a national survey, that in 32% of hospitals a podiatrist was specifically available for the care of diabetic patients.[6] There are thought to be 250,000 diabetic patients in the Netherlands, and 20 hospitals have multidisciplinary diabetic foot clinics.[6]

Although Belgium does not have such a well-developed podiatry program, a national training program in diabetic foot care for all doctors treating diabetic patients (including GPs) was established in 1997, and a well-attended course was conducted in 1998. This is led by the group from Antwerp: the same group previously participated in the European Study of Risk Factors for Foot Ulcers that demonstrated no major differences between northern and southern European clinics.[60] Multidisciplinary foot clinics are established in Antwerp, Brussels, Charleroi, and approximately the six other centers in this country of population 10 million.

Scandinavia

In comparison with other European countries, standards of screening and educational foot care are generally high in all Scandinavian countries. Qualified podiatrists are available in all countries although, as reported by Sparre et al.,[53] even in Stockholm, only a minority of diabetic patients have access to chiropody (podiatry) services. Multidisciplinary diabetic foot clinics are established in many other cities across the four countries and a number of important studies have been published by diabetic foot experts in Scandinavia.[4, 36, 51, 54]

Other Western European Countries

Austria, with a population of approximately 8 million, has no fully trained podiatrists, but at least ten foot clinics have been established in recent years.

There is no structured diabetic foot service in Greece, whose population is approximately 10 million. There are two overseas trained podiatrists in Greece, and a multidisciplinary diabetic foot service was established in Athens in 1998. However, in most centers, foot ulcer patients are referred directly to surgeons and amputation rates are high.

Structured foot care programs are now established in some Spanish cities including Madrid and Barcelona. In a community-based study in the Barcelona region, however, a high prevalence of diabetic foot problems was reported, with 10% of 2,595 type 2 diabetic patients being identified.[25]

Much work on the team approach and the importance of patient education has originated from Geneva, Switzerland, where a structured educational program for footwear has been established for many years. As demonstrated in a recent presentation, reulceration rates can be significantly reduced by regular foot clinic attendance and medical supervision.[45]

Eastern Europe

There is no organized foot care system in Russia, nor are there any major publications on this topic. There are no podiatrists or specialist footwear suppliers, but multidisciplinary diabetic foot centers have been established in Moscow,[1] St. Petersburg, and several other major cities. The first center to be formed in Moscow is training ten teams from other cities each year, and has presented data on their activity.[1] A federal program for diabetes and diabetic foot problems has been established but is experiencing difficulties because of economic hardship.

Immense problems in diabetic foot care are still experienced in former Soviet countries, and amputation rates remain depressingly high. However, some progress is being made, and diabetic foot clinics are now established in Kiev, Kharkov, and Lviv (Ukraine), Minsk (Byelorussia), and Tblisi (Georgia). Among former Soviet countries, however, the Baltic States (Lithuania, Latvia, and Estonia) probably have the best foot care systems. The main Lithuanian diabetic foot clinic in Kaunas was trained by two British teams. Subsequently, seven other centers have been established in this country of population 3.7 million. Presentations and publications have resulted on diabetic foot problems and long-term follow-up of high-risk patients.[18, 19] The main center now trains foot care teams from other Eastern European countries. In neighboring Latvia, foot care personnel have received training in Lithuania and the United Kingdom.

Former Warsaw Pact countries are developing organized foot care programs in many cities. However, major difficulties remain in many countries. In former Yugoslavia, organized foot care programs are being established in Slovenia (population 2 million), Bosnia (4 million), and Macedonia (2 million), but reliable data were not available for Serbia (10 million), Croatia (4 million), or Montenegro (1 million). Most progress has been made in Slovenia: some form of foot care is available in 15 centers, with four centers having specialized diabetic foot clinics. During a period of 16 months, over 700 patients were screened in Ljubljana, and 9% had a history of foot ulcers, and only 14% had healthy feet.[58] Foot clinics are also being established in many other countries including Bulgaria, Czech Republic, Slovakia, Poland, and Hungary.

Asia

Considering the vast population of this continent, there are sparse data on diabetic foot problems from this part of the world. As for Europe, some countries will be discussed as individual sections, but for many others, reliable information was unavailable.

China

China is the world's most populated country, and the prevalence of diabetes has risen from 0.5% to 2.5% in the adult population in the 5 years until 1995. It was then estimated that 15 million Chinese had diabetes and that a further 18 million had impaired glucose tolerance.[55] Until recently, most diabetic patients lived in rural communities, and had access to a three-tier health care system where, in the first level, village physicians received less than a year's training after junior high school level, whereas physicians in district health centers and county hospitals had full medical school training.[55] Realizing the challenge of providing appropriate care for over 15 million patients, the Ministry of Health has taken the first steps through the development of a national program for diabetes. With this background, it is not surprising that foot care problems are common in Chinese diabetic patients. There is no podiatry program for diabetic patients and amputations are common. However, interest in the diabetic foot is increasing and some centers have established multidisciplinary teams for foot care.[62]

Japan

Although there are no major publications on the prevalence of foot problems in Japan, foot ulceration and amputations are increasingly being reported as significant problems, with multidisciplinary foot teams being established. These patients, when admitted to hospital, often come under the care of dermatologists or surgeons rather than the diabetologists. There is no podiatry, but several study groups comprising diabetologists, surgeons, and nurses exist. One of the main centers in Tokyo has recently reported on the high incidence of vascular foot lesions and diabetic dialysis and predialysis patients.[29] Such patients are seen by the diabetic foot care team.

Philippines

Most physicians' concept of a diabetic foot in the Philippines is of gangrene or severe ulceration requiring amputation. Until recently, there were no statistics, no podiatrists, and minimal preventative care. A few years ago, two Australian podiatrists started a program of education and training, and subsequently a few diabetic foot care centers have been set up. Physicians from one such center have now been traveling to other parts of the country and providing educational courses under the auspices of the Philippines Diabetic Association. Thus it appears that much progress is being made in this country.

India

The population of India is approximately 1 billion, and with a prevalence of type 2 diabetes of between 1% and 5%, it is estimated that there are 30 million Indians with type 2 diabetes, or 60 million potential diabetic feet (C. V. Krishnaswami, personal communication, 1998). Although there are no major differences in risk factors, the clinical features of diabetic foot problems do vary in developing countries because of regional factors.[42] The hallmark of diabetic foot problems in India is gross infection: major contributing factors for late presentation include the frequency of barefoot gait, attempts at home surgery, trust in faith healers, and often undetected diabetes. Certain atypical features peculiar to this part of the world include rodents (usually rats) nibbling at insensitive feet while the patients sleep on the floor, maggots pouring out of open wounds, and red ants swarming inside dressings.

Sandal-induced ulcers (from the use of "chappals," with a single thong between the hallux and the second toe) are not infrequent, as the result of pressure from the thong, and pressure points on the tips of the toes from extra pressure exerted whilst trying to keep the shoe on.[43, 44]

Apart from a few specialist centers in major cities, care of the diabetic foot is not organized, a problem compounded by a lack of podiatrists and orthotists.

Other Countries

In Singapore, a number of hospitals have established diabetic foot services, with the services of podiatrists, many of whom were trained in Australia. In a survey of causes of ulcers in a podiatry clinic, the causes were mainly related to barefoot gait, sandals, and other inappropriate footwear.[21]

A number of centers in Taiwan have established specialist diabetic foot clinics, and studies have been reported on the variable risk factors for levels of amputation.[30]

Other Asian countries with historical connections with European countries have benefited from educational visits and training by overseas experts. Thus, for example, teams of diabetologists, podiatrists, and surgeons from the Netherlands have visited Indonesia to assist in the formation of the diabetic foot service in Jakarta.

Australasia

Although this continent covers a vast area, it has a relatively low population per square mile: the main nations are Australia and New Zealand, but there are also many other countries including a large number of Pacific island communities. The prevalence of type 2 diabetes is generally high among the native populations of these areas, such as the Aborigines in Australia and the Maoris in New Zealand.

Australia

Australia has a well-developed health care system, and podiatrists are available in many centers. However, until recently, there have been few multidisciplinary diabetic foot clinics: this problem is now being addressed by the establishment of a national diabetes foot care network under the auspices of the national diabetes strategy, which is endorsed by the Australian government. With funding from this source, the Sydney group has piloted this program in 14 sites, most of which have a doctor, a nurse, and a podiatrist.[38] After training in Sydney, each team has arranged teaching sessions and practical workshops for local physicians, surgeons, GPs, nurses, and podiatrists. Common protocols are being developed, and ultimately it is hoped to extend the system of foot care to all regions of Australia.

New Zealand

As for Australia, there is a well-developed health care system in New Zealand, and although podiatrists are available, the level of service remains well below the recom-mended 0.5 full-time equivalence per 100,000 of the population.[41] A recently published study reported on hospital discharges for diabetic foot disease and for a 13-year period until 1993; during this time the national number of discharges actually increased from 14 per 100,000 total population in 1980 to 26 per 100,000 in 1993.[41] Translated into costs for this country with a population of 3.3 million, this equates to an inpatient management cost for diabetic foot disease in 1993 of $7.7 million (US dollars). It is suggested that strategies that should be adopted include more ongoing education of health care professionals, development of national guidelines, improving the level of podiatry service, and the establishment of a national screening program.

Other Countries

The prevalence of diabetes in Fiji is high, greater than 10%. Until recently, the commonest cause for surgical admission to one hospital was diabetic foot ulcers, and in a 3-month period before the establishment of a foot clinic, the number of diabetic amputations at the Suva Hospital was a staggering 39. With such statistics and a grant from the Australian government in collaboration with the Fijian government, the diabetes center at a Sydney hospital established high-risk diabetic foot clinics in the three main centers of Fiji. The clinic in Suva now sees 155 patients per month with ulceration or infection, and the number of admissions has been reduced to three or four per month with a dramatic reduction in amputations (M. McGill, personal communication 1998). These dramatic results demonstrate the positive effect of a national training program, and the Sydney group can feel gratified by their major contribution to diabetic foot care in Fiji.

Another Pacific island, Nauru, which once had the dubious distinction of having the highest national prevalence of diabetes in the world, has been the focus of a study of amputations in diabetes.[31] The incidence of first amputation in Nauru in type 2 diabetic patients was 7.6 per 1,000 person-years (Table 10–1), but a decrease was seen after the introduction of a national foot care health education and prevention campaign in 1992.[31]

Africa

Of 98 presentations on the diabetic foot at the 1997 International Diabetes Meeting in Finland, only one originated from the continent of Africa. We were able to gather some information from countries in South and the north of Africa.

In South Africa, there have been no significant publications on the diabetic foot for about 30 years. The general level of diabetic foot care varies immensely across the country, mainly due to the past inequalities in the provision of health care for the majority of the population. Not all hospitals have podiatrists, resulting in the greater likelihood of surgical rather than conservative care. Most hospitals have nurse educators, providing some form of screening and education.

There are fewer than 200 podiatrists for a population of 40 million, of whom approximately 10% are thought to have diabetes. Despite these statistics, there has been a great deal of improvement in the last few years. Diabetes societies (both professional and lay) are actively involved in trying to improve the standard of diabetic foot care. There have been presentations on diabetic foot problems at national and international meetings in recent years,[14, 59] attempting to assess the extent of the diabetic foot problem and help plan improvements in screening and treatment.

Turning to north Africa, data were available from Morocco and Algeria. In Morocco, with a population of 30 million, the prevalence of diabetes is high, being 13% of the population over 30 years of age. There are estimated to be 67,000 diabetic patients in the capital city of Rabat, and 2,000 with active foot ulcers.[26] In Casablanca, 67% of foot ulcer patients are male, 88% are type 2 diabetes, and 47% of lesions are shoe induced, with 15% secondary to traditional "healing" methods.[52] The authors of this study concluded that special education is required for those patients with poor knowledge, especially those who rely on traditional healing methods.

Lastly, a study from Algeria in 1996 reported on 865 patients from 14 centers[7] (Table 10–1). Over half of the sample had experienced foot problems, including 15.5% with symptomatic neuropathy, 12% with infected ulcers, and 6.7% who had already undergone amputation. There is clearly a major need for an educational program for diabetic foot care in this country.

South and Central America

The prevalence of diabetes is high throughout this region: a recent study from Paraguay reported an age-standardized prevalence of 6.5% in the urban Hispanic population, with a further 11% with impaired glucose tolerance.[33] Similar prevalence rates of around 7% have been reported in Argentina, Brazil, Uruguay, and Venezuela: the rate in Chile is slightly lower at about 5%.

In Brazil, foot problems are common and may coexist with leprosy (Hansen's disease) in northern regions. A specific "Save the Foot in Diabetes—Brazil Project" has been established in the DF (Distrito Federal) region around the capital, Brasilia, with government backing.

Farther north, multidisciplinary teams for wound care have been set up in Costa Rica that have had a major impact on diabetic foot care.[32] A number of presentations in this region were made at the 1997 International Diabetes Meeting.[24, 49]

Conclusions

In this brief global tour we have attempted to review the standards of foot care and to identify what research is progressing, worldwide. There are many developments that encourage optimism for future improvement in diabetic foot care; however, it is important for those readers based in Western countries to acknowledge that much of what is known as the management of the insensitive diabetic foot was derived from observations many years ago on the management of foot problems secondary to leprosy in countries such as India and Brazil. It was, for example, Dr. Milroy Paul, working in Ceylon (now Sri Lanka), who first used walking below-knee plaster casts for his leprosy patients with foot ulcers over 60 years ago.[13, 20] So successful was this treatment that it spread to other leprosy centers and later to diabetes clinics.[9] Thus it now behooves us to attempt to improve matters by disseminating worldwide the key areas of knowledge in the screening, education, and management of diabetic patients at risk of foot problems.

ACKNOWLEDGMENTS

We wish to thank many friends and colleagues worldwide who have provided information for this chapter, but in particular we wish to thank: J.-L. Richard, G. Va-Han (France); H. Reike, M. Spraul (Germany); L. Uccioli (Italy); K. Bakker (Netherlands); I. Dumont, K. Van-Acker (Belgium); J. Apelqvist, K. Brismar (Sweden); T. Pieber (Austria); N. Tentolouris, D. Voyatzoglou (Greece); I. Gourieva (Russia); V. Dargis (Lithuania); A. Helds (Latvia); V. Urbancic-Rovan (Slovenia); X. Zhangrong (China); K. Hosokawa (Japan); M. T. P. Que (Philippines); C. V. Krishnaswami, S. Pendsey (India); M. McGill, J. E. Shaw (Australia); A. Clarke, K. Huddle (South Africa); Z. Slaoui (Morocco); O. Jaramillo (Costa Rica); and H. Pedrosa (Brazil).

REFERENCES

1. Ametov A, Gourieva I, Voronin A, et al: The four year activity of the diabetic foot centre in Moscow: Cooperation and partnership. Diabetes Nutr Metab 10(Suppl 1):33, 1997.
2. Anonymous: Diabetes care and research in Europe: The St. Vincent Declaration. Diabet Med 7:360, 1990.
3. Anonymous: An audit of amputations in a rural health district. Pract Diabetes Int 14:175–178, 1997.
4. Apeqvist J, Larsson J, Agardh CD: Long-term prognosis for diabetic patients with foot ulcers. J Intern Med 233:485–491, 1993.
5. Apelqvist J, Ragnarson-Tennvall G, Persson U, Larsson J: Diabetic foot ulcers in a multi-disciplinary setting: An economic analysis of primary healing and healing with amputation. J Intern Med 235:463–471, 1994.
6. Bakker K, van Houtum WH, Schaper NC: Diabetic foot care in the Netherlands: An evaluation. Pract Diabetes Int 15:41–42, 1998.
7. Belhadj M: La place du pied diabétique. Diabetes Metab 24(Suppl 1):LXVII, 1998.
8. Borssen B, Bergenheim T, Lithner F: The epidemiology of foot lesions in diabetic patients age 15–50. Diabet Med 7:438–444, 1990.
9. Boulton AJM: Diabetic foot ulceration: The leprosy connection. Pract Diabetes Dig 3:35–37, 1990.
10. Boulton AJM: The annual review—here to stay [editorial]. Diabet Med 9:887, 1992.
11. Boulton AJM, Gries FA, Jervell J: International guidelines on the diagnosis and out-patient management of diabetic neuropathy. Diabet Med 15:508–516, 1998.
12. Bouter KP, Storm AJ, Groot RRM, et al: The diabetic foot in Dutch hospitals: Epidemiological features and clinical outcome. Eur J Med 2:215–218, 1993.
13. Brand PW: Insensitive Feet: Practical Handbook on Foot Problems in Leprosy. London: Leprosy Mission, 1981.
14. Clarke A: The prevalence of foot problems in black South Africans with diabetes: A pilot study. Presented at 7th Meeting on the Diabetic Foot, Malvern, UK, May 1998.
15. Carpentier B, Benhamou PY, Pradines S, et al: Le coût économique du pied diabétique: étude analytique. Diabetes Metab 24(Suppl 1):XXIV, 1998.
16. Carrington AL, Abbott CA, Kulkarni J, et al: Can mass screening and education prevent foot problems? Diabetologia 39(Suppl 1):A3, 1996.
17. Cavanagh PR (ed): The Foot in Diabetes: A Bibliography, Vol. 2. State College, PA: Penn State University, 1995.
18. Dargis V, Pantelejeva O, Janushaite A, et al: Studies of diabetic amputations in Lithuania: Scope for prevention. Diabetologia 40(Suppl 1):A472, 1997.
19. Dargis V, Pantelejeva O, Jonushaite A, et al: Benefits of a multidisciplinary approach in the management of recurrent diabetic foot ulceration in Lithuania. Diabetes Care 22:1428–1431, 1999.
20. Duffy JC, Patout CA: Management of the insensitive foot in leprosy: Lessons learned from Hansen's disease. Mil Med 155:575–579, 1990.
21. du Perez DC, Walsh J: Clinical observations of the distribution of foot ulcerations in Asian patients. Diabetologia 40(Suppl 1):A466, 1997.
22. Edmonds ME, Blundell MP, Morris HE, et al: Improved survival of the diabetic foot: The role of a specialist foot clinic. Q J Med 232:763–771, 1986.
23. Edmonds ME, Boulton AJM, Buckenham J, et al: Report of the Diabetic Foot and Amputation Group. Diabet Med 13(Suppl):S27–S42, 1996.
24. Gamboa AY, Salazar S, Mora S, Arguedas C: Evaluation and classification of the diabetic foot in a rural community in Costa Rica. Diabetologia 40(Suppl 1):A466, 1997.
25. Gimbert RM, Mendez A, Llussa J, et al: Diabetic foot in primary health care: Catalan community-based study. Diabetologia 40(Suppl 1):A467, 1997.
26. Got I: Le pied diabetique: rapport sur la table ronde d'Alfadiem, Marrakesh, Mars 1998. Diabetes Metab 214(in press), 1998.
27. Greener M: Counting the cost of diabetes. Cost Opinions Diabetes 10:4–6, 1996.
28. Heurtier A, Danan JP, Ha Van G, et al: Bilan d'une strategie thérapeutique pluridisciplinaire du pied diabétique dans une unité de podologie. Diabetes Metab 24(Suppl 1):LXVI, 1998.
29. Hosokawa K, Atsumi Y, Mokubo A, et al: Vascular disease of the lower extremities in renal dysfunction patients. Diabetologia 40(Suppl 1):A477, 1997.
30. Hseih S-H, Chang H-Y, Chen J-F, et al: Risk factors for high level amputation in diabetic foot in Taiwan. Diabetologia 40(Suppl 1):A473, 1997.
31. Humphrey ARG, Thoma K, Dowse GK, Zimmet PZ: Diabetes and nontraumatic lower extremity amputations: Incidence, risk factors and prevention—a 12 year follow-up study in Nauru. Diabetes Care 19:710–713, 1996.
32. Jaramillo O, Elizondo J, Jones P, et al: Practical guidelines for developing a hospital-based wound and ostomy clinic. Wounds 9:94–102, 1997.
33. Jiminez JT, Palacia SM, Canete F, et al: Prevalence of diabetes mellitus and associated risk factors in an adult urban population in Paraguay. Diabet Med 15:334–338, 1998.
34. Johnson FN, Williams DRR: Economic aspects of diabetic neuropathy and related complications. In Boulton AJM (ed): Diabetic Neuropathy. Carnforth: Marius Press, 1997, pp 77–96.

35. Kumar S, Ashe H, Parnell L, et al: The prevalence of foot ulceration and its correlates in type 2 diabetic patients: A population-based study. Diabet Med 11:480–484, 1994.

36. Larsson J, Apelqvist J, Agardh CD, Sternstrom A: Decreasing incidence of major amputation in diabetic patients: A consequence of a multidisciplinary foot care team approach? Diabet Med 12:770–776, 1995.

37. LEA Study Group: Comparing the incidence of lower extremity amputations across the world: The global lower extremity amputation study. Diabet Med 12:14–18, 1995.

38. McGill M, Bolton T, Yue DK: Modern approaches to the management of diabetes foot disease. Treating Diabetes 1998 (in press).

39. McKeown KC: The history of the diabetic foot. Diabet Med 12:19–23, 1995.

40. Moss S, Klein R, Klein B: The prevalence and incidence of lower extremity amputation in a diabetic population. Am Intern Med 152:610–616, 1992.

41. Payne CB, Scott RS: Hospital discharges for diabetic foot disease in New Zealand 1980–1993. Diabetes Res Clin Pract 39:69–74, 1998.

42. Pendsey S: Epidemiolgical aspects of the diabetic foot. Int J Diabetes Dev Countries 2:37–38, 1994.

43. Pendsey S: The diabetic foot in India [editorial]. Int J Diabetes Dev Countries 14:35–36, 1994.

44. Pendsey S: Neuropathic foot ulcers: An Indian experience. *In* Hotta N, Greene DA, Ward JD, et al (eds): Diabetic Neuropathy: New Concepts and Insights. Amsterdam: Elsevier Science, 1995, pp 217–219.

45. Peter-Reisch B, Assad J-PH, Reiber GE: Foot reulceration in diabetes: Which important markers for effective prevention? Diabetologia 40(Suppl 1):A473, 1997.

46. Pryce TD: A case of perforating ulcers of both feet associated with diabetic and ataxic symptoms. Lancet 2:11–12, 1887.

47. Reike H: Amputationen der unteren extremitäten bei patienten mit diabetes in Deutschland. *In* Berger M, Trautner C (eds): Die Forderunger von St Vincent—Stand 1996 in Deutchland. Mainz: Kirchheim-Verlag, 1996, pp 80–93.

48. Richard J-L, Merle-Dubourg D: Comment reconnaître en pratique courante le risque d'ulcération d'un pied chez le diabétique. J Plaies Cictrisation 7:80–82, 1997.

49. Salazar S, Mora C, Arquedas C: Preventive care of the diabetic foot; proposal of a Costa Rica attention model. Diabetologia (Suppl 1):A472, 1997.

50. Holzer SE, Camerota A, Martens L, et al: Costs and duration of care for foot ulcers for people with diabetes. Clin Ther 20:169–181, 1998.

51. Siitonen OI, Niskanen LK, Laasko M, et al: Lower extremity amputation in diabetic and non-diabetic patients: A population-based study in Eastern Finland. Diabetes Care 16:16–20, 1993.

52. Slaoui Z, Arabou MR: Evaluation des facteurs déclenchants des lésions de pied chez le diabétique. Diabetes Metab 24(Suppl 1):LXVI, 1998.

53. Sparre K, Avered B, Matero M, et al: More than half of the diabetes population has increased risk to develop chronic foot ulcers. Diabetologia 40(Suppl 1):A476, 1997.

54. Stiegler H, Standl E, Frank S, Mendler G: Failure of reducing lower extremity amputations in diabetic patients: Results of two subsequent population-based surveys 1990 and 1995 in Germany. Vasa 27:10–14, 1998.

55. Tan MH, Freeman T, Mancuso L, et al: Diabetes care in China: Observation from project Hope. Pract Diabetes Int 15:38–40, 1998.

56. Thomson FJ, Veves A, Ashe H, et al: The team approach to diabetic foot care—the Manchester experience. Foot 1:75–82, 1991.

57. Uccioli L, Faglia E, Monticone G, et al: Manufactured shoes in the prevention of diabetic foot ulcers. Diabetes Care 18:1376–1378, 1995.

58. Urbancic-Rovan V, Slak M: Results of 16 months foot screening in Ljubljana, Slovenia. Paper presented at 7th National Meeting on Diabetic Foot, Malvern, UK, May 1998.

59. van Rensberg G, Kalk WJ: Lower extremity complications in black and other diabetic patients. Paper prestented at annual SEMDSA Meeting, Bloemfontein, South Africa, March 1995.

60. Veves A, Uccioli L, Manes C, et al: Comparison of risk factors for foot problems in diabetic patients attending teaching hospital outpatient clinics in four different European states. Diabet Med 11:709–711, 1994.

61. Vozar J, Adamka J, Holéczy P, Seilingerova R: Diabetics with foot lesions and amputations in the region of Horny Zitny Ostrov 1993–1995. Diabetologia 40(Suppl 1):A465, 1997.

62. Zhangrong XU, Yuzheng W, Xiancong W, et al: Chronic diabetic complications and treatments in Chinese diabetic patients. Natl Med J China 77:119–122, 1997.

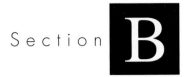

Section **B**

EVALUATION TECHNIQUES AND NONSURGICAL MANAGEMENT

AN IMPROVED METHOD FOR STAGING AND CLASSIFICATION OF FOOT LESIONS IN DIABETIC PATIENTS

■ James W. Brodsky

Classification of wounds of the diabetic foot is needed for many purposes. Among the most important is our need to be able to describe the lesions that we treat in order to study our outcomes, as well as to further our understanding of the diabetic foot. Likewise, we need a method to communicate with one another, and to compare treatments and results of those treatments from one place to another, and even one time to another.

What attributes should the ideal classification system have? First of all, it should be easy to use. It should be practical, and clear. It should be based, as much as possible, on objective criteria and measurements, and minimize subjective assessments, in order to enhance its reproducibility in time (intraobserver) and in space (interobserver). Lastly, it should be relevant. Each different class or stage should signify a different diagnostic and/or therapeutic intervention, so that it serves as a guide in clinical decision making.

Classification Systems

Numerous authors in recent years have grappled with the need for a better classification system for the diabetic foot. Each has contributed significantly to our understanding of the diabetic foot and our methodology or assessment and treatment.

Shea (1975) described a method of grading pressure ulcers. It has the clinical validity that it differentiates based upon depth of the wounds, and which structures are exposed. However, this early classification system gave no consideration of the role of ischemia or vascularity in the healing process. However, this set a precedent for evaluation of the physical characteristics of the wound.[13]

Forrest and Gambor-Neilsen (1984) proposed a wound evaluation system[6] that was similarly clinically sensible but had the disadvantage that it also gave no consideration of ischemia. Some authors have noted that it was not comprehensive, because it did not account for severe wounds.[10, 12]

Knighton et al. (1986) proposed a complex method of wound evaluation that is added together to create a single "wound score" for the purpose of evaluating the effectiveness of platelet-derived growth factors in wound healing.[9] While the single wound score made comparisons easy, other authors noted the disadvantage that it blankets the details, which obfuscates rather than illuminates the *source* of the severity. These same authors noted that many of the factors included in the score are cumbersome or subjective, while others are difficult to measure.[10, 12]

Pecoraro and Reiber (1990) described an elegant wound classification system with ten grades.[12] This classification was also used in their research to track the outcome of these wounds and their contribution to the ultimate cause of amputation. They identified factors that ultimately were associated with more severe outcomes as well as the characteristics that led to amputation. Other authors have noted that some of the terminology describing the wounds was subjective and difficult to interpret.[10] Many of the ten classes require the same diagnostic and therapeutic intervention, making the purpose of their distinction unclear. This classification allows some of the same paradoxical combinations as the original Wagner-Meggitt classification (see below) (e.g., class 1 with intact skin, but also class 9 [partial gangrene]).

Lavery, Armstrong, and Harkless (1996) described an excellent classification system in which the wound gradations were based on the Wagner-Meggitt system.[10] They separately identified and classified the ischemia and the infection, making it the closest to the system of the depth-ischemia classification (1992 and 1993) However, it is more complex to use because of the additional divisions, and the differences among the different grades do not necessarily change the diagnostic and therapeutic actions required.

All of these authors and others[2-4, 6, 9-16] have successfully striven to be more descriptive, more practical, and more comprehensive, and each has contributed significantly to the field of the care of the diabetic foot. Needless to say, further work of many kinds and in many places will continue to refine our understanding in the future.

The greatest challenge to the use of a classification system for diabetic foot wounds is the classic tension between giving the classification sufficient simplicity to make it practical and giving it sufficient detail to make it meaningful. On one hand, the fear of an overly simplified classification is that it will fail to adequately describe the difference among different kinds of wounds (or patients), so that too many lesions with too much variation among them will be "lumped" together. On the other hand, an excessively complex system that "splits" the lesions into too many groups may make the various splinters unrecognizable as a part of the whole. Any system that cannot be practically applied may retard rather than advance the main purpose of all of our efforts, which is our ability to use this knowledge in the daily treatment of actual patients.

Etiology

For purposes of tracing factors that may be predictive of outcome, there is a genuine need to consider the many etiologic factors that contribute to the development of diabetic foot wounds. These many factors include, but are not limited to, perfusion, presence and extent of gangrene, location and severity of vascular disease, location of the lesion, shape of the wound, wound size, wound depth, duration, infection, depth of infection, infecting organism(s), nutrition, immunosuppression, effect of other chronic diseases, multisystem involvement, neuropathy, underlying bony deformity, presence of active neuroarthropathy, nutrition, history of previous lesions, infections and surgeries, gait abnormalities, abnormalities of pressure under the foot, and joint stiffness. For research purposes, much work remains to be done to determine the relative effect of each of these factors, and combinations thereof. In the absence of so much definitive data, we must content ourselves with trying to narrow the scope to areas of a practical nature—factors that we can reliably and reproducibly observe or measure, and factors that have a direct effect on present-day decision making. As our base of knowledge expands, so will our classification systems expand to reflect changes in treatment.

Wagner Classification

Wagner and Meggitt developed a classification system in the 1970s at Rancho Los Amigos Hospital in California, which has been known ever since by both names, but most commonly in this country, as the "Wagner classification."[11, 14, 15] It has been the most widely accepted and universally used grading system for lesions of the diabetic foot.[5, 14, 15] Numerous authors and investigators have since worked to improve our understanding of wounds, and of diabetic foot wounds in particular, and much progress has been made. Recent work on classification has reflected this intense further thought and research as noted above.[1-4, 6, 8-10, 12, 13, 16]

However, the Wagner classification, both in practice and owing to its simplicity, has provided the most widely quoted and widely utilized system. It has been a foundation upon which the subsequent work has been built, and has functioned for the purpose of communication among investigators and clinicians and for the purpose of comparison among patients in many different locales. The original system has six grades of lesions. The first four grades (grades 0, 1, 2, and 3) are based upon the physical depth of the lesion in and through the soft tissue of the foot. The last two grades (grades 4 and 5) are completely distinct because they are based upon the extent of the loss of perfusion in the foot. The vast majority of diabetic foot wounds that are treated in everyday clinical practice are described by the first four grades: grades 0, 1, 2, and 3. Of these grades, the majority of nonhospital treatments are applied to grade 0 and grade 1 lesions, while the deeper (and more advanced) grade 2 and grade 3 lesions typically require hospitalization and/or surgery. The treatment of grades 4 (partial foot gangrene) and 5 (gangrene of the entire foot) as described, are rather direct, viz., amputation of the gangrenous portion of the foot or limb with concomitant considerations of limb revascularization and treatment of concomitant infection, when present.

We owe a debt of gratitude for the original Rancho Los Amigos classification by Wagner and Meggitt because it provided the first easily applied classification of diabetic foot lesions. However, there are two concepts in this classification that now deserve revision based upon the extensive and widespread experience of the last 20 years.

The first is the concept that all the grades of lesions of the diabetic foot from grade 1 ulcers to grade 5 gangrene occur along a naturally progressive continuum. While this may frequently be the case for a grade 1 lesion (superficial ulcer), which advances to a grade 2 lesion (deeper ulcer) and then to a grade 3 lesion (osteomyelitis or abscess), this is not the case with grades 4 and 5. Grades 4 and 5 are ischemic lesions that describe the diminished vascular status of the foot. They are fundamentally unrelated to the nature or progression of the wounds described by the lesser grades. Moreover, the ischemic lesions of grades 4 and 5 may exist in the absence of any of the lesser grades of lesions. Conversely, grades 4 or 5 may coexist with any of them, so that the inclusion of all of these grades in a single longitudinal classification is not only illogical, it obscures our complete understanding of the status of the foot.

For example, a grade 4 foot (partial gangrene) could also be a forefoot that is otherwise grade 0 (no break in the skin and soft tissue) or grade 1 (i.e., a superficial lesion), or even grade 2 or 3. Another example is the problem of classifying the foot that has osteomyelitis, but is also partially gangrenous: Is it a grade 3 or a grade 4 foot? Even more confusing is the following example: Compare a foot with chronic osteomyelitis of the calcaneus with a foot with gangrene of all the toes. By the old Wagner classification, the former is a grade 3 lesion, and the latter is a grade 4. Yet these grades seem inverted when we attempt to understand them as a single progression that mixes wound severity with ischemia. In this example the grades fail to appropriately depict the relative severity, since the patient with this grade 3 lesion needs a transtibial amputation, while the patient with the grade 4 lesion only needs a transmetatarsal amputation.

Vascular pathology absolutely must and can be graded as well, but there is no dependable relationship between the depth of ulcerative lesions (i.e., grades 0, 1, 2, and 3) and the ischemia of the foot or lower limb (i.e., grades 4 and 5). Moreover, the grade 5 foot ceases to be a foot problem and becomes a problem of salvage of the proximal portion of the leg.

The second concept that needs to be refined, while obvious, needs to be stated, viz., that contrary to the diagrams of the original classification, there are not necessarily pathways backwards and forwards from each grade of lesion (e.g., grade 4 feet [partial gangrene] cannot be reversed to grade 3).

Depth-Ischemia Classification

The "depth-ischemia" classification[3, 4] is a modification of the Wagner-Meggitt[11, 14, 15] classification and is offered in Table 11–1 and Figure 11–1. The purposes of this modified classification are first to make the classification more rational and easier to use by separating the evaluation of the wound from the evaluation of the perfusion of the foot; second, to clarify the distinctions among the grades, especially between grades 2 and 3; and third, to simplify the task of correlating appropriate treatments to the proper grade of lesion. This revision of the classification of the lesions of the diabetic foot, combined with the treatment flowchart (Fig. 11–2) make the decision-making path more clear and make this information more accessible than the old Wagner algorithms,[15] which contain a great deal of repetition of the basic diagnostic work-up from one to the other.

The depth-ischemia classification is utilized in the following manner. Each foot is given both a number and a letter grade. The combination of the two describe the physical extent of the wound (number) and the vascularity or ischemia of the foot and limb (letter). First, the soft tissue is inspected, palpated, and graded with a number grade that represents the physical extent of the lesion. Second, the limb and foot are evaluated for perfusion.

The first step is based primarily upon examination of the foot and its wound or ulcer. The grade 0 foot is a foot "at risk" (Fig. 11–3). This is a foot that either has had a previous ulceration, or which has the characteristics that make future ulcerations likely. Those two characteristics are peripheral neuropathy, and an area of pressure, usually due to a bony prominence. Because neuropathy cannot currently be reversed, the decision making for a grade 0 foot is to intervene with a technique of pressure relief, in order to re-

---

Table 11–1 ■ THE "DEPTH-ISCHEMIA" CLASSIFICATION OF DIABETIC FOOT LESIONS*

GRADE/DEFINITION	INTERVENTION
Depth Classification	
0	
The "at-risk" foot: previous ulcer or neuropathy with deformity that may cause new ulceration	Patient education, regular examination, appropriate shoe wear and insoles
1	
Superficial ulceration, not infected	External pressure relief: total-contact cast, walking brace, special shoe wear, etc.
2	
Deep ulceration exposing a tendon or joint (with or without superficial infection)	Surgical debridement, wound care, pressure relief if the lesion closes and converts to grade 1 (prn antibiotics)
3	
Extensive ulceration with exposed bone and/or deep infection (i.e., osteomyelitis, or abscess)	Surgical debridements; ray or partial foot amputation, IV antibiotics, pressure relief if wound converts to grade 1
Ischemia Classification	
A	
Not Ischemic	Observation
B	
Ischemia without gangrene	Vascular evaluation (Doppler, $TcPo_2$ arteriogram, etc.), vascular reconstruction prn
C	
Partial (forefoot) gangrene of the foot	Vascular evaluation, vascular reconstruction (proximal and/or distal bypass or angioplasty), partial foot amputation
D	
Complete foot gangrene	Vascular evaluation, major extremity amputation (TTA, TFA) with possible proximal vascular reconstruction

* Modified from Brodsky J: The diabetic foot. *In* Coughlin MJ, Mann RA (eds): Surgery of the Foot and Ankle, 7th ed. Philadelphia: Mosby, 1999, with permission.
TTA, transtibial, below-knee amputation; TFA, transfemoral amputation, above-knee amputation.

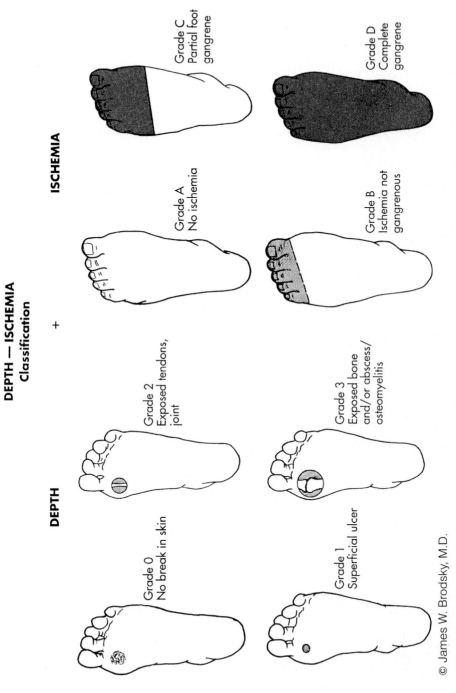

DEPTH — ISCHEMIA
Classification

DEPTH   +   **ISCHEMIA**

Grade 0
No break in skin

Grade 1
Superficial ulcer

Grade 2
Exposed tendons, joint

Grade 3
Exposed bone and/or abscess/osteomyelitis

Grade A
No ischemia

Grade B
Ischemia not gangrenous

Grade C
Partial foot gangrene

Grade D
Complete gangrene

© James W. Brodsky, M.D.

Figure 11–1 ■ The depth-ischemia classification. Each foot is graded both for wound depth (number) and for foot vascularity (letter). (Illustration © James W. Brodsky, M.D.)

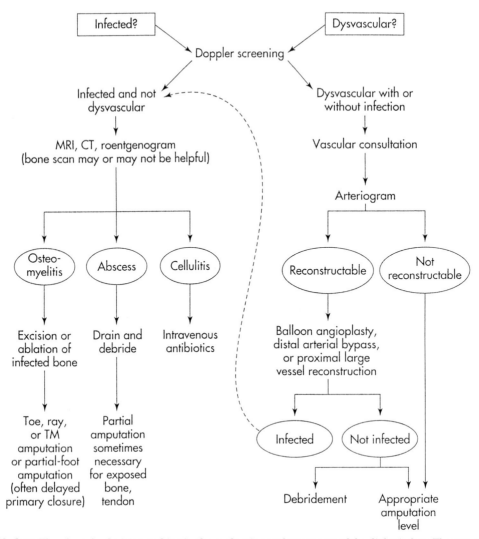

Figure 11–2 ■ Flowchart for decision making in the evaluation and treatment of the diabetic foot. The two columns represent the two major issues of infection and ischemia. Once the ischemic limb has been revascularized, the infection can be treated definitively. (From Brodsky J: The diabetic foot. *In* Couglin MJ, and Mann RA [eds]: Surgery of the Foot and Ankle, 7th ed. Philadelphia: Mosby, 1999, with permission).

duce the likelihood of ulceration. Examples might be the use of a deeper shoe with an accommodative, cushioning insole. A grade 1 lesion is a superficial wound without exposure to sight or to probing of any deep structure (Fig. 11–4). This lesion will be treated usually with some form of pressure relief. Classically, this would be a total-contact cast, to unweight the area of the high pressure if it is on the plantar surface of the foot. If the lesion were on the dorsum or border of the foot (a lesion attributable to shoe pressure), then shoe modification might be the intervention. Either way, the decision making in a grade 1 lesion is to relieve the under-

lying pressure that causes the lesion. If there is accompanying infection, this may also be treated appropriately. But regardless of the use of oral or intravenous antibiotics, the lesion will not heal without relief of the etiologic pressure.

Grade 2 lesions are deeper, with exposure of underlying tendon or joint capsule, with or without infection (Fig. 11–5). Determination of infection is secondary at this point, because it does not change the decision-making algorithm. If there is exposed deep structures, then this patient is no longer a candidate for outpatient pressure relief, and requires hospitalization for wound debride-

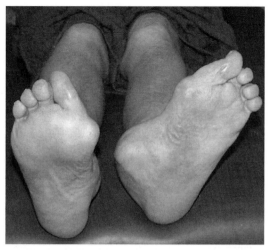

Figure 11–3 ■ Grade 0 foot. Although there is no current lesion in the soft tissue envelope, this patient's foot is "at risk" for ulceration, because of the underlying neuropathy combined with the extreme deformity caused by a Charcot joint.

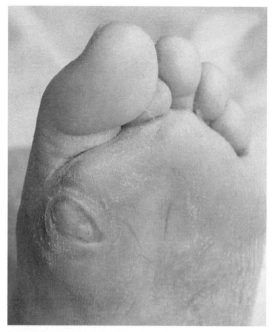

Figure 11–5 ■ Grade 2 foot. The plantar wound is intermediate in depth. The full thickness of skin and subcutaneous pressure is necrotic and the capsule of the first metatarsophalangeal joint is involved.

ment, usually with antibiotics. This decision is the same whether the ulcer is deemed infected or not.

Grade 3 lesions are the deepest, comprised of exposed bone, and/or deep infection, either

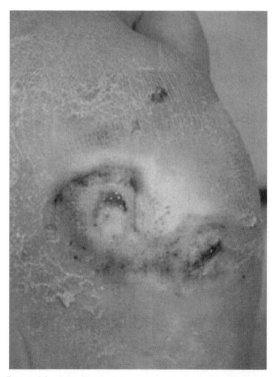

Figure 11–4 ■ Grade 1 foot. The plantar ulcer is superficial and granulating well. There is no deep exposed structure or infection.

abscess or osteomyelitis (Figs. 11–6, 11–7, and 11–8). Determination of these three basic wound grades is based upon the simple physical examination consisting of visualization *and* gentle probing of the wound with a sterile, blunt instrument. If the bone can be palpated through the wound, there is a very high likelihood that osteomyelitis is present.[7]

Once the examiner has described the extent ("depth") of the wound, signified by the numeric grade noted above, then the second step is to assign the letter grade by evaluating the limb perfusion. This "ischemia" portion of the classification is signified by a letter grade A, B, C, or D. While this may be obvious on the basis of examination alone, vascular studies such as Doppler ultrasound or transcutaneous oxygen tension may be required. For example, if the patient has bounding dorsalis pedis and posterior tibial pulses, the foot is almost certainly a grade A. Grade A is the foot without clinically significant ischemia. This is the foot with excellent pulses, color, capillary refill, and hair growth. Grade A lesions do not require vascular evaluation or intervention. If there is obvious gangrene of part (grade C) or all (grade D) of the foot, then these grades are equally facile to assign. The largest category of lesions encountered

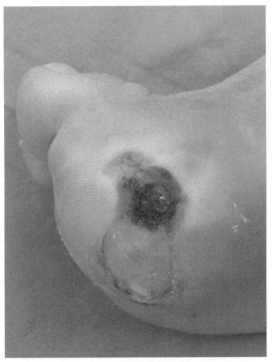

Figure 11–6 ■ Grade 3 foot. This patient has a deep abscess and septic arthritis of the hallux metatarsophalangeal joint. First ray amputation was required.

clinically are those that fall into grade B (i.e., ischemic but not gangrenous). While this is a wide band within the spectrum, it is internally consistent, and consistent as related to the ultimate decision-making algorithm that the classification supports. The grade B foot is the foot with diminished perfusion but which is not gangrenous. While there is a variation within this grade, it is a rational grouping based upon the intervention merited because these feet require vascular evaluation. It is critical in these patients to know both the wound depth and the vascularity in order to formulate a proper and successful treatment plan. Grade B feet therefore need a screening test such as that mentioned above. Depending on the result of those screening tests, vascular reconstruction might be indicated. These are the feet in which we must know if there is sufficient perfusion for either an external pressure-relieving device or an internal pressure-relieving surgery to be successful. If we are uncertain, we can proceed with neither.

Grade C feet have partial gangrene and grade D feet have complete gangrene. Patients with grade C and D lesions also require vascular evaluation to determine the level of perfusion and the level of potential healing, and to assess the need for revascularization procedures to achieve healing of that amputation.

The utility of this classification system is that it is straightforward and can be applied to the decision-making process in a sensible fashion (see Fig. 11–2). The most immediate necessary decisions are included in this algorithm. The advantage of the depth-ischemia classification is that it is succinct, and once the foot is graded the first step in the treatment decision making is clear and concise.

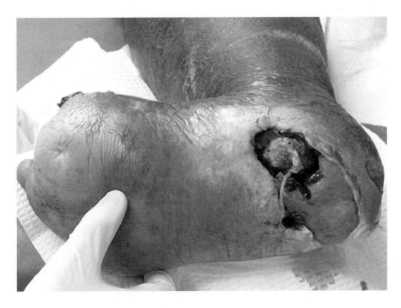

Figure 11–7 ■ Another grade 3 foot. Deep infection with exposed bone, and obvious osteomyelitis and abscess.

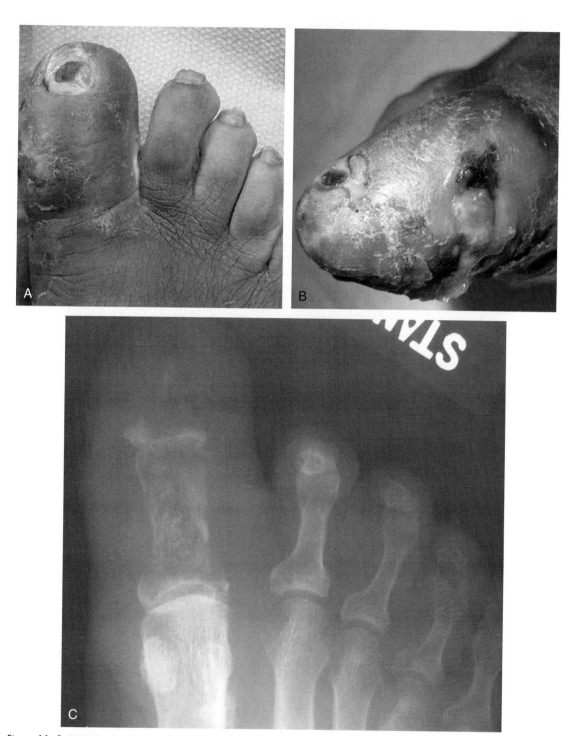

Figure 11–8 ■ A third patient with a grade 3 lesion. There are several "clues" for more extensive lesion than might be apparent at first glance. The toe is diffusely enlarged (*A*), there are multiple draining ulcers (*B*), and the "nail" lesion is actually the exposed distal phalanx. Radiographic correlation reveals the extensive bone involvement (*C*).

While much attention has been given to the depth of the diabetic foot lesion, as expressed in old and new grading systems, relatively little has been investigated regarding the important issue of the anatomic location of the lesion.[8] In general, lesions of the forefoot, especially distal to the distal third of the metatarsal, have a much lower associated mortality and much higher limb salvage than more proximal lesions of the foot, even though the actual healing time of the proximal and distal lesions may be similar.[8] This type of prognostic generalization puts into perspective the increased seriousness of lesions of the midfoot and hindfoot and should aid the treating physicians and surgeons in her/his counseling of the patients. It also points to the multifactorial nature of the wounds and the feet of diabetics that can never be entirely summarized by a single classification system.

REFERENCES

1. Alvarez DM, Gilson G, Auletta MJ: Local aspects of diabetic foot ulcer care: Assessment, dressings, and topical agents. *In* Levin ME, O'Neal, LW, Bowker JH (eds): The Diabetic Foot, 5th ed. St. Louis, Mosby Year Book, 1993.
2. Armstrong DG, Lavery LA, Harkless LB: Treatment-based classification system for assessment and care of diabetic feet. J Am Podiatr Med Assoc 86: 311–316, 1996.
3. Brodsky JW: The diabetic foot. *In* Mann RA, Coughlin MJ (eds): Surgery of the Foot and Ankle. St. Louis: Mosby, 1992, pp 877–958.
4. Brodsky JW: Outpatient diagnosis and management of the diabetic foot. Instructional Course Lectures, AAOS, 1993, p 43.
5. Calhoun J, et al: Treatment of diabetic foot infections: Wagner classification, therapy and outcome. Foot Ankle 9:101–106, 1988.
6. Forrest R, Gamborg-Neilssen P: Wound assessment in clinical practice: A critical review of methods and their applications. Acta Med Scand 687:69–74, 1984.
7. Grayson ML, Balogh K, Levin E, Karchmer AW: Probing to bone in infected pedal ulcers. A clinical sign of underlying osteomyelitis in diabetic patients. JAMA 273:721–723, 1995.
8. Kaufman J, Breeding L, Rosenberg N: Anatomic location of acute diabetic foot infections. Am J Surg 53:109–112, 1987.
9. Knighton D, et al: Classification and treatment of chronic nonhealing wounds: Successful treatment with autologous platelet-derived wound healing factors (PDWHF). Ann Surg 204:322–330, 1986.
10. Lavery L, Armstrong D, Harkless L: Classification of diabetic foot wounds. J Foot Ankle Surg 356:528–531, 1996.
11. Meggitt B: Surgical management of the diabetic foot. Br J Hosp Med 16:227–332, 1976.
12. Pecoraro RE, Reiber GE: Classification of wounds in diabetic amputees. Wounds 2:65–73, 1990.
13. Shea J: Pressure sores: Classification and management. CORR 112:89–100, 1975.
14. Wagner F: A classification and treatment program for diabetic, neuropathic and dysvascular foot problems. American Academy of Orthopaedic Surgeons. Instructional Course Lectures, 1979, 28, pp 143–165.
15. Wagner FJ: The diabetic foot and amputations of the foot. *In* Mann R (ed): Surgery of the Foot. St. Louis: Mosby-Year Book, 1986, pp 421–455.
16. Yarkony G, et al: Classification of pressure ulcers. Arch Dermatol 126:1218–1219, 1990.

DIABETIC FOOT ULCER CARE: ASSESSMENT AND MANAGEMENT

■ Diane L. Krasner and R. Gary Sibbald

The holistic care of diabetic foot ulcer patients requires a team approach. Not only must consideration be given to offloading, infection, vascularity, diabetic control, and systemic factors, but these factors must be continuously reevaluated in addition to topical treatment selections. (Prior to local wound management, diabetic patients with foot ulcers must have adequate vasculature to heal, bacterial balance in the wound, and pressure downloading of the surrounding area.) So, for example, the person whose orthotic was well fitting prior to the development of the metatarsal head ulceration, may now need reevaluation, not only for offloading of the area but also for the accommodation of the selected local wound dressing. Healability will also be determined by proper diabetic control and diet as well as treatment of coexisting medical conditions.

Due to the complexity of the diabetic foot ulcer itself, as well as the paradigm shift in the treatment of chronic wounds,[29] the assessment and topical treatment of diabetic foot ulcers is no simple, straightforward matter. The art of wound care is a virtual necessity at this time, but evidence-based science continues to evolve. Expert practitioners hone their skills by becoming proficient at

ulcer assessment, which then helps them to tailor their treatment decisions to the wound, the patient, and the setting.[58]

This chapter will describe initial skin and wound assessment and continuous monitoring of the wound. Considerations for healability and individual specific goals and outcomes will be outlined. The plan of care must address the need for timely, aggressive, and adequate ulcer debridement as well as achieving hemostasis following debridement.[25] The role of wound cleansing, irrigation, and topical antibacterials will be defined. Providers must determine whether sterile or nonsterile wound care is appropriate for a given individual by weighing the risk factors and environmental considerations. Based on these considerations, the providers must then select from the myriad of topical and adjunctive treatments, recommendations for which will be detailed in this chapter. Conventional as well as advanced wound dressings will be reviewed.[38, 59] Even if the underlying causes have been addressed and local wound care optimized, some diabetic foot ulcers do not heal. There is then a role for biologic agents: human skin equivalents (skin substitutes), growth factors (see Chapter 18), and various grafting techniques.

Over the past 30 years, dressing technologies have evolved from passive plug and conceal methods used for millennia,[12, 33] to the use of interactive and bioactive materials.[29, 50] Today, moist wound healing is considered the sine qua non of chronic wound care.[19, 55–57]

Optimizing the wound environment facilitates healing, but this is more complex than simply maintaining a moist wound environment. For example, exuding wounds need a moisture-absorbing dressing, desiccated wounds require moisture-donating dressings, and wounds without enough blood supply to heal may warrant the use of otherwise cytotoxic topical antiseptic agents or may be left dry to demarcate gangrene.

Dressing selection is just one part of a holistic approach. Careful attention to ulcer assessment and topical treatment is one—albeit very important—part of a quality, interdisciplinary coordinated plan of care.[2, 13]

The foot ulcer precedes amputation in the majority of diabetic patients.[44] The St. Vincent Declaration states that best practices should achieve a 40 to 50% reduction in nontraumatic diabetic foot amputations by the year 2000.[37] Best practices suggest that the optimal way to heal a diabetic ulcer is through the combined expertise of an interdisciplinary diabetic foot ulcer team.[13] Most importantly, patients and their significant others should be an integral part of the identification of individualized goals, treatment plan, and outcomes. These goals and outcomes must be realistic and not idealistic for the treatment setting and resource availability. Standards of care, guidelines, and algorithms are useful but must be interpreted and implemented based on local expertise, resource availability, and the individualized patient care plan. We refer to this as Advanced Wound Caring,[23] and we believe that such caring can optimize healing outcomes and improve the quality of life for people with diabetic foot ulcers.

Initial Wound and Skin Assessment and Continuous Monitoring

There are three main causes for diabetic foot ulcers: pressure, infection, and circulation (PIC). The vast majority are due to increased pressure secondary to neuropathy. Typically, neurotropic pressure-induced ulcers develop over pressure points on the plantar aspects of the feet, particularly over the metatarsal heads, beneath the great toe, and on the heel. In deformed, Charcot-type feet, midfoot ulceration on the boney prominences is common and challenging to manage. These ulcers often start with a callus or thickening of the stratum corneum, local hemorrhage, blistering, and then skin breakdown. A skin ulcer is a complete loss of epidermis with a dermal, subcutaneous, or underlying structure in the base. It should be distinguished from an erosion that still has an epidermal base, often accompanied by local hemorrhage. Pressure downloading is essential for optimal care. This includes aggressive debridement of callus, appropriate deep-toed shoes, and orthotics combined with continuous, frequent monitoring, redebridement, and modification of the orthotic when necessary.

Infection

The second most common association of diabetic foot ulceration is infection. The longer the ulcer is present, the more likely the surrounding tissue will acquire an increased bacterial load. Local signs and symptoms of infection may be masked in the diabetic patient. Increased abnormal bacterial bioburdens can significantly delay wound healing because they compete for wound oxygen and nutrients.[47] When local signs of infection are present, increased discharge usually precedes frank purulence and local malodor. The surrounding tissue may become edematous, erythematous, and can be painful in an otherwise painless foot. The average number of organisms found in the previous studies is as high as 4.8 species per ulcer from quantitative bacterial skin biopsies,[47] indicating the need for broad-spectrum antibiotics.

If the ulcer probes to bone, there is a high incidence of osteomyelitis, and prompt referral to specialists is important for limb salvage. It is particularly concerning if the erythema around the ulcer extends more than 2 cm,[8] the patient is systemically unwell, or there is a worsening of their diabetic control. Routine x-rays are often initially negative due to relative osteopenia in the neurotropic foot, but they still have clinical utility because they may demonstrate foreign bodies, fractures associated with Charcot foot, or gas in the tissue. A follow-up x-ray 2 to 4 weeks later may demonstrate the boney erosion of osteomyelitis or periosteal new bone formation associated with healing. Routine bone scans are only helpful if positive, but are often negative. Magnetic resonance imaging (MRI) or other specialized tests, when available, may have greater diagnostic accuracy. When in doubt about the presence or absence of infection, the use of an infrared thermometry device[35] may help diagnostically. The thermometer should be used on four quadrants surrounding the ulcers and compared to the opposite foot in the same locations. Differences of 4° to 5°F or more suggest infection,[5] but an acute Charcot arthropathy (more often without skin ulceration) or asymmetric vascular lesions can also cause temperature variation.

Surface bacterial cultures of the wound are often misleading and may not represent the organisms within the underlying granulation tissue of the wound. While the "gold standard" is a punch or tissue biopsy, these approaches are invasive and specialized microbiologic processing is not always available. Therefore, a culturing method should be chosen which cleanses, removes debris first, and systematically cultures the deep portion of the ulcer base, avoiding frank collections of pus. For the treatment of infection, see Chapter 22.

Circulation

It is important that health care professionals ensure that the diabetic foot ulcer has enough blood supply to heal. If a palpable pulse is present, the pressure is approximately 80 mm Hg. The Doppler ankle-brachial index (ABI) is often used to diagnose arterial disease. A ratio of 0.8 and higher indicates an absence of significant arterial disease, with a ratio of below 0.5 suggesting severe arterial compromise. In diabetics, calcification of the vessels often leads to non-compressible vessels and a falsely high ABI value. Transcutaneous oxygen saturation ($TcSo_2$) of greater than 30% or toe photophlethysmography of greater than 50 mm Hg are more reliable indicators of blood supply sufficient for healing. Bypass procedures or balloon dilation should be considered in all patients with symptoms such as claudication or rest pain. These procedures may not be beneficial in the presence of extensive distal arterial disease, but a number of diabetic patients will benefit from newer revascularization techniques.

Diabetes Control/General Health

Healability of the diabetic foot ulcer also depends on correcting other coexisting medical conditions and risk factors such as smoking. Optimal blood sugar control should be monitored every 3 months with a gycosylated hemoglobin (HbA_{1c}). If the HbA_{1c} is high[2] (e.g., >12%), there may be impairment of the host response to infection. Other diabetic complications may coexist with neuropathy and foot ulceration. Eye changes, cardiac disease (especially coronary artery problems), kidney disease, hypertension, and peripheral vascular disease should all be considered as increased risk factors in the medical assessment.

Wound Assessment

Optimal assessment of the diabetic wound requires consistent documentation of wound characteristics and is critical for continuing monitoring, identifying complications, and appropriate management. The precise location of the ulcer should be noted or mapped on a foot diagram. We believe that wound tracings and photography help the provider and patient to monitor changes in the ulcer. Measurement of length (usually the longest diameter) and the maximum width at right angles to the diameter is usually documented in centimeters. The maximum depth should be measured with a probe and any probing to bone, sinus formation, or undermining should be documented. The wound characteristics should be described in detail, preferably using a flowchart documentation of change.

The base of the ulcer should be characterized; it may be black (necrotic), yellow (fibrous), pink (granulation tissue), or a combination of these colors. Black devitalized tissue (eschar) may be soft or firm. If wound healing is the goal, this tissue needs to be removed to stage the ulcer and promote healing. In selected cases, where palliation or conservative management have been established as the goal, stable eschar may be left intact and carefully monitored (watchful waiting). Yellow fibrous bases may be firm or sloughy, indicating deep structures such as fascia, immature granulation, insufficient vasculature, or tissue destroyed by infection. Several variations of granulation tissue are often seen. Healthy granulation tissue (blood vessels and collagen) is salmon pink, firm, and moist. With an increased bacterial load, granulation tissue may become darker, exuberant, friable, or malodorous. Hypergranulation tissue should be documented because it may require removal to facilitate reepithelialization.

Exudate is usually described by its quantity (scant, moderate, copious) and characteristics (serous, sanguineous, pustular, or combinations) and its odor (presence or absence).

Wound margin treatment is critical to the successful healing of diabetic ulcers. The wound margin should be checked for callus formation, excess moisture, maceration of keratin, edema, erythema, or increased warmth, which may be signs of infection. On the plantar aspect of the foot, the stratum corneum or keratin layer is normally extremely thick. Hyperkeratotic callus increases local pressure over boney prominences, compromising the underlying tissue and frequently leading to local hemorrhage. Aggressive debridement will be discussed in the section "Debridement," below. With proper pressure downloading, callus formation usually decreases.

There are general and diabetic-specific tools for grading and staging ulcers (see Chapter 11 for a detailed discussion of staging and classification of foot lesions). The Wagner system[51] is commonly used, the National Pressure Ulcer Advisory Panel/Agency for Health Care Policy and Research (NPUAP/AHCPR) staging system[40] is sometimes used when pressure alone is the primarily etiology, and partial/full-thickness distinctions are commonly used with large data sets or in studies of ulcers of mixed etiologies. All of these tools are systems for documenting the initial assessment of wounding. Other descriptors should be used to describe the healing process.[30]

While the neuropathic diabetic foot is characteristically not painful, pain should be routinely assessed and documented using the patient's own self-report. The 10-cm visual analogue scale is the gold standard for quantitative pain assessment.[28] The patient is asked to grade their pain by placing a mark along a 10-cm line, where zero is no pain and the 10-cm mark represents the worst pain ever experienced. The presence of new or increasing pain in the diabetic patient with a foot ulcer often signals complications such as infection, Charcot arthropathy, or vascular compromise.

Goals and Outcomes

The identification of goals and outcomes should be a joint venture of the provider team and the patient and his or her significant other(s). Healing is the ideal outcome that most providers and patients strive to achieve. In the diabetic population, healing is not always possible in a significant percentage of patients. Healability will depend on a combination of general medical conditions, diabetic control, and lifestyle issues (e.g., smoking). Significant local factors in the foot include pressure, infection, and circulation (PIC), foot deformity and rigidity, and previous ulceration and amputation (both being statistically significant risk factors).[32]

If the underlying causes are addressed and best management practices are implemented in the patient who is expected to heal, evidence of healing should be noted in 4 to 12 weeks. If there is no progress or if there is deterioration, it is appropriate to refer patients to specialized wound and/or diabetic teams.

In patients with inadequate blood supply, gross deformity, nonhealing infections (especially chronic osteomyelitis), or compliance problems, healing of the ulcer may not be an achievable outcome. This assessment should be carefully documented and supported by appropriate investigations and colleague opinion. The conclusion should be shared diplomatically with the patient and his or her significant other(s). Even if healing is not the goal, there are appropriate outcomes for this patient group. These include maintaining bacterial balance, preventing systemic complications, and controlling pain. Dressings and treatments that might *not* be used when healing is the expected outcome may be appropriately utilized for these patients to control bacterial load. These include antiseptics that are cytotoxic to viable healing cells: povidone-iodine, hydrogen peroxide, sodium hypochlorite, and scarlet red. Aggressive debridement of these wounds may lead to larger nonhealing wounds (bigger holes). Dry gangrene may be best left to demarcate and autoamputate; in these cases, avoiding debridement and the autolytic activity of moist interactive dressings is the best approach.

It is important that care be patient focused. Quality-of-life tools, both general and disease specific, help us to adequately address the fears, concerns, and everyday issues of the patient with a diabetic foot ulcer and his or her significant other(s). The use of quality-of-life tools has to date been predominantly a research activity, but it needs to become part of everyday, routine practice. Measuring activities of daily living, including pain and compliance/adherence, will help the provider and patient monitor progress towards the stated goals and achieve the best possible outcomes.

Debridement

Diabetic foot ulcers are often chronic and nonhealing. Steed et al.[49] demonstrated that aggressive, ongoing surgical debridement converts a chronic nonhealing ulcer into an acute, healing wound. Adequate debridement of necrotic tissue (eschar, slough) is needed before adequate assessment and staging can be accomplished. There are several methods for wound debridement, including sharp surgical, mechanical, enzymatic, and autolytic with modern moist, and interactive dressings. Truly, it is a continuum, from flushing away debris with low-pressure irrigation, to wide excision. The following factors must be taken into consideration when selecting a method of debridement:

1. Selective versus nonselective method.
2. Presence or absence of pain.
3. Arterial insufficiency (dry gangrene).
4. Drugs that may increase bleeding (e.g., Coumadin, acetylsalicylic acid, nonsteroidal anti-inflammatory drugs [NSAIDs]).
5. Resources and setting.

Sharp Surgical Debridement

The most selective and efficacious method of debridement is sharp surgical debridement. It is important to heal the diabetic wound as quickly as possible to avoid secondary infection. Therefore, we believe that sharp surgical debridement of the hyperkeratotic rim and ulcer base, to bleeding, is the optimal method of debridement for the patient with a diabetic foot ulcer.

Other Methods of Debridement

When sharp surgical debridement is not feasible, such as when the patient is in excruciating pain or when a qualified practitioner is not available, other methods should be considered:

- autolytic
- mechanical
- enzymatic

A patient with excruciating pain may require topical, intralesional, oral or intravenous anesthetic agents prior to debridement. Topical EMLA (eutectic mixture of local anesthetic), 2.5% Xylocaine, and 2.5% prilocaine[17, 20] may be used off-label in the United States, but it is licensed in other countries, such as Canada, for open wounds. A thick coat is applied and completely occluded with an adhesive transparent film dressing or plastic wrap for 30 to 60 minutes prior to the procedure.

Autolytic Debridement

Autolytic debridement with moist interactive dressings (hydrogels, alginates, transparent films, hydrocolloids) is selective and liquefies slough and eschar as well as promotes granulation tissue formation. The tissue autolysis should be initiated in 24 to 72 hours; otherwise, another method of debridement should be tried. Scoring of eschar with a scalpel blade involves making superficial parallel grooves on the eschar surface in a grid pattern. Using this technique prior to application of the moist interactive dressing facilitates local penetration and debridement. The grooves should not reach viable tissue and bleeding should be minimal or absent.

Mechanical Debridement

Mechanical debridement may be accomplished with wet-to-dry gauze dressings, irrigation, pulsatile lavage, or whirlpool. These methods are the least selective of all methods of debridement and are potentially damaging to healthy granulation tissue and new epithelium. Wet-to-dry dressings are often used to pack large necrotic wounds that may occur with nonhealing surgical wounds. Irrigation will be discussed in the section "Wound Cleansing and Irrigation Techniques," below. Whirlpool treatment has its proponents, while other health care experts question its value. Immersing the entire foot can lead to maceration of the skin and bacterial seeding of areas of lost skin integrity (e.g., toe webs, nail folds, fissures). The addition of cytotoxic antiseptics in low concentrations to whirlpool solutions decreases their clinical effectiveness as well as the probable harmful effects on the wound base. We believe whirlpool has a limited use in diabetic foot ulcers.

Enzymatic Debridement

Historically, enzymes (collaginase, papain, urokinase, etc.) have been used as debriding agents for eschar and slough. They have a selective action, but they are slow, costly, and labor intensive. Frequently they can increase local infections in the liquefied debris and they may increase or cause local pain. We believe the role of enzymes should largely be replaced by sharp surgical debridement or the autolytic action of modern dressings.

Hemostasis Following Debridement

Hemorrhage is often desirable after surgical debridement of diabetic foot ulcers, indicating a viable ulcer base. Hemorrhage needs to be contained to avoid local hematoma, eschar, and underlying inflammatory response. Local pressure and elevation may be supplemented by application of calcium alginates that possess hemostatic properties. Calcium alginate ropes, in our experience, perform hemostasis more effectively than wafers because they have vertical wicking. The alginates may donate calcium to facilitate local hemostasis and in turn accept sodium converting a calcium alginate fiber into a sodium alginate gel, promoting moist interactive healing. Other practitioners use silver nitrate, electrocautery, absorbable gelatin sponge (e.g., Gelfoam), or chemical cauterants to control bleeding. Some of these methods may damage underlying granulation tissue or cause pain. It is important that the debridement remove all overhanging edges so that the epithelium can be seen in contact with the granulation tissue base. All sinuses or tracts should be opened or marsupialized

to allow healing from the edges. Exposed bone often requires local surgical removal of the infected focus to promote healing. Following debridement, calcium alginates, moist gauze, or other dressings should be left in place for 24 hours. Adherent dressings should be presoaked prior to removal. The availability of surgical debridement may depend on qualified health care professionals and an appropriate practice setting. It is not appropriate for some procedures to be done in ambulatory settings where equipment may not be available to control postprocedure bleeding.

Wound Cleansing and Irrigation Techniques

Wound cleansing and irrigation are used to remove surface debris and exudate, allowing for proper assessment of the wound base and facilitating wound healing. Removal of debris should help to decrease bacterial load. Complete cleansing of the wound bed allows visualization of subtle signs of wound infection or other significant changes in wound status.

Foot soaks have traditionally been used for diabetic foot care, but present the same concerns related to bacterial load transfer as whirlpool treatment (bacterial soup). Overuse of foot soaks may cause overhydration, which can lead to maceration, particularly at the toe webs, nail folds, and heel tissues. The seeded bacteria in these sites can then serve as an entry point for lower leg cellulitis and other infections. The presence of exposed bone or joints or deep sinuses is an absolute contraindication for foot soaks, whirlpool, or other immersion therapies.

Cleansing Techniques

Most diabetic foot ulcers are relatively small and are easily cleansed with each dressing change. Saline is the solution of choice. The use of tap water is controversial. In immunocompromised patients it is contraindicated because of the possibility of introducing unwanted pathogens. Individual assessment of the patient, the environment, and water source is warranted prior to the use of tap water for cleansing diabetic foot ulcers.[31]

The use of commercial wound cleansers is also highly controversial. Most experts agree that nonionic surfactants do the least harm. Rodeheaver et al.[47] have recently measured the toxicity indexes for 16 wound or skin cleansers, which can provide direction for clinical practice (Table 12–1). All commerical cleansers have a greater toxicity than saline.

Cleansing is usually accomplished by one of the following methods:

- Compressing or soaking with saline-soaked gauze.
- Pouring the solution over the wound (e.g., saline from a container, syringe, or plastic ampule).
- Pushing or squeezing a piston or bulb syringe.

The pressure exerted on the wound surface is measured in pounds per square inch (psi) and is typically up to 5 psi for simple cleansing.

Irrigation Techniques

For diabetic foot ulcers requiring removal of exudate or debris, irrigation may be selected instead of simple cleansing. Irrigation involves the delivery of directed stream at higher pressures, usually 5 to 15 psi. Pressures over 15 psi may be harmful, causing tissue destruction and edema.[47] Irrigation is usually accomplished by one of the following methods:

- A 30-mL syringe with 18- to 20-gauge Angiocath.
- Commerical wound irrigation kit.
- Water-pik on low setting.

Important variables that have not been fully studied to date and for which evidence-based practices are not available at this time include:

- the optimal distance of the device from the wound surface
- the total volume of the irrigation solution over what time period.

There are almost more questions than answers. Some experts are concerned about health care provider risk from irrigant splash-back and aerosolization. Appropriate, common sense protective precautions should be instituted. Despite all these concerns, effective wound care can be facilitated by effective wound cleansing or irrigation.

Topical Antibacterials

There is a lack of consensus on the use of topical antibacterial therapy for local wound care. If a wound has associated signs of infection (septicemia, osteomyelitis, cellulitis), systemic antibacterials should be used. If increased local discharge and odor are present without skin surface temperature change, a

---

Table 12–1 ■ TOXICITY INDEXES FOR SIXTEEN WOUND OR SKIN CLEANSERS*

CLEANSER	INTENDED PRIMARY USE	TOXICITY INDEX
Shur Clens (ConvaTec, Princeton, NJ)	Wound	10
Biolex (Bard Medical Division, Covington, GA)	Wound	
Saf Clens (ConvaTec, Princeton, NJ)	Wound	100
Cara Klenz (Carrington Laboratories, Inc., Irving, TX)	Wound	
Ultra Klenz (Carrington Laboratories, Inc., Irving, TX)	Wound	
Clinical Care (Carrington Laboratories, Inc., Irving, TX)	Wound	1,000
Uni Wash (Smith & Nephew United, Inc., Largo, FL)	Skin	
Ivory Soap (0.5%) (Proctor & Gamble, Cincinnati, OH)	Skin	
Constant Clens (Sherwood-Davis & Geck, St. Louis, MO)	Wound	
Dermal Wound Cleanser (Smith & Nephew United, Inc., Largo, FL)	Wound	
Puri-Clens (Coloplast SweenCorp., Marietta, GA)	Wound	10,000
Hibiclens (Stuart Pharmaceuticals, Wilmington, DE)	Skin	
Betadine Surgical Scrub (Purdue Frederick, Norwalk, CT)	Skin	
Techni-Care Scrub (Care-Tech Laboratories, St. Louis, MO)	Skin	
Bard Skin Cleanser (Bard Medical Division, Covington, GA)	Skin	100,000
Hollister Skin Cleanser (Hollister Incorporated, Libertyville, IL)	Skin	

* From Rodeheaver GT: Wound cleansing, wound irrigation, wound disinfection. *In* Krasner D, Kane D (eds): Chronic Wound Care: A Clinical Source Book for Healthcare Professionals, 2nd ed. Wayne, PA: Health Management Publications, Inc., 1997, p 98, with permission.

short course of a topical antibacterial agent can be instituted with careful daily monitoring of the ulcer for signs of infection. Still other ulcers may have an increased bacterial burden ($\geq 1.0 \times 10^6$ organisms/gm of tissue) without any localized symptoms or signs. These ulcers may also benefit from a short course of topical or systemic antibacterials.

The ideal topical antibacterial:

- has a broad spectrum of antibacterial coverage,
- allows good penetration of the topical agent,
- is not used systemically,
- is not a sensitizer, and
- is wound-friendly, promoting moist interactive healing.

The antibacterial coverage of commonly used agents is listed in Table 12–2.

Good penetration has been demonstrated from a topical agent mupirocin polyethylene glycol ointment. Studies have shown it has equivalent or superior local antibacterial coverage to oral erythromycin or cloxacillin.[16, 52]

Topical agents that are also used systemically will help select resistant organisms, making the systemic agents less effective. This may be a concern for gentamicin and fusidic acid (occasionally used systemically). Sensitization is common from topical ulcer preparations.[24] The skin processes antigens through sensitized Langerhans cells migrating to regional lymph nodes. Common allergens are neomycin, lanolin, and fragrances. Neomycin contains two allergens[45]: the neosamine sugar and the deoxystreptomine backbone. The neosamine sugar is shared with framycetin (Sofra-Tulle) and the deoxystreptomine is also part of the aminoglycosides that includes gentamicin. Sensitization to the aminoglycosides eliminates a very important class of systemic antibiotics. Fusidic acid ointment and some tulle dressings contain lanolin.

With increased antibacterial use, the emergence of methicillin-resistant *Staphylococcus aureus* (MRSA) and other multiantibiotic-resistant staphylococcal organisms has become an increasing problem. Mupirocin is effective against MRSA, and for this reason some institutions are restricting this agent for use only against resistant staphylococcus, including MRSA.

Three additional products have been developed for wound care that promote moist healing and have a broad antibacterial spectrum including MRSA. Cadexomer iodine is a slow-release iodine product available in a paste or wafer.[3] The product absorbs wound exudate, forming a protective gel that is nonocclusive and nonadherent. Arglaes[54] is an elemental silver product in a glass-like structure. Acticoat consists of ionized silver in an absorptive dressing.[60] Slow release of silver provides a broad-spectrum antibacterial coverage as well. These three products need more study to determine their role as primary dressings in diabetic foot ulcers.

Topicals may provide good local penetration of antibacterial agents. An increased bacterial burden may not always show clinical signs of infection but can delay healing. The use of these agents can decrease bacterial burden, exudate, or wound odor. Topical antibacterial agents should be reviewed at regular intervals. A suggested review time would be every 2 weeks. Prolonged use of these agents can lead to the emergence of resistant strains both in the laboratory and in clinical practice, although laboratory resistance does not always equate with the clinical ineffectiveness of these agents.

Topical antibacterial agents have a definite indication in chronic wounds, but their indiscriminate use and lack of close monitoring is to be discouraged. They do not act as a substitute for systemic antibacterials and should be discontinued when bacterial balance has been established.

Dressings: Conventional and Advanced

Research of the late 1950s and early 1960s demonstrated that a moist wound environment provides the best microenvironment for wound regeneration and repair and optimizes wound healing.[19, 55–57] Since then, hundreds of wound care products have become available that promote moist wound healing.[27, 29] Many of these advanced wound care products are appropriate for the care of the diabetic foot ulcer. However, it remains true that many conventional dressings are efficient and cost effective as well. This section will address the advantages and disadvantages of the major dressings categories for care of diabetic foot ulcers. Dressings must

Table 12-2 ■ TOPICAL ANTIBACTERIALS*

AGENT	VEHICLE	STAPHYLOCOCCUS AUREUS	STREPTOCOCCUS	PSEUDOMONAS	COMMENTS
Cadexomer iodine	Yellow-brown powder/paste/ointment	✓	✓	✓	Releases iodine slowly, making it less toxic to granulating tissue Broad spectrum, including virus and fungus
Fusidic acid†	Glycerin cream or lanolin‡ ointment	✓	✓		Lanolin in ointment base may act as a sensitizer
Gentamicin sulphate†	Alcohol cream base or petrolatum ointment	✓	✓	✓	Good broad spectrum vs. gram-negatives
Metronidazole	Wax–glycerin cream and carbogel 940/propylene glycol gel				Good anaerobe coverage and wound deodorizer
Mupirocin 2%	Polyethylene glycol ointment, paraffin-based nasal preparation and mineral oil–based cream	✓	✓		Good for MRSA, and other resistant staphylococcus bacteria Excellent topical penetration
Polymyxin B sulfate–bacitracin zinc	White petrolatum ointment (cream contains gramicidin instead of bacitracin for gram-positive bacteria)	✓	✓	✓	Broad spectrum Low cost
Polymyxin B sulfate–bacitracin zinc–neomycin‡	White petrolatum ointment	✓	✓	✓	Neomycin is a potent sensitizer and may cross-react in 40% of cases to aminoglycosides
Silver sulfadiazine	Water-miscible cream	✓	✓	✓	Do not use in sulfa-sensitive individuals
Silver	Ionized in an absorptive dressing or silver impregnated item	✓	✓	✓	Silver chloride is formed when mixed with saline. Use water for wound cleansing and moistening dressings.

* © R. Gary Sibbald, used with permission.
† Used systemically.
‡ Contains common sensitizer.

291

be matched to the patient, the wound, and the setting. As wound healing progresses, the dressing should be changed to optimize wound healing. The days of using wet-to-dry dressings for the entire wound healing process are over. Table 12–3 lists the characteristics of an ideal dressing as outlined by T. D. Turner.[50] Table 12–4 lists the major wound dressing categories, with several examples by trade name to illustrate each generic category.

Conventional Dressings

Conventional dressings, such as gauze, nonadherent gauze, impregnated gauze, and packing strips, are particularly well suited for care of certain diabetic ulcers, particularly those that are infected or have tunneling or sinus tracks, because of the following performance parameters:

• They are absorbent.
• They are easily impregnated with topical agents.
• They prevent premature wound contraction.
• They are effective for packing sinus tracts and tunneling areas.
• They reduce maceration.
• They are readily available.
• They are user friendly.

Washed gauze, which is low-linting, is particularly well suited for packing larger cavities after nonhealing amputations. Packing strips (plain or impregnated with iodoform) are commonly used for packing sinus tracts

---

Table 12–3 ■ CHARACTERISTICS OF AN IDEAL DRESSING

• To remove excess exudate and toxic components
• To maintain a high humidity at wound/dressing interface
• To allow gaseous exchange
• To provide thermal insulation
• To afford protection from secondary infection
• To be free from particulate or toxic contaminants and
• To allow removal without trauma at dressing change

---

* From Turner TD: The development of wound management products. *In* Krasner D, Kane D (eds): Chronic Wound Care: A Clinical Source Book for Healthcare Professionals, 2nd ed. Wayne PA: Health Management Publications, Inc, 1997, p 127, with permission.

and tunneling areas. Iodoform-impregnated and other antiseptic products should be reserved for use with wounds demonstrating clinical signs of infection or increased bacterial burden and only for a short course of treatment, because these agents have been shown to be cytotoxic in vitro to healing cells, such as fibroblasts.[47]

Advanced Dressings

Advanced dressings include the following major categories, with new combinations and categories appearing on the market regularly: alginates, collagen, composites, films, foams, hydrocolloids, and hydrogels.

It is important to note that there is a wide range of performance parameters within and between categories: all hydrocolloids are not equal. Generally speaking, the advanced dressings maintain an ideal moist wound environment by either absorbing exudate (e.g., alginates, collagen, foams, hydrocolloids) or donating or maintaining moisture (e.g., hydrogels).[13, 27, 49]

Performance parameters that should be weighed when selecting among these categories for the diabetic foot ulcer include:

1. Ability to absorb exudate versus donate or maintain moisture.
2. Adherence versus nonadherence.
3. Occlusion versus nonocclusion.
4. Frequency of dressing change required.
5. Cost and reimbursability.

Other important factors to consider include user friendliness, cost effectiveness, and reimbursement potential. Dressing bulk is another important consideration and sometimes the "thin" version of an advanced dressing, such as a thin hydrocolloid or thin sheet hydrogel, can be used without requiring an adjustment in footwear and with a lower cost as well.

Primary and Secondary Dressings

The traditional distinction between primary dressings (that fill or touch the wound) and secondary dressings (that secure the primary dressing) still apply.[7, 39] What has become complicated is the fact that many of the advanced dressings can perform either function. Providers should carefully specify the following parameters when writing orders for dressing changes in order to optimize wound care:

- method of cleansing or irrigation (including the PSI) and solution type and quantity
- sterile, no-touch, clean, or nonsterile technique to be utilized
- type and amount of primary dressing
- type and amount of secondary dressing
- frequency of dressing change

In addition, any patient particulars or "tricks of the trade" that can be shared with other providers can help to optimize a dressing change.

Sterile Versus Nonsterile Wound Care

While the research base to support a decision regarding sterile versus nonsterile wound care is shaky at best,[31] we believe that best practice at this time involves the use of sterilized products and sterilized solutions when treating immunocompromised patients, such as diabetics with foot ulcers.

In our opinion, the potential for increased bacterial load when using products, especially gauze products, that have not been sterilized does not warrant the pennies saved. Until research studies are published and replicated that show identical outcomes in all settings for all patient populations, we suggest that following the gold standard of sterile wound care is the reasonably prudent thing to do.

Occlusive Versus Nonocclusive Environments

Because diabetic wounds are prone to infection and diabetic patients may not muster a visible immune response, many wound care experts avoid using occlusive dressings (e.g., films, hydrocolloids, ointments) with diabetic wounds, unless they are reasonably certain that the ulcers are being monitored frequently by a knowledgeable wound care provider. Occlusion refers to the relative ability of a wound dressing to transmit water vapor and gases from the wound surface into the environment. The rationale for this caution about occlusion is that exudates typically will pool in the wound bed in an occlusive environment and can become a breeding ground for microorganisms. As mentioned previously, Robson has concluded that tissue organism loads in excess or equal to 1.0×10^6 colony-forming units (CFUs) per gram of tissue can impair healing.[46] Some other research suggests that occlusive environments do not negatively impact on the healing of certain chronic dermal wounds.[21] In pressure and venous ulcers, where bacterial counts of 10^6 to 10^8 with a shift to less virulent gram-negative flora was observed, the wounds did not show clinical signs of infection and continued to heal at an apparently normal rate. Organism count along with virulence and host resistance are all important in determining bacterial-wound interaction.[9, 46] The final word on occlusive versus nonocclusive environments is not yet out. In the meantime, we suggest following this advice from the fifth edition of *The Diabetic Foot*:

Occlusion, however, must be carefully controlled. In diabetic patients, it should be limited to the management of superficial wounds or full-thickness wounds that exhibit healthy granulation tissue. Diabetic patients whose foot ulcers are managed with occlusive dressings need to be followed closely (at least once weekly) and with more frequent dressing changes (at least once daily). The same environment that enhances healing may enhance pathogenic growth. Thus, occlusion is contraindicated in infected and draining wounds. The benefits and potential dangers of occlusive wound therapy are listed below:

Advantages (over conventional, nonocclusive dressings):

- Reduced pain
- Rapid healing
- Selective autolytic debridement
- Increased granulation and reepithelialization
- Reduced friction and shear

Disadvantages (over conventional, nonocclusive dressings):

- Increased potential for periwound maceration
- Accumulation of wound exudates on the wound surface
- If adhesive, adherence to healthy/new granulation tissue with potential for harm
- [Potential] increased numbers of microorganisms on the wound surface (pp. 265–266)[1]

Table 12–4 ▪ A QUICK REFERENCE GUIDE TO WOUND CARE PRODUCT CATEGORIES*†
(January 1999)

This listing of wound care products highlights the importance of generic product categories. Under each generic product category, *up to four product examples are given* (*a mix of old and new products*), to help familiarize the reader with each category. No endorsement of any product or manufacturer is intended. Within each category, products must be individually evaluated. All products within a category do not necessarily perform equally. Combination products may be listed in more than one category. Refer to manufacturers' instructions for specifics regarding product usage.

1. Antimicrobial Dressings
  Acticoat (Westaim Biomedical)
  Arglaes Film/Island (Medline Industries)
  Iodosorb Gel (Healthpoint/Smith & Nephew)
  Iodoflex Gel Pad (Healthpoint)

2. Alginate Dressings
  Cutinova alginate (Beiersdorf-Jobst)
  Restore CalciCare (Hollister)
  Seasorb (Coloplast Sween)
  Sorbsan (Dow Hickam Pharmaceuticals)

3. Biosynthetic Dressings
  BiobraneII (Dow Hickam Pharmaceuticals)
  Silon (BioMed Sciences)

4. Cleansers
  Saline (Multiple)
  Skin Cleansers
    Peri-Wash (Sween)
    Sensi-Care (ConvaTec)
    Skin Cleanser (Mentor)
    Prevacare (Johnson & Johnson Medical)
  Wound Cleansers
    Clinical Care (Care-Tech Laboratories)
    Curasol (Healthpoint Medical)
    Dermagran Spray (Derma Sciences)
    RadiaCare Klenz (Carrington Laboratories)

5. Collagen Dressings
  BGC Matrix (collagen/beta-glucan) (Brennen
    Medical)
  ChroniCure (Derma Sciences)
  Fibracol (collagen/alginate) (Johnson & Johnson
    Medical)
  Medifil/Skin Temp (BioCore)

6. Composite Dressings
  Alldress (SCA Mölnlycke)
  CombiDERM ACD (ConvaTec)
  CovaDerm/CovaDerm Plus (DeRoyal)
  OsmoCyte Island (ProCyte Corporation)

7. Compression Bandages/Wraps
  Coban (3M Health Care)
  Dome Paste (Miles)
  Elastoplast (Beiersdorf-Jobst)
  Setopress (ConvaTec)
  Multi-layered systems
    Circulon System (ConvaTec)
    Dyna-Flex (Johnson & Johnson Medical)
    Profore (Smith & Nephew)
    Unna-Pak (Glenwood)

8. Conforming/Wrapping Bandages
  Dutex/Duform (Dumex Medical)
  Elastomull (Beiersdorf-Jobst)

  Kerlix Lite (Kendall Healthcare)
  SOF-KLING (Johnson & Johnson Medical)

9. Contact Layers
  Mepitel (SCA Mölnlycke)
  Profore (Smith & Nephew)
  Tegapore (3M Healthcare)
  Ventex Vented Dressing (Kendall Healthcare)

10. Creams/Oils
  Biafine (KCI)
  Decubitene Oxygenated Oil (Ferndale Labs)
  Eucerin Cream (Beiersdorf-Jobst)
  Sween Cream (Coloplast Sween)

11. Devices
  THBO (topical hyperbaric oxygen) (GWR Medical
    LLP)
  The V.A.C. (KCI)
  Warm-Up (Augustine Medical)

12. Enzymes/Debriding Agents
  Accuzyme (Papain-Urea) (Healthpoint)
  Elase (Fibrinolysin/desoxyribonuclease) (Fugisawa)
  Panifil Ointment (Papain) (Rystan)
  Santyl (Collagenase) (Knoll/Smith & Nephew)

13. Foam Dressings
  Allevyn (Smith & Nephew)
  Flexzan/thin (Dow Hickam Pharmaceuticals)
  Lyofoam/Lyofoam C/Lyofoam T (ConvaTec)
  PolyMem (Ferris Manufacturing)

**14. Gauze Dressings (see also Composite
   Dressings)**
  Woven (Multiple)
  Nonwoven
    EXCILON (Kendall Healthcare)
    NATURALON (Kendall Healthcare)
    NU GAUZE General Use (Johnson & Johnson
      Medical)
    SOF-WICK (Johnson & Johnson Medical)
  Packing/packing strips (Nonimpregnated)
    Dumex Pak-Its (Dumex Medical)
    Kerlix (Kendall Healthcare)
    NU-BREDE (Johnson & Johnson Medical)
    TENDERSORB (Kendall Healthcare)
  Debriding
    NU-BREDE (Johnson & Johnson Medical)
    TENDERSORB (Kendall Healthcare)
  Impregnated—sodium chloride
    Mesalt (SCA Mölnlycke)
  Impregnated—Other
    Dermagran Wet Dressing (Saline) (Derma
      Sciences)
    Dumex Wet Dressings (Saline) (Dumex
      Medical)
    Dumex Pak-It Hydrogel (Dumex Medical)
    Gentell Hydrogel Dressing (MKM Healthcare)

Table 12–4 ■ A QUICK REFERENCE GUIDE TO WOUND CARE PRODUCT CATEGORIES*†
(January 1999) (*Continued*)

Nonadherent gauze
  Primapore (Smith & Nephew)
  Release (Johnson & Johnson Medical)
  Telfa (Kendall Healthcare)
Specialty absorptive gauze
  EXU-DRY (Smith & Nephew)
  SURGIPAD Combine Dressings (Johnson & Johnson Medical)
  TENDERSORB Wet-Pruf Abdominal Pad (Kendall Healthcare)
  TOPPER (Johnson & Johnson Medical)

15. Growth Factors
Procuren (autologous) (Curative Health Services)
Regranex Gel (becaplermin 0.01%) (Ortho-McNeil Pharmaceutical)

16. Human Skin Equivalents (HSE)/Skin Substitutes
Apligraf (Graftskin) (Organogenesis/Novartis)
Dermagraft (Advanced Tissue Sciences/Smith & Nephew)

17. Hydrocolloid Dressings
DuoDERM/CGF/Extra Thin (ConvaTec)
Hydrocol (Dow Hickam Pharmaceuticals)
Restore CX/Extra Thin (Hollister)
Tegasorb/Extra Thin (3M Healthcare)

18. Hydrogel Dressing (see also Impregnated Gauze Dressings)
Sheet
  CarraSorb M (Carrington Laboratories)
  Elasto-Gel (Southwest Technologies)
  Gentell (MKM)
  Vigilon (Bard)
Amorphous
  Carrington Gel Wound Dressing (Carrington Laboratories)
  Confeel Purilon Gel (Coloplast)
  DuoDERM Hydroactive Gel (Hydrogel/ Hydrocolloid) (ConvaTec)
  IntraSite Gel (Smith & Nephew)

19. Skin Sealants
Preppies (Kendall Healthcare)
Skin Prep (Smith & Nephew United)

Skin Shield (Mentor)
3M No Sting Skin Protectant (3M)

20. Transparent Film Dressings
BIOCLUSIVE/MVP (Johnson & Johnson Medical)
Flexfilm (Dow Hickam Pharmaceuticals)
OpSite/Flexifix/Flexigrid/3000 (Smith & Nephew)
Tegaderm/HP (3M Health Care)

21. Wound Fillers: Pastes, Powders, Beads, Strands
AcryDerm Strands (AcryMed)
Bard Absorption Dressing (Bard)
OsmoCyte Pillow wound Dressing (Procyte)
Multidex (DeRoyal Industries)

22. Wound Pouches
Wound Drainage Collector (Hollister)
Wound Manager (ConvaTec)
Adult and pediatric sized ostomy pouches (Multiple)

Not Otherwise Classified (NOC) Product Categories
23. Adhesives
24. Adhesive Removers
25. Adhesive Skin Closures
26. Adhesive Tapes
27. Antibiotics
28. Antimicrobials
29. Antiseptics
30. Bandages
31. Dressing Covers
32. Health Care Personnel Handrinses
33. Lubricating/Stimulating Sprays
34. Moisture Barrier Ointments/Creams/Skin Protectant Pastes
35. Moisturizers
36. Ointments
37. Perineal Cleansing Foams
38. Sterile Fields
39. Surgical Scrubs
40. Surgical Tapes
41. Miscellaneous

* © Diane Krasner, 1999.
Used with permission.
† All product names should be considered copyrighted or trademarked regardless of the absence of an ® or ™.

Biologicals: Human Skin Equivalents (Skin Substitutes, Growth Factors, and Skin Grafts)

It is important to emphasize once again best clinical practices for every patient with diabetic foot ulcers. Despite treating the cause (adequate vasculature, control of bacterial burden, appropriate pressure downloading) and good moist interactive local wound care, a significant number of diabetic foot ulcers do not heal. Steed et al. emphasized the importance of aggressive local debridement.[49] The nonhealing wound may have a deficiency growth factor or nonresponsive cells (fibroblasts, epidermal cells). Biologicals can help to stimulate some nonhealing wounds. Growth factors are discussed in Chapter 18. Platelet-derived growth factor has been marketed in a gel vehicle (Regranex) to treat non-healing diabetic neuropathic foot ulcers (see Chapter 18.)

Recent advances in tissue culture techniques have made it possible to culture cells from human foreskin donors. Donated newborn foreskins are used to extract epidermal precursor cells and fibroblasts to a master cell bank. Both the cells and mothers are extensively and repeatedly screened for possible infectious agents. Very few donors are needed because these cells are transferred to working cell banks and can produce enough skin substitute to cover four to six football fields.

Dermagraft (Advanced Tissue Sciences/ Smith & Nephew) is an in vitro bioengineered dermal skin construct consisting of a bioabsorbable polyglactin mesh (Vicryl, Ethicon Inc.) and seeded fibroblasts. The seeded fibroblasts proliferate and spread through the mesh, producing cytokines (growth factors), glycosaminoglycans (GAGs) and other matrix proteins, including collagen, fibronectin, and tenascin.[41] After the construct has matured, it is cryopreserved to −70°C in a bioreactor and then thawed prior to patient application. In the rat aorta ring assay, enhancement of wound tissue expansion and angiogenesis was linked to hepatocyte growth factor/scatter factor produced by the cells.[22] A pilot study protocol in nonhealing diabetic neuropathic foot ulcers implanted Dermagraft weekly for 8 weeks. There was a 12-week healing rate of 50%, compared to 8% in the control group.[14] In a follow-up, multicenter study, there were 129 patients in the control group and 109 in the Dermagraft group.[22] At the interim analysis, it was discovered that the therapeutic range for Dermagraft should be narrower than the original release criteria. Testing before and after cryopreserving is performed to determine a therapeutic range. The MTT (3-[4,5,-dimethylthiazol-2-y-1]-2,5,diphenyltetrazolium bromide) assay result was compared to healing rates following application and it was found that both very low and very high levels inhibited healing.[36] The 12-week healing rate of all Dermagraft in the multicenter study was 38.5% (40 of 109), but increased to 50.8% (31 of 61) if therapeutic range product was given for the majority of applications, compared to control 31.7% ($p = 0.007$).[22] Complete healing at week 32 for all Dermagraft patients was 57.5%; therapeutic range patients only, 57.7%; and control, 42.4% ($p = 0.022$ and 0.39, respectively). This study is now being repeated with the more precise therapeutic range release criteria for Dermagraft.

Apligraft (Human Skin Equivalent, Graftskin) (Organogenesis/Novartis) is a skin substitute composed of an epidermis (epidermal cells, stratum corneum) and dermis (bovine collagen, dermal fibroblasts).[48] In this construct, bovine collagen is acid dissociated and added to a transwell with fibroblasts from newborn donors. After 5 to 6 days, epidermal cell precursors are added, and when a number of epithelium are formed, the construct is raised to the air-liquid interphase to facilitate the production of a stratum corneum. This skin equivalent is also currently being tested for nonhealing diabetic foot ulcers. Besides the technology, we also need to determine the optimal clinical technique to use for these products and if bacterial burden of the wound needs to be corrected for optimal results.

In the future, many new generations of skin substitutes will become available. The dermis can be manipulated with GAGs that can enhance wound healing, and the transplanted cells can be transfected with extra copies of genes that promote the wound healing process such as platelet-derived growth factor. For widespread use, however, these products have to demonstrate not only clinical effectiveness but cost effectiveness.

Adjunctive Treatments

A number of adjunctive therapies are currently being utilized for care of diabetic foot ulcers. These include electrical stimulation, topical oxygen, ultrasound, vacuum-assisted closure, and warmth therapy. Generally speaking, the evidence for use of these therapies is limited at present, but growing. Randomized controlled clinical trials are difficult to do. The experience of expert clinicians varies from mild enthusiasm to strong support, depending on the modality. Thus, lacking strong evidence and community consensus, the onus is on each provider of care to critically evaluate the literature and the potential candidate for the therapy and to proceed with caution. Each of these therapies will be briefly addressed below.

Electrical Stimulation

Electrical stimulation is usually considered a physical therapy modality in North America. Claims for its efficacy for decreasing wound bioburden, debridement, promoting granulation tissue formation, improving tensile strength, and reducing pain have been made.[6, 15] While the body of research to support the use of electrical stimulation for wound healing is growing,[26] there is no consensus to date as to which voltages, currents, waveforms, or polarities produce which effects. Electrode placement is also an area of debate.

Topical Oxygen

Topical oxygen, also referred to as THBO, is the topical application of oxygen to a wound. It should not be confused with systemic hyperbaric oxygen therapy, which involves administration of oxygen in monoplace or multiplace chambers under greater than normal atmospheric pressure. Topical oxygen is a modality utilized primarily by physical therapists and podiatrists at this time. Advocates claim that topical oxygen dissolves in tissue fluids, is bacteriostatic, and stimulates angiogenesis and wound healing.[18, 43] Clinical trials comparing topical oxygen and hyperbaric oxygen are currently being undertaken in several centers in the United States.

Ultrasound

Therapeutic ultrasound, which is primarily a physical therapy modality, has been advocated for wound management.[10, 11] This form of ultrasound may stimulate the rate of wound healing, particularly if used during the inflammatory or proliferative phases of wound healing. Ultrasound has also been used diagnostically to monitor healing rates. Consensus has yet to be reached as to whether the indirect, direct, or underwater techniques are most efficacious for promoting wound healing and whether pulsed or continuous treatment should be utilized.

Vacuum-Assisted Closure (The V.A.C.)

Vacuum-assisted closure, represented in the marketplace by KCI's The V.A.C., is a method for applying negative pressure via suction to chronic wounds. It provides an alternative to traditional wound closure with sutures, skin grafts, flaps, or by secondary intention. This form of therapy has been shown in the laboratory and clinically to enhance granulation tissue formation, and to reduce bioburden and edema.[4, 34] The V.A.C. is also credited with enhancing cellular migration, promoting moist wound healing, and increasing blood flow and oxygenation to the area.[4, 34] The therapy is particularly useful for large chronic and exudating wounds, but it has been used successfully in diabetic foot ulcers and in preparing foot ulcer beds for flap closure. It is contraindicated with fistulas to organs or body cavities, necrotic tissue, untreated osteomyelitis, and malignancy. The V.A.C. system includes a powered therapy unit (a rental item), a collection canister, a sponge dressing which is cut to fit the wound bed, and film drape.

Warmth Therapy (Warm-Up)

Warmth therapy, represented in the marketplace by Warm-Up Active Wound Therapy from Augustine Medical, Inc., is a system for warming, humidifying, and protecting wounds. The Warm-Up raises the temperature of the environment around the wound to 38°C. Laboratory and clinical findings[42, 53] suggest that Warm-Up therapy brings the wound bed temperature into the normothermic range, increases local perfusion, and thereby stimulates the healing process. Decreased local wound pain has also been noted clinically. The system includes a battery-powered infrared heater (a rental or purchase item) and a noncontact bandage. It received Food and Drug Administration (FDA) approval in 1997 and is available by prescription at this time in the United States and Canada.

Conclusion

Diabetic foot ulcer care is a challenge for both providers and patients. A team approach is necessary to identify and treat general medical conditions and local foot problems. The holistic approach to the assessment and management of the diabetic foot ulcer is summarized in the care algorithm (Fig. 12–1). It reflects best practices and evidence-based literature when available. The interpretation of these principles requires an interdisciplinary team approach. Helpful tools for standardized care include:

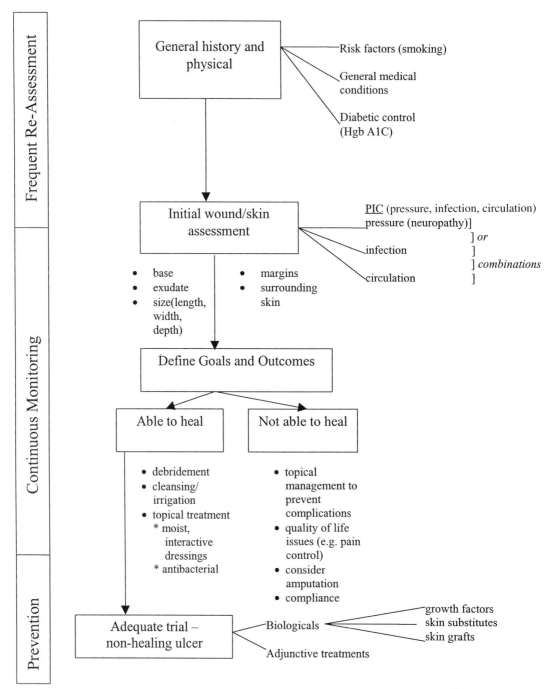

Figure 12–1 ■ The diabetic foot ulcer: Assessment and management algorithm.

- common case record or chart and precise ulcer monitoring/documentation;
- a combined clinic or meeting of the interdisciplinary team for networking, member education, and coordinating patient care;
- strategic linkage of institution and community services across the health care continuum; and

- a diabetes education program that includes diabetic sugar control and preventive foot care education.

In the future, diabetic patients will have a longer lifespan. With an aging population, the incidence of diabetes will further increase. It is important to optimize holistic care of these patients to improve outcomes. Despite correction of the underlying cause and best practice wound care, a proportion of these ulcers do not heal in a timely manner. The introduction of biologic alternatives (growth factors, human skin equivalents) and adjunctive treatments has increased the potential healability. In the future, more of our best practices will be validated with evidence-based science and we will have genetically altered skin substitutes to increase the percentage and shorten the time of healing in resistant ulcers. Advanced wound caring is just beginning!

REFERENCES

1. Alvarez OM, Gilson G, Auletta MJ: Local aspects of diabetic foot ulcer care: Assessment, Dressings, and Topical Agents. *In* Levin ME, O'Neal LW, Bowker JH (eds): The Diabetic Foot, 5th ed. St. Louis: Mosby Year Book, 1993, pp 265–266.

2. American Diabetes Association: Consensus Development Conference Report on Diabetic Foot Wound Care. Diabetes Care 22:1354–1360, 1999.

3. Apelqvist J, Ragnarson Tenvall G: Cavity foot ulcers in diabetic patients: A comparative study of cadexomer iodine ointment and standard treatment. An economic analysis alongside a clinical trial. Acta Derm Venereol 76:231–235, 1996.

4. Argenta LC, Morykwa MJ: Vacuum-assisted closure: A new method for wound control and treatment: Clinical experience. Ann Plast Surg 38:563–576, 1997.

5. Armstrong DG, Lavery LA, Liswood PL, Todd WF: Infrared dermal thermometry of the high risk diabetic foot. Diabetologia 39(Suppl):1013, 1996.

6. Brown M: Electrical stimulation for wound management. *In* Gogia PP (ed): Clinical Wound Management. Thorofare, NJ: Slack Incorporated, 1995, pp 175–184.

7. Bryant R: Acute and Chronic Wound Management. St. Louis: Mosby, 1992.

8. Caputo GM, Cavanagh PR, Ulbrecht JS, et al: Assessment and management of foot disease in patients with diabetes. N Engl J Med 331:854–860, 1994.

9. Dow G, Browne A, Sibbald RG: Infection in chronic wounds: Controversies in diagnosis and treatment. Ostomy/Wound Management 45:23–40, 1999.

10. Dyson M: Role of ultrasound in wound healing. *In* Kloth LC, McCulloch JM, Feedar JA (eds): Wound Healing: Alternatives in Management. Philadelphia: FA Davis, 1990, pp 259–285.

11. Dyson M: Ultrasound for wound management. *In* Gogia PP (ed): Clinical Wound Management. Thorofare, NJ: Slack Incorporated, 1995, pp 197–206.

12. Elliott IMZ: A Short History of Surgical Dressings. London: Pharmaceutic Press, 1964.

13. Ferris F, Krasner D, Sibbald RG: 12 Toolkits for Successful Wound Care. Copyright 1999.

14. Gentzkow GC, Iwasaki SD, Hershon KS, et al: Use of Dermagraft, a cultured human epidermis, to treat diabetic foot ulcers. Diabetes Care 4:350–354, 1996.

15. Gogia PP: Physical therapy intervention in wound management. *In* Krasner D, Kane D (eds): Chronic

16. Gratton D: Topical mupirocin versus oral erythromycin in the treatment of primary and secondary skin infections. Int J Dermatol 26:472–473, 1987.

17. Hansson C, Holm J, Lillieborg S, Syren A: Repeated Treatment with lidocaine/prilocaine cream (EMLA®) as a topical anaesthetic for the cleansing of venous leg ulcers. A controlled study. Acta Derm Venereol (Stockh) 73:231–233, 1993.

18. Heng MCY: Topical hyperbaric therapy for problem skin wounds. J Dermatol Surg Oncol 19:784–793, 1993.

19. Hinman CD, Maibach HI: Effect of air exposure and occlusion on experimental human skin wounds. Nature 200:377–378, 1963.

20. Holst RG, Kristofferson A: Lidocaine-prilocaine cream (EMLA Cream®) as a topical anaesthetic for cleansing of leg ulcers. The effect of length of application time. Eur J Dermatol 8:245–247, 1998.

21. Hutchinson JJ: Prevalence of wound infection under occlusive dressings: A collective survey of reported research. Wounds 1:123–133, 1989.

22. Jiang WG, Harding K: Enhancement of wound tissue expansion and angiogenesis by matrix-embedded fibroblast (Dermagraft), a role of hepatocyte growth factor/scatter factor. Int J Mol Med 2:203–210, 1998.

23. Kane D, Krasner D: Wound healing and wound management. *In* Krasner D, Kane D (eds): Chronic Wound Care: A Clinical Source Book for Healthcare Professionals, 2nd ed. Wayne, PA: Health Management Publications, Inc, 1997, pp 1–4.

24. Katsarou-Katsari A, Armenaka M, Katsenis K, et al: Contact allergens in patients with leg ulcers. J Eur Acad Dermatol Venereol 11:9–12, 1998.

25. Kennedy KL, Tritch DL: Debridement. *In* Krasner D, Kane D (eds): Chronic Wound Care: A Clinical Source Book for Healthcare Professionals, 2nd ed. Wayne, PA: Health Management Publications, Inc, 1997, pp 227–235.

26. Kloth LC, Feedar JA: Electrical stimulation in tissue repair. *In* Kloth LC, McCulloch JM, Feedar JA (eds): Wound Healing: Alternatives in Management. Philadelphia: FA Davis, 1990, pp 221–256.

27. Krasner D: Resolving the dressing dilemma: Selecting wound dressings by category. Ostomy Wound Management 35:62–70, 1991.

28. Krasner D: Chronic wound pain. *In* Krasner D, Kane D (eds): Chronic Wound Care: A Clinical Source Book for Healthcare Professionals, 2nd ed. Wayne, PA: Health Management Publications, Inc, 1997, pp 336–343.

29. Krasner D: Dressing decisions for the twenty-first century: On the cusp of a paradigm shift. *In* Krasner D, Kane D (eds): editors: Chronic Wound Care: A Clinical Source Book for Healthcare Professionals, 2nd ed. Wayne, PA: Health Management Publications, Inc, 1997, pp 139–151.

30. Krasner D: Pressure ulcers: Assessment, classification and management. *In* Krasner D, Kane D (eds): Chronic Wound Care: A Clinical Source Book for Healthcare Professionals, 2nd ed. Wayne, PA: Health Management Publications, Inc, 1977, pp 152–157.

31. Krasner D, et al: Sterile versus nonsterile wound care: An interactive monograph for healthcare pro-

fessionals. Toronto: Dumex Medical Surgical Products Ltd, 1998.

32. Lavery LA, Armstrong DG, Vela SA, et al: Practical criteria for screening patients at high risk for diabetic foot ulceration. Arch Intern Med 158:157–162, 1998.

33. Majno G: The Healing Hand. Cambridge, MA: The Harvard University Press, 1975.

34. Morykwas MJ, Argenta LC, Shelton-Brown EI, McGuirt W: Vacuum-assisted closure: A new method for wound control and treatment: Animal studies and basic foundation. Ann Plast Surg 38:553–562, 1997.

35. Murff RT, Armstrong DG, Lanctot D, et al: How effective is manual palpation in detecting subtle temperature differences. Clin Podiatr Med Surg 15:151–154, 1998.

36. Naughton G, Mansbridge J, Gentzkow G: A metabolically active human dermal replacement for the treatment of diabetic foot ulcers. Artif Organs 21:1203–1210, 1997.

37. New JP, McDowell D, Burns E, Young RJ: Problem of amputations in patients with newly diagnosed diabetes mellitus. Diabet Med 15:760–764, 1998.

38. Ovington LG: The well-dressed wound: An overview of dressing types. Wounds 10(Suppl A):1A–11A, 1998.

39. Ovington LG: Dressings and Adjunctive Therapies: AHCPR Guidelines Revisited. Ostomy Wound Management 45(Suppl):94S–106S, 1999.

40. Panel for the Prediction and Prevention of Pressure Ulcers in Adults. Pressure ulcers in adults: Prediction and Prevention. Clinical Practice Guideline, Number 2. AHCPR.

41. Pollak RA, Edington H, Jensen JJ: A human dermal replacement for the treatment of diabetic foot ulcers. Wounds 9:175–183, 1997.

42. Rabkin JM, Hunt TK: Local heat increases blood flow and oxygen tension in wounds. Ach Surg 122:221–225, 1987.

43. Rehm KB, Goudberg D, Longobardi JJ, Tinwell G: THBO: Putting pressure on non-healing wounds. Podiatry Today 54–65, 1997.

44. Reiber GE, Boyko EJ, Smith DG: Lower extremity foot ulcers and amputations in diabetes. In Harris MI, Cowie CC, Stern MP, et al (eds): Diabetes in America, 2nd ed. Washington, DC: U.S. Government Printing Office 408-28, DHSS Pub No. 95-1468, 1995.

45. Rietschel RL, Fowler JF Jr: Reactions to topical antimicrobials in Fisher's contact dermatitis, Vol 4. Baltimore: Williams & Wilkins, 1995, pp 205–208.

46. Robson MC: Wound infection. A failure of wound healing caused by an imbalance of bacteria. Surg Clin North Am 77:637–650, 1997.

47. Rodeheaver GT: Wound Cleansing, Wound Irrigation, Wound Disinfection. In Krasner D, Kane D (eds): Chronic Wound Care: A Clinical Source Book for Healthcare Professionals, 2nd ed. Wayne, PA: Health Management Publications, Inc, 1997, pp 97–108.

48. Sabolinski ML, Alverez O, Auletta M, et al: Cultured skin as a 'smart' material for healing wounds: Experience in venous ulcers. Biomaterials 17:311–320, 1996.

49. Steed DL, Donohoe D, Webster MW, Lindsley L: Effect of extensive debridement and treatment on the healing of diabetic foot ulcers. Diabetic Ulcer Study Group. J Am Coll Surg 183:61–64, 1996.

50. Turner TD: The development of wound management products. In Krasner D, Kane D (eds): Chronic Wound Care: A Clinical Source Book for Healthcare Professionals, 2nd ed. Wayne PA: Health Management Publications, Inc, 1997, pp 124–139.

51. Wagner FW: The dysvacular foot: A system for diagnosis and treatment. Foot Ankle 2:64–122, 1998.

52. Welsh O, Saenz C: Topical mupirocin compared with oral ampicillin in the treatment of primary and secondary skin infections. Curr Ther Res 41:114–120, 1987.

53. West JM, Hopf HW, Hunt TK: A radiant-heat bandage increases abdominal subcutaneous oxygen tension and temperature. Wound Repair Regeneration 4:134, 1996.

54. Williams C: Arglaes controlled release dressing in the control of bacteria. Br J Nurs 6:114–115, 1997.

55. Winter GD: Formation of the scab and the rate of epithelisation of superficial wounds in the skin of the young domestic pig. Nature 193:293–294, 1962.

56. Winter GD: Healing of skin wounds and the influence of dressings on the repair process. In Harkiss KJ (ed): Surgical Dressings and Wound Healing. London: Crosby Lockwood, 1971, pp 46–60.

57. Winter GD, Scales JT: Effect of air drying and dressings on the surface of a wound. Nature 197:91–92, 1963.

58. Wiseman DM, Rovee DT, Alverez OM: Wound dressings: Design and use. In Cohen IK, Diegelmann RF, Lindblad WJ (eds): Wound Healing: Biochemical & Clinical Aspects. Philadelphia: WB Saunders Company, 1992, pp 562–580.

59. van Rijswijk L, Beitz J: The traditions and terminology of wound dressings: Food for thought. J WOCN 25:116–122, 1998.

60. Wright JB, Hansen DL, Burrell RE: The comparative efficacy of two antimicrobial controlled release of silver dressings. Wounds 10:179–188, 1998.

Chapter 13

TOTAL-CONTACT CASTING IN THE TREATMENT OF NEUROPATHIC ULCERS

■ David R. Sinacore and Michael J. Mueller

Total-contact casting is the "gold standard" among methods used to heal diabetic foot ulcers. Numerous clinical reports[3, 6, 9, 17, 19, 21, 28, 31, 35, 36, 38, 41, 43, 48] and one controlled clinical trial[34] over the past 25 years, suggest that no treatment is as effective as total-contact casting (TCC) in healing Meggitt-Wagner grade 1 or 2 neuropathic ulcers. Total-contact casting and other off-loading methods remain the "cornerstone" for healing diabetic pedal ulcers, and may be used in conjunction with other methods.

The specific methods of application have undergone several modifications and refinements as the technique of contact-casting has gained popularity over the past two decades. Currently, the emphasis has been placed on utilizing newer materials with improved technology that continues to demonstrate the value of pressure-relief in healing neuropathic ulcers. The purpose of this chapter remains, as in previous editions, to summarize the indications and contraindications of total-contact casting and to detail the basic method of application. Several variations in the casting procedure and alternative pressure-relieving methods are now available and discussed. These alternatives may be used when TCC is either contraindicated or when certain patient characteristics are present and when more appropriate circumstances warrant their use. In addition, the effectiveness and expected outcomes of TCC are discussed, as well as some of the factors that directly impact healing times and eventual therapeutic outcomes. Finally, a typical case example is outlined that underscores the utility of TCC for healing neuropathic ulcers.

History and Theory

Total-contact casting to heal diabetic neuropathic ulcers is not a new method. It has been time-tested over many years, though there has been a general reluctance on the part of the medical community to embrace its use. The earliest published report of casting for trophic ulcerations dates back to the 1930s.[25] Dr. Joseph Kahn in India described an ambulatory technique for the treatment of plantar ulcers occurring in patients with Hansen's disease (leprosy) as an alternative to prolonged, expensive periods of bed rest in the hospital. Dr. Paul Brand and his associates refined and popularized the current technique in the early 1960s at the Gillis W.

Long Hansen's Disease Center in Carville, Louisiana.[14] Total-contact casting as a treatment for neuropathic plantar-surface ulcerations has since been applied to a variety of conditions involving insensitivity of the feet, including patients with diabetes mellitus, myelomeningocele, Charcot-Marie-Tooth disease, tabes dorsalis, chronic alcoholism, and herniated nucleus pulposus resulting in S1 motor and sensory neuropathy.[12, 41] More recently, immobilization with TCC has been used effectively for acute Charcot arthropathies of the ankle and foot with or without accompanying pedal ulceration.[1, 42, 44]

It is now well recognized that the primary factor in the cause of diabetic plantar surface ulcerations is the presence of peripheral neuropathy leading to diminished or absent sensation. This insensitivity allows excessive and prolonged stresses and pressures to occur in the diabetic foot, which ultimately results in tissue breakdown.[10, 11, 16] If the tissue breakdown (ulcer) goes unnoticed or untreated, infection is imminent and major amputation is likely.[37]

The main purpose of treating neuropathic plantar ulcerations by total-contact casting is to reduce excessive mechanical forces (including vertical pressure and horizontal shear) on the plantar surfaces of the feet as advocated by Brand and his associates,[10, 11, 16] while maintaining ambulation. The reduction of these pressures in the areas of ulceration allows healing to occur. The cast is fabricated to reduce excessive pressure at the ulcer site by spreading forces over an increased surface area of the foot and leg, thus allowing the ulcer to heal rapidly and completely. Two studies report TCC can increase the surface area of the foot between 15 and 24%.[15, 32] These modest increases in foot surface area result in dramatic reductions in peak plantar pressures throughout the foot. On average, peak plantar pressures are reduced 40 to 80% with casting compared to walking in therapeutic footwear[15, 30, 32] or normal street shoes.[7] One study reported a 75 to 84% reduction in peak pressure at the first and third metatarsal heads, respectively, when a person walked in the total-contact cast compared to normal shoes.[7] Therefore, the utility of contact-casting is in reducing peak plantar pressures, through increasing the surface area of the foot.

Depending on the presence and degree of foot deformity present, TCC causes the greatest and most consistent reductions in peak plantar pressures in the forefoot compared to the midfoot or the hindfoot.[7, 32] Total-contact casting appears to be least effective in reducing peak pressures in the hindfoot.[32] This may help explain why plantar ulcers located in the hindfoot take considerably longer to heal with casting than either forefoot or midfoot ulcers.[45] Fortunately, the metatarsal head region and great toe are the most frequent and susceptible areas to develop ulcerations in the diabetic patient.[41] Therefore, TCC is well-suited for ulcers of the forefoot and midfoot because peak plantar pressures are effectively reduced, allowing these pedal ulcers to heal rapidly and thoroughly.

Effectiveness and Expected Outcomes of TCC

Total-contact casting is the most effective ambulatory method in reducing excessive plantar pressures, and also has been shown to be the most effective method for healing diabetic neuropathic ulcers.[43] Several studies report the average time of healing to be 36 to 43 days.[3, 6, 9, 12, 14, 17, 19, 21, 25, 28, 31, 34-36, 38, 41, 45, 48] Many patients report having had a plantar surface ulcer for a number of years that would not heal until a total-contact cast was applied (Fig. 13–1). Two studies[39, 41] report healing in patients who had chronic plantar ulcers for an average of 11 months (ranging from 1 week to 13 years!) despite other forms of treatment, including daily dressing changes, antibiotic therapy, frequent callus shaving and debridement, and multiple skin grafts.

We have conducted a controlled clinical trial that compared TCC to a control group receiving traditional treatments including daily wound care, dressing changes, and footwear modifications.[34] Nineteen of 21 (91%) ulcerations treated with TCC healed in a mean time of 42 days compared to a healing rate of 32% in a mean time of 65 days in the control group. In addition, none of the casted ulcers developed an infection, while 26% (5 of 19 patients) of the traditional therapy group developed serious infection that required hospitalization. Of the five hospitalized patients, two required a subsequent forefoot amputation. The results of this prospective study confirm earlier descriptive studies and support our contention that TCC is superior to traditional treatment methods in the rates

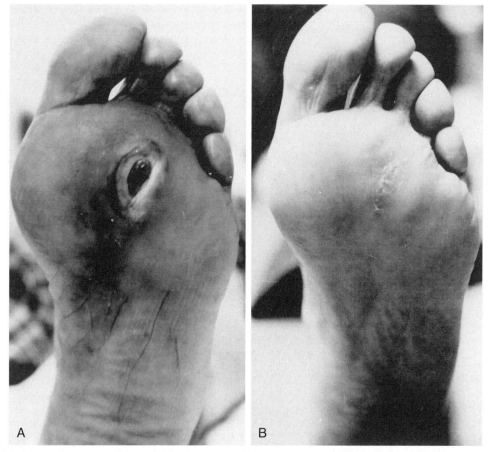

Figure 13–1 ■ *A*, Ulcerated region over third metatarsal head of a 68-year-old man. This patient has been diabetic for 25 years. Ulcer had been present for 36 months despite daily dressing changes. *B*, Ulcer closed after 49 days in total-contact cast. After fitting with Plastazote inserts and rocker-bottom shoes, foot shows no signs of ulceration.

of healing and the prevention of serious infection.

There have been no studies directly comparing the healing rates of total-contact casting to other methods used to treat diabetic neuropathic foot ulcers. Figure 13–2 shows the average healing time (in days) and the percentage (%) of diabetic foot ulcers healed for each of several popular treatment methods described in the literature. Clearly, total-contact casting has the most rapid (i.e., shortest number of days) healing time and consistently reports the greatest percentage of ulcers healed (mean 90%).[43] Other methods take longer than an average of 43 days and report a considerably greater percentage of the ulcers that fail to heal.[8, 20, 22, 23, 50] Comparisons of healing times and the percentage of ulcers healed among the various methods help underscore the importance of maximizing pressure relief through casting to promote neuropathic ulcer healing.

Indications and Contraindications

The indications and contraindications to total-contact casting are outlined in Table 13–1. The indication for total-contact casting is a grade 1 or 2 plantar ulcer[48] in the presence of insensitivity. For the purposes of this chapter, we define insensitivity as the inability to sense the 5.07 (10 gm) Semmes-Weinstein monofilament on any portion of the plantar surface of the foot. Some ulcerations, although not technically on the plantar surface of the foot, may actually be weight-bearing ulcers and respond well to this pressure-relieving therapy. For example, the patient with an ulcer on the lateral border of the foot secondary to a severe varus deformity would respond well to this form of therapy.

Absolute contraindications and relative contraindications to TCC exist that either

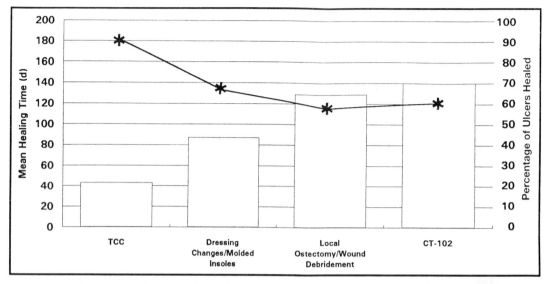

Figure 13-2 ■ Comparison of mean healing times (in days) and average percentage of ulcers healed for various methods described for healing diabetic foot ulcers. Bar heights correspond to the left ordinate; *—* corresponds to right ordinate. Total-contact casting (TCC) represents the average from several studies (references 3, 6, 9, 17, 19, 21, 34–36, 38, 41, 48, 49), values from dressing changes/molded insoles from references 23 and 34 combined; values for local ostectomy/wound debridement are from references 20 and 50 combined; values for CT-102 (a combination of several platelet-derived wound growth factors) are from reference 22. The bar height for CT-102 is the *median* time to healing not mean healing time. (From Sinacore DR: Total contact casting for diabetic neuropathic ulcers. Phys Ther 76:296,1996. With the permission of the APTA.)

can delay healing or lead to a poor outcome.[47] Adherence to the guidelines listed in the box will maximize success and minimize potential side effects. In the presence of a deep infection such as osteomyelitis or deep sepsis (wound grades 3 to 5), the foot should not be casted.[48] Antibiotic therapy and bed rest until the acute infection has subsided has been recommended.[11] Surgical debridement

of infected and necrotic soft tissue and bone may be required.

A relative contraindication is the size (area of surface opening) to depth ratio of the wound. If the ulcer depth is greater than the ulcer width (surface opening), it may be necessary to open the ulcer prior to casting to allow the deeper layers to heal and prevent premature superficial closing. Packing the superficial opening with loose-mesh gauze will help ensure that the deeper layers heal before the wound closes over.

Another relative contraindication is the patient with excessively fragile skin (such as seen with chronic steroid use or stasis ulcers) on the dorsum of the foot or leg. In our experience, these patients are more likely to develop skin breakdown or abrasions with TCC compared to patients without excessively fragile skin. Patients with excessively dry, cracked skin as occurs with severe autonomic nervous system neuropathy are more susceptible to additional skin breakdown with casting.[47] In these patients, total-contact walking splints might be a better alternative.[5]

Excessive and fluctuating edema in the foot or lower limb presents a challenge for full-contact casting. Because snug-fitting, uniform contact between the cast and the

Table 13-1 ■ INDICATION AND CONTRAINDICATIONS FOR TOTAL-CONTACT CASTING

Indication
    Grade 1 or 2 plantar ulcerations in the presence
        of insensitivity
Contraindications
    Absolute
        Active or acute deep infection, sepsis or gangrene
            (grades 3–5).
    Relative
        Ulcer depth greater than ulcer width
        Fragile skin
        Excessive leg or foot swelling
        Patient unwilling to have cast on extremity
        Patient unable to comply with follow-up visits or
            wearing precautions
        Patient unsafe in mobility while in cast
        Doppler pressure <0.4

lower limb is an essential element to a successful outcome, the presence of edema should be considered prior to casting. Frequently, the edema in the foot and leg reduce rapidly after only a few days of TCC, causing the cast to loosen. Any loosening of the cast may allow excessive shearing pressure as the cast moves on the skin. This can delay ulcer healing and may cause additional skin breakdown. Therefore, any patients with significant lower limb edema may require more frequent cast changes (i.e., every 3 to 7 days) until the edema has stabilized or subsided.

Any patient who is unable to keep regularly scheduled follow-up visits or is opposed to having a cast on their lower limb, or is unable to adhere to the cast precautions and instructions, should not be treated with TCC. For these patients, alternative methods of therapy should be explored.

Advantages

The major advantages to total-contact casting are outlined in Table 13–2. Above all, total-contact casting allows the patient to remain ambulatory and reduces the need for lengthy and expensive hospital stays associated with complete bed rest and nursing care. In most cases, below-knee TCC allows the patient to remain working, thereby minimizing income loss for the individual.

The cast is fabricated to reduce excessive pressures on the plantar surface of the foot by spreading the peak forces uniformly throughout the leg and entire foot. The even distribution of plantar pressure also helps eliminate or reduce edema in the lower limb. Immobilization in a cast may help to localize any minor infection and prevent the spread to adjacent tissues.[34] In addition, casting will protect the insensitive foot from additional trauma while healing occurs.

Finally, total-contact casting requires little daily effort by the patient or family members to care for their pedal ulcer. There is no need for daily wound care and dressing changes, so there is relatively little burden to the health care team. Daily or weekly office visits (e.g., to podiatrists or foot care nurse) or home visits for wound care are unnecessary. The cost of an entire period of casting (usually 6 weeks) is often less than the cost of one overnight admission to the hospital, and one cast application is roughly equivalent to the cost of an office visit with dressing supplies, topical antiseptic agents, and growth factor applications.[43]

Disadvantages

The major disadvantages of total-contact casting are listed in Table 13–3. The major disadvantage of the cast is that it impairs the patients's mobility and makes it difficult to carry on normal activities of daily living. The bulky nature of the below-knee cast, while allowing ambulation, can significantly impair balance and coordination, thereby placing the patient at greater risk for secondary injury due to falls. Combined with peripheral and motor neuropathies, the sensory ataxia present in patients with chronic diabetes[40] may make walking in the cast difficult. For all of our patients, we recommend using assistive devices such as walkers or crutches to prevent falls or loss of balance.

If immobilization with casting is prolonged, side effects such as joint stiffness and muscular atrophy can ensue. These side effects can be minimized with proper flexibility and strengthening exercises at cast changes and when the cast is removed. One study reported minimal deficits in ankle and subtalar joint range of motion before and after TCC immobilization.[17] Other side effects, such as bone demineralization and neuropathic (Charcot) joints have been reported, al-

Table 13–2 ■ ADVANTAGES OF TOTAL-CONTACT CASTING

1. Maintains ambulation
2. Reduces excessive plantar pressures
3. Protects foot from further trauma
4. Immobilization helps localize and prevent spread of infection
5. Controls edema
6. Requires "minimum" patient compliance

Table 13–3 ■ DISADVANTAGES OF TOTAL-CONTACT CASTING

1. Impairs mobility (i.e., walking, performing basic and instrumental activities of daily living, balance, coordination)
2. Joint stiffness and muscle atrophy if immobilization is prolonged
3. Possible skin abrasions or new ulcerations if cast is poorly applied or not monitored
4. Possible foul odor if drainage is excessive

though it is not clear if these changes are consequent to the immobilization or are osseous sequelae to diabetes mellitus.[1] We and others have not observed any acute fractures or arthropathies following immobilization with TCC for pedal ulcers.[29, 45]

Frequently, patients who do not limit their ambulation and remain full weight-bearing seem to be more susceptible to skin abrasions in the cast. Similarly, if care is not taken when applying and removing the cast, skin breakdown and new ulcerations can occur, particularly around bony prominences or bony deformities. New skin abrasions from the cast rubbing can be minimized through proper application and removal of the cast, by providing patients precise cast wearing instructions, and adhering to regularly scheduled follow-up visits. Even with optimal application of the cast and adherence to precautions by the patient, skin abrasions and fungal infections can develop.[9, 34] In our experience, skin abrasions as a result of TCC typically occur on non–weight-bearing areas and heal quickly with cessation of casting. Superficial fungal infections (most commonly *Trichophyton rubrum*) on the foot or leg occur in approximately 15% of casted patients[34] and should be treated immediately with topical antifungal cream such as Lotrimin cream (Schering Corp, Kenilworth, NJ). These minor complications do not appear to delay healing of the primary ulcer. Casting should be discontinued when severe fungal infections occur. Ulcers with moderate amounts of drainage can have foul odors that are socially unacceptable with prolonged casting. Delaying casting until drainage is minimal, or frequent cast changes (i.e., 3 to 5 days) and cleaning the ulcer will minimize this problem.

Cast Application

Patient Preparation

The ulcer must be thoroughly assessed for any evidence of sinuses or penetrating tracts. If the ulcer is deeper than it is wide, it may be opened to the width equal to its depth to ensure adequate drainage and healing of the wound's inner layers and prevent premature superficial healing. Alternatively, the deep ulcer can be packed loosely with wide-mesh gauze to prevent superficial healing. The ulcer should be cleaned and all necrotic tissue

removed. The surrounding callus should be removed or pared to reduce pressure at the margins of the ulcer. Young et al. have demonstrated that removing callus can reduce dynamic plantar pressures in the forefoot by 30% during barefoot walking.[51]

The ulcer size and depth are measured by a millimeter ruler or depth gauge. The perimeter of the ulcer also may be traced onto clear radiographic film using an indelible ink marker and later placed in the patient's record for subsequent comparison measurements (Fig. 13–3). We have found this a reliable method of quantifying the size of the ulcer[18] and very useful, because it gives the patient visual feedback regarding the effectiveness of TCC. This method also is helpful in convincing the reluctant patient to continue the casting procedure.

After the ulcer has been evaluated, a saline-soaked wide-mesh gauze is placed over the ulcer, covered with a dry thin dressing, and secured with paper tape (Fig. 13–4). The dressing should be kept as thin and small as possible to avoid excessive pressures from the dressing on the ulcer in the cast. If the ulcer is deep, a loosely packed gauze may be used to fill the ulcer to the surface, and then the thin dressing is applied.

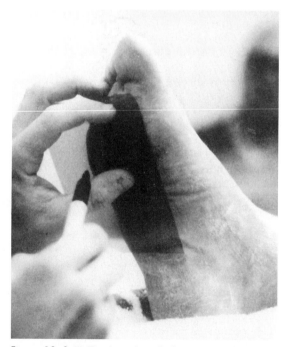

Figure 13–3 ■ Tracing size of ulcer on sterilized exposed radiographic film for permanent record of size of the ulcer.

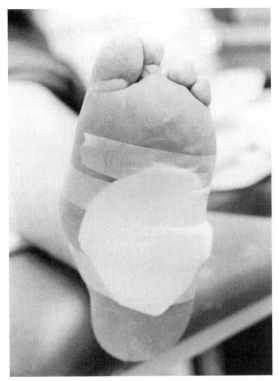

Figure 13–4 ■ Thin dressing is used to cover the ulcer in the cast.

To apply a total-contact cast, place the patient in the prone position with the involved limb's knee and ankle flexed to 90 degrees (the plantar surface of the ulcerated foot should be parallel to the floor). This position prevents further edema, takes the stretch off the gastrocnemius muscle, and allows the extremity to be held up easily while the inner layers of the cast are forming, thus preventing dents or other high-pressure areas in the cast. Patients often are unable to comfortably assume the prone position because of hip flexor tightness or low back pain. In these patients, it is necessary to modify the position by placing a number of pillows under the abdomen or pelvis. If necessary (though not ideal), the cast may be applied with the patient in the long-sitting position. We have found that adjustable tables, which allow half of the table to be lowered, thus accommodating slight hip flexion, afford a comfortable position during the casting procedure (Fig. 13–5).

A small amount of cotton padding is placed loosely between adjacent toes to absorb any moisture and prevent maceration. A 3-inch-wide, closely-fitting cotton stockinette is rolled over the foot and leg up to the knee. The toe-end of the stockinette should be sewn closed or can be folded into the toe sulcus

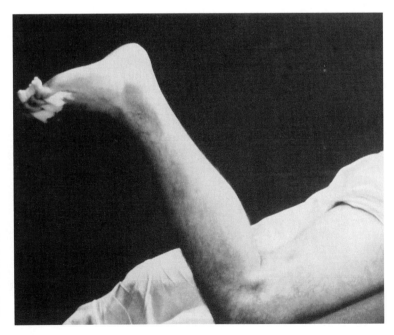

Figure 13–5 ■ Cast is applied with patient in prone position with ulcerated limb flexed at knee and dorsiflexed at ankle. Adjustable tables modify prone position for patients unable to maintain complete hip extension. Note cotton padding placed between adjacent toes.

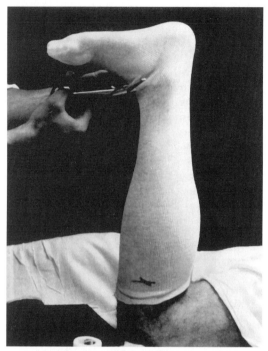

Figure 13–6 ■ Wrinkles in stockinette over dorsum of ankle are cut and edges are overlapped and taped.

Next, a layer of foam (½-inch adhesive-backed Sifoam [Omni Medical Specialties, San Diego, CA]) or felt is applied to cover and protect all the toes. This foam layer should be placed over the closed stockinette and extended dorsally from the metatarsophalangeal area around the toes to the toe sulcus on the plantar surface (Fig. 13–7). The edges of the foam should be trimmed medially and laterally and beveled to minimize pressure. The toes in the total-contact cast are enclosed in plaster to protect the insensitive foot and prevent damage to the toes from striking objects or from objects being lodged in the cast.

The leg should now be supported by an assistant and the foot and ankle held stable in the neutral position (90 degrees at the ankle), with the toes passively dorsiflexed only slightly. Many diabetic patients are unable to achieve the neutral, or 90-degree, position of the ankle joint secondary to joint or muscle limitations. Attempts to achieve this position passively may result in abnormal pronation and a prominent talus or navicular bone medially. Bony prominence in the abnormally pronated foot may cause areas of high pressure in the cast, so excessive pressure to achieve the neutral position is not recommended. A small amount of equinus can be accommodated in the cast by building up the posterior portion of the sole of the cast with plaster to level the weight bearing surface.

and taped closed. The stockinette is pulled so it is wrinkle-free. Wrinkles, occurring at the dorsum of the ankle, are cut and the edges are overlapped then taped to prevent a seam (an area of high pressure) when applying the plaster (Fig. 13–6).

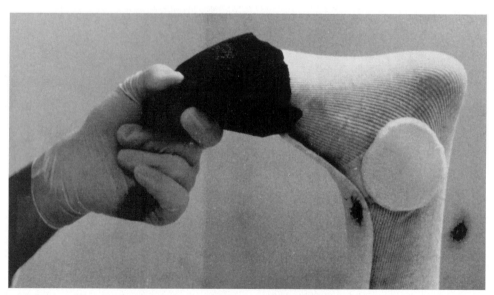

Figure 13–7 ■ Foam layer covers toes. Toes are enclosed in cast for protection. Felt padding is applied over malleoli and tibial crest to protect bony prominence. Felt strip along tibia facilitates cast removal.

Next, two circular pieces (approximately 2 inches in diameter) of ⅛ to ¼-inch adhesive-backed felt are placed over the malleoli on the stockinette. The felt pieces should be beveled along the edges to reduce the pressure along the felt-to-plaster interface. Another felt pad 18 to 20 inches long and 2 inches wide is beveled along the edges and placed along the anterior aspect of the leg and dorsum of the foot from just below the tibial tuberosity distal to the metatarsal heads (Fig. 13–7). This felt pad protects the prominent tibial crest and facilitates cast removal. Felt pads prevent the cast from rubbing on bony prominences. Occasionally, additional bony prominences such as the styloid process of the fifth metatarsal or talonavicular area may be padded, depending on the foot type. No other padding is used.

One to two layers of fast-setting, creamy plaster bandage (Gypsona II [National Patent Development Corp, Dayville, CT; Chaston Med, Melville, NY]) are wrapped loosely around the leg and foot from the proximal to the distal aspect. The plaster bandage should commence approximately 1 to 1½ inches below the previously marked fibular head and continue distally to beyond the metatarsal heads. Care must be taken to avoid any wrinkles in the plaster. The plaster bandage should be rolled quickly without tension. The bandage is then rubbed continuously to conform to the shape of the foot and leg until it has set. The plaster is molded into every crevice and around bony prominence and pads (Fig. 13–8). Particular attention should be given to molding the plaster to the contours of the sole of the foot. This thin layer of plaster is the most critical part of the contact cast. The patient should be instructed not to move the foot or leg once this "eggshell" layer has been applied. The assistant supporting the leg and foot should not move the foot or apply pressure to the plaster, which could distort or dent it and cause potential areas of high pressure. The inner layer should be allowed to fully set before any more plaster is applied.

Once the inner eggshell layer of plaster has set (approximately 3 minutes), additional layers should be added for reinforcement. Plaster splints (five layers thick) approximately 30 inches long are applied anteriorly to posteriorly (Fig. 13–9A) from the dorsal surface of the toes around to the plantar aspect of the foot and up to posterior aspect of the leg. A second set of splints are

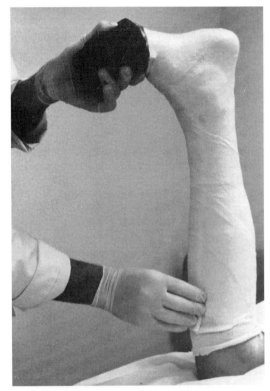

Figure 13–8 ■ First layer of plaster is continuously molded around bony prominence to conform to foot and leg until it has set.

wrapped in a medial to lateral direction around the calcaneus and up the proximal side of the leg (Fig. 13–9B). These splints reinforce the plantar and posterior portions of the cast.

To complete the cast, we usually incorporate a rubber walking heel on the plantar surface of the cast. A ¼-inch plywood board is used between the walking heel and the cast to minimize the danger of cracks in the sole of the cast from pressure on the heel. The ¼-inch plywood board should be cut smaller than the length of the foot (Fig. 13–10). It should extend from the heel to the toe sulcus and be slightly narrower than the foot's width. The area between the contoured sole of the foot and the board should be filled with a plaster roll to level the plantar surface.

When the walking heel is used, the placement of the heel is critical for balance. The walking heel should be placed on the board just behind the midline of the foot (Fig. 13–11). Placing the heel too far forward on the foot will cause the patient to have difficulty with balance and may cause excessive move-

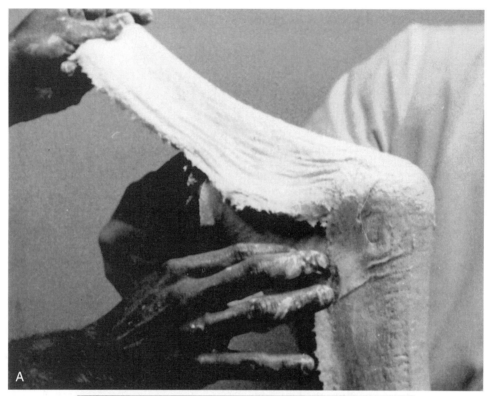

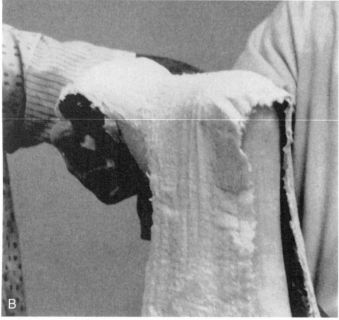

Figure 13–9 ■ *A* and *B*, Layers of plaster splints are applied to medial, lateral, posterior, and plantar walls of the cast for strength.

ment of the foot and leg in the cast. Placing the heel too far posteriorly will cause the patient to roll forward onto the toe of the cast and may contact the ground, breaking the toe region of the cast. The walking heel is attached to the cast, and the toes are fully enclosed by an additional one or two rolls of plaster. Every attempt should be made to keep the anterior portion of the cast thin to facilitate removal. We use a fiberglass tape

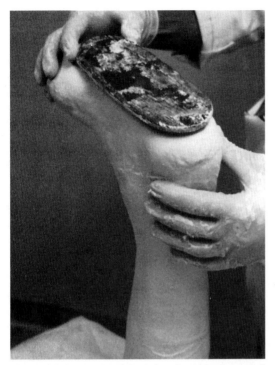

Figure 13–10 ■ A ¼-inch board is placed between walking heel and cast. Space between board and contoured cast is filled with plaster for support and to level plantar surface for walking.

(3M Orthopedic Products, Irving, CA) to attach the heel and complete the outer layers (Fig. 13–12). This material is lightweight, durable, quick-setting, and water-resistant, though the fiberglass tape is not molded as easily to the foot. We recommend the use of this material, particularly with patients who may need to bear weight soon after application.

In some cases, the rubber walking heel may not be appropriate to use because the patient's balance is very unsteady or if temporary casting may cause a sudden onset of back pain due to unequal limb lengths. In these cases, we prefer to use a postoperative cast boot over the cast while ambulating (Fig. 13–13). Postoperative cast boots with rigid, slightly rocker-bottom soles are most easily tolerated. In all cases the ¼-inch plywood board should be used to strengthen the plantar aspect of the cast and prevent damage to the inner layers during weight-bearing.

The completed cast should now be allowed to dry thoroughly. As an added precaution, the patient is instructed not to bear weight for at least 24 hours after application to allow the inner layers to harden. Before dismissing the patient, the cast should be checked for proper fit and the patient instructed in proper cast care and precautions.

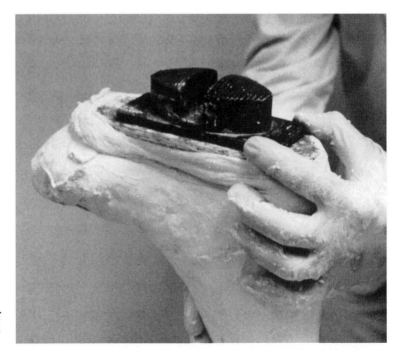

Figure 13–11 ■ Placement of walking heel on board just behind midline of foot.

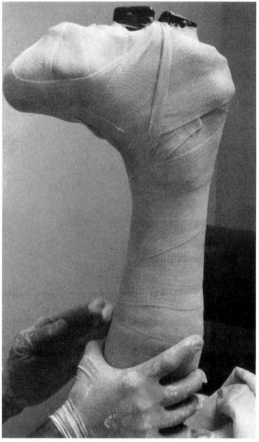

Figure 13-12 ▪ Completed cast. Weight-bearing should be delayed 24 hours to allow inner layers to thoroughly set.

Instructions to Patients

The patient with a total-contact walking cast should be given meticulous instruction in the care and monitoring of their cast. Since the patient's foot lacks protective sensation, the patient must be instructed to watch for signs of intolerance and problems. We routinely obtain written informed consent prior to casting to ensure the patient understands the purpose of TCC, and to explain the risks and precautions involved with the application. We have found that providing detailed, written instructions, including an explanation of the purpose of the casting procedure and how it differs from an ordinary below-knee cast, has been useful for patients. An emergency telephone number to contact should problems occur must be provided to all patients. An example of these written instructions and some helpful reminders regarding the care of the cast are provided in Table 13-4. If the patient experiences any one or a combination of the following signs, the cast should be removed and the ulcer inspected immediately:

1. Excessive swelling of the leg or foot, causing the cast to become too tight.
2. Loosening or excessive mobility of the foot in the cast.
3. Drainage on the outside of the cast.
4. Deep cracks or soft spots in the cast.
5. Sudden tenderness in the inguinal lymph nodes.

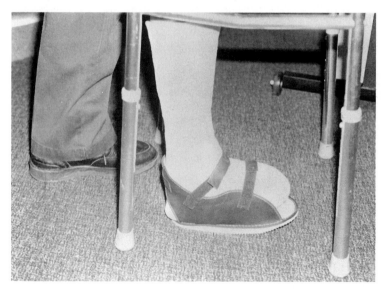

Figure 13-13 ▪ A postoperative cast boot covers the TCC (instead of a rubber walking heel). The cast boot has a rigid rockered sole to assist walking in the cast.

Table 13-4 ■ TOTAL CONTACT CAST INSTRUCTIONS GIVEN TO EACH PATIENT AT THE INITIAL VISIT

You have a total-contact cast applied to your foot for the purpose of healing the ulcer (sore) on your foot. These ulcers do not heal because of the extremely high pressures on the sole of the foot during walking. The cast is made to decrease the pressure on the ulcer, thereby allowing the ulcer to heal. In addition to the pressure relief, the cast is designed to be very snug-fitting with the toes enclosed for protection.

In order for the total contact cast to be effective, you must know how to take care of your cast. The following is a list of what to do and *Not* to do.

- *Do not* bear weight or walk on your cast until you are told to do so by the person putting the cast on your foot. Usually, no weight bearing is allowed for 24 hours after the cast is applied. This allows the inner layers of plaster to dry thoroughly.
- After 24 hours, you may resume walking. We recommend you limit your walking to one third of the normal daily walking distance.
- Never use the cast to strike or hit objects. Dents, cracks, or softened areas of the cast may cause excessive pressure on your foot in the cast and should be reported immediately.
- Keep the cast dry at all times. Water will destroy your cast. Sponge bathing is recommended while your cast is on. *Do not* shower. If the cast does become wet, dry it immediately with a towel, or hair dryer set to "cool." If it rains, cover the cast with a plastic bag.
- Your cast may be inconvenient and you may have difficulty sleeping. This is not uncommon. You may try wrapping your cast in a towel or placing it on a pillow while in bed. You may also want to wear a cotton, athletic sock on your noncasted foot and leg to prevent the cast from causing abrasions or rubs.
- After wearing the cast several days, perspiration and dirt may cause itching of the skin inside the cast. This is common. You must ignore it. *Do not* stick pencils or coat hangers or other objects in the cast to scratch the skin.
- Inspect the entire cast daily. Look and feel for deep cracks or soft spots on the cast. Use a small hand mirror to inspect the sole of the cast.
- Never attempt to remove your cast by yourself.

REMOVING YOUR CAST

We have a specially designed saw to remove the cast with little discomfort. It should be removed only by a health care professional. After removal, your skin may be flaky and dry, and your joints may feel stiff. Apply a thick cream or oil for several days to moisten and soften the skin. Your therapist will show you exercises to decrease the stiffness in your foot. You will need to have your specially made shoes ready to wear *immediately* after the cast is removed to prevent your foot from getting another ulcer. You should continue to use crutches or a walker for several weeks after the ulcer is healed to help protect your foot. Be sure and talk to your doctor or therapist about protecting the foot after the cast is removed.

WARNING SIGNS

If any of the following signs or symptoms occur call (phone number).

1. Excessive swelling of the leg or foot if the cast becomes too tight.
2. If the cast becomes too loose and your leg can move up or down in the cast greater than 1/4 inch.
3. If the cast has any deep cracks or soft spots.
4. Any drainage of pus or blood on the outside of the cast. This will appear brownish or dark yellow in color.
5. Any foul-smelling odor of the cast.
6. If you experience any excessive tenderness in your groin or the casted foot.
7. Any excessive leg pain or annoying pressure in the ankle or foot that will not go away.
8. If you notice any sudden onset of fever or increase in body temperature.

If any of the above conditions occur, do the following:

1. Notify appropriate professional personnel as soon as possible at (phone number).
2. *Do not* walk on your cast. Keep your leg elevated.
3. Use crutches or a walker and keep the casted foot off the ground until seen by professional personnel.

---

6. Sudden increase in body temperature (fever) or chills.
7. Complaints of discomfort or pain.

In addition to instruction in the warning signs, the patient should be instructed in proper ambulation. It must be emphasized that both walking distance and frequency must be limited. The less the patient walks, the less the pressures on the foot. In the ab-
sence of excessive pressure, the ulcer will heal quickly. The patient is encouraged to shorten their stride length, avoid fast walking and excessive push-off in the late-stance phase of the gait cycle, and to limit ambulation to one third of their normal daily routine. We routinely issue crutches or walkers to patients to help decrease weight-bearing and improve their balance. If patients develop low back pain or leg pain, a temporary lift

may be added to the opposite shoe to level the pelvis. Alternatively, the walking heel may be eliminated and replaced with a postoperative cast boot.

Follow-up Visits

The initial cast is left on no more than 5 to 7 days. The cast should be changed earlier if excessive edema or drainage was present when applying the initial cast. The cast is removed using a standard cast saw and spreaders. Cuts are made along the anterior surface from proximal to distal along the felt strip, then medial to lateral at the level of the ankle (Fig. 13–14). It should be remembered that the anterior wall of the cast is thin compared to the other walls, so caution must be taken to prevent injury from the saw to the insensitive skin.

At the first cast change, the ulcer is reevaluated. The perimeter of the ulcer is retraced on the radiographic film to document any change in ulcer size. The first cast change also provides the opportunity to evaluate the patient's response to the cast.[12] Skin temperature checks will detect any local inflammation caused by the cast rubbing on the skin,[12] so future modifications can be made.

This first cast change also provides the opportunity to begin preparation for definitive footwear for the diabetic patient. Custom shoes and insole fabrication require a negative mold of the foot. Since edema should be resolved, the foot can be casted at this time to allow time for fabrication. Although this practice is somewhat time consuming, it will ultimately save time and expense and provide protection when the ulcer is healed.

The cast may now be reapplied as described previously. The next cast may be left in place for up to 2 weeks. Casts should be changed more frequently in the presence of significant edema or drainage. At each cast change, the ulcer should be evaluated and the cast reapplied if healing is incomplete. For individuals whose compliance is dubious, more frequent monitoring and cast changes are recommended.

If the ulcer is healed, the patient should be placed immediately in appropriate therapeutic footwear (see Chapter 34). Custom-molded insoles with rigid rocker-bottom shoes are recommended for forefoot ulcers.[4, 10] In addition to the appropriate footwear, the patient must be carefully instructed in monitoring the newly healed ulcer. Brand[11] indicates that the newly healed ulcer is particularly susceptible to reulceration within the first month after healing. This is because of the poor capacity of scar tissue to accommodate shear stress.[11] Several studies have documented that recurrence rate after TCC is approximately 30%,[43] with two studies suggesting that as many as 50% of the ulcers recur.[28, 38] Mueller and colleagues reported that 27% of foot ulcers recur within the first 3 months following transmetatarsal amputation and 48% of these ulcers reopen within the first month.[33] These data underscore the critical period after initial healing. The diabetic patient with a newly healed ulcer should be instructed to increase weight-bearing activities slowly, continue using ambulatory aids, and frequently check skin temperature to identify local warm spots on the feet that may indicate inflammation. Frequent follow-up visits *after* the cast is removed are mandatory to educate the patient and reinforce the roles of excessive pressure and insensitivity.

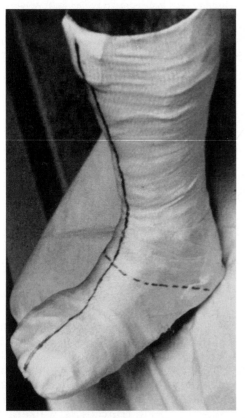

Figure 13–14 ■ Lines on cast indicate where cuts should be made when removing cast. Single cut is made along felt strip. Additional cuts (if necessary) may be made on either side of ankle.

Precautions

The methods of cast application described in this chapter are detailed enough to replicate; however, caution is necessary. Thorough training and practice in the cast application is requisite to ensure early success and to minimize the potential side effects and sequelae of immobilizing an insensitive foot. We recommend visiting a facility or medical center that regularly performs TCC to observe, learn, and practice the application of these casts before one attempts them alone. An excellent videotape depicting this method is available on a loan basis from the U.S. Public Health Service.* The treatment of diabetic neuropathic ulcers by this method requires a strong commitment and willingness on the part of the diabetic foot care team members (or individuals applying the cast) to respond quickly to patients' complaints or problems at any time.

The keys to minimizing potential side effects and successful management by this method are close and frequent monitoring of the ulcer and the patient's tolerance to the casting procedure. Strict patient compliance with subsequent follow-up visits is paramount. If patients are unable or unwilling to be followed-up regularly as outpatients, complications from the casts are inevitable, and this method should not be employed.

Alternatives and Modifications of the Below-Knee Walking Cast

Several modifications to the original total-contact below-knee walking cast have been suggested.[5, 8, 13, 19] The molded double-rocker plaster shoe is one such modification[19] (Fig. 13–15). The plaster shoe is molded over the entire foot but ends at the ankle (below the malleoli). The wooden double-rocker platform is attached to the molded foot, and the medial and lateral arches are filled with plaster to complete the weight-bearing surface. As with the below-knee cast, placement of the double rocker platform on the sole is critical. It should be placed so that the center of the posterior rocker bar is aligned with the

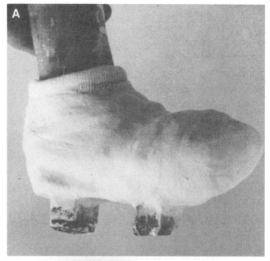

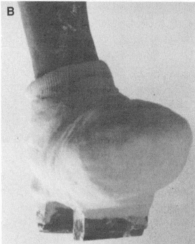

Figure 13–15 ■ A molded double-rocker shoe. A, Lateral view. B, Oblique view.

center of the medial malleolus and the front edge of the anterior rocker bar is immediately behind the first metatarsal head.

We believe the primary indication for using the rocker-bottom plaster shoe is for patients with superficial plantar ulcers who have fragile skin or concomitant stasis ulcers on the lower leg and who may not tolerate the below-knee cast (Fig. 13–16). Several descriptive studies report favorable healing rates and quick healing times with this method.[19, 24, 39] These reports also are quick to point out that the molded double-rocker plaster shoes were more socially acceptable, less costly to fabricate, and may have less risk associated with them than the below-knee cast.

---

* The videotape is available from Gillis W. Hansen's Disease Center, Department of Education and Training, 5445 Point Clair Rd, Carville, LA 70721–9607.

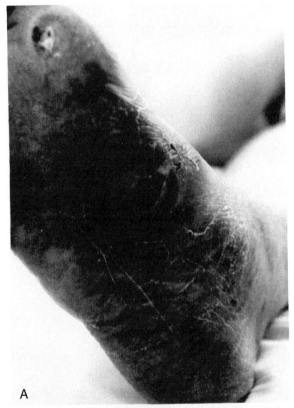

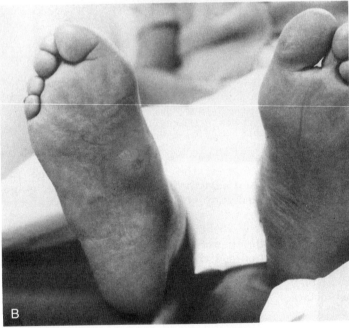

Figure 13–16 ■ *A*, An example of chronic neuropathic ulcer in cuneiform metatarsal region of a 66-year-old diabetic woman. Ulcer had been present for 10 months before casting. Ankle-arm index of ulcerated limb was 0.43. *B*, Same ulcer after 39 days in a molded double-rocker plaster shoe. Ulcer is well-healed.

Another alternative to TCC is a walking splint or a padded ankle-foot orthosis.[5] A walking splint is fabricated using a method similar to the TCC, except the anterior portion of the cast is removed. The splint is se-cured to the foot and leg with elastic bandages. Birke et al. indicate that use of the walking splint is advisable in patients with hypotrophic skin, active infection, poor circulation, or patients fearful of being casted.[5]

The obvious advantage of the walking splint is that it can be removed to observe the skin and ulcer frequently and easily. A potential disadvantage is that the patient may not comply with proper reapplication of the splint.

An alternative to a plaster walking splint is a custom-fabricated padded ankle-foot orthosis (AFO) (Fig. 13–17A and B). One commercially available AFO (DH Pressure-Relief Walker, Royce Medical/Centec Orthopaedics, Camarillo, CA) has several features that make it a potentially useful alternative to the TCC (Fig. 13–17B). Lavery and colleagues recently showed the DH Pressure-Relief Walker can reduce (vertical) plantar pressures in the forefoot to the same extent as a TCC.[30] In addition, the removable closed-cell padded insole of the DH Pressure-Relief Walker can be modified to accommodate any size ulcer or dressing. This is readily accomplished by removing any number of Velcro-fastened, multidensity rubber plugs from the insole as necessary. Another feature is the rigid rocker-bottom sole (toe and heel), which limits plantar pressures in the forefoot during the late stance (i.e., push-off) phase of gait.[26] The rigid bilateral uprights of the AFO help to limit talocrural, subtalar, and midtar-sal joint movement. The innermost layers of the DH Pressure-Relief Walker are adjustable and snug-fitting, providing a degree of uniform, total-contact pressure. These alternative methods to below-knee TCC are indicated when complicating factors are present or when patients are unable or unwilling to have a full-contact cast. In our experience, alternative pressure-relieving methods should be used when TCC is contraindicated because they provide some degree of immobilization and pressure reduction. A potential drawback is that the rapid healing rates observed with TCC may not be observed with these alternative methods,[8] since most patients can freely remove them. Further research is needed to determine if healing rates with removable splints and other alternative methods are comparable to healing rates using below-knee TCC.

Compliance

Total-contact casting offers an element of forced-compliance, since the cast is not easily removed. Without doubt, this forced-compliance contributes to the rapid healing times observed with TCC compared to re-

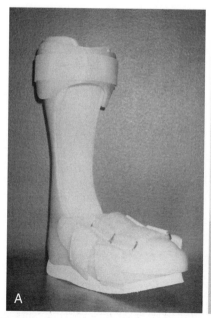
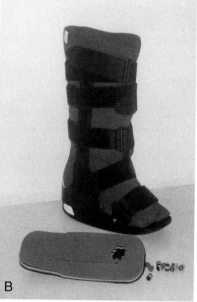

Figure 13–17 ■ Custom-made bivalved ankle foot orthosis (AFO) and commercially available DH Pressure-Relief Walker are alternative weight-distributing methods to heal neuropathic plantar ulcers. A, The custom-made bivalved AFO is lined with Plastazote or Aliplast to reduce plantar pressures. B, The DH Pressure-Relief Walker has removable, multidensity rubber plugs in the insole that can be customized to reduce pressures around the ulcerated region.

movable healing AFOs despite similar reductions in plantar pressures.[8] If patients have the opportunity to remove an AFO while sleeping, they are more apt to stand or walk unprotected around their homes (e.g., night trips to the bathroom or standing in the shower) since their feet are insensitive. Even these brief exposures to high plantar pressures are adequate stimuli to delay wound healing. For these reasons, and when compliance is dubious, TCC is the better treatment choice to ensure quicker healing times.

Compliance with partial weight-bearing prescription is a difficult task. We advocate the use of partial weight-bearing (PWB) on the casted limb, using an assistive device (walker or bilateral crutches) at all times during ambulation to help unload the casted limb and further reduce pedal pressures, thereby facilitating ulcer healing. Using PWB with assistive devices decreases the ambulatory patient's walking speed, shortens their step length, thereby further reducing plantar pressures. Not all authorities agree that PWB and assistive devices are necessary (or even practical!) for patients with diabetes, peripheral neuropathy, and a pedal ulcer.[2, 35] Although the major pressure reduction is afforded by the cast in response to increasing the surface area of the foot, we believe further reduction in plantar pressures using an assistive device will promote a faster healing time.

In addition to encouraging use of PWB with assistive devices, the patient should be encouraged to reduce the amount of daily weight-bearing activities and walking. Based on the classic works of Kosiak[27] and Brand,[10] ulcer formation and delayed wound healing are directly related to magnitude of peak plantar pressures as well as the duration and number of repetitions that peak plantar pressures are applied. Even modest plantar pressures applied continuously throughout the day may delay ulcer healing. Therefore, any combination of strategies to limit plantar pressures should hasten healing time and reduce unnecessary complications such as skin abrasions or cast rubs. Adherence to PWB instructions are problematic for patients with diabetes and a neuropathic pedal ulcer. Typically, only 30% of all patients are compliant with instructions for PWB using assistive devices and reducing their frequency of weight-bearing activities.[44] When patients are compliant with PWB and reduced ambulation, we have observed significantly shorter healing times,[44] fewer complications from casting (i.e., less skin abrasions), and less pedal pressures during walking. Therefore, our results suggest using PWB with an assistive device while ambulating is beneficial to those patients who strictly follow the recommendations. Additional research is needed to determine if adherence to PWB and limited ambulation in the cast contribute to faster healing times.

■ CASE STUDY

A 55-year-old male with type 2 diabetes mellitus (reported 22 years' duration) presented with bilateral plantar ulcerations beneath the right first metatarsal head and left third metatarsal head (Fig. 13–18A and B). Each grade 1 ulcer measured approximately 5 cm² in area and was 1 to 2 mm deep. Reported duration of both ulcers was 18 months. This patient demonstrated severe sensory neuropathy in both feet, as evidenced by an inability to sense the 6.10 (75-gm) Semmes-Weinstein monofilament. Peripheral pulses were present and palpable on both feet. Bilateral Doppler ankle-arm indices were 1.0. We typically cast the foot with the larger ulcer first, since patients do not tolerate bilateral casts, because of the difficulty with ambulation.[46] A total-contact cast was applied initially to the right foot, while dressing changes were continued on the left foot. He was instructed in the use of a walker. The initial cast was changed in 1 week. Subsequent casts were changed every 2 weeks, with complete healing in 65 days (Fig. 13–18B). He immediately was fit with a rigid-rocker-bottom shoe containing an accommodative, total-contact insert for the newly healed ulcer.

The ulcer on the left foot did not change significantly in size during casting of the right foot. Casting then was begun on the left foot following a similar procedure as the right foot. Healing of the ulcer on the left foot was complete in 42 days. After the left plantar ulcer healed (Fig. 13–18C), the patient was fit with another rocker-bottom shoe and total-contact accommodative insert. After both plantar ulcers were healed, we encouraged him to continue to use the walker and to remain partial weight-bearing on the left foot for an additional 2 weeks to allow further maturation of the recently healed ulcer. After 2 weeks, this patient ambulated independently without ulcers or an assistive device in his therapeutic shoes.

Summary

Total-contact casting is the most effective, rapid, and ambulatory therapy for healing

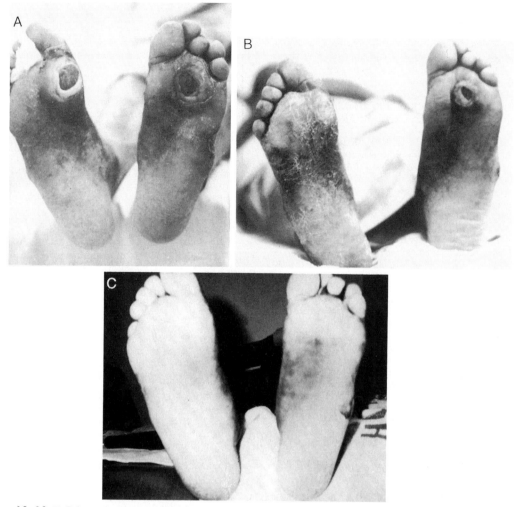

Figure 13-18 ■ Bilateral plantar-surface ulcers in a 55-year-old patient with type 2 diabetes mellitus. *A,* Prior to TCC. *B,* After 65 days of TCC to right foot only. *C,* After 42 days of TCC to left foot. See text for case history.

the diabetic neuropathic plantar ulcer. We believe the methods of cast application are worth mastering, since the reported benefits greatly outweigh potential complications. Given the current emphasis for shortened hospital stays, total-contact casting provides an effective and cost-prudent alternative to prolonged, expensive periods of bed rest in the hospital.

ACKNOWLEDGMENT

The authors gratefully acknowledge the early guidance and support of Steven J. Rose, Ph.D., P.T.

REFERENCES

1. Armstrong DG, et al: The natural history of acute Charcot's arthropathy in a diabetic foot specialty clinic. Diabet Med 14:357–363, 1997.

2. Armstrong DG, Lavery LA, Bushman TR: Peak foot pressures influence healing time of diabetic foot ulcers treated with total contact casts. J Rehabil Res Dev 35:1–5, 1998.

3. Baker RE: Total contact casting. J Am Podiatr Med Assoc 85:172–176, 1995.

4. Bauman JH, Girling JP, Brand PW: Plantar pressures and trophic ulceration: An evaluation of footwear. J Bone Joint Surg 45:652, 1963.

5. Birke JA, et al: Methods of treating plantar ulcers. Phys Ther 71:116–122, 1991.

6. Birke JA, Novick A, Patout CA, Coleman WC: Healing rates of plantar ulcers in leprosy and diabetes. Lepr Rev 63:365–374, 1992.

7. Birke JA, Sims DA, Buford WL: Walking casts: Effect of plantar foot pressures. J Rehabil Res Dev 22:18–22, 1985.

8. Boninger ML, Leonard JA: Use of bivalved ankle foot-orthosis in neuropathic foot and ankle lesions. J Rehabil Res Dev 33:16–22, 1996.

9. Boulton AJM, et al: Use of plaster casts in the management of diabetic neuropathic foot ulcers. Diabetes Care 9:149–152, 1986.

10. Brand PW: The insensitive foot. *In* Jahss MM (ed): Disorders of the Foot, Vol 2. Philadelphia: WB Saunders Company, 1982.

11. Brand PW: The diabetic foot. *In* Ellenberg M, Rifkin H (eds): Diabetes Mellitus. Garden City, NY: Medical Examination Publishing Co, Inc, 1983.

12. Brenner MA: An ambulatory approach to the neuropathic ulceration. J Am Podiatry Assoc 64:862, 1974.

13. Burden AC, et al: Use of the "Scotchcast boot" in treating diabetic foot ulcers. Br Med J 286:1555, 1983.

14. Coleman WC, Brand PW, Birke JA: The total contact cast: A therapy for plantar ulceration on insensitive feet. J Am Podiatry Assoc 74:548, 1984.

15. Conti SF, Martin RL, Chaytor ER, et al: Plantar pressure measurements during ambulation in weight bearing conventional short leg casts and total contact casts. Foot Ankle Int 17:464–469, 1996.

16. Ctercteko GC, et al: Vertical forces acting on the feet of diabetic patients with neuropathic ulceration. Br J Surg 68:608, 1981.

17. Diamond JE, Mueller MJ, Delitto A: Effect of total contact cast immobilization of subtalar and talocrural joint motion in patients with diabetes mellitus. Phys Ther 73:310–315, 1993.

18. Diamond JE, Mueller MJ, Delitto A, Sinacore DR: Reliability of a diabetic foot evaluation. Phys Ther 69:797–802, 1989.

19. Diamond JE, Sinacore DR, Mueller MJ: Molded double-rocker plaster shoe for healing a diabetic plantar ulcer. Phys Ther 67:1550–1552, 1987.

20. Griffiths GD, Wieman TJ: Meticulous attention to foot care improves the prognosis in diabetic ulceration of the foot. Surg Gynecol Obstet 174:49–51, 1992.

21. Helm PA, Walker SC, Pullium G: Total contact casting in diabetic patients with neuropathic foot ulcerations. Arch Phys Med Rehabil 65:691–693, 1984.

22. Holloway GA, Steed DL, DeMarco MJ, et al: A randomized, controlled multicenter dose response trial of activated platelet supernatant, topical CT-102 in chronic, nonhealing diabetic wounds. Wounds 5:198–206, 1993.

23. Holstein P, Larsen K, Sager P: Decompression with the aid of insoles in the treatment of diabetic neuropathic ulcers. Acta Orthop Scand 47:463–468, 1976.

24. Joseph B, Joshua S, Fritschi EP: The molded double-rocker plaster shoe in the field treatment of plantar ulcer. Lepr Rev 54:39, 1983.

25. Kahn JS: Treatment of leprous trophic ulcers. Lepr India 11:19, 1939.

26. Kelly VE, Mueller MJ, Sinacore DR: Gait characteristics associated with peak plantar pressures. Phys Ther 78:S, 1998.

27. Kosiak M: Etiology and pathology of ischemic ulcers. Arch Phys Med Rehabil 40:62–69, 1959.

28. Laing PW, Cogley DJ, Klenerman L: Neuropathic foot ulceration treated by total contact casts. J Bone Joint Surg Br 74-B:133–136, 1992.

29. Lavery LA, Armstrong DG, Walker SC: Healing rates of diabetic foot ulcers associated with midfoot fracture due to Charcot's arthropathy. Diabet Med 14:46–49, 1997.

30. Lavery LA, Vela SA, Lavery DC, Quebedaux TL: Reducing dynamic foot pressures in high risk diabetics with foot ulcerations: A comparison of treatments. Diabetes Care 19:818–821, 1996.

31. Lee EH, Bose K: Orthopedic management of diabetic foot lesions. Ann Acad Med 14:331, 1985.

32. Martin RL, Conti SF: Plantar pressure analysis of diabetic rocker bottom deformity in total contact casts. Foot Ankle Int 17:470–472, 1996.

33. Mueller MJ, Allen BT, Sinacore DR: Incidence of skin breakdown and higher amputation following transmetatarsal amputation: Implications for rehabilitation. Arch Phys Med Rehabil 76:50–54, 1995.

34. Mueller MJ, et al: Total contact casting in treatment of diabetic plantar ulcers: Controlled clinical trial. Diabetes Care 12:384–388, 1989.

35. Myerson M, Papa J, Eaton K, Wilson K: The total contact cast for management of neuropathic plantar ulceration of the foot. J Bone Joint Surg Am 74-A:261–269, 1992.

36. Nawoczenski DA, Birke JA, Graham SL, Koziatek E: The neuropathic foot—a management scheme: A case report. Phys Ther 69:287–291, 1989.

37. Pecoraro RE, Reiber GE, Burgess EM: Pathways to diabetic limb amputation: Basis for prevention. Diabetes Care 13:513–521, 1990.

38. Pollard JP, LeQuesne LP: Method of healing diabetic forefoot ulcers. Br Med J 286:436–437, 1983.

39. Pring DJ, Casiebanca N: Simple plantar ulcers treated by below-knee plaster and molded double-rocker plaster shoe—a comparative study. Lepr Rev 53:261, 1982.

40. Simoneau GG, et al: Postural instability in patients with diabetic sensory neuropathy. Diabetes Care 17:1411–1421, 1994.

41. Sinacore DR, et al: Diabetic neuropathic ulcers treated by total contact casting. Phys Ther 67:1543–1549, 1987.

42. Sinacore DR: TCC: An old therapy with new indications. Biomechanics 3:71–74, 1996.

43. Sinacore DR: Total-contact casting for diabetic neuropathic ulcers. Phys Ther 76:296–301, 1996.

44. Sinacore DR: Acute neuropathic (Charcot) arthropathy in patients with diabetes mellitus: Healing times by foot location. J Diabetes Complications 12:287–293, 1998.

45. Sinacore DR: Healing times of diabetic foot ulcers in the presence of fixed foot deformities using total contact casting. Foot Ankle Int 19:613–618, 1998.

46. Sinacore DR: Neuropathic plantar ulcers in patients with diabetes mellitus. PT: Magazine of Physical Therapy 6:58–66, 1998.

47. Sinacore DR, Mueller MJ: Total-contact casting for wound management. *In* Gogia PP (ed): Clinical Wound Management. Thorofare, NJ: Slack Inc, 1995, pp 147–162.

48. Wagner FW: Treatment of the diabetic foot. Compr Ther 10:29, 1984.

49. Walker SC, Helm PA, Pullium G: Total contact casting and chronic diabetic neuropathic foot ulcerations: Healing rates by wound location. Arch Phys Med Rehabil 68:217–221, 1987.

50. Wieman TJ, Griffiths GD, Polk HC: Management of diabetic midfoot ulcers. Ann Surg 215:627–632, 1992.

51. Young MJ, Cavanagh PR, Thomas G, et al: The effect of callus removal on dynamic plantar foot pressures in diabetic patients. Diabet Med 9:55–57, 1992.

Chapter 14

ALTERNATIVE WEIGHT REDISTRIBUTION METHODS IN THE TREATMENT OF NEUROPATHIC ULCERS

■ Nancy Elftman

Increasing awareness of the complications of diabetes mellitus has provided the impetus for research and development in product and material designs. In the past decade, these products have opened state-of-the-art methods of evaluation, treatment, and prevention of neuropathic complications. Many of these complications do not involve ischemia or infection and can be treated by nonsurgical methods. Mild deformities can usually be managed by partial or complete off-loading of the affected area to decrease local trauma. Moderate to severe deformities may require surgical correction prior to long-term orthotic management.[3] By far, the most common mechanism causing ulceration in diabetics is repetitive stress to the plantar surface, with the most vulnerable locations being the metatarsal heads and the great toe. The presence of corns or calluses reveals increased mechanical pressure and shear, which must be decreased to avoid primary or recurrent skin breakdown.[6] This chapter describes both custom orthoses, off-loading techniques, and readily available products that specifically involve treatment of these complica-

tions and their long-term management. Because skin that is traumatized and/or ulcerated is often inflamed, surface temperature scanning devices are valuable for tracking progression of healing, since a gradual decline in temperature at the site defines primary healing.[8]

The Semmes-Weinstein sensory monofilaments are useful for determining the presence of protective sensation, a key element in defining the foot at risk.

Total-Contact Cast

The neuropathic ulcer has historically been successfully healed with the total-contact casting method. The total-contact cast (TCC) significantly off-loads forefoot lesions, decreases edema, and reduces shear forces.[6] Plantar forces are transferred into leg forces to prevent further trauma to existing ulcers and bone structure.[7] First metatarsal head lesions are most common, with pressures from the sesamoids a contributing factor.[18] The larger medial sesamoid is most com-

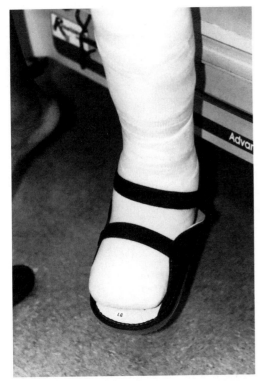

Figure 14–1 ■ The total-contact cast. Fabricated for intimate fit to the lower extremity to reduce plantar pressures. It may be made from plaster or fiberglass or a combination. Limited ambulation may be permitted by an attached walking pad or cast shoe.

monly associated with ulcerations. The total contact cast, made with plaster or fiberglass wrap, is not removable, forcing the patient to be compliant (Fig. 14–1). Alternative methods may be preferred, however, for patients fearful of confinement within the TCC.[2] The frequent (weekly) initial applications of the TCC increase cost.[5, 6] Nonetheless, the total contact cast remains the standard against which all other methods must be compared.[7, 17]

Orthotic Dynamic System Splint

For ulcerations that require daily inspections and wound care, the orthotic dynamic system (ODS) splint has been of benefit due to its bivalve construction and custom plantar insert. While the total-contact cast may need to be changed weekly in some cases, the ODS splint must be refabricated only when decreasing limb volume cannot be compensated for by additional socks. Construction of the splint is similar to the TCC, except that

there is an integral plantar insert, additional padding, and a lining of cotton stockinette. The cast is bivalved into anterior and posterior halves and closed with integral straps (Fig. 14–2). A rocker bottom cast shoe is strapped to the plantar surface to allow ambulation. Throughout the healing process, the plantar insert may be removed for adjustment and returned to the splint. Following wound healing, the ODS splint is retained by the patient for immediate application when necessary to prevent progression of future ulceration.

Posterior Splint

The posterior splint covers the posterior lower leg and plantar foot and is held in place with elastic wraps. This splint is not total contact, but acts to protect the plantar foot surface. It may be chosen for the patient whose limb is compromised by poor circulation.[2] It is also useful for patients who cannot tolerate the confinement of a total-contact cast. For ulcerations in non–weight-bearing

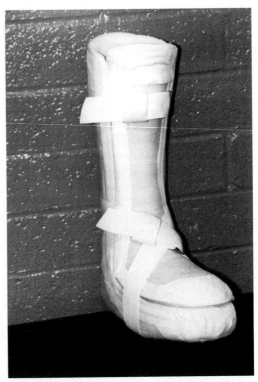

Figure 14–2 ■ The ODS splint. Similar to the TCC but has a plantar insert and is bivalved. A cast shoe will allow ambulation. The plantar insert is removable for adjustments.

areas (posterior heel, the malleoli, dorsal foot) this soft ankle foot orthosis (AFO) is constructed of foam and a rigid posterior support. It is easily donned and readily modified with heat (Fig. 14–3).

Neuropathic Walker

For long-term management of the neuropathic limb, the custom copolymer total contact AFO allows the patient to ambulate without excessive trauma to the high-risk limb. The patient who has chronic recurrent ulceration or bony deformities that cannot be accommodated in ready-made indepth or custom shoes may be well served by the device. It is the treatment of choice for stage II (subacute) and stage III (chronic) neuroarthropathy to support the hindfoot and ankle.[17] This custom bivalved AFO incorporates total contact, plantar insert, and rocker bottom features (Fig. 14–4). The contralateral shoe will require a lift to compensate for the height of the orthosis.

Variations of the neuropathic walker design include the axial resist total contact AFO and the total contact AFO, both of which function within a shoe for ambulation.[11] The axial resist design is patella-tendon bearing to reduce plantar pressures. The patient must wear the orthosis continually except for

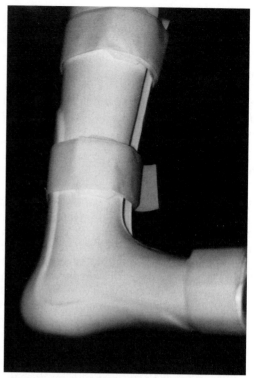

Figure 14–3 ■ Soft AFO. The soft AFO is heat adjustable and an inexpensive option for non–weight-bearing ulcerations. The posterior heel, malleoli, anterior tibial crest, etc., are protected and relieved from shear stresses.

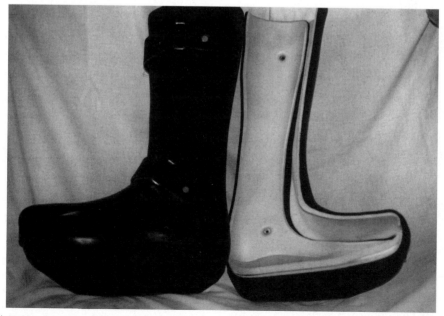

Figure 14–4 ■ Neuropathic walker. A total-contact custom AFO with full padding and plantar insert. The rocker bottom construction allows for easier ambulation.

bathing, sleeping, or wound care. The copolymer construction can be reinforced to accommodate obese patients who may experience skin breakdown in traditional casts and splints.[14]

Standard posterior AFO designs that are not lined and do not contain a plantar insert have been used when the patient's protective sensation is intact.

Prefabricated Walkers

Although prefabricated walkers are not custom-made to provide total contact, they contain features that will assist in reducing movement of the limb within the walker by means of adjustable or inflatable pads (Fig. 14–5). These walkers are preferable to the TCC when the foot has vascular compromise and/or requires device removal for frequent treatment.[1] They can be improved in function with the addition of a wide base, rocker sole, and custom off-loading insert.[5] They are very convenient, being easily donned and doffed by the patient. The low-risk patient does well in the orthosis, but healing may be assisted by providing a total contact plantar insert. The high-risk patient without protective sen-

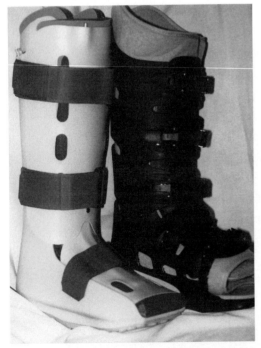

Figure 14–5 ■ Prefabricated walkers. They reduce movement of the limb by means of adjustable or inflatable pads. The rocker sole aids in ambulation.

sation may be better served by custom-made devices such as a total-contact cast, ODS splint, or neuropathic walker. The cast walker can be modified to off-load and reduce plantar pressures, but it will not significantly control edema or reduce shear forces.[6]

Weight Relief Shoes

These temporary shoes are designed to allow ambulation for activities of daily living while treating an ulcer or postoperative wound. They effectively off-load the area being treated, instead of simply redistributing pressures. They also protect the wound from further trauma, are easily removed for dressing changes, and are very cost-effective if used consistently (i.e., for *all* weight-bearing activities). They must also be individually fitted and modified as necessary to ensure an effective, safe fit. The patient should be evaluated for limitations of standing balance and may require the use of a cane or walker for ambulation. A temporary heel and sole lift on the opposite shoe can be used to equalize limb length if back pain is a complaint.

Since over 90% of diabetic foot ulcers occur on the plantar forefoot (Rancho Los Amigos Medical Center), a type of forefoot-relief shoe is most commonly used. Although healing time is greatly increased compared to the TCC if the patient uses it inconsistently or improperly, it has shown success with hallux ulcerations.[5]

The forefoot-relief shoes have a wedged-negative heel to enhance load-reduction or total off-loading of the forefoot by increasing the load on the heel (Figs. 14–6 and 14–7). This type of shoe is contraindicated if the ankle dorsiflexion range is less than the angle of inclination of the shoe. Although the wedge makes roll-over difficult, the patient must be carefully instructed to stay on the heel and avoid forefoot contact at the end of stance phase.

The heel-relief shoe reduces direct and shear forces on the posterior aspect of the heel by transferring weight-bearing forces to the midfoot and forefoot (Fig. 14–8). Both of these shoes are commercially available. Midfoot ulcers are seen over bony prominences secondary to Charcot neuroarthropathy. They can be successfully managed with a "bridge" shoe modified from a wedge shoe to provide midfoot unloading between anterior and posterior heels. To prevent sag under

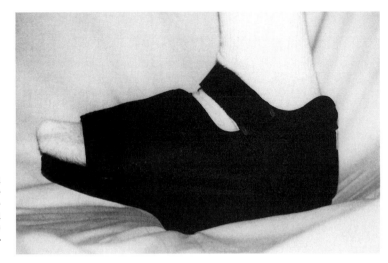

Figure 14–6 ■ Wedged shoe with forefoot load-reduction. The inclination angle reduces forefoot pressures, yet the sole is in contact with the foot. The severe rocker construction allows rolling proximal to metatarsal heads.

the ulcerated area, a "tie-bar" sole is used to join the two heels (Fig. 14–9).

Custom Sandals

The custom Plastazote sandal was developed to treat neuropathic ulcers on the plantar surface of the foot. The construction combines a rigid rocker sole that is lightweight, stable, and reusable.[1] The sandal continues to be used successfully for lesions on the plantar surface of the toes.[12] This device is low cost and can be modified after molding to decrease pressures at ulcer sites. The perim-

eter and dorsal surface of the foot must be examined carefully for shoe border, strap, and environmental trauma to the unprotected surface.[2]

Healing Shoe with Orthosis

The healing shoe, like the sandal, contains a plantar surface insert that can be adjusted to reduce pressure on the healing area. The Plastazote contacts the plantar surface as well as the dorsal surface of the foot. As a closed shoe, it protects the toes much better than the sandal, while its volume is designed

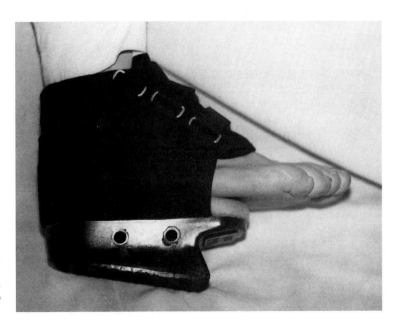

Figure 14–7 ■ Wedged forefoot relief shoe. The foot is non–weight-bearing under the forefoot and the inclination angle loads the heel to promote healing of forefoot ulcers.

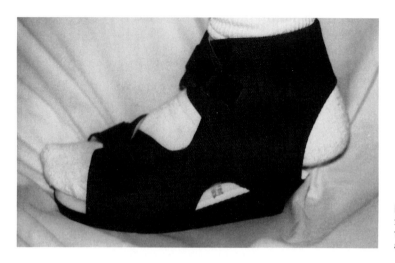

Figure 14–8 ■ Heel relief shoe. The inclination angle loads the forefoot with no contact at the heel to encourage heel ulceration healing.

to accommodate wound dressings (Fig. 14–10).

In-depth Shoe with Orthosis

The in-depth shoe is not designed to heal wounds.[5] Its therapeutic role is the prevention of future trauma.[1] After a wound has healed, the foot must be adequately protected by the shoe to prevent recurrence. The shoe must have adequate depth to provide sufficient room for the toes and dorsal foot surface while accommodating an insert of suitable thickness to properly distribute forces on the plantar surface of the foot (see Chapter 34).

Postoperative/Cast Shoe

Many facilities treating neuropathic wounds do not have access to orthotic, prosthetic, pedorthic, or casting expertise. In these situations, a commercially available rigid sole postoperative shoe or moderately flexible cast shoe may be the only options (Figs. 14–11 and 14–12). These standard shoes support, protect, and accommodate the foot during the healing process.[15] When an immediate off-loading device is required as part of the wound dressing protocol, a modified postoperative shoe may be used short term (Fig. 14–13). The temporary shoe should con-

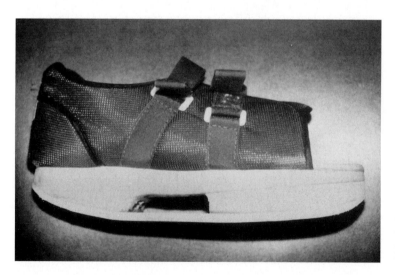

Figure 14–9 ■ Bridge shoe. This is customized from the shoe shown in Figure 14–6 by removing the portion of the heel beneath the midfoot lesion and adding an anterior "heel." A "tie-bar" sole is added to prevent sagging of the sole. (Courtesy J.H. Bowker, M.D.)

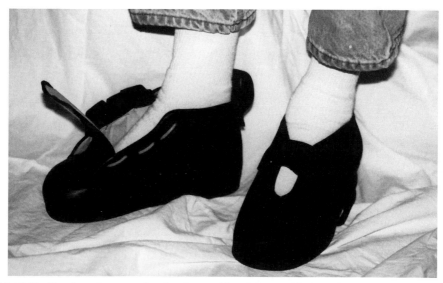

Figure 14–10 ■ Healing shoe. Accommodate bandages with soft internal lining. The plantar inserts can be adjusted to reduce pressures on ulcerations.

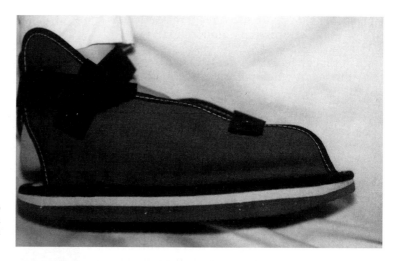

Figure 14–11 ■ Cast shoe. Velcro closure on a canvas cast shoe with high heel counter. The heel is open to reduce heel ulcer contact.

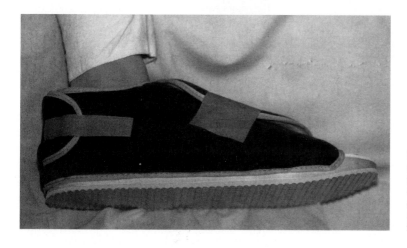

Figure 14–12 ■ Postoperative shoe. Laces allow more control of foot within the shoe. Rigid construction is more suitable to postoperative condition, but rocker sole can be added for wound healing orthosis.

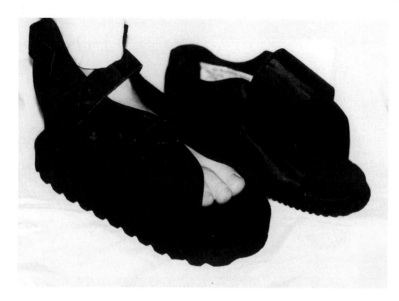

Figure 14–13 ■ Padded wound shoe. The shoe incorporates a rocker sole, soft padded upper, and site reduction of weight-bearing forces. Straps allow for girth and heel adjustment.

tain materials that will protect the plantar surface and area of ulceration from excessive pressures. The most functional of these prefabricated shoes will also have a rocker sole, allow girth of dressings, and relieve ulcerations with an insert. The cost is minimal and, although less than ideal, the patient has an immediate temporary functional orthosis.[6]

should never be worn because of rough repair edges that can irritate the skin. Tube socks do not contour to the foot, leaving folds that can abrade the skin. It is important that socks are changed regularly with care to apply them without wrinkles. The patient who has dysvascularity should not wear stockings with any constricting material.

Toe Sock

Maceration of skin between the toes is common in the neuropathic population. This moist environment encourages growth of fungus and may lead to ulceration and bacterial infection. Separation of the toes with lamb's wool or tube foam has been the standard treatment protocol for many years. A newer and very convenient treatment option is the toe sock, which is fitted to the foot and toes much as a glove fits the hand and fingers. The wicking properties of the material keep the area between the toes dry (Fig. 14–14). The seamless construction helps reduce the overlapping of lesser toes and shear from the shoe. Patients with a history of severe maceration wear the sock regularly with shoes sized to fully accommodate toe girth, thus relieving both pressure and interdigital maceration.

Socks for Diabetics

The neuropathic foot requires socks that are free of seams, ridges, and holes. Darned socks

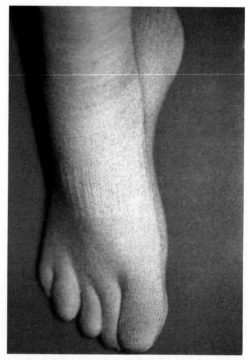

Figure 14–14 ■ Toe sock. Wicks moisture to prevent maceration between toes and allow healing at interdigital spaces.

The patient with excessive moisture will require a sock other than pure cotton, that will wick away moisture. Conversely, the patient with loss of sweat production due to autonomic neuropathy can use pure cotton socks safely. It is preferable that the patient wear light colors so that drainage or bleeding can be easily noticed. When the shoe is new, it is recommended that the patient wear two thin socks on each foot for the break-in period. The two socks will reduce the incidence of blisters by absorbing shear forces between the socks and protect the skin.

Partial-Foot Socks

The partial-foot sock has a highly elastic construction that allows a single size to conform to any length of transverse partial foot ablation from Chopart disarticulation to a long transmetatarsal amputation without wrinkles, seams, or extra distal material. It is woven of a blend that will wick away moisture.

Compression Therapy Stockings

The purpose of compression therapy is to prevent pooling of blood in leg veins with incompetent valves. The highest compression must be applied at the metatarsal head level and gradually reduces as the distance to the heart diminishes.[4]

Prior to fitting compression stockings, a vascular evaluation must be done to determine that the limb has venous and not arterial deficiency. The ankle/brachial index will determine the safe compression that can be used to reduce and maintain limb volume (Table 14–1). The lymphedema patient without arterial compromise will require a high compression treatment of 60 mm Hg.

Venous stasis ulcerations are commonly located over the medial malleolus due to the close proximity of the veins to the skin. These ulcerations are treated with wound dressings and compression wraps to reduce edema. When the wound has healed, healing can be maintained by compression stockings.

Prosthetic shrinker socks, used after major lower limb amputation, reduce edema of the limb by applying both circumferential and vertical (distal to proximal) compression.[4]

Common Materials

Orthoses designed for the neuropathic patient require stability during stance and gait, protection of high-risk locations, and prevention of skeletal breakdown.[9] Materials used in neuropathic lower limb orthoses combine open and closed cell properties to meet these design goals. The materials are combined to provide both deformity accommodation and off-loading of ulcerations in high-risk locations, thus complementing wound care protocols. When pressures are removed from an area of injury, they are redistributed to locations that are capable of sustaining higher pressures. The foot orthosis must provide total contact (moldable) as well as shear stress distribution.[13]

Closed cell polyethylene foam materials such as Plastazote are used as an interface when wound exudate is present. These closed cell materials do not absorb fluids and may be easily cleaned. Open cell materials, such as Spenco or Poron, are important as an intermediate layer to provide shock absorption and shear reduction but will absorb exudate so they cannot be used in contact with a wound surface. When no drainage is present, however, the open cell materials can be used as an interface with the foot.

The highest performance for the neuropathic limb is achieved with a tridensity insert. The combination will typically include a top layer of moldable polyethylene foam (Plastazote), an intermediate layer for shock absorption (Poron), and a base of semirigid material (EVA, cork, neoprene, Aliplast) for stability and support.

All materials will compress with time and follow-up is necessary. Adjustments may be required to better distribute weight-bearing forces. Depending on the individual activity level and weight of patients, the accommodative insert will usually require replacement within 8 to 12 months.

Table 14–1 ■ ANKLE-BRACHIAL INDEX FOR COMPRESSION CRITERIA

ABI	INDICATION	COMPRESSION
0.8–1	Venous	30–40 mm Hg
0.6–0.8	Venous and arterial	20–30 mm Hg modified
<0.6	Arterial	No compression

Summary

Orthotic treatment of the neuropathic limb requires accommodation, relief of pressure/shear forces, and shock absorption.[19] The role of the orthotic, prosthetic, and pedorthic practitioner is to redistribute weight-bearing forces by use of footwear and a variety of orthoses.[10] This includes the use of products to prevent complications such as socks and other specialty products as discussed above (see Appendix 1).

Molding techniques as well as material selection and design must be applied on an individual basis to protect the limb and preserve function for ambulation.[10] Patient education must be an integral part of the process of follow-up and prevention of limb loss by all members of the treatment team.

REFERENCES

1. Armstrong DG, Lavery LA, Harkless LB, et al: Healing the diabetic wound with pressure off-loading. Biomechanics VII:67–73, 1997.
2. Birke J, Novick A, Graham S, et al: Methods of treating plantar ulcers. Phys Ther 71: 41–47, 1991.
3. Bowker JH: Identifying the limits of nonsurgical management of diabetic foot problems. Biomechanics IV:73–74, 1997.
4. Field M: The use of garments to create compression. Biomechanics Desk Reference IV:139–140, 1997.
5. Fleischli JG, Laughlin TJ: TCC remains gold standard for off-loading plantar ulcers. Biomechanics V:43–53, 1998.
6. Giacalone VF: Diabetic foot care: Pressure-relief modalities. Podiatry Today 10:18–20, 1998.
7. Harkless LB, Quebedeaux-Farnham T: Total contact casting: Why, when, and how to. Biomechanics II:81–82, 1995.
8. Horzic M, Bunoza D, Maric K: Three-dimensional observation of wound temperature in primary healing. Ostomy/Wound Management 42:38–47, 1996.
9. Ishii S: Orthotic materials must match needs of neuropathic patient. Biomechanics V:65–84, 1998.
10. Levin ME, O'Neal LW, Bowker JH (eds): The Diabetic Foot, 5th ed. St. Louis: Mosby Year Book, 1993.
11. Marzano R: Bivalve AFO for Charcot arthropathy. Biomechanics III:69–71, 1996.
12. Nawoczenski DA, Birke JA: Management of the neuropathic limb in the elderly. Geriatr Rehabil 7:36–48, 1992.
13. Sanders JE, Greve J, Mitchell S, et al: Material properties of commonly-used interface materials and their coefficients of friction with skin and socks. J Rehabil Res Dev 35:161–176, 1998.
14. Schaepper H: Thinking big, Gentle giant's equinovarus deformities call for innovation. Biomechanics V:47–51, 1998.
15. Schoenhaus HD: Post-operative footwear. Biomechanics III:99–100, 1996.
16. Sibbald RG: Leg ulcers and the diabetic foot: A practical approach to diagnosis and treatment. Satellite Symposium Conference/ Dermatology Update: Vancouver, BC, October 24, 1996.
17. Sinacore DR: TCC, an old therapy with new indications. Biomechanics III:71–74, 1996.
18. Stephenson KA, Brodsky JW: Management strategies for diabetic ulcers of the first metatarsal head, Biomechanics IV:55–61, 1997.
19. Sussman C, Bates-Jensen BM: Wound Care, A Collaborative Practice Manual for Physical Therapists and Nurses. Gaithersburg, MD: Aspen Publishers, Inc, 1998.

RESOURCE LIST

Compression Supplies

Active International
Acor Orthopedic
Aircast, Inc.
AliMed, Inc.
Apex Foot Health
Bauerfeind USA, Inc.
Benson's Surgical Supply
Juzo-Julius Zorn, Inc.
Moore Medical Corp.

Materials for Custom Off-Loading

Active International
Acor Orthopedic
AliMed, Inc.
Apex Foot Health
Esko Orthopedic Specialties
Hapad, Inc.
Riecken's Orthotic Lab.
Roden Leather Co.
Theradynamics
UCO International
Verne Bintz Co, Inc.

Postoperative and Cast Shoes

Active International
Acor Orthopedic
AliMed
Apex Foot Health
Benson's Surgical Supply
Darco International
Esko Orthopedic Specialties
Hands on Foot
IPOS North America
Moore Medical Corp.
Pedifix Footwear Co.

Riecken's Orthotic Lab.
Russo Co.
Verne Bintz Co., Inc.

Prefabricated Splints and Orthoses

Active International
Acor Orthopedic
Aircast, Inc.
AliMed
Apex Foot Health
Bauerfeind USA, Inc.
Benson's Surgical Supply
Boston Brace International, Inc.
Darco International
Esko Orthopedic Specialties
Hapad, Inc.
IPOS North America
JMS Plastics Supply, Inc.
Moore Medical Corp
Pedifix Footcare Co.
Riecken's Orthotic Lab
Russo Co.
Verne Bintz Co. Inc

Socks

Bauerfeind USA, Inc.
Benson's Surgical Supply
Comfort Products
Esko Orthopedic Specialties
Hands on Foot
Juzo-Julius Zorn, Inc.
Pedifix Footcare Co
Silipos Inc.
Verne Bintz Co. Inc.

These companies represent a sample of resources. Check with your local representatives for other options.

Acor Orthopedic, 18530 South Miles Pk., Cleveland, OH 44128 800 237-2267 fax 216 662-4547

Active International, 1256 Liberty Ave., Hillside, NJ 07066 800 782-5678 fax 908 687-8787

Aircast, Inc., 92 River Road, Summit, NJ 07940 800 526-8785 fax 800 457-4221

AliMed, Inc., 297 High St., Dedham, MA 02026 800 225-2610 fax 800 437-2966

Apex Foot Health, 170 Wesley St., South Hackensack, NJ 07606 800 526-2739 fax 800 526-0073

Bauerfeind USA, 55 Chastain Rd #112, Kennesaw, GA 30144 800 423-3405 fax 770 429-8477

Benson's Surg. Supply, 1025 Kenmore Ave., Buffalo, NY 14217 800 876-1113 fax 716 873-5557

Boston Brace International, 20 Ledin Dr., Avon, MA 02322 800 262-2235 fax 800 634-5048

Comfort Products, Inc. 705 Linton Ave., Croydon, PA 19021 800 822-7500 fax 215 785-5737

Darco International, Inc, 1327 7th Ave., Huntington, WV 25701 800 999-8866 fax 304 522-0037

Esko Orthopedic Spec. 907 Prairie Trail, Austin, TX 78758 800 252-2739 fax 512 837-3597

Hands on Foot, 2076 Bonita Ave., La Verne, CA 91750 909 506-7674 fax 909 596-5211

Hapad, Inc., 5301 Enterprise Blvd., Bethel Park, PA 15102 800 544-2723 fax 412 835-6460

IPOS N.A. 2045 Niagra Falls Blvd #8, Niagra Falls, NY 14304 800 626-2612 fax 716 297-0153

JMS Plastics, 3535 Route 66, Bld #4, Neptune, NJ 07753-2625 800 342-2602 fax 732 918-1131

JUZO-Julius Zorn, Inc., P.O.B. 1088, Cuyahoga Falls, OH 44223 800 222-4999 fax 800 645-2519

Moore Medical, 389 John Downey Dr., New Britian, CT 06050 800 234-1464 fax 800 944-6667

Pedifix Footwear Co., 4 Columbus Ave., Mt. Kisco, NY 10549 800 424-5561 fax 914 241-1650

Riecken's Ortho. Lab, 5115 Oak Grove, Evansville, IN 47715 812 476-8006 fax 812 476-4271

Roden Leather, 1725 Crooks Rd., Box 555, Royal Oak, MI 48068 800 521-4833 fax 800 685-0955

Russo Company, 1460 E. 4th St., Los Angeles, CA 90033, 323 261-0391 fax 323 266-3985

Silipos, Inc., 2150 Liberty Drive, Niagra Falls, NY 14304 800 224-4404 fax 716 283-0600

Theradynamics, 7283 W. Appleton Ave., Milwaukee, WI 53216 800 803-7813 fax 414 438-1051

UCO Intern., 16 E. Piper Ln #130, Prospect Heights, IL 60070 800 541-4030 fax 847 541-4144

Verne Bintz Co. Inc., 333 So. Cross St., Wheaton, IL 60187 800 235-8480 fax 630 653-5077

Chapter 15

IMAGING OF THE DIABETIC FOOT

■ Andrew J. Fisher, Louis A. Gilula, and Kevin W. McEnery

A variety of imaging studies may significantly contribute to the evaluation and treatment of diseases of the diabetic foot. Imaging is a valuable adjunct to physical examination of the foot, helping to demonstrate the distribution and severity of the disease process. Common indications for imaging evaluation of the diabetic foot include gangrene or soft tissue ulceration. Such dermatologic changes may be caused by vascular insufficiency, diabetic neuropathy, infection, or a combination of these factors. Skeletal changes in diabetic feet may be manifested by several findings, including generalized demineralization, focal osteolysis, Charcot joint, or infection. Although conventional radiography is the most cost-effective and readily available modality for imaging the diabetic foot, other modalities, particularly scintigraphy and magnetic resonance imaging (MRI), are very useful in resolving specific clinical problems in selected cases.

Plain Radiography

Skeletal Changes Not Directly Associated with Diabetes Mellitus

Causes of foot pain that are not related to diabetes are occasionally discovered when patients with suspected diabetic skeletal changes are evaluated. Although usually clinically apparent, hallux valgus deformity (Fig. 15–1) may produce secondary changes in the metatarsophalangeal joint and the surrounding bursae, producing both pain and redness. Diffuse idiopathic skeletal hyperostosis (DISH) is relatively common in diabetic and obese patients.[19, 26, 32] Although the process is most commonly associated with spinal abnormalities, osseous excrescences of the foot and heel are present in most patients or may be seen in diabetic patients without DISH.[65]

Additionally, subungual exostoses (Fig. 15–2) and spurs of the calcaneus (Fig. 15–3) are particularly important causes of foot pain not directly attributable to diabetes. Subungual exostoses may produce ulceration of the nail bed or the surrounding tissue and may simulate tumor.[57] Chronic infection has been reported in 34 to 60% of patients with subungual exostoses. Even without ulceration or redness, the pain of a subungual exostosis may simulate vascular insufficiency.[39] The pain produced by calcaneal spurs is well known.

Another cause of foot pain seen in both diabetic and nondiabetic patients is a stress fracture (Fig. 15–4). These are usually lo-

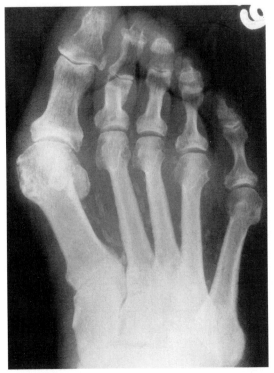

Figure 15–1 ■ Hallux valgus deformity and vascular calcification in a diabetic foot with medial bowing at first metatarsophalangeal joint. The joint has mild degenerative changes. Parallel linear densities between the metatarsal shafts are typical arterial calcifications.

cated in the second through fourth metatarsal or the calcaneus. The presence of periosteal reaction can confound the diagnosis.

Generalized Demineralization and Focal Osteolysis

While interpreting the plain film examination, remember that avascular bone cannot be resorbed. When osseous destruction underlies impending or actual gangrene, Phemister noted that sufficient osseous vascular supply must be present to produce the observed resorption.[59] Therefore, the destructive bone changes associated with diabetes are found in patients with an adequate vascular supply to the foot.

Bone resorption has a variety of forms. All of the foot bones may be diffusely demineralized, and this change can be entirely independent of disuse (Fig. 15–5). Alternatively, osteolysis may begin as a focal forefoot defect. The defect is typically sharply marginated and local, measuring 1 to 5 mm in diameter

and most often located in the phalanges and the metatarsal heads (Fig. 15–6A). It may remain stable for years or progress to massive osteolysis relatively rapidly (Fig. 15–6B–D). The osteolysis generally begins in the metaphysis as an ill-defined loss of cortex and spreads through the remaining metaphysis and subsequently into the epiphysis, sparing the diaphysis. The end of the diaphysis may at first be ragged, but as the lesion progresses, it becomes pointed, producing a penciling or candlestick-like configuration (Fig. 15–6B–D). Later, the surface becomes smooth and the remaining bone, sclerotic (Fig. 15–6C and D).

The etiology of erosive or resorptive changes about the phalangeal tufts and the metatarsal heads remains uncertain. Some authors[83] believe these changes are present only in diabetic patients with peripheral neuropathy, foot ulcerations, and soft tissue and bone infections. There is no question, however, that these changes may be noninfectious in etiology. Localized forefoot osteolysis

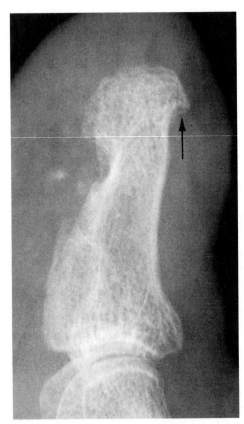

Figure 15–2 ■ Subungual exostosis in great toe (arrow) was source of pain in this diabetic patient. (Courtesy of O.L. Lippard, M.D., St. Louis.)

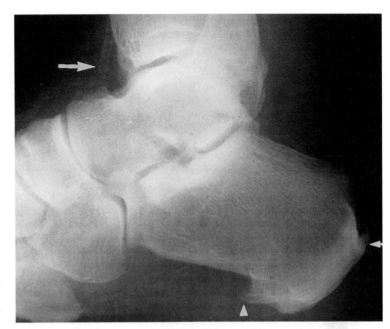

Figure 15–3 ■ Spurs extend from the calcaneus at the insertion of the Achilles tendon (*small arrow*) and plantar fascia (*arrowhead*). Vascular calcifications are also noted in this diabetic patient (*large arrow*).

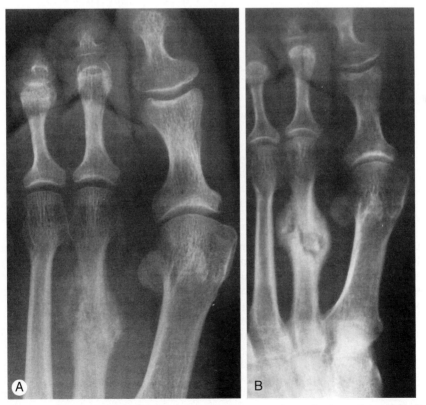

Figure 15–4 ■ Stress fracture. *A,* The diaphysis of the second metatarsal contains irregular periosteal proliferation. *B,* Three weeks later, there has been mild osseous resorption, making the fracture line evident. The callus has assumed a mature, organized appearance.

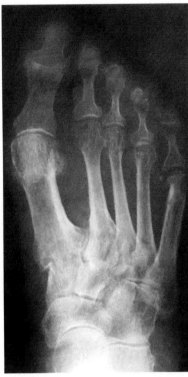

Figure 15–5 ■ Diffuse demineralization in diabetic foot.

is poorly understood yet likely related to ischemia, infection, or neurologic deficiency, either alone or in combination. In some patients, the condition will be found without proof of any of these conditions.[64]

The osteolysis may be self-limiting, destroying a single bone and producing a shortened digit with a pencil-like base of a proximal phalanx and a slightly irregular metatarsal head (Fig. 15–6C–D). Usually the articular surface is the last to be resorbed.

Similarly, the tips of the phalanges may be resorbed (Fig. 15–6E). When associated with soft tissue infection in the tip of a digit, the acroosteolysis may be difficult to differentiate from osteomyelitis. Again, radiographic demonstration of bone destruction should not be the sole basis of a decision concerning amputation of a digit or an extremity.

Meltzer et al.[48] reviewed the foot radiographs of 32 diabetic patients with soft tissue necrosis. Without any further history, they placed 17 patients with no radiographic evidence of osseous resorption into an ischemic limb category. Of these 17, only three had palpable dorsalis pedis and posterior artery pulses. Intermittent claudication was present in 70%, and two had clinical diabetic neuropathy. All of these patients with soft tissue necrosis but no bone resorption required major amputation within 1 week to 3 months because the soft tissue lesions persisted or progressed.

The other 15 patients had bone resorption and were classified as nonischemic. The ankle pulses were palpable in 13 patients, and claudication was found in only two patients. Eleven patients had gangrene of one or more toes, and four patients had trophic ulcers, abscesses, and cellulitis. None of these patients required a major amputation despite radiographic evidence of bone resorption. Conservative management such as debridement, oscillating bed, antibiotic therapy, and diabetic control produced healing in seven patients. Minor surgery, usually amputation of the phalanx, affected adequate healing in the remainder, as indicated in clinical follow-up.

Diabetic Neuropathy

The radiographic appearance of the diabetic neuropathic joint cannot be differentiated from the neuropathic joint (Charcot joint) of syringomyelia, syphilis, or congenital insensitivity to pain. Conversely, there are clinical and radiographic findings that indicate the diabetic joint destruction is neuropathic in origin (Fig. 15–7). The classic radiographic appearance of a neuropathic joint is one of extensive osseous destruction with little or no demineralization. In fact, the bones may be sclerotic. Localized, mature periosteal proliferation along the proximal second through fourth metatarsals is very common in diabetic patients.[10] The precise cause is uncertain but believed to be secondary to neuropathic changes.[23, 37] There may be massive destruction with the joint greatly swollen and small osseous fragments scattered throughout the soft tissue (Fig. 15–7C and D).

Histologic examination shows these osseous fragments embedded within the synovium of the distended joint. The ligaments and capsule contain areas of fibroblastic and small round cell infiltration and edema. The articular cartilage shows varying degrees of degeneration replaced by fibrous tissue. The subchondral bone is necrotic, fragmented,

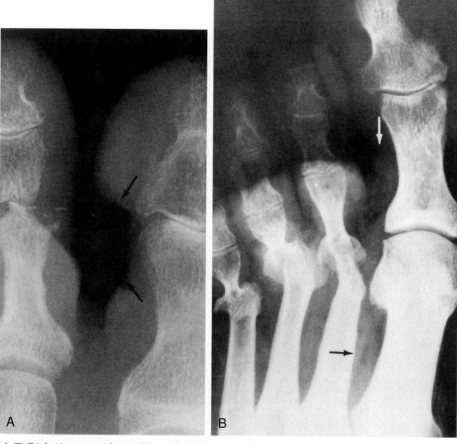

Figure 15–6 ■ Diabetic osteopathy. *A,* The proximal interphalangeal joint of the second toe is involved with diabetic osteopathy. The base of the middle phalanx shows early penciling, and both sides of the head of proximal phalanx are eroded. The skin over second toe is intact but the medial aspect of first toe is ulcerated (*arrows*). *B,* The second and fourth metatarsal heads are eroded, and the second and fourth toes are dislocated ventrally at the metatarsophalangeal joints. The shaft of the second metatarsal has early penciling. Lucency in the webspaces is subcutaneous air secondary to infection (*arrows*).

Illustration continued on following page

and avascular. Separate fragments of necrotic bone may be present.[60]

Severe joint pain is not characteristic in the neuropathic joint. In fact, the patient with such a joint often has been walking on the extremity. Therefore, the bone is well-mineralized despite severe destruction because no bone atrophy from disuse has occurred. Neuropathic arthropathy and destruction by pigmented villonodular synovitis are the primary conditions in which severe destruction fails to produce demineralization of associated structures.

The subtalar joint may be similarly affected. The findings may be more subtle yet identical to those found in other joints. The opposing joint surfaces become fragmented with the fragments potentially extruded to the calcaneal or talar margin (Fig. 15–8).

The neuropathic foot is predisposed to fractures and dislocations. Small periarticular fractures are a common early manifestation of diabetic neuroarthropathy. When the neuroarthropathic changes become severe with resultant alteration of normal biomechanical function, fractures, subluxations, or dislocations may occur.[54] This may be in the absence of any definite abnormality in the underlying osseous structure.[15, 38] Fractures of the calcaneus, for example, have been reported in diabetics who have not sustained any injury.[12] In addition, large avulsion fractures

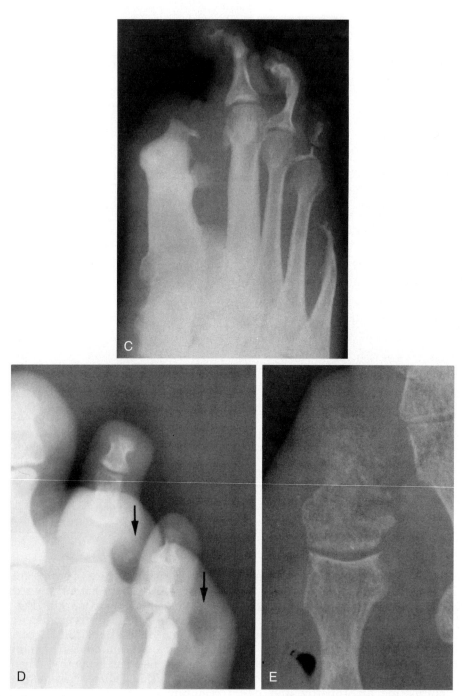

Figure 15–6 *Continued* ■ *C,* Penciling of the fourth toe proximal phalanx and the fifth metatarsal is present. The first and fifth toes were amputated because of infection. *D,* Both penciling and sclerosis involves the third metatarsal. Large portions of the second and fourth proximal phalanges have been resorbed. Soft tissue lucencies adjacent to the metatarsal heads are trophic ulcers on the plantar aspect of the foot (*arrows*). *E,* Parts of the little toe distal and middle phalanges have been resorbed. (Courtesy of Dr. O.L. Lippard, M.D., St. Louis.)

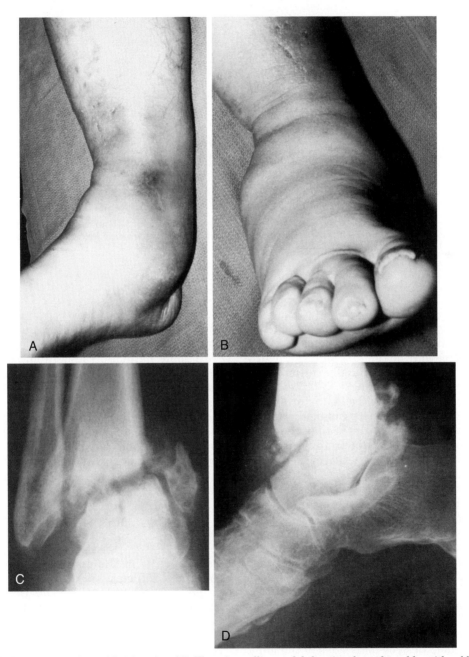

Figure 15–7 ■ Neuropathic ankle joint. *A* and *B,* There is swelling and deformity about the ankle, with subluxation of foot. *C* and *D,* Multiple fragments of the distal tibia are present with some fragments embedded in the synovium. The bone has increased density, contrary to osseous lucency generally seen in severe injuries in nondiabetic patients.

Illustration continued on following page

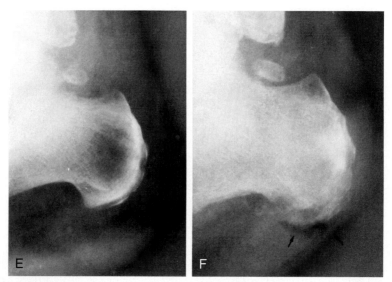

Figure 15–7 *Continued* ■ *E,* The soft tissue about the calcaneus was normal. *F,* Four weeks later, a trophic ulcer had developed on the heel (*arrows*). Disruption and loss of soft tissue thickness are evident. (Courtesy of Edward Lansche, M.D., St. Louis.)

of the posterosuperior tuberosity of the calcaneus are characteristic of diabetes.[33]

Fractures may be the first sign of a neuropathic joint and may actually initiate neuroarthropathic joint changes.[11, 31] These neuropathic changes may be a factor in the etiology of avascular necrosis of the fourth metatarsal head, known as Freiberg's infraction.[56] Insensitivity to pain probably is a contributing factor[3] and repetitive exercise is likely the most common cause of this fracture. Fractures that develop in diabetic patients without a history of significant trauma have a poor prognosis.

It is common for a patient with neuropathic joint to seek medical attention because of dissatisfaction with the deformed extremity rather than pain. Radiographs of some of these patients have been misinterpreted as showing a malignant tumor because of the extensive destruction; however, malignant primary bone tumors, even when large, seldom destroy both sides of the joint. Furthermore, an extensive malignant lesion should be accompanied by considerable pain. Even though pain is present in approximately 50% of patients with a Charcot joint, it is seldom of any great severity. Disuse of the extremity with a malignant tumor produces diffuse demineralization directly adjacent to the lesion in contrast to the bones of

the neuropathic joint, which frequently show osteosclerosis.

In some patients, radiographic examination will be performed after diabetic neuropathic arthropathy has healed. Features that suggest healed diabetic arthropathy in the foot include well-corticated deformity of the metatarsal heads, shortening of the first proximal phalanx (usually as a result of prior articular destruction or fracture deformity), and ankylosis of joints (especially the interphalangeal joints).[63]

Infection

Osteomyelitis in the distal foot may be exceedingly difficult to differentiate radiographically from diabetic osteopathy. The destruction of diabetic osteopathy may appear radiographically identical to osteomyelitis in a bone underlying ulcerated skin. If the skin is intact, the destruction is more likely to be diabetic osteopathy than osteomyelitis. Asymptomatic patients with foot ulcer have underlying osteomyelitis in 68% of cases.[55]

An example of diabetic osteopathy appearing radiographically identical to osteomyelitis is shown in Figure 15–6A. The 60-year-old patient had been diabetic for 10 years. The skin of the second through fourth toes

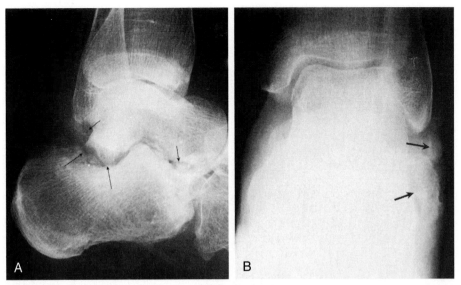

Figure 15–8 ■ Neuropathic subtalar joint. *A,* Lateral view. The posterior articular facet of the calcaneus is eroded (*long arrows*). Bone fragments have extruded anteriorly and posteriorly (*short arrows*). *B,* Anteroposterior view. Bone fragments have been extruded laterally (*arrows*).

was intact but reddened. The radiograph showed destructive changes at the proximal interphalangeal joint of the second toe. The base of the middle phalanx of this toe was slightly pointed. The lack of skin ulcerations makes it unlikely that the changes were caused by osteomyelitis, although hematogenous osteomyelitis cannot be entirely excluded. This lesion healed with bed rest and skin protection. He had no antibiotic therapy.

On the other hand, the 64-year-old woman whose toe is shown in Figure 15–9 had developed a skin ulceration of the medial aspect of her left great toe. A small erosion had developed in the metaphyseal cortex of the proximal phalanx. Three weeks later this ulcer had deepened with severe osseous destruction. These findings suggested osteomyelitis, which was confirmed following amputation of the toe. Similar changes are seen in the heads of the third and fourth metatarsals in the patient in Figure 15–11. The erosive changes over the metatarsal heads, soft tissue ulceration, and swelling had developed in approximately 6 weeks.

Pathologic fractures through areas of osteomyelitis, often in the distal portions of the first or second proximal phalanges, may also occur in patients with diabetes. Frequently

there is no history of significant trauma in these individuals.[49]

Soft tissue infection can be seen radiographically as edema, ulceration, or subcutaneous emphysema. Edema separates the subcutaneous fat into lucent globules, producing a reticulated pattern and widening the subcutaneous tissues (Figs. 15–10 and 15–11). Ulcerations are demonstrated radiographically as defects or irregularities in the skin surface and are usually visible on routine foot films (see Figs. 15–6*A,* 15–9*A,* and 15–11). Specific soft tissue technique is unnecessary, as bright lighting routine films will make the soft tissues radiographically apparent. When the skin is ulcerated, infection caused by gas-forming organisms may extend from the ulcer and produce subcutaneous emphysema (see Figs. 15–6*B* and 15–12).

The 60-year-old man whose foot is shown in Figure 15–12 had a 15-year history of diabetes mellitus. Several weeks before seeing his physician, he developed a painful sore on his foot. On examination, the lateral aspect of the red, swollen foot contained an ulcer that resulted in osteomyelitis of the fourth and fifth metatarsal heads.

In the diabetic patient, coliform organisms are the most common cause of subcutaneous emphysema. In some patients the gas collec-

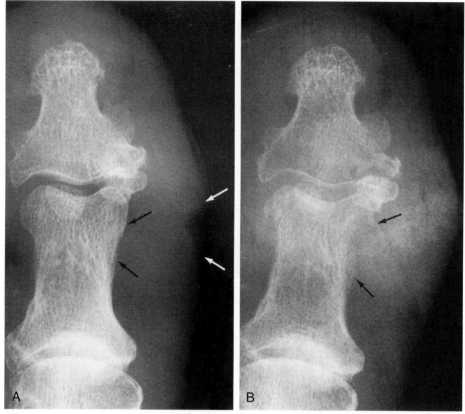

Figure 15–9 ■ Osteomyelitis. *A,* A small soft tissue ulceration (*white arrows*) is present over the medial aspect of proximal phalanx, which contains a small erosion (*black arrows*). *B,* Three weeks later, the proximal phalangeal erosion has enlarged (*arrows*). The medial aspect of the distal phalangeal base has also been destroyed. The toe is swollen.

tion may not be caused by infection but rather air sucked in through the skin defect. Localized osseous destruction directly adjacent to a soft tissue ulceration may be caused by osteomyelitis or diabetic osteopathy. Radiographically this differentiation may be difficult, and a trial of conservative therapy should be made. Again, the degree of vascularization of the remaining part of the foot should be a consideration in the proper treatment of osteomyelitis.

Advanced Imaging

In the presence of active infection, the bone changes of osteomyelitis may not be apparent on radiographs for 10 to 14 days. Magnification radiography, scintigraphy, computed tomography (CT), and MRI are employed to increase the accuracy of imaging for the presence of infection.[81] The distinction between simple cellulitis and osteomyelitis is important for patient prognosis as well as clinical management. With the use of MRI, diagnostic imaging can not only distinguish between cellulitis and osteomyelitis but can detect abscess formation, which necessitates surgical drainage.

In addition to selection of the appropriate imaging modality, diabetic patients pose other imaging dilemmas. The safety of intravascular contrast in patients taking metformin (Glucophage) has been questioned. Patients who develop contrast-induced renal failure while on the drug may develop metformin-associated lactic acidosis, which carries a high morbidity. However, these patients generally have contributing comorbid factors. In fact, only 7 of 110 cases of metformin-associated lactic acidosis reported worldwide followed intravasacular

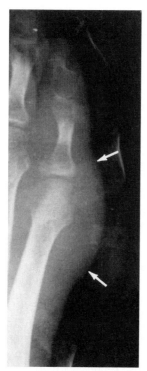

Figure 15-10 ■ Edema lateral to fifth metatarsal head. Soft tissue thickening is prominent (*arrows*).

ment of microfocal spot x-ray tubes. A small (100- to 150-μm) focal spot produces a magnified image of unusual clarity and definition, particularly in delineating the fine detail of bone structures in which early osteomyelitis or, less commonly, neuropathic change is suspected.[40] They may prove useful in detecting focal areas of cortical erosion in an area of suspected osteomyelitis; however, the presence of focal cortical erosion is not specific, because early neuropathic change can have a similar appearance. Magnification radiographs can monitor response to therapy with healing periosteal reaction, reflecting a response to therapy (Fig. 15-13). Magnification radiographs can also demonstrate otherwise subtle trabecular disruptions associated with insufficiency fracture.

The imaging characteristics of magnification radiography also enhance soft tissue detail. An image enlarged up to four times can

iodinated contrast administration.[71] Consequently, the American College of Radiology's Committee on Drugs and Contrast Media recommend holding metformin 48 hours prior to and following a contrast study; however, the committee also recommends that a patient with normal renal function who is taking metformin can have an urgent contrast study if metformin is held for the 2 days following the study.[9] Reevaluation of renal function should be performed before reinstating metformin therapy.

While contrast-induced renal failure is uncommon, it can pose significant problems in the diabetic patient. Therefore, administration of iodinated contrast is generally withheld in patients with a serum creatinine greater than 1.5 to 2.0 mg/dL. Although preliminary studies have shown that adenosine-receptor blockade with theophylline may attenuate contrast-induced nephrotoxicity, it is not yet clinically practiced and further studies are warranted.[34]

Magnification Radiography

Direct radiographic magnification techniques have been improved by the develop-

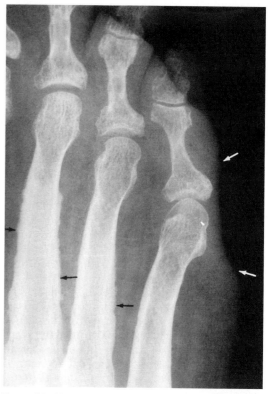

Figure 15-11 ■ Soft tissue ulceration near fifth metatarsal head (*white arrows*). Dense, nonaggressive periosteal new bone formation is identified about the third and fourth metatarsal diaphyses. This is caused by chronic vascular insufficiency (*black arrows*). Subtle erosions are present in the third and fourth metatarsal heads (*arrowheads*).

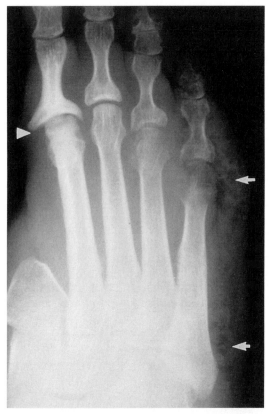

Figure 15–12 ▪ This 60-year-old diabetic man has extensive subcutaneous gas (*arrows*) and soft tissue infection along the lateral aspect of the foot. There is rarefaction of the fifth metatarsal head and, to a lesser extent, the fourth metatarsal head. Osteomyelitis was found at surgery. The patient has also undergone prior great toe transmetatarsal amputation for osteomyelitis. A pencil-in-cup deformity of the metatarsophalangeal joint of the second digit is present (*arrowhead*).

be readily obtained on commercially available equipment.[20, 21] Direct radiographic magnification results in a fourfold increase in skin dose when compared with conventional radiographic techniques and therefore should be used in only selected cases.[20] The role of magnification radiography may be the evaluation of equivocal plain film findings, where focal cortical erosions or inflammatory periosteal changes may be demonstrated in the setting of a strong clinical suspicion for focal osteomyelitis underlying soft tissue ulceration.

Radionuclide Imaging

Bone scintigraphy with technetium-99m (^{99m}Tc) phosphonates, indium-111 (^{111}In)–

labeled leukocytes, and gallium-67 (^{67}Ga) citrate has been reported as useful in the detection of acute osteomyelitis in the diabetic foot.[17, 24, 35] In patients with equivocal radiographs, scintigraphy may identify subradiographic osteomyelitis (Fig. 15–14).[58] In the diabetic patient, neuropathic osseous change, manifest as increased radiopharmaceutical uptake on both technetium and gallium scans, decreases the specificity of these examinations for the detection of osteomyelitis.

Technetium-99m is the most widely employed agent in scintigraphic imaging. It is ideally suited for clinical imaging, with a short half-life (6 hours) and an optimal photopeak (140 keV) for gamma cameras. Readily available portable molybdenum radioisotope generators provide a reliable source of ^{99m}Tc. It is intravenously administered, bound to either methylene diphosphonate or hydroxymethylene diphosphonate.

In a patient with suspected osteomyelitis, a ^{99m}Tc bone scan is performed in three phases: flow, blood pool, and delayed. Dynamic flow imaging begins at the moment of intravenous radiopharmaceutical injection. A series of 3-second image acquisitions is obtained at the site of suspected osteomyelitis. Static blood pool images are obtained approximately 5 minutes following injection. Static delayed images are acquired approximately 2 to 3 hours following injection.

Technetium diphosphonate localizes in areas of increased osseous metabolism as well as regions of increased vascularity. Focally increased osseous metabolism occurs in both diabetic neuropathy and osteomyelitis. Thus, scintigraphic images in a diabetic patient with cellulitis and neuropathic change will appear similar to those of a diabetic patient with cellulitis, neuropathic change, and superimposed osteomyelitis.

Processes that can demonstrate increased activity on both flow and blood pool images include cellulitis, septic synovitis, and abscess.[70, 79] In both soft tissue inflammation and osteomyelitis hyperemia is present and results in increased radiopharmaceutical accumulation on flow and blood pool images. In soft tissue processes, the delayed images typically demonstrate decreased soft tissue activity without focal abnormal bone uptake. In osteomyelitis, there is focally increased osseous activity on delayed images. A four-phase scan involving additional imaging 24 hours following radiopharmaceutical

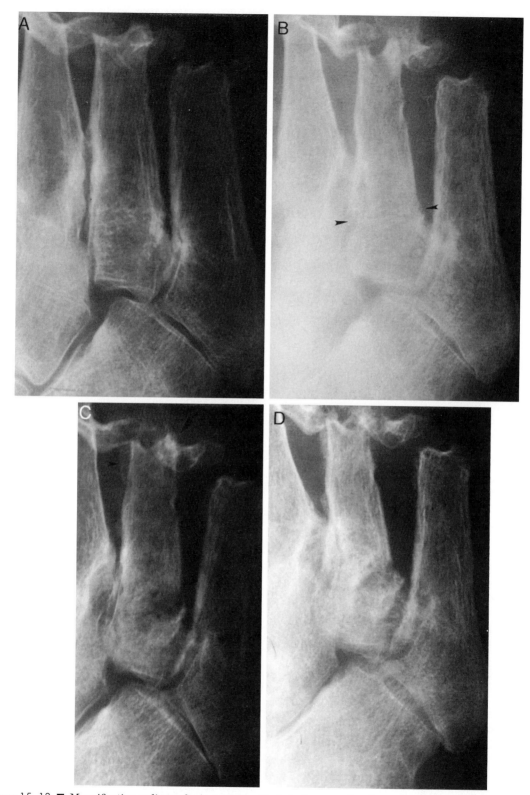

Figure 15–13 ■ Magnification radiographs in patient with foot ulcer over fourth metatarsal head. *A,* The original examination shows metatarsal amputation defects. *B,* At 4 weeks, a linear density is seen in the base of the fourth metatarsal, suggesting a stress fracture. *C,* At 8 weeks, the fourth metatarsal is osteopenic with resorption along the suspected stress fracture. Periosteal reaction distally with focal stump erosion is present. There is new periosteal reaction at the distal end of the fifth metatarsal. These findings are suspicious for superimposed osteomyelitis at the distal end of the metatarsal and possibly the fracture site. *D,* Four months later after extended course of antibiotics, the periosteal changes have matured with increased ossification, indicating healing response.

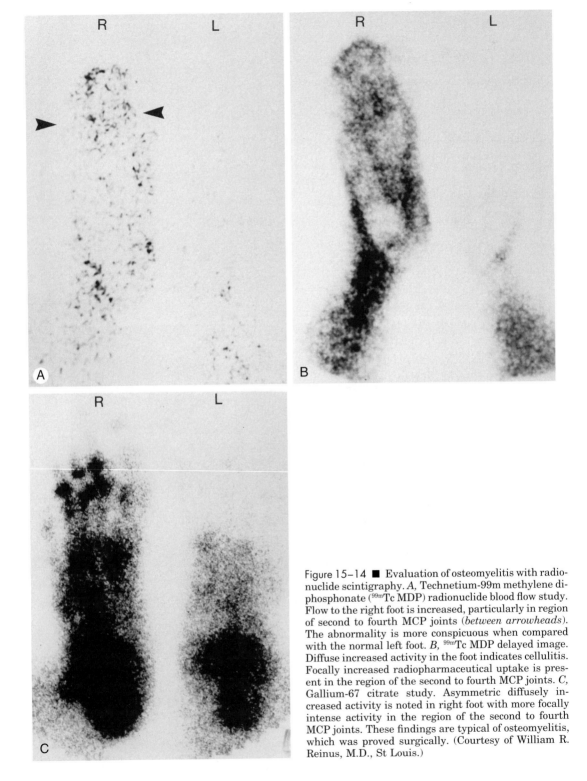

Figure 15–14 ■ Evaluation of osteomyelitis with radio-nuclide scintigraphy. *A,* Technetium-99m methylene diphosphonate (⁹⁹ᵐTc MDP) radionuclide blood flow study. Flow to the right foot is increased, particularly in region of second to fourth MCP joints (*between arrowheads*). The abnormality is more conspicuous when compared with the normal left foot. *B,* ⁹⁹ᵐTc MDP delayed image. Diffuse increased activity in the foot indicates cellulitis. Focally increased radiopharmaceutical uptake is present in the region of the second to fourth MCP joints. *C,* Gallium-67 citrate study. Asymmetric diffusely increased activity is noted in right foot with more focally intense activity in the region of the second to fourth MCP joints. These findings are typical of osteomyelitis, which was proved surgically. (Courtesy of William R. Reinus, M.D., St Louis.)

injection has been proposed.[1] It has been reported to raise the specificity of the examination in those patients with vascular insufficiency, including diabetics. In osteomyelitis, there is further sequestration of activity on the delayed images. The use of four-phase bone scintigraphy is not widespread.[66]

In a review by Schauwecker,[66] the sensitivity of bone scintigraphy for osteomyelitis is 94% and the specificity is 95%. However, in patients with complicating conditions including diabetes, the specificity decreases to 33%; the sensitivity remains at 95%. The limitation of scintigraphy is in patients with neuropathic change as the increased uptake on delayed images is scintigraphically similar to the appearance of osteomyelitis. The low specificity of ^{99m}Tc for differentiation of neuropathic bone change from superimposed osteomyelitis limits the clinical usefulness of bone scintigraphy in the diabetic patient.

Gallium-67 citrate has been employed in the imaging of acute osteomyelitis. The predominant mechanism of ^{67}Ga localization is by increased vascular permeability as well as transferrin and lactoferrin binding. Granulocytic and bacterial uptake are less significant contributors. ^{67}Ga also localizes nonspecifically in areas of increased bone remodeling. Therefore, it demonstrates the same lack of specificity as ^{99m}Tc, accumulating nonspecifically in areas of diabetic osteoarthropathy. Some authors have reported increased specificity of ^{67}Ga imaging by computer subtraction of concurrent ^{99m}Tc bone imaging. Increased ^{67}Ga activity out of proportion to ^{99m}Tc activity supports the presence of infection.[22, 25, 27, 77] Some authors[1] have proposed a role for ^{67}Ga in the imaging of chronic osteomyelitis.

Indium-111 white blood cell (WBC) imaging relies on the localization of WBCs within areas of leukocyte sequestration. ^{111}In WBCs also localize to areas of active bone marrow, which is not normally present in adult feet. Therefore, any sequestration of ^{111}In WBCs within the mature foot is indicative of infection.[2, 46, 50, 62]

Although ^{111}In WBCs is currently the most specific radiopharmaceutical agent for acute inflammation, a major disadvantage is the labor-intensive protocol to label the leukocytes. For this reason, some centers rely on commercial laboratories to perform the labeling. The entire process is beyond our scope. In general, the labeling procedure involves drawing 50 mL of the patient's blood, followed by repeated centrifuging to isolate the WBC portion, which is labeled with ^{111}In and then reinjected into the patient. Routine ^{111}In imaging is performed at 4 and 24 hours after tracer injection. The labeling process and the costly cyclotron-produced ^{111}In contribute to make ^{111}In WBCs one of the more expensive scintigraphic imaging procedures.

^{111}In oxine is an agent that relies on sequestration of WBCs and does not respond to altered bone metabolism. In several studies, WBCs labeled with ^{111}In oxine have been demonstrated to be the radiopharmaceutical of choice for imaging suspected osteomyelitis in the diabetic patient.[35, 41, 46, 55, 67, 69] In these studies, sensitivity of ^{111}In WBC scanning for the detection of osteomyelitis was reported at 75 to 100%. The specificity ranged from 73 to 89% and can be increased to an 86% sensitivity and 94% sensitivity if combined with ^{99m}Tc bone scintigraphy.[36] The false-positive results of ^{111}In scans have been noted in patients with rapidly progressive osteoarthropathy.[69]

^{111}In scans generally have poor spatial resolution. Although sensitive for infection, ^{111}In scanning may not allow the separation of soft tissue uptake from uptake in adjacent bone.[46, 47] This makes it difficult to distinguish cellulitis from osteomyelitis, potentially resulting in a false-positive interpretation. To increase the anatomic sensitivity of the ^{111}In images, concurrent ^{99m}Tc and ^{111}In imaging has been performed. Computer image manipulation can provide better discrimination between soft tissue and bone uptake.[30, 67, 74] Yet in one series, ^{111}In scanning alone was performed with similar specificity for distinguishing cellulitis from osteomyelitis as studies that employed both modalities.[35]

More recent studies have centered about other techniques. These include ^{99m}Tc HMPAO-labeled leukocytes, antigranulocyte antibodies, and ^{99m}Tc macroaggregated albumin.[7, 53, 68, 75] These remain of limited availability and utility at most centers.

Computed Tomography

The role of CT is to assess subtle plain film abnormalities such as periosteal or cortical erosion, which may indicate underlying osteomyelitis.[84] It can also provide precise imaging of cortical articular surfaces.[72, 73] CT should be directed to the area of specific clinical concern such as a scintigraphic abnormality or a foot ulcer (Fig. 15–15). CT technique consists of thin-section, high-resolution images perpendicular to the bone cortex. This will provide the greatest sensitivity for subtle erosions. CT can show the presence of an abnormal medullary space and areas of soft tissue abnormality; however, MRI is more sensitive for these abnormalities.

The role of CT to provide detailed views of subtle erosions has been supplanted to a degree by MRI, especially because of the value of MRI to examine medullary spaces and soft tissues. CT may be useful in demonstrating the relationship of osseous fragments, particularly in the setting of neuroarthropathy. In those patients who have a cardiac pacemaker or other contraindication to MRI, CT continues to serve as a primary cross-sectional imaging modality.

Magnetic Resonance Imaging

MRI has become incorporated into routine management of many clinical problems, including the diabetic foot. It offers direct multiplanar imaging and excellent soft tissue contrast to provide detailed anatomic images superior to other imaging modalities.[6, 82] The presence and extent of both bone marrow and soft tissue inflammatory processes can accurately be evaluated.[18, 51, 76]

For image contrast and detail, MRI relies on free protons in the tissues which, in general, are proportional to the tissue water content. Water demonstrates decreased signal on T1-weighted images and increased signal on T2-weighted images. Magnetic resonance images of the foot are usually acquired in at least two planes, often the coronal and sagittal planes. Most MRI scanners employ the head surface coil for foot imaging. Spin echo images of T1, proton density, and T2 weighting are standard (Fig. 15–16). With the clinical question of osteomyelitis, spin echo images are usually supplemented with short-tau inversion recovery (STIR) images, which null fat signal so that normal bone marrow is absent of signal.[85] These images are consequently very sensitive to marrow edema (Fig. 15–17).

On MRI, the diagnosis of osteomyelitis is made by detection of focal bone marrow edema, an indication of osteomyelitis. Usual criteria for osteomyelitis are focally decreased signal on T1-weighted images and focally increased marrow signal on T2 or STIR images.[28, 85] Some have suggested STIR images may have a decreased specificity compared with T2-weighted images due to extreme sensitivity for marrow edema that may be caused by noninfectious entities.[16, 52, 85] Heavily T2-weighted images, although very sensitive for the presence of fluid, sometimes do not allow definite anatomic distinction between soft tissue and marrow processes.

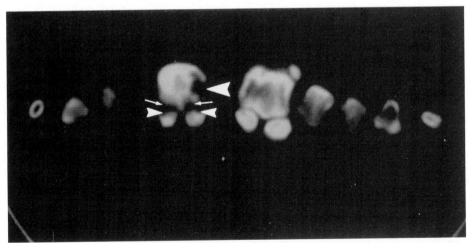

Figure 15–15 ■ Evaluation of osteomyelitis with CT. A CT scan at the level of the first metatarsal head demonstrates an unsuspected erosion of the plantar (*arrows*) and medial cortical surfaces (*large arrowhead*) of the first metatarsal head along with apposing articular surfaces of two adjacent sesamoid bones (*small arrowheads*). Contralateral first metatarsal head and sesamoid bones are normal. In this case, CT demonstrates the true extent of osseous disease with these findings poorly delineated on conventional radiography.

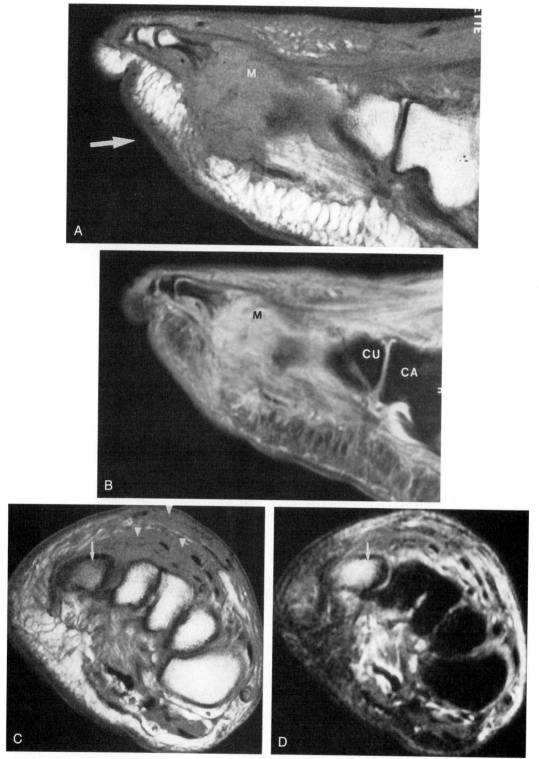

Figure 15–16 ■ MRI in a patient with a nonhealing foot ulcer adjacent to the left fifth metatarsal. *A,* T1-weighted sagittal image (TR 760, TE 20) shows destruction of the fifth metatarsal and proximal phalanx by a phlegmonous mass (*M*). Low signal (*arrow*) in the subcutaneous fat represents cellulitis and ulcer site. *B,* Proton density-weighted image with fat saturation (TR 3500, TE 16) shows increased signal in the regions of edema and inflammation (*M*). Normal marrow signal is present in the calcaneus (*CA*) and cuboid (*CU*). *C,* T1-weighted axial image (TR 760, TE 20) shows decreased marrow signal in the fifth metatarsal (*arrow*) compared with the adjacent metatarsals. There is marked dorsal soft tissue edema (*arrowheads*). *D,* T2-weighted axial image with fat saturation (TR 3500, TE 98) shows increased marrow signal in the fifth metatarsal (*arrow*).

Illustration continued on following page

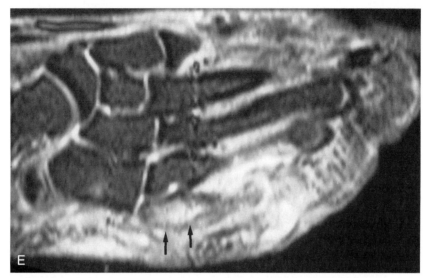

Figure 15–16 *Continued* ■ *E,* STIR (inversion recovery) images (TR 3600, TE 20) demonstrate increased signal within the fifth metatarsal base (*arrows*). Findings on all pulse sequences are compatible with osteomyelitis of the fifth metatarsal and proximal phalanx.

The sensitivity of MRI for the presence of osteomyelitis has been reported at 99 to 100%, with a specificity exceeding 80%.[4, 29, 78, 80, 82, 85] The specificity decreases in the presence of septic arthritis, occult bone fracture, and recent surgery including bone biopsy.[16] Rapidly progressive, noninfected osteoarthropathy can demonstrate bone marrow edema on MR. Therefore, as with ^{111}In WBC imaging, acutely evolving noninfected neuropathic osteoarthropathy may be indistinguishable from osteomyelitis on MRI.[4, 45, 69] Soft tissue signal changes and subtle cortical and periosteal alterations may be clues to osteomyelitis. In these patients, biopsy may be considered for diagnosis.

Focal edema localized to the soft tissues does not necessarily indicate cellulitis. Diffuse soft tissue edema, fluid in tendon sheaths, and joint effusions have been noted with regularity in asymptomatic diabetic patients.[4, 52] Increased soft tissue fluid has been demonstrated secondary to neuropathic change. MRI can be useful for the noninvasive detection of focal abscess formation demonstrated as pockets of fluid within the soft tissues.[5, 13, 29, 42, 61] MR has been reported to be over 92% accurate in the depiction of these soft-tissue abscesses.[5] These abscesses could be treated with local incision and drainage, with MRI providing anatomic information to focus the surgical incision.[61] Ultrasound can also be useful in abscess localization for drainage.

MRI is increasingly the modality of choice for the detection of osteomyelitis at many institutions. Its sensitivity generally exceeds scintigraphy with a comparable specificity.[14] The ability to clearly identify potentially surgically treatable soft tissue processes and provide exquisite anatomic detail are advantageous. MRI has become widespread and, while costs vary greatly, it may be comparable to or less expensive than three-phase bone scintigraphy.

Summary

Examination of the diabetic foot has benefited through the use of advanced imaging. The presence of concurrent pathologic conditions continues to hamper consistently accurate diagnosis. The following algorithm for the diabetic patient with suspected osteomyelitis could serve as a general guideline, but individual institutions may have local factors that make standardization impractical.[8, 28, 43, 44] Some have suggested that an empiric 10-week antibiotic course is more cost-effective than imaging in patients with suspected osteomyelitis yet no systemic toxicity.[14]

The work-up of the diabetic foot with suspected infection should begin with plain radiographs. This, if for no other reason, can establish a baseline for the patient. With unremarkable plain films, a ^{99m}Tc bone scan is an appropriate and economical test, al-

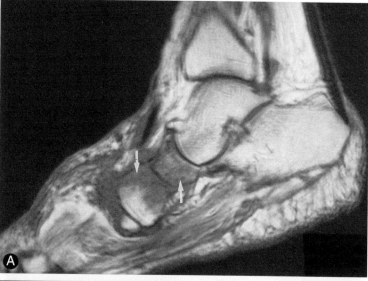

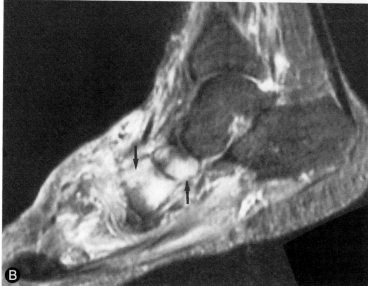

Figure 15–17 ■ A, T1-weighted sagittal image (TR 700, TE 14). Normal bright marrow signal of the navicular and medial cuneiform is replaced with abnormal lower intensity signal (*arrows*). B, Inversion recovery sagittal image (TR 5100, TE 30). Marrow signal in the navicular and medial cuneiform is brighter and less uniform (*arrows*) than that of the lower-intensity normal talus and calcaneus included on the same image. Findings are characteristic of osteomyelitis of the navicular and medial cuneiform bones.

though it suffers from low specificity. However, a negative bone scan essentially excludes acute or chronic osteomyelitis. With abnormal plain films, detailed views using CT, magnification radiography, or both may clarify cortical destruction.

MRI and ^{111}In scanning have similar specificities, although MRI has a greater sensitivity in diagnosing osteomyelitis. Consequently, MRI is preferred at an increasing number of centers, especially given the ease of the procedure, the higher imaging resolution, and the ability to differentiate between bone and soft tissue infection. With current imaging methods, it may still be impossible to differentiate rapidly progressive osteoarthritis from acute osteomyelitis. Future comparative studies may further define the specific role of these various important imaging modalities.

REFERENCES

1. Alazraki N, Fierer J, Resnick D: Chronic osteomyelitis: Monitoring by 99mTc phosphate and 67-gallium imaging. AJR Am J Roentgenol 145:767–771, 1985.
2. Al-Sheikh W, Sfakianakis GN, Mnaymneh W, et al: Subacute and chronic bone infections: Diagnosis using In-111, Ga-67, and Tc-99m MDP bone scintig-

raphy and radiography. Radiology 155:501–506, 1985.

3. Baldwin SC, Black JR: Pedal stress fracture associated with diabetic peripheral neuropathy. J Am Podiatr Med Assoc 76:30–32, 1986.

4. Beltran J, Campanini DS, Knight C, et al: The diabetic foot: Magnetic resonance imaging evaluation. Skeletal Radiol 19:37–41, 1990.

5. Beltran J, McGhee RB, Schaffer PB, et al: Experimental infections of the musculoskeletal system: Evaluation with MR imaging and TC-99m MDP and Ga-67 scintigraphy. Radiology 167:167–172, 1988.

6. Berquist TH, Brown ML, Fitzgerald RH, et al: Magnetic resonance imaging: Application in musculoskeletal infection. Magn Reson Imaging 3:219–230, 1985.

7. Blume PA, Dey HM, Daley LJ, et al: Diagnosis of pedal osteomyelitis with Tc-99m HMPAO labeled leukocytes. J Foot Ankle Surg 36:120–126, 1997.

8. Brower AC: What is the preferred method for diagnosing osteomyelitis in the foot of a patient with diabetes? Question/Answer. AJR Am J Roentgenol 163:471–472, 1994.

9. Bush WH, Bettmann MA: Metformin (Glucophage) therapy and the risk of lactic acidosis. Am Coll Radiol Bull 53:18–19, 1997.

10. Clouse ME, Gramm HF, Legg M, et al: Diabetic osteoarthropathy: Clinical and roentgenographic observations in 90 cases. AJR Am J Roentgenol 121:34, 1974.

11. Connolly JF, Jacobsen FS: Rapid bone destruction after a stress fracture in a diabetic (Charcot) foot. Nebr Med J 70:438–440, 1985.

12. Coventry MB, Rothacker GW Jr: Bilateral calcaneal fractures in a diabetic patient. J Bone Joint Surg 61A:462, 1979.

13. Durham JR, Lukens ML, Campanini DS, et al: Impact of magnetic resonance imaging on the management of diabetic foot infections. Am J Surg 162:150–153, 1991.

14. Eckman MH, Greenfield S, Mackey WC, et al: Foot infections in diabetic patients. Decision and cost-effectiveness analyses. JAMA 273:712–720, 1995.

15. El-Khoury GY, Kathol MH: Neuropathic fractures in patients with diabetes mellitus. Radiology 134:313–316, 1980.

16. Erdman WA, Tamburro F, Jayson HT: Osteomyelitis: Characteristics and pitfalls of diagnosis with MR imaging. Radiology 180:533–539, 1991.

17. Eymontt MJ, Alavi A, Dalinka MK, et al: Bone scintigraphy in diabetic osteoarthropathy. Radiology 140:475–477, 1991.

18. Fletcher BD, Scoles PV, Nelson AD: Osteomyelitis in children: Detection by magnetic resonance. Radiology 150:57–60, 1984.

19. Forestier J, Lagier R: Ankylosing hyperostosis of the spine. Clin Orthop 74:65, 1971.

20. Genant HK, Resnick D: Magnification radiography. In Resnick D (ed): Diagnosis of Bone and Joint Disorders, 3rd ed. Philadelphia: WB Saunders Company, 1995, pp 72–102.

21. Genant HK, Doi J, Mall JC: Optical versus radiographic magnification for fine detail skeletal radiology. Invest Radiol 2:160, 1975.

22. Gilday DL: Problems in the scintigraphic detection of osteomyelitis. Radiology 135:791, 1980.

23. Griffiths HJ: Diabetic osteopathy. Orthopedics 8:398–406, 1985.

24. Gupta NC, Prezio JA: Radionuclide imaging in osteomyelitis. Semin Nucl Med 18:287–299, 1988.

25. Handmaker H: Acute hematogenous osteomyelitis: Has the bone scan betrayed us? Radiology 135:787–789, 1980.

26. Harris J, Carter AR, Glick EN, et al: Ankylosing hyperotosis: I. Clinical and radiological features. Ann Rheum Dis 31:69, 1972.

27. Hetherington VJ: Technetium and combined gallium and technetium scans in the neurotrophic foot. J Am Podiatr Assoc 72:458–463, 1982.

28. Hochman MG, Min KK, Zilberfarb JL: MR imaging of the symptomatic ankle and foot. Orthop Clin North Am 28:659–683, 1997.

29. Horowitz JD, Durham JR, Nease DB, et al: Prospective evaluation of magnetic resonance imaging in the management of acute diabetic foot infections. Ann Vasc Surg 7:44–50, 1993.

30. Jacobson AF, Harley JD, Lipsky AF, et al: Diagnosis of osteomyelitis in the presence of soft tissue infection and radiologic evidence of osseous abnormalities: Value of leukocyte scintigraphy. AJR Am J Roentgenol 157:807–812, 1991.

31. Johnson JTH: Neuropathic fractures and joint injuries: Pathogenesis and rationale of prevention and treatment. J Bone Joint Surg 49A:1–30, 1967.

32. Julkunen H, Karava R, Viljanen V: Hyperostosis of the spine in diabetes mellitus and acromegaly. Diabetologia 2:123, 1966.

33. Kathol MH, El-Khoury GY, Moore TE, et al: Calcaneal insufficiency avulsion fractures in patients with diabetes mellitus. Radiology 180:725–729, 1991.

34. Katholi RE, et al: Nephrotoxicity from contrast media: Attenuation with theophylline. Radiology 195:17–22, 1995.

35. Keenan AM, Tindel NL, Alavi A: Diagnosis of pedal osteomyelitis in diabetic patients using current scintigraphic techniques. Arch Intern Med 149:2262–2266, 1989.

36. Kolindou A, Liu Y, Ozker K, et al: In-111 WBC imaging of osteomyelitis in patients with underlying bone scan abnormalities. Clin Nucl Med 21:183–191, 1991.

37. Kraft E, Spyropoulos E, Finby N: Neurogenic disorders of the foot in diabetes mellitus. AJR Am J Roentgenol 124:17–24, 1975.

38. Kristiansen B: Ankle and foot fractures in diabetics provoking neuropathic joint changes. Acta Orthop Scand 51:975–979, 1980.

39. Landon GC, Johnson KA, Dahlin DC: Subungual exostoses. J Bone Joint Surg 61A:256, 1979.

40. Lee SM, Lee RGL, Wilinsky J, et al: Magnification radiography in osteomyelitis. Skeletal Radiol 15:625–627, 1986.

41. Lipinsky B, Pecoraro R, Harley J. Diagnosis of bone lesions in the diabetic feet: Osteomyelitis or osteoarthropathy? In Abstract of the 29th Interscience Conference on Antimicrobial Agents and Chemotherapy. Houston, TX: American Society for Microbiology, 1989, abstract 913.

42. Longmaid HE III, Kruskal JB: Imaging infections in diabetic patients. Infect Dis Clin North Am 9:163–182, 1995.

43. Loredo R, Metter D: Imaging of the diabetic foot. Emphasis on nuclear medicine and magnetic resonance imaging. Clin Podiatr Med Surg 14:235–264, 1997.

44. Mader JT, Ortiz M, Calhoun JH: Update on the diagnosis and management of osteomyelitis. Clin Podiatr Med Surg 13:701–724, 1996.

45. Marcus CD, Ladam-Marcus VJ, Leone J, et al: MR imaging of osteomyelitis and neuropathic osteoarthropathy in the feet of diabetics. Radiographics 16:1337–1348, 1996.

46. Maurer AH, Millmond SH, Knight LC, et al: Infection in diabetic osteoarthropathy: Use of indium-labeled leukocytes for diagnosis. Radiology 161:221, 1986.

47. McCarthy K, Velchik MG, Mandell GA, et al: Indium-111-labeled white blood cells in the detection of osteomyelitis complicated by a pre-existing condition. J Nucl Med 29:1015–1021, 1988.

48. Meltzer AD, Skuersky N, Ostrum BJ: Radiographic evaluation of soft tissue necrosis in diabetics. Radiology 90:300, 1968.

49. Mendelson EB, Fisher MR, Deschler TW, et al: Osteomyelitis in diabetic foot: A difficult diagnostic challenge. Radiographics 3:248–261, 1983.

50. Merkel KD, Brown ML, Dewanjee MK, et al: Comparison of indium-labeled-leukocyte imaging with sequential technetium-gallium scanning in the diagnosis of low-grade musculoskeletal sepsis: A prospective study. J Bone Joint Surg 67A:465–476, 1985.

51. Modic MT, Feiglin DH, Piraino DW, et al: Vertebral osteomyelitis: Assessment using MR. Radiology 157:157–166, 1985.

52. Moore TE, Yoh WTC, et al: Abnormalities of the foot in patients with diabetes mellitus: Findings on MR imaging. AJR Am J Roentgenol 157:813–816, 1991.

53. Moriarty KT, Perkins AC, Robinson AM, et al: Investigating the capillary circulation of the foot with 99mTc-macroaggregated albumin: A prospective study in patients with diabetes and foot ulceration. Diabet Med 11:22–27, 1994.

54. Newman JH: Non-infective disease of the diabetic foot. J Bone Joint Surg 63B:593–596, 1981.

55. Newman LG, Waller J, Palestro CJ, et al: Unsuspected osteomyelitis in diabetic foot ulcers: Diagnosis and monitoring by leukocyte scanning with indium-111 oxyquinoline. JAMA 266:1245–1251, 1991.

56. Nguyen VD, Keh RA, Daehler RW: Freiberg's disease in diabetes mellitus. Skeletal Radiol 20:425–428, 1991.

57. Pambor M, Neubert H: Tumorartige begleitreaktionen der haut bei exostoses der zehenendphalangen. Dermatol Monatsschr 157:532, 1971.

58. Park E, Wheat LJ, Siddiqui AR, et al: Scintigraphic evaluation of diabetic osteomyelitis: Concise communication. J Nucl Med 23:569–573, 1982.

59. Phemister DB: Lesions of bones and joints arising from interruption of circulation. J Mt Sinai Hosp N Y 15:55, 1948.

60. Pogonowska MJ, Collins LC, Dobson HL: Diabetic osteopathy. Radiology 89:265, 1967.

61. Quinn SF, Murray W, Clark RA, Cochran C: MR imaging of chronic osteomyelitis. J Comput Assist Tomogr 12:113–117, 1988.

62. Raptopoulos V, Doherty PW, Goss TP, et al: Acute osteomyelitis: Advantage of white cells in early detection. AJR Am J Roentgenol 39:1077–1082, 1982.

63. Reinhardt K: The radiological residua of healed diabetic arthropathies. Skeletal Radiol 7:167–172, 1981.

64. Resnick D: Disorders of other endocrine glands and of pregnancy. In Resnick D (ed): Diagnosis of Bone and Joint Disorders, 3rd ed. Philadelphia, WB Saunders Company, 1995 pp 2076–2104.

65. Resnick D, Niwayama G: Diffuse idiopathic skeletal hyperostosis (DISH): Ankylosing hyperostosis of Forestier and Rotes-Querol. In Resnick D (ed): Diagnosis of Bone and Joint Disorders, 3rd ed. Philadelphia, WB Saunders Company, 1995, pp 1463–1495.

66. Schauwecker DS: The scintigraphic diagnosis of osteomyelitis. AJR Am J Roentgenol 158:9–18, 1992.

67. Schauwecker DS, Park HM, Burt RW, et al: Combined bone scintigraphy and indium-111 leukocyte scans in neuropathic foot disease. J Nucl Med 29:1651–1655, 1988.

68. Scheidler J, Leinsinger G, Pfahler M, Kirsch CM: Diagnosis of osteomyelitis. Accuracy and limitations of antigranulocyte antibody imaging compared to three-phase bone scan. Clin Nucl Med 19:731–737, 1994.

69. Seabold JE, Flickinger FW, Kao SCS, et al: Indium-111-leukocyte/technetium-99m-MDP bone and magnetic resonance imaging: Difficulty of diagnosing osteomyelitis in patients with neuropathic osteoarthropathy. J Nucl Med 31:539–556, 1990.

70. Seldin DW, Heiken JP, Alderson PO: Effect of soft-tissue pathology on detection of pedal osteomyelitis in diabetics. J Nucl Med 26:988–993, 1985.

71. Sirtori CR, Pasik C: Re-evaluation of a biguanide, metformin: Mechanism of action and tolerability. Pharmacol Res 30:187–228, 1994.

72. Solomon MA, Gilula LA, Oloff LM, et al: CT scanning of the foot and ankle: Part 1, normal anatomy. AJR Am J Roentgenol 146:1192–1203, 1986.

73. Solomon MA, Gilula LA, Oloff LM, et al: CT scanning of the foot and ankle: Part 2, clinical applications and review of the literature. AJR Am J Roentgenol 146:1204–1214, 1986.

74. Splittgerber GF, Spiegelhoff DR, Buggy BP: Combined leukocyte and bone imaging used to evaluate diabetic osteoarthropathy and osteomyelitis. Clin Nucl Med 14:156–160, 1989.

75. Sturrock NDC, Perkins AC, Wastie ML, et al: A reproducibility study of technetium-99m macroaggregated albumin foot perfusion imaging in patients with diabetes mellitus. Diabet Med 12:445–448, 1995.

76. Totty WG: Radiographic evaluation of osteomyelitis using magnetic resonance imaging. Orthop Rev 18:587–592, 1989.

77. Tumeh SS, Aliabadi P, Weissman BN, et al: Chronic osteomyelitis: Bone and gallium scan patterns associated with active disease. Radiology 158:685–688, 1986.

78. Ulger E, Moldofsky P, Gatenby R, et al: Diagnosis of osteomyelitis by MR imaging. AJR Am J Roentgenol 150:605–610, 1988.

79. Visser JH, Oloff L, Jacobs AM, et al: The use of differential scintigraphy in the clinical diagnosis of osseous and soft tissue changes affecting the diabetic foot. J Foot Surg 23:74–85, 1984.

80. Wang A, Weinstein D, Greenfield LM, et al: MRI and diabetic foot infections. Magn Reson Imaging 8:805–809, 1990.

81. Wegener WA, Alavi A: Diagnostic imaging of musculoskeletal infection. Orthop Clin 22:401–418, 1991.

82. Weinstein D, Wang A, Chambers R, et al: Evaluation of magnetic resonance imaging in the diagnosis

of osteomyelitis in diabetic foot infections. Foot Ankle 14:18–22, 1993.

83. Whitehouse FW: On diabetic osteopathy: A radiographic study of 21 patients. Diabetes Care 1:303, 1978.

84. Williamson BRJ, Treates CD, Phillips CD, et al: Computed tomography as a diagnostic aid in diabetic and other problem feet. Clin Imag 13:159–163, 1989.

85. Yuh WTC, Corson JD, Baraniewski HM, et al: Osteomyelitis of the foot in diabetic patients: Evaluation with plain film, 99m-Tc-MDP bone scintigraphy, and MR imaging. AJR Am J Roentgenol 152:795–800, 1989.

NONINVASIVE VASCULAR TESTING: BASIS, APPLICATION, AND ROLE IN EVALUATING DIABETIC PERIPHERAL ARTERIAL DISEASE

■ Joseph J Hurley, Matthew Jung, John J. Woods, Jr., and Falls B. Hershey

Correct utilization and interpretation of non-invasive testing in the evaluation of lower extremity arterial disease (LEAD) in diabetic individuals requires a knowledge of its inter-relationships with the medical history, physical examination findings, and angiographic results. In each of these areas clear differences exist in comparing diabetic to nondiabetic persons. In attempting mastery of non-invasive testing in diabetic patients, it is worthwhile emphasizing noninvasive studies do not stand alone but rather supplement information accumulated by methodical history-taking and careful physical examination. Likewise, knowing the results of noninvasive (physiologic) testing allows a more thorough examination of angiogram (anatomic) results. This chapter defines the role of noninvasive examinations in assessing the status and prognosis of potential LEAD in diabetic individuals.

The burden LEAD places upon diabetic individuals, whether insulin-dependent or non–insulin-dependent, is remarkable for its implications regarding not only limb-threatening morbidity but also potential mortality. While only 5 to 6% of the population in this country is suspected of having diabetes mellitus, they constitute 15 to 17% of patients diagnosed with intermittent claudication, 30 to 50% of patients undergoing lower extremity arterial surgery[14, 38] (60 to 70% having bypass grafts to arteries below the popliteal artery),[19] and as many as 50 to 60% of those persons undergoing major lower extremity amputations. Symptoms are more likely to appear at an earlier age in diabetic persons as reported by Reunaneu,[37] where he noted intermittent claudication in 4.3% of diabetic persons aged 30 to 59 years versus only 2.0% of nondiabetics in the same age group.

Beach et al.,[5] evaluating 50- to 70-year-old volunteers, noted LEAD was much more prevalent in the type 2 patients (22%) than in controls (3%). In these same type 2 patients, the incidence (14%) of new LEAD over a 2-year period was lower than the incidence (87%) of LEAD progression determined by noninvasive testing (ankle-arm index [AAI] < 0.95, abnormal Doppler-derived waveforms, or a decrease of 0.15 in the AAI from previous testing). Finally, type 2 patients with LEAD also demonstrated a high incidence of mortality, 22% compared with those without LEAD (4%) during this same study period.

Another prospective, minimal 24-month follow-up study conducted by Bendick et al.[6] also employing noninvasive evaluation in diabetic patients seemingly confirms these results. Using the noninvasive criteria of an AAI of less than 0.9, monophasic waveforms, or evidence of progression as indicated by a drop in the AAI of greater than or equal to 0.15, they likewise determined that less than 10% of patients initially considered to have a normal study developed any criteria of LEAD during the study period. In contrast, 76% of those identified as having LEAD at the start of the trial revealed progression of their arterial disease. The strongest indicator of LEAD progression is the presence of preexisting arterial disease. This progression had a high likelihood to occur in a relatively short time.

The magnitude of discovering LEAD in diabetic persons is also seen in a collected series of 2,323 patients undergoing major lower extremity amputation,[13] in which 54% were diagnosed as having diabetes mellitus. In this same series, 20% of these individuals had incurred a previous contralateral amputation, while only 37% of the entire series, diabetic and nondiabetic alike, survived for 5 years.

Patients with severe or symptomatic large-vessel peripheral vascular disease have a sharply increased probability of clinically important coronary and cerebrovascular atherosclerosis risk. Criqui et al.[12] found that moderately severe to even asymptomatic LEAD in the posterior tibial artery would increase the risk of coronary artery disease three- to sixfold. Patients who became symptomatic or harbored severe lower extremity vascular disease had a 10-year risk of death due to coronary heart disease 10 to 15 times greater than for subjects free of large-vessel arterial disease.

McDaniel and Cronenwett[29] noted that even with only the diagnosis of intermittent claudication, mortality was significant after 5 years, revealing a 23% mortality rate in nondiabetic persons, which jumps to a 49% mortality rate in those persons diagnosed with diabetes mellitus.

The implications of diagnosing LEAD in a diabetic individual are enormous and should lead to a more vigorous patient assessment and management of cardiovascular risk factors.

Clinical Diagnosis

An extensive history, followed by a thorough physical examination, provides the initial suggestions of the possibility of LEAD. The level and severity of this occlusive disease can usually be determined at a surprisingly accurate level with the use of history and physical examination in experienced hands. Historically, the natural progression of arterial insufficiency commences with intermittent claudication. The claudication onset distance decreases until patients start experiencing pain even at rest. The final stage in this progression is the appearance of gangrene or failure of even minor cuts and abrasions to heal, while at the same time becoming extremely painful. Unfortunately, since many diabetic individuals have some element of peripheral neuropathy, the stage of rest pain is often lacking, and even lesions at the gangrenous stage can be relatively nonirritating. Commonly a history of claudication in diabetic patients leads directly to the unheralded appearance of nonhealing wounds or gangrene.

The presence of a critical narrowing in the peripheral artery is related to the severity of the stenosis (fixed) and the volume of crossing blood flow (variable). Claudication occurs when muscular limb activity increases the blood flow by up to 20-fold over the resting state. While the delivery of oxygen and removal of lactic acid and other metabolic products is adequate at resting flows, a critical stenosis prevents these exchanges at increased demand, resulting in onset of muscle discomfort. Cessation of exercise allows a correction of this situation and disappearance of the symptoms, which will reappear at virtually the same distance given the identical angle of terrain and gait. Increasing the elevation of terrain (including stairs) or the briskness of gait normally would result in a shortened claudication onset distance. For convenience and patient communication sake, we often relate this distance to blocks (i.e., 4- to 6-blocks claudication, 1/2-block claudication, etc.) It is, likewise, important to understand that claudication, a word derived from the Latin verb *claudicatio,* meaning "to limp," while usually described as painful can also be described as weakness, heaviness, or even cramping of the leg muscles. The level of the discomfort often gives a clue to the probable level of arterial narrowing or occlusion. Thigh and buttock claudication suggests an aortoiliac location if bilateral or iliac if unilateral, while calf claudication points to femoral or popliteal involvement. Impotence in nondiabetic persons is highly suggestive of aortoiliac artery involvement when combined with claudication (Leriche's syndrome), but because of the high prevalence of neuropathy in diabetic males, it is much less helpful diagnostically. The appearance of rest pain usually implies multilevel disease that is severely stenotic or of a totally occlusive nature. When present, the typical pain associated with rest pain is likely to be described with onset an hour or two after assuming a supine position. It classically involves the distal forefoot, can be relieved by dangling the foot over the side of the bed, short distance ambulation, or sleeping in a sitting position, and it is repetitive with resuming a supine position. Rest pain occurs as a result of arterial pressures at the ankle level inadequate to force blood against gravity to the now upright foot, with the toes and distal forefoot most vulnerable.

Physical findings require observation and palpation. The ischemic foot will display changes in color with elevation and dependency as a result of ischemia-induced deranged autonomic autoregulation. A ruborous foot on dependency blanches rapidly when elevated to 45 degrees above the examination table. The hypoxemia resulting from insufficient blood flow due to LEAD is a potent stimulus to vasodilatation, probably the strongest known. Rubor results from the dilated vessels attempting to trap blood for increased oxygen extraction. Two ways of evaluating this in a more objective fashion are "capillary refill time" and "venous refill time." In the supine position, pressure is applied to the skin and, once removed, the

reappearance of the usual skin color in this area is timed. Capillary refill time is usually considered abnormal where it takes longer than 5 seconds to return to baseline. Venous refill time can be determined by identifying a prominent vein in the foot in a supine patient. The leg is then elevated 45 degrees for 1 minute, following which the patient sits up and hangs the leg over the side of the examination table. The time in seconds between assuming the upright position and the reappearance of the vein bulging above the skin level is recorded. Normal venous refill time is considered to be 20 seconds or less.[34]

Assessment of pulses at the femoral, popliteal, and pedal (dorsalis pedis and posterior tibial) locations should be graded as normal, diminished, or absent. The occurrence of congenital absence of these vessels is rare. Where doubt occurs as to whether one is feeling one's own pulse or the patient's, a check against the patient's radial pulse quickly settles the issue. Auscultation of the femoral and aortoiliac region for a bruit should be performed. Bruits occur at areas of arterial narrowing, with onset around 50% stenosis and disappearance around 90% stenosis. They provide a clue as to the presence, location, and severity of LEAD. Changes in skin, hair, and nails may be a sign of critical ischemia and should be sought. Skin atrophy or rubor, nail thickening, or hair loss all tend to occur with progressive LEAD.

Boyko et al.[9] examined the utility of clinical history-taking and physical examination in evaluating LEAD in diabetic patients. Using multivariate analysis, the highest probability for finding severe LEAD was obtained with the following parameters: patient age (>65 years old), a self-reported history of physician-diagnosed LEAD (or <1-block claudication), peripheral pulse deficit, and abnormal venous filling time. Additionally, they noted that greater than 85% of patients with an AAI of less than or equal to 0.5 had a history of tobacco abuse. Diminished peripheral foot pulses and delayed venous filling time were associated with the highest likelihood of having severe (AAI ≤0.5) LEAD.

Pathophysiology

In the resting state only high-grade stenosis or total occlusion of a vessel results in abnormal changes recorded at the ankle level (Fig. 16–1). Arterial narrowing or obstruction forces the blood to follow collateral arteries, which are usually high-resistance pathways. The greater the number of sequential critical stenoses or occlusions, the greater the degree of total impairment that will be detected at the most distal assessment point.

Besides a generalized yes or no answer regarding the presence of arterial obstructive disease, segmental pressure measurements allow some attempt at accurate identification of the anatomic location of the obstruction (Fig. 16–2). Strandness and Bell,[41] however, caution that inaccuracies are most likely to occur when there is multilevel involvement. They further note the following specific problems: (1) high thigh pressures may be abnormally low in the presence of an occluded proximal superficial femoral artery, and (2) gradients between high thigh and low thigh may be "normal" in patients with superficial femoral obstructions when there is significant aortoiliac disease; and (3) disease below

the knee will not be recognized consistently unless the obstruction is quite severe and involves all three vessels. The authors mention these problems not to condemn this approach but to point out that pressure measurements may be more reliable than arteriograms as a guide to the surgeon in selecting therapy, because they more accurately reflect the physiologic magnitude of the disease.

Even more information can be obtained when the response to a demand for maximum flow in the limb is obtained. The data of Strandness and Bell[42] and others demonstrate that exercise in the presence of occlusive arterial disease proximal to the blood supply of the calf muscles results in a transient decrease in blood pressure at the ankle. Furthermore, it has been shown that this fall in the ankle pressure may be used as an objective test for assessing and following the course of the disease in patients with obliterative arterial disease of the lower extremities. Increases in heart rate, systolic blood

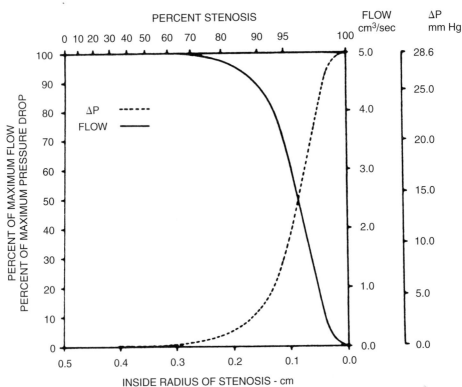

Figure 16–1 ■ Effect of increasing stenosis on blood flow and pressure drop across the stenotic segment. Collateral and peripheral resistances are considered to be fixed. (From Strandness DE, Sumner DS: Hemodynamics for Surgeons. New York: Grune & Stratton, 1975, with permission.)

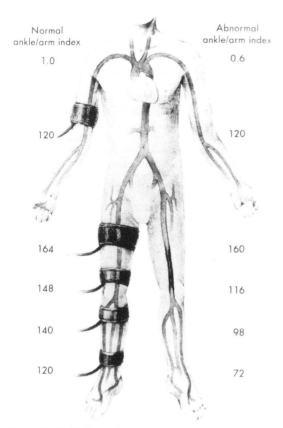

Figure 16–2 ■ Normal condition on right side of body with ankle systolic pressure equal to brachial systolic pressure. Ankle pressure divided by arm pressure determines AAI, in this case 1.0. On left side, AAI is 0.6, indicating only 60% of expected normal flow at rest. In addition, any gradient greater than 30 mm Hg between two successive cuffs indicates high-grade stenosis or occlusion. Here 44 mm Hg high thigh gradient localizes diseased segment to superficial femoral artery. (From Arizona Heart Institute: Cerebrovascular and peripheral vascular disease: Advanced noninvasive diagnostic techniques, with permission.)

pressure, cardiac output, oxygen consumption, and limb blood flow are the normal responses to exercise. The magnitude of these changes is a direct function of the work performed. In addition, the duration of increased blood flow after exercise (reactive hyperemia) is a valuable mark of the amount of work performed and a mark of the vascular system's ability to respond adequately to such demands (Fig. 16–3). Normal individuals display postexercise reactive hyperemia of very short duration, lasting only a few minutes in response to normal exercise loads. In contrast, those patients with critical arterial stenosis or occlusions display markedly prolonged periods of decreased blood flow in re-

sponse to even minimum exercise demands. The magnitude of the decrease in ankle pressure and its time course are rough guides to the extent of the impairment to blood flow after exercise or induced hyperemia.[40] Reactive hyperemia can be assessed in those individuals unable to exercise by inflating a thigh cuff 50 mm Hg greater than systolic pressures for 3 minutes and then recording the serial pressures on release of the cuff. This is referred to as "induced reactive hyperemia."

Progression of arteriosclerotic lesions or recurrent distal embolism will increase stenosis or cause occlusion of the vascular tree. Hypertension, diabetes mellitus, hyperlipidemia, and tobacco use clearly encourage atherosclerotic disease. Control of the first three conditions and total cessation of smoking, on the other hand, when coupled with a walking program and the passage of time, can lead to collateral channel development. Although collateral pathways are high-resistance pathways, their development can improve distal blood flow. This is usually detected

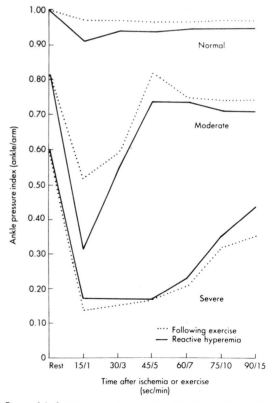

Figure 16–3 ■ Effect of increasing blood flow demands on normal patients and those with moderate and severe peripheral arterial disease. Note correlation between exercise measured in minutes and reactive hyperemia measured in seconds.

Table 16–1 ▪ DETERMINATION OF CRITICAL STENOSIS*

CONDITION OF MEASUREMENT	AVERAGE BLOOD FLOW (mL/min)	CRITICAL STENOSIS DETERMINED BY 10% DROP IN FLOW (%)	CRITICAL STENOSIS DETERMINED BY 10% DROP IN PRESSURE (%)
Iliac artery	144	85	86
Iliac artery + 1 AV fistula	456	75	74
Aorta + 1 AV fistula	314	86	86
Aorta + 2 AV fistulas	593	79	79
Aorta + 3 AV fistulas	886	73	73

* This table demonstrates the pathophysiology of arterial stenotic disease. Increasing the flow by opening a progressively larger number of arteriovenous (AV) fistulas causes a progressively lesser amount of stenosis necessary to initiate a 10% drop in flow. The validity of using noninvasive pressure measurements to determine flow changes is seen by comparing the last two columns. (Courtesy of Dr. Wesley Moore, Tucson, AZ.)

first by exercise testing after a prolonged period of ambulatory therapy. Positive signs are a smaller drop in pressure after exercise and a more rapid rise of the pressures to preexercise baselines. Moore and Malone,[32] in a series of canine experiments using multiple in-line arteriovenous fistulas, which provided a wide range of iliac artery blood flow, demonstrated that (1) the percentage of decrease in blood pressure was the same as the percentange of decrease in blood flow (i.e., blood pressure and blood flow vary directly), and (2) the greater the flow the less stenosis necessary to create the same incremental decrease in pressure (Table 16–1). One additional difficulty in interpreting angiography is the relationship between the actual three-plane cross-sectional area changes and the lumen size as determined by two-plane angiograms (Table 16–2).

Noninvasive Evaluation

Over the past quarter of a century a progression of new instrumentation has been introduced in an effort to develop the ideal single or combination of noninvasive tests allowing an ability to predict spontaneous wound healing, need for revascularization, or the appropriate level for minor or major amputation in diabetic individuals. Initial endeavors were the measurement of segmental pressures and qualitative waveform assessment at the ankle and toe level. Subsequent progression has given us transcutaneous oxygen determination, laser Doppler velocimetry, and duplex and now magnetic flow arterial imaging. A review of the methods, benefits, costs, and role of these various testing modalities follows.

Some individuals question any role for noninvasive testing in the clinical assessment and management of diabetic patients with LEAD. In 1979, Gibbons et al.,[15] employing ankle systolic blood pressure measurements, evaluated 150 diabetic patients seeking a decisive number to predict the success in selecting an amputation level. The conclusion, "In the diabetic patient, clinical judgement continues to provide the most accurate and reliable information by which the type of amputation and the likelihood of its success can be judged" was well supported

Table 16–2 ▪ CORRELATION BETWEEN DIAMETER, AREA, AND FLOW REDUCTION FOR ARTERIAL STENOSIS*

$2/5 \times 100 = 40\%$ OR 60% STENOSIS BY DIAMETER (%)	$(2/5)^2 \times 100 = 16\%$ OR 84% STENOSIS BY AREA (%)	30% REDUCTION OF FLOW (%)
0	0	0
30	51	>0
40	64	≤20
60	84	~30
70	91	~40
85	98	~70

* A lateral, two-dimensional 60% stenosis actually represents an 84% cross-sectional area obliteration. This nevertheless results in only a 30% reduction of resting flow.

by their clinical material. Mehta et al.[30] confirmed the fallibility of ankle pressures in predicting healing of transmetatarsal amputations in diabetes, whereas Barnes et al.[4] did likewise for the healing of below-knee amputations. The latter favored the presence of a popliteal pulse. Bone and Pomajzl[7] suggested the value of indexing the potential of healing forefoot amputations using toe pressures derived photoplethysmographically. In their study, eight limbs with digital pressures of less than 45 mm Hg failed to heal. Two of eight (25%) failed to heal in the range of 45 to 55 mm Hg, and all 14 patients subjected to forefoot amputation with a pressure greater than 55 mm Hg healed. They also demonstrated the unreliability of ankle systolic blood pressure (ASBP) in predicting amputation success. These and other investigators had a twofold impact: (1) the need for careful clinical evaluation was reemphasized, and (2) the need for better noninvasive testing was suggested.

Instrumentation

We use several pieces of equipment to determine the hemodynamic status of our patients in an entirely noninvasive fashion: the photoplethysmograph, Doppler velocity flow meters and probes, and a set of 12-cm blood pressure cuffs. An automatic cuff insufflator and a strip chart recorder increase the ease of performance and provide a permanent hard copy of the waveform for the patient's file.

More recently we have added duplex scanners, which help clarify proximal superficial femoral artery occlusions, as well as provide information on the number and status of nonstenotic or occluded tibial vessels.

Photoplethysmography

Photoplethysmography employs a transducer that transmits infrared light from an emitting diode into the tissue. Part of the transmitted light is reflected back from the blood within the cutaneous microcirculation and is received by an adjacent phototransistor. The amount of reflected light varies with the blood content of the microcirculation. The output of the phototransistor is A/C, coupled to an amplifier for recording as a pulsatile analog waveform. This phototransducer is taped to the end of the toe with a double-faced cellophane tape while a small digital blood pressure cuff is placed at the base of the digit. Figure 16–4 demonstrates the instrumentation. The pressure at which the waveform obliterates corresponds to the digital systolic pressure. The pressure may also be measured using a digital strain gauge or a peripherally placed Doppler probe.

Doppler Ultrasound

The Doppler ultrasound device consists of two piezoelectric crystals mounted in a probe. By stimulating one of the crystals with

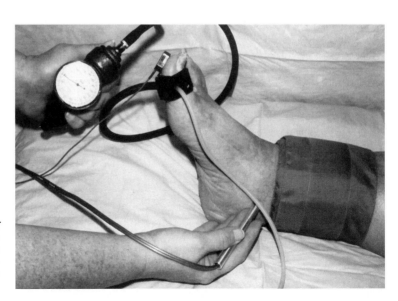

Figure 16–4 ■ Measurement of both posterior tibial ankle pressure and great toe pressure is demonstrated using Doppler ultrasound device and photoplethysmography.

an electrical charge, sound waves of various frequencies (all beyond the range of human hearing) are emitted. The second crystal receives the sound waves reflected from moving particles, producing a voltage change. This change can be amplified and converted to analog waveforms or sound. The higher the frequency emitted by the crystal, the less the depth of penetration and the narrower the width investigated. A frequency of 5 MHz or lower gives deep penetration and comparatively broad beam especially suited for monitoring deep blood vessel flow in the vena cava or iliac veins or for examining peripheral veins. An operating frequency of 10 MHz is less penetrating but permits a sharper focus and is ideal for blood velocity detection in arteries and veins of limbs and digits. The Doppler probe is coupled to the skin with acoustic gel and held at an appropriate angle to the vessel being examined. This angle varies in accordance with the specifications of the individual manufacturers, ranging from 38 to 52 degrees.[3] A good seal between the probe and the skin is critical because the sound waves travel poorly through the air. Because there is no ideal probe angle for optimum recording, using a large amount of acoustic coupling gel allows one to vary the angle of insonation to find that point where the audible sound is clearest. A beam of ultrasound travels to the underlying vessel where it is reflected from red blood cells and shifted in frequency by an amount proportional to the flow velocity of erythrocytes in that vessel. The pitch of the audiofrequency signal produced by the receiving crystal is, therefore, proportional to the average velocity of the blood flowing within the vessel under study. The Doppler does not record the flow velocity itself but a phase shift. The recorded Doppler signal is used in two ways: (1) to measure segmental systolic pressure and (2) to produce flow velocity waveform patterns for analysis.

Segmental Pressures

Pressure cuffs 12 cm wide are placed at the high thigh level, above the knee, below the knee, and at the ankle level. By listening with the Doppler probe over one of the pedal vessels (dorsalis pedis, posterior tibial, or lateral tarsal arteries), one can obtain the pressure at the level of the inflated cuff. An AAI is obtained by dividing the segmental systolic

pressure by the brachial systolic pressure. The usual index recorded is that of the ankle (ankle pressure/brachial pressure), which should be 1 or just slightly higher. Pressure changes correlate directly with flow as previously discussed; thus an index of 0.5 represents only 50% of the expected blood flow. A gradient of 40 mm Hg or greater between the levels being compared suggests an occlusion or highly stenotic segment. In normal situations, the high thigh pressure is 1.3 times the brachial systolic pressure.

Toe Pressures

The role of toe pressures with or without pulse waves in predicting the clinical course of rest pain, skin ulcerations, and gangrene in diabetic patients has been extensively examined.[20, 21] Holstein et al.[17] feel that absolute toe pressures provide a highly accurate method for determining the likelihood of success in the healing of an ulcer or in minor amputation, thus preventing a more proximal, major, potentially disabling amputation. Barnes et al.[3] seemingly concur with this assessment in diabetic persons for the likelihood for minor amputation healing. Bowers et al.[2] likewise found a role for toe pressure measurements to predict the likelihood of clinical deterioration. Defining clinical deterioration as rest pain, tissue loss, or gangrene, they found a toe systolic pressure (TSP) of 40 mm Hg or less to have significance. Patients with diabetes in this group had even a significantly higher risk of developing critical ischemia. Carter and Tate,[11] meanwhile, validated the significance of toe systolic pressure and added pulse wave measurements in an attempt to increase accuracy. They felt toe pressure reflected the overall obstruction in the arterial tree proximal to the digits and was not affected by arterial incompressibility. Study conditions were stressed with patients resting supine for at least 20 minutes, bodies and extremities covered with a heating blanket in a room with an ambient temperature of approximately 23°C. The presence of diabetes mellitus increased the odds ratio for rest pain, skin lesions, or both after controlling for systolic pressures and wave amplitude. Further lower toe pulse wave amplitude was significantly related to the occurrence of rest pain, skin breakdown, or both. In summary, rest pain, skin lesions, or both were present in approximately 50% of limbs with toe pressures less than or equal to 30 mm Hg, in 16% of those with pressure of 31 to 40 mm Hg, and in 5% of limbs with arterial disease and toe pressure greater than 40 mm Hg. They believe measurement of wave amplitude may help identify those with good prognosis for spontaneous healing among limbs with toe systolic pressure less than or equal to 30 mm Hg.

Waveform Evaluation

Many approaches to quantitative analysis of waveforms have been suggested, but all have seemingly added little, if any, value over a subjective or qualitative evaluation.[27] The waveform in the normal state shows a rapid systolic upstroke and usually a peaked appearance. The actual magnitude of the waveform can be affected by the depth of the artery (e.g., decreased in obese persons), by probe pressure that actually compresses a thin patient's artery, by the probe angle in relation to the artery, or even by the consistency of the vessel being evaluated (e.g., a prosthetic graft will give a distorted picture even when fully patent). Thus, no comparisons of the heights of the peak should be attempted. In addition, a normal peripheral waveform will usually show a reversed component as the initial diastolic portion, followed by a small second forward component (Figs. 16–5, 16–6, and 16–7). The reverse segment is the result of distal resistance, followed by the elastic recoil of the vessel wall. This can sometimes be absent in the normal subject at the ankle level. Deterioration of the waveform can be seen just proximal to an obstructing lesion; distal to the lesion the waveform is always abnormal with a loss of the normal rapid systolic upstroke so that the slope is the same as that of the downstroke. In addition, even before these changes, earlier milder stenosis will cause loss of the diastolic components at the popliteal or femoral levels. As the flow deteriorates, waveforms become flattened and then undulating before they totally disappear.

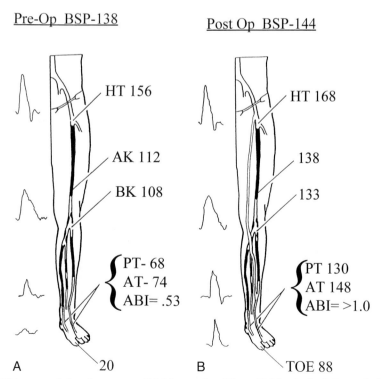

Pre-Op BSP-138   Post Op BSP-144

Figure 16–5 ■ *A*, This example involves a superficial femoral and three tibial arteries being occluded. A toe pressure of 20 mm Hg makes spontaneous healing of an ulcer of the second toe unlikely. *B*, After a common femoral–to–distal anterior in situ saphenous vein bypass graft the ABI is now greater than 1.0 and the great toe pressure has risen to 88 mm Hg.

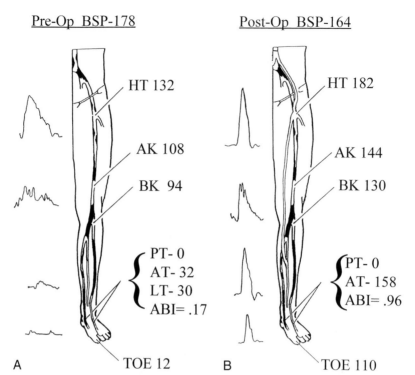

Pre-Op BSP-178

HT 132

AK 108

BK 94

PT- 0
AT- 32
LT- 30
ABI= .17

A   TOE 12

Post-Op BSP-164

HT 182

AK 144

BK 130

PT- 0
AT- 158
ABI= .96

B   TOE 110

Figure 16–6 ■ *A,* This example displays multilevel disease with occlusion of the common iliac, superficial femoral, popliteal, and anterior and posterior tibial arteries. The ABI is 0.16 and the toe pressure is 12 mm Hg. *B,* After both an aortobifemoral as well as a femoral-to-peroneal in situ saphenous vein bypass graft the ABI is now 1.0 and the toe pressure is 110 mm Hg.

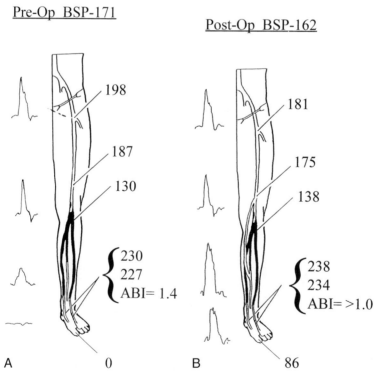

Pre-Op BSP-171

198

187

130

230
227
ABI= 1.4

A   0

Post-Op BSP-162

181

175

138

238
234
ABI= >1.0

B   86

Figure 16–7 ■ *A,* In this example, the classic pattern of distal severe occlusive arterial disease is found with total occlusion of the distal popliteal; tibial peroneal; and the proximal anterior tibial, posterior tibial, and peroneal arteries. A toe pressure of 0 mm Hg in spite of an ABI of 1.4 makes healing of severe foot ulcers unlikely. *B,* After a popliteal-to-peroneal in situ saphenous vein bypass the toe pressure is now 86 mm Hg and the ABI remains at 1.4. Total healing of the ulcers occurred within 3 weeks.

Flow and viability may exist despite absent waveforms, because the Doppler probes rarely detect flow at less than 6 mL/min. Comparing pressures with waveforms helps to avoid errors in interpretations, especially at the high thigh level.

Exercise Stress Testing

Exercise can lead to a 10- to 20-fold increase in blood flow through the peripheral arteries. As is apparent in Figure 16–8, increased flows can lower the degree of stenosis necessary to create a given drop in flow or pressure. In addition, limiting factors other than claudication are sometimes demonstrated. A standard treadmill test is done on an incline of 12 degrees at 2 mph.[1] The treadmill test is limited to a maximum of 5 minutes or the onset of chest discomfort, shortness of breath, dizziness, or severe leg pain. The cuffs placed before stress to determine the resting ankle pressure remain in place during the study. Immediately when the stress is stopped, at 2½ minutes and again at 5

minutes, ankle pressures are determined. The level of exercise necessary to validate claudication is much less than would be routinely encountered in cardiac stress testing. Nevertheless, caution is urged in patients who have coronary artery disease, and it is our policy to have a well-trained nurse or technician in attendance at all times.

In patients with recent contralateral amputations, painful infections, ulcers, digital necrosis, or recent surgery, reactive hyperemia can be induced. The high thigh pressure cuff is inflated to 50 mm Hg over the previously determined resting high thigh pressure. The patient is supine for this study and the cuff remains inflated for 3 minutes. Ankle pressures are again measured immediately after release of the high thigh pressure cuff and at 15-second intervals for 3 to 5 minutes. Figure 16–3 shows the configuration of curves obtained in this way for cases with moderate and severe arterial obstruction compared with normal individuals. Although the curves are similar in shape, note that the response is rapid with reactive hyperemia (seconds) and slow (minutes) after exercise testing.

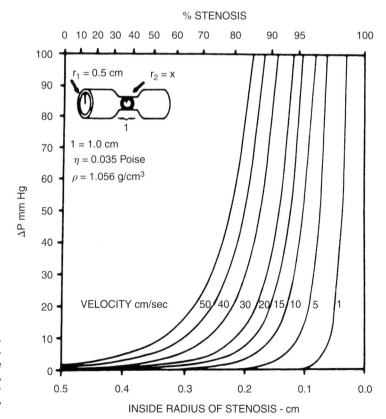

Figure 16–8 ■ Relationship of pressure drop across a stenosis to the radius of the stenotic segment and the flow velocity. (From Strandness DE, Sumner DS: Hemodynamics for Surgeons. New York: Grune & Stratton, 1975, with permission.)

Ouriel et al.[35] performed a critical evaluation of stress testing in the diagnosis of peripheral vascular disease. They studied 218 patients (372 limbs) and 25 normal subjects (50 limbs) with resting ankle index (RAI), treadmill exercise (TE), and postocclusive reactive hyperemia (PORH) to determine reliability and discrimination. They concluded that RAI was a simple, accurate, and reproducible test and that routine stress testing was not cost effective, adding little diagnostic information whether one is dealing with claudicants or patients harboring rest pain, ulceration, or gangrene. They suggested that stress testing should be reserved for the small subset of symptomatic patients with normal RAI. They also noted that walking distance was not a reproducible measure and that only a weak correlation existed between walking distance and the severity of disease as assessed by RAI.

A gradual decrease in the use of stress testing has been experienced. It nevertheless can prove useful in those situations where symptoms seemingly contradict physical findings and resting AAI. At times, other etiologies (e.g., pulmonary, cardiac, arthritic) for decreased ambulatory ability are clearly elucidated when the patient reproduces symptoms while undergoing testing.

Ankle-Toe Pressures

We reviewed the predictive value of AAIs and absolute digital systolic pressures in diabetic and nondiabetic patients. In 120 limb salvage patients, the average AAI preoperatively in diabetics was 0.53, increasing to 0.97 postoperatively, with a very wide scatter. This index appeared more reliable in nondiabetic persons: 0.34 preoperatively (Fig. 16–9A) and rising to 1.03 postoperatively, with a narrower scatter (Fig. 16–9B). Photoplethysmographically derived digital pressures (PDDPs) were much more predictable and precise in both diabetic and nondiabetic patients. In the diabetic population, only four patients demonstrated a pressure greater than 40 mm Hg preoperatively (Fig. 16–10A), whereas only five remained below this range (only one <30 mm Hg) after successful revascularization (Fig. 16–10B). More recently, McCollum et al.[28] confirmed the value of PDDP in the assessment of severe ischemia but cautioned that appropriate warming of the foot permitting adequate foot vasodilation was essential to allow accurate conclusions to be drawn and to allow meaningful interpretation of results. Appropriate testing conditions are critical to every method of noninvasive testing to be reported

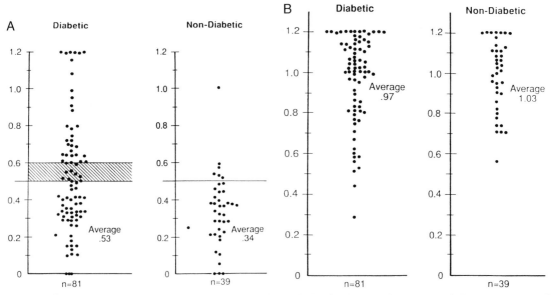

Figure 16–9 ■ A, Preoperative ankle-arm pressure indices (AAIs) display a wide range in diabetic as compared with nondiabetic patients, because of medial calcinosis of the vessels causing incompressibility. (Incompressibility >1.2 AAI recorded as 1.2.) B, Postoperative indices in nondiabetic patients display a significant change from preoperative levels. The same change to a lesser degree is seen with diabetic individuals.

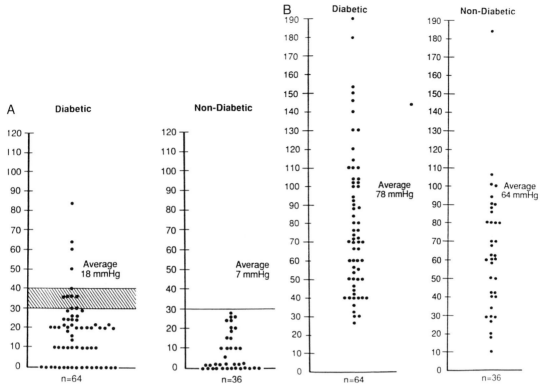

Figure 16-10 ■ *A,* Absolute toe pressure measurements obtained photoplethysmographically in preoperative diabetic and nondiabetic limb salvage patients reveal only four patients with a value >40 mm Hg in the diabetic group and none with >30 mm Hg in nondiabetic patients. *B,* Absolute photoplethysmographically obtained pressure measurements in postoperative assessment reveal three patients with values <30 mm Hg and only five patients with <40 mm Hg in the diabetic group. This degree of improvement is not observed in the nondiabetic patient.

on. Vincent et al.[43] reported on the use of PDDP toe-brachial index, noting in patients with chronic ulcerations, toe pressures were higher in diabetics than in nondiabetics. They believed that during pressure measurements attention must be directed to the patient's state of relaxation, digital skin temperature, and toe position relative to the level of the heart. They emphasized that systolic pressures fluctuated with respiration and activity (e.g., talking). Nielson[33] demonstrated that skin temperature variation from 33° to 24°C caused an average change of 10 mm Hg in toe systolic pressures secondary to changes in vasomotor tone. Finally, the same authors revealed diminished toe pressure as a result of hydrostatic forces when measurements were obtained with the patient supine.

Regional Tissue Perfusion Measurements

Efforts to improve noninvasive evaluation after ankle and toe pressure testing have centered on regional microcirculation using transcutaneous oximetry.

Tissue oxygen tension, a reflection of the adequacy of the circulatory system, is an absolute number on which a possible etiology of symptoms and the likelihood of healing can be based. The transcutaneous oxygen pressure ($TcPo_2$) monitors containing a chemical electrode are placed in a peripheral (10 cm above the knee, 5 cm below the knee, and on the dorsum of the foot) and central or reference positions (5 cm below the middle left clavicle) to obtain readings. After patients have remained supine 10 to 15 minutes to allow equilibration, readings are then obtained at 3- to 5-minute intervals with the patient standing. Accuracy in testing depends on multiple systemic (fractional concentration of oxygen in inspired gas [FIo_2], lung function, blood hemoglobin level, and cardiac output) and local (skin thickness, capillary formation and density, and the presence of inflammation or edema) factors.

The ability to discriminate severity of disease, likelihood of ulcer healing, or the appropriate amputation level was claimed for transcutaneous oximetry by Hauser et al.[16] in 1984. They employed positional changes of the foot. They derived a region perfusion index (RPI) for each limb as the ratio of foot to chest measurements $TcPo_2/TcPo_2 \times 100$. These were determined in the supine, standing, and leg-elevated positions. They found claudicants could be discerned from normal patients best with leg elevation, but with rest pain and gangrene, RPI values were quite similar in the supine and elevated positions, diverging in the dependent position. They compared transcutaneous oximetry to ankle systolic blood pressure measurements and found superiority at a statistically significant ($p < 0.001$) level. They believed regional transcutaneous oximetry to be the only noninvasive test of limb perfusion consistently accurate in diabetics.

Subsequent to attempts to use transcutaneous oximetry, the employment of laser Doppler velocimetry (LDV) alone or in conjunction with $TcPo_2$ was reported. The LDV device emits a monochromic helium-neon laser beam at a frequency of 632.8 nm that is conducted to the skin through a plastic fiberoptic probe. The basis of LDV is that a collimated beam becomes diffusely scattered, absorbed, and broadened when applied to the skin, resulting in Doppler shifts that may be detected by a sensitive photodetector. The Doppler shift is linearly related to the mean velocity of red blood cells (RBCs) within skin capillaries and varies with the angle of the probe to the tissue being monitored. Measurements reflect an average over a semisphere of skin approximately 1 mm in radius. The photo-detected reflected signal is fed into an analog signal processor, and values are expressed in millivolts. The normal LDV tracing is fairly characteristic, whereas ischemic tissues generate pulse waves of lesser magnitude and amplitude. Kram et al.[23] performed LDV measurements in 29 patients (16 diabetic individuals) before they underwent below-knee amputations. Anterior and posterior calf LDV values greater than or equal to 20 mV were associated with successful below-knee amputation wound healing in 25 of 26 patients; all three patients with either anterior or posterior calf LDV values less than 20 mV had below-knee amputations that failed to heal. Karanfilian et al.[21] combined $TcPo_2$ and LDV measurements in predicting healing of ischemic forefoot ulcerations and amputa-

tions in diabetic and nondiabetic patients. Fifty-nine limbs, 63% of which were nondiabetic patients, were studied. Either transmetatarsal amputation or debridement with or without skin grafting was performed. Criteria for successful healing included a $TcPo_2$ value of more than 10 mm Hg, laser Doppler pulse wave amplitude of more than 4 mV, and an ankle systolic pressure of more than 30 mm Hg. With these criteria, the outcome was predicted correctly in 53 of 56 limbs (95%) by $TcPo_2$, in 46 of 53 limbs (87%) with LDV, and in 31 of 59 limbs (52.5%) with Doppler ankle pressures. They concluded that the estimation of skin blood flow by the $TcPo_2$ and LDV is significantly better than Doppler ankle pressure measurements in predicting the healing of forefoot ulcerations and amputations in diabetic and nondiabetic patients.

More recently, Bacharach et al.[2] at the Mayo Clinic looked at $TcPo_2$ to predict amputation site healing in lower limbs with arterial occlusive disease. Fifty-eight percent of their patients had diabetes and testing was obtained with accurate calibration of the equipment in the supine and limb elevated modes. They found that a $TcPo_2$ value greater than or equal to 40 mm Hg was associated with primary or delayed healing in 50 of 52 limbs (98%), and a $TcPo_2$ value of less than 20 mm Hg was universally associated with failure. Measurement of $TcPo_2$ during limb evaluation improved predictability in limbs with borderline supine $TcPo_2$ values.[2]

Sheffer and Rieger[39] looked at the role of oxygen inhalation and leg dependency in predicting the need for revascularization or the likelihood of successful amputation. While they did not discriminate results based on the presence or absence of diabetes, one third of the patients were diabetic. Satisfactory results were achieved by combining limits for, first, supine (10 mm Hg) and sitting (45 mm Hg) $TcPo_2$; as well as, second, ankle arterial pressure (60 mm Hg) and supine $TcPo_2$ (10 mm Hg). Oxygen inhalation proved to be of no significant help.

Duplex Scanning of Peripheral Arterial Tree

Duplex scanning combines B-mode capabilities of revealing the anatomic situation and the Doppler-derived velocity recordings, indicating the degree of vessel lumen stenosis.

Gating the Doppler signal on the B-mode imagery allows the arterial blood flow to be analyzed at selective levels within the lumen, as well as at progressive sites along the vessel course. Introduction of color imaging has greatly aided the interrogation of vessels, allowing easier, more rapid identification of high-flow (hence, stenotic) areas. Duplex imaging requires the use of probes capable of deeper insonation, such as 2.25- and 3.5-MHz as well as 5- and 8-MHz heads, for more shallowly placed vessels. Low-megahertz, high-penetrance probes are necessary for interrogation of vessels deep in obese patients. These studies are significantly impeded by increased depth of penetration needed, bone, intestinal gas, and cutaneous problems, preventing the direct application of the probes. Duplex imaging, much like arteriograms, can give the anatomic assessment of the arterial tree, as well as the severity of multiple areas of stenosis, but fail to give a bottom-line evaluation of the severity of distal ischemia. Hence, this study is an adjunct but realistically cannot stand alone in determining the severity of ischemia in the lower limbs.

Moneta et al.[31] discussed the accuracy of lower limb arterial duplex mapping (LLADM) from the aortic bifurcation to the ankle in 150 consecutive patients. They compared the noninvasive results to angiography in a standard fashion. The LLADM visualized 99% of arterial segments proximal to the tibial vessels, with overall sensitivities for detecting a 50% or greater lesion ranging from 89% in the iliac vessels to 67% at the popliteal artery. Stenosis was successfully distinguished from occlusion in 98% of cases. In the tibial vessels, LLADM was better at visualizing anterior tibial and posterior tibial arterial segments (94% and 96%) than peroneal artery segments (83%) ($p < 0.001$).

In a study from the Netherlands,[22] a meta-analysis of 16 studies compared duplex ultrasonography versus angiography in detection of a stenosis of greater than or equal to 50% or occlusion in the lower arterial tree. Pooled estimates of the above ability in the aortoiliac tract were 86% (80 to 91%) sensitivity and 97% (95 to 99%) specificity. The results for the femoropopliteal tract compared with this, with a sensitivity of 80% (74 to 85%) and a specificity of 98% (94 to 98%). The accuracy of detection of a stenosis greater than or equal to 50% or an occlusion in the infrageniculate vessels was lower with a sensitivity of 83% (59 to 96%) and a specificity of 84% (69 to 93%).

Another European study comparing digital subtraction angiography with color duplex sonography in determining the dominant distal lower leg arterial segment suitable for femorocrural bypass surgery in patients with femoropopliteal occlusions was not as favorable.[26] While they were able to determine the presence of a hemodynamically relevant arterial lesion (100% in the posterior tibial artery, 78% in the anterior tibial artery, and 92% in the peroneal artery), it could not replace an accurate preoperative angiogram for the routine clinical practice. They concluded that color flow Doppler was limited in the accurate judgment of the morphologic features of the runoff arteries in their full length in patients with LEAD. They felt it might play a role in special circumstances such as history of impaired renal function or history of contrast allergy.

Lai et al.[24] found similar results comparing color duplex ultrasonography (CDS) to angiography but did suggest that the high negative predictive value of CDS may be used in excluding hemodynamically significant disease. This approach in high-risk patients, where the potential for significant morbidity and even mortality with angiography is present, should be considered. Unfortunately, with increased incidence of vessel calcification in diabetic individuals, even this use would be less accurate.

We have in the past, however, made use of CDS of the iliac vessels to determine an actual pressure gradient. Using the modified Bernoulli equation ($P = 4V_{max}$), a pressure gradient can be calculated.[25] Close correlation with arterial pull-through pressures obtained at the time of angiography is established. In those circumstances where interpretation of the significance of angiography findings is in question, a gradient of 30 mm Hg alerts the interpreter to the fact that a significant stenosis does in fact exist. Percutaneous transluminal angioplasty or correction at the time of a surgical procedure can be performed.

Magnetic Resonance Flowmetry

As additional studies accumulate, the role of magnetic resonance angiography (MRA) in evaluating LEAD and revascularization potential becomes clearer. A relative newcomer in the noninvasive arena, beginning development in 1979 and with the first commercial units appearing in 1984, it is proving reliable in comparison to contrast angiography. Basic units included a 0.1 tesla filled producing magnet, weighing 5,300 lb in an electric or magnetic shielded work environment. Temperature control between 17.8° and 29°C is critical. Any patient having a significant metal implant, including hip prosthesis and cardiac pacemaker, are excluded. Huber et al.[18] evaluated the ability of magnetic resonance arteriography for distal lower extremity revascularization. In a comparison study of preoperative contrast angiography and intraoperative angiography (IOA), they found the combination of MRA and IOA provided an accurate, cost-effective, and potentially safer strategy for visualization of the infrageniculate vessels before revascularization procedures. A similar though slightly less enthusiastic evaluation of MRA versus contrast angiography (CA) was provided by Cambria et al.[10] in a prospective study. They felt MRA and CA were nearly equivalent examinations in the demonstration of infrainguinal vascular anatomy. Inability of MRA to assess the significance of inflow disease and inadequate detail of tibial/pedal vessels were the principal deficiencies. Again, consideration of this technique in specific circumstances where CA is more risky may be worthwhile. Further discussion of MRA in this volume can be found in Chapter 17. This modality bridges noninvasive CDS and CA and, as such, is mentioned briefly in this chapter.

Peripheral Noninvasive Investigation

Two questions are raised with regard to noninvasive evaluation in diabetic patients. First, which patients should undergo these studies? Second, which studies should be employed in these investigations? A set of guidelines developed by an international workshop addressed the first question, whereas the second requires understanding of the effectiveness, cost, and effort required of each study.

At an international meeting addressing the assessment of peripheral vascular disease in diabetics, the following recommendations for the detection and follow-up of lower extremity arterial occlusive disease

(LEAOD) in diabetic subjects being seen in a primary care setting were made.[34] The first criterion is claudication. On an annual basis diabetic patients should be asked about the presence of exercise-induced calf leg pain not present at rest. Patients with lifestyle-limiting, exercise-induced calf pain should be referred to a specialist, a vascular laboratory, or both for special vascular assessment (SVA). Second, the presence of any potential signs of critical ischemia (i.e., foot or limb ulceration), the presence of skin changes (nail or skin atrophy or dependent rubor), or the detection of gangrene should lead to a referral for SVA. Third, palpation of the dorsalis pedis or posterior tibial pulses should be performed on an annual basis for all adult (>18 years old) diabetic patients. An absent or diminished pedal pulse is an indication for performing an ankle-brachial index (ABI) or referral to a vascular laboratory for evaluation if an ABI cannot be determined by the primary care physician. It is further recommended that, whenever possible, the presence of diminished or absent pulses be confirmed by a second observer or repeat examination before referral. Fourth, auscultation for femoral bruits on an annual basis is recommended for all adult diabetic patients. The detection of femoral bruits is an indication for performing an ABI or, if not available, referral to a vascular laboratory. Furthermore, it is recommended that all physician offices providing routine care to adult diabetic patients should be able to measure ankle-brachial blood pressures to detect LEAOD. Additional recommendations for obtaining an ABI are: any diabetic patient who has newly detected diminished pulses, femoral bruits, or a foot ulcer; any diabetic patient with leg pain of unknown etiology; at baseline examination in all IDDM patients greater than 35 years of age or with greater than 20 years' duration of diabetes; and at baseline examination in all type 2 patients greater than 40 years old. Follow-up for ABI greater than 0.9 are every 2 to 3 years; 0.5 to 0.9 every 3 to 4 months; and less than 0.5 referral to a vascular specialist, vascular laboratory, or both. If an incompressible artery with an ankle pressure greater than 300 mm Hg or ankle pressure 75 mm Hg above arm pressure is found, repeat in 3 months. If still present, refer these patients for SVA.

The foregoing has answered which patients should be evaluated, even suggesting the initial test. While the ABI is easy and inexpensive to perform, it lacks the ability to allow a more specific assessment of the severity of LEAOD. This leads to the question of what is the best noninvasive study to employ in investigating LEAOD in diabetic subjects? The study employed depends upon the clinical circumstances of the patient. Assessing hemodynamically significant iliac artery stenosis versus the likelihood of digital amputation success are two vastly different situations requiring different noninvasive procedures. Overall, severity of LEAOD can be determined with TSP or $TcPo_2$ assessment, which helps determine the greatest likelihood of healing ulcers, or success in digital amputations without concomitant limb revascularization. Normally CDS, segmental pressure measurements, or exercise testing can give reliable information on iliac and femoral popliteal arterial occlusive disease, discerning stenosis from occlusion as well as assessing collateral circulation and location of the lesions. In certain circumstances (contrast dye allergy, renal artery insufficiency), CDS or MRA may supplant CA in preoperative assessment. They may also prove useful in evaluating ambiguous CA results.

Careful attention to testing conditions, including ambient temperature, patient's state of relaxation, and limb positioning, coupled with experienced application of noninvasive techniques, is critical for most of these noninvasive studies. Likewise, physician understanding of the limitations of these noninvasive studies is necessary for applying the results to clinical situations. Unrecognized ischemia occurs for two reasons: patient error or physician error. Patient error centers around physical findings often in hard to examine areas (plantar surface, heel, interdigital spaces) or where significant tissue damage is obscured by severe peripheral neuropathy as discussed by Pfeifer.[36] Diabetic retinopathy can frequently deprive the patient of their backup sense of vision. Reliance upon spouse, family member, or friend on a regular basis to examine the feet is recommended in this situation.

Physician error can stem from inappropriate interpretation of noninvasive testing as a result of a lack of knowledge in their limitation. Most often near normal or extremely high ankle pressures are equated with no risk of distal ischemia. As you should be aware by now and to be demonstrated in the examples, extremely high ABIs can be associated with limb-threatening ischemia. Secondly, diabetic individuals deserve a methodical examination of their feet to include the interdigital spaces, plantar surface, and heels of both feet with every visit. The Foot Council of the American Diabetes Association reminds all physicians to remove the shoes and socks of all diabetic patients and inspect the feet whenever they are seen in consultation. To this wise admonition should be added, also understand the applications and limitations of noninvasive testing.

Summary

The enormous cost of diabetic foot problems has been aptly described in preceding chapters. Prevention and early detection of LEAOD should be the cornerstone in managing diabetic foot lesions. Correct application and reliability of noninvasive testing has been described. Examples of common clinical situations and the noninvasive test findings illustrate the vagaries in the evaluation and management of these problems. These examples, while straightforward, illustrate the essence of LEAOD in diabetic subjects and should be understood. The greater question involves the implication for progressive LEAOD and mortality associated with the finding of significant arterial lesions in diabetic subjects. Clearly, this group of patients requires careful, frequent, and methodical following, which is often aided by use and understanding of noninvasive testing. It is hoped that to that end, this chapter will prove beneficial to all who have read it.

REFERENCES

1. Ad Hoc Committee on Reporting Standards, Society for Vascular Surgery, North American Chapter. International Society for Cardiovascular Surgery: Suggested standard for reports dealing with lower extremity ischemia. J Vasc Surg 4:80, 1986.
2. Bacharach JM, Rooke TW, Osmundson PJ, Gloviczki P: Predictive value of transcutaneous oxygen pressure and amputation success by use of supine and elevation measurements. J Vasc Surg 15:558–563, 1992.
3. Baker WH, Barnes RW: Minor forefoot amputation in patients with low ankle pressure. Am J Surg 133:331, 1977.

4. Barnes RW, Thornhill B, Nix L, et al: Prediction of amputation wound healing. Arch Surg 116:80, 1981.
5. Beach KW, Bedford GR, Bergelin RO, et al: Progression of lower extremity arterial occlusive disease in type II diabetes mellitus. Diabetes Care 11: 464–472, 1988.
6. Bendick PJ, Glover JL, Kuebler TW, et al: Progression of atherosclerosis in diabetes. Surgery 93: 834, 1983.
7. Bone GE, Pomajzl MJ: Toe blood pressure by photoplethysmography: An index of healing in forefoot amputations. Surgery 16:834, 1983.
8. Bowers BL, Valentine RJ, Myers SI, et al: The natural history of patients with claudication with toe pressures of 40 mmHg or less. J Vasc Surg 18:506–511, 1993.
9. Boyko EJ, Ahroni JH, Davingnon D, et al: Diagnostic utility of the history and physical examination for peripheral vascular disease among patients with diabetes mellitus. J Clin Epidemiol 50:659–668, 1997.
10. Cambria RP, Kaufman JA, L'Italien GL, et al: Magnetic resonance angiography in the management of lower extremity arterial occlusive disease: A prospective study. J Vasc Surg 25:389–389, 1997.
11. Carter SA, Tate RB: Value of toe pulse waves in addition to systolic pressures in the assessment of the severity of peripheral arterial disease and critical limb ischemia. J Vasc Surg 24:258–265, 1996.
12. Criqui MH, Langer RD, Fronek A, et al: Mortality over a period of 10 years in patients with peripheral arterial disease. N Engl J Med 326:381–386, 1992.
13. DeFrang RD, Taylor LM, Porter JM: Basic data related to amputations: Basic data underlying clinical decision-making in vascular surgery. Ann Vasc Surg 2:62, 1988.
14. Duj JJ, Jimes RA: The role of diabetes in the development of degenerative vascular disease: With special reference to the incidence of retinitis and peripheral vasculitis. Assn Intern Med 14:1902, 1941.
15. Gibbons GW, Wheeloch FC, Siembreda C, et al: Noninvasive predictions of amputation level in diabetic patients. Arch Surg 114:1253, 1979.
16. Hauser CJ, Klein SR, Hehringer CM, et al: Superiority of transcutaneous oximetry in noninvasive vascular diagnosis in patients with diabetes. Arch Surg 119:690, 1984.
17. Holstein P, Noer I, Tonneses KH, et al: Distal blood pressure in severe arterial insufficiency. In Bergan J, Yao J (eds): Gangrene and Severe Ischemia of the Lower Extremities. New York: Grune & Stratton, 1978.
18. Huber TS, Back MR, Ballinger RJ, et al: Utility of magnetic resonance arteriography for distal lower extremity revascularization. J Vasc Surg 26:415–424. 1997.
19. Hurley JJ, Auer AI, Hershey FB, et al: Distal arterial reconstruction: Patency and limb salvage in diabetics. J Vasc Surg 5:796, 1987.
20. Jonason T, Ruggvist I: Diabetes mellitus and intermittent claudication: Relation between peripheral vascular complications and location of the occlusive atherosclerosis. Acta Med Scand 218:217, 1985.
21. Karanfilian RG, Lynch TG, Zirul VT, et al: The value of laser Doppler velocimetry and transcutaneous oxygen tension determination in predicting healing of ischemic forefoot ulcerations and amputations in diabetics. J Vasc Surg 4:511, 1986.
22. Koelemay MJW, denHarlog D, Prins MH, et al: Diagnosis of arterial disease of the lower extremities with duplex ultrasonography. Br J Surg 83:404, 1996.
23. Karm HB, Appel PL, Shoemaker WC: Prediction of below-knee amputation wound healing using noninvasive laser Doppler velocimetry. Am J Surg 158:29, 1989.
24. Lai DTM, Glassont R, Grayndler V, et al: Colour duplex ultrasonography versus angiography in the diagnosis of lower extremity arterial disease. Cardiovasc Surg 4:384–388, 1996.
25. Langsfeld M, Nepute J, Binnington HB, et al: The use of deep duplex scanning to predict hemodynamically significant aorto-iliac stenosis. J Vasc Surg 7:395, 1988.
26. Larch E, Minar E, Ahmadi R, et al: Value of color duplex sonography for evaluation of tibioperoneal arteries in patients with femoropopliteal obstruction: A prospective comparison with antegrade intraarterial digital subtraction angiography. J Vasc Surg 25:629, 1997.
27. Marinelli MR, Beath KW, Glass MJ, et al: Noninvasive testing vs. clinical evaluation of arterial disease: A prospective study. JAMA 241:2031, 1979.
28. McCollum PT, Stanley ST, Kent P, et al: Assessment of arterial disease using digital systolic pressure measurements. Ann Vasc Surg 5:349, 1991.
29. McDaniel MD, Cronenwett JL: Basic data underlying history of intermittent claudication: Basic data underlying clinical decision making in vascular surgery. Ann Vasc Surg 2:1, 1988.
30. Mehta K, Hobson RW, Jamil Z, et al: Fallibility of Doppler ankle pressures in predicting healing of transmetatarsal amputations. J Surg Res 28:466, 1980.
31. Moneta GL, Yearger RA, Antonovic R, et al: Accuracy of lower extremity arterial duplex mapping. J Vasc Surg 5:275, 1991.
32. Moore WS, Malone JM: Effect of flow rate and vessel caliber on clinical arterial stenosis. J Surg Res 26:1, 1979.
33. Nielson PE: Digital blood pressure in normal subjects and patients with peripheral arterial disease. Scand J Clin Lab Invest 36:731, 1976.
34. Orchard TJ, Strandness DE: Assessment of peripheral vascular disease in diabetes. Diabetes Care 16:1199–1209, 1993.
35. Ouriel K, McDonnell AE, Metz CE, et al: A critical evaluation of stress testing in the diagnosis of peripheral vascular disease. Surgery 91:686. 1982.
36. Pfeifer M, Green D: Neuropathy in the diabetic foot: New concepts in etiology and treatment. In Bowker JH, Pfeifer M (eds): The Diabetic Foot, 6th ed. Philadelphia: WB Saunders Company, 2000.
37. Reunanen A, Takkuneu H, Aromaa A: Prevalence of intermittent claudication and its effects on mortality. Acta Med Scand 211:249, 1982.
38. Rosenblood MS, Flanigan DP, Schuler JJ, et at: Risk factors affecting the natural history of intermittent claudication. Arch Surg 123:867, 1988.
39. Sheffer A, Rieger H: A comparative analysis of transcutaneous oximetry (TcP$_{o_2}$) during oxygen inhalation and leg dependency in severe peripheral

arterial occlusive disease. J Vasc Surg 16:218–224, 1992.
40. Strandness DE: Abnormal exercise response after successful reconstructive arterial surgery. Surgery 59:325, 1966.
41. Strandness DE, Bell IW: An evaluation of the hemodynamic response of the claudicating extremity to exercise. Surg Gynecol Obstet 59:325, 1966.
42. Strandness DE, Priest RE, Gibbons GE: Combined clinical and pathologic study of diabetic and non diabetic peripheral arterial disease. Diabetes 13:366, 1964.
43. Vincent DG, Salles-Cunha SX, Bernnhard VM, et al: Noninvasive assessment of toe systolic pressures with special reference to diabetes mellitus. J Cardiovasc Surg 24:22, 1983.

Chapter 17

RADIOLOGIC INTERVENTION IN DIABETIC PERIPHERAL VASCULAR DISEASE

■ Karl S. Chiang and Michael D. Tripp

Peripheral vascular disease (PVD) is a significant complication in diabetic patients and occurs twice as frequently as in the general population. Fifty percent of all nontraumatic amputations in the United States are related to vascular complications of diabetes.[12] Despite advances in improved surveillance and management, the incidence of the disease continues to increase steadily at 3% annually,[11] creating greater numbers of patients with vascular complications requiring ongoing medical care. Clearly, emphasis should continue on the prevention of the complications. The vascular interventional radiologist plays an integral role in the continuity of care in these patients by diminishing the consequences of existing vascular complications.[12]

Peripheral vascular imaging allows for accurate assessment of hemodynamically significant vascular disease and serves as a guide for planning appropriate therapy. The experienced vascular radiologist is then better able to help triage the patient for either percutaneous interventional revascularization and/or surgical bypass revascularization.

Angiography and Contrast Agents

Angiography is the "gold standard" for assessment of the diabetic patient with peripheral vascular disease. The primary emphasis of this discussion will be the performance of diagnostic angiography and related intervention (i.e., percutaneous revascularization and minimally invasive therapy).

The financial pressure of managed health care has dictated a shift from costly inpatient service to cost-effective outpatient therapy. Interventional radiology has led the transition, allowing complex procedures to be performed under conscious sedation requiring only a short convalescence. Our practice reflects these changes and now consists of 70% outpatients compared to 90% inpatients during the late 1980s. Neither safety nor quality of patient care has been sacrificed to accomplish this change.

Safe performance of diagnostic angiography and interventions requires a thorough review of the patient's condition. The combination of appropriate laboratory analysis, noninvasive studies, and physical examination allows for a tailored approach to the individual patient. Patients with diabetes should have a comprehensive evaluation, due to the significant incidence of comorbid disease, to anticipate and avoid complications.

A team approach is important during the performance of minimally invasive therapy to fully utilize the special talents of not only the physician, but also the radiologic technical and nursing staffs. The physician benefits in several ways: from double checking of adverse reactions, from the reassurance to the patient, and from assistance during conscious sedation or resuscitation if it should become necessary. Secondary benefits include optimal safety, diminished risks, and a grateful patient.

The nurses' responsibilities serve as an example of the characteristic team player. A certified radiologic nurse assesses the patient, ensures adequate intravenous access for hydration, reassures the patient, provides conscious sedation, and constantly updates the physician on the patient's status. Physiologic monitoring is one of the most vital functions in the modern angiographic suite. Up-to-the-minute data on vital signs, oxygen saturation, and cardiac rhythm are important to avoid untoward events.

Special attention should be given to hemodynamic monitoring during the procedures (also performed by the nurse), which allows the radiologist to determine which diseased segment of vasculature is significant and also serves as an affirmation of successful intervention.

Frequent additions to the team include the nephrologist and vascular surgeon, both of whom provide valuable consultation and appropriate backup. This ensures comprehensive evaluation and safety for the patient and promotes optimal patient care. Timely consultation also expedites same-day patient care.

Due to advances in technology, film screen angiography has largely been replaced by digital subtraction angiography (DSA)[17] (Fig. 17–1). DSA provides superior contrast resolution, rapid data archiving, and shorter exam time, while avoiding many technical problems associated with film screen systems. DSA also provides the capability of postprocessing data once the patient has left the exam room. The goal is to achieve the optimum visualization of the symptomatic vessels, maximize the guidance for minimally invasive therapy, and use the least amount of contrast. Digital subtraction angiography fulfills all these requirements. It is no coincidence that many of the advances in minimally invasive therapy and interventional radiology occurred concomitantly with digital angiography.

Research and development in interventional radiology has targeted the equipment used in vivo in patients to accomplish minimally invasive therapy: catheters in all shapes and sizes, balloon and stent develop-

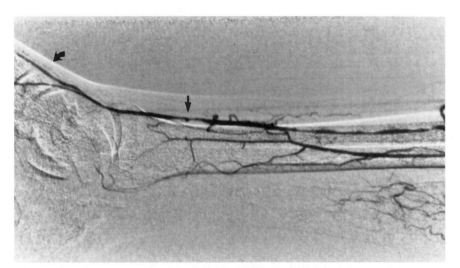

Figure 17–1 ■ Digital subtraction angiography (DSA). Diabetic patient with posterior tibial occulusion and severe anterior tibial stenosis distally (*straight arrow*), but with a patent dorsalis pedis artery (*curved arrow*). DSA images are more conspicuous than ordinary film angiography (see Fig. 17–19).

ment, and steerable guidewires with slippery hydrophilic coatings. Advances have also been made in contrast media, which is fundamental to the production of radiographic images.

The nephrotoxicity of iodinated contrast, particularly in diabetic patients, has compelled research into contrast media. Currently, iodinated contrast is the most widely used form in angiography. Contrast media–associated nephrotoxicity (CM-AN) is an unusual event in the absence of a predisposing condition. However, CM-AN is of great concern in diabetics, particularly when associated with renal insufficiency. Several recent articles emphasize the importance of prophylaxis to prevent CM-AN.[2, 31, 33, 39] The pathogenesis occurs at the microscopic level with endothelial cell dysfunction and the release of various mediators including endothelin.[24]

Preprocedural hydration is one of the most important factors in prophylaxis of CM-AN. A recent controlled trial was completed in high-risk patients undergoing coronary angiography.[33] In this trial, low-osmolality contrast media (LOCM) was shown to be superior to higher osmolality contrast media (HOCM) in patients with diabetes, both with and without azotemia. LOCM is superior to mannitol and Lasix, which have been utilized for this purpose.[2] Though not widely utilized, theophylline has been proposed for prophylaxis of CM-AN.[16]

Special consideration should be given to diabetic patients on metformin (Glucophage). The drug, produced by Bristol-Myers-Squibb (Princeton, NJ), originally came with the package insert requiring cessation for 48 hours before and after the use of iodinated contrast media. This was felt to be indicated due to an unusual occurrence of lactic acidosis that could be fatal. Due to its short half-life (6 hours) and wider acceptance, the insert has been revised. The current recommendation is to stop metformin on the day of the exam, thus avoiding unnecessary delays in procedures. The drug can be restarted in 48 hours if the renal function is normal.

Development of innovative contrast agents that are not associated with nephrotoxicity continues. Carbon dioxide[20] and gadopentetate[18] have been advocated in patients with renal insufficiency. These have been shown to be safe and effective and require special imaging techniques, reiterating the utility of digital angiography.

Newer Imaging Techniques

Technical refinements in ultrasound, computed tomography (CT), and magnetic resonance imaging (MRI) allow noninvasive modalities to play an expanded clinical role in the evaluation of peripheral vascular disease. In addition to standard Doppler arterial exams performed in vascular laboratories, radiologists now have focused duplex ultrasound scanning to evaluate specific arterial segments to determine the type and severity of disease. Duplex color flow ultrasound is frequently used to diagnose aneurysms in femoral and popliteal arteries. Duplex ultrasound surveillance of distal bypass grafts is highly sensitive to abnormalities that might lead to graft thrombosis.[14] The marriage of ultrasound transducers to catheters has created a completely new modality, intravascular ultrasound (IVUS), which can evaluate vessels "from inside out." IVUS makes precise vessel measurements, determines percentage of stenosis, confirms dissections, evaluates vessel walls and plaques, and diagnoses uncommon entities such as cystic adventitial disease.[28] IVUS may have an adjunctive role in complex endovascular interventions involving angioplasty, stents, and stent-grafts[28] (Fig. 17–2).

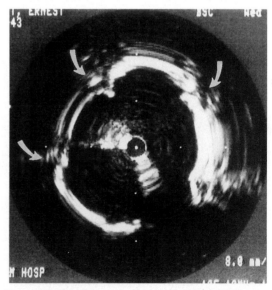

Figure 17–2 ■ Intravascular ultrasound (IVUS) cross-section of a stent-graft as seen with IVUS. Graft material is echogenic along the periphery; stent struts cause shadowing (*arrows*).

Spiral CT has replaced conventional CT imaging in most hospitals. One advantage, besides the speed of scanning, is its ability to generate three-dimensional (3-D) images from the overlapping transaxial images. CT arteriography (CTA) is an important application of the 3-D capabilities of spiral CT and is most useful in large arteries such as the thoracic or abdominal aorta in the evaluation of aneurysmal disease (Fig. 17–3). Disadvantages include the intravascular administration of iodinated contrast and the inability to accurately assess small vessel disease.[30] Immediate applications are very limited in smaller leg arteries infrainguinally.

The most important imaging development of this decade is the introduction of magnetic resonance angiography (MRA). MRA has been extensively evaluated in the extra- and intracranial cerebral circulation, but has been vastly ignored in the peripheral arterial circulation until recently. This bias was based on the notion that MRA was impractical and fraught with artifacts, and inferior to the gold standard for peripheral imaging, which was contrast angiography. Contrast angiography, though usually a benign procedure with qualified operators, does carry a significant morbidity rate of about 3% in older patients with severe peripheral vascular disease.[9] The potential complications include puncture site thrombosis, pseudoaneurysms, arteriovenous fistulae, dissections, contrast-induced renal failure, and allergic reactions. Despite the high degree of sensitivity, DSA contrast angiography (CA) may fail to opacify distal peripheral arteries, especially when advanced PVD is present, as seen in diabetics who might otherwise be candidates for distal vascular bypass.[26] Additionally, CA may be anxiety provoking and is sometimes avoided by some patients due to its invasive nature,[34] and also requires either outpatient or inpatient convalescent bedrest.

In light of these factors, a simple, quick, noninvasive, nonrenal toxic, relatively inexpensive test would be a logical replacement for CA as a screening exam. In the near future, MRA may be a primary imaging exam for peripheral vascular disease, with CA reserved for percutaneous interventions and equivocal findings.[29] Patients with severe occlusive disease who are not candidates for percutaneous revascularization may directly proceed to vascular bypass surgery after MRA[6] (Fig. 17–4). MRA may be very sensitive in identifying distal pedal arteries for surgical bypass in diabetics with tibial occlusions[6, 7] (Fig. 17–5).

Originally, peripheral MRA employed 2-D time-of-flight technique, which allowed flowing blood to be a natural contrast agent in the background suppressed by repeated, frequent radiofrequency pulses.[19] Unfortunately, the complexity of acquisition and interpretation and the long examination time prevented widespread acceptance until the recent introduction of gadolinium (Gd) as a positive contrast agent. Further refinements in technique, namely, bolus chasing with the patient moving during the exam, dynamic Gd injection, and digital subtraction which resembles DSA CA, have decreased scanning time to less than 4 minutes currently[13]

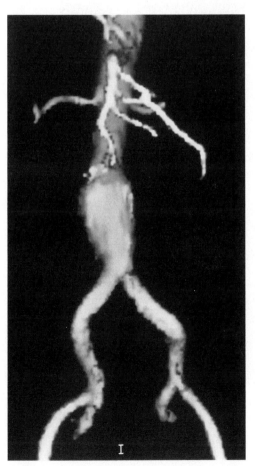

Figure 17–3 ■ 3-D CT angiography. 3-D reconstruction images of an abdominal aortic aneurysm with visualization of the superior mesenteric and renal arteries.

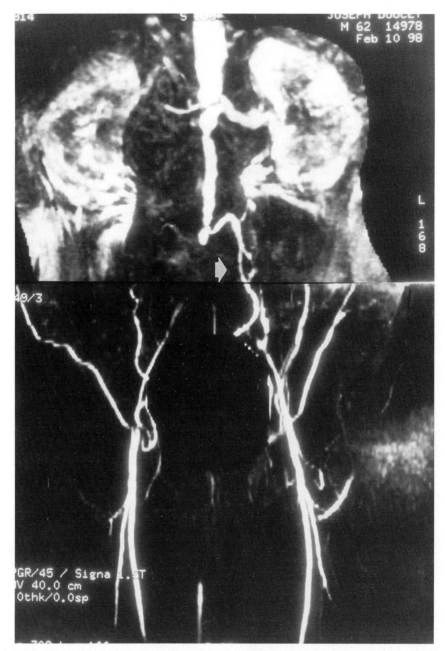

Figure 17–4 ■ Magnetic resonance angiography (MRA). 3-D MRA with gadolinium enhancement shows bilateral common iliac occlusions with collaterals (*arrow*).

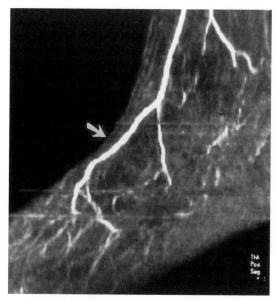

Figure 17–5 ■ MRA of foot. 2-D TOF MRA demonstrates a patent dorsalis pedis artery (*arrow*), which is a possible bypass artery.

(Fig. 17–6). Peripheral MRA exams may be commonplace in the future high-field MRI units when peripheral hardware and software packages become readily available.

A General Overview of Vascular Intervention

Percutaneous transluminal angioplasty (PTA) is the standard for interventional revascularization treatment of vascular disease. PTA was first introduced in 1964 by Dr. Charles Dotter, who used dilators to serially increase the diameter of the lumen of narrowed atherosclerotic arteries.[8] In 1978, Dr. Andreas Gruntzig developed the modern-day balloon catheter (Fig. 17–7), which could be inflated to predetermined pressures and diameters.[10] Further refinements have allowed smaller balloon catheters to be used in very small vessels such as the coronary arteries and in the tibial arteries. The exponential growth of PTA procedures is due in part to the demonstrated safety and medical benefit to patients with atherosclerotic disease. PTA, as compared to surgery, is minimally invasive, and not only reduces morbidity, mortality, and length of hospital stay, but also preserves saphenous veins for possible distal extremity or coronary artery bypass at a later date. Even though the most common

indication is severe claudication, PTA is also used as an adjunct to distal revascularization bypasses to improve inflow and as a limb-salvaging procedure in nonsurgical situations. Generally, PTA is performed by qualified vascular interventional radiologists with surgical backup. Consultation with the referring physician and the patient's informed consent are standard before PTA is per-

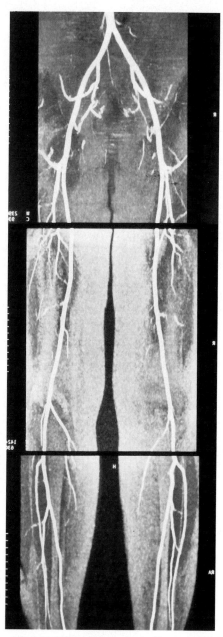

Figure 17–6 ■ MRA of lower limb. Dynamic Gd-MRA gives good visualization of all the patent leg arteries in a normal patient.

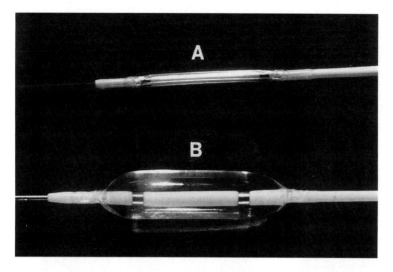

Figure 17–7 ■ Angioplasty balloon catheters. Typical 5-Fr angioplasty balloons in closed (*A*) and open (*B*) configurations. Metallic marker bands delineate the length of the balloons.

formed. Adequate angiographic assessment before angioplasty will help determine the balloon catheter size and length. As a rule, a 50% diameter stenosis corresponds to a 75 to 80% area stenosis and is probably hemodynamically significant.[36] Angioplasty can be performed after placement of a femoral sheath and administration of a bolus of 3,000 to 5,000 units of heparin. After a guidewire is used to traverse the lesion, a balloon catheter is inflated across the lesion for 30 to 60 seconds from 5 to 12 atm, usually two to three times until the stenotic "waist" disappears (Fig. 17–8). Actual technique is very opera-

tor and situation dependent. A follow-up angiogram should not reveal a residual stenosis of greater than 30% or a resting systolic pressure gradient greater than 10 mm Hg.[36] The lesion is usually slightly overdilated, approximately 10 to 20%, but this is not recommended for large vessels such as the aorta, which may rupture.[5] Postangioplasty recuperation is usually 8 hours of bedrest and patients are placed on low-dose aspirin daily afterward.

The mechanisms of angioplasty-induced vessel wall enlargement are actually complex. It is speculated that there is plaque

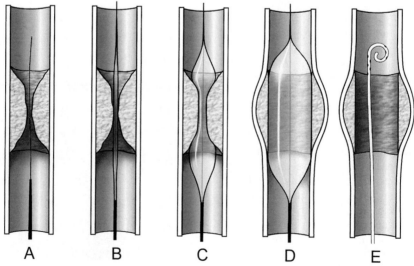

Figure 17–8 ■ Diagram of angioplasty technique. *A*, Wire traverses stenosis. *B*, Balloon catheter is positioned within lesion over wire. *C*, Balloon expanding with "waist" outlining the stenotic lesion. *D*, Balloon fully inflated. *E*, Postangioplasty result with enlarged lumen.

compression and fracture with localized wall dissection and concomitant arterial wall stretching[36] (Fig. 17–9). In essence, PTA is a controlled injury to the diseased vessel wall which then heals and remodels, but with a larger lumen. However, excessive repair (intimal hyperplasia) can again narrow the lumen within months and cause late PTA failure.[36] However, dissection, thrombosis, spasm, and vessel recoil can cause acute PTA failure or suboptimal results.[36]

Predictors of angioplasty success are dependent on the morphology and character of stenotic lesions. As a general rule, short, concentric, nonstial, noncalcified lesions respond best to angioplasty. Long, occluded, heavily calcified, eccentric, ostial lesions have lower primary patency rates with angioplasty alone.[5]

With the advent of endovascular stents, approximately 10 years ago, suboptimal angioplasty can now be treated with a metal "buttress" (Fig. 17–10). Lesions with severe dissections or significant residual stenosis after angioplasty would be ideal stent candidates. The Palmaz stent (Fig. 17–11) was the first endovascular stent approved for use in the iliac arteries.[27] The Palmaz stent is a single stainless steel tube with etched rectangular slots cut out which is deployed by balloon expansion. It has high radial outward strength, but can crimp. The newer and longer versions are somewhat flexible (Fig. 17–11). The Wallstent (Fig. 17–12) also has recently been approved by the Food and Drug Administration (FDA) for use in the iliac arteries.[21] The Wallstent differs from the Palmaz stent in that it is self-expanding, very flexible, and also comes in many lengths and predetermined diameters. Newer nitinol stents are being evaluated clinically. Covered stents (Fig. 17–11) are being evaluated with the hope that they will more closely mimic surgical grafts and be resistant to restenosis.

Mechanical atherectomy devices and laser-assisted angioplasty have fallen out of favor, since the devices are much more expensive than angioplasty catheters and have shown no better long-term patency rates than angioplasty or stents.[3] Investigators are applying gene therapy and radiation therapy to angioplasty sites to reduce the incidence of restenosis from intimal hyperplasia.[3] Pharmacologic strategies and induction of collateral angiogenesis also appear promising.

Chronic arterial insufficiency treatment differs significantly from acute lower extremity ischemia. Acute occlusion of native arteries can occur with thrombosis in situ or from embolization, usually from the heart. Prosthetic or vein grafts may thombose from intimal hyperplasia or technical failures. Tradi-

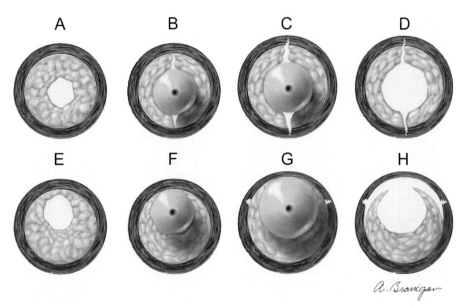

Figure 17–9 ■ Cross-section of angioplasty mechanism on concentric (A–D) and eccentric (E–H) atherosclerotic stenosis. Angioplasty causes plaque compression and fracture, as well as arterial wall stretching and some dissection. As expected, concentric lesions have better morphologic results from angioplasty.

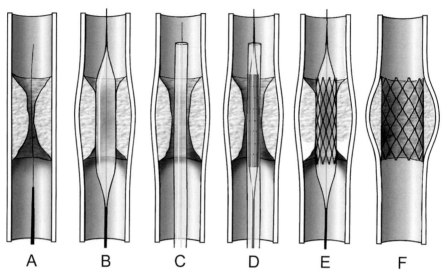

Figure 17–10 ■ Diagram of angioplasty and stent technique. After suboptimal angioplasty (*A–C*) a stent mounted on a balloon is deployed to maintain a larger arterial lumen (*D–F*).

tionally, surgical Fogarty thrombectomy can revascularize a threatened extremity rapidly with a salvage rate of 62 to 96%, but with a mortality of 17% and complications of 44%.[15] Thrombolytic therapy has proven to be a viable alternative unless the extremity is immediately threatened with neuromuscular dysfunction. Streptokinase and recombinant tissue plasminogen activator (rt-PA) have been used as thrombolytic agents but can be associated with systemic bleeding complications.[40] Urokinase, a direct plasminogen activator with a half-life of approximately 16 minutes, produces a more regional lytic effect on the fibrin in thrombus, but can still be associated with bleeding complications, the most serious being intracranial hemorrhage.[25] Multiple dose regimens and delivery

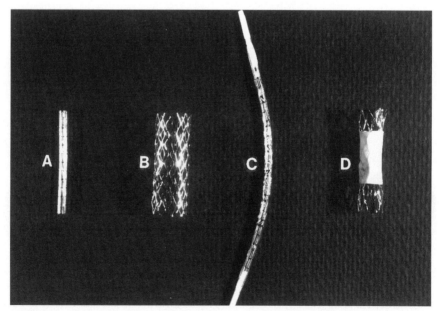

Figure 17–11 ■ Balloon expandable Palmaz stents. *A,* Unopened stent. *B,* Fully expanded stent. *C,* New longer, flexible Palmaz stent. *D,* Stent-graft, Palmaz stent covered with thin-wall PTFE material.

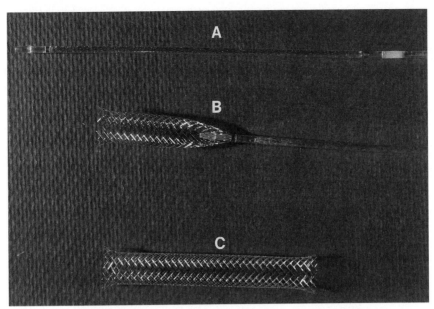

Figure 17–12 ▪ Self-expanding Wallstents. *A*, Constrained Wallstent within 7-Fr delivery device. *B*, Partially opened Wallstent. *C*, Fully deployed and expanded Wallstent.

catheters have been employed, but the average time for complete lysis in the intensive care unit is approximately 24 hours.[5] After successful lysis, the uncovered stenotic lesion can be treated with either angioplasty or surgical revision (Fig. 17–13). A recent multicenter randomized trial found that urokinase thrombolysis was an effective alternative treatment that reduced the number of open surgical procedures without an increased risk of amputation or death.[25] Newer thrombectomy catheters undergoing clinical evaluations can actually remove thromboembolic material atraumatically in minutes even in small vessels or grafts.[37]

Peripheral Arterial Interventions

Patients undergoing peripheral arteriograms and possible percutaneous revascularization can be admitted to an outpatient observation bed. A pertinent history and physical and recent labs which include creatinine and prothrombin time (PT)/partial thromboplastin time (PTT) are mandatory. Patients may have a clear liquid diet after midnight before the procedure and should take their usual medications. Diabetic patients are usually instructed to take one half of their usual morning insulin dose.

A satisfactory diagnostic aortobifemoral arteriogram should include the renal arteries and the distal abdominal aorta with oblique views of the iliac arteries, and both lower extremities in addition to the vessels of the ankles and feet. A focal stenotic lesion in the abdominal aorta, which is more common in female smokers, can be readily treated percutaneously, often with a single balloon (Fig. 17–14), with results comparable to surgical bypass.[23] More commonly, aortic lesions are distally located and involve the bifurcation. Those bifurcation lesions involving the common iliac arteries are best treated with simultaneous bilateral balloon inflations ("kissing" balloon technique) (Fig. 17–15).

Isolated common and external iliac stenoses can also be treated percutaneously with balloon angioplasty, with results rivaling surgical bypass. A 5-year primary patency rate of 54 to 92% with an average of 72% can be expected.[4] With the advent of stents, many practitioners have opted for primary stenting (stenting before angioplasty), hoping to achieve a higher patency rate. However, this has not been proven in a randomized clinical trial and, in fact, one recent abstract suggested that there was not a significant clinical difference within a 2-year follow-up period between primary stenting and selective stenting for suboptimal angioplasty.[35] There

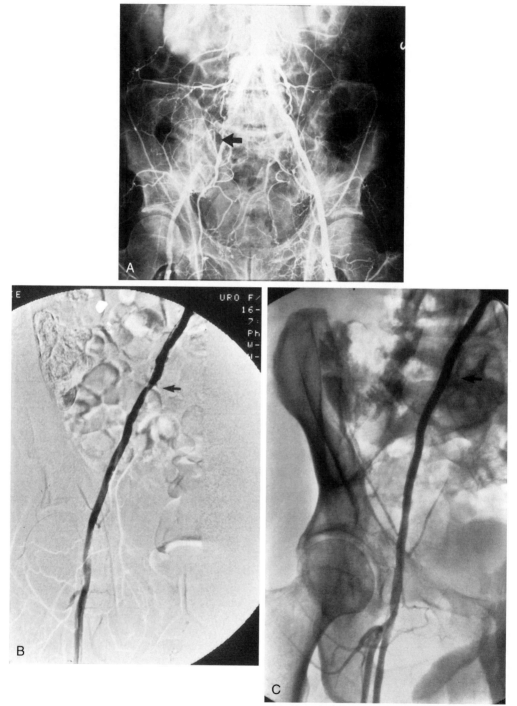

Figure 17–13 ■ Thrombolysis of acute iliac occlusion. *A,* Acute thrombosis of distal common and proximal external iliac artery (*arrow*). *B,* Thrombolysis uncovers the stenotic lesion (*arrow*), which is (*C*) treated successfully with balloon angioplasty.

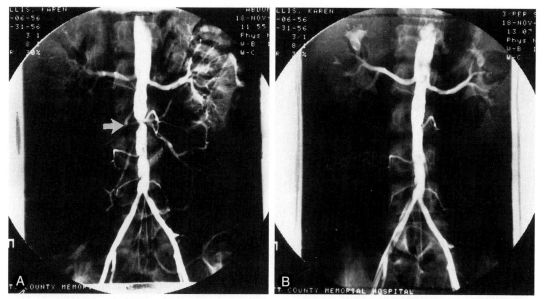

Figure 17–14 ■ Aortic angioplasty. *A*, Severe symptomatic stenosis of abdominal aorta (*arrow*). *B*, Postangioplasty (12-mm balloon) result.

may be a considerable cost savings if stents (average of $1,000) are used selectively. Primary stenting may be indicated in the treatment of iliac occlusions (Fig. 17–16), long segment disease, severely calcified eccentric lesions, and in those vessels in which distal bypass is contemplated. Chronic iliac occlusions may also be treated with urokinase thrombolysis first, followed by angioplasty and stent placement.

Femoropopliteal angioplasty has enjoyed a success similar to that of iliac interventions. Usual indications for femoropopliteal angioplasty include rest pain and ischemic ulcers, lifestyle-limiting claudication, blue-toe syndrome, and the use of adjunctive distal bypass. Ideal angioplasty lesions with high technical and clinical success are short (<2 to 3 cm), concentric, not heavily calcified and have at least two patent outflow vessels distally[22] (Fig. 17–17). Technical success is very high (83 to 98%) for femoropopliteal angioplasty, even in occlusions.[22] Clinical patency results are very encouraging with 1-year rates of 60 to 80% and 5-year rates of 50 to 60%.[22] This compares very favorably with femoropopliteal bypass surgery results of 50 to 70% 5-year patency rates.[22] There are obvious advantages of angioplasty over surgery. Angioplasty can be performed as an outpatient procedure at lower cost and morbidity with fewer complications. Angioplasty can also salvage the peripheral veins for future

heart bypass or leg bypass. Stents are rarely used in the femoropopliteal segments unless there is suboptimal result such as an immediate, severe restenosis or flow-limiting PTA-induced dissection[22] (Fig. 17–18).

After the introduction of small-vessel balloons and guidewires, infrapopliteal angioplasties became feasible, and it is generally agreed by vascular surgeons and interventional radiologists that limb salvage is the primary indication for below-the-knee tibial angioplasties even though it can be performed in conjunction with femoropopliteal PTA or in patients with severe claudication.[1] Most patients (63 to 91%) undergoing tibial angioplasty are diabetics.[1] This is not surprising, since diabetics have a twofold risk for gangrene and a fourfold risk for amputation as compared to nondiabetics.[1] Unfortunately, diabetic peripheral vascular disease has a predilection for the tibioperoneal arteries and frequently all the tibial arteries are occluded with distal reconstitution of a dorsalis pedis or common plantar artery (Fig. 17–19). Tibial angioplasty is most successful in arteries with short focal (<1 cm) stenosis and with good in-line distal runoff (Fig. 17–20). Technical success has been reported as high as 97%, and clinical response with a 2-year limb salvage rate has ranged from 75 to 83%.[1]

Percutaneous interventions in peripheral bypass grafts deserve special attention. Leg

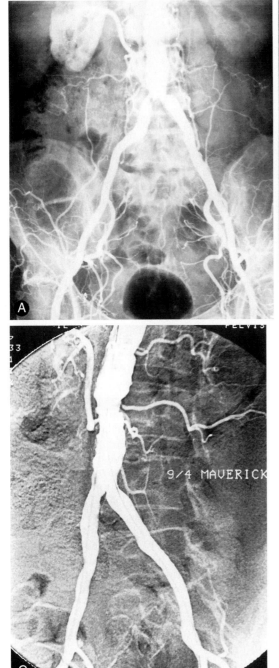

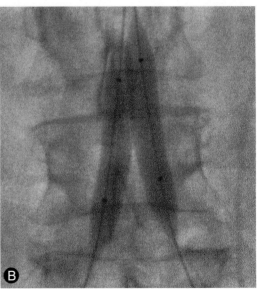

Figure 17–15 ■ ■ "Kissing" balloon angioplasty. A, Severe, bilateral, common artery stenoses. B, Simultaneous "kissing" balloon angioplasty. C, Postangioplasty result.

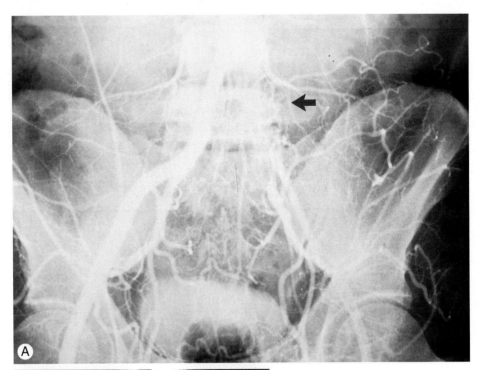

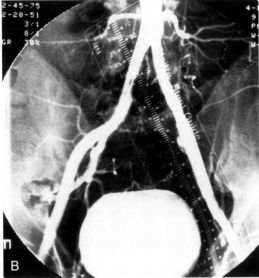

Figure 17–16 ■ Primary iliac stenting. *A*, Chronic common iliac artery occlusion (*arrow*) with collaterals. *B*, Poststenting and angioplasty result.

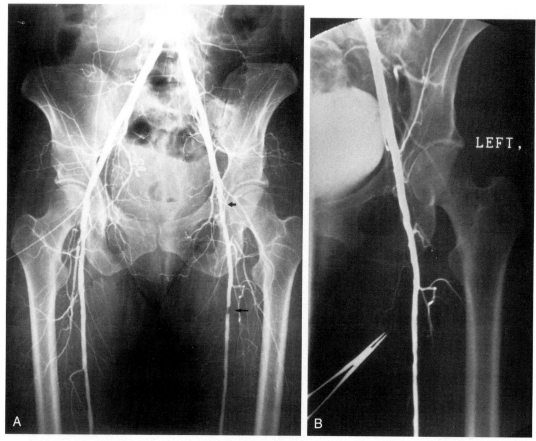

Figure 17–17 ■ Common femoral and superficial femoral angioplasty. *A,* Significant stenosis (*arrows*) of both common and superficial femoral arteries. *B,* Postangioplasty results.

bypass grafts are either synthetic polytetrafluoroethylene (PTFE) or saphenous veins. Femoropopliteal PTFE grafts have a greater predilection for thrombosis, and those occlusions can be treated surgically or with thrombolysis with similar results.[25, 40] After urokinase thrombolysis, balloon angioplasty or patch angioplasty is performed to treat the underlying stenosis, usually of the distal anastomosis from intimal hyperplasia.[40] Vein grafts have a higher patency rate than synthetic grafts, but must undergo regular duplex surveillance, since more than 10% develop flow-limiting stenosis within 2 years of surgery.[40] Depending on the preference of the vascular surgeon, vein graft stenoses can receive a surgical revision or balloon angioplasty if the lesion is less than 1.5 cm long in grafts at least 3 mm in diameter[40] (Fig. 17–21). A primary patency rate of 66% in 2 years has been reported in vein graft

stenoses treated with PTA, but this does not surpass most surgical revision results.[32]

Summary

Percutaneous vascular intervention and surgical bypass serve complementary roles in the treatment of peripheral vascular disease in the diabetic patient. Through the process of informed consent, patients are guided to the specific therapy best suited to treat their disease. Minimally invasive techniques serve as useful adjuncts to the diagnostic angiographic examination, allowing contemporaneous treatment following surgical consultation. Percutaneous revascularization using angioplasty and/or stents does not interfere with subsequent surgery and may avoid amputation of an ischemic limb. The use of these techniques in the

Text continued on page 393

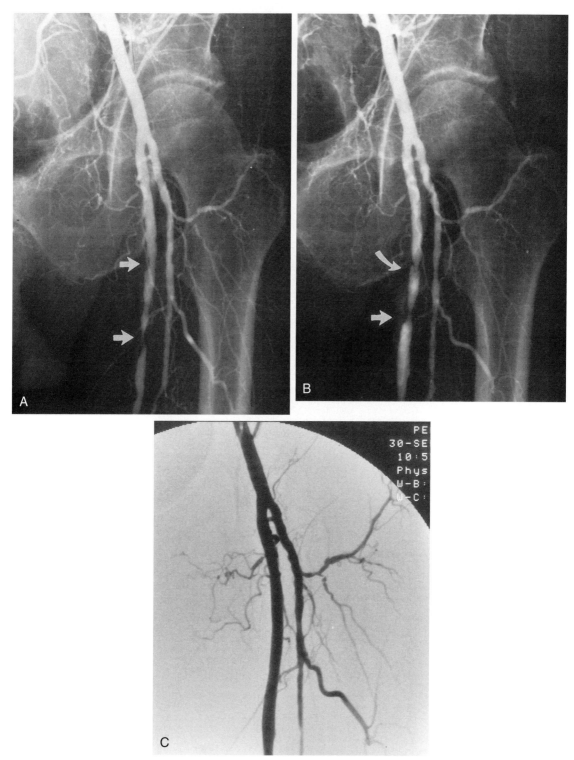

Figure 17–18 ■ SFA angioplasty and stent. *A,* Recurrent severe SFA stenoses (*arrows*) following endarterectomy. *B,* Residual stenosis (*straight arrow*) with dissection (*curved arrow*) after angioplasty. *C,* Post-Wallstent placement.

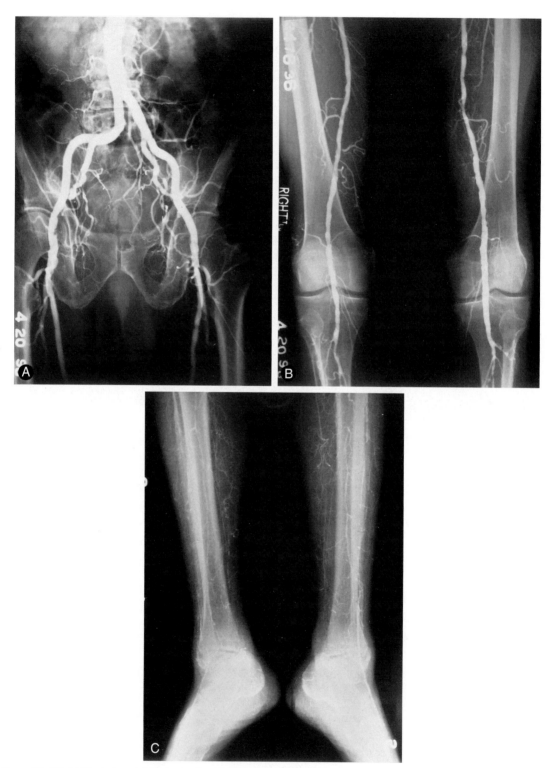

Figure 17–19 ■ Typical peripheral vascular disease in diabetes. Iliac arteries are normal, but early atherosclerotic disease is seen in the superficial femoral arteries. Tibial arteries are occluded bilaterally with collateral reconstitution of the dorsalis pedis arteries.

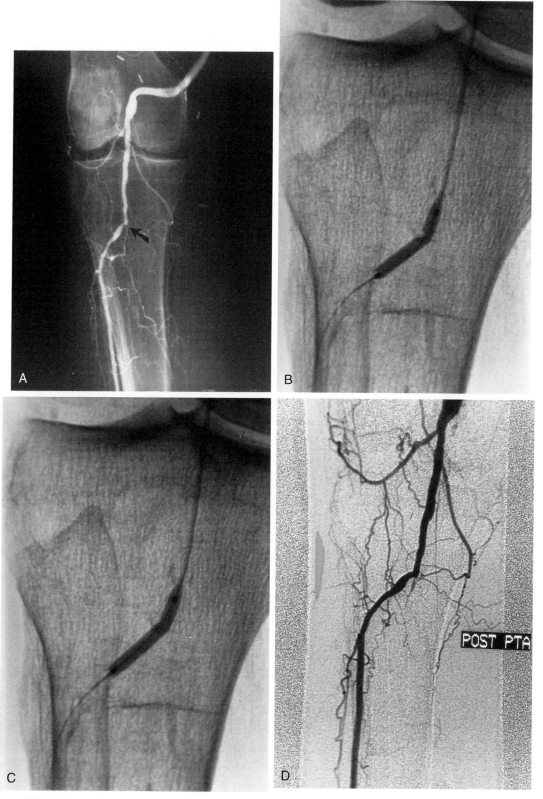

Figure 17–20 ▪ Tibial angioplasty. *A,* Severe stenosis (*arrow*) at origin of single anterior tibial runoff artery. *B,* Small 3-mm balloon PTA with "waist," (*C*) which disappears with successful angioplasty, and (*D*) with excellent morphologic results.

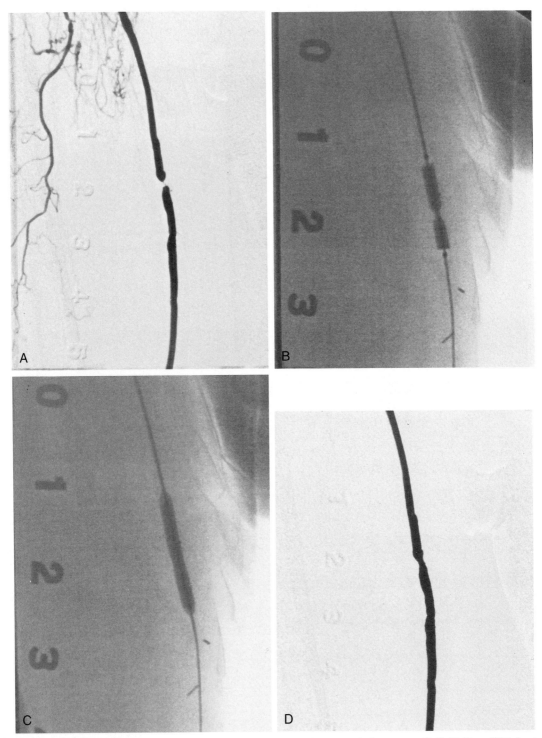

Figure 17–21 ■ Vein graft angioplasty. *A*, Tight stenosis of saphenous vein bypass graft. *B*, Balloon PTA "waist" (*C*) disappears with (*D*) good results.

outpatient setting creates a cost-effective medical environment without sacrificing quality care. Close cooperation between physicians and technical and nursing staff creates a team approach, which optimizes care in the diabetic patient.

REFERENCES

1. Bakal CW: Subtrifurcation percutaneous transluminal angioplasty: Techniques and results. *In* Darcy MD, LaBerge JM (eds): Peripheral Vascular Interventions. Fairfax, VA: Society of Cardiovascular and Interventional Radiology, 1994.
2. Barrett BJ, Carlisle EJ: Metaanalysis of the relative nephrotoxicity of high and low osmolality iodinated contrast media. Radiology 188:171–178, 1993.
3. Baum S, Pentecost MJ (eds): Abrams' Angiography. Interventional Radiology, Vol III. Boston: Little, Brown & Co, 1997.
4. Becker GJ, Katzen BT, Dake MD: Noncoronary angioplasty. Radiology 170:921–940, 1989.
5. Braun MA, Nemcek AA, Vogelzang RL: Interventional Radiology Procedure Manual. New York: Churchill Livingstone, 1997.
6. Carpenter JP, Baum RA, Holland GA, Barker CF: Peripheral vascular surgery with magnetic resonance angiography as the sole preoperative imaging modality. J Vasc Surg 20:861–871, 1994.
7. Carpenter JP, Golden MA, Barker CF, et al: The fate of bypass grafts to angiographically occult runoff vessels detected by magnetic resonance angiography. J Vasc Surg 23:483–489, 1996.
8. Dotter DT, Judkins MP: Transluminal treatment of arteriosclerotic obstruction: Description of a new technique and preliminary report of its application. Circulation 3:654–670, 1964.
9. Egglin TKP, O'Moore PV, Feinstein AR, et al: Complications of peripheral arteriography: A new system to identify patients at increased risk. J Vasc Surg 22:787–794, 1995.
10. Gruntzig A: Transluminal dilation of coronary artery stenosis [letter to editor]. Lancet 1:263, 1978.
11. Helms RB: Implications of population growth on prevalence of diabetes. Diabetes Care 15(Suppl 1E):6–9, 1992.
12. Hirsch IB: Approach to the patient with diabetes undergoing a vascular or interventional procedure. J Vasc Interv Radiol 8:329–336, 1997.
13. Ho KY, Leiner T, de Haan, et al: Peripheral vascular tree stenoses: Evolution with moving bed infusion tracking MR angiography. Radiology 206:683–692, 1998.
14. Idu MM, Blankenstein JD, deGier P, et al: Impact of a color-flow Doppler surveillance program on infrainguinal vein graft patency: A five year experience. J Vasc Surg 17:42–53, 1993.
15. Johnson JA, Cogbill TA, Strutt BJ: Late results after femoral artery embolectomy. Surgery 103:289–293, 1988.
16. Katholi RE, Taylor GJ, McCann WP, et al: Nephrotoxicity from contrast media attenuation with theophylline. Radiology 193:17–22, 1995.
17. Katzen BT: Current status of digital angiography in vascular imaging. Radiol Clin North Am 3:1–14, 1995.
18. Kaufman JA, Stuart CG, Waltman AC: Renal insufficiency: Gadopentetate dimeglumine as a radiographic contrast agent during peripheral vascular interventional procedures. Radiology 198:579–581, 1996.
19. Keller PJ, Saloner D: Time-of-flight flow imaging. *In* Potchen EJ, Siebert JE, Haake EM, Gottschalk A (eds): Magnetic Resonance Angiography Concepts and Applications. St. Louis: Mosby, 1993.
20. Kern SR, Hawkins IF: Carbon dioxide angiography: Expanding applications and evolution of technique. AJR Am J Roentgenol 164:735–741, 1995.
21. Martin EC, Katzen BT, Benenati JF, et al: Multicenter trial of the Wallstent in the iliac and femoral arteries. J Vasc Interv Radiol 6:843–849, 1995.
22. Marx MV: Superficial femoral and popliteal angioplasty: Techniques and results. *In* Darcy MD, LaBerge JM (eds): Peripheral Vascular Interventions. Fairfax, VA: Society of Cardiovascular and Interventional Radiology, 1994.
23. Odurny A, Colapinto RF, Sniderman KW, Johnston KW: Percutaneous transluminal angioplasty of abdominal aortic stenoses. Cardiovasc Intervent Radiol 12:1–6, 1989.
24. Oldroyd S, Slee SJ, Haylor J, et al: Role for endothelin in the renal responses in radiocontrast media in the rat. Clin Sci 87:427–434, 1994.
25. Ouriel K, Veith EJ, Sasahara AA: A comparison of recombinant urokinase with vascular surgery as initial treatment for acute arterial occlusion of the legs. N Engl J Med 338:1105–1111, 1998.
26. Owen RS, Carpenter JP, Baum RA, et al: Magnetic resonance imaging of angiographically occult runoff vessels in peripheral arterial occlusive disease. N Engl J Med 436:1577–1581, 1992.
27. Palmaz JC, Richter GM, Noeldge G, et al: Intraluminal stents in atherosclerotic iliac artery stenosis: Preliminary report of a multicenter study. Radiology 168:727–731, 1998.
28. Perler BA, Becker GJ (eds): Vascular Intervention: A Clinical Approach. New York: Thieme, 1998.
29. Prince MR: Peripheral vascular MR angiography: The time has come. Radiology 206:592–593, 1998.
30. Rubin GD, Dake MD, Napel S: Spiral CT of renal artery stenosis: Comparison of three-diminsional rendering techniques. Radiology 190:181–189, 1994.
31. Rudnick MR, Goldfarb S, Wexler L, et al: Nephrotoxicity of ionic and nonionic contrast media in 1195 patients. Kidney Int 47:254–261, 1995.
32. Sanchez LA, Suggs WD, Marin ML, et al: Is percutaneous balloon angioplasty appropriate in the treatment of graft and anastomotic lesions responsible for failing vein bypasses? Am J Surg 168:97–101, 1994.
33. Soloman R, Werner C, Mann D, et al: Effects of saline, mannitol and furosemide on acute decreases in renal function induced by radiocontrast agents. N Engl J Med 331:1416–1420, 1994.
34. Swan JS, Fryback DG, Lawrence WF, et al: MR and conventional angiography: Work in progress toward assessing utility in radiology. Acad Radiol 4:475–482, 1997.
35. Tetteroo E, DeGraaf YV, Bosch JL, et al: Randomized comparison of primary stent placement versus angioplasty with selective stent placement in pa-

tients with iliac artery obstruction disease. Radiology 205(Suppl):254, 1997.

36. Vesely TM: General percutaneous transluminal angioplasty techniques: Clinical aspects. *In* Darcy MD, LaBerge JM (eds): Peripheral Vascular Interventions. Fairfax, VA: Society of Cardiovascular and Interventional Radiology, 1994.

37. Wagner HJ, Muller-Hulsbeck S, Pitton MB, et al: Rapid thrombectomy with a hydrodynamic catheter:

Results from a prospective multicenter trial. Radiology 205:675–681, 1997.

38. Wang Y, Lee HM, Khilnani NM, et al: Bolus-chase MR digital subtraction angiography in the lower extremity. Radiology 207:263–269, 1998.

39. Wilcox CS: Management of the diabetic or azotemic patient, categorical course, SCVIR, 1998.

40. Wojtowycz M: Handbook of Interventional Radiology and Angiography. St. Louis: Mosby, 1995.

18

MODULATING WOUND HEALING IN DIABETES

■ David L. Steed

Diabetic foot ulcers are a serious problem that may lead to infection and loss of limb. There are between 11 and 16 million patients with diabetes in the United States. Ten percent of diabetic patients may be at risk for the development of foot ulcers. Although 6 to 10% of hospitalizations in diabetic patients are for management of foot ulcers, these admissions account for nearly 25% of the hospital days in this patient group. There are 50,000 to 60,000 amputations performed in diabetic patients each year in the United States. The cost to society of caring for these patients is billions of dollars.

Diabetic foot ulcers occur because of neuropathy and peripheral vascular disease. Sixty to 70% of diabetic patients with foot ulcers have peripheral neuropathy as the etiology, while 15 to 20% have peripheral vascular disease as the cause, and another 15 to 20% have both. The neuropathy occurs as a complication of prolonged glucose elevation. It may be present in as many as 10% of patients when diabetes is diagnosed and nearly half of diabetic patients who have had their disease for more than 20 years. Peripheral neuropathy has both sensory and motor components. The sensory neuropathy leads to a loss of protective sensation in the foot. The motor neuropathy affects the nerves that control motion of the foot. Paralysis of the

intrinsic muscles of the foot leads to a "claw" deformity of the foot where the toes are pulled up and do not touch the ground. This causes the metatarsal heads to become more prominent on the plantar surface and reduces weight bearing from the toes. The metatarsal heads are a common site of plantar ulceration in diabetic patients. This is especially true for the areas beneath the first and fifth metatarsal heads. The patients can also develop midfoot collapse with loss of the plantar arch due to fractures and fracture dislocations. This Charcot neuroarthropathy may result in a markedly abnormal shape to the foot, which coupled with the sensory neuropathy, makes the diabetic patient at risk for skin breakdown.

There are other factors that lead to ulceration in diabetic patients. The patients commonly have peripheral vascular disease. Diabetes is a commonly accepted risk factor for atherosclerosis as are smoking, hyperlipidemia, and hypertension. Although there was once debate as to whether diabetic patients had "small vessel disease" with occlusion of very small vessels, that theory has not been upheld. Most would agree that diabetic patients are at increased risk for typical atherosclerosis. They do seem to develop a pattern of disease commonly involving the tibial arteries. Other problems in diabetic patients also complicate the problem of foot ulceration such as some thinning of the skin of the plantar surface of the foot and an inability to deal well with infection.

Wound Healing

Wound healing is the process by which tissues respond to an injury. The biologic process is complex and involves chemotaxis, cell replication, production of proteins, neovascularization, maturation, and wound remodeling. Wound repair and regeneration occur in an orderly and predictable manner and are under the control of growth factors, which though present in the body in only small amounts, exert a strong influence on wound repair.[13] Growth factors are polypeptides that regulate the growth, differentiation, and metabolism of cells and direct the process of tissue repair.

Wound healing occurs in three phases: inflammation, fibroplasia, and maturation. Each of these phases is controlled by growth factors. The inflammatory response begins immediately after injury. Vasoconstriction limits hemorrhage within the site of wounding.[28] Damage to the endothelial surface of arteries and veins allows blood to leak from the vessel wall, exposing platelets to collagen within the media of the vessel wall. The coagulation cascade is initiated by these platelets. Serotonin and thromboxane are released to enhance vasoconstriction locally to keep healing factors within the wound space. At nearly the same time, vasodilatation occurs at adjacent sites to allow new factors to be brought into the wound. This vasodilatation is mediated by histamine, and released by platelets, mast cells, and basophils. Vascular permeability increases to allow these blood-borne factors to enter the site of wounding.

Platelets activate the coagulation cascade through both the intrinsic and extrinsic response. The intrinsic response is mediated through Hageman factor, factor XII, as it comes into contact with collagen. In the presence of kininogen, a precursor of bradykinin and prekallikrein, factor XII activates factor XI then factor IX, then factor VIII. The extrinsic system is activated through thromboplastin formed when phospholipids and glycoproteins are released by blood coming into contact with the injured tissues. In the presence of calcium, factor VII is activated. Both the intrinsic and extrinsic systems stimulate the final common pathway leading to fibrin production and polymerization. Simultaneously, the fibrinolytic system is activated to monitor clotting so as to prevent coagulation from extending beyond the wound space.[27] It is controlled by the same factors that initiate coagulation and thus serves as a regulator of the process. Arachidonic acid is produced and serves as an intermediate for the production of prostaglandins and leukotrienes.

These intense vasodilators act with histamine, bradykinin, and complement to increase vascular permeability. Thromboxane also increases platelet aggregation and local vasoconstriction. The complement cascade is activated at the same time by platelets and neutral proteases to produce very potent anaphylotoxins, which cause mast cells to degranulate and release histamine. This process leads to margination and then migration of white blood cells into the wound space. The neutrophils are phagocytes for bacteria. Although wounds can heal without white blood cells, the risk of infection is increased. Other substances released by the inflammatory process are also chemoattractants for neutrophils, which produce free oxygen radicals and lysosomal enzymes for host defense. The neutrophils are later removed from the wound by tissue macrophages.

Monocytes migrate into the wound space by the third day and become tissue macrophages. Wounds cannot heal without the macrophage. These cells control and regulate the wound environment through the production and regulation of growth factors. These growth factors control the cellular composition of the wound as well as matrix formation and remodeling. Extracellular matrix is a variety of proteins in a polysaccharide gel composed of glycosaminoglycans and proteoglycans produced by fibroblasts. Matrix proteins may be structural such as collagen and elastin, while others such as fibronectin and laminin regulate cell adhesion. Thrombospondin, von Willebrand factor, and laminin are also adhesion molecules. Fibronectin is also a chemoattractant for circulating monocytes and stimulates their differentiation into tissue macrophages.[11]

Macrophages and fibroblasts enter the wound to begin the process of fibroplasia, the second phase of wound healing. This process begins around the fifth day following injury and may continue for 2 weeks. The inflammatory response lessens as the mediators of inflammation are no longer produced, and those present are inactivated or removed by diffusion or by macrophages. Fibroplasia is the process of matrix formation including collagen synthesis. Angiogenesis is critical to this phase of wound healing to bring a blood supply into the wound. Fibroblasts are attracted to the wound and replicate in response to fibronectin, platelet-derived growth factor (PDGF), fibroblast growth factor (FGF), transforming growth factor (TGF), and C5a, a product of the complement system. These fibroblasts produce proteoglycans and structural proteins necessary for wound healing. This matrix is composed of hyaluronate and fibronectin, which allow for cellular migration stimulated by chemotactic factors formed in the wound. Fibronectin is also important in epithelialization and angiogenesis.

Collagen, the major structural protein in the wound, is the most common protein in the mammalian world. Produced by the fibroblast, it is a family of at least 12 proteins, rich in glycine and proline and bound in a tight triple helix. Cross-linking between the three strands results in a very stabile molecule resistant to breakdown. The production and release of collagen from fibroblasts is controlled by growth factors such as PDGF, epidermal growth factor (EGF), FGF, and TGF-β produced by the tissue macrophage. Once deposited in the wound, collagen is then remodeled for several years. Elastin is another structural protein in the wound present in much smaller amounts than collagen. It contains proline and lysine. It is configured as random coils, allowing both stretch and recoil. Angiogenesis is the process of capillary formation from the budding of existing capillaries after stimulation by FGF.[9, 22] These capillaries are composed of endothelial cells that migrate through the healing wound. Connections are developed between the capillaries to form a network in the wound space. This capillary network provides a pathway for new healing factors to enter the wound. The process ceases when the wound has an adequate blood supply. It appears as if the process of angiogenesis is controlled by oxygen tension and is stimulated by hypoxia. Epithelialization occurs only after granulation tissue is established. Cells migrate from the edge of the wound over the collagen-fibronectin surface. This process results in mature skin covering the wound.

Scar contracture occurs as the wound matures. During the maturation process, the scar becomes less hyperemic as blood supply is reduced. Although remodeling and wound strengthening increase for up to 2 years following injury, the total collagen content of the wound does not change. Hyaluronidase, collagenase, and elastase are key elements in wound remodeling. Hyaluronate is replaced by dermatan sulfate and chondroitin sulfate, which reduce cell migration and allow those cells already in the wound space to differentiate. Plasmin formed from plasminogen degrades fibrin. Collagenase is secreted by macrophages, fibroblasts, epithelial cells, and white blood cells and is able to break the collagen triple helix to allow remodeling. Urokinase, produced by leukocytes, fibroblasts, endothelial cells, and keratinocytes, activates collagenase and elastase.

Growth Factors

The process of wound healing is controlled by growth factors, polypeptides that initiate cell growth and proliferation and protein production by binding to specific high-affinity receptors on the cell surface. They have the ability to stimulate mitosis of quiescent cells. They commonly have endocrine, paracrine, and autocrine function. Some are transported in plasma bound to large carrier proteins, while others affect nonadjacent cells or may have a self-regulating effect. They are produced by platelets, macrophages, epithelial cells, fibroblasts, and endothelial cells. Although growth factors are present in only minute amounts, they modulate the process of wound repair. The growth factors most commonly involved in wound healing include PDGF, TGF, EGF, FGF, and insulin-like growth factor (IGF).

Platelet-Derived Growth Factor

Platelets that initiate the coagulation cascade in the wound are the initial source of growth factors including PDGF, TGF-β, EGF, and IGF-l. Other cells drawn into the wound space such as inflammatory cells, fibroblasts, and epithelial cells are also involved in growth factor production. Growth factors are chemoattractants for neutrophils, macrophages, fibroblasts, and endothelial cells. Macrophages release factors such as tumor necrosis factor (TNF). Wound remodeling occurs under the control of collagenase, which is produced in response to EGF, TNF, interleukin-1 (IL-1), and PDGF. Thus, the complete process of wound repair is controlled directly or indirectly by growth factors.

PDGF is the most widely studied growth factor clinically. It is produced by platelets, macrophages, smooth muscle cells, vascular endothelium, and fibroblasts.[18] PDGF has a molecular weight of 24,000 daltons and is composed of two chains, A and B, held together by disulfide bonds in three dimeric forms, AA, AB, and BB. There is a 60% amino acid homology between the two chains. Human platelets contain all three forms of PDGF in a ratio of about 12% AA, 65% AB, and 23% BB.[3] The B chain is quite similar to the transforming gene of the simian sarcoma virus. The human proto-oncogene C-sis is similar to the viral oncogene V-cis and encodes for the B chain of PDGF. There are two PDGF receptors, an α- and a β-receptor.[33] The α-receptor recognizes both the A and B chains of PDGF and thus can bind to the AA form, the AB form, and the BB form. The β-receptor recognizes only the B chain, and thus binds only to the BB form and weakly to the AB form. Most cells have many times more β-receptors than α-receptors. Cells with PDGF receptors include fibroblasts, vascular smooth muscle cells, and some microvascular endothelial cells.

PDGF is a mitogen for cells of mesenchymal origin. PDGF is a potent chemoattractant and mitogen for fibroblasts, smooth muscle cells, and inflammatory cells. It also acts with TGF-β and EGF to stimulate mesenchymal cells. Although PDGF is produced by endothelial cells, they do not respond to PDGF but work in a paracrine manner to stimulate adjacent vascular smooth muscle. Smooth muscle cells also act in an autocrine fashion and produce PDGF.

PDGF is stabile to extremes of heat, a wide range of pH, and degradation by proteases. Platelets are the largest source of PDGF in the human body. There are no cases of a human PDGF deficiency state, perhaps suggesting that PDGF is critical to the survival of the individual.

PDGF has been isolated from the α-granules of platelets and has been produced through recombinant DNA technology. In animal models, it has been shown to improve the breaking strength of incisional wounds in rats when applied topically even as a single dose.[23] PDGF accelerates wound healing; however, by 3 months, there is no difference in wound healing as compared with untreated wounds, suggesting that wound healing stimulated by PDGF is quite similar to normal healing. Wounds treated with PDGF had a marked increase in neutrophils, monocytes, and fibroblasts in an animal model.[21] This cellular response leads to an increase in granulation tissue production. Similar findings were observed in a rabbit ear excisional wound model. Despite the fact that PDGF does not have a direct effect on keratinocytes, wounds in animals were shown to have an increase in epithelialization. This is due to the influence of macrophages and fibroblasts attracted into the wound by PDGF. Wounds in animals treated topically with PDGF have an increase in neovascularization, although PDGF does not directly stimulate endothelial cells. Again, this is likely related to the influence of other cells attracted into the wound by PDGF. Thus it appears that PDGF accelerates wound healing by accelerating the normal responses. The healed wounds appear to be normal in all aspects.

PDGF has been studied in several clinical trials. The effectiveness of recombinant human PDGF-BB in healing decubitus ulcers was evaluated in patients treated and followed for 28 days.[24] There appeared to be greater reduction in wound closure in patients treated with PDGF. In another trial, patients with decubitus ulcers were treated with PDGF or placebo for 1 month.[20] The ulcer volume was significantly reduced in the PDGF-treated patients. No significant toxicity related to PDGF was noted in either study. A randomized, prospective, double-blind trial of recombinant human PDGF-BB was performed in patients with diabetic neurotrophic foot ulcers.[29] Patients were treated with PDGF (at a dose of 2.2 $\mu g/cm^2$ of ulcer area) in vehicle, carboxymethylcellulose, or vehicle alone for up to 20 weeks or until complete wound closure had been achieved. All wounds had been present for at least 8 weeks. All patients were free of infection and had an adequate blood supply as demonstrated by a transcutaneous oxygen tension (TcPo$_2$) of a least 30 mm Hg. Wounds were debrided prior to entry into the study and as needed during the trial. Forty-eight percent healed using PDGF, while only 25% healed using vehicle alone ($p < 0.01$). The median reduction in wound area was 98.8% for PDGF-treated patients but only 82.1% for those treated with vehicle. There were no significant differences in incidence or severity of adverse events in either group. This was the first study to suggest that a growth factor, and specifically PDGF, could be applied topically and be effective and safe in promoting the healing of chronic wounds in humans. In another trial using recombinant human PDGF in the treatment of patients with diabetic foot ulcers, PDGF-BB was found to increase the incidence of complete wound closure by 43% as compared with placebo ($p = 0.007$).[34] It also decreased the time to achieve complete wound closure by 32% ($p = 0.013$) when compared with the placebo gel. Over 1,000 patients treated with PDGF have been reported. It appears to be safe and efficacious and is now approved for use in the treatment of diabetic foot ulcers. It has been noted that those patients receiving the best wound care healed better when treated with PDGF. Debridement was found to be critically important.[30] The benefits from PDGF will not be achieved if the wounds are not treated properly.

Vascular Endothelial Growth Factor

Vascular endothelial growth factor (VEGF) is quite similar to PDGF. It has a molecular weight of 45,000 daltons. Although it has a 24% amino acid homology to the B chain of PDGF, it binds different receptors than PDGF and has different actions.[17] VEGF is a potent mitogen for endothelial cells but not for fibroblasts or vascular smooth muscle cells as is PDGF. Thus, VEGF is angiogenic and plays a role in wound healing through this mechanism. There has been interest in using VEGF to stimulate the development of collateral vessels in patients with symptomatic arterial ischemic disease. VEGF may be delivered to the ischemic area as a protein or through gene transfer.

Fibroblast Growth Factor

Fibroblast growth factor is a series of heparin-bound growth factors.[10] There are two forms of this growth factor, acidic FGF (aFGF) and basic FGF (bFGF). Both are single-strand molecules with molecular weights of 15,000. There is a 50% amino acid

homology between the two molecules. The binding of these molecules to heparin or heparan sulfate may protect them from enzymatic degradation. Both aFGF and bFGF are found in the extracellular matrix in the bound form. Matrix degradation proteins may act to release aFGF or bFGF. Acidic FGF is similar to endothelial cell growth factor, while bFGF is similar to endothelial cell growth factor II. Both aFGF and bFGF are similar to keratinocyte growth factor. FGFs are produced by fibroblasts, endothelial cells, smooth muscle cells, and chondrocytes and are mitogens for cells of mesodermal and neuroectodermal origin. FGFs are also potent mitogens for endothelial cells and act as angiogenesis factors by stimulating growth of new blood vessels through proliferation of capillary endothelial cells.[8] In addition to endothelial cells, FGFs can stimulate fibroblasts, keratinocytes, chondrocytes, and myoblasts. Multiple different FGF receptors have been identified. They appear to have a similar function. To date, there are no clinical trials that have proven FGF to be of benefit in clinical wound healing.

Keratinocyte Growth Factor

Keratinocyte growth factor (KGF) is related to the FGFs. It is a protein with a molecular weight of 28,000 and has a significant amino acid homology with the FGFs.[6] Although KGF is found only in fibroblasts, it stimulates keratinocytes, not fibroblasts. It may share a receptor with FGF. At this time, there are no clinical trials reported using KGF, and its role in human wound healing remains to be defined.

Transforming Growth Factors

TGFs are composed of two polypeptide chains, α- and β.[26] TGF-α has a 30% amino acid homology with EGF. It received its name because of its ability to reversibly stimulate the growth of cells. Cancer cells do this as well. TGF-α is produced by macrophages, keratinocytes, hepatocytes, eosinophiles, and other cells. TGF-α and EGF are mitogens for keratinocytes and fibroblasts but TGF-α is a more potent angiogenesis factor. Both TGF-α and EGF bind to the EGF receptor but their specific actions may be different partly due to differences in their binding to the receptor. To date there have been no clinical trials of wound healing with TGF-α.

TGF-β has no amino acid homology with TGF-α or any other growth factor. TGF-β is a molecule with many different functions and can stimulate or inhibit the growth or differentiation of many different cells. It is, thus, in some respects a master growth factor. There have been three different forms of TGF-β isolated, TGF-βl, TGF-β2, and TGF-β3.[19] Just as there are three forms of TGF-β, there are three receptors, although the three are not equally important. The actions of the three different forms of TGF-β are very similar although not exactly the same. TGF-βs have a molecular weight of approximately 25,000. TGF-β is a group of proteins that can reversibly inhibit growth of cells, especially those of ectodermal origin. TGF-β is produced by a variety of cells including platelets, macrophages, fibroblasts, keratinocytes, and lymphocytes. Nearly all cells have receptors for TGF-β and have the potential to respond to it. It appears as if TGF-β is the most widely acting of the growth factors. The TGF-βs are potent stimulators of chemotaxis in inflammatory cells and stimulate cells to produce extracellular matrix. These characteristics make the family of TGF-βs important to the wound healing process. There have been trials of TGF-β in the treatment of psoriasis, but as yet, there are no trials reported using TGF-β in human wound healing.

Epidermal Growth Factor

EGF is a small molecule quite similar to TGF-α, with a molecular weight of 6,200 daltons. EGF is produced by the platelet and is present in large amounts in the early stages of wound healing. EGF is produced by the kidney, salivary glands, and lacrimal glands; therefore, it is found in high concentrations in urine, saliva, and tears.[7] EGF promotes epidermal regeneration and corneal epithelialization, and increased the tensile strength of wounds in animals. EGF increases wound healing by stimulating the production of proteins such as fibronectin and the migration of epithelial cells. Although EGF does not stimulate collagen production, it increases the number of fibroblasts in the wound. These cells produce collagen and improve the wound strength. EGF has a common receptor

with TGF-α. EGF has been studied in a randomized trial of skin graft donor site healing. Treatment of donor sites with silver sulfadiazine containing EGF accelerated epidermal regeneration compared with sites treated with silver sulfadiazine alone.[5] EGF reduced the healing time by 1.5 days. Although these results may not be clinically significant, this was the first trial to suggest a benefit from treatment with an isolated growth factor in human wounds. EGF was also used in a prospective open label trial in patients with chronic wounds.[4] Chronic wounds were treated with silver sulfadiazine. In this crossover dosing, those who did not heal were then treated with silver sulfadiazine containing EGF. Many of the patients improved. The results from these studies suggest that EGF may be beneficial in wound healing, although there is not adequate proof as yet to confirm this premise.

Insulin-Like Growth Factors

IGFs, also called somatomedins, are proteins sharing a 50% amino acid homology with proinsulin. They have insulin-like activity. The two forms of this growth factor, IGF-1 and IGF-2, are both secreted as large precursor molecules, which are cleaved to an active form.[25] IGF-1 is also called somatomedin-C while IGF-2 is simply somatomedin. Many tissues synthesize these growth factors. IGF-1 can be found in the liver, heart, lung, pancreas, brain, and muscle.[2] Although produced by a number of tissues, IGF-2 is particularly prominent during fetal development and plays a significant role in fetal growth. IGF-1 and IGF-2 have separate receptors. The actions of pituitary growth hormone are mediated through IGF-1. Pituitary growth hormone stimulates cell differentiation and the production of IGF-1. IGF-1 then causes cell division. IGF-1 is produced mainly in the liver. It is found in high concentrations in platelets and is released into the wound space when clotting occurs. Levels of IGF-1 and IGF-2 depend on multiple factors, such as age, gender, nutritional status, and hormone level. Growth hormone regulates IGF-1 and IGF-2 levels as does prolactin, thyroid hormone, and the sex hormones. Elevated levels of somatomedins have been identified in patients with acromegaly.

IGF-1 and IGF-2 are anabolic hormones that stimulate the synthesis of glycogen, protein, and glycosaminoglycans. They increase the transport of glucose and amino acids across cell membranes. They also increase collagen synthesis by fibroblasts. There is no clinical evidence to suggest these growth factors are of benefit in treating wounds.

As previously described, the process of wound healing is complex and involves platelets and macrophages. In the first 2 days following injury, platelets control the wound space by way of growth factors that they produce and release. Following this period, this function is taken over by macrophages. Within the α-granules of the human platelet are multiple growth factors that are released when platelets are activated and degranulate. These include PDGF, TGF-β, FGF, EGF, platelet factor 4, platelet-derived angiogenesis factor, and β-thromboglobulin.

Platelet Releasates

A purified platelet releasate has been prepared by stimulating human platelets to release the contents of their α-granules by using thrombin. Use of a platelet releasate in wound healing has several advantages. First, the growth factors that are released are identical to and in the same proportion as the growth factors normally brought in the wound space by the platelet. Second, preparation of a platelet releasate is relatively easy and inexpensive, as the platelets can be harvested from peripheral blood. They readily release the contents of their α-granules when stimulated with thrombin. As growth factors are preserved in banked blood, large amounts can be retrieved from the platelets of pooled human blood. There are, however, disadvantages to using a platelet releasate. Not all growth factors promote healing of a wound. It seems reasonable to assume that there is a signal for wound healing to stop. It is likely that this, too, is growth factor related. Since the proper concentration of a platelet releasate is uncertain, a platelet releasate might concentrate factors promoting healing as well as those that trigger the wound healing process to end. Another major disadvantage of such a preparation is that there is the possibility of transmission of an infectious agent from the platelet donor. This could be minimized if the releasate were harvested from a single donor.

Clinical Trials

There have been several reports using a platelet releasate in wound healing. A preliminary report described the use of an autologous platelet releasate in six patients with chronic lower extremity ulcers from connective tissue diseases with minimal benefit. A homologous platelet releasate was used to treat 11 patients with leg ulcers from diabetes and eight patients with leg ulcers secondary to chronic venous insufficiency.[31] No benefit was observed from the treatment with a platelet releasate. In managing these patients, treatment of the underlying disease was not addressed. Growth factors cannot be expected to improve wound healing unless they are applied in a comprehensive wound care program that addresses the underlying etiology of these wounds such as diabetes, venous hypertension, or ischemia. In another trial, 49 patients with chronic nonhealing cutaneous wounds were treated with an autologous platelet releasate.[15] There was some improvement in achieving complete wound healing. This was the first clinical trial to suggest a benefit from a platelet releasate applied topically to promote the healing of chronic wounds. A randomized trial comparing platelet releasate versus a placebo was conducted in patients with ulcers secondary to diabetes, peripheral vascular disease, venous insufficiency or vasculitis.[14] Although this study suggested a benefit from the treatment, the growth factor preparation was added to microcrystalline collagen, a potent stimulator of platelets. The exact contribution from the collagen to the healing of these wounds was not clear. Two other trials suggested a benefit from a platelet releasate. In one trial, patients were treated for 3 months with saline and silver sulfadiazine. Only 3 of the 23 lower extremity wounds healed; however, when the platelet releasate was then applied, the remaining ulcers healed.[1] Thirteen patients with diabetic neurotrophic ulcers were enrolled in a randomized trial of a platelet releasate versus saline placebo.[32] A benefit was seen in those treated with the platelet releasate. By 20 weeks of therapy, five of seven patients healed using the platelet releasate, whereas only two of six patients healed using the saline placebo. By 24 weeks of treatment, another three of six patients in the control group healed, suggesting that the platelet releasate stimulated more rapid healing but did not result in a greater proportion of healed wounds. Another study of 70 patients suggested a similar benefit from a platelet releasate.[12]

Despite this evidence that platelet releasates are of benefit, another trial observed very different results using a homologous platelet releasate. In a randomized, prospective, double-blind, placebo-controlled trial, topical platelet releasate was applied to leg ulcers due to diabetes, peripheral vascular disease, or chronic venous insufficiency. Wounds treated with the platelet releasate worsened, while wounds in the control group improved.[16] This study not only suggested no benefit from a platelet releasate over standard care in the management of lower extremity ulcers, but in fact intimated that a platelet releasate might be detrimental to wound healing.

Although the results of the clinical trials using platelet releasates have been varied, there is some evidence to suggest that they may be of benefit applied topically to lower extremity wounds. However, the inconsistency of the results as well as the concern about transmission of infectious agents in using a homologous preparation leaves their role in human wound healing undefined. Molecules other than growth factors may play a role in the healing of wounds, especially in patients with diabetes. Mice deficient in inducible nitric oxide synthase (iNOS) had a slower rate of healing of full-thickness wounds than normal animals.[35] When given iNOS, the rate of healing returned to normal.

Conclusion

In conclusion, growth factors control the growth, differentiation, and metabolism of cells. Thus they control wound repair and maturation, although there are only a limited number of reports where growth factors have improved wound healing. One isolated growth factor, PDGF, does improve healing in diabetic ulcers and is approved for that indication. It is likely that the actions and benefits of growth factors will be defined further. This will allow health care providers to control the wound environment to achieve complete and durable wound healing in patients.

REFERENCES

1. Atri SC, Misra J: Use of homologous platelet factors in achieving total healing of recalcitrant skin ulcers. Surgery 108:508–512, 1990.
2. Baxter R: The somatomedins: Insulin like growth factors. Adv Clin Chem 25:49–115, 1986.
3. Bennett N, Schultz C: Growth factors and wound healing: Biochemical properties of growth factors and their receptors. Am J Surg 165:728–737, 1993.
4. Brown GL, Curtsinger L: Stimulation of healing of chronic wounds by epidermal growth factor. Plast Recontr Surg 88:189–194, 1991.
5. Brown GL, Nanney LB: Enhancement of wound healing by topical treatment with epidermal growth factor. N Engl J Med 321:76–80, 1989.
6. Cook P, Mattox P, Keeble W: A heparin sulfate regulated human keratinocyte autocrine factor is similar or identical to amphiregulin. Mol Cell Biol 11:2547–2557, 1991.
7. Fisher D, Lakshmanan J: Metabolism and effects of epidermal growth factor and related growth factors in mammals. Endocr Rev 11:418–442, 1990.
8. Folkman J, Klagsburn M: Angiogenic factors. Science 235:442–447, 1987.
9. Folkman T, Lansburn M: Angiogenic factors. Science 235:442–447, 1987.
10. Gospodarowicz D: Fibroblast growth factor: Chemical structure and biologic function. Clin Orthop 257:231–243, 1990.
11. Grinnel F: Fibronectin and wound healing. Am J Dermatopathol 4:185–192, 1982.
12. Holloway GA, Steed DL, DeMarco MJ: A randomized controlled dose response trial of activated platelet supernatant topical CT-102 (APST) in chronic nonhealing wounds in patients with diabetes mellitus. Wounds 5:198–206, 1993.
13. Hunt TK, LaVan EB: Enhancement of wound healing by growth factors. N Engl J Med 321:111–112, 1989.
14. Knighton DR, Ciresi K: Stimulation of repair in chronic, nonhealing, cutaneous ulcers using platelet-derived wound healing formula. Surg Gynecol Obstet 170:56–60, 1990.
15. Knighton DR, Ciresi KF: Classifications and treatment of chronic nonhealing wounds. Ann Surg 104:322–330, 1986.
16. Krupski WC, Reilly LM: A prospective randomized trial of autologous platelet-derived wound healing factors for treatment of chronic nonhealing wounds: A preliminary report. J Vasc Surg 14:526–532, 1991.
17. Leung D, Chaines G, Kuang W, et al: Vascular endothelial growth factor is a secreted angiogenic mitogen. Science 246:1306–1309, 1989.
18. Lynch SE, Nixon JC: Role of platelet-derived growth factor in wound healing: Synergistic effects with growth factors. Proc Natl Acad Sci U S A 84:7696–7697, 1987.
19. Massague J: The transforming growth factor-β family. Annu Rev Cell Biol 6:597–641, 1990.
20. Mustoe T, Cutler N: A phase II study to evaluate recombinant platelet-derived growth factor-BB in the treatment of stage 3 and 4 pressure ulcers. Arch Surg 129:212–219, 1994.
21. Mustoe T, Pierce G, Morishima C, Deuel T: J Clin Invest 87:694–703, 1991.
22. Pevec WC, Ndoye A, Brinsky JL: New blood vessels can be induced to invade ischemic skeletal muscle. J Vasc Surg 24:534–544, 1996.

23. Pierce G, Mustoe T, Senior R, et al: J Exp Med 167:974–987, 1988.
24. Robson M, Phillips L: Platelet-derived growth factor BB for the treatment of chronic pressure ulcers. Lancet 339:23–25, 1992.
25. Spencer EM, Skover G, Hunt TK: Somatomedins: Do they play a pivotal role in wound healing? In Barbul A, Pines E, Caldwell M (eds): Growth Factors and Other Aspects of Wound Healing: Biological and Clinical Implications. New York: Alan R Liss, 1988.
26. Sporn MB, Robert AB: Transforming growth factor. JAMA 262:938–941, 1989.
27. Steed DL: Hemostasis and coagulation. In Simmons RL, Steed DL (eds): Basic Science Review for Surgeons. Philadelphia: WB Saunders Company, 1992, pp 30–37.
28. Steed DL: Mediators of inflammation. In Simmons RL, Steed DL (eds): Basic Science Review for Surgeons. Philadelphia: WB Saunders Company, 1992, pp 12–29.
29. Steed DL, Diabetic Ulcer Study Group: Clinical evaluation of recombinant human platelet-derived growth factor for the treatment of lower extremity diabetic ulcers. J Vasc Surg 21:71–81, 1995.
30. Steed DL, Donohoe D, Webster MW: Effect of extensive debridement and treatment on the healing of diabetic foot ulcers. J Am Coll Surg 183:61–64, 1996.
31. Steed DL, Goslen B, Hambley R: Clinical trials with purified platelet releasate. In Barbul A (ed): Clinical and Experimental Approaches to Dermal and Epidermal Repair: Normal and Chronic Wounds. New York: Alan R Liss, 1990, pp 103–113.
32. Steed DL, Goslen JB, Holloway GA: CT-102 activated platelet supernatant, topical versus placebo: A randomized prospective double blind trial in healing of chronic diabetic foot ulcers. Diabetes Care 15:1598–1604, 1992.
33. Westermark B: The molecular and cellular biology of platelet derived growth factor. Acta Endocrinol 123:131–142, 1990.
34. Wieman J, Smiel J, Nacht J, Su Y: Efficacy and safety of recombinant human platelet derived growth factor-BB (Becaplermin) in patients with nonhealing lower extremity diabetic ulcers: A phase III randomized double blind study [abstract]. Poster Am Coll Surg 1997.
35. Yamasaki K, Edington H, McCloskey C, et al: Reversal of impaired wound repair in iNOS deficient mice by topical adenoviral mediated iNOS gene transfer. J Clin Invest 101:967–971, 1998.

ADJUNCTIVE HYPERBARIC OXYGEN THERAPY IN THE TREATMENT OF THE DIABETIC FOOT WOUND

■ Paul Cianci and Thomas K. Hunt

Diabetes mellitus affects 5 to 6% of the population (half are undiagnosed).[2] The annual cost of care exceeds $92 billion.[2] Recent data from a study at a major health maintenance organization (HMO) involving more than 175,000 patients showed the diabetics consumed 2.4 times more health care dollars than nondiabetic controls ($480,660,718 vs. $197,948,887).[100] The federal government is becoming increasingly aware of this problem. "Diabetics account for 27% of the federal medical budget" (Newt Gingrich, Chairman, House of Representatives in an address to the AMA, March 9, 1998). At any given time perhaps 1 million diabetic patients have lower limb ulcers. Twenty percent of hospital admissions of diabetics are because of lower limb problems.[9] The incidence of amputation is 6 per 1,000. Diabetics accounted for 50 to 70% of the 118,000 amputations performed in the United States in 1983. From 1993 to 1995 about 67,000 amputations were performed yearly among people with diabetes.[116] Nine percent required amputation of a foot, 31% of the lower leg, and 30% lost at or above the knee.[72] The cost of a primary amputation in 1986 was reported to be in excess of $40,000.[79] Medicare reimbursement for primary amputation is approximately $12,500.[28] The morbidity and mortality associated with amputation are significant. Ipsilateral, often higher amputation will occur in 22% of cases. Contralateral amputation occurs at a rate of approximately 10% a year. Sixty-eight percent of elderly amputees will be alive at 4 years.[36] Only 40 to 50% of elderly amputees will be rehabilitated.[31] The length of hospital stay for primary amputation varies widely but has been reported to average 22 days.[23, 47] Six to 9 months may be necessary to maximize walking ability.[69] In 1997 dollars, the cost of amputation is in excess of $2.7 billion yearly.[77] Readmission within 2 years for stump modification or reamputation may represent an additional $1.5 billion expenditure.[24] Mortality associated with amputation at a major teaching hospital was recently reported as 4%. Morbidity, including myocardial infarction, arrhythmia, or congestive heart failure requiring therapy, was 14%.[47]

Clearly, these data show that primary amputation is far from an expeditious solution to the problem of foot wounds in diabetics. Total costs for patients who achieved primary healing and did not have critical ischemia were $16,000 compared to $63,000 for patients who had required major amputation.[3] An aggressive, multidisciplinary team approach to diabetic foot management can result in improved salvage and significant cost savings.[28, 47, 72, 74, 105] We have utilized this regimen at our community hospital since 1983. Patients are quickly evaluated, seen by appropriate specialists, revascularized aggressively, and, when indicated, receive hyperbaric oxygen (HBO) therapy as an adjunct to their medical and surgical care. This chapter is a comment on this experience.

The Diabetic Foot

The "diabetic foot" is characterized by sensory, motor, and autonomic neuropathy and macrovascular disease. These may lead to ulceration, infection, gangrene, and amputation. Motor neuropathy may cause alteration of pressure distribution. Foot deformities and altered sensation can result in ulceration. The classic plantar ulcer is caused by the loss of sensation and painless trauma. This can occur in the absence of ischemia and frequently heals with conservative measures such as unweighting and aggressive wound management (see Chapter 9). Primary management is directed to patient education and foot care. Autonomic neuropathy may cause alterations in blood flow and diversion of nutritive flow, resulting in cutaneous ischemia.[37] Ulcers associated with ischemia may be associated with pathophysiologic alterations involving small cutaneous vessels in addition to the contribution of arterial insufficiency. Many diabetics have areas of low flow and hypoxia in their feet and ankles, even in the presence of palpable pulses. Contributing factors may be increased blood viscosity, platelet aggregation, excessive adherence of leukocytes to capillary endothelial cells, and accelerated capillary endothelial growth.[1, 4, 83] Recently, it has been suggested that capillary hyperfusion and vasodilation lead to injury via subendothelial deposition of macromolecules.[127] Progressive capillary wall hyalinization leads to small vessel obstruction.[46, 117] Surgical revascularization can often provide the necessary substrate for wound healing. Some wounds, however, fail to heal, even in the presence of

restored circulation and when tissue perfusion appears adequate.[122] Defective wound healing is a major factor contributing to limb loss.[93] Thrombosis also predisposes to ulceration and gangrene. "In the diabetic, response to local tissue stresses is by thrombosis and necrosis as opposed to inflammatory response in nondiabetics."[66] There is evidence that tight control of diabetes mellitus can delay the onset or prevent the progression of microvascular complications.[89, 98, 110] The crucial role of the endothelium in the regulation of local microvascular hemodynamics is now apparent. Injury to the endothelium due to increased pressure and flow ultimately leads to sclerosis.[44, 103, 113] The role of nitric oxide and white cell adherence in this process is beginning to be elucidated.[114] Recent data suggest that HBO has a direct beneficial effect on the endothelium by preventing or treating white cell adherence. This effect is mediated, in part, through increased levels of endothelial nitric oxide.[12, 17–19, 81] These findings are in agreement with observed clinical results. Regardless of mechanisms, however, the net result of this excessive adherence is hypoxia that involves focal regions of the foot or ankle, often toes, or the lateral side of the foot. Hyperbaric oxygen therapy, therefore, may favorably influence outcome.

HBO therapy is not new, having been used since 1943.[32] Modern therapy dates to the early 1960s, when Dutch investigators demonstrated the efficacy of HBO therapy in gas gangrene and anemic states.[10, 14] Hyperbaric oxygen therapy is presently used as primary treatment for decompression sickness (the bends), air embolism, and severe carbon monoxide poisoning.[49, 68, 112, 123] Adjunctive indications include clostridial myonecrosis,[14, 59, 62] crush injury and traumatic ischemias,[13, 104, 108, 109] enhancement of healing in selected problem wounds,[34] necrotizing soft tissue infections,[6, 51, 99] refractory osteomyelitis,[33, 34, 80, 85, 104] radiation damage to soft or hard tissue,[39–42, 82, 87] compromised skin grafts or flaps,[67, 109, 126, 127] and burns.[23, 25, 26, 56] All of these conditions have focal hypoperfusion, hypoxia, or both in common.

Rationale for Therapy: Role of Oxygen in Healing

Injuries damage microvasculature and initiate several chemoattractant and growth factor pathways, including coagulation and complement generation. Consequently, inflammatory cells (which consume large amounts of oxygen) collect at the site. In this manner, most injuries and infections create "energy-poor" environments characterized by poor local perfusion, low oxygen tensions, increased oxidant production, low pH, and high lactate concentrations. Macrophages sense this environment and because of it, release potent growth factors resulting in a brisk angiogenesis and multiplication of fibroblasts at the wound margins.[71] High lactate also stimulates growth factor secretion by inflammatory cells and appears to be a sufficient stimulus to maintain wound healing when oxygen tension increases. As macrophages move into the injured area, fibroblasts begin to multiply and migrate after them. Endothelial buds then follow, largely from venules, and follow fibroblasts into the hypoxic, highly lactated area. Under the influence of the lactate and growth factors, fibroblasts transcribe collagen genes and synthesize collagen.

Most, and perhaps all, events thus far in the healing sequence can proceed in very low oxygen tensions.[76] A variety of mechanisms, clotting, complement activation, oxidant re-lease, and others, stimulate release of growth factors. However, fibroblasts must modify the collagen they synthesize so that it can be secreted into the extracellular space and polymerized. This vital step can be accomplished only when oxygen is present at rather high partial pressures (Fig. 19–1).[95]

Thus, collagen is deposited most rapidly when both lactate and oxygen concentrations are high. The idea that this process can be initiated by lactate as a signal of "energy deficit" and accelerated by hyperoxia is not paradoxic because macrophages release lactate, even in well-oxygenated environments and continue to produce it in well-oxygenated wounds. The stimulus to collagen production, lactate, remains, therefore, even during hyperoxia. The need for oxygen persists well into the healing process because "new collagen" must be deposited as "old collagen" is lysed. Production must accommodate to degradation if wounds are to heal and maintain strength.

The mechanism of the oxygen effect rests at least partly on one important step in collagen biosynthesis, the hydroxylation of proline and lysine residues in procollagen. In the synthetic pathway of collagen, proline and lysine are incorporated into the growing

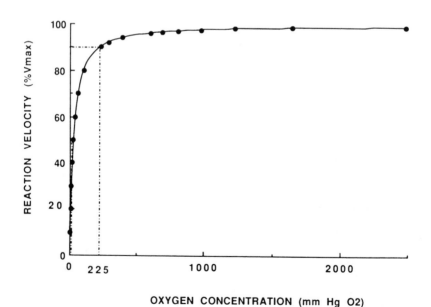

Figure 19–1 ■ Kinetics of prolyl hydroxylase (Km = 25 mm Hg). Reaction velocity of prolyl hydroxylase depends on the concentration of oxygen in the endoplasmic reticulum, with half maximal velocity (Km) at about 20 mm Hg. Normally, the Po_2 there varies between a few to perhaps 50 mm Hg. Normal mean probably is in the region of 30 to 40 mm Hg. In foot lesions in diabetics the number of focal areas at which Po_2 is zero increases markedly, and the mean may fall close to zero. Clearly, there is better collagen deposition at somewhat higher levels.

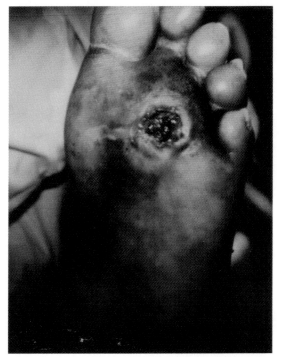

A

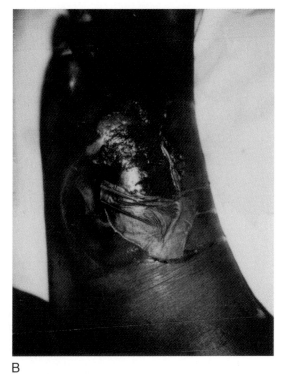

B

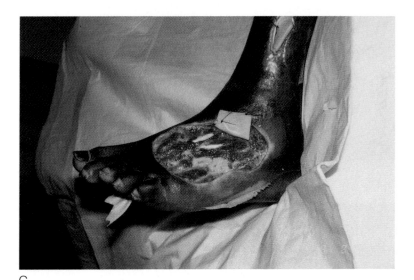

C

Plate 20 ■ *A,* Malperforans ulcer in a 57-year-old insulin-dependent diabetic. *B,* Dorsum view showing cellulitis and desquamation of overylying skin. *C,* Wound has been débrided and drained; patient has received 1 week of hyperbaric oxygen therapy.

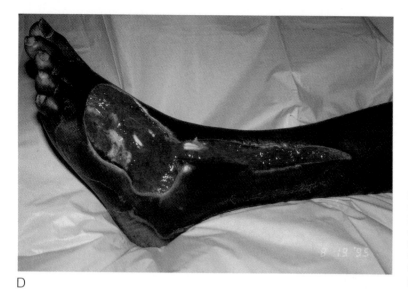

D

Plate 20 ■ *D,* Eleven days later with further débridement and hyperbaric oxygen therapy; note exuberant granulation tissue, even over exposed tendons. *E,* Patient 9 days later shows excellent take of split-thickness mesh graft. *F,* Patient 21 days later; excellent coverage; intact foot.

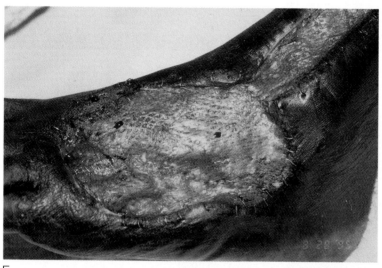

E

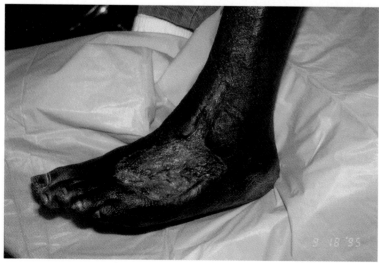

F

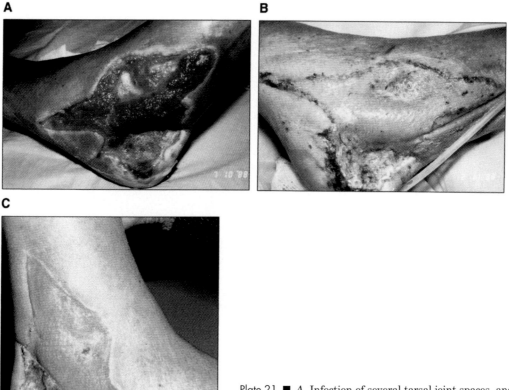

Plate 21 ■ *A,* Infection of several tarsal joint spaces, and lateral skin necrosis. In the subsequent débridement these spaces were opened and expanded. Cartilage was not debrided. *B,* Much of this wound healed during a period in which the patient breathed oxygen at sea level pressure. After several weeks of HBO therapy, skin grafts were placed. *C,* Wound remains healed and the patient ambulant 20 months later.

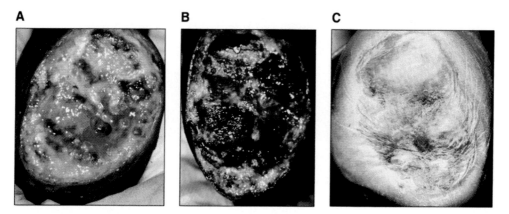

Plate 22 ■ *A,* Unhealed transmetatarsal wound in a 55-year-old man 5 weeks after extensive débridement and successful revascularization of viable tissue. Standard wound care was provided but failed. *B,* Angiogenesis after 10 days of wound care and HBO treatment. *C,* Wound remains healed after split-thickness mesh grafting at 27 months' follow-up. The contralateral limb was paralyzed.

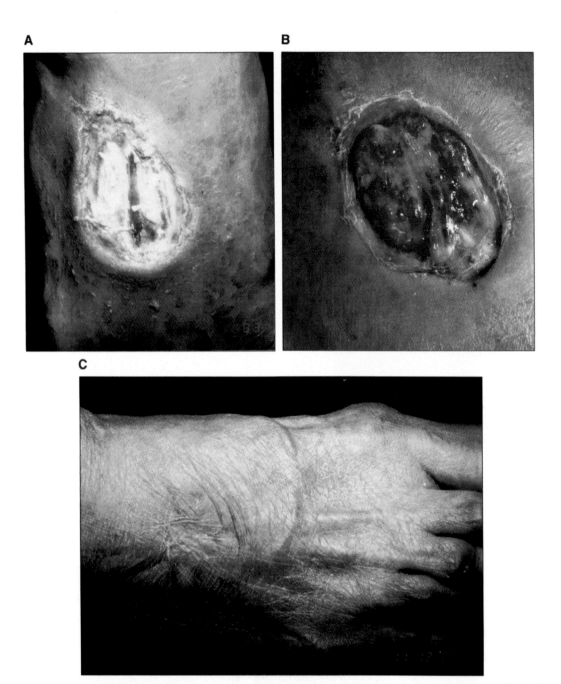

Plate 23 ■ *A*, Unhealed, painful dorsal foot lesion in a 70-year-old woman 6 weeks after successful revascularization. Wound showed no evidence of healing with standard care. *B*, 3 weeks later after 38 hyperbaric treatments. Note extensive granulation tissue. *C*, Lesion closed without further surgical intervention and remained healed at 4-year follow-up.

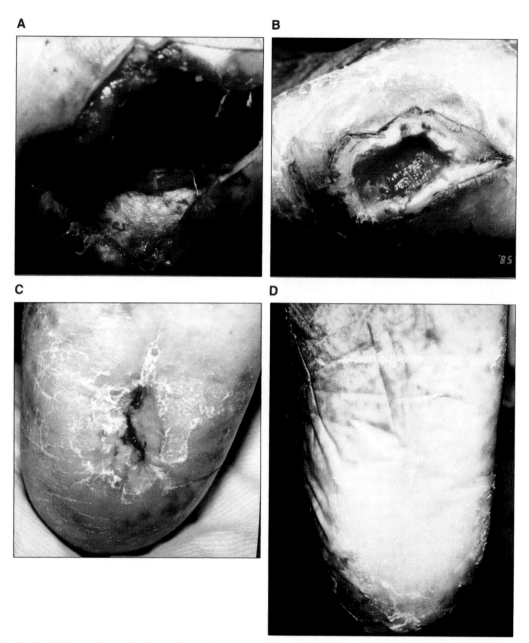

Plate 24 ■ *A,* Deep calcaneal lesion 2 days after successful revascularization and débridement of necrotizing heel lesion. Because of infection, compromised host, and a limb-threatening lesion, adjunctive HBO therapy was initiated early. *B,* 50% reduction of wound diameter and volume after 27 days of wound care and adjunctive HBO treatment. *C,* Healed lesion after 28 HBO treatments. *D,* At 4-year follow-up, lesion remains healed. Patient lost opposite limb during interim.

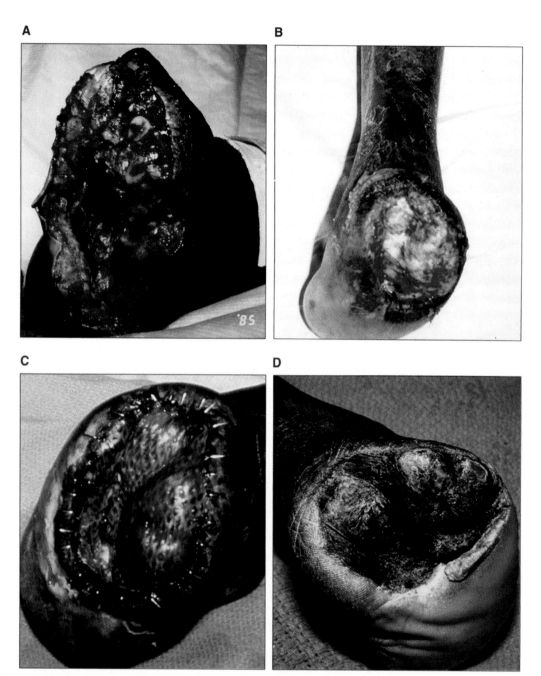

Plate 25 ■ *A,* Forefoot amputation status after revascularization in a 70-year-old man with diabetes mellitus, renal failure, and necrotizing infection. Because of limb-threatening lesion and prior contralateral limb amputation, adjunctive HBO therapy was initiated in the postoperative period. *B,* Lesion 3 weeks later, after 21 HBO treatments and aggressive wound care. Note extensive healing. *C,* Lesion 50 days after radical débridement and split-thickness mesh graft was placed. *D,* Foot remains healed at 1-year follow-up.

peptide chain and are hydroxylated later when the peptides enter the endoplasmic reticulum. These hydroxylations are necessary for polymerization and cross-linkage of procollagen strands and transport of collagen molecules to the extracellular space. This process proceeds at one half maximal rate at Po_2 20 mm Hg and 90% maximal rate at about 200 mm Hg (see Fig. 19–1). Thus, collagen *deposition,* the process that fills tissue defects and supports new blood vessels, proceeds in proportion to local oxygen tensions throughout and even beyond the entire physiologic range.[91] Transcutaneous Po_2 ($TcPo_2$) is a reasonable indication of local Po_2 in cutaneous ulcers.

Cell replication also requires oxygen. Fibroblast and vascular endothelial cells have been reported to replicate most rapidly at about 40 mm Hg, whereas epidermal cells replicate best at about 700 mm Hg![84]

Hehenberger et al. have recently reported that diabetic fibroblasts showed diminished cell turnover when compared to normal controls.[61] Hyperbaric oxygen exposure results in dramatic increases in cell proliferation, which appears to be proportional to O_2 tensions, maximum effect being seen at 2.5 atm (the pressure equivalent of breathing 100% oxygen at 45 ft of seawater) (Figs. 19–2 and 19–3).

Any interference with oxygen delivery to wounds also increases susceptibility to infection. Raising Po_2 levels, conversely, confers resistance. In a sense, this has been obvious to surgeons for centuries. Wounds of the extremities are often infected, whereas those in tissues that have higher blood flow and tissue oxygen tensions, such as the tongue or face, rarely are infected. The difference between these sites is blood flow and consequently the Po_2 in the wounds. Blood flow may be low in the extremities due to regional arterial obstructions, small vessel disease, and sympathetic nervous system activation by cold, pain, or dehydration. Leukocytes kill bacteria most effectively when supplied with abundant oxygen (Fig. 19–4).[80] Phagocytosis stimulates a huge, often 50-fold increase in oxygen consumption, the so-called respiratory burst. At least 98% of this oxygen is converted to superoxide, peroxide, and other active oxygen species (oxygen radicals) which, when released into phagosomes, are lethal to many bacteria. This oxidative mechanism is at its best in high oxygen tensions, even up to several hundred mm Hg.[96] The

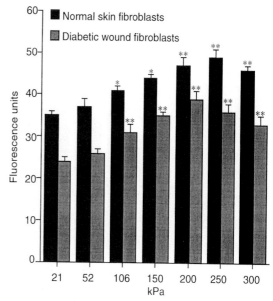

Figure 19–2 ■ DNA content, expressed as fluorescence units, of human fibroblasts derived from normal skin (*filled bars*) and from chronic diabetic wounds (*shaded bars*) 24 hours after a 1-hour treatment at multiple oxygen pressures. Values represent the mean ± standard deviation of five different patients, each assayed in triplicate. Significant difference (*$p < 0.05$, **$p < 0.01$) compared with 21 kPa (untreated cells). (From Hehenberger K, et al: Dose-dependent hyperbaric oxygen stimulation of human fibroblast proliferation. Wound Repair Regen 5:147–150, 1997, with permission.)

key enzyme that converts oxygen to superoxide has kinetics similar to those of prolyl hydroxylase, but the Km is even higher (Km ~50). It fails rapidly as tissue oxygen tensions fall to less than 30 to 40 mm Hg. Oxidative killing and antibiotic killing of bacteria are independent mechanisms and are additive in wounds (Fig. 19–5).[63, 73]

Well-perfused and oxygenated myocutaneous flaps are resistant to infection and infectious gangrene. Random flaps, which have low distal oxygen tensions (analogous to the low oxygen tensions measured near diabetic foot ulcers),[101] are susceptible to infection and suffer a high degree of necrosis secondary to infection.[21, 50, 65, 94] Oxygen administration to elevate Po_2 values to more than 100 mm Hg minimizes infectious necrosis. Borer et al.[11] have shown improvement in diabetic white cell function when exposed to HBO. This effect seems to be mediated by both adherence molecules (intracellular adhesion molecule [ICAM]), etc., and increased levels of nitric oxide.

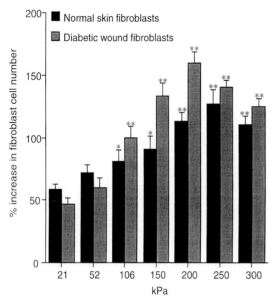

Figure 19–3 ■ Percentage increase in fibroblast cell number, DNA content, 24 hours after a 1-hour treatment at multiple oxygen pressures as compared with untreated cells. Normal skin (*filled bars*) and chronic diabetic wounds (*shaded bars*). Values represent the mean ± standard deviation of five different patients, each assayed in triplicate. Significant difference (*$*p < 0.05$, **$**p < 0.01$) compared with 21 kPa (untreated cells). (From Hehenberger K, et al: Dose-dependent hyperbaric oxygen stimulation of human fibroblast proliferation. Wound Repair Regen 5:147–150, 1997, with permission.)

Angiogenesis

Stimulation and regulation of angiogenesis are similar in principle to that of collagen synthesis and deposition. In short, increased lactate concentration and probably production of oxidants such as NO, H_2O_2, and O_2^- stimulate macrophages to produce angiogenic substances that are both chemattractic and growth factors to endothelial cells. The most important of these in wounds appears to be vascular endothelial growth factor (VEGF). VEGF secretion responds to mild exposure to oxidants and lactate. These stimuli are not inhibited by hyperoxia; in fact, they may be enhanced; notably, hyperoxia does not lower lactate in wounds. From both clinical observation and laboratory experiment, there is no longer any doubt that angiogenesis occurs most rapidly in well-oxygenated animals.[43, 48, 72] In the latest of these, anti-VEGF antibody was found to abrogate the effects of hyperbaric oxygen on angiogenesis in a Matrigel model (Fig. 19–

6).[48] HBO therapy stimulates angiogenesis and leads to an increase in new vessel concentration. As this occurs, $TcPo_2$ increases. This increase seems to be long lasting, perhaps "permanent."[38]

Hyperbaric Oxygen Therapy

The Undersea and Hyperbaric Medical Society, an international scientific organization and the leading authority for diving and hyperbaric medicine in the United States, defines HBO therapy as the intermittent ad-

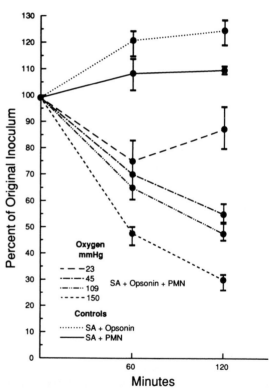

Figure 19–4 ■ This study reinforces the validity of the kinetic approach noted in Figure 19–1. Mean (± SE [brackets]) phagocytic killing of *Staphylococcus aureus* (SA) under different oxygen tensions. SA, rabbit peritoneal leukocytes (PMN), and opsonin (10% normal human serum) were tumbled for 30 minutes at 40°C in a total volume of 1 mL. Each tube was decanted into a culture dish so that the suspension was 1 mm thick; an aliquot was removed for determination of the number of colony-forming units (CFUs) of SA. Dishes were placed under different oxygen tensions at 37°C, and removed after 60 or 120 minutes, when the number of CFUs of the initial inoculum was counted. At least six separate experiments at each oxygen tension were performed, each in duplicate. As oxygen tension increases, staphylococcal survival decreases, reflecting increased killing by PMNs. (Courtesy of Jon Mader, M.D.)

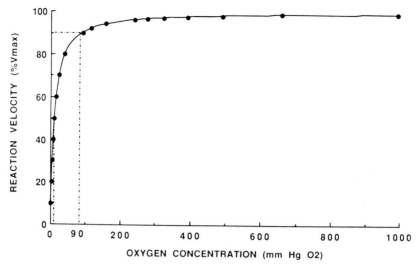

Figure 19–5 ■ Kinetics of NADPH-linked oxidase of leukocytes. Curve describing NADPH-linked oxidase conversion of molecular oxygen of superoxide (O_2^-) (compare with Figure 19–1). Km is variously estimated at 8 and 25 mm Hg. Thus, the V_{max} will vary from approximately 80 to 250 mm Hg. The oxidative antibacterial system is particularly directed at the usual wound pathogens, such as *Staphylococcus, Streptococcus,* and *Escherichia coli.*

ministration of 100% oxygen *inhaled* at pressure greater than sea level. The technique may be implemented in a walk-in (multiplace) chamber (Fig. 19–7) compressed to depth with air while the patient breathes 100% oxygen via head tent, face mask, or endotracheal tube (Fig. 19–8). Alternatively, the patient may be treated in a one-person (monoplace) chamber (Fig. 19–9) pressurized to depth with oxygen. In either case,

the arterial partial pressure of oxygen will approch 1,500 mm Hg at the pressure equivalent of 33 ft of seawater (2 atm absolute [ATA], 10 m).

Topical Oxygen Therapy

Topical oxygen therapy rendered in limb-encasing devices is not considered to be hy-

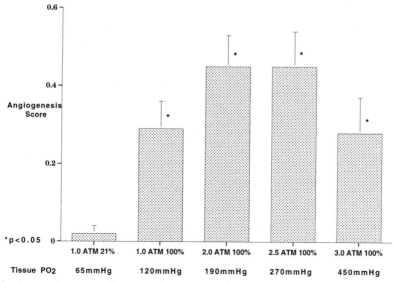

Figure 19–6 ■ Angiogenesis score with nonsupplemented Matrigel under increasing oxygen tensions. *$p < 0.05$ compared to control at 1 atm (1.0 ATA), 21% oxygen. Fisher's LSD Mean ± SE. (From Gibson JJ, Angeles AP, Hunt TK: Increased oxygen tension potentiates angiogenesis. Surg Forum 48:696–699, 1997, with permission.)

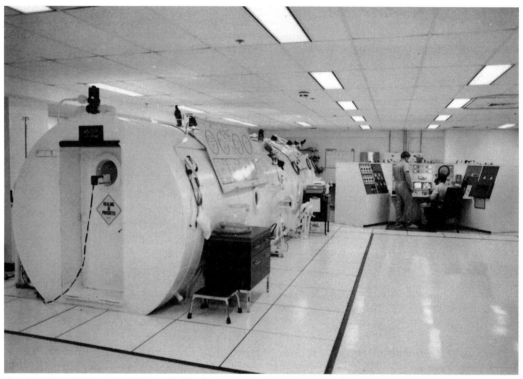

Figure 19–7 ■ Multiplace chamber with capacity for concurrent treatment of multiple patients. Hands-on capability and provision of critical care are advantages in this type of unit. (Courtesy of Dean Heimbach, M.D., Ph.D., San Antonio, TX.)

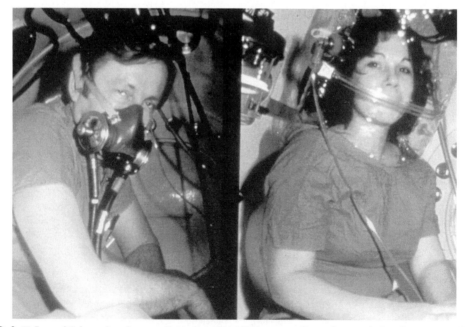

Figure 19–8 ■ In multiplace chambers, patients breathe 100% oxygen through a mask, head tent, or endotracheal tube. Chamber is pressurized to treatment depth with compressed air.

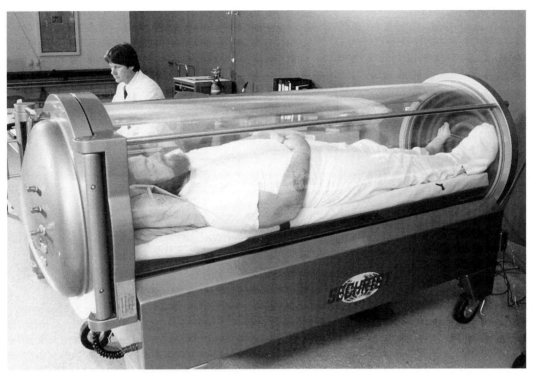

Figure 19-9 ■ Patient being treated in a monoplace chamber pressurized with 100% oxygen. No mask or head tent is necessary.

perbaric oxygen therapy. "A hyperbaric chamber is a device that is intended to increase the environmental oxygen pressure to promote the movement of oxygen from the environment to a patient's tissues by means of pressurization that is greater than atmospheric pressure. This device does not include topical oxygen chambers for extremities."[45] Several groups have demonstrated that topical oxygen chambers are ineffective and may even reduce blood flow and oxygen delivery to the affected extremity.[30, 75]

Mechanisms of Action

Oxygen inhaled at pressure dissolves in plasma. At the pressure equivalent of 3 atm (66 ft of seawater), an arterial Po_2 of nearly 2,200 mm Hg may be achieved. Up to 6.9 vol% of oxygen may be forced into solution, a quantity sufficient to maintain life in the absence of hemoglobin.[10]

With HBO therapy, tissue oxygen tensions can often be raised to the relatively moderate levels necessary for fibroblast replication, de-velopment of a collagen matrix, and the ingress of capillaries into avascular areas. This can occur because wounds actually consume relatively little oxygen. Diffusion of oxygen away from functional capillaries is mainly a function of Po_2, independent of hemoglobin, and is increased two- to fourfold at the pressure equivalent of 3 atm. This may be of vital importance in preserving marginally viable tissue and enhancing collagen deposition, angiogenesis, and bacterial killing in wounds. A marked increase in tissue oxygen tension may be achieved only with HBO therapy (Table 19–1).[15, 64, 80, 111, 119]

Neovascularization

Restoration of abnormally low tissue oxygen tensions to physiologic values assists in capillary proliferation and advancement into the wound space. The reasons are not entirely clear. The effect may be due to oxidant-induced VEGF production or support of endothelial growth and/or migration[48] (see Fig. 19–6).

Table 19–1 ■ TISSUE OXYGEN TENSION WITH INCREASING INSPIRED OXYGEN PRESSURE*

ATA O_2 (mm Hg)	SUBJECT					
	Rat Brain[66]	Rabbit Tibia[56]		Man[67] (Clostridial Myonecrosis)	Man (Subcutaneous)[68]	
		Normal	Osteo	Phlegmon[67]	Muscle	Tissue
0.2	34	45	21	50	29 + 3	37 + 6
1.0	90	—	—	110	59 + 13	53 + 10
2.0	244	321	104	250	221 + 72	221 + 72
3.0	452	—	—	330	—	—

* From Thom SR, Stephen R: Hyperbaric oxygen therapy. J Intensive Care Med 4:58–74, 1989, with permission.
ATA, 1 atmosphere; O_2 oxygen.

Enhancement of White Cell Killing Ability

Control of infection is an important aspect of caring for diabetic foot ulcers. When HBO therapy is effective, diminution of inflammation is an early feature. Doctor et al.[35] have shown rapid sterilization of diabetic wounds using HBO and appropriate antibiotics.

Vasoconstriction

Exposure to oxygen at pressure results in a 20% reduction in blood flow in normal tissue. This effect is offset by the 10- to 15-fold increase in oxygen content of plasma. This vasoconstriction may favorably affect the neurogenic edema seen in the feet of diabetics.[8] Hyperoxia probably does not cause vasoconstriction in ischemic or hypoxic tissues.[101]

Toxicity and Side Effects

Risks involved in the use of HBO therapy are related to pressure changes and the toxic effects of oxygen. They include barotrauma to the ears or sinuses, pulmonary overpressure accidents with pneumothorax, and pulmonary toxicity. Trauma to the ears or sinuses can be averted by slow compression, the use of decongestants, and patient education. Occasionally, myringotomy is necessary. Pulmonary overpressure accidents are very rare, perhaps 1 in 50,000 treatments (P. Cianci, personal survey), and can be avoided by careful pretreatment screening for pulmonary blebs; air trapping caused by bronchospasm or secretions; and the presence of preexisting pneumothorax secondary to chest compression, central lines, ventilatory support, or other forms of trauma.[86] An undetected pneumothorax at sea level can be converted to a tension pneumothorax on ascent from a hyperbaric treatment as ambient pressure decreases. Treatment is immediate insertion of a chest tube. Additional minor side effects are a transient change in visual acuity that reverts to baseline within a few weeks to months after treatment. There is no evidence that the protocols presently used in the United States predispose to cataract formation.[20, 70, 92]

Oxygen Toxicity

Oxygen has definite toxic effects as a result of overdosage, usually affecting the brain or lungs. Exposure to oxygen at depth may cause grand mal seizures, possibly related to interference with γ-aminobutyric acid (GABA) metabolism.[120, 121, 124] Susceptibility varies widely. As the Po_2 value rises, so does the risk of seizures. For this reason, oxygen treatments are usually limited to a maximum depth of 2.8 ATA (60 ft of seawater, 18.2 m) (Fig. 19–10). Fever and certain medications can predispose this complication, and careful attention to potential drug enhancement is mandatory. Oxygen seizures are, in fact, rare, occurring in perhaps 1 in 10,000 to 12,000 treatments.[32] They are self-limited and treated by cessation of oxygen therapy. Hyperbaric oxygen treatment may be reestablished after seizure activity has ceased.

Damage to lung tissue, manifested by irritation to the large airways and a decrement in vital capacity, is a predictable complication of oxygen exposure at depth. The mechanism is believed to be loss of surfactant and

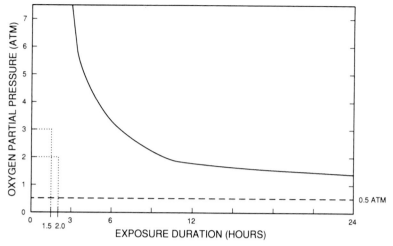

Figure 19–10 ■ Central nervous system and pulmonary toxicity as a function of depth and time of exposure. Treatment protocols are designed to stay within acceptable limits of tolerance. Oxygen is not administered at depths greater than 66 ft. Most clinical exposures are 2 to 2.4 atm for 90 minutes once or twice daily.

changes in the pulmonary macrophages.[5, 49] Because toxicity is related to the depth and duration of exposure, treatment protocols are designed to use the shallowest depth consistent with the desired results (see Fig. 19–10). In practice, pulmonary toxicity from currently used wound healing protocols is virtually unheard of.[32, 57]

Confinement Anxiety

Although not a complication of treatment, claustrophobia may be a problem for patients being treated in hyperbaric chambers. Sedation and reassurance usually remedy the problem. A small percentage of patients cannot tolerate treatment.

Use of Hyperbaric Oxygen Therapy in the Treatment of the Diabetic Foot

Restoration of $TcPo_2$ to normal or slightly raised levels enhances epithelialization, fibroplasia, collagen deposition, angiogenesis, and bacterial killing. Controversy remains as to whether specific cellular immunity is diminished in diabetics in the absence of hyperglycemia, but no one argues that hypoxia increases morbidity of infection, resulting in sepsis, loss of life or limb, or both.

Hyperbaric oxygen greatly increases tissue oxygen levels, and even though treatment is brief (2 to 3 hours daily), oxygen tension values may remain elevated for some time after the cessation of therapy (Fig. 19–11).[88, 119] Davidson et al. have demonstrated elevation of subcutaneous tissue oxygen tensions for several hours after exposure (Fig. 19–12).[102]

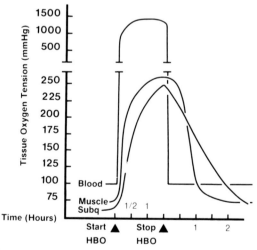

Figure 19–11 ■ Rapidity of rise of oxygen tension after the onset of HBO is proportional to the capillary density of the organ at which the oxygen is transferred, either in the blood or to the peripheral tissue. The decline also is proportional to the height of the peak and to the rate of oxygen consumption. Subcutaneous tissue consumes little oxygen. Height of the peak is lower and the decline rather more rapid in inflamed tissue. (Courtesy of George Hart, M.D.)

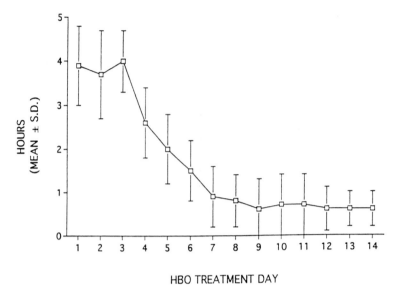

Figure 19–12 ■ Time required for the $Psco_2$ to return to baseline after termination of each hyperbaric oxygen treatment ($n = 22$ ears). Of note, the mean value for day 14 was 3.4 ± 0.8 hours compared with 0.7 ± 0.6 hours for the treatment group ($p < 0.005$). (From Siddiqui A, Davidson JD, Mustoe TA: Ischemic tissue oxygen capacitance after hyperbaric oxygen therapy: A new physiologic concept. Plast Reconstr Surg 99:148–155, 1997, with permission.)

In the long run, the effect on angiogenesis may be the fundamental one. Sheffield[101] has elegantly demonstrated the improvement in capillarity, measuring transcutaneous oxygen levels over healing tissue in diabetic feet. His experience clearly documents the slow improvement in blood flow over the first 3 weeks of therapy as evidenced by rising oxygen tensions in the tissue, especially during HBO therapy sessions. Faglia et al. have shown a highly significant and apparently permanent increase in transcutaneous oxygen values in diabetic patients who benefited from hyperbaric oxygen therapy.[38] Marx et al.[82] have demonstrated the same changes in ischemic irradiated tissues.

Clinical Experience

Several groups have reported increased limb salvage with HBO.[22, 90, 107] Baroni et al.[8] reported a statistically significant reduction in morbidity (amputation) in HBO-treated patients. Sixteen of 18 patients in their treated group healed, whereas only one in ten in the controls did. The amputation rate was 40% in the controls versus 12.5% in the treated group ($p < 0.001$). HBO-treated patients were improved sufficiently to be discharged in 62 days, and 16 went on to complete healing. Nine of ten of the controls had not healed 82 days later. In a continuation of this study,[90] 62 patients in the treated group were compared with 18 controls. A 95% salvage rate was achieved in the HBO-treated group in which there were three amputations (4.8%). The control group suffered six amputations (33%, $p < 0.001$). The incidence of amputation in the untreated group was essentially unchanged from a historical control group of patients treated nearly 10 years earlier without adjunctive HBO therapy. There were no statistical differences in any of the groups relating to age, glycemic control, or diabetic complications. In 1988, we[24] reported a series of 19 diabetics as a subset of 39 patients with lower limb lesions. We noted a salvage rate of 89%. Forty-two percent of these patients had undergone successful revascularization and were referred to us because of infection or nonhealing wounds. Salvage was defined as bipedal ambulation (if two limbs were originally present) and wound coverage for at least 1 year. Hyperbaric oxygen costs were $12,668 and were reflected in total hospital charges of $34,370, with an average stay of 35 days.

More recently we reported a longitudinal outcome study of 41 diabetic patients averaging 63.1 years in age. All patients had limb-threatening lesions. Twenty patients (49%) had undergone revascularization. The average Wagner score was 4 (gangrene of the toes or forefoot). Thirty-five patients' extremities were salvaged (85%). Hyperbaric charges were $15,000, total hospital

Table 19–2 ■ INITIAL PATIENT PROFILE*†

Average Age	63.6 yr
Average Wagner score	4
Patients with limb-threatening lesions	41 (100%)
Patients undergoing vascular surgery	20 (49%)
Average length of stay	27 days
Mean hospital charges (including HBO charges)	$31,264
HBO charges	$15,000
Patients with salvaged limbs, initially	35 (85%)

* From Cianci P, Hunt TK: Long-term results of aggressive management of diabetic foot ulcers suggest significant cost effectiveness. Wound Repair Regen 5:141–146, 1997, with permission.
† Values determined from a patient population of 41.

Table 19–4 ■ SUMMARY OF THE 1993 FOLLOW-UP OF INITIAL PATIENT POPULATION*†

Follow-up obtained	22 (81%)
Patients deceased	6 (27%)
Average age of deceased patients	72.6 yr
Average duration of repair of deceased patients	3.4 yr (42 mo)
Patients still living	16 (73%)
Average age	68.3 yr
Patients with below-the-knee amputation	1 (6%)
Patients with limb intact	15 (94%)
Duration of repair	4.6 yr (55 mo)

* From Cianci P, Hunt TK: Long-term results of aggressive management of diabetic foot ulcers suggest significant cost effectiveness. Wound Repair Regen 5:141–146, 1997, with permission.
† Values are based on a patient population of 27.

charges were $31,264, and the average length of stay was 27 days.[28] These costs compare favorably with the cost of primary amputation, which has been reported as more than $40,000 in 1986.[79] Avoidance of perhaps another $40,000 to $50,000 in rehabilitation costs[24] and the additional savings involved in prevention of reamputation or stump revision have been an additional benefit. Follow-up at two points in time, 1991 and 1993, has shown durability of 32 and 55 months, respectively (Tables 19–2, 19–3, and 19–4). Even in those patients who had died, the average durability of repair was 42 months.[28]

Stone has reported a large series showing 70% salvage in hyperbaric-treated patients vs. 53% in control patients with similar wounds who did not received HBO ($p < 0.002$).[106] Faglia in a prospective, randomized, and blinded study showed an 8.6% amputation rate in HBO-treated patients versus 33.3% in the controls ($p < 0.016$). Transcutaneous oxygen measurements significantly improved with the treated group

(14.0 ± 11.8 vs. 5.0 ± 5.4) over the nontreated group ($p < 0.0002$). They concluded that hyperbaric oxygen therapy in conjunction with an aggressive multidisciplinary protocol is effective in severe, ischemic diabetic foot lesions.[38] In a prospective study, Zamboni reported more rapid healing of diabetic wounds when compared to nonhyperbaric treated controls (Table 19–5 and Fig. 19–13).[125]

These studies are encouraging, but as with all other therapeutic interventions in the diabetic foot, adequacy of control data remains

Table 19–3 ■ SUMMARY OF 1991 FOLLOW-UP OF THE ORIGINAL 41 PATIENTS WITH DIABETES*†

Patients contacted	28 (80%)
Average age	67.3 yr
Patients with limb intact	27 (96%)
Patients with below-the-knee amputation	1 (4%)
Mean durability of repair	2.63 yr (32 mo)

* From Cianci P, Hunt TK: Long-term results of aggressive management of diabetic foot ulcers suggest significant cost effectiveness. Wound Repair Regen 5:141–146, 1997, with permission.
† Values based on a patient population of 35.

Table 19–5 ■ BASELINE PATIENT CHARACTERISTICS* (MEAN ± SEM)

CHARACTERISTICS	CONTROL (N = 5)	HBO THERAPY (N = 5)
Age (yr)	53.8 ± 3.50	63.6 ± 3.96
Gender: male/female	4 : 1	4 : 1
Baseline wound area (cm²)	4.4 ± 1.50	6.02 ± 1.73
TcPo₂ (mm Hg)		
Reference (room air)	60.0 ± 2.12	53.4 ± 4.35
Wound at:		
Room air	35.3 ± 2.30	12.0 ± 2.91
100% mask O₂	80.0 ± 16.34	71.2 ± 25.23
HBO 2.0 ATA	N/A	562.4 ± 55.79
Osteomyelitis	60% (3/5)	80% (4/5)

* From Zamboni WA, Wong HP, Stephenson LL, Pfeifer MA: Evaluation of hyperbaric oxygen for diabetic wounds: A prospective study. J Hyperbar Med 24:175–179, 1997, with permission.
TcPo₂, transcutaneous oxygen tension; mm Hg, millimeters of mercury; HBO, hyperbaric oxygen; ATA, atmospheres absolute.

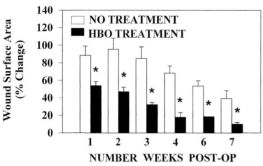

Figure 19–13 ■ Weekly mean wound area as a percentage of the initial baseline pretreatment wound area for control and hyperbaric oxygen (HBO) patient treatment groups (*$p < 0.05$ vs. controls) (From Zamboni WA, Wong HP, Stephenson LL, Pfeifer MA: Evaluation of hyperbaric oxygen for diabetic wounds: A prospective study. J Hyperbar Med 24:175–179, 1997, with permission.)

a problem.[52, 94] One cannot escape, however, the reality that there is no such thing as a "control chronic wound" in humans. Fortunately, the large number of controlled studies and firm mechanistic data in animals are convincing, and the recent clinical reports confirm these animal data.

Patient Selection

Shallow ulcers, particularly of neuropathic origin, unless grossly infected, will usually respond to more conservative treatment. Patients with Wagner class 3, 4, or 5 lesions are considered for treatment based on assessment of blood flow. Patients without adequate arterial flow are referred for angiograms and revascularization as indicated.

TcPo$_2$ values are increasingly recognized as the most reliable, useful noninvasive method for evaluation of perfusion and selecting patients for vascular referral.[7, 16, 55, 60] This measurement is widely available and can be helpful in patient selection for HBO therapy. Pecoraro and Reiber have shown that low TcPo$_2$ confers a high risk of amputation.[94, 97] Patients with transcutaneous periwound TcPo$_2$ values greater than 30 to 40 mm Hg on room air may heal without intervention. Patients with readings less than 20 mm Hg while breathing air have a poor prognosis.[93] An increase to 40 mm Hg or greater while breathing 100% oxygen by tight-fitting mask or while in the hyper-

baric chamber at 1 atm indicates perfusion is adequate for oxygen therapy to benefit.[101] If periwound TcPo$_2$ levels are low and unresponsive, angiography may be helpful in selecting those patients who might benefit from revascularization. In cases where TcPo$_2$ level is low and revascularization is not possible, the prognosis is very guarded. In these instances, a trial of therapy may be indicated on a case-by-case basis if limb loss is the only alternative. More recently, Wattel et al.[118] have reported that patients who show transcutaneous oxygen values of 100 mm Hg in the vicinity of the wound while breathing pure oxygen at 2.5 ATA heal 75% of the time, whereas patients with lower values will go on to amputation (Fig. 19–14). Hart et al.[58] have reported data that support this hypothesis. An additional benefit of transcutaneous oxygen measurements is the determination of when a patient may have obtained maximum benefits of therapy with normalization of periwound TcPo$_2$ values.[29] As more data become avail-

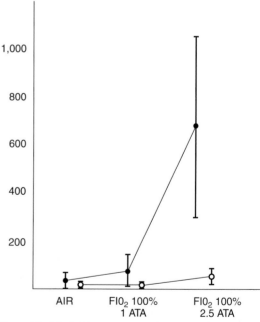

Figure 19–14 ■ Measurement of periwound transcutaneous oxygen level while one breathes 100% oxygen in a hyperbaric chamber appears to be a good predictor of healing. Patients who healed are represented by the *open circles*; *solid circles* represent healing failures. (From Wattel F, Mathieu D, Coget J-M, Billard V: Hyperbaric oxygen therapy in chronic vascular wound management. Angiology 41:59–65, 1990, with permission.)

able, patient selection criteria will become even more precise.

Treatment Protocols

Treatment protocols vary depending on the severity of the problem and the type of chamber used. In larger, multiplace chambers, treatments are rendered at 2 to 2.4 atm for 90 to 120 minutes once or twice daily. In monoplace, single-person configurations, most centers use treatment at 2 atm.

Patients with serious infections are hospitalized for intravenous antibiotics and tight diabetes control. Hyperbaric oxygen treatment in such cases is usually rendered twice daily for 90 minutes. As soon as feasible, patients are transferred to an in-house skilled nursing facility or to home health care where daily wound care, debridement, and HBO treatments can be continued in the outpatient setting. In such instances, HBO is administered once daily for 2 hours, usually right after whirlpool or debridement. After a suitable capillary bed has been established, split-thickness mesh grafts or other plastic techniques are used to effect rapid wound closure. In our experience, early application of grafts, when appropriate, can significantly shorten morbidity, hospital stay, and cost of care. With proper coordination, this program has proved cost effective, even in this era of severe fiscal constraint.[24, 27, 28] It is ironic that the federal reimbursement for amputation, which involves a much greater long-term cost, is 30% greater than that provided for attempts at limb salvage.[28, 53, 78]

Future Trends

Recent data suggest that in selected cases wound growth factors and HBO therapy may be synergistic and lead to even further shortening of healing times (J. Dunn et al., personal communication, 1992).[129] Zhao et al.[128] have demonstrated synergism when used in conjunction with hyperbaric oxygen therapy.

Two additional recent studies are worthy of comment. Haapaniemi and Nylander showed markedly improved healing in a well-designed ischemic animal model. Hyperbaric-treated animals healed faster than nontreated ischemic controls and also faster than nonischemic controls![115] Hammarlund et al. have shown in a randomized, double-blinded, controlled clinical study that HBO increased healing (decreased wound sizes over time) when compared to nontreated controls.[54]

Summary

Hyperbaric oxygen therapy rendered in specially designed chambers is an adjunct to current medical and surgical treatment of frequently discouraging and difficult problems of healing failure in diabetics. Recent investigations have demonstrated that adequate tissue oxygen tension is an essential factor in wound healing. Frequently, adequate levels can be reached only through adjunctive HBO treatment. This results in more normal fibroblast proliferation, angiogenesis, collagen deposition, epithelization, and enhancement of bacterial killing. Although HBO therapy is costly, the ability to preserve a functional extremity can reduce the high cost of disability resulting from amputation. The shortened healing time for chronic wounds will reduce the cost of frequent, repeated surgical procedures. As part of a multidisciplinary program of wound care, it can be cost effective and durable. Indeed, the Consensus Development Conference of the American Diabetes Association has recognized the value of adjunctive hyperbaric oxygen in difficult cases, stating that it is reasonable to use this modality to treat severe or life-threatening wounds that have not responded to other treatments, particularly if ischemia that cannot be corrected by vascular procedures is present.[130]

Case Illustrations (Plates 20 to 25)

Revascularization often can provide the substrate necessary for healing. However, historically limbs have been lost to necrotizing infections, even in the presence of adequate circulation and excellent wound care. We use adjunctive HBO therapy early when there is extensive soft tissue infection, which often necessitates extensive radical debridement. Adjunctive HBO therapy can speed the healing process in the severely compromised limb.

REFERENCES

1. Aagenaes O, Moe H: Light- and electron-microscope study of skin capillaries of the diabetic. Diabetes 10:253–259, 1961.
2. American Diabetes Association: Diabetes 1996 Vital Statistics, 1996.
3. Apelquist J, et al: Long-term costs for foot ulcers in diabetic patients in a multidisciplinary setting. Foot Ankle Int 16:388, 1995.
4. Arenson OJ, et al: Neuropathic angiopathy and sepsis in the diabetic foot. Part 2. Angiopathy JAPA 71:661–665, 1981.
5. Armbruster S: Surfactant in pulmonary oxygen toxicity. Adv Exp Med Biol 215:345–349, 1987.
6. Bakker DJ: Pure and mixed aerobic and anaerobic soft tissue infections. Hyperbaric Oxygen Rev 6:65–96, 1985.
7. Ballard JL, et al: A prospective evaluation of transcutaneous oxygen measurements in the management of diabetic foot problems. J Vasc Surg 22:485–492, 1995.
8. Baroni G, et al: Hyperbaric oxygen in diabetic gangrene treatment. Diabetes Care 10:81–86, 1987.
9. Block P: The diabetic foot ulcer: A complex problem with a simple treatment approach. Mil Med 146:644, 1981.
10. Boerema I, et al: Life without blood: A study of the influence of high atmospheric pressure and hypothermia on dilution of blood. J Cardiovasc Surg 1:133–146, 1960.
11. Borer RC: Neutrophil adhesion and the diabetic. Hyperbaric Medicine 1998 Advanced Symposium, University of South Carolina School of Medicine, 1998.
12. Borer RC, Gamble JR: Hyperbaric oxygen therapy (HBO) corrects impaired neutrophil adhesion in patients with non-insulin dependent diabetes mellitus (NIDDM). Undersea Hyperbar Res 24(Suppl): 15, 1997.
13. Bouachour G, et al: Hyperbaric oxygen therapy in the management of crush injuries: A randomized double-blind placebo-controlled clinical trial. J Trauma 41:333–339, 1996.
14. Brummelkamp WH: Considerations on hyperbaric oxygen therapy at three atmospheres absolute for clostridial infections type welchii. Ann N Y Acad Sci 117:688–699, 1965.
15. Brummelkamp WH, Hoogendijk J: Borerema: Treatment of anaerobic infections (clostridial myositis) by drenching the tissues with oxygen under high atmospheric pressure. Surgery 49:299–302, 1961.
16. Bunt TJ, et al: TcPo$_2$ as an accurate predictor of therapy in limb salvage. Ann Vasc Surg 10:224–227, 1996.
17. Buras J: HBO regulation of ICAM 1 in an endothelial cell model of ischemia/reperfusion injury. Hyperbaric Medicine 1998 Advanced Symposium, University of South Carolina School of Medicine, 1998.
18. Buras JA, Reenstra WR, Svoboda KKH: Hyperbaric oxygen down-regulates hypoxia/hypoglycemia-stimulated endothelial cell surface ICAM-1 protein expression. Mol Biol Cell 8:230A, 1997.
19. Buras JA, Reenstra WR, Svoboda KKH: HBO decreases endothelial cell intercellular adhesion molecule-1 (ICAM-1) protein expression and neutrophil adhesion in an in-vitro model of ischemia/reperfusion. Undersea Hyperbar Med 25 (Suppl): 51, 1998.
20. Butler FK: Diving and hyperbaric ophthalmology. Surv Ophthalmol 39:347–365, 1995.
21. Chang N, Mathes SJ: Comparison of the effect of bacterial inoculation in musculocutaneous and random-pattern flaps. Plast Reconstr Surg 70:1–10, 1982.
22. Cianci P: Adjunctive hyperbaric oxygen in the treatment of problem wounds an economic analysis. In Kindwall E (ed): Proceedings of the Eighth International Congress on Hyperbaric Medicine. San Pedro, CA: Best Publishing, 1984, pp 213–216.
23. Cianci P, et al: Adjunctive hyperbaric oxygen reduces the need for surgery in 40–80% burns. J Hyperb Med 3:97–101, 1988.
24. Cianci P, et al: Salvage of the problem wound and potential amputation with wound care and adjunctive hyperbaric oxygen therapy: An economic analysis. J Hyperbar Med 3:127–141, 1988.
25. Cianci P, et al: Adjunctive hyperbaric oxygen reduces length of hospitalization in thermal burns. J Burn Care Rehabil 10:432–435, 1989.
26. Cianci P, et al: Adjunctive hyperbaric oxygen in the treatment of thermal burns—an economic analysis. J Burn Care Rehabil 11:140–143, 1990.
27. Cianci P, et al: Adjunctive hyperbaric oxygen in the salvage of the diabetic foot. Undersea Biomed Res 18(Suppl):108, 1991.
28. Cianci P, Hunt TK: Long-term results of aggressive management of diabetic foot ulcers suggest significant cost effectiveness. Wound Repair Regen 5:141–146, 1997.
29. Clarke D: Transcutaneous oxygen. Interpretation and reporting. Hyperbaric Medicine Symposium, University of South Carolina School of Medicine, 1994.
30. Cotto-Cumba C, et al: Transcutaneous oxygen measurements in normal subjects using topical HBO control module. Undersea Baromed Res 18(Suppl):109, 1991 (presented at the UHMS Annual Scientific Meeting, San Diego).
31. Couch NP, et al: Natural history of the leg amputee. Am J Surg 133:469–473. 1977.
32. Davis JC: Refractory osteomyelitis. In Davis JC, Hunt TK (eds): Problem Wounds: The Role of Oxygen. New York: Elsevier, 1988, pp 125–142.
33. Davis JC: Hyperbaric oxygen therapy. Intensive Care Med 4:55–57, 1989.
34. Davis JC, et al: Chronic non-hematogenous osteomyelitis treated with adjuvant-hyperbaric oxygen. J Bone Joint Surg 68A:1210–1217, 1986.
35. Doctor N, Pandya S, Supe A: Hyperbaric oxygen therapy in diabetic foot. J Postgrad Med 38:112–114, 1992.
36. Ebskov G, Josephsen P: Incidence of reamputation and death after gangrene of the lower extremity. Prosthet Orthot Int 4:77–80, 1980.
37. Edmonda ME, et al: Improved survival of the diabetic foot: The role of the specialized foot clinic. Q J Med 60:763–771, 1986.
38. Faglia, et al: Adjunctive systemic hyperbaric oxygen therapy in treatment of severe prevalently ischemic diabetic foot ulcer. Diabetes Care 19:1338–1343, 1996.
39. Feldmeier JJ, et al: Hyperbaric oxygen as an adjunctive treatment for severe laryngeal necrosis: A report of nine consecutive cases. Undersea Hyperbar Med 20:329–335, 1993.

40. Feldmeier JJ, et al: Hyperbaric oxygen as an adjunctive treatment for delayed radiation injury of the chest wall: A retrospective review of twenty-three cases. Undersea Hyperb Med 22:383–393, 1995.

41. Feldmeier JJ, et al: Hyperbaric oxygen as a prophylaxis for radiation-induced delayed enteropathy. Radiother Oncol 35:138–144, 1995.

42. Feldmeier JJ, et al: Hyperbaric oxygen an adjunctive treatment for delayed radiation injuries of the abdomen and pelvis. Undersea Hyperbar Med 23:205–213, 1996.

43. Feng JJ, et al: Angiogenesis in wound healing. J Surg Pathol 3:1–7, 1998.

44. Flynn MD, Tooke JE: Diabetic neuropathy and the microcirculation. Diabet Med 12:298–301, 1995.

45. Foreman C: The FDA and HBO. Hyperbaric Medicine 1998 Advanced Symposium, University of South Carolina School of Medicine, 1998.

46. Friederici HHR, Tucker WR, Schwartz TB: Observations on small blood vessels of skin in the normal and in diabetic patients. Diabetes 15:233–250, 1960.

47. Gibbons GW, et al: Improved quality of diabetic foot care, 1984 vs 1990. Arch Surg 128:576–581, 1993.

48. Gibson JJ, Angeles AP, Hunt TK: Increased oxygen tension potentiates angiogenesis. Surg Forum 48:696–699, 1997.

49. Goodman MW, Workman RP: Oxygen-breathing approach of treatment of decompression sickness in divers and aviators. Bureau of Medicine and Surgery, BuShips Project SF0110606, Task 11513-2, Research Report 5-65, 1965.

50. Gottrup F, et al: Dynamic properties of tissue oxygen in healing flaps. Surgery 95:527–536, 1984.

51. Gozal D, et al: Necrotizing fasciitis. Arch Surg 121:233–235, 1986.

52. Grunfield C: Diabetic foot ulcers: Etiology, treatment, and prevention. In Stollerman GH, et al (eds): Advances in Internal Medicine, Vol 37. St. Louis: Mosby-Year Book, 1991, pp 103–132.

53. Gupta SK, Veith FJ: Inadequacy of diagnosis related group (DRG) reimbursements for limb salvage lower extremity arterial reconstructions. J Vasc Surg 22:348–357, 1990.

54. Hammarlund C, Sundberg T: Hyperbaric oxygen reduced size of chronic leg ulcers: A randomized double-blind study. Plast Reconstr Surg 93:829–834, 1994.

55. Hanna GP, et al: Infrapopliteal transcatheter interventions for limb salvage in diabetic patients: Importance of. J Am Coll Cardiol 30:664–669. 1997.

56. Hart GB, et al: Treatment of burns with hyperbaric oxygen. Surg Gynecol Obstet 139:693–696, 1974.

57. Hart GB, et al: Vital capacity of quadraplegic patients treated with hyperbaric oxygen. J Am Paraplegia Soc 7:91–92, 1984.

58. Hart GB, et al: Transcutaneous partial pressure of oxygen measured in a monoplace hyperbaric chamber at 1, 1.5 and 2 atm abs oxygen. J Hyperbar Med 5:223–229, 1990.

59. Hart GB, Lamb RC, Strauss MB: Gas gangrene. 2 parts. J Trauma 23:991–1000, 1983.

60. Hauser CJ, et al: Assessment of perfusion in the diabetic foot by regional transcutaneous oximetry. Diabetes 33:527–531, 1984.

61. Hehenberger K, et al: Dose-dependent hyperbaric oxygen stimulation of human fibroblast proliferation. Wound Repair Regen 5:147–150, 1997.

62. Heimbach RD: Gas gangrene: Review and update. Hyperbaric Oxygen Rev 1:41–61, 1980.

63. Hunt TK: The physiology of wound healing. Ann Emerg Med 17:1265–1273, 1988.

64. Jamieson D, Van Daen Brenk HAS: Measurement of oxygen tensions in cerebral tissues of rats exposed to high pressures of oxygen. J Appl Physiol 18:869–876, 1963.

65. Johnsson K, Hunt TK, Mathes SJ: Effect of environmental oxygen on bacterial-induced tissue necrosis in flaps. Surg Forum 35:589–591, 1984.

66. Joseph WS, LeFrock JL: The pathogenesis of diabetic foot infection—immunopathy, angiopathy, and neuropathy. J Foot Surg 26:S7–S11, 1987.

67. Kaelin CM, et al: The effects of hyperbaric oxygen on free flaps in rats. Arch Surg 125:607–609, 1990.

68. Kindwall EP: Carbon monoxide and cyanide poisoning. Hyperbaric Oxygen Rev 1:115–122, 1980.

69. Kihn RB, et al: The geriatric amputee. Ann Surg 176:305–314, 1972.

70. Kindwall EP: Contraindications and side effects to hyperbaric oxygen treatment. In Kindwall EP (ed): Hyperbaric Medicine, 1994, Best Publishing Company, pp 45–56.

71. Knighton DR, et al: Oxygen tension regulates the expression of angiogenesis factor by macrophages. Science 221:1283–1285, 1983.

72. Knighton DR, et al: Amputation prevention in an independently reviewed at-risk diabetic population using a comprehensive wound care protocol. Am J Surg 160:466–472, 1990.

73. Knighton DR, Halliday B, Hunt TK: Oxygen as an antibiotic: The effect of inspired oxygen on infection. Arch Surg 119:199–204, 1984.

74. Larsson J, et al: Decreasing incidence of major amputation in diabetic patients: A consequence of a multidisciplinary foot care team approach? Diabet Med 12:770–776, 1995.

75. Leslie CA: Randomized controlled trial of topical hyperbaric oxygen for treatment of diabetic foot ulcers. Diabetes Care 11:111–115, 1988.

76. Levene CI, et al: The activation of protocollagen proline hydroxylation by ascorbic acid in cultured 3T6 fibroblasts. Biochem Biophys Acta 338:29, 1974.

77. Levin ME: Diabetic foot lesions: Pathogenesis and management. J Enterostomal Ther 17:29–34, 1990.

78. Lorenz EW: The Physician's DRG Working Guidebook 1988, 1988, St. Anthony's Hospital Publications.

79. Mackey WC, et al: The cost of surgery for limb-threatening ischemia. Surgery 99:26–35, 1986.

80. Mader JT, et al: A mechanism for the amelioration by hyperbaric oxygen of experimental staphylococcal osteomyelitis in rabbits. J Infect Dis 142:915–922, 1980.

81. Martindale VE: Nitric oxide as therapeutic mechanism in HBO therapy? Hyperbaric Medicine 1998 Advanced Symposium, Univeristy of South Carolina School of Medicine, 1998.

82. Marx RE, et al: Relationship of oxygen dose to angiogenesis induction in irradiated tissue. Am J Surg 160:519–524, 1990.

83. McMillan DE, et al: Forearm skin capillaries of diabetic, potential diabetic and non-diabetic subjects: Changes seen by light microscopy. Diabetes 15:251–257, 1966.

84. Medawar PB: The cultivation of adult mammalian skin epithelium. Q J Microbiol Sci 89:187, 1948.

85. Morrey BF, et al: Hyperbaric oxygen and chronic osteomyelitis. Clin Orthop 144:121–127, 1979.

86. Murphy DG, et al: Tension pneumothorax associated with hyperbaric oxygen therapy. Am J Emerg Med 9:176–179, 1991.

87. Myers RAM, Marx RE: Use of hyperbaric oxygen in postradiation head and neck surgery. NCI Monogr 9:151–157, 1990.

88. Niinikoski J, Aho AJ: Combination of hyperbaric oxygen, surgery, and antibiotics in the treatment of clostridial gas gangrene. Infect Surg 2:23–37, 1983.

89. Ohkubo Y, et al: Intensive insulin therapy prevents the progression of diabetic microvascular complications in Japanese patients with non-insulin-dependent diabetes mellitus: A randomized prospective 6-year study. Diabetes Res Clin Pract 28:103–117, 1995.

90. Oriani G, et al: Hyperbaric oxygen therapy in diabetic gangrene. J Hyperbar Med 5:171–175, 1990.

91. Pai MP, Hunt TK: Effect of varying oxygen tensions on healing of open wounds. Surg Gynecol Obstet 135:756–758, 1972.

92. Palmquist BM, Philipsson B, Barr PO: Nuclear cataract and myopia during hyperbaric oxygen therapy. Br J Ophthalmol 68:113–117, 1984.

93. Pecoraro RE: The nonhealing diabetic ulcer—a major cause for limb loss. Prog Clin Biol Res 365:27–43, 1991.

94. Pecoraro RE, et al: The chronology and determinants of tissue repair in diabetic lower extremity ulcers. Diabetes 40:1305–1313, 1991.

95. Prokop DJ, et al: Biosynthesis of collagen and its disorders. N Engl J Med 301:13–23, 1979.

96. Rabkin J, Hunt TK: Infection and oxygen. In Davis JC, Hunt TK (eds): Problem Wounds: The Role of Oxygen. New York: Elsevier, 1987, pp 1–16.

97. Reiber GE, Pecoraro RE, Koepsell TD: Risk factors for amputation in patients with diabetes mellitus. Ann Intern Med 117:97–105, 1992.

98. Reichard P, Nilsson BY, Rosenqvist U: The effect of long-term intensified insulin treatment on the development of microvascular complications of diabetes mellitus. N Engl J Med 329:304–309, 1993.

99. Riseman JA, et al: Hyperbaric oxygen therapy for necrotizing fasciitis reduces mortality and the need for debridements. Surgery 108:847–850, 1990.

100. Selby JV, et al: Excess costs of medical care for patients with diabetes in a managed care population. Diabetes Care 20:1396–1402, 1997.

101. Sheffield PJ: Tissue oxygenation measurements. In Davis JC, Hunt TK (eds): Problem Wounds: The Role of Oxygen. New York: Elsevier, 1988, pp 17–51.

102. Siddiqui A, Davidson JD, Mustoe TA: Ischemic tissue oxygen capacitance after hyperbaric oxygen therapy: A new physiologic concept. Plast Reconstr Surg 99:148–155, 1997.

103. Skalak TC, Price RJ: The role of mechanical stresses in microvascular remodeling. Microcirculation 3:143–165, 1996.

104. Slack WK, Thomas DA, Perrins JD: Hyperbaric oxygenation in chronic osteomyelitis. Lancet 1:1093–1094, 1965.

105. Stone JA, Cianci P: The adjunctive role of hyperbaric oxygen therapy in the treatment of lower extremity wounds in patients with diabetes. Diabetes Spectrum 10:118–123, 1997.

106. Stone JA, et al: The role of hyperbaric oxygen therapy in the treatment of the diabetic foot. Diabetes 44(Suppl 1):71A, 1995.

107. Strauss MB, et al: Salvaging the difficult wound through a combined management program. In Kindwall E (ed): Proceedings of the Eighth International Congress on Hyperbaric Medicine. San Pedro, CA: Best Publishing, 1984.

108. Strauss MB, Hart GB: Crush injury and the role of hyperbaric oxygen. Topics Emerg Med 6:9–24, 1984.

109. Tan CM, et al: Effects of hyperbaric oxygen and hyperbaric air on the survival of island skin flaps. Plast Reconstr Surg 73:27–28, 1984.

110. The Diabetes Control and Complications Trial Research Group: The effect of intensive treatment of diabetes on the development and progression of long-term complications in insulin-dependent diabetes mellitus. N Engl J Med 329:977–986, 1993.

111. Thom SR: Hyperbaric oxygen therapy. J Intensive Care Med 4:58–74, 1989.

112. Thom SR, et al: Delayed neuropsychologic sequelae after carbon monoxide poisoning: Prevention by treatment with hyperbaric oxygen. Ann Emerg Med 25:474–537, 1995.

113. Tooke JE: Microvascular function in human diabetes. A physiological perspective. Diabetes 44:721–726, 1995.

114. Tooke JE, Morris SJ, Shore AC: Microvascular functional abnormalities in diabetes: The role of the endothelium. Diabetes Res Clin Pract 31 (Suppl):S127–S132, 1996.

115. Uhl E, et al: Hyperbaric oxygen improves wound healing in normal and ischemic skin tissue. Plast Reconstr Surg 93:835–841, 1994.

116. U.S. Dept of Health and Human Services: National Diabetes Fact Sheet. Centers for Disease Control and Prevention, National Center for Chronic Disease Prevention and Health Promotion, November 1, 1997.

117. Vracko R, Strandness DE Jr: Basal lamina of abdominal skeletal muscle capillaries in diabetics and nondiabetics. Circulation 35:690–700, 1967.

118. Wattel F, et al: Hyperbaric oxygen therapy in chronic vascular wound management. Angiology 41:59–65, 1990.

119. Wells CH, et al: Tissue gas measurements during hyperbaric oxygen exposure. In Smith G (ed): Proceedings of the 6th International Conference on Hyperbaric Medicine, 1977, Aberdeen University Press, pp 118–124.

120. Wood JD: GABA and oxygen toxicity: A review. Brain Res Bull 6:777–780, 1980.

121. Wood JD, et al: Sensitivity of GABA synthesis in human brain to oxygen poisoning. Aviat Space Environ Med 46:1155–1156, 1975.

122. Wyss CR, et al: Relationship between transcutaneous oxygen tension, ankle blood pressure, and clinical outcome of vascular surgery in diabetic

and nondiabetic patients. Surgery 101:56–62, 1987.

123. Yarbrough OB, Behnke AR: The treatment of compressed air illness utilizing oxygen. J Ind Hygiene Toxicol 21:6, 1939.

124. Yoneda Y, et al: Modulation of synaptic GABA receptor binding by membrane phospholipids: Possible role of active oxygen radicals. Brain Res 333:111–122, 1985.

125. Zamboni WA, et al: Evaluation of hyperbaric oxygen for diabetic wounds: A prospective study. J Hyperbar Med 24:175–179, 1997.

126. Zamboni WA, et al: The effect of acute hyperbaric oxygen therapy on axial pattern skin flap survival when administered during and after total ischemia. J Reconstr Microsurg 5:343–347, 1989.

127. Zatz A, Brenner BM: Pathogenesis of diabetic microangiopathy: The hemodynamic view. Am J Med 80:443–453, 1986.

128. Zhao LL, et al: Effect of hyperbaric oxygen and growth factors on rabbit ear ischemic ulcers. Arch Surg 129:1043–1049, 1994.

129. Zhao LL, et al: Total reversal of hypoxic wound healing deficit by hyperbaric oxygen plus growth factors. Surg Forum 43:711–714, 1992.

130. American Diabetes Association: Consensus development conference on diabetic foot wound care, 7–8 April 1999, Boston, Massachusetts. Diabetes Care 22:1354–1360, 1999.

FOOTWEAR FOR INJURY PREVENTION: CORRELATION WITH RISK CATEGORY

■ William C. Coleman

The most successful diabetic foot programs in the United States concentrate their efforts on injury prevention. In many medical centers, foot care for the diabetic patient begins with treatment of the first injury. In an ideal situation, however, the possibility of the first foot injury should have been anticipated. Proper care for diabetic foot problems should always include an aggressive program of injury prevention. Every medical practitioner treating persons with diabetes needs to inspect the feet of these patients regularly. All diabetic patients need education on footwear selection and foot inspection. As soon as changes due to diabetes are noted on the feet, persons who sell, modify, or construct medically indicated shoes need to be included as contributing consultants.

With the proper use of appropriate footwear and instruction related to foot care, most diabetic patients can expect to avoid a skin wound on their feet. Providing appropriate footwear for the diabetic patient who has never had a foot injury continues to be a difficult problem. It is often difficult to convince a person who feels no foot discomfort and who has never had a foot injury with neuropathy to severely restrict themselves to only the types of footwear they can safely wear. Few medical practitioners have sufficient training regarding the applications and prescription of protective footwear. Most shoe modifications are recommended as the result of trial-and-error experience and training that is based on the empiric findings of shoemakers of previous generations. There are few objective, experimentally derived data to support most shoe therapy.[33]

Unlike many European countries, the United States is in the early stages of developing a formal training program for shoemakers or shoe-fitters. In Europe, representatives of large-scale, regional companies that manufacture prescription footwear are present at clinics to contribute to the decision-making process and become familiar with the clinical goals for each patient who is prescribed shoes.

A person with an insensitive foot should never walk with an open foot wound or fracture. Shoes are not reliable as part of wound or fracture management and usually will prolong the time needed to heal.[6]

Even if a shoe is perfectly fitted to the foot and relieves stress to an open ulcer, the shoe will be removed by the patient at home. Many diabetics need to urinate in the middle of the night. When they walk to and from the bathroom they seldom wear their protective shoes. One unguarded step on an insensitive foot with an ulceration, fracture, or infection can be devastating to the prognosis of that foot.[6] Shoes have their best utility as a means of injury prevention and not as a means of treating active injuries. If the patient with neuropathy must walk, then casts or splints are a more effective means of protection.[9]

Frequently, diabetic patients cannot afford the proper, medically indicated footwear. Many "third-party" reimbursement systems do not cover shoes intended for the prevention of injury to the feet of a diabetic. As of May 1993, persons at risk from complications related to diabetes and covered by the United States Medicare program are entitled to reimbursement for a pair of shoes and three pairs of insoles a year. The study conducted to evaluate the cost of this provision found that this benefit increased the possibility that a person with diabetes would obtain and use prescribed footwear.[43]

This chapter is formatted according to a prevention program that was developed at the Gillis W. Long Hansen's Disease Center. The basic concept for the program was presented by Joseph Reed, RPT, in 1982.[28] He felt it was easier to anticipate possible injuries if patients could be classified according to their potential risk of injury. Patients with the highest risk would need the most protective footwear and return for evaluation more often than patients who have less chance of damaging their feet as a result of diabetes.

Risk Determination

This system of risk determination is based on the ability of a clinician to determine the presence or absence of protective levels of sensation. Protective levels of sensation, for the purpose of this chapter, are present when a person can perceive and react to a threatening stimulus to effectively minimize or prevent injury. In a recent survey of factors that place a person with diabetes at higher risk of experiencing a foot ulceration, neuropathy

was determined to be the most prevalent complication. Other factors that contribute to higher risk are the presence of diabetes for more than 10 years, poor blood sugar control, male gender, foot deformity, higher pressures under the feet, and a history of amputation.[22]

People with diabetes were not found to be at higher risk of developing an ulceration if they also had peripheral vascular disease, a lower level of formal education, retinopathy, obesity, or had a history of ethanol abuse or tobacco use.[22]

Sensory Examination

Historically, clinicians would observe diabetic patients walking on open foot wounds without limping. This would be occurring despite a "normal" sensory examination as determined by using the accepted tests for that time. As a result sensory examination was not routinely performed. Their tests were incapable of revealing the presence or absence of protective sensation.[21] A more precise, quantifiable system of sensory testing was needed for diabetic patients. After extensive reliability testing and clinical trials, Semmes-Weinstein monofilaments seem to provide reproducible quantification to differentiate patients who have protective sensation from those who cannot feel that damage has occurred.[4, 13] In a study to screen 1,001 patients for risk at two clinics in the United Kingdom, Klenerman et al. found that 21.8% of their patients with diabetes displayed a loss of protective sensation.[20]

Semmes-Weinstein monofilaments (Fig. 20–1) are a set of progressively thicker nylon filaments each attached at right angles to a small handle. They are a modification of a sensory testing system described by von Frey in 1925.[41] Pressure is applied to the skin with the filament until it bends. A series of filaments graduated in diameter is used. Larger diameter filaments require more force to bend them. Sensations of light touch and deep pressure can be determined finding the threshold between filaments that can be and cannot be felt by the patient.[2] For use on the feet, loss of protective sensation has been described at the level when the patient cannot feel the Semmes-Weinstein monofilament which bends at a linear force of 10 gm.[4] Sets of filaments

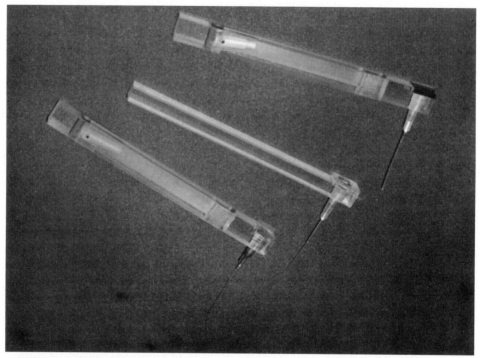

Figure 20–1 ■ A set of three Semmes-Weinstein monofilaments is used for sensory testing on feet. Here the monofilaments are attached to the end of lucite rods. Each of the three filaments is a different thickness. The middle thickness bends with a force of 10 gm. The smaller filament bends with 1 gm force and the larger at 75 gm.

that bend with the forces of 1, 10, and 75 gm are frequently used clinically. These filaments can easily be differentiated by a test subject with normal sensation. The 1-gm filament can be felt by most persons with normal sensation. A person with protective sensory loss may have some sensation remaining and the 75-gm filament can help determine the presence of this sensation. In a comparison of Semmes-Weinstein monofilaments to the Biothesiometer (a device to test sensation with quantifiable vibration), Klenerman et al. found only the monofilaments to have sufficient reproducibility in a screening program.[20]

Clinics that have incorporated new programs of foot examination and patient education, managed by professionals trained to manage foot problems, have dramatically reduced amputation rates and hospital days for foot-related problems. At Atlanta's Grady Memorial Hospital the amputation rate was decreased by 50%.[19] The County Health Department in Memphis reduced the number of days spent in the hospital by 68%.[31] The University Hospital in Geneva, Switzerland,

was able to reduce the transtibial amputation rate by 85%.[1]

Vascular Examination

Vascular evaluation is essential to develop a complete impression of a patient's ability to heal foot pathology and to identify their risk of developing ischemic changes (see Chapter 16). Clinicians may be disproportionately focused, however, on the problems created by vascular disease and, as a result, are often unprepared to manage neuropathic complications.

Although the knowledge of an individual's vascular status is very important, it needs to be kept in perspective. One still must help protect patients with severe arterial occlusion. Some of these persons may never meet the criteria for the interventions to improve their vascular status.[23] The potential for catastrophic consequences, as the result of small injury, is very high in this group of patients and they need close observation and reinforcement to remain vigilant against the occurrence of an injury.

Risk Categorization

The risk categories presented here can all be included within grade 0 (intact skin) of the ulcer classification system described by Wagner.[42]

Risk Category 0

Category 0 (Table 20–1) of risk includes all patients who have been diagnosed as having diabetes who retain protective levels of sensation. Sensory systems within the foot and vascular supply to the foot, however, can be lost during any stage of the disease. Since this loss may be so gradual that it is not

Table 20–1 ■ RISK AND MANAGEMENT CATEGORIES

RISK	MANAGEMENT
Category 0	
Protective sensation present	Foot clinic once/yr
No history of plantar ulcer	Patient education to include proper shoe style selection
May have foot deformity	
Has a disease which could lead to insensitivity	
Category 1	
Protective sensation absent	Foot clinic every 6 mo
No history of plantar ulceration	Review all footwear the patient wears
No foot deformity	Add soft insoles— Spenco*, nylon covered PPT†
Category 2	
Protective sensation absent	Foot clinic every 3–4 mo
No history of plantar ulcer	Custom-molded orthotic devices usually necessary
Foot deformity present	Prescription footwear are often required
Category 3	
Protective sensation absent	Foot clinic every 1–2 mo
There is a history of foot ulceration and/ or vascular laboratory findings indicate significant vascular disease	Custom orthotic devices are necessary Prescription shoes are often required

* Spenco Medical Corporation, Waco, TX.
† Professional Protective Technology, Deer Park, NY.

Table 20–2 ■ INSENSITIVE FOOT EXAMINATION*

EXAMINATION	JUSTIFICATION
General	Inspect for possible ulceration, areas of inflammation, or other skin changes related to vascular disease
Sensory	Test vibratory sensation and perform a quantifiable sensory test to determine level of protective sensation
Temperature	With no sensation, a localized skin temperature increase $> 2°C$ in a localized area indicates an area of inflammation
Shoes	Identify the characteristics of the footwear that because of wear or style pose a threat to the feet
Muscle	Diseases that result in sensory loss can also lead to muscle paralysis; in the feet, intrinsic paralysis is the most frequent early involvement and results in clawed toe deformities

* Patient education for self-examination should be provided to expand or reinforce the patient's active participation in his or her own care on every visit.

noticed by the patient, a periodic, objective evaluation of sensation should be done to help prevent tissue damage. A standardized record of foot risk factors should be maintained for the duration of the patient's life (Table 20–2).

Risk Category 1

Patients in category 1 have not had ulcers of their feet but have lost protective levels of sensation. This places them at a higher risk of injury. The repetitive stress of walking alone can result in damage to their feet. Veves et al. reported that 39% of all patients with diabetic neuropathy had higher than normal pressures under their feet.[39]

For most patients, an inability to feel the Semmes-Weinstein monofilament that bends with a pressure of 10 gm (5.07) would place them in this category.

Risk Category 2

Patients included in category 2 have lost sensation and also have a deformity in their foot, but have not had ulcers. Deformity results in the concentration of stress in a small area of the foot. The added stress usually occurs in a part of the foot that is not accustomed to additional pressure resulting in injury. Surgical correction of deformity can result in moving a diabetic patient to a lower risk category.

Risk Category 3

Persons in category 3 not only have lost sensation but have a history of previous foot ulceration. Human skin and underlying soft tissues are more easily reinjured in areas where previous damage has occurred.

Patient Management

As the risk of ulceration rises, so does the need for more frequent foot examination. With deformity or previous ulceration, these vulnerable areas need footwear modifications to limit stress even further. Also, as risk increases, the patient needs ever-increasing levels of education to ensure that only protective footwear is worn and that the patient identifies possible sites of injury early. In a survey of patients with diabetes at Kings College Hospital in London, the recurrence rate of ulceration was 26% among those with special footwear and 83% among those who returned to using their regular footwear.[14]

It is extremely difficult to indoctrinate most diabetic patients adequately in foot care and ulcer prevention before extensive damage has taken place. Many injuries can be prevented with a regular schedule of clinic visits and minimal guidelines for shoe modification. With this in mind, management categories have been established to complement the risk categories (Table 20–1).

Assisting a population of persons with diabetes in preventing ulcerations can be very frustrating. Diabetes can result in psychological change in the diabetic patient that interferes with successful injury prevention or management.[1] Despite careful patient education and examination, careless action on the part of the neuropathic person often results in foot injury. Over a 4-year period of time, King's College Diabetic Foot Clinic in London reported 86 preventable foot injuries among persons with diabetes who had received education on foot care.[17] These injuries resulted from wearing inappropriate footwear, picking at skin, or walking barefoot.

Education is essential at every visit for evaluation of the feet. It is also essential not to overwhelm the person with information. Each patient should be educated in accordance to their risk of developing a foot problem. As their risk increases, foot care education should also increase. To ensure that every patient obtains complete instructions, this form of education can be provided on videotape. The patient should view the tape and then any questions would be answered by the clinical personnel. If a specific behavior is required of the patient, this behavior should be rehearsed by the patient under supervision of the clinical staff.

Management Category 0

Patients in risk category 0 need to receive education on footwear selection. The feet of patients in this group could lose sensation before their next visit. They should begin to wear only shoes that pose no threat to their feet if loss of sensation develops. A person with insensitive feet can no longer trust the "feel" of a shoe to determine proper fit. To obtain the same "feel" on feet that now have lost sensation, the diabetic may prefer to buy a smaller sized shoe. Diabetics should always inform shoe-fitters of their disease. A publication of the National Shoe Retailers Association estimates that only 5% of all persons who sell shoes have any significant training or experience in fitting footwear.[29]

Since insensitivity or vascular disease can occur at any time, the peripheral sensory and circulatory status of each diabetic should be reevaluated each year.

Management Category 1

A patient in this category has exhibited loss of protective sensation. Since the only internal system providing protection has been lost, external behavioral changes have to be taught. Persons in this category need more complete information on common foot problems such as callus formation, redness, and swelling. Once protective sensation is lost, that person is 15 times more likely to develop a foot ulceration than a person with diabetes and normal sensation.[22]

A multidisciplinary clinic for the management of diabetic feet should have a reliable means of determining the pressures under a person's foot as they walk.[39] Ideally, the device would have the ability to record these pressures within the shoe as a person walks. Persons with insensate feet often experience higher pressures under their feet than normally sensate people.[40] There seems to be a threshold of pressure that can increase a person's risk from walking. The actual threshold has not yet been definitively established. Young et al. report that they have not noted any ulcers on patients who had pressures of less than 112 N/cm^2 under their feet as they walked.[44] Lavery reports the threshold to be at 81.9 N/cm^2.[22]

Due to glycosylation of tissues around the joint structure, the range of motion of the major joints of the foot can become reduced.[16] This has been established as a contributing factor that results in higher pressures under the feet of diabetics.

A study in England has shown that callus tissue and the areas under the foot where callus forms are subjected to greater pressures than other tissues.[45] Periodic reduction of callus reduces these pressures.

Patients with sensory loss in their feet should never walk barefoot. After stepping on a sharp object the person with an insensitive foot will keep walking as though the foot was not injured. This often results in added injury, delayed healing, or abscess formation. Pressures are reduced under the feet when wearing most forms of low-heeled footwear as compared to walking barefoot or in socks.[32]

Patients with insensitive feet need to maintain vigilance for possible dangerous circumstances at all times. Occasionally, injuries occur because of objects that have fallen into the shoe since it was last worn. Before putting a shoe on, the inside should be inspected for foreign objects by the patient, then turned upside down and shaken to be sure nothing is inside.

As a person walks, the bottom of the foot is subjected to repetitive stress. To minimize the effects of repetitive stress, persons in category 1 should have soft insoles made of materials such as microcellular rubber or polyurethane foam in all shoes they wear. These materials are available in precut insoles or in sheets of material that can be cut to the proper size. A nylon covering helps to minimize shear between the insole and the foot and the soft cushion helps to reduce vertical (normal) stress.

As sensation is lost the use of dress shoes becomes a risk factor among women. Frey has reported that 88% of women in the United States wear shoes an average of 1.2 cm narrower than their feet.[18] Several studies have reported on the increase of pressure under the metatarsal heads when high-heeled shoes are worn. Snow correlated the pressure increase to heel height.[35] A 1.9-cm heel resulted in a 22% higher pressure, a 5-cm heel led to a 57% higher pressure, and a 8.3-cm heel increased the pressure by 76%. Also, as a higher-heeled shoe is worn, the pressure under the forefoot shifts from the middle of the metatarsal heads region to the first metatarsal head.[11]

Studies with rats have shown that the likelihood of damage from repetitive stress increases as the number of steps increases.[7] If walking is gradually increased over a long period the tissues will adapt, thereby increasing the tissue's ability to remain undamaged by repetitive stress. If the number of steps per day is significantly increased over a short period, however, tissue damage can develop. These studies should make the clinical staff aware that a patient leaving for vacation or expecting guests is about to enter a high-risk situation. The patient needs to be aware that they should not significantly increase the amount of daily walking or use new footwear during these times.

Bergtholdt described the use of thermometry in determining the presence of inflammation on insensitive feet. This technique is particularly helpful in preventing injury to the feet when shoes are new and have not yet conformed to the shape of the foot.[3] The surface skin temperature will be elevated at the site of inflammation. The temperature can be used to identify areas where the stress is beginning the process of injury.

Being at a higher risk of injury, people in this category need to visit their foot-care physician more frequently than those in category 0. A visit every 6 months can help detect developing problems such as claw-toe deformity.

Management Category 2

Deformity in the foot sometimes requires custom footwear to accommodate the shape (Fig. 20–2). Many custom shoes are made from a plaster model of the foot that is sent to a manufacturer for last construction and

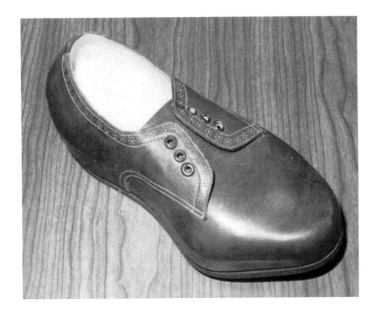

Figure 20-2 ■ This shoe was custom made to accommodate a bunion deformity.

shoe fabrication. This process creates a communication gap between the foot-care providers and the shoe fabricators. The person who actually sees the foot needs to inform the shoemaker of any special observation that may need to be considered in the construction of the shoe. When the shoemaker sees a unique bulge on the plaster model of a foot he does not know if that bulge is soft, and therefore can be compressed, or if it is rigid and the upper of the shoe needs to be molded around it. This communication gap often results in less than ideal footwear.

Most of the patients in category 2 do not require custom footwear. Depth footwear appropriately fit and modified by a prescription shoe-fitter will provide the necessary accommodations for most common deformities, such as clawed toes. Clawed toes are a common finding because, as the denervation progresses, the toes contract as the result of paralysis of the intrinsic foot muscles.[42] After the toes claw, the pressure under the metatarsal heads increases. Studies have shown that ulcerated patients have reduced pressures under their toes.[12, 36]

Persons in this category need to visit a foot specialist at least every 4 months and probably more often until the problem is fully protected by shoes or the deformity is corrected by surgery.

Management Category 3

Patients in category 3 have insensate feet that have been previously ulcerated. Ulcers

occur most frequently under the insensate foot at the location of previous ulcers.[6] Scarring makes tissues less flexible and more likely to break down, particularly as the result of shear, a force applied parallel to the skin surface. Soft tissues withstand shear through the process of one layer of tissue gliding over adjacent tissues. Scar binds tissue layers together and prevents this gliding action. With this greater degree of susceptibility, these patients need a higher level of protection within their footwear.

Also in category 3 are patients with significant peripheral vascular disease. These patients have tissues that are more friable that, once injured, have a much more difficult time healing. Often, when peripheral vascular disease and neuropathy coexist, the injury occurs in a manner typical of neuropathic lesions but requires much more protection and time to heal because of poor tissue perfusion.

These patients require the most intense efforts of the medical community. With proper footwear and no current injury these persons should routinely be seen by a foot specialist, with education reinforcement, every 1 to 2 months. In a study of patient compliance reported from Germany in 1993, 51 previously ulcerated patients who were compliant with regular foot clinic visits and used prescribed footwear were free of recurrent ulcers after 20 months. Thirty-eight percent of the patients who were not compliant with visits or footwear reulcerated. After 40 months 54% of the compliant patients had reulcerated, whereas 100% of the noncompliant patients had developed another open wound. The authors attributed most of the new ulcers on the feet of the compliant patients to failures in the footwear materials to maintain the original levels of protection. They concluded that footwear needs to be renewed every 2 years.[8]

Footwear

When a shoe is too tight, ulcers usually develop medial to the first metatarsal head and lateral to the fifth metatarsal head (Fig. 20–3). The ulceration is due to pressure ische-mia. This pressure is the result of tension within the leather that applies the greatest stress in areas of smallest circumference.[7] This breakdown is also related to the length of time a shoe is worn. For damage to occur, pressure from a shoe that is too tight must be maintained for hours with no relief. A diabetic patient should be taught to change their shoes at midday and perhaps again in the evening. By doing this, the patient does not allow pressures to remain in one place on the foot for an excessive period of time.

The number given for a shoe size by a manufacturer can only be used as a general guideline for fitting a particular foot. Shoes of the same numbered size vary greatly in width

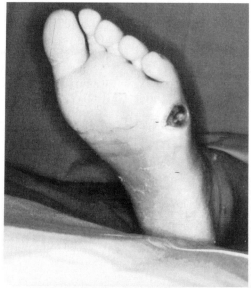

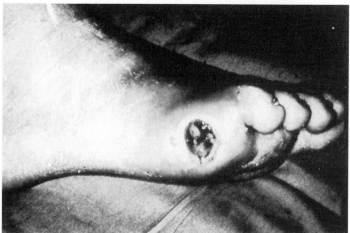

Figure 20–3 ■ These ulcerations were on the feet of patients whose shoes were too tight.

and length due to differences in shoe lasts. Shoes, for an insensitive patient, should never be purchased just by asking for a specific numbered size.

The fit of a shoe should be determined by an experienced shoe-fitter, such as a certified pedorthist, while the patient is standing in the shoe (see Chapter 34). The shoe should be ½ to ⅝ inch longer than the longest toe.[30] Length is only one of many factors that need to be evaluated to achieve good fit. "Guesswork" can result in permanent damage to the foot.

As previously stated, heel heights greater than 2 inches, in particular, shift the body weight towards the forefoot, particularly onto the first and second metatarsal heads.[30, 34] This shift of body weight increases pressure under the metatarsal heads increasing the risk of foot ulceration. Actual heel height is a vertical measurement from the top of the insole under the metatarsal heads to the top of the insole under the heel.

Pressure-sensitive socks are available to help a shoe-fitter to objectively evaluate fit (Fig. 20–4).[5] These socks are coated with wax capsules containing dye that fracture when a certain pressure threshold is exceeded. The dye will stain the sock in areas of high pressure (Fig. 20–5) in the shoe as the person walks.

Shoe Inserts

Well-molded, custom inserts are usually required to adequately distribute forces around foot deformities. If a shoemaker, orthotist, or pedorthist wants to redistribute plantar forces with shoe inserts, the means of doing so fall into four general categories:

1. Pressure under one part of the foot can be relieved by increasing the pressure (elevating the insole) on an adjacent part. Metatarsal "cookies," build-ups or depressions in the insole are included into this group. These techniques are imprecise and can result in foot injury by greatly increasing local pressure on insensitive skin. Therefore, the following techniques are preferred.

2. Pressure under one part can also be reduced by exactly molding an insole to the plantar shape. Since pressure is equal to force (body weight) divided by the area (amount of foot in contact with the insole), exact molding reduces pressure under ev-

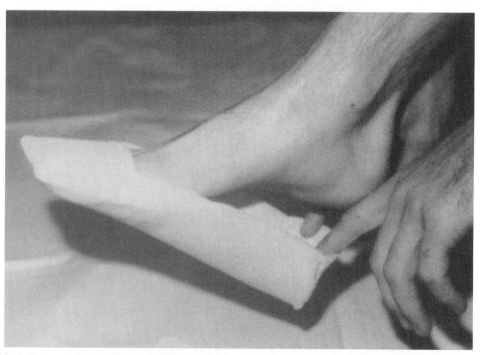

Figure 20–4 ■ Pressure-sensitive socks can be worn on the foot, within the shoe, to assist the clinician or shoe-fitter in determining proper fit for a diabetic patient with insensitive feet.

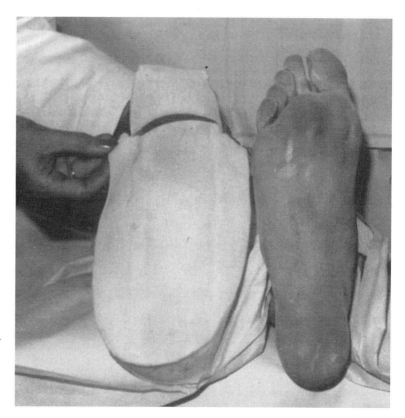

Figure 20–5 ■ Pressure-sensitive socks will localize areas of higher pressure within the shoe. Wax capsules within the sock fracture with high pressures and release a dye which stains the fabric.

ery part of the foot by increasing the area of contact.

3. The effects of pressure can be spread over time. Soft materials take time to compress. This compression slows the foot as it presses down into the insole. Thicker foam insoles are more effective than thinner insoles of the same material but, as the material used becomes thicker, the foot will begin developing blisters due to rubbing up and down against the side of the shoe.

4. In theory, dynamic functional foot orthoses can reduce the pressure in one part of the foot by altering internal motions of the bones within the foot. If properly constructed, these inserts can successfully control the effects of mild to moderate pronatory deformities. Excessive pronation results in localized forces under one or two metatarsal heads and, in some cases, the first toe.[29] Effective control of pronation reduces these localized pressures by allowing all metatarsal heads to share the force of each step.

The toe region of an insole should not be molded under an insensitive foot. The foot elongates with pronation and the toes must be free to slide forward as this motion occurs. Ridges created by molding often result in distal toe ulceration.

There are a great variety of insole materials available from medical suppliers. Softer materials, such as polyethylene, polyurethane or microcellular rubber foams, help to cushion the foot but cannot fully replace all capabilities of human soft tissues. These materials are molded and trimmed more easily. Unfortunately, this is often the only reason they are selected for insole construction. These materials are best used as a temporary or trial device.[15] Softer materials will not hold their molded shape for a long time because repetitive compression and decompression breaks down the cellular structure.

The current preferences in insole design, for long-term wear, are a lamination of different materials or a single firm material. By combining materials in one insole the manufacturer can take advantage of the good properties of one material while minimizing its weaknesses by using a second material with different mechanical characteristics (Figs. 20–6 and 20–7). Rigid materials generally hold their shape for longer periods of time

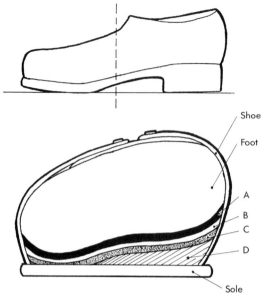

Figure 20-6 ■ This cross-section shows layers of different materials in one type of laminated orthotic device. Layer A is nylon-covered PPT or Spenco. Layer B is Pelite. Layer B is Suborthalene (JMS Berkshire Resource, Inc. Clifton, NJ). Layer D is neoprene crepe. The nylon covering reduces shear stress and the underlying foam allows for cushioning. The Pelite molds well to the shape of the positive model and is then reinforced by the rigid Suborthalene. The neoprene crepe provides a firm support for the other materials.

and are not as easily deformed as a person walks.

A laminated insole of Plastazote, cork, polyurethane foam, and leather was used in a study in Germany.[8] Patients who routinely wore the molded inserts greatly reduced their chance of developing foot ulceration when compared to persons who returned to nonmolded footwear occasionally. This study reinforces the concept that a properly made insole must be worn all the time. A person cannot even occasionally wear shoes that are not especially designed to protect their feet.

Whenever possible, it is preferable to utilize the person's own soft tissue structures as a cushion. Human soft tissues have viscoelastic properties that provide more effective injury protection than any man-made materials. To hold soft tissues in place under bony prominences, frequently the site of localized pressure, firmer materials are usually needed.

Rigid materials are more effective in functional control of the foot. Since they retain a molded shape for longer periods of time, rigid materials are preferred when the intent is to hold a foot in a particular position or to resist motion in a given direction. The more rigid the material used as the upper surface of an insole, the more precision and expertise regarding foot insensitivity is needed by the insole manufacturer, because rigid materials that are not properly formed can quickly result in severe injury to an insensitive foot.

Many insole devices require extra vertical room within the shoe because of the additional space needed for the insole. To accommodate these inserts, several shoe companies manufacture depth footwear. These shoes are ¼ to ⅝ inch deeper than conventional oxford shoes (Fig. 20–8).

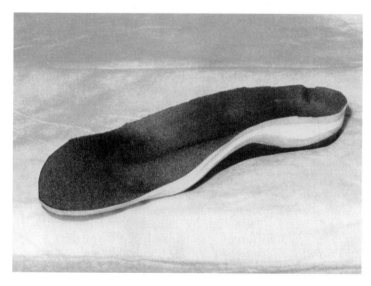

Figure 20-7 ■ A molded insert constructed of the materials illustrated in Figure 20–6.

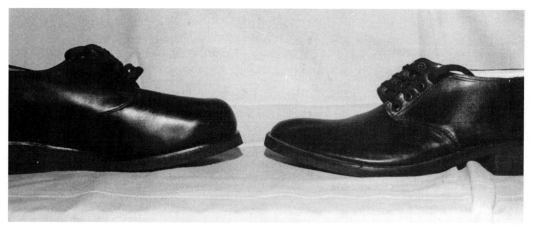

Figure 20–8 ■ A conventional oxford shoe is on the right and a shoe with extra vertical depth is on the left.

Shoe Sole Modifications

Common external shoe modifications such as metatarsal bars, Mayo crescent, anterior heels,[25] and Hauser bars are not recommended for insensitive feet. These devices are intended to mold the inside of the shoe against the foot by applying pressure against the bottom of the sole (Fig. 20–9). This type of molding is not precise and can result in injury to an insensitive foot.

The most frequent location of plantar ulceration on an insensitive foot is beneath the first metatarsal head with the interphalangeal joint of the first toe and second metatarsal head almost as frequent.[36] Later studies

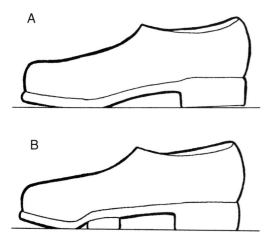

A

B

Figure 20–9 ■ Shoe A is a conventional shaped shoe and shoe B shows the effect of a properly constructed metatarsal bar. The metatarsal bar molds the shoe sole behind the metatarsal heads to relieve stresses in this region. These are not recommended for insensitive feet.

correlated the location of ulcers under the feet of diabetics with the region's higher vertical pressures.[12]

Studies have also shown that a rigid shoe sole can reduce shear stress on the foot.[26] Rigid soles also limit the damage to toes, which have limited motion at the metatarsophalangeal joint. An added sole rocker creates a fulcrum under the foot (Fig. 20–10). As the shoe rotates over the fulcrum during walking, pressures on the metatarsal heads are reduced.

With a curved or roller sole (Fig. 20–11), as the heel is lifted, the shoe will roll forward keeping the heel of the shoe against the foot.[24] The rocker style is more effective than the roller at reducing forefoot pressures. As much as 50% of the pressure can be reduced by use of a rigid rocker sole.[10]

Shoes and insoles need periodic professional evaluation to maintain the proper shape as wear occurs. The temperature of the foot skin should also be tested during these visits. Elevation of the surface skin temperature is often the first clinical evidence of inflammation due to an emerging injury on an insensitive foot.

Constant reinforcement concerning the essential use of appropriate footwear needs to be provided by all of the patient's health care providers.

Shortened Feet

Feet that have been shortened by destruction or amputation are a particularly difficult problem. A shortened foot has to compensate

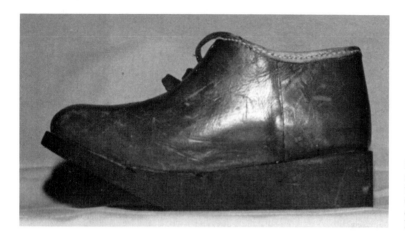

Figure 20–10 ■ The rocker style sole is rigid and as a person walks the shoe rotates over a ridge (fulcrum) in the sole, which is located posterior to the metatarsal heads.

for the loss of length by performing more work. From a mechanical perspective, the shorter foot is a shorter lever. More force has to be applied to a shorter lever, compared to one of more length, to do the same amount of work. On a short foot, this additional force is concentrated under what has become the front of the foot (Fig. 20–12).

For cosmetic reasons, people want to wear shoes of equal length. In order to have shoes of equal length when one foot is much shorter, the shoe on the shorter foot will be excessively long. In this case, the short foot must do even more work by having a poor mechanical advantage to push down on the long shoe. The end of the foot will press against the middle of the shoe rather than provide stability at the distal end of the shoe.

The skin of the shortened foot will tend to ulcerate under the front surface. Because the foot is a shorter lever, additional work is needed for walking. Eventually the muscles in the back of the leg will accommodatively shorten, resulting in equinus. Both of these complications lead to greatly increased pressure under the front of the foot.

Shoes for shortened feet should fit the foot in length. The sole of the shoe should be of a roller or rocker design to minimize the distal pressures under the forefoot.

To further redistribute the forces of body weight, a boot that fits snugly to the exact shape of the lower leg can be constructed. This boot, known as a fixed-ankle-brace walking boot (Fig. 20–13) or FAB walker, has lacing in front of the leg. These laces allow for daily adjustment to compensate for variances in leg volume and to ensure snug fit at all times.

If the patient insists on a long shoe for a short foot, the sole should be rigid with a rocker fulcrum that is behind the distal end

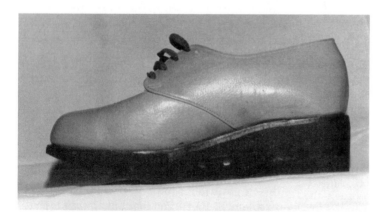

Figure 20–11 ■ A roller style sole is also rigid but does not have a ridge like the rocker style. As the person walks and lifts their heel the shoe rolls forward on the curved sole. This prevents pressures from remaining in one location under the foot by having the point of contact with the ground constantly moving forward as the heel is lifted.

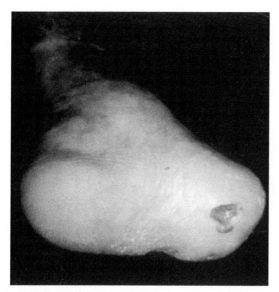

Figure 20–12 ■ Pressures under a shortened foot are much greater than under a foot of normal length. Extra protective measures need to be taken to prevent plantar, forefoot soft tissue destruction.

of the foot. The distal end of the shoe should not touch the ground as the person walks.

Temporary Footwear

The person with an insensate foot and/or significant peripheral vascular disease should never take an unprotected step. There are times, usually when shoes are being ordered, repaired, or modified, when the feet need some sort of interim protective shoes. These shoes need to be readily available. They should be custom molded to the individual's feet and made of materials that allow rapid construction. Since these shoes are not intended for definitive long-term use, they do not need to have long-term wear capability. When the definitive footwear is available these shoes can continue to be useful as house shoes or shower sandals.

Currently, ideal materials for these temporary shoes are thermoplastic polyethylenes such as Plastazote. Being water resistant, the closed cell structure can be washed and will not absorb fluids.

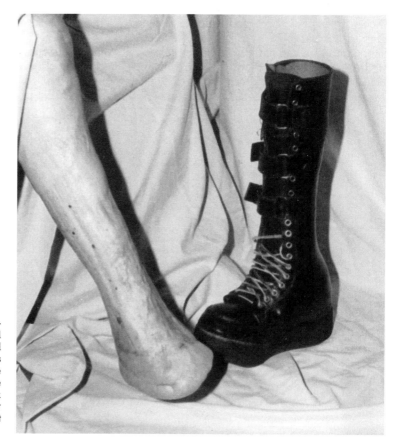

Figure 20–13 ■ This fixed-ankle-brace walking boot has been used by this patient with a shortened foot for over 20 years. The boot is made over a positive model of the patient's lower leg. The back of the boot is reinforced with ⅛-inch-thick polypropylene. The lacing allows for daily adjustment of fit over the foot and leg.

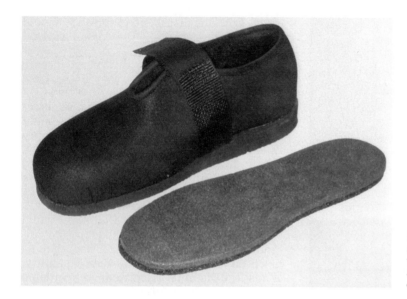

Figure 20–14 ■ A commercially available total Plastazote shoe with a polyethylene insert is available for temporary protection until definitive footwear is available.

A commercially available, total Plastazote shoe (Fig. 20–14), in most cases, can be used for temporary use.[28] These shoes have soft uppers and enough space internally for the addition of a molded insole.

For severely deformed feet, during times when shoes are being repaired or before shoes have been provided, custom-molded Plastazote sandals can be constructed.[27] These sandals consist of an upper layer of medium-density Plastazote (which is actually the softest), reinforced beneath with a firmer Plastazote. A neoprene crepe sole and straps of either leather or cotton webbing complete the sandal (Figs. 20–15 and 20–16).

Conclusion

If clinical programs of injury prevention for insensitive feet are going to be successful, medical professionals will have to insist that people who fit and modify medically indicated footwear be knowledgeable, professional, and precise in their work. Shoes are

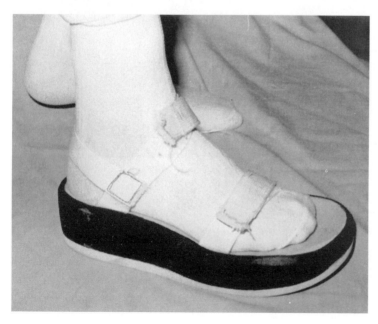

Figure 20–15 ■ A custom-made Plastazote sandal with cotton webbing for straps and Velcro closures.

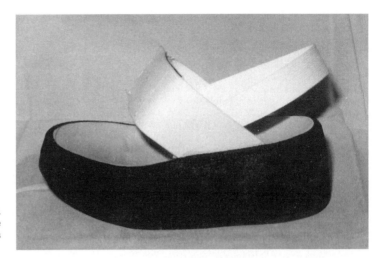

Figure 20–16 ■ For shorter feet a single strap can be used but should be wider to prevent excessive pressures over the dorsal surface of the foot.

the primary means of protecting insensitive feet. The responsibility to ensure proper shoe applications must rest with the physician.

Several publications have emphasized the need to develop multidisciplinary teams to adequately manage the foot problems of many diabetics.[1, 14, 19, 33] The best published data for developing programs to benefit patients with diabetic foot problems and reducing amputation rates have come from endocrinologists who have brought teams together (see Chapter 9).

The primary day-to-day management of the vast majority of persons with diabetes must be under the supervision of medical professionals familiar with pathology and mechanics of the foot. Because foot problems can develop quickly and unexpectedly in the patient with diabetes, they must be readily available. Medical as well as surgical expertise is needed on the team to make comprehensive diabetic foot care as seamless as possible.

Physicians who accept the responsibility for the foot care of diabetic patients should be familiar with every aspect of shoe modification for therapeutic use. They should also accept the fact that the patient with an insensitive foot will always need life-long assistance to prevent tissue damage.

REFERENCES

1. Assal JP, Muhlhauser I, Pernat A, et al: Patient education as the basis for diabetic foot care in clinical practice. Diabetologia 28:602, 1985.
2. Bell JA: Light touch-deep pressure testing using Semmes-Weinstein monofilaments. In Hunter JM, Schneider LH, Mackin EJ, Callahan AD (eds): Rehabilitation of the Hand. St. Louis: CV Mosby, 1984.
3. Bergtholdt HT: Thermography on insensitive limbs. In Uematsu S (ed): Medical Thermography, Theory and Clinical Applications. Los Angeles: Brentwood Publishing Corporation, 1976.
4. Birke J, Sims D: Plantar sensory threshold in the ulcerative foot. Leprosy Rev 57:261, 1986.
5. Brand PW, Ebner JD: Pressure sensitive devices for denervated hands and feet. J Bone Joint Surg 51A:109, 1969.
6. Brand PW: Insensitive Feet, A Practical Handbook on Foot Problems in Leprosy. London: The Leprosy Mission, 1981.
7. Brand PW: The insensitive foot (including leprosy). In Jahss MH (ed): Disorders of the Foot and Ankle, 2nd ed. Philadelphia: WB Saunders Company, 1991.
8. Chantelau E, Haage P: An audit of cushioned diabetic footwear: Relation to patient compliance. Diabet Med 10:114, 1993.
9. Coleman WC, Brand PW, Birke JA: The total contact cast. J Am Podiatr Med Assoc 74:548, 1984.
10. Coleman WC: The relief of forefoot pressures using outer shoe sole modifications. In Patil KM, Srinivasan H (eds): Proceedings of the International Conference on Biomechanics and Clinical Kinesiology of Hand and Foot. Indian Institute of Technology, Madras, India, 1985.
11. Corrigan JP, Moore DP, Stephens MM: Effect of heel height on forefoot loading. Foot Ankle 14:148, 1993.
12. Ctercteko GC, Dhanendran MK, Hutton WC, et al: Vertical forces acting on the feet of diabetic patients with neuropathic ulceration. Br J Surg 68:608, 1981.
13. Dellon AL: Evaluation of Sensibility and Reeducation of Sensation in the Hand. Baltimore: Williams & Wilkins, 1981.
14. Edmonds ME, Blundell MP, Morris ME, et al: Improved survival of the diabetic foot: The role of a specialised foot clinic. Q J Med 232:763, 1986.
15. Enna CD, Brand PW, Reed JP Jr, et al: The orthotic care of the denervated foot in Hansen's disease. Orthot Pros 30:33, 1976.
16. Fernando DJS, Hutchison A, Veves A, et al: Relationship of limited joint mobility to abnormal foot pressures and diabetic foot ulceration. Diabetes Care 14:8, 1991.
17. Foster AVM, Snowden S, Grenfell A, et al: Reduction of gangrene and amputations in diabetic renal

transplant patients: The role of a special foot clinic. Diabet Med 12:632, 1995.

18. Frey C, Thompson F, Smith J, et al: American Orthopedic Foot and Ankle Society women's shoe survey. Foot Ankle 14:78, 1993.

19. Hobgood E: Conservative therapy of foot abnormalities infections and vascular insufficiency. *In* Davidson JK (ed): Clinical Diabetes Mellitus. New York: Thieme Publishers, 1986.

20. Klenerman L, McCabe C, Cogley D, et al: Screening patients at risk of diabetic foot ulceration in a general diabetic outpatient clinic. Diabet Med 13:561, 1996.

21. Lang-Stevenson AI, Sharrard WJW, Betts RP, et al: Neuropathic ulcers of the foot. J Bone Joint Surg 67-B:438, 1985.

22. Lavery LA, Armstrong DG, Vela SA, et al: Practical criteria for screening patients at high risk of diabetic foot ulceration. Arch Intern Med 158:157, 1998.

23. Logerfo FW, Gibbons GW: Ischemia in the diabetic foot: Modern concepts and management. Clin Diabetes 7:72, 1989.

24. Milgram JE: Office measures for relief of the painful foot. J Bone Joint Surg 46-A:1095, 1964.

25. Miller WE: The anterior heel for metatarsalgia in the adult foot. Clin Orthop 123:55, 1977.

26. Price EW: Studies on plantar ulceration in leprosy, VI. The management of plantar ulcers. Leprosy Rev 31:159, 1960.

27. Reed JK Jr: Plastazote insoles, sandals, and shoes— for insensitive feet. *In* McDowell F, Enna CD (eds): Surgical Rehabilitation in Leprosy. Baltimore: Williams & Wilkins, 1974.

28. Reed JK Jr: Footwear for the diabetic. *In* Levin ME, O'Neal LW (eds): The Diabetic Foot, 3rd ed. St. Louis: CV Mosby, 1983.

29. Root ML, Orien WP, Weed JH: Normal and Abnormal Function of the Foot, Vol II. Los Angeles: Clinical Biomechanics Corporation, 1977.

30. Rossi WA, Tennant R: Professional Shoe Fitting. New York: National Shoe Retailers Association, 1984.

31. Runyan JW: The Memphis Chronic Disease Program. JAMA 231:264, 1975.

32. Sarnow MR, Veves A, Guirini JM, et al: In-shoe foot pressure measurements in diabetic patients with at-risk feet and in healthy subjects. Diabetes Care 17(9):1002, 1994.

33. Schaff PS, Cavanagh PR: Shoes for the insensitive foot: The effect of a "rocker bottom" shoe modification of plantar pressure distribution. Foot Ankle 11:29, 1990.

34. Schwartz RP, Heath AL: A quantitative analysis of recorded variables in the walking pattern of "normal" adults. J Bone Joint Surg 46A:324, 1964.

35. Snow RE, Williams KR, Holmes GB: The effects of wearing high heeled shoes on pedal pressure in women. Foot Ankle 13:85, 1992.

36. Stokes IAF, Faris IB, Hutton WC: The neuropathic ulcer and loads on the foot in diabetic patients. Acta Orthop Scand 46:839, 1975.

37. Veves A, Fernando DJS, Walewski P, et al: A study of plantar pressures in a diabetic clinic population. Foot 1:75, 1991.

38. Veves A, Masson EA, Fernando DJS, et al: Use of experimental padded hosiery to reduce foot pressures in diabetic neuropathy. Diabet Med 7:324, 1990.

39. Veves A, Murray HJ, Young MJ, et al: The risk of foot ulceration in diabetic patients with high foot pressure: A prospective study. Diabetologia 35:660, 1992.

40. Veves A, Van Ross ERE, Boulton AJM: Foot pressure measurements in diabetic and non-diabetic amputees. Diabetes Care 15:905, 1992.

41. von Frey M: Gibt es tiefe Druckempfindungen. Dtsch Med Wochenschr 51:113, 1925.

42. Wagner FW Jr: A classification and treatment program for diabetic, neuropathic, and dysvascular foot problems. AAOS Instuctional Course Lecture, Vol XXVIII. St. Louis: CV Mosby, 1979.

43. Wooldridge J, Moreno L: Evaluation of the costs to Medicare of covering therapeutic shoes for diabetic patients. Diabetes Care 17:541, 1994.

44. Young MJ, Breddy JL, Veves A, et al: The prediction of diabetic neuropathic foot ulcerations using vibration perception thresholds. Diabetes Care 16:557, 1994.

45. Young MJ, Cavanagh PR, Thomas SG, et al: The effect of callus removal on dynamic plantar foot pressure in diabetic patients. Diabet Med 9:55, 1992.

21

CHARCOT NEUROARTHROPATHY OF THE FOOT

■ Lee J. Sanders and Robert G. Frykberg

The Charcot foot is a poorly understood and frequently overlooked complication of diabetes mellitus that poses a formidable diagnostic and treatment challenge for all members of the health care team. The probability of successful management is greatly increased with heightened awareness and thorough understanding of the pathogenesis, natural history, and anatomic patterns of neuropathic osteoarthropathy. Identification of high-risk individuals facilitates early implementation of management strategies directed toward prevention and minimization of foot deformity, joint instability, ulceration, disability, and surgery. Early recognition and timely treatment will often result in a more satisfactory outcome. The key to treatment is prevention, with avoidance of further trauma until the bone and soft tissues heal. The aim of treatment should be to obtain stability of the foot and to avoid excessive pressure on the skin from a bony prominence. Since William Reily Jordan's linkage of neuropathic arthropathy of the foot and ankle with diabetes mellitus in 1936, the number of case reports has steadily increased.[29–32, 50, 73, 125] The growing number of cases reflects the seriousness of this disorder, as well as increased recognition of Charcot joints.

Charcot's Perspective

During the last third of the 19th century, Jean-Martin Charcot's clinicoanatomic studies of patients with tabes dorsalis at the Salpetriere enabled him to describe a distinct pathologic entity, the arthropathy of ataxia.[26–28] He noted that "among the diverse conditions that may develop in the extremities as a result of certain traumatic or spontaneous lesions of the peripheral nerves, some as we know, have a predilection for the joints. This group of arthropathies . . . is frequently discussed today as an example of various nutritional disturbances that sometimes affect the distribution of nerve trunks affected by some alteration of a greater or lesser degree. . . . To begin with, we shall note one more time the absence of any external cause, traumatic or otherwise. . . . As for the site, the arthropathy . . . showed no preference to one side. . . . It always started unexpectedly, rather suddenly, without precipitating cause."

Charcot[26–28] believed that lesions of the spinal cord, particularly of the gray matter, were responsible for disorders of the skin, the muscles, and the bones and joints commonly associated with the tabetic arthropathies.[63] "The irritative lesions of the spinal cord . . . react sometimes on the periphery, and determine various nutritive disorders. . . . The bones and articulations do not appear to escape this law. It follows that the arthropathies of locomotor ataxia would be . . . one of the forms of these articular affections, developed under the more or less direct influence of the spinal centre."[26] His concept of a nutritive trophic regulation of bones and joints, mediated by the spinal cord, became the basis of the French theory, for the etiology of arthropathy seen in ataxic patients.[16–18, 26–28, 63] Charcot's theory was vehemently opposed by the German surgeons Volkmann and Virchow, who believed that the arthropathy of ataxia was nothing more than a "traumatic arthritis caused by the manner of locomotion peculiar to these patients."[26] Their concept became known as the German, mechanical, or neurotraumatic theory.

Charcot described his observations of a sudden and unexpected arthropathy, which often began without apparent cause. Lancinating pains in the limbs often preceded the joint affection. He described a sudden onset of generalized tumefaction of the limb with rapid changes in the articular surfaces of the joint. Crepitations in the joint would occur within a few days after the onset and would normally precede the development of the characteristic motor incoordination of tabes. He argued that these arthropathies did not result exclusively from the distention of the ligaments and capsules of the joints or from the awkward gaits of these patients. "Anatomically the enormous wear and tear shown by the heads of the bones, the extensive looseness of the ligaments of the joints, and the frequent occurrence of luxations seem to distinguish these arthropathies from the ordinary type of osteoarthritis."[26]

Charcot's contribution to the understanding of spinal arthropathies was recognized in the *Rapport du Congrès* (Transactions of Congress) published in London in 1882, where it was written that "these bone changes constitute a distinct pathological entity. They deserve the name of 'Charcot's joint.'"[63] Accordingly, this term has been perpetuated to describe the bone and joint changes associated with all of the neuropathic arthropathies.

Charcot reasoned that "behind the disease of the joint there was a disease far more important in character, which in reality dominated the situation."[26] This reasoning applies equally well to diabetes mellitus with its neuropathic influence and ravaging effects on the bones and joints of the foot and ankle.

Disorders Producing Charcot Joint

A variety of disorders affecting the spinal cord and peripheral nerves have been reported to destroy the protective mechanisms of joints and interfere with the "nutritive" trophic regulation of bone.[16–18, 26–28, 36, 63, 126, 131] The mechanisms of destruction may be precipitated by a single injury or by repetitive moderate stress applied to the bones and joints of an insensate foot and ankle. The results are fractures, effusions, and ligamentous laxity, followed by erosion of articular cartilage, fragmentation, luxation, disintegration, and collapse of the foot. The presence of peripheral neuropathy and the clinical and laboratory evidence of diabetes mellitus,[60, 54, 58, 59, 94, 102] tabes dorsalis,[20, 106, 127] leprosy,[16, 54, 65, 132] syringomyelia,[20, 54, 72, 106, 107] meningomyelcoele,[16, 106, 107] congenital insensitivity to pain,[54, 106] chronic alcoholism,[11, 106] spinal cord injury and compression,[26–28, 54, 63, 72] and peripheral nerve injuries[77, 106] complete the picture of neuroarthropathy, or bona fide Charcot joint. The key characteristic that all of these disorders have in common is the absence or decrease of pain sensation in the presence of uninterrupted physical activity.

As the number of cases of tabes dorsalis has declined, diabetes mellitus has emerged as the leading cause of neuropathic arthropathy today.[54, 58–60, 94, 99] The importance of the diabetic form of neuropathic arthropathy was established in 1955 in a report by Miller and Lichtman[94] at the Cook County Hospital and Chicago Medical School. They noted that "whereas tabes of syphilitic origin was formerly the usual cause of these painless deformities of the feet, with complicating soft tissue infections, ulcers and osteomyelitis, the diabetic neuropathic foot is now showing the higher incidence. Perhaps there is greater alertness in recognition."

Prevalence and Patient Characteristics

The prevalence of diagnosed neuropathic bone and joint disease associated with diabetes mellitus has been reported to be from

0.08% to 7.5%.[6, 50, 104, 125] Pogonowska et al.[104] reported on a clinical and radiologic survey of 242 patients in Houston, Texas. They noted 6.8% of the cases had bone abnormalities classified as "diabetic osteopathy." Forgacs in a comprehensive literature review of data on 237 patients estimated that diabetic neuropathic osteoarthropathy (DNOAP) occurs in 0.3% to 0.5% of all diabetic patients.[50] Radiographic evidence of lower limb bone and joint changes was found in 29% of 333 diabetics with peripheral neuropathy, reported by Cofield et al.[32] It is very likely that there are many more cases of DNOAP that go undetected or misdiagnosed.[54, 55, 58–60]

The average age reported for the onset of DNOAP is approximately 57 years, with the majority of patients in their sixth and seventh decades.[4, 6, 30–32, 50, 94, 113, 125] Of greater significance, the average duration of diabetes at the time of diagnosis of neuropathic bone changes is approximately 15 years, with 80% of the patients being diabetic for more than 10 years and 60% more than 15 years.[4, 6, 30–32, 50, 113, 125] Clohisy and Thompson[30] reported on a homogeneous group of 18 adult juvenile-onset diabetics with neuropathic arthropathy, an average age of 33.5 years, and a 20-year history of diabetes mellitus. Age therefore does not appear to be as important a factor in the development of DNOAP as the duration of diabetes mellitus (Table 21–1).

Bilateral involvement has been reported to occur in 5.9 to 39.3% of the heterogeneous cases.[31, 94, 113, 125] Seventy-five percent of the cases reported by Clohisy and Thompson[30] had bilateral involvement, with a very high incidence of serious fractures of the ankle and the tarsal bones. There does not appear to be a significant difference in sex distribution, with men and women affected equally.[55, 112]

Natural History of Charcot Foot

Various descriptions of the course of bone and joint changes associated with neuropathic arthropathies have appeared in the literature over the last century. The terms atrophic, destructive, and hyperemic have been used to describe acute or early radiographic findings. Hypertrophic, reparative, proliferative, sclerotic, and quiescent all are terms used to describe chronic or late findings.[54, 58–60, 81, 112, 119, 127] These descriptions are based on clinical, radiologic, and histologic observations, as well as the chronicity of disease. Norman et al.[102] suggested that neuropathic joints be classified as acute or chronic, on the basis of the suddenness of their onset and speed of development. They believed that "since both reaction to injury and repair

Table 21–1 ■ REPORTED CHARACTERISTICS OF DIABETICS WITH NEUROPATHIC OSTEOARTHROPATHY*

REFERENCE	NO. OF CASES REPORTED	AGE (YR) (RANGE)	DURATION DM (YR) (RANGE)	% BILATERAL INVOLVEMENT
Bailey and Root[6]	17	56 (30–69)	11.5	23.5 4/17
Miller and Lichtman[94]	17	53		5.9 1/17
Sinha et al.[125]	101	2/3s 50s–60s (20–79)	83% > 10 65% > 15	23.8 24/101
Clouse et al.[31]	90	55 (25–78)	18 (1.5–43)	18
Forgács[50]	23	63 (48–79)	14.8 (2–32)	
Cofield et al.[32]	96	56 (27–79)	81% > 10 16 (1–40)	21 20/96
Clohisy and Thompson[30]	18	33.5 (25–52)	20	75 14/18
Sanders and Mrdjenovich[113]	28	79% 50s–60s 57.2 (36–70)	78% > 10 59% > 15 15.1 (1–27)	39.3 11/28

* Modified from Sanders LJ, Frykberg R: Diabetic neuropathic osteoarthropathy: The Charcot foot. *In* Frykberg RG (ed): The High Risk Foot in Diabetes Mellitus. New York: Churchill Livingstone, 1991, with permission.
DM, diabetes mellitus.

occur simultaneously in the joint two separate phases of development do not take place." What seems to link these opposite states is the process of bony resorption and repair, as determined by the balance of osteoclastic and osteoblastic activity (Fig. 21–1).[62]

The acute phase of neuroarthropathy is often precipitated by minor trauma and is characterized by swelling, local heat, erythema, laxity of ligaments, joint effusion, and bone resorption. Early findings may be indistinguishable from those of osteoarthritis and infection. Skin temperature elevation on the affected foot has been reported to be approximately 5°C.[4] Nearly all reports confirm the role of trauma in initiating the evolution of neuropathic osteoarthropathy in patients with an underlying neurologic deficit.[54, 55, 65, 72, 112]

Newman[100] suggested that the earliest changes in the evolution of neuropathic joints involve the soft tissues. He postulated that gross neuropathic changes in the ligaments were responsible for spontaneous dislocation of the foot, which he observed in five cases occurring without bone destruction. In those cases of neuropathic osteoarthropathy that do not begin with spontaneous fractures, ligamentous lesions may be of paramount importance, leading to spontaneous dislocation of the foot. Ligaments and joint capsule are thought to be stretched by the abnormal stresses applied to the joints, allowing them to go beyond their normal range of motion. They may be further weakened at their insertions into bone by hyperemic resorption, allowing complete dislocation to take place.[72]

Eichenholtz[44] divided the disease process into three radiographically distinct stages: development, coalescence, and reconstruction. The stage of development represents the acute, destructive period, which is distinguished by joint effusions, soft tissue edema, subluxation, formation of bone and cartilage debris (detritus), intra-articular fractures, and fragmentation of bone. This phase of bone and joint destruction is induced by minor trauma and aggravated by persistent ambulation on an insensitive foot. The consequence of trauma is a hyperemic response, which promotes additional resorption of bone and increases the susceptibility to further

| **MINOR TRAUMA** | **STAGE OF DEVELOPMENT** | **REST AND IMMOBIL- IZATION** | **STAGES OF COALESCENCE AND RECONSTRUCTION** |

Swelling and Joint Effusion
Local Elevation in Skin Temperature
Bone Resorption & Softening from Hyperemia
Osteolysis and Osteopenia
Ligaments Weakened by Hyperemic Resorption
Abnormal Joint Alignment (subluxation)
Increased Joint Mobility
Erosion of Cartilage & Subchondral Bone
Dislocation and Fragmentation of Bone
Bone and Cartilage Debris (detritus)
Hemorrhage into Periarticular Tissues

Absorption of Fine Debris
Periosteal New Bone Formation
Fusion and Rounding of
Large Fragments
Exuberant (metaplastic) Bone
Decreased Joint Mobility
*** Increased Stabilization ***
Increased Bone Density and Sclerosis
Deformity

RESORPTION OF BONE

REPAIR

ATROPHIC PHASE
(DESTRUCTIVE OR HYPEREMIC CHANGES)
ACUTE (EARLY) FINDINGS
ACTIVE

HYPERTROPHIC PHASE
(REPARATIVE OR SCLEROTIC CHANGES)
CHRONIC (LATE) FINDINGS
QUIESCENT

LJS '92

Figure 21–1 ■ Natural history of Charcot foot.

injury and progressive deterioration. Non–weight bearing must be initiated during this acute phase of the disease process.[54, 55]

The stage of coalescence is noted by a lessening of edema, absorption of fine debris, and healing of fractures. Clinical and radiographic evidence of coalescence indicates that the reparative phase of healing has begun. The final phase of bone healing is the stage of reconstruction, wherein further repair and remodeling of bone take place in an attempt to restore stability and homeostasis (see Fig. 21–1). Neuropathic osteoarthropathy can be arrested during the stage of development if diagnosed before the disease has had a chance to mature. Early identification and treatment will ideally result in minimal joint destruction and deformity.

Late neuropathic bone and joint changes are an exaggeration of those seen in osteoarthritis: cartilage fibrillation, loose body formation, subchondral sclerosis, and marginal osteophytes.[54] These lesions often heal with the formation of hyperplastic dense bone, especially in the midfoot. The early phase of healing is distinguished by the gradual absorption of fine debris and hematoma, with callus formation and the coalescence and reattachment of loose fragments of bone or cartilage. Proliferative changes are characteristic of this phase, with usual findings being intra-articular and extra-articular osteophytes, exostoses, ossification of ligaments and joint cartilage, and marginal lipping at contact points.[36] Proliferation of new bone is often evidenced by exuberant overgrowth, "florid ossification" with decreased joint mobility, and increased stabilization of the foot. Fusion and rounding of large fragments are late findings.

Pathogenesis of Charcot Foot

Multiple factors appear to contribute to the development of bone and joint destruction in persons with diabetes. Peripheral neuropathy with loss of protective sensation, mechanical stress, autonomic neuropathy with increased blood flow to bone, and trauma have emerged as the most important determinants. Other factors possibly relevant in the development of diabetic neuropathic osteoarthropathy include metabolic perturbations, renal disease, renal transplantation, corticosteroid-induced osteoporosis, osteoclastic-osteoblastic imbalance, decreased

cartilage growth activity, and nonenzymatic glycosylation of bone proteins and extra-articular soft tissues (Fig. 21–2). Notwithstanding, the mechanism for development of neuropathic bone and joint lesions is not completely understood.

Two mechanisms have been described for the development of bony resorption (osteolysis); one mechanism is mediated by increased blood flow to bone and the other through unbalanced osteoclastic activity.[1, 62, 135] Infection may cause increased blood flow to bone through granulation tissue as is often the case with a mal perforans ulcer. The resultant radiographic changes in bone are usually nonspecific. What initially appears to be bone destruction consistent with osteomyelitis may not be caused by direct extension of infection to the bone but may instead represent osteolysis secondary to increased peripheral blood flow, inflammatory hyperemia, granulation tissue, or soft tissue infection.

Bone resorption and joint deformity, especially in the metatarsophalangeal joints, may be exaggerated by the presence of trophic ulceration and infection.[76, 129] The diagnostic dilemma in these cases is which came first, the osteoarthropathy or the infection. The differentiation of osteoarthropathy from osteomyelitis is often difficult in the presence of overlying soft tissue infection and ulceration; however, newer imaging modalities can aid in making this important distinction.[9, 12, 71, 93, 124] Because the presenting symptoms of ulceration and infection often precede radiographic evaluation of the foot, it is invariably construed that pathologic bone and joint changes must have occurred secondary to infection. In their discussion of the role of infection in the pathogenesis of the Charcot foot and ankle, Lippman et al.[88] determined that in 4 of their 12 patients, collapse preceded infection. In four other cases it seemed likely that ulceration and bacterial invasion occurred after the Charcot lesion had been established for some time. Other authors[90, 91] have reported similar observations. The role of infection in many of these patients should be viewed as a complication and not an etiologic factor.[104]

The relationship that exists between certain lesions of the spinal cord and the peripheral nerves and the subsequent development of neuropathic joints has been well documented.[15, 17, 18, 20, 26–28, 63, 72, 73, 77, 81, 91, 122, 127, 135] The presence of peripheral sensorimotor neurop-

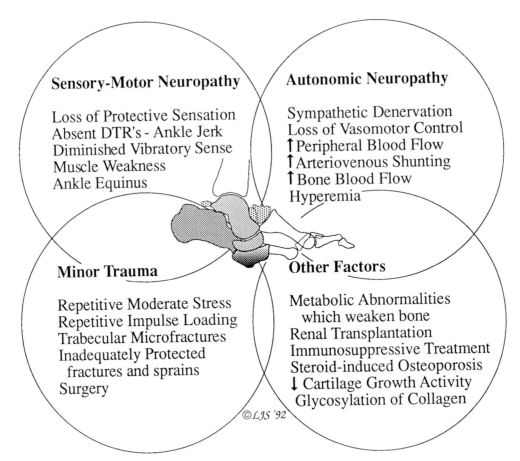

Sensory-Motor Neuropathy

Loss of Protective Sensation
Absent DTR's - Ankle Jerk
Diminished Vibratory Sense
Muscle Weakness
Ankle Equinus

Autonomic Neuropathy

Sympathetic Denervation
Loss of Vasomotor Control
↑ Peripheral Blood Flow
↑ Arteriovenous Shunting
↑ Bone Blood Flow
Hyperemia

Minor Trauma

Repetitive Moderate Stress
Repetitive Impulse Loading
Trabecular Microfractures
Inadequately Protected
   fractures and sprains
Surgery

Other Factors

Metabolic Abnormalities
   which weaken bone
Renal Transplantation
Immunosuppressive Treatment
Steroid-induced Osteoporosis
↓ Cartilage Growth Activity
Glycosylation of Collagen

©LJS '92

Figure 21–2 ■ Pathogenesis of Charcot foot. (Modified from Sanders LJ, Frykberg RG: Diabetic neuropathic osteoarthropathy: The Charcot foot. *In* Frykberg RG [ed]: The High Risk Foot in Diabetes Mellitus. New York: Churchill Livingstone, 1991, with permission.)

athy characterized by loss of protective sensation, absent deep tendon reflexes, diminished vibratory perception, and muscle weakness sets into motion a series of events that eventually result in the development of Charcot joint. The following discussion is directed at understanding the neurovascular etiology of DNOAP, as well as the possible roles of other important factors, that may be less well known.

Increased Peripheral Blood Flow

Autonomic nervous system dysfunction has been noted as an associated finding in patients with neuropathic osteoarthropathy.[2, 18, 28, 39, 42, 52, 89, 94, 131, 135] Support for the hypothesis that increased blood flow and active bone resorption are responsible for the development of Charcot joint is evidenced by several case reports and experimental data.[16–18, 39, 40, 41, 88, 90, 91, 119, 131, 133] Schwarz et al.[119] described the case of a 61-year-old diabetic who developed severe whittling down of the metatarsal bones and proximal phalanges of the left foot after a left lumbar sympathectomy 22 years earlier. Edelman et al.[39] reported three cases where neuropathic osteoarthropathy developed within 2 to 5 years after successful lower limb revascularization. Lippman et al.[88] suggested that excess local arterial flow can be a contributing factor to osseous breakdown under stress.

A neurally initiated vascular reflex leading to increased blood flow and active bone resorption has been proposed as an important etiologic factor in the development of bone and joint destruction in neuropathic patients.[16–18, 39, 112, 131] Wartenberg[131] noted a possible role of the sympathetic nervous system in the manifestations of tabes dorsalis and in the production of tabetic joints. He observed local disturbances in sympathetic vessel innervation in unilateral tabetic arthropa-thies, in proximity to the affected joints. "The following pathologic disturbances were found: elevation of the local temperature, rise in the arterial and venous blood pres-sure, increase in the oscillometric index, anomalies of the sweat secretion and distur-bances in the pilomotor reflex."[131]

Normal circulation with palpable pedal pulses have consistently been reported in di-abetic patients with neuropathic osteoar-thropathy.[4, 6, 52, 73, 125] "Pedal pulses in most of our patients were accentuated. The feet were warm with bounding dorsalis pedis and pos-terior tibial pulses."[125] The existence of auto-nomic neuropathy in patients with diabetic neuropathic arthropathies has likewise been reported with regularity.[52, 91, 94, 119, 135]

Evidence exists that autonomic neuropa-thy with sympathetic denervation resulting in high peripheral blood flow is common in patients with diabetes mellitus.[2, 13, 15, 35, 40, 42, 51, 133, 135] Archer et al.,[2] at the King's College Hospital, measured resting foot blood flow in 22 diabetic patients with severe sensory neuropathy using mercury strain gauge plethysmography and Doppler sonogram techniques. They found blood flow to be in-creased on the average five times greater than normal at 20° to 22°C. They noted that foot skin temperature was also elevated, re-flecting the increased circulation.

Edmonds et al.,[40] also from King's College Hospital, studied the uptake of methylene diphosphonate labeled with technetium-99m (^{99m}Tc) in 13 neuropathic diabetics and eight nondiabetic controls. Bone scans were per-formed, and uptake of radiopharmaceutical was monitored in three phases. Uptake in all three phases (2 minutes after injection, at 4 minutes, and at 4 hours) was markedly elevated and confined to the feet in all neuro-pathic subjects. Increased uptake at 2 and 4 minutes indicated increased blood flow. These investigators concluded that the most likely explanation for their findings was in-creased bony blood flow secondary to sympa-thetic denervation. They also noted that se-verely abnormal autonomic function occurs in association with neuropathic ulceration.[40] High blood flow, vasodilatation, and arterio-venous shunting, which result from sympa-thetic denervation, could lead to abnormal venous pooling.[133] Young et al.[135] corrobo-rated the importance of autonomic neuropa-thy in promoting diminished bone mineral density in patients with peripheral neuropa-thy. Those patients with active Charcot feet had significantly greater deficits in auto-nomic parameters than their non-Charcot neuropathic counterparts. Furthermore, bone mineral density in both lower limbs of Charcot patients was lower than that found in matched non-Charcot subjects. Although bone density was lower in the affected limb of Charcot patients in contrast to the contra-lateral side, we must consider that a treat-ment effect might be responsible rather than a true causative effect.[135] These results aug-ment those of Forst et al.,[51] who also de-scribed diminished bone mineral density (BMD) in the lower extremities of type 1 dia-betic patients as compared to age- and sex-matched controls. Additionally, a link be-tween decreased BMD and neuropathy was found in the femoral neck. Investigating markers of osteoclast and osteoblastic activ-ity in osteoarthropathy, Gough et al.[62] deter-mined that patients with acute Charcot feet had significantly higher levels of osteoclastic activity than those found in patients with chronic deformities, diabetic controls, and healthy subjects. There were no significant elevations for the osteoblastic marker in any of the groups. Although the excess osteoclas-tic activity certainly cannot be considered as causative for osteoarthropathy, the authors suggest that there is an uncoupling of bone absorption and deposition during the active stage of this process and that such markers might be used to monitor disease activity.

Mean venous Po_2 in the feet of neuropathic subjects with ulcers was found to be signifi-cantly higher than in controls by Boulton et al.[13] They frequently observed the presence of prominent pedal arteries and distended dorsal foot veins in their diabetic patients who had noninfected neuropathic foot ulcers. These observations led them to believe that arteriovenous (AV) shunting with increased venous oxygenation was important in the pathogenesis of ulceration.

Mechanical Stress

Mechanical elements have long been recog-nized in the etiology of osteoarthritis. Situa-tions that impose chronically increased stress on articular cartilage can act as the inciting primary cause. The repetitive me-chanical stress of ambulation with impulsive loading of bone, applied to a foot that has lost protective sensation, results in soft tissue injury (ulcers) and tensile fatigue of cartilage and bone. Trabecular microfractures in the subchondral cancellous bone are the earliest ultrastructural evidence of cartilage damage.[105] The result of healing of these microfractures and remodeling is an increase in the stiffness of the subchondral bone,[107] which reduces the bones' normal resilience and ability to absorb shock. Total collapse of the neuropathic foot can occur over a very short period and may be evidenced clinically by depression of the medial longitudinal arch and complaints by the patient that "my arch has fallen."[114]

Any disturbance of the bones and joints of the neuropathic foot resulting in a change of shape, bony deformity, or alteration of foot mechanics has the potential for causing skeletal and soft tissue lesions.[55] Patients with Charcot arthropathy will also typically be found to have elevated peak plantar pressures.[3] The consequence of increased vertical force and shear stress directed on the soft tissues overlying prominent bone is ulceration, followed by infection and further collapse of the foot. The degree of injury is determined by the extent of sensory loss, amount of stress on the joint; duration of the inflammatory process; and the patient's persistent ambulation in spite of the swelling, redness, and deformity. Cavanagh et al.[24] determined that foot deformity rather than body mass is a major determinant for high peak plantar pressures and subsequent ulceration in patients with peripheral neuropathy. A deformed Charcot foot, therefore, significantly places the limb at risk for ulceration and attendant complications.[22]

Fractures

Fractures of significant magnitude were responsible for initiating or increasing joint changes in the majority of the 118 cases of neuroarthropathy reported by Johnson.[72] He concluded that "the behaviour of the bones and joints in neuroarthropathy can be explained on the basis of the usual responses of these tissues to trauma modified by the presence of decreased protective sensation." Lack of attentive recognition and a cavalier attitude with regard to protection of fractures, sprains, and effusions sustain the atrophic phase and result in bone and joint destruction. As long as the trauma of repetitive stress and weight bearing continues, resorption outpaces new bone formation, and this destructive cycle continues. Figure 21–3 illustrates a simplified diagram of the pathogenesis and perpetuation of the acute stage from unaltered weight bearing.

Eleven percent of the cases reported by Newman[99] had spontaneous fractures and dislocations. These cases presented the greatest therapeutic problems compared

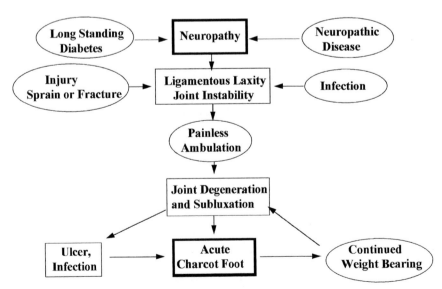

Figure 21–3 ■ The pathogenesis and destructive cycle of the acute Charcot foot. If the trauma of weight bearing continues, the acute stage is perpetuated and further deformity will result. Ulcers with subsequent infection complicate this process and contribute to joint disintegration.

with other noninfective diseases of bone. Newman stressed the importance of recognizing these conditions and distinguishing them from osteomyelitis. Holmes[68] has reported on a series of diabetic patients sustaining foot and ankle fractures. Where there was a delay in diagnosis and treatment, a high incidence of Charcot changes developed. Many such fractures of a minor nature in patients with neuropathy may go undetected and lead to lesser degrees of osteoarthropathy that is diagnosed randomly during routine radiography.[25]

Autonomic neuropathy with loss of vasomotor control and increased peripheral blood flow to bone, coupled with an inflammatory hyperemia of the soft tissues, results in resorption of bone with further weakening. Atrophic bone is easily fractured or fragmented. Frequent spontaneous fractures in neuropathic patients has led some authors[45, 51, 135] to believe that intrinsic bone disease may be an etiologic factor.

Equinus Deformity

Weakness of the anterior group muscles of the leg (ankle dorsiflexors) may result in a compensatory contracture of the gastrocnemius-soleus muscles, with equinus deformity.[3, 7, 56, 111, 117] Although there are no data confirming a direct causal relationship between equinus deformity and the development of neuroarthropathy, intuitively this appears to be a reasonable assumption, especially at the tarsometatarsal and midtarsal joints. Weight bearing on a neuropathic foot with weak ankle dorsiflexors causes the triceps surae to forcefully plantarflex the foot, resulting in increased pressure over the metatarsophalangeal joints, a slapping gait, and stress at the tarsometatarsal, naviculocuneiform, and midtarsal joints once calf contracture occurs. Conversely, equinus of the rearfoot (hind foot) may develop *after* midfoot collapse due to some other type of external trauma. Since most reports on this topic measure equinus after the Charcot deformity has already manifested, we cannot exclude the possibility of a secondary triceps surae contracture. Only longitudinal studies of a large diabetes population will be able to determine the true role of equinus, if any, in the etiology of osteoarthropathy.

Renal Transplantation

Isolated reports have shown an association between renal transplantation with long-term corticosteroid or other immunosuppressive treatment and the subsequent development of neuropathic osteoarthropathy.[30] These reviews show that after renal transplantation, diabetics have a much higher incidence of neurotrophic joint disease than the nontransplanted diabetic population. Clohisy and Thompson[30] reported on 18 patients with juvenile-onset diabetes and severe neuropathic arthropathy of the ankle and tarsus. Fourteen of these patients had received a renal transplant before the fracture was diagnosed, and none had a history of major trauma. It remains unclear whether corticosteroid-induced osteoporosis or some other metabolic abnormality, which tends to weaken bone, was the underlying factor responsible for the development of bone and joint destruction in these patients. Further discussion of this subject follows in the section, "Pattern V: Calcaneus," below.

Glycosylation of Collagen

The synthesis of abnormal collagen types not usually found in cartilage, bone, ligaments, or other soft tissues may be another possible factor in the development of DNOAP. Nonenzymatic glycosylation of proteins associated with chronic hyperglycemia, in particular hemoglobin and dermal collagen, has been reported in several publications.[14, 19, 21, 95] Digital sclerosis and joint contractures were found affecting the hands in 18% of children with insulin-dependent diabetes mellitus.[21] Biopsies of patients with limited joint mobility have shown increased cross-linking and glycosylation of collagen.[14] Limited joint mobility (LJM) of the ankle, subtalar, and metatarsophalangeal joints has been studied in cross sections of diabetic and nondiabetic patients by several authors.[37, 48, 97] Characteristically, those patients with a history of neuropathic ulceration had significantly less mobility than those without ulceration or nondiabetic controls, although LJM was not restricted to patients with neuropathy. Fernando[48] also correlated LJM with higher plantar foot pressures. Sixty-five percent of those subjects with both LJM and neuropathy had a history of ulceration. Studies are lacking, however, in patients with Charcot arthropathy, and it is intuitively difficult to correlate limited joint mobility with the severe hypermobility frequently observed in this disorder.

Abnormal (type 1) collagen has been found by immunohistochemical assays in the immediate vicinity of chondrocytes in osteoarthritic cartilage.[69] Diminution of chondroitin sulfate content relative to the collagen matrix is a feature common to osteoarthritic alteration of joint cartilage. Hough and Sokoloff[69] suggest that this change might alter the material properties of cartilage with respect to wear and tear.

Decreased Cartilage Growth Activity

Skeletal integrity may be affected by insulin deficiency through its effect on insulin-like growth factor 1 (IGF-1). Insulin growth factor 1, also known as somatomedin C, is synthesized in response to growth hormone influence and acts directly to produce cartilage proliferation and skeletal growth. Data suggest that IGF-1 serves as a mitogenic signal to cause mitosis of newly differentiated chondrocytes.[118] The induction of streptozotocin-induced diabetes in rats has been shown to result in a significant decrease in serum somatomedin and cartilage growth activity.[87]

Patterns of Bone and Joint Destruction

Five characteristic anatomic patterns of bone and joint destruction have been observed to occur in diabetics with DNOAP or osteopathy.[112, 113] Sanders and Frykberg[112] compiled information on the distribution of bone and joint involvement in neuropathic diabetics, reported in the English literature, as well as cases from a Veterans Administration retrospective study, and developed the following anatomic classification: pattern I, forefoot; pattern II, tarsometatarsal joints; pattern III, naviculocuneiform, talonavicular, and calcaneocuboid joints; pattern IV, ankle and/or subtalar joint; and pattern V, calcaneus. Two of these patterns, I and II, are frequently associated with bony deformity and ulceration. The most frequent joint involvement is seen in patterns I, II, and III, with the most severe structural deformity and functional instability seen in patterns II and IV. Pattern V osteopathy is the least common and may

be seen as an isolated fracture of the calcaneus or in association with involvement of other tarsal bones.[74] These anatomic patterns may be seen singly or in combination in any given individual (Fig. 21–4).

Pattern I: The Forefoot

This commonly occurring pattern of osteoarthropathy is characterized by involvement of the forefoot; in other words, the interphalangeal joints, phalanges, metatarsophalangeal joints, or distal metatarsal bones. Radiographic findings in this location are typically atrophic and destructive in nature, characterized by osteopenia, osteolysis, juxta-articular cortical bone defects, subluxation, and destruction. Pattern I involvement has been reported to occur in 26 to 67% of all affected sites.[12, 32, 94, 113] Of the affected joints (10 of 21) in Miller and Lichtman's[94] study, 47.6% involved the metatarsophalangeal and interphalangeal joints. Sanders and Mrdjenovich[113] found pattern I involvement in 30% of affected sites (20 of 66); Cofield et al.[32] reported metatarsophalangeal and interphalangeal joint involvement in 67% of 116 affected limbs. Sinha et al.[125] reported metatarsophalangeal joint involvement in 26.8% (34 of 127) of all affected sites.

Plantar ulceration is a common finding associated with osteopathy of the forefoot. Cofield et al.[32] reported that 91% of their patients with radiographic evidence of metatarsophalangeal joint involvement had underlying ulcers. It may not be readily apparent whether the bone and joint changes preceded or developed as a result of the ulceration. The presence of neuropathic plantar ulceration should be considered a serious finding, which may lead to major disability. This finding may, in fact, be a cutaneous marker for neuropathic arthropathy of the forefoot. Newman et al.[101] assessed the prevalence of osteomyelitis in 35 diabetic patients with 41 foot ulcers (38 classic mal perforans ulcers). As determined by bone biopsy and culture, these investigators found osteomyelitis to underlie 68% of the foot ulcers. All patients with ulcers exposed to bone had osteomyelitis. Digital findings include concentric resorption of bone that may be seen to affect the phalangeal diaphyses with a characteristic hourglass appearance. Broadening of the bases of the proximal phalanges occurs, with the

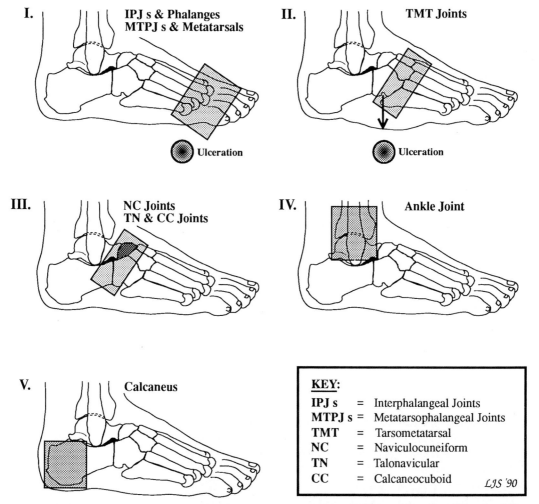

I. IPJ s & Phalanges
MTPJ s & Metatarsals
Ulceration

II. TMT Joints
Ulceration

III. NC Joints
TN & CC Joints

IV. Ankle Joint

V. Calcaneus

KEY:

IPJ s	=	Interphalangeal Joints
MTPJ s	=	Metatarsophalangeal Joints
TMT	=	Tarsometatarsal
NC	=	Naviculocuneiform
TN	=	Talonavicular
CC	=	Calcaneocuboid

LJS '90

Figure 21–4 ■ Anatomic patterns of bone and joint destruction reported in diabetics with neuropathic osteoarthropathy of the foot and ankle. Patterns I and II are frequently associated with bony deformity and ulceration. The most frequent joint involvement is seen in patterns I, II, and III, with the most severe structural deformity and functional instability associated with patterns II and IV. (From Sanders LJ, Frykberg RG: Diabetic neuropathic osteoarthropathy: The Charcot foot. *In* Frykberg RG [ed]: The High Risk Foot in Diabetes Mellitus. New York: Churchill Livingstone, 1991, with permission.)

formation of a cup around the metatarsal head (Fig. 21–5).[82, 119]

Resorption of the distal metatarsal bones and phalanges is characteristic of atrophic, destructive diabetic osteopathy. This is evidenced, on anteroposterior radiographs, as a pencil-like tapering of the metatarsal bones with a licked peppermint stick, or sucked candy, appearance (Fig. 21–6). The histopathologic picture reveals erosion of articular cartilage, periarticular fibrosis, increased vascularity, synchronous resorption of bone, and new bone formation. There is disorganization of subchondral bone, with bony resorption and a fatty marrow. Chronic ulceration and infection may be associated with these changes.

Pattern II: Tarsometatarsal Joints

Pattern II osteoarthropathy is distinguished by affection of the tarsometatarsal (Lisfranc's) joints and is often associated with plantar ulceration at the apex of the collapsed cuneiforms or cuboid. Tarsometatarsal involvement has been reported to occur in 15 to 48% of the cases of DNOAP.[4, 5, 32, 94, 106, 125] This pattern of osteoarthropathy occurs spontaneously and with greater frequency in diabetics than in patients with leprosy (Hansen's disease). Unlike the tarsometatarsal joint pattern associated with Hansen's disease, this pattern is rarely caused by "definite violence."[65]

The normal anatomic relationships of the tarsometatarsal joints are illustrated in Figure 21–7. The second metatarsal base is securely recessed in the intercuneiform mortise. This tenon-in-mortise relationship creates a very stable keystone for the midfoot. Disturbance of this relationship weakens the foot and allows for dorsolateral displacement of the metatarsal bones on the cuneiforms and cuboid followed by their architectural collapse.

Early changes in the tarsometatarsal joints may be subtle and consistent with incipient osteoarthritis; there may be slight dorsal prominence of the metatarsal bases with local swelling and increased skin temperature on the dorsum of the foot. Late changes reveal degenerative arthritis with fragmentation and subluxation of the cuneiform bones and the metatarsal bases. The metatarsal bases often override the cuneiforms. There may be evidence of total disintegration of the cuneiforms, with collapse of

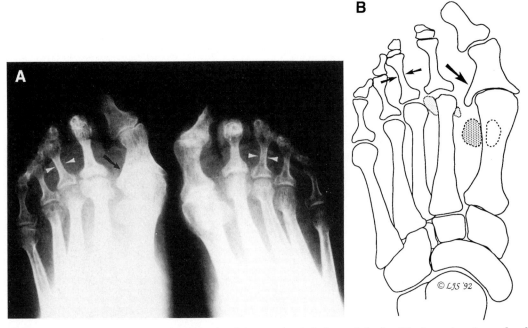

Figure 21–5 ■ *A,* Concentric resorption of bone involving proximal phalangeal shafts of the lesser toes (*arrowheads*). Note hour-glass appearance of the phalanges. Note also, broadening of the phalangeal base of the hallux and cupping of the first metatarsal head (*arrow*). Proliferative changes of the second metatarsal head are also noted. *B,* Graphic illustration of radiographic findings.

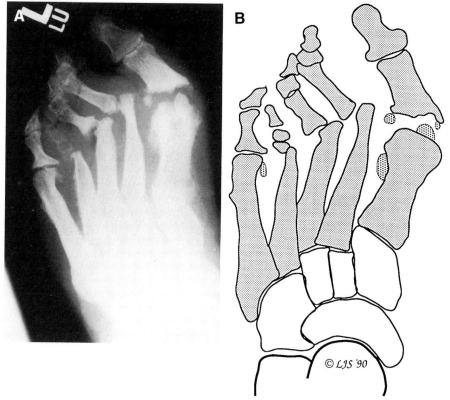

Figure 21-6 ■ *A,* Anteroposterior radiograph reveals osteolytic destruction of all metatarsophalangeal joints, with pencil-like tapering of the metatarsal shafts resembling "sucked candy" or "licked peppermint stick." *B,* Graphic representation of radiographic findings. (From Sanders LJ, Frykberg RG: Diabetic neuropathic osteoarthropathy: The Charcot foot. *In* Frykberg RG [ed]: The High Risk Foot in Diabetes mellitus. New York: Churchill Livingstone, 1991, with permission.)

the midfoot and a resultant rocker bottom foot deformity.

A fracture or minimal subluxation of the base of the second metatarsal, even from ostensibly insignificant trauma, may precede collapse of the tarsometatarsal joints, as seen in the following case. A 66-year-old neuropathic diabetic man had mild swelling and erythema on the dorsum of his right foot after a fall in his kitchen. Radiographs revealed a laterally displaced fracture of the second metatarsal base (Fig. 21-8). The patient was placed in a plaster cast, non–weight bearing, with crutches for 6 weeks. During this time he was poorly compliant and refused further treatment. Within 8 months the patient's midfoot collapsed. Diabetic patients may have an erythematous, hot, painful, swollen foot, with no recognizable history of antecedent injury.[4, 55] The clinical picture may be nonspecific, resembling an acute gouty arthritis, septic arthritis, or cellulitis. Patients are usually afebrile with no clinical or laboratory evidence of infection. There may, however, be a mildly elevated erythrocyte sedimentation rate (ESR) with normal white blood cell (WBC) count. Sanders and Mrdjenovich[113] reported a mean ESR of 32 ± 6.7 mm/hr (range, 22 to 41) in a group of 13 neuropathic diabetics with bone and joint changes and normal WBC counts. The radiographic picture, however, is quite remarkable, revealing subluxation or fracture dislocation of Lisfranc's joint.[5] The base of the second metatarsal is laterally displaced from its normal recessed position in the intercuneiform mortise, and all of the metatarsals are shifted laterally on the lesser tarsus.

The following case represents an acute neuropathic osteoarthropathy affecting the tarsometatarsal articulations. The patient, a 63-year-old neuropathic diabetic man with a 15-year history of diabetes mellitus, poorly controlled with insulin, was admitted to the emergency room with acute erythema, swelling, increased skin temperature, and defor-

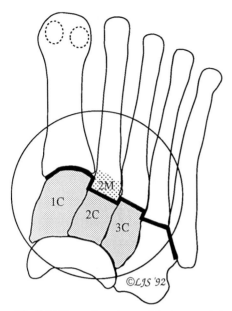

Figure 21–7 ■ Normal anatomy of the tarsometatarsal (Lisfranc's) joints. Note recessed position of the second metatarsal base (*stippled area*) in the intercuneiform mortise. M, metatarsal; C, cuneiform.

mity of the right foot. He reported having mild pain and no history of trauma. The patient, a unilateral transtibial amputee, was afebrile with an elevated blood glucose level of 447 mg/dL. Radiographs revealed a tarsometatarsal joint dislocation, with all of the metatarsal bases shifted laterally on the lesser tarsus. The lateral radiograph revealed plantar dislocation of the cuneiforms and navicular, with dorsal displacement of the metatarsal bases. The patient was admitted to the hospital for conservative management of the right foot, an unsuccessful attempt at closed reduction of the dislocation, and control of diabetes mellitus. In spite of efforts to immobilize the limb and to limit weight bearing, this unilateral amputee continued to walk on his right lower limb. Within 6 months total collapse of the foot occurred, along with extrusion of the medial cuneiform. Ulceration developed from shear stress over the prominent medial cuneiform (Fig. 21–9).

Pattern III:
Naviculocuneiform, Talonavicular, and Calcaneocuboid Joints

This pattern of osteoarthropathy involves the naviculocuneiform and midtarsal joints.

Pattern III is frequently characterized by dislocation of the navicular or by disintegration of the naviculocuneiform joints. Sanders and Mrdjenovich[113] reported naviculocuneiform, talonavicular, or calcaneocuboid involvement in approximately 32% of the affected joints (21 of 66 sites) in 28 cases. Very early radiographic changes of impending Charcot's joint destruction may be evidenced by osteolysis of the naviculocuneiform joints. Typical fragmentation, osteolysis, and sharply defined osseous debris are visible on the lateral radiograph (Fig. 21–10). Observation of this finding signals the need for non–weight-bearing cast immobilization of the foot. Ignoring this finding may result in progressive deterioration of the lesser tarsal bones and ultimately in collapse of the midfoot.

Isolated midtarsal joint dislocations associated with neuropathic diabetics have been reported by several authors.[72, 86, 100] Lesko and Maurer[86] reported their experience with eight talonavicular dislocations, in which dislocations of the navicular were described as either inferomedial, mediodorsal, or medial. Fragmentation of bone frequently accompanies these dislocations. Talonavicular dislocation may be seen alone or in associa-

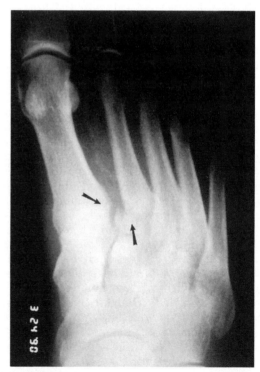

Figure 21–8 ■ Laterally displaced fracture of the second metatarsal base (*arrows*).

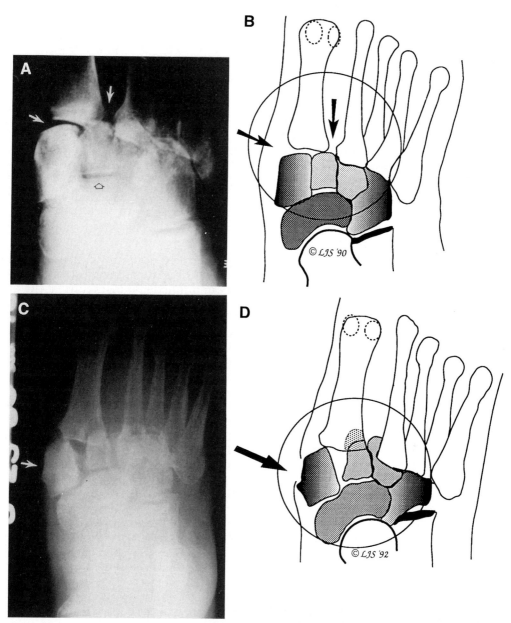

Figure 21–9 ■ *A,* Anteroposterior radiograph reveals dislocation of the tarsometatarsal joints, with lateral displacement of the metatarsal bases on the cuneiforms and cuboid. Second metatarsal base is completely displaced from the intercuneiform mortise, with the first metatarsal base articulating with the medial half of the second cuneiform (*arrows*). Note distal migration of the second cuneiform (*arrowhead*). *B,* Graphic illustration of radiographic findings in *A. C,* Anteroposterior radiograph taken 6 months after initial presentation. There has been extensive deterioration of the tarsometatarsal, navicular cuneiform, and midtarsal joints. Note extrusion of the medial cuneiform (*arrow*). The second cuneiform has eroded its way into the plantar-lateral aspect of the first metatarsal base. *D,* Graphic illustration of radiographic findings in *C.* (From Sanders LJ, Frykberg RG: Diabetic neuropathic osteoarthropathy: The Charcot foot. *In* Frykberg RG [ed]: The High Risk Foot in Diabetes Mellitus. New York: Churchill Livingstone, 1991, with permission.)

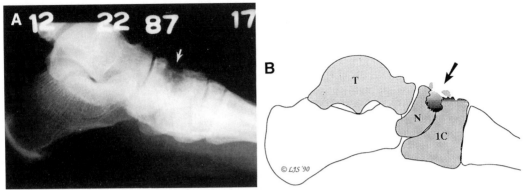

Figure 21–10 ■ *A,* Osteolytic destruction of the naviculocuneiform joints (*arrow*). Fragmentation, osteolysis, and sharply defined osseous debris are noted. *B,* Graphic illustration of radiographic findings. *1C,* first cuneiform bone; *N,* navicular bone; *T,* talus. (From Sanders LJ, Frykberg RG: Diabetic neuropathic osteoarthropathy: The Charcot foot. *In* Frykberg RG [ed]: The High Risk Foot in Diabetes Mellitus. New York: Churchill Livingstone, 1991, with permission.)

tion with involvement of the naviculocuneiform joints, disintegration of the cuneiform bones, or with deterioration of the head and neck of the talus (Fig. 21–11).

A combination of patterns II and III is represented in Figure 21–12. Note the dramatic collapse of the midfoot with a rocker bottom appearance. Ulceration of the skin occurred at the apex of the rocker. The tarsometatarsal, naviculocuneiform, talonavicular, and calcaneocuboid joints all are involved.

Pattern IV: Ankle and Subtalar Joints

Ankle joint with or without subtalar joint involvement accounts for only 3 to 10% of

the reported cases,[32, 94, 113, 125] yet this pattern invariably results in severe structural deformity and functional instability of the ankle. Charcot joint affecting the ankle may develop suddenly without any appreciable external cause, with spontaneous swelling and localized redness of the foot and ankle. Patients will initially notice swelling and deformity of the affected ankle, with little pain. They often continue to walk on the affected limb until the collateral ligaments stretch or tear, and there is erosion of bone and cartilage with collapse of the joint. Steindler's[127] observations of foot and ankle fractures in patients with tabetic joints caused him to conclude that "the greatest pathological changes correspond to the maximum of mechanical

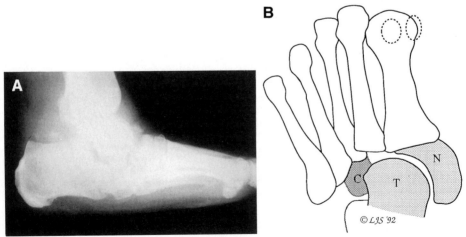

Figure 21–11 ■ *A,* Disorganization of the talonavicular and calcaneocuboid joints. *B,* Graphic illustration of talonavicular dislocation with inferomedial displacement of the navicular bone.

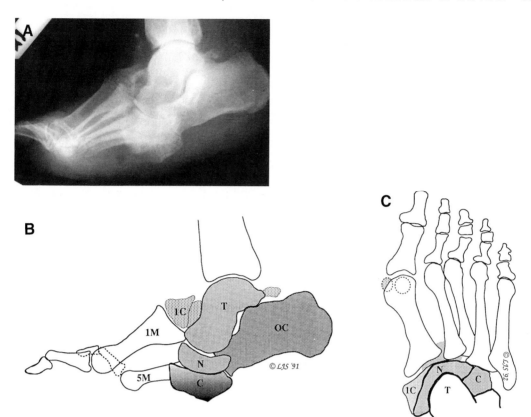

Figure 21–12 ■ *A*, Lateral radiograph demonstrates collapse of the tarsometatarsal, naviculocuneiform, talonavicular, and calcaneocuboid joints (combination of patterns II and III). *B* and *C*, Graphic illustrations of radiographic findings, with identification of involved structures. *C*, cuboid; *N*, navicular; *T*, talus; *OC*, calcaneous; *1C*, medial cuneiform; *M*, metatarsal. (*A* and *B* from Sanders LJ, Frykberg RG: Diabetic neuropathic osteoarthropathy: The Charcot foot. *In* Frykberg RG [ed]: The High Risk Foot in Diabetes Mellitus. New York: Churchill Livingstone, 1991, with permission.)

stress . . . in the direction of the greatest weight-bearing." He noted two types of destruction: one in the direction of the long axis of the leg, breaking down the talus and calcaneus; the other evidenced by collapse of the forefoot and tarsus. Free bodies were seen in the ankle joint in 8 of 21 cases.

Harris and Brand[65] noted that if during weight bearing "the posture of the foot is disturbed by external forces or paralysis an abnormal position results, and the new weight stream will cross the trabecular lines so that minor fractures occur more readily and ligaments may rupture." They described "a relatively rapid and catastrophic disintegration of the proximal tarsal bones allowing the tibia to grind its way through the foot to the ground."

Even trivial trauma associated with an ankle sprain or a relatively minor fracture may result in instability of the ankle joint, with resultant collapse and disintegra-

tion.[65, 72, 94] Miller and Lichtman[94] described a case in which total destruction of the ankle joint resulted after surgical intervention for a fractured medial malleolus. Johnson[72] reported the case of a 55-year-old woman who 8 weeks after a sprained left ankle developed complete displacement of the medial malleolus with grinding away of one half of the talus and part of the distal end of the tibia.

Rapid disintegration of the ankle joint occurred in a 59-year-old neuropathic woman with a 15-year history of diabetes mellitus. Her chief complaints were pain, redness, and swelling of her left foot and ankle of 1 week's duration. There was no history of trauma; however, she had recently been treated by her family physician for "an infected blister" on her left fifth toe. Infection resolved promptly, but shortly thereafter pain and swelling developed over the lateral aspect of her foot and ankle. The patient had bounding pedal pulses and a dense peripheral neuropathy. Radiographs revealed osteopenia of the tarsal bones, with evidence of osteoarthritis of the tarsometatarsal joints. Radionucleotide scan with methylene diphosphonate labeled with ^{99m}Tc revealed very high uptake in the left ankle and tarsal bones, as well as marked uptake in the asymptomatic right ankle. Blood cultures and ankle joint aspirate obtained on admission grew *Staphylococcus aureus*. The opinion of an infectious disease consultant was that a septic arthritis was overlying a diabetic neuropathic arthropathy.[109] In spite of appropriate treatment with parenteral antibiotics, bed rest, elevation of the limb, and non–weight-bearing casts, progressive deformity of the left ankle ensued. The clinical picture was characterized by lateral bulging and instability of the ankle, with medial displacement of the foot and fragmentation of bone. Radiographs and clinical photographs revealed extensive joint destruction with dislocation of the foot to the medial side of the leg (Fig. 21–13).

Pattern V: Calcaneus

Calcaneal Insufficiency Avulsion Fractures

Pattern V osteopathy involves fractures of the calcaneus, characterized by avulsion of the posterior tubercle, and has been the least frequently reported pattern of bone destruction seen in neuropathic diabetics.[10, 30, 33, 45, 74] (Although we appropriately include these neuropathic fractures as a pattern of bone and joint destruction in the diabetic foot, we realize that since they do *not* involve a joint they cannot truly be considered osteoarthropathy.) Kathol et al.[74] reported on 21 diabetic patients with calcaneal fractures, of which 18 were nontraumatic and 14 were limited to the posterior third of the calcaneus. This fracture pattern occurs in the same plane as a fatigue-type calcaneal fracture, with displacement and rotation of the posterior tuberosity. The term "calcaneal insufficiency avulsion fracture" was coined by Kathol's group to describe this specific pattern.[74]

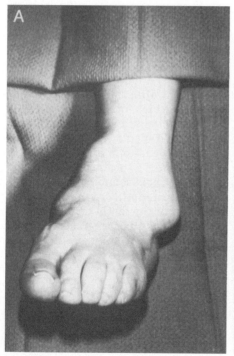 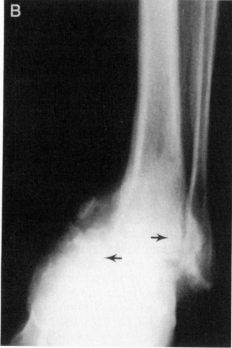

Figure 21–13 ■ *A,* Unstable neuropathic left ankle, with lateral bulging. *B,* Anteroposterior radiograph reveals extensive joint destruction with fragmentation of bone. Note dislocation of the joint (*arrows*), with the foot displaced medially. (From Sanders LJ, Frykberg RG: Diabetic neuropathic osteoarthropathy: The Charcot foot. *In* Frykberg RG [ed]: The High Risk Foot in Diabetes Mellitus. New York: Churchill Livingstone, 1991, with permission.)

Harris and Brand[65] attributed increased vulnerability of the calcaneus in an insensitive foot to (1) increased force on the heel caused by the patient's landing more heavily on an insensitive foot, (2) continued walking on a fractured bone, and (3) previous or concurrent ulceration "which may have weakened the bone by hyperaemic decalcification or may allow infection and osteomyelitis to complicate the fracture."

A bilateral calcaneal fracture was reported by Coventry and Rothacker[33] in a 45-year-old neuropathic woman with juvenile-onset diabetes. El-Khoury and Kathol[45] reported on four patients with spontaneous, unusual avulsion fractures of the posterior tubercle of the calcaneus, "where the avulsed fragment migrated superiorly due to the constant pull of the achilles tendon." These patients had diminished pain and vibratory perception. Clohisy and Thompson[30] reported 19 calcaneal fractures in 18 neuropathic juvenile-onset diabetics who had no history of major trauma to their limbs. Five of these patients had bilateral calcaneal fractures. In 17 limbs the calcaneal fractures were seen together with fractures of more than one other tarsal bone. Fourteen of the patients in this study underwent renal transplant surgery before the fracture was diagnosed.

Thompson et al.,[128] in a retrospective review of 55 neuropathic kidney transplant patients, found a 20% incidence of skeletal disease among diabetic patients, with the highest incidence occurring in the third and fourth years after transplantation. They reported seeing three calcaneal fractures in 11 patients with neurotrophic joint disease. The initial manifestation in all patients was a pathologic fracture, usually in a metaphyseal area near a joint. Only later did they see actual joint destruction that seemed to result from the subchondral collapse associated with the initial fracture.

A calcaneal insufficiency avulsion fracture of the posterior tubercle of the right calcaneus occurred spontaneously in an active 53-year-old neuropathic diabetic woman with a 5-year history of diabetes mellitus. She reported hearing a loud crack and feeling a sharp pain in the back of her right heel while walking in the hallway at work. Lateral radiographs revealed posterior and superior displacement of the posterior process of the calcaneus (Fig. 21–14). In addition to the calcaneal insufficiency avulsion fracture, radiographs of the asymptomatic left foot revealed concentric resorption of the proximal phalanges, a cup-shaped proximal phalangeal base of the hallux, and fragmentation of the second metatarsal head.

Diagnostic Studies

The diagnosis of DNOAP depends primarily on the physician's clinical suspicion of the disease. Medical history, clinical manifestation, and radiographic findings should help to narrow down the differential diagnosis. This disorder should be suspected when bone and joint pathologic conditions are found in

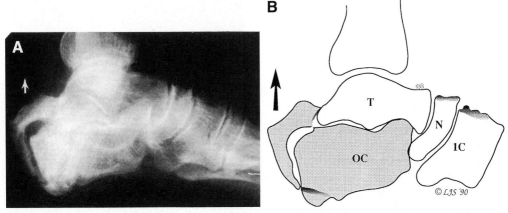

Figure 21–14 ■ *A*, Lateral radiograph demonstrates an avulsion fracture of the posterior tubercle of the calcaneus. *Arrow* points in the direction of pull of the Achilles tendon. Early osteolytic changes are seen to affect the naviculocuneiform joint. *B*, Graphic illustration of radiographic findings. (From Sanders LJ, Frykberg RG: Diabetic neuropathic osteoarthropathy: The Charcot foot. *In* Frykberg RG [ed]: The High Risk Foot in Diabetes Mellitus. New York: Churchill Livingstone, 1991, with permission.)

a diabetic patient with loss of protective sensation, absent deep tendon reflexes, and diminished vibratory sense.

The most specific diagnostic tools for distinguishing between DNOAP and osteomyelitis in the diabetic foot are careful clinical, radiographic, radionucleotide, and magnetic resonance imaging (MRI) examinations, followed by bone biopsy, bone cultures, and histopathologic examination. Bone biopsy should be reserved for those cases that are equivocal, when there has been a chronic nonhealing wound or soft tissue infection contiguous to bone. Radiographs may occasionally be unremarkable during the early manifestation of the Charcot foot. At this time, the clinical picture may be very subtle, with only mild inflammation of the soft tissues and radiographic findings consistent with incipient osteoarthritis or osteolysis. In cases where there is a clear history of injury but the initial plain films are negative, radiographic studies should be repeated within 2 to 3 weeks to rule out stress fractures, fragmentation of bone, and periosteal new bone formation. During this time a cautious approach to treatment should be taken with a high index of suspicion. Affected limbs of neuropathic individuals should be immobilized and kept non–weight bearing. Serial radiographs are beneficial in following the course of this disease through the stage of reconstruction.[54, 58]

Computed tomography (CT) and MRI are valuable adjuncts in the evaluation of the diabetic Charcot foot. Williamson et al.,[134] at the University of Virginia Medical School, reported CT scans correctly predicted the presence or absence of osteomyelitis in all of a series of seven patients. Nuclide bone scans had one false-positive and one false-negative result. Beltran et al.[9] found MRI to be particularly helpful in differentiating neuroarthropathy from osteomyelitis. They identified a distinctive pattern for Charcot's joints consisting of low signal intensity on T1- and T2-weighted images within the bone marrow space adjacent to the involved joint. Others[34, 120] have made similar observations but question the ability of MR imaging to reliably distinguish rapidly progressing osteoarthropathy from osteomyelitis.

The following example demonstrates the use of MRI for evaluation of a 54-year-old woman with collapsed midfoot and associated plantar ulcer. The sagittal image clearly demonstrates the talus and calcaneus with

no alteration of signal intensity to suggest edema or active osteomyelitis. The MRI scan allows clear visualization of the soft tissue structures demonstrating ulceration penetrating through the plantar aponeurosis (Fig. 21–15).

Positive technetium and gallium bone scans may be seen with osteomyelitis, but they may also be false-positive because of neuropathic bone disease.[71, 115] Diffuse and focal uptake of technetium has been reported in neuropathic feet by several authors in areas of active bone turnover and increased bony blood flow, as seen in patients with osteoarthropathy.[40, 41, 47, 66] Positive scans have been reported to sometimes precede radiographic changes.[47] Gallium-67 citrate, which accumulates in sites of infection, has also been reported to localize in noninfected neuropathic bone.[61, 67]

Leukocyte scanning with indium-111 (^{111}In) has been shown to have a high specificity and a very high negative predictive value for osteomyelitis.[75, 92, 108, 115, 116, 136] Newman et al.[101] from the Mount Sinai Medical Center in New York compared the results of radiographs, leukocyte scans with ^{111}In oxyquinolone, and bone scans with bone biopsy

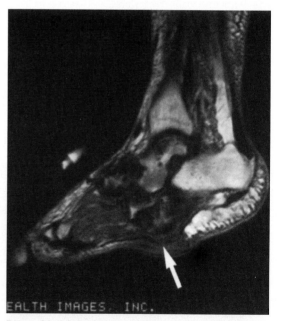

Figure 21–15 ■ MRI scan in a 54-year-old diabetic woman with collapsed midfoot and associated plantar ulcer. Note defect in the plantar aponeurosis (*arrow*) secondary to chronic ulceration. There is no alteration in signal intensity of the bones to suggest edema or active osteomyelitis. (Courtesy of Health Images, Inc., Atlanta Magnetic Imaging, and John A. Ruch, D.P.M.)

and culture results. Of all imaging tests, the leukocyte scan had the highest sensitivity, 89%. The specificity for osteomyelitis with ^{111}In has been reported to be from 78 to 89%[75, 92, 116] compared with 38 to 75% for three-phase bone scans.[75, 108] Schauwecker et al.[115, 116] found that in the absence of infection, ^{111}In-labeled leukocytes do not usually accumulate in neuropathic bone. However, false-positive results do occur in the presence of noninfected osteoarthropathy, making this modality less specific in its ability to distinguish osteomyelitis from neuroarthropathy.[71, 92, 120] Although the utility of ^{99m}Tc hexamethyl propylenamine oxime (HMPAO)–labeled leukocytes in this regard is still under investigation, one study reported no accumulation of the labeled WBCs in subjects with noninfected Charcot joints.[12]

Management Strategies

Management of the Charcot foot should be based on the acuteness of symptoms, the anatomic pattern of bone and joint destruction, the degree of involvement (e.g., deformity, fractures, bone fragmentation, and instability), and presence of infection. Surgery should be contemplated only when attempts at conservative care have failed to establish a stable, plantigrade foot or prevent recalcitrant plantar ulceration. Steindler in 1931 recognized the necessity for early detection of the neuropathic joint and the importance of immediate protection to prevent further deterioration of the articulation.[127] He stated that "early and adequate splinting, preservation of protecting musculature by physical therapy and, above all, earliest stabilization and alinement by conservative or operative means furnish the best prospects of extending the usefulness of these joints for many years." Johnson,[72] in his classic 1967 article, reiterated the need for protection sufficient enough to prevent further damage, ranging from a brace or plaster cast to complete bed rest. Healing would be indicated by lessened edema, reduced local temperature, and radiographic evidence of repair rather than absorption. Harris and Brand were of the similar opinion, also recognizing the possible need for surgical stabilization should cast immobilization be ineffective in arresting the complete disintegration of the involved joints.[65]

An objective rationale of treatment based on the chronicity of injury, anatomic alignment, and associated degree of deformity has been outlined by Lesko and Maurer[86] at the University of California, San Francisco. For acute injuries with acceptable alignment, they suggest immobilization and protective weight bearing to prevent further progression of neuropathic joint destruction. For acute dislocation with marked deformity and little bone fragmentation, reduction and surgical arthrodesis may be indicated. For chronic dislocation with severe deformity and bone fragmentation, surgical treatment is recommended only as a last resort if soft tissue breakdown cannot be prevented by therapeutic footwear and bracing. Armstrong et al.[4] recently reviewed the natural history of the Charcot foot and provided a treatment algorithm encompassing the aforementioned principles of management (Fig. 21–16).

Diabetics with acute symptoms of neuropathic osteoarthropathy, as evidenced by erythema, swelling, and bone and joint destruction, may be best treated by early hospitalization, bed rest, non–weight bearing, and cast immobilization. Compliant patients with supportive family members or friends may be efficiently managed on an outpatient basis. Hospitalization, although not often necessary, may be required to establish the diagnosis of the Charcot foot or to facilitate the treatment of poorly compliant or high-risk individuals. Unfortunately, in the current era of managed care such admissions may not be deemed allowable.

Surgical intervention during the atrophic phase should be avoided, because it may accelerate the destructive process.[65, 72] If the acute injury goes unnoticed and unprotected, luxation, fragmentation, architectural collapse, hypertrophic bone formation, and deformity will follow. The aim of treatment should be to *obtain stability* of the foot with no excessive pressure on the skin from a bony prominence.[55, 72, 100, 102, 112] The key to treatment is *prevention* of further trauma and deformity, thereby allowing the active process to convert to the reparative (quiescent) stage.

Progressive destruction of the neuropathic foot can be halted if recognized early enough.[65, 88, 112] The appropriate way to treat the Charcot foot is first to prevent its occurrence. Careful history and physical examination directed toward risk assessment and stratification will help to identify individuals

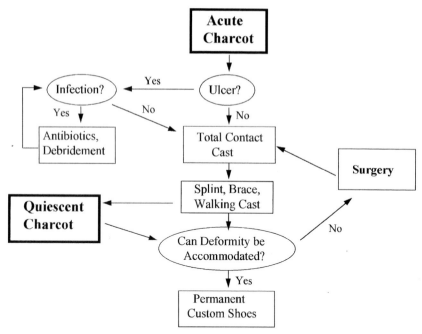

Figure 21–16 ■ Generalized treatment algorithm for the acute Charcot foot. (From Armstrong DG, Todd WF, Lavery LA, et al: The natural history of acute Charcot's arthropathy in a diabetic foot specialty clinic. Diabet Med 14:357–363, 1997, with permission.)

at greatest risk. Patients in their sixth or seventh decade, who have been diabetic for more than 10 years, and who demonstrate peripheral neuropathy with loss of protective sensation are prime candidates for the development of neuropathic osteoarthropathy. A stated history of trauma or suspicion of unrecognized injury complete this picture. Added risk factors include the presence of nephropathy and retinopathy.[30, 125]

Early recognition of DNOAP with a high index of suspicion is vitally important. The physician and patient must look for areas of mild swelling, increased skin temperature, deformity, or instability of the foot and ankle. Local temperature assessment is valuable for monitoring tissue damage in the insensitive foot.[4, 65, 72, 112] Areas of increased warmth correspond to areas of inflammation in the insensitive limb that are at risk for bony resorption and ulceration. A hand-held infrared digital thermometer is a useful tool for the physician to monitor the inflammatory response in insensate patients. Any increase in skin temperature greater than 2°C should be considered a significant finding indicating impending osteoarthropathy or preulcerative inflammation.[4, 65, 112, 114, 135] Degenerative changes in any foot with proven peripheral

sensory impairment are indicative of neuropathic arthropathy.[76]

In contrast to Charcot's description of a painless arthropathy, pain is often an associated feature but appears to be less severe than would normally be expected in view of the pathologic changes present. One report indicated that 76% of patients with acute neuroarthropathy complained of pain on initial presentation.[4] Elevation of the limb to reduce edema, cessation of weight bearing, prolonged cast immobilization, and comprehensive patient education are basic components of effective treatment.

Immobilization

A general rule of thumb to follow in managing patients with neuropathic osteoarthropathy is that at least 3 months of non–weight-bearing cast immobilization is required before the resumption of partial weight bearing in a therapeutic shoe or walking brace.[55, 103] The duration of immobilization should be determined by assessment of skin temperature, as well as by radiographic evidence of consolidation of fractures and fragmented bone. Warmth of the skin indicates persistent inflammation, which requires continued immobilization. This period may be as short as 2 to 3 months or perhaps as long as 4 to 6 months, depending on the anatomic pattern and extent of involvement.[80, 98] Armstrong et al.[4] reported an average total-contact casting (TCC) duration of 18.5 weeks in their study of 55 patients with acute Charcot feet. No mention, however, is made of non–weight bearing. After ambulatory TCC, the patients were weaned into a removable cast walker prior to wearing accomodative footwear. Recent evidence from Shaw et al.[123] indicates that approximately one third of the total load applied to the casted extremity is transmitted to the leg via the walls of the cast. However, pressure was reduced least in the midfoot while total force-time integral in the heel was actually increased compared to walking in shoes and barefoot. These data therefore suggest that ambulatory casting might not be as effective as once thought and that non–weight bearing should indeed be initially prescribed. Attention should also be directed to the "asymptomatic" limb with respect to the development of bilateral osteoarthropathy. Clohisy and Thompson[30] observed that when the patient with an affected limb was prevented from weight bearing, involvement of the contralateral limb became evident after an average of 4.5 months. They therefore recommend prophylactic immobilization of the contralateral limb with a protective cast or orthosis.

Orthoses and Shoes

A patellar tendon-bearing (PTB) orthosis used together with therapeutic shoes may effectively decrease load on the foot.[30, 64, 86, 110] Clohisy and Thompson[30] suggest short-term prophylactic protection of the "uninvolved" limb with a PTB cast or orthosis during the period of cast immobilization of the involved limb. For long-term protection of the affected limb they institute a calf-containment PTB orthosis. Saltzman et al.[110] at the Mayo Clinic measured mean peak force transmitted to the foot in six diabetics with neurotrophic arthropathy. They found that use of a properly fitted standard PTB orthosis with a free ankle and an extra-depth shoe reduced mean peak force to the entire foot by 15%. The addition of extra padding to the orthosis decreased the force by 32%. Interestingly, these investigators found that although load trans-

mission was reduced in the hindfoot, it was not reduced in the midfoot or forefoot.

Alternative pressure-reducing modalities to casting or PTB bracing include prefabricated walking braces and custom fabricated ankle-foot orthoses (AFO). Several studies have indicated that commercially available walking braces can be as effective as TCC in reducing dynamic peak plantar pressures.[8, 49, 85] Greatest reductions were found in the forefoot, while pressure-time integrals, a measure of pressure and contact duration, were actually increased in the heel region compared to both cast and shoe.[8] Landsman recently reported on the use of a custom-fabricated padded AFO in a small series of patients with ulceration and midfoot Charcot arthropathy.[83] The orthoses provided a reduction in peak pressure at the midfoot ulcer sites ranging from 70 to 92%, allowing ulcerations to heal in an average of 9 weeks. A variation on both of these modalities is the custom fabricated Charcot restraint orthotic walker (CROW).[96] The authors describe this device as a custom, bivalved, total-contact, full-foot enclosure AFO consisting of a polypropylene outer shell, rocker sole, and well-padded inner lining. The benefits of this modality, used after an initial period of non–weight bearing, are stated to be edema control, effective ankle and foot immobilization, near-normal ambulation, and excellent patient satisfaction. Cost comparisons, including cost/benefit analyses between these various modalities, have not yet been made.

Prescription footwear and foot orthoses should be considered essential for the management of diabetics with loss of protective sensation. Cavanagh et al.[23] reported a significant reduction in the incidence of plantar lesions after the provision of special footwear to a group of high-risk neuropathic patients. Both Uccioli et al.[130] and Lavery et al.[84] have more recently corroborated the effectiveness of specially designed shoes with customized insoles, wherein the former authors prospectively found a reduction in the incidence of foot ulcer relapses after 1 year of use. Extra-depth, super-extra-depth, and thermal moldable shoes with soft leather uppers and well-molded insoles are a cost-effective approach to management of patients with mild to moderate deformity. Shoes should be employed only after adequate conservative management with initial non–weight-bearing immobilization of the limb. Most often, such patients will subsequently be treated with one of the aforementioned pressure-reducing ambulatory modalities prior to progressing to protective footwear. Ulcers should be healed or very shallow before ambulation is allowed. An interim healing shoe can be fabricated using a custom-molded orthosis in a surgical shoe as dictated by the patient's clinical circumstances.[55, 57] More comprehensive coverage of this subject follows in the chapters on footwear (Chapters 20 and 34).

Bisphosphonates

Recent interest has developed in the possible use of bisphosphonate compounds for the treatment of acute osteoarthropathy.[121] This premise is supported by findings previously discussed wherein patients with acute Charcot arthropathy have been found to have reduced bone density in their affected lower extremity and elevated markers for osteoclastic activity.[62, 135] Bisphosphonates, which are potent inhibitors of osteoclastic activity, have been most commonly used for the treatment of diseases typified by increased bone turnover such as osteoporosis, Paget's disease, hyperparathyroidism, and hypercalcemia. Structurally related to endogenous pyrophosphates, these analogs are selectively taken up on the skeletal surface at sites of bone resorption and become attached to exposed calcium hydroxyapatite crystals.[79, 121] When ingested by migrating osteoclasts, the bisphosphonate molecules effectively inactivate the cells' ability to produce acid and proteolytic enzymes, thereby preventing bone absorption. At appropriate doses, the inhibition of osteoclastic activity has no effect on osteoblastic bone formation, which proceeds normally.[79] Several bisphosphonate compounds have been investigated including pamidronate, etidronate, clodronate, and alendronate. Although pamidronate has been the subject of study in patients with acute Charcot joints,[121] alendronate (Fosamax) is an oral compound widely used in the United States for the treatment of osteoporosis.

In 1994, Selby et al. reported on a small uncontrolled series of six diabetic patients with acute neuroarthropathy treated with pamidronate.[121] A total of six intravenous infusions of the bisphosphonate were administered at 2-week intervals, and changes in temperature between the affected and non-Charcot foot were recorded to assess Charcot activity. However, no mention was made of other concurrent treatments such as off-loading or casting which might have also modified the active stage of this disorder. Two weeks after the first infusion, there was a rapid and significant fall in the temperature differential between the feet that remained within a normal 2°C for the remainder of the study. Alkaline phosphatase activity, a marker for bone turnover, also significantly diminished by 25% by the end of the 12-week investigation. Again, while this study might be considered as hypothesis generating, it is limited by the lack of a control group and the likely confounding of these results by concurrent off-loading of the extremity.[121] It is hoped that prospective, randomized, controlled study currently in progress by this same group will elucidate the value of this therapy in modifying the disease process.

Surgical Management

Instability, deformity, chronic ulceration, and progressive joint destruction, despite rest and immobilization, are the primary indications for surgical intervention in diabetic individuals with neuropathic osteoarthropathy.[4, 7, 72, 78, 111, 112] Once the acute inflammatory stage has subsided, unstable joints and deformities that predispose to shearing stress and ulceration can be considered for surgical correction. This approach is fully discussed in Chapter 27.

ACKNOWLEDGMENTS

We thank Barbara E. Deaven and Roxanne Felli, Medical Library Service, VA Medical Center, Lebanon, Pennsylvania; Paul Vagainas, Medical Librarian, Beth Israel Deaconess Medical Center, Boston, for assistance in searching the medical literature; and Patricia Whitehead and the Lebanon VA Medical Center podiatry staff for support during preparation of this chapter.

REFERENCES

1. Aegerter E, Kirkpatrick JA: Metabolic diseases of bone. *In* Aegerter E, Kirkpatrick JA (ed): Orthopedic Diseases. Philadelphia: WB Saunders Company, 1983, p 33.
2. Archer AG, Roberts VC, Watkins PJ: Blood flow patterns in diabetic neuropathy. Diabetologia 27:563, 1984.

3. Armstrong DG, Lavery LA: Elevated peak plantar pressures in patients who have Charcot arthropathy. J Bone Joint Surg 80A:365–369, 1998.

4. Armstrong DG, Todd WF, Lavery LA, et al: The natural history of acute Charcot's arthropathy in a diabetic foot specialty clinic. Diabet Med 14:357–363, 1997.

5. Arntz CT, Veith RG, Hansen ST: Fractures and fracture-dislocations of the tarsometatarsal joint. J Bone Joint Surg 70A:173, 1988.

6. Bailey CC, Root HF: Neuropathic foot lesions in diabetes mellitus. N Engl J Med 236:397, 1947.

7. Banks AS, McGlamry ED: Charcot foot. J Am Podiatr Med Assoc 79:213, 1989.

8. Baumhauer JF, Wervey R, McWilliams J, et al: A comparison study of plantar foot pressure in a standardized shoe, total contact cast, and prefabricated pneumatic walking brace. Foot Ankle Int 18:26–33, 1997.

9. Beltran J, Campanini S, Knight C, et al: The diabetic foot: Magnetic resonance imaging evaluation. Skeletal Radiol 19:37, 1990.

10. Biehl WC, Morgan JM, Wagner WF, Gabriel R: Neuropathic calcaneal tuberosity avulsion fractures. Clin Orthop 296:8–13, 1993.

11. Bjorkengren AG, Weisman M, Pathria MN, et al: Neuroarthropathy associated with chronic alcoholism. Am J Radiol 151:743, 1988.

12. Blume PA, Dey HM, Daley LJ, et al: Diagnosis of pedal osteomyelitis with Tc-99m HMPAO labeled leukocytes. J Foot Ankle Surg 36:120–126, 1997.

13. Boulton AJM, Scarpello JHB, Ward JD: Venous oxygenation in the diabetic neuropathic foot: Evidence of arteriovenous shunting? Diabetologia 22:6, 1982.

14. Brink SJ: Limited joint mobility as a risk factor for diabetes complications. Clin Diabetes 5:122, 1987.

15. Brooks AP: The neuropathic foot in diabetes: Part II, Charcot's neuroarthropathy. Diabet Med 3:116, 1986.

16. Brower AC, Allman RM: Neuropathic osteoarthropathy in the adult. In Taveras JM, Ferrucci JT (eds): Radiology: Diagnosis—Imaging—Intervention. Vol 5. Philadelphia. JB Lippincott, 1989, p 1.

17. Brower AC, Allman RM: Pathogenesis of the neurotrophic joint: Neurotraumatic vs. neurovascular, Radiology 139:349, 1981.

18. Brower AC, Allman RM: The neuropathic joint: A neurovascular bone disorder. Radiol Clin North Am 19:571, 1981.

19. Brownlee M, Cerami A, Vlassara H: Advanced glycosylation end products in tissue and the biochemical basis of diabetic complications. N Engl J Med 318:1315, 1988.

20. Bruckner FE, Howell A: Neuropathic joints. Semin Arthritis Rheum 2:47, 1972.

21. Buckinham BA, Uitto J, Sanborg C, et al: Scleroderma-like changes in insulin-dependent diabetes mellitus: Clinical and biochemical studies. Diabetes Care 7:163, 1984.

22. Caputo GM, Cavanagh PR, Ulbrecht JS, et al: Assessment and management of foot disease in patients with diabetes. N Engl J Med 331:854–860, 1994.

23. Cavanagh PR, Sanders LJ, Sims DS: The role of pressure distribution measurement in diabetic foot care: Rehabilitation R&D progress reports 1987. J Rehabil Res Dev 25:53, 1988.

24. Cavanagh PR, Sims DS, Sanders LJ: Body mass is a poor predictor of peak plantar pressure in diabetic men. Diabetes Care 14:750–755, 1991.

25. Cavanagh PR, Young MJ, Adams JE, et al: Radiographic abnormalities in the feet of patients with diabetic neuropathy. Diabetes Care 17:201–209, 1994.

26. Charcot JM: Lectures on the diseases of the nervous system: Lecture IV, on some visceral derangements in locomotor ataxia, arthropathies of ataxic patients [edited and translated by Sigerson G.] London: New Sydenham Society, 1881.

27. Charcot JM: On some arthropathies apparently related to a lesion of the brain or spinal cord [by Charcot JM, January 1868; translated and edited by Hoché G, Sanders LJ]. J Hist Neurosci 1:75–87, 1992.

28. Charcot JM: Sur quelques arthropathies qui paraissent dépendre d'une lésion du cerveau ou de la moelle épinière. Arch Physiol Norm Pathol 1:161, 1868.

29. Classen JN: Neuropathic arthropathy with ulceration. Ann Surg 159:891, 1964.

30. Clohisy DR, Thompson RC: Fractures associated with neuropathic arthropathy in adults who have juvenile-onset diabetes. J Bone Joint Surg 70A:1192, 1988.

31. Clouse ME, Gramm HF, Legg M, et al: Diabetic osteoarthropathy: Clinical and roentgenographic observations in 90 cases. AJR Am J Roentgenol 121:22, 1974.

32. Cofield RH, Morison MJ, Beabout JW: Diabetic neuroarthropathy in the foot: Patient characteristics and patterns of radiographic change. Foot Ankle 4:15, 1983.

33. Coventry MB, Rothacker GW: Bilateral calcaneal fracture in a diabetic patient. J Bone Joint Surg 61A:462, 1979.

34. Craig JG, Amin MB, Wu K, et al: Osteomyelitis of the diabetic foot: MR imaging–pathologic correlation. Radiology 203:849–855, 1997.

35. Cundy TF, Edmonds ME, Watkins PJ: Osteopenia and metatarsal fractures in diabetic neuropathy. Diabetic Med 2:461, 1985.

36. Delano PJ: The pathogenesis of Charcot's joint. AJR Am J Roentgenol 56:189, 1946.

37. Delbridge L, Perry P, Marr S, et al: Limited joint mobility in the diabetic foot: Relationship to neuropathic ulceration. Diabet Med 5:333–337, 1988.

38. Drennan DB, Fahey JJ, Maylahn DJ: Important factors in achieving arthrodesis of the Charcot knee. J Bone Joint Surg 53A:1180, 1971.

39. Edelman SV, Kosofsky EM, et al: Neuro-osteoarthropathy (Charcot's joints) in diabetes mellitus following revascularization surgery: Three case reports and a review of the literature. Arch Intern Med 147:1504, 1987.

40. Edmonds ME, Clarke MB, Newton S, et al: Increased uptake of bone radiopharmaceutical in diabetic neuropathy, Q J Med (New Ser) 57:843, 1985.

41. Edmonds ME, Morrison N, Laws JW, et al: Medial arterial calcification and diabetic neuropathy. Br Med J 284:938, 1982.

42. Edmonds ME, Nicolaides KH, Watkins PJ: Autonomic neuropathy and diabetic foot ulceration. Diabet Med 3:56, 1986.

43. Edmonds ME: The neuropathic foot in diabetes: Part I, blood flow. Diabet Med 3:111, 1986.

44. Eichenholtz SN: Charcot Joints. Springfield, IL: Charles C Thomas, 1966.

45. El-Khoury GY, Kathol MH: Neuropathic fractures in patients with diabetes mellitus. Radiology 134:313, 1980.

46. Ellman MH: Neuropathic joint disease (Charcot joints). *In* McCarty DJ (ed): Arthritis and Allied Conditions: A Textbook of Rheumatology. Philadelphia: Lea & Febiger, 1989, p 1255.

47. Eymont MJ, Alavi A, Dalinka MK, et al: Bone scintigraphy in diabetic osteoarthropathy. Radiology 140:475, 1981.

48. Fernando DJS, Masson EA, Veves A, Boulton AJM: Relationship of limited joint mobility to abnormal foot pressures and diabetic foot ulceration. Diabetes Care 14:8, 1991.

49. Fleischli JG, Lavery LA, Vela SA, et al: Comparison of strategies for reducing pressure at the site of neuropathic ulcers. J Am Podiatr Med Assoc 87:466–472, 1997.

50. Forgács S: Clinical picture of diabetic osteoarthropathy. Acta Diabetol Lat 13:111, 1976.

51. Forst T, Pfutzner A, Kann P, et al: Peripheral osteopenia in adult patients with insulin-dependent diabetes mellitus. Diabet Med 12:874–879, 1995.

52. Foster DB, Bassett RC: Neurogenic arthropathy (Charcot joint) associated with diabetic neuropathy: Report of two cases. Arch Neurol Psychiatry 57:173, 1947.

53. Friedman SA, Rakow RB: Osseous lesions of the foot in diabetic neuropathy. Diabetes 20:302, 1971.

54. Frykberg RG, Kozak GP: Neuropathic arthropathy in the diabetic foot. Am Fam Physician 17:105, 1978.

55. Frykberg RG, Kozak GP: The diabetic Charcot foot. *In* Kozak GP, Campbell DR, Frykberg RG, Habershaw GM (eds): Management of Diabetic Foot Problems, 2nd ed. Philadelphia: WB Saunders Company, 1995, pp 88–97.

56. Frykberg RG: Biomechanical considerations of the diabetic foot. Lower Extremity 2:207–214, 1995.

57. Frykberg RG: Diabetic foot ulcerations. *In* Frykberg RG (ed): The High Risk Foot in Diabetes Mellitus. New York: Churchill Livingstone, 1991, pp 151–195.

58. Frykberg RG: Diabetic osteoarthropathy. *In* Brenner MA (ed): Management of the Diabetic Foot. Baltimore: Williams & Wilkins, 1987, p 75.

59. Frykberg RG: Osteoarthropathy. Clin Podiatr Med Surg 4:351, 1987.

60. Frykberg RG: The diabetic Charcot foot. Arch Podiatr Med Foot Surg 4:15, 1978.

61. Glynn TP: Marked gallium accumulation in neuropathic arthropathy. J Nucl Med 22:1016, 1981.

62. Gough A, Abraha H, Li F, et al: Measurement of markers of osteoclast and osteoblast activity in patients with acute and chronic diabetic Charcot neuroarthropathy. Diabet Med 14:527–531, 1997.

63. Guillain G: J.M. Charcot 1825–1893 his life—his work [edited and translated by Pearce Bailey]. New York: Paul B. Hoeber, 1959.

64. Guse ST, Alvine FG: Technique tip: Treatment of diabetic foot ulcers and Charcot neuroarthropathy using the patellar tendon-bearing brace. Foot Ankle Int 18:675–677, 1997.

65. Harris JR, Brand PW: Patterns of disintegration of the tarsus in the anaesthetic foot. J Bone Joint Surg 48B:4, 1966.

66. Hart TJ, Healey K: Diabetic osteoarthropathy versus diabetic osteomyelitis. J Foot Surg 25:464, 1986.

67. Hartshorne MF, Peters V: Nuclear medicine applications for the diabetic foot. Clin Podiatr Med Surg 4:361, 1987.

68. Holmes GB, Hill N: Fractures and dislocations of the foot and ankle in diabetics associated with Charcot joint changes. Foot Ankle Int 15:182–185, 1994.

69. Hough AJ, Sokoloff L: Pathology of osteoarthritis. *In* McCarty DJ (ed): Arthritis and Allied Conditions: A Textbook of Rheumatology. Philadelphia: Lea & Febiger, 1989, p 1571.

70. Jacobs RL: Charcot foot. *In* Jahss MH (ed): Disorders of the Foot and Ankle: Medical and Surgical Management, 2nd ed. Philadelphia: WB Saunders Company, 1991, p 2156.

71. Johnson JE, Kennedy EJ, Shereff MJ, et al: Prospective study of bone, indium-111-labeled white blood cell, and gallium-67 scanning for the evaluation of osteomyelitis in the diabetic foot. Foot Ankle Int 17:10–16, 1996.

72. Johnson JTH: Neuropathic fractures and joint injuries: Pathogenesis and rationale of prevention and treatment. J Bone Joint Surg 49A:1, 1967.

73. Jordan WR: Neuritic manifestations in diabetes mellitus. Arch Intern Med 57:307, 1936.

74. Kathol MH, El-Koury GY, Moore TE: Calcaneal insufficiency avulsion fractures in patients with diabetes mellitus. Radiology 180:725–729, 1991.

75. Keenan AM, Tindel NL, Alavi A: Diagnosis of pedal osteomyelitis in diabetic patients using current scintigraphic techniques. Arch Intern Med 149: 2262, 1989.

76. Kelly PJ, Coventry MB: Neurotrophic ulcers of the feet: Review of forty-seven cases. JAMA 168:388, 1958.

77. Kernwein G, Lyon WF: Neuropathic arthropathy of the ankle joint resulting from complete severance of the sciatic nerve. Ann Surg 115:267, 1942.

78. Kidd JG: The Charcot joint: Some pathologic and pathogenetic considerations. South Med J 67:597, 1974.

79. Kirk JK, Spangler JG: Alendronate: A bisphosphonate for treatment of osteoporosis. Am Fam Physician 54:2053–2060, 1996.

80. Klenerman L: The Charcot joint in diabetes. Diabet Med 13:S52–S54, 1996.

81. Knaggs LR: Charcot joints. *In* Knaggs RL (ed): Inflammatory and Toxic Diseases of Bone. Bristol, John Wright and Sons, 1976, p 105.

82. Kraft E, Spyropoulos E, Finby N: Neurogenic disorders of the foot in diabetes mellitus. AJR Am J Roentgenol 124:17, 1975.

83. Landsman AS, Sage R: Off-loading neuropathic wounds associated with diabetes using an ankle-foot orthosis. J Am Podiat Med Assoc 87:349–357, 1997.

84. Lavery LA, Vela SA, Fleischli JG, et al: Reducing plantar pressure in the neuropathic foot; a comparison of footwear. Diabetes Care 20:1706–1710, 1997.

85. Lavery LA, Vela SA, Lavery DC, Quebedeaux TL: Reducing dynamic foot pressures in high-risk diabetic subjects with foot ulcerations. Diabetes Care 19:818–821, 1996.

86. Lesko P, Maurer RC: Talonavicular dislocations and midfoot arthropathy in neuropathic diabetic

feet: Natural course and principles of treatment. Clin Orthop 240:226, 1989.

87. Levin ME: Diabetes and bone. Compr Ther 4:63, 1978.

88. Lippman HI, Perotto A, Farrar R: The neuropathic foot of the diabetic. Bull N Y Acad Med 52:1159, 1976.

89. Lister J, Maudsley RH: Charcot joints in diabetic neuropathy. Lancet 2:1110, 1951.

90. Martin MM: Charcot joints in diabetes mellitus. Proc R Soc Med 45:503, 1952.

91. Martin MM: Diabetic neuropathy: A clinical study of 150 cases. Brain 76:594, 1953.

92. Maurer AH, Millmond SH, Knight LC, et al: Infection in diabetic osteoarthropathy: Use of indium-111 labeled leukocytes for diagnosis. Radiology 161:221, 1986.

93. Milgram JW: Osteomyelitis in the foot and ankle associated with diabetes mellitus. Clin Orthop 296:50–57, 1993.

94. Miller DS, Lichtman WF: Diabetic neuropathic arthropathy of feet. Arch Surg 70:513, 1955.

95. Monnier VM, Vishwanath V, Frank KE, et al: Relation between complications of type I diabetes mellitus and collagen-linked fluorescence. N Engl J Med 314:403, 1986.

96. Morgan JM, Biehl WC, Wagner FW: Management of neuropathic arthropathy with the Charcot restraint orthotic walker. Clin Orthop 296:58–63, 1993.

97. Mueller MJ, Diamond JE, Delitto A, Sinacore DR: Insensitivity, limited joint mobility, and plantar ulcers in patients with diabetes mellitus. Phys Ther 69:453–462, 1989.

98. Myerson MS, Henderson MR, Saxby T, Short KW: Management of midfoot diabetic neuroarthropathy. Foot Ankle Int 15:233–241, 1994.

99. Newman JH: Non-infective disease of the diabetic foot. J Bone Joint Surg 63B:593, 1981.

100. Newman JH: Spontaneous dislocation in diabetic neuropathy. J Bone Joint Surg 61B:484–488, 1979.

101. Newman LG, Waller J, Palestro CJ, et al: Unsuspected osteomyelitis in diabetic foot ulcers: Diagnosis and monitoring by leukocyte scanning with indium In 111 oxyquinoline. JAMA 266:1246, 1991.

102. Norman A, Robbins H, Milgram JE: The acute neuropathic arthropathy—a rapid, severely disorganizing form of arthritis. Radiology 90:1159, 1968.

103. Pinzur MS, Sage R, Stuck R, et al: A treatment algorithm for neuropathic (Charcot) midfoot deformity. Foot Ankle 14:189–197, 1993.

104. Pogonowska MJ, Collins LC, Dobson HL: Diabetic osteopathy. Radiology 89:265, 1967.

105. Radin EL: Mechanical aspects of osteoarthrosis. Bull Rheum Dis 26:862, 1976.

106. Resnick D: Neuroarthropathy. In Resnick D, Niwayama G (eds): Diagnosis of Bone and Joint Disorders with Emphasis on Articular Abnormalities, Vol 3. Philadelphia: WB Saunders Company, 1981, p 2422.

107. Rodnan GP: Neuropathic joint disease (Charcot joints). In Hollander JL, et al (eds): Arthritis and Allied Conditions. Philadelphia: Lea & Febiger, 1985, p 1095.

108. Rosenblatt S: Principles of evaluation and treatment of osteomyelitis in the diabetic foot. Clin Diabetes 7:85, 1989.

109. Rubinow A, Spark EC, Canoso JJ: Septic arthritis in a Charcot joint. Clin Orthop 147:203, 1980.

110. Saltzman CL, Johnson KA, Goldstein RH, et al: The patellar tendon-bearing brace as treatment for neurotrophic arthropathy: A dynamic force monitoring study. Foot Ankle 13:14, 1992.

111. Sammarco GJ: Diabetic arthropathy. In Sammarco GJ (ed): The Foot in Diabetes. Philadelphia: Lea & Febiger, 1991.

112. Sanders LJ, Frykberg RG: Diabetic neuropathic osteoarthropathy: The Charcot foot. In Frykberg RG (ed): The High Risk Foot in Diabetes Mellitus. New York: Churchill Livingstone, 1991.

113. Sanders LJ, Mrdjenovich D: Anatomical patterns of bone and joint destruction in neuropathic diabetics. Diabetes 40(Suppl 1):529A, 1991.

114. Sanders LJ, Murray-Leisure K: Infections of the diabetic foot. In Abramson C, McCarthy DJ, Rupp M (eds): Infectious Diseases of the Lower Extremity. Baltimore: Williams & Wilkins, 1991.

115. Schauwecker DS, Park HM, Burt RW, et al: Combined bone scintigraphy and indium-111 leukocyte scans in neuropathic foot disease. J Nucl Med 29:1651, 1988.

116. Schauwecker DS: Osteomyelitis: Diagnosis with in-111-labeled leukocytes. Radiology 171:141, 1989.

117. Schoenhaus HD, Wernick E, Cohen R: Biomechanics of the diabetic foot. In Frykberg RG (ed): The High Risk Foot in Diabetes Mellitus. New York: Churchill Livingstone, 1991.

118. Schwartz ER: Chondrocyte structure and function. In McCarty DJ (ed): Arthritis and Allied Conditions: A Textbook of Rheumatology. Philadelphia: Lea & Febiger, 1989, p 289.

119. Schwarz GS, Berenyi MR, Siegel MW: Atrophic arthropathy and diabetic neuritis. AJR Am J Roentgenol 106:523, 1969.

120. Seabold JE, Flickinger FW, Kao S, et al: Indium-111 leukocyte/technetium-99m-MDP bone and magnetic resonance imaging: Difficulty of diagnosing osteomyelitis in patients with neuropathic osteoarthropathy. J Nucl Med 31:549–556, 1990.

121. Selby PL, Young MJ, Boulton AJM: Bisphosphonates: A new treatment for diabetic Charcot neuroarthropathy? Diabet Med 11:28–31, 1994.

122. Shands AR: Neuropathies of the bones and joints: Report of a case of an arthropathy of the ankle due to a peripheral nerve lesion. Arch Surg 20:614, 1930.

123. Shaw JE, Hsi W-L, Ulbrecht J, et al: The mechanism of plantar unloading in total contact casts: Implications for design and clinical use. Foot Ankle Int 18:809–817, 1997

124. Shih W-J, Purcell M: Diabetic Charcot joint mimicking acute osteomyelitis in radiography and three-phase radionuclide bone imaging study. Radiat Med 9:47–49, 1991.

125. Sinha S, Munichoodappa C, Kozak GP: Neuro-arthropathy (Charcot joints) in diabetes mellitus: Clinical study of 101 cases. Medicine (Baltimore) 52:191, 1972.

126. Soto-Hall R, Haldeman KO: The diagnosis of neuropathic joint disease (Charcot joint): An analysis of 40 cases. JAMA 114:2076, 1940.

127. Steindler A: The tabetic arthropathies. JAMA 96:250, 1931.

128. Thompson RC, Havel P, Goetz F: Presumed neurotrophic skeletal disease in diabetic kidney transplant recipients. JAMA 249:1317, 1983.

129. Treves F: Treatment of perforating ulcer of the foot. Lancet 2:949, 1884.
130. Uccioli L, Faglia E, Monticone G, et al: Manufactured shoes in the prevention of diabetic foot ulcers. Diabetes Care 18:1376–1378, 1995.
131. Wartenberg R: Neuropathic joint disease. JAMA 111:2044, 1938.
132. Wastie ML: Radiological changes in serial x-rays of the foot and tarsus in leprosy. Clin Radiol 26:285, 1975.
133. Watkins PJ, Edmonds ME: Sympathetic nerve failure in diabetes. Diabetologia 25:73–77, 1983.
134. Williamson B, Treates CD, Phillips CD, et al: Computed tomography as a diagnostic aid in diabetic and other problem feet. Clin Imaging 13:159, 1989.
135. Young MJ, Marshall A, Adams JE, et al: Osteopenia, neurological dysfunction, and the development of Charcot neuroarthropathy. Diabetes Care 18:34–38, 1995.
136. Zeiger LS, Fox IM: Use of indium-111 labeled white blood cells in the diagnosis of diabetic foot infections. J Foot Surg 29:46, 1990.
137. Zlatkin MB, Pathria M, Sartoris DJ, et al: The diabetic foot. Radiol Clin North Am 25:1095, 1987.

Chapter 22

INFECTIOUS PROBLEMS OF THE FOOT IN DIABETIC PATIENTS

■ Benjamin A. Lipsky

Infections of various types may be more common and are often more severe in patients with diabetes mellitus.[3, 20] Foot infections are probably the most common and important of these infections. Diabetic foot infections pose a potentially serious acute medical problem, usually requiring immediate medical attention, appropriate diagnostic evaluations, various therapeutic modalities, and sometimes hospitalization. These infections may also be associated with long-term morbidity, including soft tissue infection recurrences, bone involvement, and the need for surgical resections and amputations. Infections that begin as a minor problem may progress to become limb- or even life-threatening disorders, especially if not managed properly.

Despite the substantial morbidity and occasional mortality that foot infections cause, there are no widely accepted guidelines for assessing and treating these lesions. Fortunately, in the past two decades additional data have become available that allow a rational approach to dealing with diabetic foot infections. Several committees in different countries have addressed recommendations for the proper approach to diabetic foot infections.[6, 17, 24] This chapter reviews the epidemiology, pathophysiology, microbiology, diagnosis and clinical presentation, and treatment of these complex infections.

Epidemiology

Anecdotal clinical experience has identified several types of infections (primarily respiratory, genitourinary, and soft tissue) that occur more frequently in diabetic patients. Only a few, however, have been shown by controlled observational studies to be statistically significantly associated with diabetes.[3] Among these are various types of foot infections. The relative frequency of foot cellulitis is more than nine times greater in diabetic compared with nondiabetic persons.[3] Similarly, osteomyelitis of the foot and ankle account for a greater proportion of hospitalizations of diabetic patients than bone infections of other locations. Furthermore, the relative proportion of hospitalization for foot osteomyelitis is almost 12 times greater in diabetic compared with nondiabetic persons.[3]

Several studies in Western countries have shown that as many as a quarter of diabetic patients will develop a foot ulceration at some time in their life. Depending on the definitions used, perhaps 40 to 80% of these ulcers will become infected. Fortunately, most infections will be superficial, but about a quarter will spread contiguously from the skin to the deeper subcutaneous tissues, including bone. Up to half of those who have one foot infection will have another within a few years. Foot ulcerations and infections are now the commonest diabetes-related cause of hospitalization in the United States, accounting for almost half of all hospital days. Clinical studies (most of which are retrospective) have reported that 25 to 50% of diabetic foot infections lead to a minor (i.e., foot-sparing) amputation, while 10 to 40% have required major amputations.[24] Other chapters in this textbook deal with the epidemiology of foot ulceration; of importance here is that about 10 to 30% of patients with a diabetic foot ulcer will eventually progress to an amputation, and about 60% of amputations are preceded by an infected foot ulcer. Thus, infection is often the proximate cause leading to this tragic outcome.[34, 38]

Pathophysiology

Why are diabetic patients so prone to developing foot infections? A variety of physiologic and metabolic disturbances conspire to cause these infections. The various predisposing factors, including metabolic derangements, faulty wound healing, neuropathy, and vasculopathy are covered in other chapters of this text. Immunologic disturbances are also an important predisposing factor for infections. Among the defects in host immune defenses associated with diabetes are impairments of polymorphonuclear leukocyte functions; these include abnormalities of migration, phagocytosis, intracellular killing, and chemotaxis. Many of these immunodeficiencies are directly related to the metabolic perturbations caused by poorly controlled diabetes. The prevalence of these defects appears to be correlated, at least in part, to the adequacy of glycemic control.[31] Ketosis in particular impairs leukocyte function.[40] Some evidence suggests that in diabetic patients cellular immune responses and monocyte function are reduced as well.[40] Hyperglycemia also appears to worsen complement function, at least in experimental situations.

Poor granuloma formation, prolonged persistence of abscesses, and impaired wound healing are further accompaniments of diabetes that may predispose to infectious complications. Diabetic patients also appear to have a higher rate of carriage of *Staphylococcus aureus* in their anterior nares, and subsequently on the skin.[4] This colonization may predispose to skin infections with this virulent pathogen when there is a break in the protective dermal surface. In addition, several types of skin disorders as well as skin and nail fungal (tenia) infections disproportionately plague diabetic patients. These also provide breaks in the cutaneous envelope that then offer potential sites for bacterial invasion.

Among the reasons that infection is potentially so serious in the foot is its unique anatomy. The structure of the various compartments, tendon sheaths, and neurovascular bundles tend to favor the proximal spread of infection. The deep plantar space of the foot is divided into medial, central, and lateral compartments. Because rigid fascial and bony structures bound these compartments, edema associated with an acute infection may rapidly elevate compartment pressures, causing ischemic necrosis of the confined tissues.[5] Infection may spread from one compartment to another at their proximal calcaneal convergence or by direct perforation of septae, but lateral or dorsal spread is a late sign of infection.[5]

Microbiologic Considerations

Definitions

The surface of the body is coated with bacteria present in a harmless association known as *colonization*, which may be transient or permanent. Primary pathogens like *Staphylococcus aureus* or β-hemolytic streptococci are rarely present on intact skin, but will rapidly colonize disrupted epithelium. When microbial multiplication ensues, with local tissue destruction and release of bacterial toxins inciting a host response, the wound is defined as *infected*. Infection may either follow colonization or occur as a primary event. Infection involves the invasion of host tissues by microorganisms (*pathogens*), with a subsequent host inflammatory response (erythema, induration, pain or tenderness, warmth, loss of function). *Superficial infection* is confined to soft tissues external to the fascia (i.e., skin and subcutaneous fat), while *deep infection* involves invasion of fascia, muscle, tendon, joint, or bone. Infection may be due to a single organism (*monomicrobial*) or more than one (*polymicrobial*).

Bacteria are broadly divided into groups defined by their cell wall reaction with *Gram's stain* (*positive* or *negative*), their requirement for oxygen (*aerobes* or obligate *anaerobes*), and their morphology (*bacilli* [or *rods*] or *cocci*). The predominant bacteria of normal skin are gram-positive aerobes, particularly the low-virulence coagulase-negative staphylococci, α-hemolytic streptococci, and the corynebacteriae (short rods). When skin is abnormal (e.g., with eczema or psoriasis), or when the patient has certain underlying diseases (e.g., diabetes), the colonizing flora become more complex; virulent aerobic gram-positive cocci, notably *Staphylococcus aureus* and β-hemolytic streptococci, may flourish. Antibiotic therapy will also alter the colonizing flora of skin or wounds, favoring organisms resistant to the agent administered. Lesions that have been infected for a short time tend to be monomicrobial, and to be caused by gram-positive pathogens.[29, 30] Chronic wounds develop complex flora, with aerobic gram-negative rods, anaerobes (gram-positive and negative), and enterococci, in addition to the gram-positive aerobes. Fungi (including *Candida* and *Tenia* species) also appear to disproportionately colonize the skin of diabetic patients.

Wound Cultures

Culturing a clinically uninfected wound is unnecessary, unless the purpose is to seek the presence of an epidemiologically significant organism (e.g., methicillin-resistant *Staphylococcus aureus* [MRSA]). When a wound is infected, a microbiologic diagnosis will usually assist subsequent management. A culture will identify the etiologic agent(s), but only if specimens are collected and processed properly. Since it is necessary to traverse the skin to obtain wound samples, they may become contaminated with microorganisms derived from the skin. Some argue that culturing a diabetic foot infection is futile, as "mixed flora" usually grow. This may be true for patients with severe, longstanding or complicated infections, or who have already received antibiotic therapy. In this situation, however, culture and sensitivity results generally help to tailor (and in many cases constrain) antibiotic regimens. In antibiotic-naive patients with an uncomplicated infection, growth of only staphylococci, streptococci, or both is the rule. But even in this situation, the rising prevalence of antibiotic-resistant organisms makes obtaining antibiotic sensitivity results potentially useful.

Culture specimens are sometimes defined by how likely the results are to be reliable.[44] Deep tissue specimens obtained aseptically at surgery are more likely to contain only the true pathogens than cultures of superficial lesions. Clinicians frequently culture superficial wounds by rolling a cotton swab across the surface, often without prior cleansing or debriding. This lesion will contain the total colonizing flora from which the infecting organisms originated, lowering the culture's specificity. Furthermore, the hostile environment of the air-filled cotton swab inhibits growth of anaerobes and fastidious organisms, lowering sensitivity. A curettage or tissue scraping from the base of a debrided ulcer provides more accurate results than a swab.[29, 39] Specimens should be promptly submitted to the microbiology laboratory and cultured for both aerobes and anaerobes. Interpreting culture results requires clinical correlation and judgment. Therapy directed against organisms grown from a swab culture is likely to be unnecessarily broad and may occasionally miss key pathogens. If multiple organisms are isolated the clinician must decide which require specifically targeted therapy. Less virulent bacteria, such as enterococci, coagulase-negative staphylococci, or corynebacteria can sometimes be ignored, although they may also represent infecting organisms. In general, organisms isolated from reliable specimens that are the sole or predominant pathogens on both the Gram-stained smear and culture are likely to be true pathogens.

Mild infections occurring in patients who have not previously received antibiotic therapy are usually caused by only one or two species of bacteria, almost invariably aerobic gram-positive cocci. *Staphylococcus aureus* is by far the most important pathogen in diabetic foot infections; even when it is not the sole isolate, it is usually a part of a mixed infection. Serious infections in hospitalized patients are often caused by three to five bacterial species, including both aerobes and anaerobes.[30, 39] Gram-negative bacilli, mainly Enterobacteriaciae, are found in many patients with chronic or previously treated infections. *Pseudomonas* species are often isolated from wounds that have been soaked or treated with wet dressings. Enterococci are commonly cultured from patients who have previously received a cephalosporin, a class of antibiotics to which they are inherently resistant. Obligate anaerobic species are most frequent in ischemic wounds with necrosis or that involve deep tissues. Anaerobes are rarely the sole pathogen, but most often participate in a mixed infection with aerobes. Antibiotic-resistant organisms, especially MRSA, are frequent in patients who have previously received antibiotic therapy; they are often (but not always) acquired during previous hospitalizations or at chronic care facilities.

Diagnosis and Clinical Presentation

Diagnosing Infection

Because all skin wounds will be colonized with microorganisms, infection cannot be defined microbiologically. Rather, it is diagnosed clinically (i.e., by the presence of purulent secretions [pus], or two or more signs or symptoms of inflammation). Infection should be suspected at the first appearance of a local foot problem (e.g., pain, swelling, ulceration, sinus tract formation, or crepitation) or a systemic infection (e.g., fever, rigors, vomiting, tachycardia, confusion, malaise) or metabolic disorder (severe hyperglycemia, ketosis, azotemia). It should be considered even when the local signs are less severe than might be expected. In rare instances inflammatory signs may be caused by such noninfectious disorders as gout or acute Charcot disease. On the other hand, some uninflamed ulcers may be associated with underlying osteomyelitis.[33] Signs of systemic toxicity generally do not accompany diabetic foot infections,[14] even in patients with limb-threatening infections.

Properly evaluating a diabetic foot infection requires a methodic approach, including those elements listed in Table 22–1. It is distressing that even in university-affiliated teaching hospitals the great majority of diabetic patients with an acute foot infection do not have even a minimally acceptable evaluation.[12] When infection is considered the diagnosis should be pursued aggressively, as these infections can worsen quickly, sometimes in a few hours. While infection is diagnosed on clinical grounds, it may be aided

Table 22–1 ■ RECOMMENDED EVALUATION OF A DIABETIC PATIENT WITH A FOOT INFECTION*

Describe lesion (cellulitis, ulcer, etc.) and any drainage (serous, purulent, etc.)

Enumerate presence or absence of various signs of inflammation

Define whether or not infection is present and attempt to determine probable cause

Examine soft tissue for evidence of crepitus, abscesses, sinus tracts

Probe any skin breaks with sterile metal probe to see if bone can be reached

Measure the wound (length × width; estimate depth); consider photograph

Palpate and record pedal pulses; use Doppler instrument if necessary

Evaluate neurologic status: protective sensation; motor and autonomic function

Cleanse and debride wound; remove any foreign material and eschar

Culture cleansed wound (by curettage, aspiration, or swab)

Order plain radiographs of the infected foot in most cases

* Listed in the approximate order in which they are to be done; not all procedures are necessary in all patients.

by laboratory investigations. The latter may include hematologic, serologic, imaging, or other tests, but most important is visualizing and culturing microorganisms from samples of tissue, blood, body fluids, or pus.

Clinical Presentation

The clinical characteristics of patients with diabetic foot infections are similar in most reported series. Their average age is about 60 years old, and most have had diabetes for 15 to 20 years. Almost two thirds of patients have evidence of peripheral vascular disease (absence of pedal pulses) and about 80% have lost protective sensation (lack of vibration sensation or perception of 10 gm of pressure with a nylon monofilament). Infections most often involve the forefoot, especially the toes and metatarsal heads, particularly the plantar surface. About half the patients in reported series have received antibiotic therapy for the foot lesion by the time they present, and up to a third have had their foot lesion for over a month. Many patients do not report pain with an infection because of their sensory neuropathy. More than half of all patients, including those with serious infections, lack a fever, elevated white blood cell count, or elevated erythrocyte sedimentation rate.[2, 14]

Assessing Severity

Several classification systems have been proposed for diabetic foot lesions, none of which is universally accepted. While the Wagner system has been the most used, it is imprecise, and only grade 3 addresses infection. The key factors in classifying a foot infection are assessing the depth of the wound (by both visually inspecting the tissues involved and estimating depth in millimeters), the presence of ischemia (absent pulses or diminished blood pressure in the foot), and the presence of infection.[1] A simple clinical classification of infections is shown in Table 22–2. Moderately severe infections may be limb-threatening, while severe infections may be life-threatening.

Assessing infection severity is essential to selecting an antibiotic regimen. This influences the route of drug administration and need for hospitalization. Severity also helps assess potential necessity and timing of surgery. The wound should be carefully explored to determine its depth and to seek foreign or necrotic material, and it should be probed with a sterile metal instrument. Because of the anatomy of the foot, deep space infections often have deceptively few signs in the plantar or dorsal aspects. Thus, it is crucial that a patient with even mild swelling of the foot but with systemic toxicity be evaluated by a knowledgeable surgeon for an occult deep space infection.[5] Evidence of systemic toxicity or metabolic instability generally signifies a serious infection. In these instances one should consider the possibility of potentially life-threatening necrotizing soft tissue infection. Clinical features that help define the severity of infection are shown in Table 22–3.

One of the first decisions the clinician must make is determining which patients with a diabetic foot infection should be hospitalized. Patients with a serious infection, or those who need parenteral therapy, should be admitted. They may require surgical interventions, fluid resuscitation, and control of metabolic derangements. Hospitalization should also be considered if the patient is unable or unwilling to perform proper wound care, or can or will not be able to off-load the affected area. Furthermore, patients thought to be unlikely to comply with antibiotic therapy, or needing close monitoring of response to treatment may need hospitalization. In the absence of these factors, most patients can be treated cautiously on an outpatient basis, with frequent reevaluation (i.e., every few days initially). Wound care and glycemic control should be optimized; antibiotics will not overcome poor foot care. This is also an opportune time to teach and reinforce how to prevent future foot complications.

Bone Infection

Diabetic patients may have destructive bone changes caused by peripheral neuropathy that are called neuroarthropathy, osteoarthropathy, or Charcot disease. These disorders may be difficult to distinguish from those caused by bone infection. Bone infection generally results from contiguous spread of a deep soft tissue infection through the cortex (osteitis) to the bone marrow (osteomyelitis). About 50 to 60% of serious foot infections are complicated by osteomyelitis. The proportion of apparently mild to moderate infections that have bone involvement is probably in the range of 10 to 20%. There are no validated or well-accepted guidelines for diagnosing or treating diabetic foot osteomyelitis. Among the important considerations are the anatomic site of infection (i.e., forefoot, midfoot, or hindfoot), the vascular supply to the area, the extent of soft tissue and bone destruction, the degree of systemic illness, and the patient's preferences.

Table 22–2 ■ SIMPLE CLINICAL CLASSIFICATION OF SEVERITY OF DIABETIC FOOT INFECTIONS

	SUPERFICIAL ULCER OR CELLULITIS PRESENT	DEEP SOFT OR BONE INVOLVED	TISSUE NECROSIS OR GANGRENE PRESENT	SYSTEMIC TOXICITY OR METABOLIC INSTABILITY PRESENT
Mild	√	—	±	—
Moderate	√	± (No gas or fasciitis)	± (Minimal)	—
Severe	√	±	±	√

√ = present; ± = may or may not be present; — = not present.

Table 22–3 ■ CLINICAL CHARACTERISTICS THAT HELP DEFINE THE SEVERITY OF AN INFECTION

FEATURE	MILD INFECTION	SERIOUS INFECTION
Presentation	Slowly progressive	Acute or rapidly progressive
Ulceration	Involves skin only	Penetrates to subcutaneous tissues
Tissues involved	Epidermis and dermis	Fascia, muscle, joint, bone
Cellulitis	Minimal (<2-cm rim)	Extensive, or distant from ulceration
Local signs	Slight inflammation	Severe inflammation, crepitus, bullae
Systemic signs	None or minimal	Fever, chills, hypotension, confusion, volume depletion, leukocytosis
Metabolic control	Mildly abnormal (hyperglycemia)	Severe hyperglycemia, acidosis, azotemia, electrolyte abnormalities
Foot vasculature	Minimally impaired (normal/reduced pulses)	Absent pulses, reduced ankle or toe blood pressure
Complicating features	None or minimal (callus, ulcer)	Gangrene, eschar, foreign body, abscess, marked edema

There are two main classification systems used for osteomyelitis.[27] That promulgated by Waldvogel and colleagues broadly divides infections into those resulting from hematogenous dissemination versus contiguous spread, with the latter category subdivided by whether or not there is attendant vascular insufficiency. The scheme proposed by Cierny and Mader combines anatomic disease types and physiologic host categories (local and systemic factors) to define 12 clinical stages. Most diabetic foot osteomyelitis is chronic, and would be classified 2Bsl (superficial, physiologically compromised host, systemic compromise [diabetes], local compromise [neuropathy or vasculopathy]).

All patients with a deep or longstanding ulcer or infection (especially if located over a bony prominence) should be clinically evaluated for possible osteomyelitis. Larger (>2 cm) and deeper (>3 mm) ulcers are more often associated with underlying osteomyelitis. A substantially elevated erythrocyte sedimentation rate (>70 mm/hr) increases the likelihood of bone infection. Clinical evaluation should include probing to bone.[22] Contacting a bony surface with a sterile metal probe has a positive predictive value of almost 90% for osteomyelitis. Plain radiographs should be ordered for most patients with a diabetic foot infection, except perhaps those with just cellulitis or an acute superficial ulcer. Roentgenographic changes generally take at least 2 weeks to be evident, giving them a sensitivity of only about 55%. Specificity of plain x-ray is about 75%, with the characteristic changes including focal osteopenia, cortical erosions, or periosteal reaction early, and sequestration of sclerotic bone late. When there is doubt about bone infection but the patient is stable, repeating a plain radiograph in a couple of weeks is probably more cost-effective than scanning procedures.

If clinical and plain radiographic findings do not confidently diagnose or exclude osteomyelitis, various imaging procedures may be useful.[27, 45] Bone (e.g., technecium-99 [^{99}Tc]) scans are sensitive (~85%), but because they show increased uptake with noninfectious bone disorders they are too nonspecific (~45%). Leukocyte (e.g., indium-111 [^{111}In] or ^{99m}Tc-hexamethyl propylenamine oxime [HMPAO]) scans are similarly sensitive, but more specific (~75%). Unlike bone scans, leukocyte scans may be useful for defining when infection has been arrested, but they are complicated and time consuming. Combining bone and leukocyte scans increases the accuracy and the localization of infection, but also the cost. Radiolabeled antigranulocyte fragments (e.g., sulesomab) also may increase the accuracy of scanning.[23] Among the newer diagnostic techniques that show promise are high-resolution ultrasound and positron emission tomography (PET). However, magnetic resonance imaging (MRI) is probably now the diagnostic procedure of choice, with a sensitivity of over 90% and specificity of over 80%.[10] Its limitations include the fact that early cortical infection may be missed, and marrow edema or evolving neuropathic osteoarthropathy can cause false-positive results. The diagnostic test characteristics of all of these procedures exhibit high variation across studies, and their interpretation is greatly influenced by the pretest probability of disease.[45]

Definitive diagnosis, and identifying the etiologic agent, requires obtaining bone for culture and histology. Specimens may be obtained by open (e.g., at the time of debridement or surgery) or percutaneous (usually image-guided) biopsy. These procedures are both easy to perform and safe in experienced hands, although somewhat expensive. To avoid contamination, specimens must be obtained without traversing an open wound. Patients who are receiving antibiotic therapy may have a negative culture, but histopathology can help diagnose infection. Bone biopsy is usually needed if the diagnosis remains in doubt after performing other diagnostic tests, or if the etiologic agent(s) cannot be predicted because of confusing culture results or previous antibiotic therapy. Microbiologic studies of diabetic foot osteomyelitis have revealed that the majority of cases are polymicrobial, and have uniformly found that S. aureus is the most common etiologic agent (isolated in about 40% of infections); S. epidermidis (~25%), streptococci (~30%), and Enterobacteriaceae (~40%) are also common isolates.[27]

Treatment

Debridement and Surgery

Minor

Almost all infected foot lesions (other than primary cellulitis) must be debrided.[26] This can safely be done by any appropriately trained health care professional. Debridement is aimed at removing any eschar (full-thickness dead skin), other necrotic tissue or foreign material, or surrounding callus. This procedure helps to fully evaluate the wound, prepare the wound for being cultured, allow penetration of any topical agents applied, and hasten wound healing. It also serves to turn a chronic wound into an acute wound, which is more likely to heal.[6] Debridement is best done mechanically (i.e., with instruments), rather than with enzymatic or chemical agents. Sharp debridement for minor foot wounds can usually be done in the clinic or at the bedside; most patients are sufficiently neuropathic that local anesthesia is not required. A scalpel or scissors are used to progressively pare away callus and remove all undermining, or to saucerize the wound. Some use tissue nippers for more aggressive debridement, sometimes including removing exposed bone. Debridement will often need to be done in more than one session, or be repeated at follow-up visits. Failure to ade-

quately debride a wound is a common cause for persistent infection and lack of healing.

Surgical

Patients with deeper infections often need surgical debridement. Early surgical intervention can reduce the duration of antibiotic therapy, decrease the need for major amputations, and more quickly restore full ambulation.[42] The presence of pus in an enclosed space requires drainage. Similarly, fulminant soft tissue infections, such as gas gangrene or necrotizing fasciitis, require urgent debridement of involved tissue. Conditions within an abscess prevent the effective function of both polymorphonuclear leukocytes and antibiotics. Ischemic tissue cannot receive leukocytes or systemic antibiotics. Finally, dead tissue (especially bone) that cannot be quickly resorbed or remodeled provides a surface to which bacteria can adhere. There they can establish complex communities of organisms enmeshed in an exocellular glycocalyx (a biofilm), which is remarkably resistant to most antibiotics.

The extent of the tissue destruction may not be apparent at first inspection. All deep compartments involved by infection must be opened. Necrotizing infections of the superficial or deeper tissues require rapid, thorough surgical debridement. Diabetic patients tolerate surgical excisions and drainage much better than they do undrained pus.[19] In the appropriate treatment setting a surgeon with knowledge of foot anatomy should drain any areas of suspected infection, regardless of the patient's circulatory status. Patients with systemic toxicity will not improve until the wound is adequately surgically debrided and thoroughly drained. While attempts should be made to conserve healthy tissue for later reconstruction, small stab wounds or inserting drains cannot usually accomplish adequate debridement and drainage.[19]

Antibiotic Therapy

Indications for Therapy

Available data suggest that about 40 to 60% of diabetic patients who are treated for a foot ulcer receive antibiotic therapy.[25] Although some practitioners believe that any foot ulcer requires administering antibiotics, either for therapy or for prophylaxis, available data do not generally support this view. In most of the published clinical trials antibiotic therapy did not improve the outcome of uninfected lesions.[9] One recent abstract,[18] however, reported that in a small randomized trial antibiotic therapy of uninfected foot ulcers increased the likelihood of healing and reduced the incidence of clinical infection, hospitalization, and amputation. While provocative, this work will need to be replicated before this strategy is adopted. Antibiotic therapy is associated with frequent adverse effects, substantial financial costs, and potential harm to the local and global microbial ecology. In view of these undesirable outcomes, for now antibiotic therapy should probably be used only to treat established infection.

Route of Therapy

Intravenous antibiotics are indicated for patients who are systemically ill, have a severe infection, are unable to tolerate oral agents, or are known or suspected to have pathogens that are not susceptible to available oral agents. After the patient is stabilized and the infection is clearly responding, most patients can be switched to oral therapy. Patients who require prolonged intravenous therapy (e.g., for osteomyelitis or infections resistant to oral agents) can often be treated on an outpatient basis when a program to provide this service is available.

Of note is that in patients with peripheral vascular disease, therapeutic antibiotic concentrations with many agents are often not achieved in the infected tissues, even when serum levels are adequate. This has led to experimentation with novel methods of antibiotic therapy. In one procedure, called retrograde venous perfusion, antibiotic solutions are injected under pressure into a foot vein while a sphygmomanometer is inflated on the thigh. High local antibiotic concentrations have been observed in anecdotal and uncontrolled reports. Some have also tried lower extremity intra-arterial antibiotic administration. For infections that have undergone surgical tissue resection, antibiotic (usually with an aminoglycoside)-loaded beads or cement have been used in some instances to fill the dead space and supply high local antibiotic concentrations. None of these therapies has been adequately evaluated and cannot currently be routinely recommended.

Oral antibiotic therapy is less expensive and more convenient than parenteral, and for patients not meeting the criteria listed above it is usually sufficient. Several newly licensed agents have expanded the spectrum of organisms that can be treated. The bioavailability of oral antibiotics is variable, and diabetic patients may absorb oral medications poorly. Fortunately, some drugs (e.g., clindamycin and the fluoroquinolones) have been shown to be well absorbed on oral dosing. Fluoroquinolones in particular usually achieve high tissue concentrations in diabetic foot infections when administered orally, even in patients with gastroparesis.

For mildly infected foot ulcers, an additional option is topical therapy. This has several theoretical advantages, including high local drug levels, avoidance of systemic antibiotic adverse effects, and the possibility of using novel agents not available for systemic use. Furthermore, this route draws the attention of both the patient and physician to the foot, and the need for good wound care. Antiseptics (e.g., povidone-iodine or chlorhexidine) are not recommended, as they are generally too harsh on the host tissues. Topical antibiotics, however, may have a role. Silver sulfadiazine, neomycin, polymixin B, gentamicin, and mupirocin have each been used for soft tissue infections in other sites, but there are no published data on their efficacy in diabetic foot infections. An investigational peptide antibiotic, pexiganin acetate 1% cream (MSI-78), has been shown in two large phase III randomized trials to be safe and nearly as effective (about 85 to 90% clinical response rate) as oral ofloxacin for mildly infected diabetic foot ulcers.[28] These results are encouraging, and other novel topical antimicrobial therapies are being explored, including an antibiotic-impregnated bovine collagen sponge.

Choice of Antibiotic Agents

Most patients will begin antibiotic therapy with an empiric regimen, pending the results of wound cultures. This therapy should aim to cover the most common pathogens, with some modification according to infection severity. Relatively narrow-spectrum agents may be used for minor infections, as there is likely to be time to modify treatment if there is no clinical response. Regimens for severe infection are broader spectrum and are often intravenously administered, because the stakes are higher. Empiric regimens must also take into consideration such factors as patient allergies, renal dysfunction, previous antibiotic therapy, and known local antibiotic sensitivity patterns.

An antibiotic regimen should almost always include an agent active against staphylococci and streptococci. Previously treated or severe cases may need extended coverage that also includes gram-negative bacilli and *Enterococcus* species. Necrotic, gangrenous, or foul-smelling wounds usually require antianaerobic therapy. When culture and sensitivity results are available, more specific therapy should be chosen. Narrower spectrum agents are preferred, but it is important to assess how the infection has been responding to the empiric regimen. If the lesion is healing and the patient is tolerating therapy, there may be no reason to change, even if some or all of the isolated organisms are resistant to the agents being used. On the other hand, if the infection is not responding, treatment should be changed to cover all the isolated organisms. If the infection is worsening despite susceptibility of the isolated bacteria to the chosen regimen, reconsider the need for surgical intervention or the possibility that fastidious organisms were missed.

While theoretical and pharmacokinetic considerations are important, the proof of an antibiotic's efficacy is the clinical trial. Agents that have demonstrated clinical effectiveness in prospective studies of diabetic foot infections include the following:

- Penicillin/β-lactamase inhibitor congeners (amoxicillin/clavulanate orally; ampicillin/sulbactam, piperacillin/tazobactam, and ticarcillin/clavulanate parenterally)
- Cephalosporins (cephalexin orally; cefoxitin and ceftizoxime parenterally)
- Clindamycin (orally and parenterally)
- Fluoroquinolones (ciprofloxacin orally and parenterally; ofloxacin orally and parenterally; trovafloxacin orally and parenterally)
- Imipenem/cilastatin (parenterally).

Overall, the clinical and microbiologic response rates have been similar in trials with the various antibiotics and no one agent or combination has emerged as most effective. New antibiotics are introduced and some older ones are made obsolete by emergence of resistance. Understanding the principles of antibiotic therapy is therefore more impor-

tant than knowing the specific agents currently in vogue. The antimicrobial spectrum of several antibiotics, grouped by class, are shown in Table 22–4. While all of the above agents (and others) are approved by the U.S. Food and Drug Administration (FDA) for treating complicated skin and soft tissue infections, the only drug specifically approved for diabetic foot infections is trovafloxacin. Unfortunately, problems with hepatotoxicity have led to this antibiotic being reserved for serious infections in hospitalized or institutionalized patients.

Cost of therapy is also an important factor in selecting a regimen. A large prospective study of deep foot infections in Sweden found that antibiotics accounted for only 3 to 5% of the total costs for treatment; costs for topical wound treatments were considerably higher.[36] Variables that explained 95% of the total treatment costs were the time between diagnosis, the final required procedure and wound healing, and the number of surgical procedures performed.[36] One American study demonstrated that therapy with ampicillin/sulbactam was significantly less expensive than with imipenem/cilastatin for limb-threatening diabetic foot infections, primarily because of the lower drug and hospitalization costs and less severe side effects associated with the former.[32] More comparative trials and economic analyses are needed. Published suggestions on specific antibiotic regimens for diabetic foot infections vary, but are more alike than different. My recommendations, by type of infection, are given in Table 22–5.

Duration of Therapy

The necessary duration of antibiotic therapy for diabetic foot infections has not been well studied. For mild to moderate infections, a 1- to 2-week course has been found to be effective,[29] while for more serious infections treatment has usually been given for 2 weeks or longer. Adequate debridement, resection, or amputation of infected tissue can shorten the necessary duration of therapy. In those few patients with diabetic foot infection who develop bacteremia, therapy for at least 2 weeks seems prudent. Antibiotic therapy can generally be discontinued when all signs and symptoms of infection have resolved, even if the wound has not completely healed. Healing of an ulcer must be understood to be a separate, albeit important, issue in treating

Table 22-4 ■ SELECTED CHARACTERISTICS OF ANTIBIOTICS THAT MAY BE USED FOR DIABETIC FOOT INFECTIONS

ANTIBIOTIC	FORMULATION		RELATIVE ACTIVITY AGAINST LIKELY INFECTION PATHOGENS*			
	Oral	IM/IV	S. aureus	Streptococci	Enterobacteriaceae	Anaerobes
Penicillins						
Penicillin G/V	Yes	Yes	+	++++	+	++
Cloxacillin, dicloxacillin	Yes	No	++++	+++	0	++
Nafcillin, oxacillin, methicillin	No	Yes	++++	+++	0	++
Ampicillin, amoxicillin	Yes	Yes	+	++++	++	++
Mezlocillin, ticarcillin	No	Yes	+	+++	+++	+++
Azlocillin, piperacillin						
Ampicillin/sulbactam	No	Yes	++++	++++	+++	++++
Piperacillin/tazobactam						
Ticarcillin/clavulanate						
Amoxicillin/clavulanate	Yes	No	+++	++++	++	+++
Cephalosporins						
Cephapirin, cefazolin, cefuroxime	No	Yes	++++	++++	++	++
Cephalexin, cefaclor, cephradine	Yes	No	++++	++++	++	++
Cefoxitin, cefotetan, ceftizoxime	No	Yes	+++	+++	+++	+++
Cefotaxime, cefoperazone	No	Yes	+++	+++	++++	++
Ceftriaxone, ceftazidime				+++	++++	
Aminoglycosides						
Gentamicin, tobramycin	No	Yes	+++	0	++++	0
Amikacin, netilmicin						
Fluoroquinolones						
Ciprofloxacin, ofloxacin	Yes	Yes	+++	++	++++	0
Levofloxacin	Yes	Yes	+++	+++	++++	+
Trovafloxacin	Yes	Yes	++++	++++	++++	+++
Others						
Doxycycline	Yes	Yes	+++	++	++	++
Trimethoprim/sulfamethoxazole	Yes	Yes	+++	++	+++	+
Rifampin	Yes	No	++++	++	0	0
Vancomycin	No	Yes	++++	++++	0	++
Imipenem–cilastatin	No	Yes	++++	++++	++++	+++
Aztreonam	No	Yes	0	0	++++	0
Anaerobic agents						
Clindamycin	Yes	Yes	+++	+++	0	++++
Metronidazole	Yes	Yes	0	0	0	+++

* Activity: ++++, high = +++, moderate = ++, some = +, little = 0, none.

476

Table 22–5 ■ SUGGESTED ANTIBIOTIC REGIMENS FOR TREATING DIABETIC FOOT INFECTIONS*

SEVERITY OF INFECTION	RECOMMENDED[†]	ALTERNATIVE[‡]
Mild/moderate (oral for entire course)	Cephalexin (500 mg qid) Amoxicillin/clavulanate (875/ 125 mg bid) Clindamycin (300 mg tid)	Ofloxacin (400 mg bid) ± clindamycin (300 mg tid) TMP/SMX (2 DS bid)
Moderate/severe (intravenous until stable, then switch to oral equivalent)	Ampicillin/sulbactam[§] (2.0 gm qid) Clindamycin (450 mg qid) + ciprofloxacin (750 mg bid)	Trovofloxacin (300 mg IV)[∥] Clindamycin (600 tid) + ceftazidime (2 gm tid)[‡]
Life-threatening (prolonged intravenous)	Imipenem/cilastin (500 mg qid)[§] Clindamycin (900 mg tid) + tobramycin§ (5.1 mg/kg/day) + ampicillin (50 mg/kg qid)	Vancomycin (15 mg/kg bid) + aztreonam (2.0 gm tid) + metronidazole (7.5 mg/kg qid)

* Given at usual recommended doses for serious infections; modify for azotemia, etc.
† Based upon theoretical considerations and available clinical trials.
‡ Prescribed in special circumstances (e.g., patient allergies, recent treatment with recommended agent, cost considerations).
§ A similar agent of the same class or generation may be substituted.
∥ Currently recommended only for serious infections in hospitalized or institutionalized patients.
TMP/SMX, trimethoprim/sulfamethoxazole.

diabetic foot infections. Some patients who cannot, or will not, undergo surgical resection, or who have surgical metalwork at the site of infection, may require prolonged suppressive antibiotic therapy.

Therapy of Osteomyelitis

Antibiotic choices should be based on bone culture results, when possible, especially because of the need for long-duration therapy. Soft tissue or sinus tract cultures probably do not accurately predict bone pathogens. If empiric therapy is necessary, the microbiology of osteomyelitis suggests one should always cover S. aureus. Because mixed infections are common, broader coverage should be considered if the history or soft tissue cultures suggest it is needed. Antibiotics generally do not penetrate well to infected bone, and the number and function of leukocytes in this environment are suboptimal. Thus, treatment of osteomyelitis should usually be parenteral (at least initially) and prolonged (at least 6 weeks). Cure of chronic osteomyelitis has generally been thought to require removing the infected bone by debridement or resection. Several recent retrospective series have shown, however, that diabetic foot osteomyelitis can be arrested for at least 2 years with antibiotic therapy alone in about two thirds of cases.[35, 43] Furthermore, oral antibiotics with good bioavailability (e.g., fluoroquinolones and clindamycin) may be adequate for most, or perhaps all, of the therapy. If all of the infected bone is removed, a shorter course of antibiotic therapy (e.g., 2

weeks) may be sufficient. In some patients long-term suppressive therapy, or intermittent short courses of treatment for recrudescent symptoms, are the most appropriate approaches.

Adjuvant Therapies

An essential question in managing most diabetic foot infections is, "Does the patient need an operation?" This may be incision and drainage, removal of dead tissue, revascularization, or a procedure to alter the mechanics and pressure distribution of the foot. These maneuvers improve the physiologic perturbations, permitting antibiotics and normal host defenses to work together to arrest infection and heal ulceration. Several additional measures have been employed to improve infection resolution, wound healing, and host response. Those for which there are published data are briefly reviewed here.

Recombinant Granulocyte Colony-Stimulating Factor

A recent small randomized controlled study showed that adding (to usual care, including antibiotic therapy) subcutaneous injections of granulocyte colony-stimulating factor (G-CSF) led to significantly more rapid infection resolution and better outcomes in diabetic patients with serious foot infections.[21] Another small randomized controlled trial found, however, that there was no significant benefit to adjuvant G-CSF in patients with limb-threatening diabetic foot infections.[11]

This expensive drug represents one of several growth factors now likely to emerge through biotechnology. Larger trials are needed to define whether, and for whom, these promising compounds can be recommended.

Hyperbaric Oxygen

This treatment is designed to increase oxygen delivery to ischemic tissue, which may help fight infection and improve wound healing in the high-risk foot. For years anecdotal and uncontrolled reports have suggested benefit in diabetic foot infections. Recently, prospective studies, including one double-blind randomized trial, have shown improved wound healing and a reduced rate of amputation with hyperbaric oxygen (HBO) therapy.[41] HBO is a high-technology and limited resource that will remain reserved for severe cases, even if it is further confirmed as effective.

Revascularization

Over the past decade, lower extremity vascular procedures, including angioplasty and bypass grafting, have been shown to be safe and effective for patients with diabetic foot infections. Feet with critical ischemia that once required amputation can now often be saved with these techniques. Improving blood flow may also be crucial to controlling infection in an ischemic foot. While initial debridement must be performed even in the face of poor arterial circulation, revascularization is generally postponed until sepsis is controlled.[7] Waiting for more than a few days in hopes of sterilizing the wound is, however, inappropriate and may result in further tissue loss.

Larval (Maggot) Therapy

"Biosurgery" with fly larvae (maggots) has been used for many years, but it is enjoying a revival recently.[35, 36] Uncontrolled trials with sterilized larvae suggest they are useful for treating infection (soft tissue and bone), debriding wounds, and controlling wound odor. Larvae are available in the United States and Europe from commercial laboratories. This low-technology and relatively inexpensive treatment is currently used with apparent benefits at several centers, but it requires proper staff training and patient acceptance.

Controlled trials are needed to define which types of infections may benefit from this therapy.

Outcome of Treatment

A good clinical response for mild to moderate infections can be expected in 80 to 90% of appropriately treated patients, and 50 to 60% of deeper or more extensive infections. When infection involves deep soft tissue structures or bone, more thorough debridement is usually needed. Bone resections or partial amputations are required in about two thirds of this patient group. Most of these amputations can be foot-sparing and long-term control of infection is achieved in over 80% of cases. Many above-ankle amputations can be avoided and the length of hospitalization substantially reduced by aggressive early minor surgical procedures and appropriate antibiotic use.[42] Infection recurs in 20 to 30% of patients, many of whom have underlying osteomyelitis. Factors that predict healing include the absence of exposed bone, a palpable popliteal pulse, toe pressure of more than 45 mm Hg or an ankle pressure of more than 80 mm Hg, and a peripheral white blood cell count of less than 12,000/mm^3.[14] The presence of edema or atherosclerotic cardiovascular disease increases the likelihood of an amputation. Patients with combined soft tissue and bone infection may require amputation more often than either type of infection alone.[15] Patients who have had one infection are at substantial risk of having another within a few years; thus, educating them on prevention techniques and prompt consultation for foot problems is critical.

Summary

Diabetic foot infections are a common, complex, and serious problem with dire financial and medical consequences. Fortunately, much progress in this field has been made in the past two decades. Prospective comparative trials have clarified the proper culture techniques, defined the differences in milder versus more severe infections, delineated the microbiology of these wounds, and shown the effectiveness of several specific antibiotic regimens in treating these infections. Careful prospective studies have shown that patients with mild, non–limb-threatening infections can be treated as outpatients with oral antibiotic therapy. The importance of debridement, surgical interventions, weight off-loading, and local foot care have been confirmed. Methods for diagnosing and treating osteomyelitis have been refined. Vascular surgical procedures have been developed and their proper role has been demonstrated. Adjuvant therapies are being added to the standard ones previously available. Accumulating evidence suggests that with proper wound care, optimal metabolic control, and early, aggressive, appropriate surgical and antibiotic therapy infection can be controlled and a functional foot preserved in the great majority of patients. The current challenge is to not only continue to develop new treatments but to marshal existing ones in a seamless, cost-effective, evidence-based, and multi-disciplinary manner.

REFERENCES

1. Armstrong DG, Lavery LA, Harkless LB: Validation of a diabetic wound classification system. The contribution of depth, infection, and ischemia to risk of amputation. Diabet Med 21:855–859, 1998.
2. Armstrong DG, Perales TA, Murff RT, et al: Value of white blood cell count with differential in the acute diabetic foot infection. J Am Podiatr Med Assoc 86:224–227, 1996.
3. Boyko EJ, Lipsky BA: Infection and diabetes mellitus. In Harris MI (ed): Diabetes in America, 2nd ed. Diabetes data compiled 1995. Bethesda, MD: National Institutes of Health. NIH publication No 95-1468, 1995, pp 485–499.
4. Breen JD, Karchmer AW: *Staphylococcus aureus* infections in diabetic patients. Infect Dis Clin North Am 9:11–24, 1995.
5. Bridges RM, Deitch EA: Diabetic foot infections. Pathophysiology and treatment. Surg Clin North Am 74:537–555, 1994.
6. Cavanagh PR, Buse JB, Frykberg RG, et al, for the American Diabetes Association: Diabetic foot wound care. Census Development Conference. Diabetes Care 22:1354–1360, 1999.
7. Caputo GM, Cavanaugh PR, Ulbrecht JS, et al: Assessment and management of foot disease in patients with diabetes. N Engl J Med 331:854–860, 1994.
8. Chang BB, Darling RC III, Paty PSK, et al: Expeditious management of ischemic invasive foot infections. Cardiovasc Surg 4:792–795, 1996.
9. Chantelau E, Tanudjaja T, Altenhöfer F, et al: Antibiotic treatment for uncomplicated neuropathic forefoot ulcers in diabetes: A controlled trial. Diabet Med 13:156–159, 1996.
10. Craig JG, Amin MB, Wu K, et al: Osteomyelitis of the diabetic foot: MR imaging-pathological correlation. Radiology 203:849–855, 1997.
11. De Lalla F, Pellizzer G, Strazzabosco M, et al: A randomized prospective controlled trial of granulocyte-colony stimulating factor (G-CSF) in limb-threatening (LT) diabetic foot infections (DFI). Abstracts of the 38th ICAAC Conference, San Diego, CA. Abstract MN-31.
12. Edelson GW, Armstrong DG, Lavery LA, Caicco G: The acutely infected diabetic foot is not adequately evaluated in an inpatient setting. Arch Intern Med 156:2373–2378, 1996.
13. Enderle MD, Coerpre S, Schweizer HP, et al: Correlation of imaging techniques to histopathology in patients with diabetic foot syndrome and clinical suspicion of chronic osteomyelitis. The role of high-resolution ultrasound. Diabetes Care 22:294–299, 1999.
14. Eneroth M, Apelqvist J, Stenstrom A: Clinical characteristics and outcome in 223 diabetic patients with deep foot infections. Foot Ankle Int 18:716–722, 1997.
15. Eneroth M, Larsson J, Apelqvist J: Deep foot infection in diabetes mellitus—an entity with different characteristics, treatment and prognosis. Abstracts of the 3rd International Symposium on the Diabetic Foot. Noordwijkerhout, The Netherlands, May 5–8, 1999, Abstract p01, p 21.
16. Estes JM, Pomposelli FB Jr: Lower extremity arterial reconstruction in patients with diabetes mellitus. Diabet Med 13:S43–S47, 1996.
17. Fong IW, for the Committee on Antimicrobial Agents: Management of diabetic foot infection: A position paper. Can J Infect Dis 7:361–365, 1996.
18. Foster AVM, Bates M, Doxford M, Edmonds ME: Should oral antibiotics be given to "clean" foot ulcers with no cellulitis? Abstracts of the 3rd International Symposium of the Diabetic Foot, Noordwijkerhout, The Netherlands, May 6, 1998, Abstract O13.
19. Gibbons GW, Habershaw GM: Diabetic foot infections. Anatomy and surgery. Infect Dis Clin North Am 9:131–142, 1995.
20. Gleckman RA, Al-Wawi M: A review of selective infections in the adult diabetic. Compr Ther 25:109–113, 1999.
21. Gough A, Clapperton M, Rolando N, et al: Randomized placebo-controlled trial of granulocyte-colony stimulating factor in diabetic foot infections. Lancet 350:855–859, 1997.
22. Grayson ML, Gibbons GW, Balogh K, et al: Probing to bone in infected pedal ulcers: A clinical sign of underlying osteomyelitis in diabetic patients. JAMA 273:721–723, 1995.
23. Harwood SJ, Valdivia S, Hung G-L, Quenzer RW: Use of sulesomab, a radiolabeled antibody fragment, to detect osteomyelitis in diabetic patients with foot ulcers by leukoscintigraphy. Clin Infect Dis 28:1200–1205, 1999.
24. International Working Group on the Diabetic Foot. International Consensus on the Diabetic Foot. Amsterdam, May 1999, pp 1–96.
25. Jaegeblad G, Apelqvist J, Nyberg P, Berger B: The diabetic foot: From ulcer to multidisciplinary team approach. A process analysis. Abstracts of the 3rd International Symposium of the Diabetic Foot, Noordwijkerhout, The Netherlands, May 6, 1998, Abstract p87, p 149.
26. Jones V: Debridement of diabetic foot lesions. Diabet Foot 3:88–94, 1998.
27. Lipsky BA: Osteomyelitis of the foot in diabetic patients. Clin Infect Dis 25:1318–1326, 1997.
28. Lipsky BA, McDonald D, Litka PA: Treatment of infected diabetic foot ulcers: Topical MSI-78 vs. oral ofloxacin [abstract]. Diabetologia 40(Suppl 1):482, 1997.

29. Lipsky BA, Pecoraro RE, Larson SA, Ahroni JH: Outpatient management of uncomplicated lower-extremity infections in diabetic patients. Arch Intern Med 150:790–797, 1990.

30. Lipsky BA, Pecoraro RE, Wheat JL: The diabetic foot: Soft tissue and bone infection. Infect Dis Clin North Am 4:409–432, 1990.

31. McMahon MM, Bistrian BR: Host defenses and susceptibility to infection in patients with diabetes mellitus. Infect Dis Clin North Am 9:1–10, 1995.

32. McKinnon PS, Paladino JA, Grayson ML, et al: Cost effectiveness of ampicillin/sulbactam versus imipenem/cilastatin in the treatment of limb-threatening foot infections in diabetic patients. Clin Infect Dis 24:57–63, 1997.

33. Newman LG, Waller J, Palestro CJ, et al: Unsuspected osteomyelitis in diabetic foot ulcers: Diagnosis and monitoring by leukocyte scanning with indium 111 oxyquinoline. JAMA 266:1246–1251, 1991.

34. Pecoraro RE, Ahroni JH, Boyko EJ, Stencil VL: Chronology and determinants of tissue repair in diabetic lower-extremity ulcers. Diabetes 40:1305–1313, 1991.

35. Pittet D, Wyssa B, Herter-Clavel C, et al: Outcome of diabetic foot infections treated conservatively. A retrospective cohort study with long-term follow-up. Arch Intern Med 159:851–856, 1999.

36. Ragnarson Tennvall G, Apelqvist J, Eneroth M: Costs of deep foot infections. An analysis of factors determining treatment costs. Abstracts of the 3rd International Symposium of the Diabetic Foot. Noordwijkerhout, The Netherlands, May 5–8, 1999, Abstract p101, p 163.

37. Rayman A, Stansfield G, Woollard T, et al: Use of larvae in the treatment of the diabetic necrotic foot. Diabet Foot 1:7–13, 1998.

38. Reiber GE, Pecoraro RE, Koepsell TD: Risk factors for amputation in patients with diabetes mellitus. A case control study. Ann Intern Med 117:97–105, 1992.

39. Sapico FL, Witte JL, Canawati HN, et al: The infected foot of the diabetic patient: Quantitative microbiology and analysis of clinical features. Rev Infect Dis 6(Suppl 1):171–176, 1984.

40. Sentochnik DE, Eliopoulos GM: Infection and diabetes. In Kahn CR, Weir GC (eds): Joslin's Diabetes Mellitus, 13th ed. Philadelphia: Lea & Febiger, 1994, pp 867–888.

41. Stone JA, Cianci P: The adjunctive role of hyperbaric oxygen in the treatment of lower extremity wounds in patients with diabetes. Diabetes Spectrum 10:118–123, 1997.

42. Tan JS, Friedman NM, Hazelton-Miller C, et al: Can aggressive treatment of diabetic foot infections reduce the need for above-ankle amputation? Clin Infect Dis 23:286–291, 1996.

43. Venkatesan P, Lawn S, Macfarlane RM, et al: Conservative management of osteomyelitis in the feet of diabetic patients. Diabetic Med 14:487–490, 1997.

44. Wheat LJ, Allen SD, Henry M, et al: Diabetic foot infections. Bacteriologic analysis. Arch Intern Med 146:1935–1940, 1986.

45. Wrobel JS, Connolly JE: Making the diagnosis of osteomyelitis. The role of prevalence. J Am Podiatr Med Assoc 88:337–343, 1998.

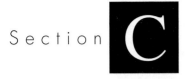

Section **C**

SURGICAL ASPECTS

Chapter 23

SURGICAL PATHOLOGY OF THE FOOT AND CLINICOPATHOLOGIC CORRELATIONS

■ Lawrence W. O'Neal

A knowledge of the anatomy of the foot is essential so that progression of pathologic changes in the diabetic foot can be understood and proper surgical treatment applied. Effective clinical evaluation and surgery are based on an understanding of gross anatomy and of alterations produced by disease. In treatment of diabetic foot problems, success is often uncertain, limited, and temporary even under the care of the most knowledgeable and diligent physician. Close attention to detail is necessary to obtain optimum results.

Anatomy of the Foot

Some of the externally visible landmarks of the foot are shown in Figure 23–1.

Skin

The skin of the dorsum of the foot is flexible and unspecialized. It contains hair follicles, sweat glands, and scanty sebaceous glands.

Over the dorsum of the foot the skin is about 2 mm thick. In the dorsum few fibrous septa penetrate to deeper fascial structures except in the areas of wrinkle in the dorsal skin, overlying the metatarsophalangeal joints and the interphalangeal joints, where fibrous septa attach the dermis to the deep fascia. The skin in these sites is relatively more fixed than at other dorsal sites.

The plantar skin is 4 or 5 mm thick, with the thickest areas covering the heel and the distal metatarsals. The skin of the plantar surface is richly innervated; it has no hair follicles or sebaceous glands but has numerous sweat glands. Throughout the plantar skin the collagenous fibers of the dermis are connected to the deep fascia by heavy fibrous septa, which separate the subcutaneous fat into firm, partly discontinuous lobules. These septa are particularly heavy at the creases. Because of this dermal fixation to deep fascia, the skin of the sole is relatively fixed. Dorsal skin will glide 2 or 3 cm, but plantar skin will glide over deeper structures only 1 cm or less.

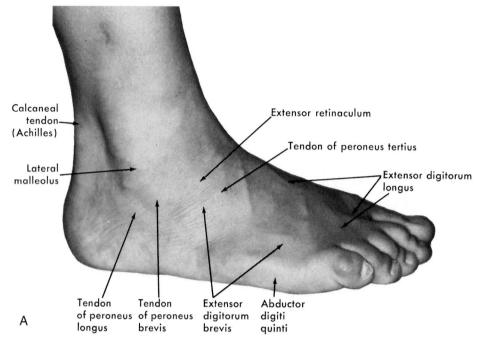

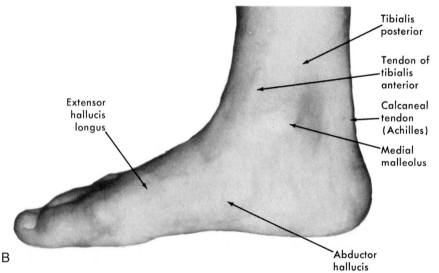

Figure 23–1 ■ Surface anatomy of lateral (A) and medial (B) aspects of foot.

Nails

The nails are specialized skin appendages. The nail itself is composed of keratinous flattened epithelial cells derived from the generative areas of the nail fold and nail bed (Fig. 23–2). The adult nail is composed of three ill-defined layers: the dorsal nail, the intermediate nail, and the ventral nail.[16]

The dorsal nail arises from the proximal half of the roof of the nail fold and from the most proximal part of the floor of the nail fold. The intermediate nail arises from the distal part of the nail fold and the proximal nail bed up to the distal margin of the lunula. The ventral nail arises from the distal half to two thirds of the nail bed up to the hyponychium (Fig. 23–3).

The nail is bedded firmly on the epithelium of the nail bed, which apparently advances with nail growth, as is seen with the forward migration of small subungual hematomas.

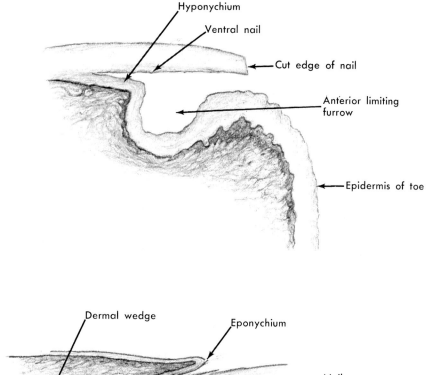

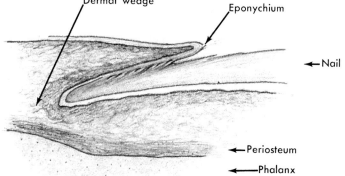

Figure 23-2 ■ Anatomy of nails with longitudinal sections of digits. (Modified from Lewis BL: Microscopic studies of fetal and mature nail and surrounding soft tissue. Arch Dermatol Syph 70:732, 1954. Copyright © Springer-Verlag, with permission.)

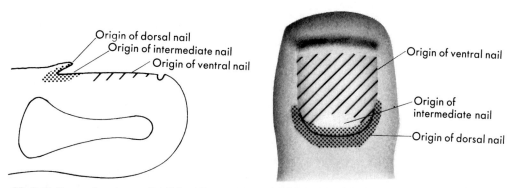

Figure 23-3 ■ Generative areas of nail lamellae. Most of nail bed and nail folds contribute some elements to ill-defined nail layers. (Modified from Lewis BL: Microscopic studies of fetal and mature nail and surrounding soft tissue. Arch Dermatol Syph 70:732, 1954. Copyright © Springer-Verlag, with permission.)

The margins of the nail are overhung with skin folds called the nail wall.

Nerves

Elements of the sciatic nerve furnish the motor and sensory innervation of the foot (Fig. 23–4). The fourth and fifth lumbar segments and the first and second sacral segments contribute. The *saphenous nerve* reaches the skin over the anteromedial side of the lower tibia and as far distally as the medial side of the first metatarsophalangeal joint. The *common peroneal* branch of the sciatic nerve reaches the leg at the fibular head. It crosses anterior to the fibular neck deep to the origin of the peroneus longus muscle. The musculocutaneous (*superficial peroneal*) branch stays at first in the peroneal compartment and supplies the motor nerves of the peroneus longus and brevis muscles. The superficial peroneal nerve then pierces the fascia in the lower one third of the leg. A medial dorsal cutaneous branch descends in front of the ankle joint to the medial side of the hallux and to the adjoining portions of the second and third toes. The intermediate dorsal cutaneous branch of the superficial peroneal nerve lies anterior to the lateral malleolus and innervates the skin of the third and fourth interdigital spaces and corresponding digital segments.

The deep branch of the common peroneal nerve enters the extensor compartment of the leg and is distributed to the extensor muscles of the ankle and toes. Its termination is a dorsal digital nerve to the first interdigital web and adjoining segments of toes (lateral half of the hallux and medial half of the second toe).

The lateral margin of the foot derives its nerve supply from the *sural nerve,* which is known in the foot as the lateral dorsal cutaneous nerve. The medial calf and medial side of the ankle are supplied by the *saphenous nerve.*

The sensory innervation of the heel is from a medial calcaneal branch of the *tibial nerve.* The tibial nerve divides deep to the plantar fascia into the medial and lateral plantar branches. The cutaneous distribution of the *medial plantar nerve* includes the medial three and one half digits and the distal two thirds of the medial sole. Small interdigital twigs from the medial plantar nerve innervate the nail beds of the medial three toes.

The *lateral plantar nerve* supplies the lateral portion of the sole of the foot and the lateral one and one half toes.

Vessels

All of the arterial supply of the foot is derived from the popliteal artery, which lies on the knee joint and on the popliteal muscle. At the lower border of the popliteal muscle the popliteal artery divides into anterior and posterior tibial arteries.

The *anterior tibial artery* penetrates the upper part of the interosseous membrane and enters the extensor compartment of the leg. Distally it lies between the tibialis anterior and extensor muscles. At the ankle it lies more medially and crosses the ankle joint anteriorly, becoming in the foot the *dorsalis pedis artery.* The dorsalis pedis artery usually lies lateral to the extensor hallucis longus muscle. Small dorsal digital arteries arise from a variable dorsal arcuate branch of the dorsalis pedis artery.

The *posterior tibial artery* accompanies the tibial nerve. The artery lies between the tibialis posterior and flexor digitorum longus muscles and the soleus muscle and tendon of the calcaneus. Near the medial malleolus it sends a branch to the heel pad along the medial calcaneal nerve.

In the plantar space the posterior tibial artery divides into medial and lateral plantar arteries. These arteries course with the medial and lateral plantar nerves. The plantar arch is formed by anastomosis between the medial and lateral plantar arteries, with a contribution from the dorsalis pedis artery at the first intermetatarsal space.

The plantar digital vessels arise from the plantar arch. The plantar arch is variable in detail but in the healthy individual provides abundant opportunity for collateral circulation in the distal foot. The arterioles to the skin form an *internal vascular belt* at the junction between the subcutaneous tissue and the dermis. Arising from this internal vascular belt are dermal plexuses that are intimately interconnected, forming a reticular network of vessels of different sizes. From this network arboreal terminal branches form a subpapillary plexus with capillary loops into the dermal papillae, integrating a number of papillae into *vascular districts,* which are also interconnected.

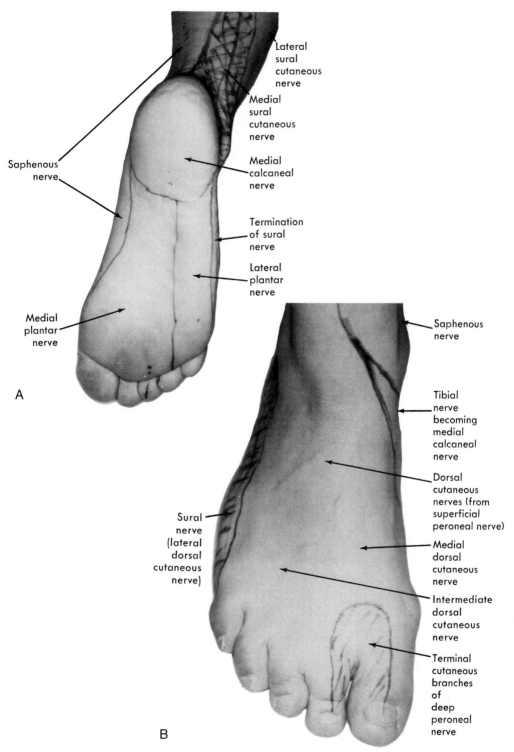

Figure 23–4 ■ Cutaneous nerve distribution of sole (*A*) and dorsum (*B*) of foot.

Muscles, Tendons, and Fascia

The muscles in the extensor group are located anteriorly in the leg. They include the tibialis anterior, the extensor hallucis longus, and the extensor digitorum longus. Laterally are the peroneal muscles. Both the anterior and the lateral muscle groups are innervated by the common peroneal nerve.

The flexors of the foot and toes are innervated by the tibial nerve. The flexors are in the posterior compartment of the leg behind the interosseous membrane.

The deep muscular fascia encloses the muscles of the superficial portion of the tibia and of the lateral malleolus. At the anterior ankle thickened areas of this fascia form the extensor retinacula (the transverse crural ligament and the cruciate crural ligament), under which the extensor tendons course. The fascia is then continuous with the thinner fascia of the dorsum of the foot and toes.

The gastrocnemius muscle arises from medial and lateral attachments on the distal posterior femur. These heads of the gastrocnemius form the distal margin of the popliteal fossa. The soleus muscle arises from the proximal tibia and fibula. Its tendon joins the tendon of the gastrocnemius and is attached to the calcaneus as the calcaneal tendon (Achilles tendon). The small plantaris muscle arises from the lateral femoral condyle. The plantaris tendon crosses between the soleus and the gastrocnemius and forms the medial portion of the calcaneal tendon. The gastrocnemius, soleus, and plantaris are innervated by branches of the tibial nerve.

Across the ankle the long tendons maintain their relative position to each other and are held in place by fascial condensations.

In the sole of the foot the plantar aponeurosis is the most superficial fascia (Fig. 23–5).[10] The dermis of the sole is attached to plantar fascia by fibrous septa that enclose the fat lobules. Its central portion is the thickest and is attached to the medial tubercle of the calcaneus. The plantar fascia spreads fan-like distally. Near the metatarsal heads the fascial fibers divide into five processes, which form bundles surrounding the metatarsal heads. Distally the plantar aponeurosis joins with transverse fibers (the superficial transverse metatarsal ligament) and anchors the dermis at the distal plantar crease. Some deeper fibers extend to the flexor sheaths near the metatarsophalangeal joints.

In the central plantar space the flexor digitorum brevis muscle arises from the proximal portion of the plantar fascia. The lateral and medial portions of the plantar fascia are thinner than the central portion. Medially the fascia covers the abductor hallucis and laterally the abductor digiti quinti muscles. The strong plantar aponeurosis forms the principal stay of the longitudinal arch.

Beneath the plantar fascia the muscles in the sole of the foot are categorized into four layers. The most superficial *first layer* (Fig. 23–6)[10] consists of the flexor digitorum brevis, the abductor hallucis, and the abductor digiti quinti muscles. The flexor digitorum brevis originates from the medial tubercle of the calcaneus and from the deep surface of the plantar aponeurosis. Its four tendons insert into the middle phalanges of the four lateral toes. The abductor hallucis arises from the medial tubercle of the calcaneus and inserts on the medial side of the base of the proximal phalanx of the hallux. The abductor digiti quinti arises from the medial and lateral tubercle of the calcaneus and inserts into the base of the proximal phalanx of the little toe.

The *second layer* is composed of the tendons of the flexor hallucis longus and the flexor digitorum longus muscles. These tendons insert in the proximal portion of the distal phalanges on their plantar aspect. The quadratus plantae, or accessory flexor, arises from the calcaneus and inserts on the flexor digitorum longus tendons. The four lumbrical muscles arise from the medial side of the tendons of the flexor digitorum longus group, pass to the hallux side of the toes, and insert on the capsule of the metatarsophalangeal joint and on the dorsal expansion of the extensor tendon of the lateral four toes. The tendons of the lumbricals lie superficial to the deep transverse metatarsal ligament. The lumbrical muscle, as in the hand, extends the proximal interphalangeal joint and assists in flexion of the metatarsophalangeal joint.

In the *third layer* (Fig. 23–7)[10] lie the flexor hallucis brevis, the flexor digiti quinti, and the two adductor hallucis muscles—the oblique and the transverse. The flexor hallucis brevis originates from the dense fibrous plantar tarsometatarsal ligaments and from the cuboid. It splits into a medial and lateral tendon, each of which encases a sesamoid bone under the metatarsal head. At their insertion on the proximal phalanx of the hallux

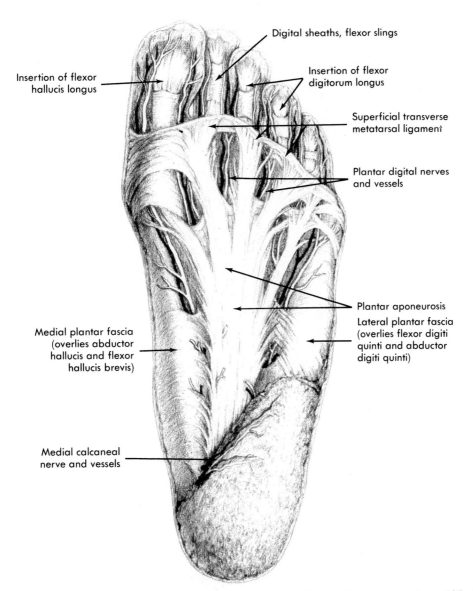

Figure 23–5 ■ Plantar fascia. Note separating bundles near metatarsal heads. (Redrawn from Grant JCB: An Atlas of Anatomy, 6th ed. Baltimore: Williams & Wilkins, 1972, with permission.)

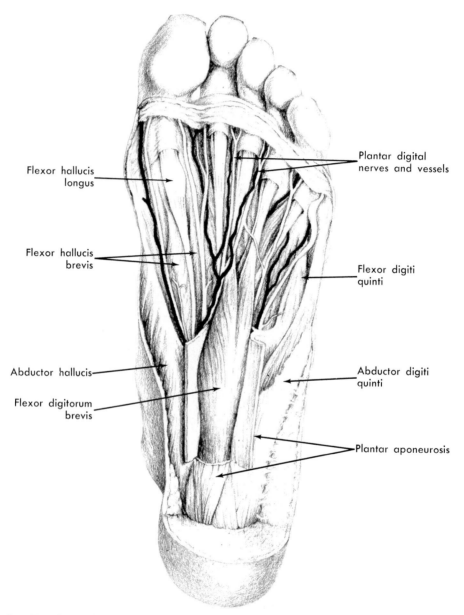

Figure 23–6 ■ First layer of plantar muscles. (Redrawn from Grant JCB: An Atlas of Anatomy, 6th ed. Baltimore: Williams & Wilkins, 1972, with permission.)

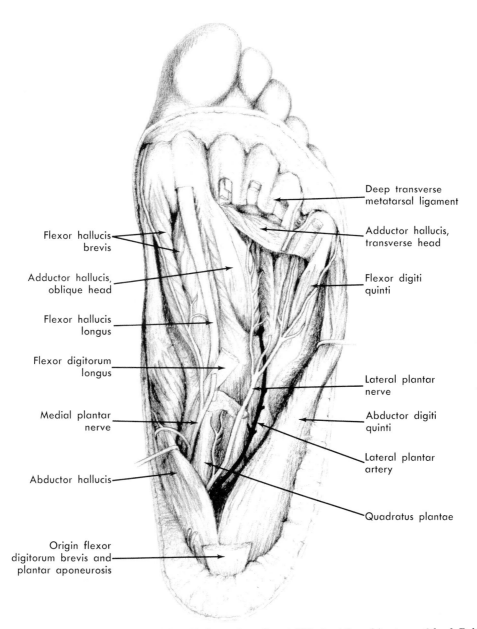

Figure 23–7 ■ Third layer of plantar muscles. (Redrawn from Grant JCB: An Atlas of Anatomy, 6th ed. Baltimore: Williams & Wilkins, 1972, with permission.)

they are joined by the tendon of the abductor hallucis medially and the tendons of the oblique and transverse heads of the adductor hallucis to form a composite flexor tendon. The oblique head arises from the bases of the second, third, and fourth metatarsal heads and from the fascial sheath of the peroneus longus. The transverse head of the adductor hallucis arises from the plantar aspect of the four lateral metatarsophalangeal joints and the deep transverse metatarsal ligament. The small flexor of the little toe arises from the base of the fifth metatarsal and inserts in the base of the proximal phalanx of the little toe.

The plantar interossei, the dorsal interossei, and the tendons of the tibialis posterior and peroneus longus muscles lie in the *fourth layer* (Fig. 23–8).[10] The three plantar interossei arise from metatarsal shafts of the third, fourth, and fifth metatarsals and insert in the medial side of the bases of the corresponding proximal phalanges. They are adductors to these toes. The four dorsal interossei muscles each arise from adjoining metatarsal surfaces in the first, second, third, and fourth intermetacarpal spaces and attach at the bases of the proximal phalanges of the second, third, and fourth toes. The dorsal interossei abduct from the axis of the sec-

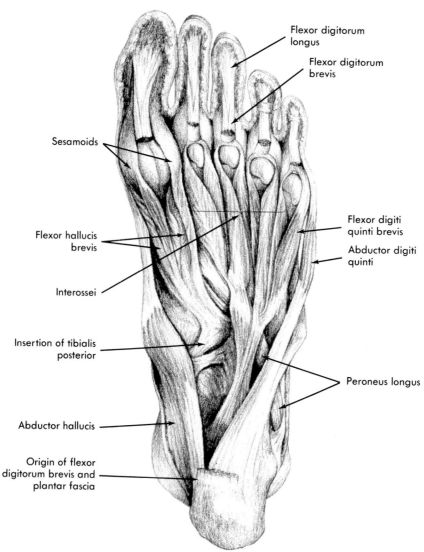

Figure 23–8 ■ Fourth layer of plantar muscles. (Redrawn from Grant JCB: An Atlas of Anatomy, 6th ed. Baltimore: Williams & Wilkins, 1972, with permission.)

ond toe. The tendon of the peroneus longus lies in a groove in the cuboid, passes deep to the flexor hallucis brevis, and inserts in the base of the first metatarsal and the first (medial) cuneiform. The tibialis posterior inserts chiefly on the medial aspect of the navicular tubercle but sends fibrous attachments to the complex ligaments of the plantar tarsus and tarsometatarsal ligaments.

The collagenous structures of the distal foot intermingle to a degree not made clear by the preceding descriptions. In the 2 cm between the heads of the metatarsals and the plantar metatarsophalangeal crease, the dermal collagen, plantar fascia, flexor sheaths, joint capsule, and periosteum of sesamoid, metatarsal, and proximal phalanges are closely approximated to one another and attached more or less by commonly used fibrous sheaths and septa. The superficial transverse metatarsal ligament is a local condensation of this fibrous tissue.

Adjacent to joint capsule and commingling with joint capsule fibers is the deep transverse metatarsal ligament.

The *bones* of the foot and some of the major tendon insertions are shown in Figure 23–9.

Fascial Compartments[15, 18]
(Fig. 23–10)

The *medial compartment* is bounded by the inferior surface of the first metatarsal dorsally, an extension of the plantar aponeurosis medially and intermuscular septum laterally. The medial compartment contains the abductor hallucis and the flexor hallucis brevis muscles and the flexor hallucis longus, peroneus longus, and posterior tibial tendons.

The *central compartment* is bounded by the plantar aponeurosis inferiorly, intermuscular septa medially and laterally, and the tarsometatarsal structures dorsally. The central compartment contains the flexor digitorum brevis muscle, the flexor digitorum longus tendons, the lumbricales, quadratus plantae, adductor hallucis muscle, and the peroneal and posterior tibial tendons.

The *lateral compartment* is bounded by the fifth metatarsal dorsally, an intermuscular septum medially, and the edge of the plantar aponeurosis laterally. The lateral compartment contains the abductor digiti quinti, the flexor digiti quinti, and the opponens muscles of the fifth toe.

The *interosseous compartment* is bounded by the interosseous fascia of the metatarsals and contains the seven interossei.

The Candidate for Foot Problems

Anyone who has diabetes for 15 years or more is a potential candidate for foot problems, because neuropathy progresses enough in that time to cause clinical problems. However, in some patients the diagnosis of diabetes is first made when the patient is examined for foot ulcers or infections. A tendency of many authors is to classify diabetic foot lesions as "ischemic" or "neuropathic." Although an ischemic or neuropathic pattern may predominate, most ulcers have an element of each. Deterioration of the pedal vessels and nerves is accompanied by other problems of diabetes, such as retinopathy and nephropathy (see Chapter 9). Changes in the foot develop so gradually that many patients are unaware of the degree of deterioration and become distressed when minor injury precipitates major disability. Although most diabetics are aware of the risk for foot infections and amputations, few understand the causes and mechanisms of the process or the measures needed to maintain an intact foot.

The Vulnerable Foot

Many deformities develop in the feet of older persons. In diabetes of long duration, foot deformities are nearly universal. In a survey of diabetic patients at a Veteran's Affairs Hospital clinic, 50% had vascular insufficiency, neuropathy, and a coexisting foot deformity, indicating a high risk for morbidity.[22] The common abnormalities were angular, usually hallux valgus and hammer digit. Less common, but significant, abnormalities were submetatarsal head calluses, interdigital soft corns, and Charcot foot. Several of the deformities of the foot in this study were ulcerated; one patient had osteomyelitis and one had gangrene of the hallux.

A recent Swedish study[4] showed that angular bony foot deformities were present in 68% of diabetic men, compared with 28% of men without diabetes.

Foot deformities in the diabetic patient have several causes. Of course some are old, long-tolerated abnormalities that become problems only when circulation and sensa-

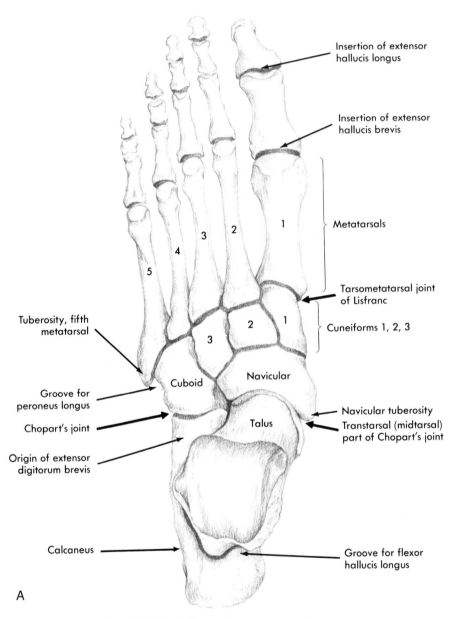

Figure 23–9 ■ *A*, Bones of foot from dorsal aspect.

Illustration continued on opposite page

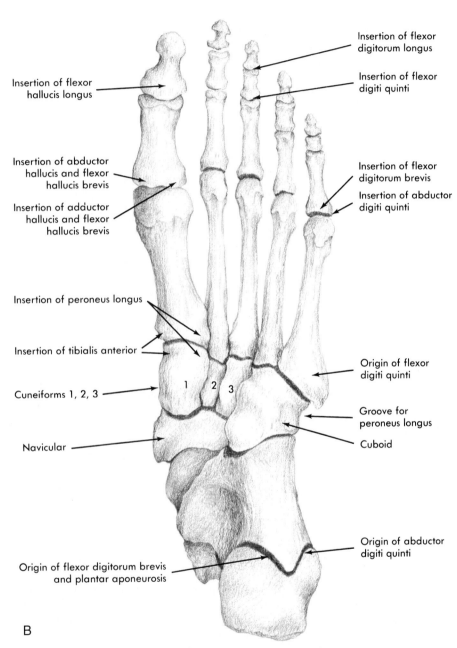

Insertion of flexor
hallucis longus

Insertion of abductor
hallucis and flexor
hallucis brevis

Insertion of adductor
hallucis and flexor
hallucis brevis

Insertion of peroneus longus

Insertion of tibialis anterior

Cuneiforms 1, 2, 3

Navicular

Origin of flexor digitorum brevis
and plantar aponeurosis

Insertion of flexor
digitorum longus

Insertion of flexor
digiti quinti

Insertion of flexor
digitorum brevis

Insertion of abductor
digiti quinti

Origin of flexor
digiti quinti

Groove for
peroneus longus

Cuboid

Origin of abductor
digiti quinti

B

Figure 23–9 *Continued* ■ *B,* Bones of foot from plantar aspect.

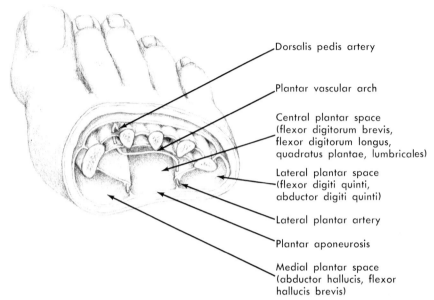

Figure 23–10 ■ Plantar spaces in distal foot.

tion diminish. At first the most distal muscles, the intrinsic muscles of the foot, seem to be affected. The loss of balancing lumbrical function results in extension of the metatarsophalangeal joint of the toes and flexion of the proximal interphalangeal joints (the "intrinsic minus foot").[5] The result of this imbalance is hammer toes. In addition, loss of abduction function of the dorsal interossei causes the toes to become crowded on the axis of the second digit, accentuating the angular prominences at the first and fifth metatarsophalangeal joints (bunion and bunionette). The neuropathic arthropathy of diabetes, or Charcot foot, eventually results in a collapse of the midfoot.[8] The subsequent rocker-bottom foot, medial tarsal subluxation, digital subluxation, and bone fragments offer additional opportunity for ulceration, including the unique midplantar ulcer. In addition to the osseous abnormalities, a loss of soft tissue mass in the sole of the foot (particularly in diabetics with plantar ulcerations) causes less padding and dispersion of mechanical forces than in the normal foot.[9]

With careful supervision, the intact foot of an educated patient can be maintained despite low blood flow. Injury, including surgery or infection, requires an increased blood flow to contain and heal the damage. The arteries and arterioles of the diabetic often cannot deliver the required relative hyperemia.[23]

The Vulnerable Patient

Walsh et al.[24] described a group of patients with newly diagnosed diabetes who had retinopathy and foot lesions at the time of diagnosis. The patients were remarkably unconcerned about their condition. Their self-neglect and lack of insight contributed to a poor prognosis.

It is well known that preventive care and education are extremely important in maintaining the intact foot.[26] These factors are, however, difficult to implement and evaluate. In the Nottingham study,[25] 93% of those interviewed (all patients previously hospitalized for diabetic foot ulceration, infection, or gangrene) later claimed that they had not been told or offered anything to read about preventing foot problems. Many of these patients were, when interviewed, using the services of the diabetic clinic or the district nurse. Few had used these services before hospitalization.

Any physician who treats diabetics with foot problems recognizes patients who are doomed to serious foot infections and amputations. The bravado of the late-stage juvenile diabetic who wants to match the activities of peers is ominous. The type 2 diabetic who "has to" walk, work, or even dance and hike with an ulcerated foot presents an educational challenge. Physicians often call these patients "noncompliant." The closer the physician can bring the patient to understanding the problems of collaborative health maintenance, the more likely the patient is to keep an intact foot.

Often medical care is inadequate. Feet are not always examined routinely, even by endocrinologists.[21] In admissions of diabetic patients with foot problems to a university teaching hospital, 31.4% did not have pedal pulses documented, 59.7% were not evaluated for neuropathy, and foot radiographs were not obtained in 32.9%.[6]

The aim of education in this field is to prevent the development of a foot ulcer, or if the patient gets one, to never get another. Unfortunately, this goal is not achieved often enough. Amputation of one leg is too often followed by the need for amputation of the other leg, which usually has the risk factors that had been seen in the amputated limb (Fig. 23–11).

A substantial number of diabetic patients at high risk of foot ulceration do not attend clinics.[14]

Mechanisms of Progression of Foot Lesions

Initial Lesions

Although the end of the process may be loss of limb or life or both, the initial event is a break in the skin somewhere in the foot followed by penetration of bacteria and local infection. Ordinarily most of the initial incidents leading to severe infections, gangrene, amputation, and disability in the diabetic seem trivial and indeed would be trivial or negligible to younger nondiabetics. The initial lesion may be *acute mechanical trauma* in which skin is torn or punctured. Frequently the poor eyesight of the diabetic patient contributes to stubbing the toes, stepping on sharp objects, or gouging the skin in trimming nails. *Thermal trauma* from foot baths and heating pads may destroy skin in the neuropathic foot (see Chapter 9). *Incessant friction* over angular prominences is often associated with improperly fitting shoes. One brief episode of walking on an insensitive foot may result in blistering and erosion. If the circulation is adequate, healing usually occurs with rest. If circulation is inadequate to deliver the hyperemic response needed for healing, a patch of gangrene may result.

Several of the deformities of the foot result in concentrated weight bearing, predisposing to callus formation and ulceration. The toes play an important part in increasing the weight-bearing area during walking. Areas of callus and ulceration correlate well with areas of maximal vertical and sheer forces (see Chapter 6).

In bedridden disabled patients the heel is vulnerable to ulceration. The simple weight of the immobile foot on the mattress will obliterate blood perfusion in skin on the posterolateral side of the heel. The consequence of these initial events, which seem minor and are often ignored or minimized, may be midthigh amputation when ulcers occur in a foot debilitated by diabetes. The degree of vulnerability of the debilitated foot is often not appreciated by the patient, who may have difficulty in understanding why "such a little thing" can result in tissue loss and progres-

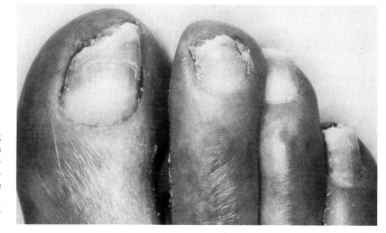

Figure 23–11 ■ Foot in patient with advanced diabetes shows shiny, thin, dry, hairless skin; dermal hemosiderin deposits; and irregular growth of nails, with evidence of poor care. This man, in his fifties, had had his left leg amputated and was nearly blind from retinopathy.

sive disability. The diabetic with severe neuropathy frequently does not know how the lesions happened.

Local Progression

The progression to major infection with necrosis of tissue results from (1) a circulation inadequate to confine the infection; (2) a neuropathy so profound that the part is not voluntarily put at rest as a foot with normal sensation would be, resulting in milking of the infection through the natural fascial pathways; and (3) more aggressive bacterial superinfection. Although the "ischemic" foot may have a somewhat different pattern than the "neuropathic" foot and one pattern or the other may predominate, both vascular lesions and nerve lesions contribute to the problem. Treatment for the predominantly ischemic foot differs substantially from that of the predominantly neuropathic foot.

Septic Arteritis and Tissue Necrosis

In tissues adjoining infection, small vessels commonly develop thrombotic occlusion. This process is seen in arterioles of the skin adjoining stasis ulcers, in small vessels in the base and margins of duodenal ulcers, and in small pulmonary arterioles in the wall of tubercular cavities. Thrombosis of small vessels is partly responsible for the necrosis of tissue in these lesions and for the frequent chronicity of these and other types of infections. Usually in tissues with otherwise normal small vessels, this process occurs only at the margin of the infection. After sloughing, draining, or other control of the infection, normal arterioles recanalize and form abundant granulation tissue, which is the first stage in wound healing.

Numerous bacteria elaborate angiotoxic (necrotizing) substances. For example, particularly injurious is the α-toxin of staphylococci, which, when injected into the skin, results in the local development of an impressive necrotic lesion. Streptokinase and streptococcal hyaluronidase have been implicated in the rapid extension of cellulitis by digestion of fibrin barriers and intracellular ground substance. In the mixed infections so common in the diabetic foot, the necrotizing toxins following the spreading factors can produce a devastating lesion.

In the already diseased small vessels in the diabetic patient,[23] the occlusive process is exaggerated, and one sees paronychia, ingrown nails, and minor injuries proceeding to ever-enlarging areas of necrosis rather than staying limited. More arterioles are obliterated, larger arterioles are obliterated, and the original lesions become converted from trivial infections to areas of gangrene. Creeping advancement of this process of infective obliterative microangiopathy (Fig. 23–12) can occur until a plane or space is reached, such as a tendon sheath, into which the bacteria will spill and spread. As more of the arterioles and small arteries become involved, the infection and necrosis progress (Fig. 23–13).

Regardless of any debate about the significance of microangiopathy in diabetes,[13] the potential virulence of infection arising in local lesions is greater in the diabetic than in other neuropathic conditions (paraplegia, syringomyelia, tabes, Hansen's disease). The greater risk to the diabetic foot may indicate that the capillaries and arterioles of diabetics are more likely to occlude when exposed to bacterial toxins.

Many authors have taken a static view toward the role of microangiopathy in the progression of foot infections. It seems ap-

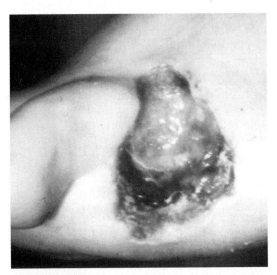

Figure 23–12 ■ Creeping gangrene after amputation of fifth toe. Small skin vessel thrombosis led to patch of gangrenous skin inferior to base of toe.

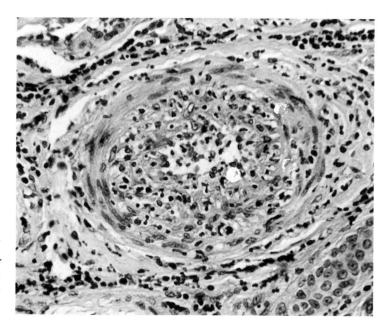

Figure 23–13 ■ Obliteration of lumen of small dermal arteriole by intimal hyperplasia and septic thrombus. Note cellular evidence of inflammation in areolar tissues near arteriole. This arteriole was about 1 mm from margin of area of dry gangrene.

parent now that the maximum vasodilator capacity of the resistance vessels and the autoregulation of blood flow are reduced in long-term diabetics.[13] Consequently, when increased blood flow is required to contain infection in the foot, it is not always readily available.

Although the plantar fascia, tendon sheaths, and other structures in and near the superficial transverse metatarsal ligament form barriers to infection when the arterial circulation is good, creeping infective microangiopathy can destroy fibrous barriers, as well as skin, and allow spread through and along structures in the distal foot that would ordinarily retard the spread of infection.

"End-Artery" Disease in the Diabetic Foot

The normally rich collateral circulation in the foot, with extensive complex communications in the plantar arches and the dorsal arch and between the two arches, as well as smaller unnamed communications everywhere in the normal foot, allows major trauma, major operations, and major infections to be tolerated in the normal foot with little attention being required for the arteries distal to the ankle.

In the diabetic, however, multiple complete and partial arteriosclerotic blockades of large, medium-sized, and small arteries result in a situation comparable with end-arteries as in the heart or kidney, where opportunity for collateral circulation is barred. If the end-artery becomes blocked, there is no replacement for its function, and the tissue supplied by the artery dies (Fig. 23–14).

Examples are seen in plantar space abscesses. After penetrating wounds of the sole of the foot (e.g., from a tack, pin, glass, or nail in shoe), the plantar space may be directly entered and an abscess formed. In the inexpansile central plantar space, infection can quickly obliterate the plantar arterial arch and its branches, to be followed by necrosis not only of tissue in the central plantar space but also of the second, third, and fourth toes, which receive most of their blood supply from the plantar arch (Fig. 23–15). The fifth toe and the hallux receive some of their circulation through the lateral and medial plantar spaces, respectively, and may survive central plantar space abscesses.

Frequently, digital and web infections will produce localized gangrene that spreads by means of septic obliterative angiopathy until the digital arteries are reached. Occlusion of these may lead to gangrene of the adjoining

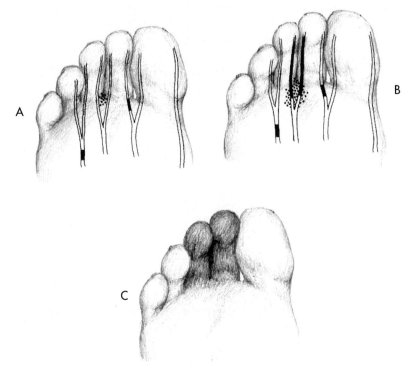

Figure 23–14 ■ Schematics of mechanisms whereby advancing infection causes obliteration of small arteries that have been converted into end-arteries by arteriosclerotic disease process, with resultant gangrene. *A*, Early web space infection in foot with patchy segmental arteriosclerotic occlusion of digital and metatarsal vessels. *B*, Thrombosis of arteries adjacent to web space infection. *C*, Gangrene of second and third toes.

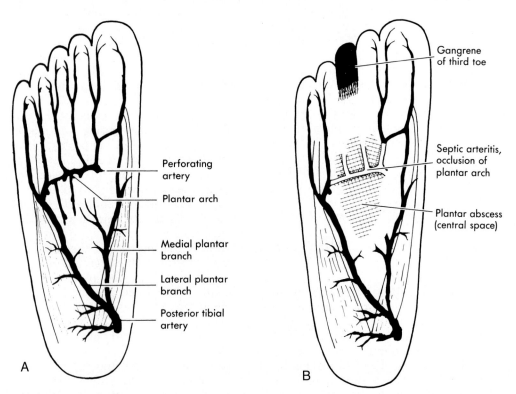

Figure 23–15 ■ *A*, Normal plantar arch receives contributions from medial and lateral plantar branches of posterior tibial artery and from dorsalis pedis via a perforating artery or arteries. *B*, If central plantar space abscess causes occlusion of plantar arch, gangrene of middle toe will result.

500

digits if the neighboring small vessels are obstructed and an end-artery situation exists (Fig. 23–16).

Histologically, there are no clear-cut differences between lower limb arteriosclerosis of diabetics and nondiabetics. The major difference is that in the diabetic limb the obstructive disease tends to spread more distally and in particular to involve the metatarsal arteries. These findings have been amply confirmed and are often seen in lower limb angiograms.

The distal arteriosclerosis occurs at an earlier age in diabetics than in nondiabetics. In type 2 diabetes, progression of lower limb arterial occlusive disease was seen in 87% of patients followed for more than 2 years.[2]

The distinctive distal patchy atherosclerosis in the diabetic with multiple blockades in capillaries, arterioles, small arteries, and named larger arteries converts tissue that in health is perfused by interlocking and alternate channels of blood flow to tissue supplied by only one artery, sometimes tenuously. The amount of tissue thus dependent on its single artery may vary from a few square millimeters of skin in a *vascular district* to the entire area of the foot or leg.

Common Foot Deformities in Diabetic Patients

Digits

The Nails (Table 23–1)

The initial break in the skin often originates near the nails. Nail deformities after trauma, fungus infection, systemic disease, and poor care are common in the general population. In the ischemic neuropathic foot of diabetics, some nail abnormality appears to be universal. Nails lead to difficulty in several ways. The reduced vision and frequent obesity of many diabetic patients make it difficult for them to reach the nails, and they may cut the adjacent skin. With neglect the nails grow too long, and a nail may gouge the skin of the neighboring toe (Fig. 23–17). Frequently in the elderly, as the nail grows long, it incurves and partly encircles the distal nail bed. Then stubbing the toe or wearing new shoes can break the skin. In some of the nail abnormalities, excess keratin and debris accumulate under the nail and in the nail folds, where bacteria might grow.

Infections beginning in the nail bed, paronychium, or nail wall spread on the dorsal

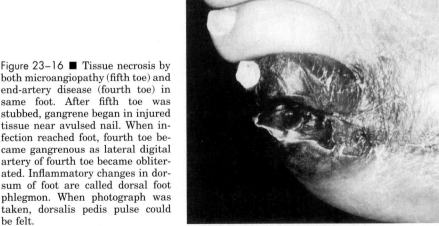

Figure 23–16 ■ Tissue necrosis by both microangiopathy (fifth toe) and end-artery disease (fourth toe) in same foot. After fifth toe was stubbed, gangrene began in injured tissue near avulsed nail. When infection reached foot, fourth toe became gangrenous as lateral digital artery of fourth toe became obliterated. Inflammatory changes in dorsum of foot are called dorsal foot phlegmon. When photograph was taken, dorsalis pedis pulse could be felt.

Table 23-1 ▪ GLOSSARY OF NAILS*

Onych-, onycho- Greek *Onyx,* meaning nail
Onychatrophy Atrophy of the nails
Onychauxis Marked overgrowth of the nails
Onychectomy Ablation of a nail
Onychia Inflammation of the matrix of the nail; onychitis
  O. lateralis Paronychia
  O. maligna Acute onychia in debilitated patients
  O. parasitica Onychomycosis
  O. periungualis Paronychia
  O. sicca Brittle nails
Onychitis Onychia
Onychodystrophy Dystrophy in the nails occurring as a congenital defect or due to any illness or injury that may cause a malformed nail
Onychogryposis Enlargement with increased curvature of the nails (Fig. 23–18)
Onycholysis Loosening of the nails, beginning at the free border and usually incomplete

Onychomadesis Complete shedding of the nails, usually with systemic disease
Onychomalacia Abnormal softness of the nails
Onychomycosis Fungus infection of the nails
  O. favus Favus of the nails
  O. trichophytina Tinea unguium
Onychonosus Any disease of the nails; onychopathy, onychosis
Onychophosis Growth of horny epithelium in the nail bed
Onychophyma Swelling or hypertrophy of the nails
Onychoptosis Falling off of the nails
Onychorrhexis Abnormal brittleness of the nails with splitting of free edge
Onychoschizia Loosening of the nail from the nail bed
Ungius incarnatus Ingrowing nail; onychocryptosis (Figs. 23–19 and 23–20)

* Adapted from Sutton RL Jr: Diseases of the Skin, 11th ed. St. Louis: Mosby-Year Book, 1956, with permission.

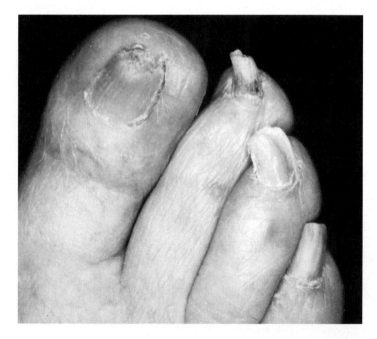

Figure 23-17 ▪ Toes of obese diabetic patient with onychomycosis of nail of hallux and incurving distal growth of all nails. Nails have grown long because of neglect. Note that nail of third toe gouges skin of second toe.

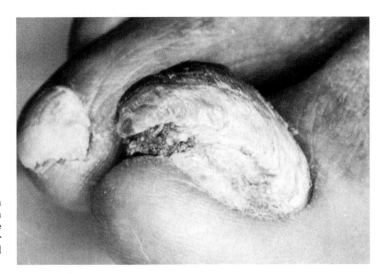

Figure 23–18 ■ Onychogryposis. In diabetic patient, infection may begin in debris covering nail bed. This type of nail easily hooks bedding, socks, or furniture, causing avulsion of nail and trauma to proximal nail fold.

and lateral aspects of the toes. Characteristically the infections spread on the dorsum of the digit to reach the dorsum of the foot by way of the lymphatics. However, if the distal digit becomes necrotic, the flexor tendon sheath may be entered.

After the initial break in the skin, the rate of spread of the infection depends on the virulence of the pathogenic bacteria and the degree of ischemia. Indolent small infections may be confined to the tissues adjacent to the nail for a long time. Relief of infections near the nails usually requires removal of a portion of the nail, which must be done cautiously, or further tissue damage may be caused.

Toes

Toe deformities seem more common in diabetics than in the general population (Fig. 23–21) in part because of neuropathy involving the nerve supply to the small intrinsic muscles of the foot. Neuropathy of motor nerves supplying the lumbrical muscles and the interossei results in claw toes, hammer toes, crowding of toes, and exaggeration of bunions and bunionettes. Less weight is borne on the toes, and more is borne on the metatarsal heads. The angular prominences are susceptible to skin-on-shoe friction. Friction is ignored in the insensitive foot, and blisters, ulcers, and ulcerated calluses appear (Fig. 23–22).

Cock-Up Deformity

Cock-up deformity is seen in the great toe. The interphalangeal joint is flexed, and the metatarsophalangeal joint is extended. The deformity appears to be caused by an imbalance between the flexor and extensor muscles of the great toe. In the diabetic patient ulceration of the callus on the dorsum of the interphalangeal joint may quickly permit the joint to become infected.

Hammer Toe

In hammer toe, the metatarsophalangeal joint of the digit is extended, and the proxi-

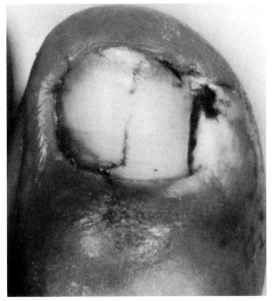

Figure 23–19 ■ Ingrowing nail with infection and granulation tissue of medial nail wall and cellulitis near base of nail.

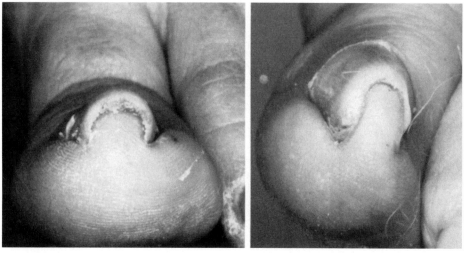

Figure 23–20 ■ Type of nail that is particularly hazardous in diabetic patient. It starts from wide base at nail root and incurves distally, pinching nail bed. These two nails form arcs of greater than 200 degrees at distal toe. If neglected, medial and lateral nail margins may meet beyond distal toe, forming full circle and brittle claw.

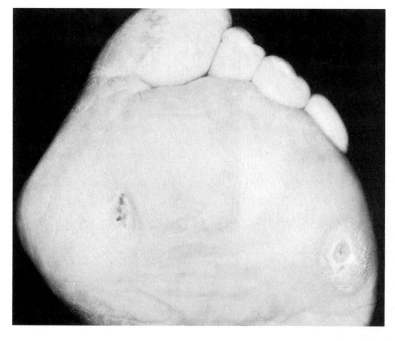

Figure 23–21 ■ Diabetic foot with crowding of toes, hammer toes (note position of nails), bunion, and distal plantar calluses.

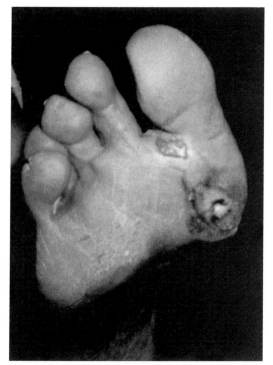

Figure 23–22 ■ Concentrated weight bearing in intrinsic minus foot with resultant ulcer over first metatarsal head.

mal interphalangeal joint is flexed. A painful corn (clavus) overlies the bony prominence of the proximal interphalangeal joint (Fig. 23–23). When the clavus ulcerates, septic arthritis of the proximal interphalangeal joint

may result. Occasionally calluses and penetrating ulcers may develop on the tips of the toe, which in the hammer toe is subject to friction on the insole of the shoe.

Varus Deformity of Toes

Varus deformity, in which the third, fourth, and fifth toes drift medially, may cause nails to gouge adjacent toes, producing small ulcers. Crowding, sometimes with overlap, causes skin friction of toe on toe.

Web Infections

Web infections are particularly hazardous, because they may occur without preexisting anatomic deformity. They may simply occur because of poor foot hygiene and accumulation of moist detritus in the webs, fissuring of skin, and entrance of infection. Infections beginning in the interdigital webs are especially dangerous because of the proximity of the digital arteries and because of ready access to the deeper structures of the foot by way of the lumbrical tendons.

Heloma Molle

Heloma molle is a soft corn between the toes caused by a combination of osteoarthritis of the toe and crowding. The most common location is on the lateral side of the base of the fourth toe from pressure and friction of the

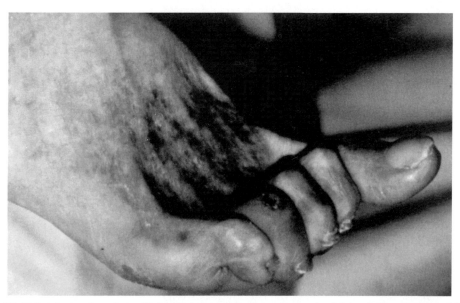

Figure 23–23 ■ Intrinsic minus foot with hammer toes and ulcer over proximal interphalangeal joint of fourth toe. Such ulcers can readily enter joint.

adjacent head of the proximal phalanx of the fifth toe. Heloma molle can occur in other areas where a knobby joint of one toe crowds in on an adjoining toe (Fig. 23–24). Heloma molle can lead to web space abscess.

Distal Foot

Hallux Valgus

Hallux valgus is a deformity of the great toe at the metatarsophalangeal joint. The hallux deviates laterally (adduction) in relation to the first metatarsal shaft and head. A bony prominence, exostosis, appears over the head of the metatarsal medially, and a swollen bursa forms. Erosion and ulceration of the skin over the bony prominence allow spread into a joint or into the lateral plantar space (Fig. 23–25).

Tailor's Bunion

Tailor's bunion (bunionette of the fifth toe) is an exostosis of the lateral part of the fifth metatarsal head often associated with varus deformity of the fifth toe. As in hallux valgus, ulceration may occur in the diabetic with this deformity, and infection may enter the bursa. Subsequently the infection may spread along the abductor hallucis and flexor hallucis bre-

vis muscles, causing lateral plantar space infections. More indolent infections can erode the metatarsophalangeal joint and enter the joint with resultant septic arthritis and osteomyelitis.

Distal Foot Calluses

Distal foot calluses are highly predictive of ulceration in the diabetic[19] (Fig. 23–26). Ulceration of the calluses causes mal perforans, which is discussed later in this chapter. The majority of foot calluses occur under the metatarsal heads. The first, second, and fifth joints are involved in that order. All of the patients with calluses exert maximum loads at the site of the ulcer. See also Chapter 6 for a discussion of detecting loads and pressure points.

Middle Part of Foot

The middle part of the foot is not as subject to calluses and deformities with ulcerations as are the toes but is frequently injured by penetrating objects. In the patient with advanced diabetes who cannot see well and cannot feel pain, infection spreads either directly to the central plantar space or along collagenous septa that connect the dermis to the

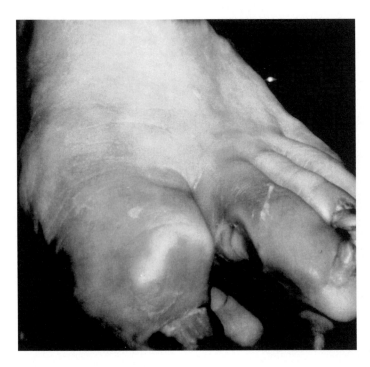

Figure 23–24 ■ Heloma molle of base of second toe from pressure of deformed adjacent interphalangeal joint of hallux.

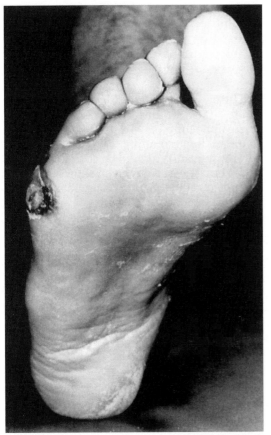

Figure 23–25 ■ Ulcerated callus at bunionette. Amputation of fifth ray was required because of penetration to joint. Ulcerated bunionette often is associated with shoes that are too snug.

plantar fascia. Inadequate circulation and failure to put the foot at rest contribute to worsening of the infection. Central plantar space abscesses can rupture in the sole of the middle part of the foot.

When Charcot foot collapses into a rocker sole, the weight on walking can be concentrated on the middle of the sole rather than on the metatarsal heads. Midsole ulcers may result.

Heel

Because of the bony prominences of the calcaneus, the heel is sometimes the site of neurotrophic ulcers. When ulceration and gangrene occur in the heel, the foot is seldom salvageable because debridement and amputations in this area often preclude functional weight bearing. Ulcers and patches of gangrene can develop on the posterolateral sur-

face of the heel as the immobile foot of the supine patient lies abducted on the mattress (Fig. 23–27). Lesions of the more posterior portion of the heel usually indicate excessive walking on the insensitive foot (Fig. 23–28). Heel lesions present exceedingly difficult surgical problems. Leg or thigh amputations are often necessary.

Question of Prophylactic Surgery

Many of the aforementioned abnormalities that can later lead to a break in the skin, infection, and progression to gangrene and major debridements and amputations are seen in younger diabetics, perhaps at a time when neuropathy is insignificant and arterial flow is adequate. Commonly these deformities are ignored at this time because they are being tolerated. Later, when they are being poorly tolerated, elective correction is hazardous and may itself precipitate disaster. Serious consideration should be given to correction of deformities early.[1] Most of them can be palliated and the difficulty deferred

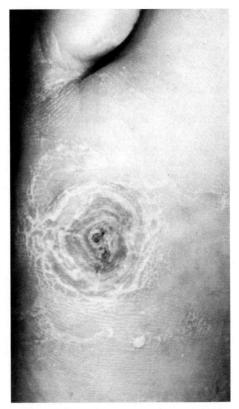

Figure 23–26 ■ Callus of distal part of lateral sole. Cracking and fissuring allow entry of bacteria.

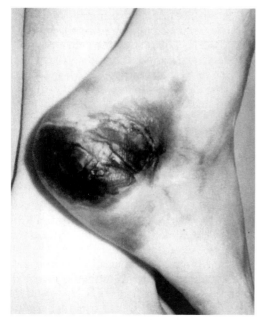

Figure 23–27 ■ Gangrene of heel in bedridden diabetic patient caused by weight of immobile neuropathic foot on mattress.

The following are requirements for prophylactic operations for toe and foot deformities in diabetes. Amputation and debridements for infection and gangrene are discussed in Chapters 28 and 29.

1. The deformity should no longer be amenable to foot maintenance techniques such as nail clipping, protuberance padding, and callus trimming.
2. The deformity should be of such a character that ulceration can be expected or may have already occurred despite a good, supervised foot maintenance program.
3. If the foot is ischemic, no procedure should be done unless revascularization has been successful (see Chapter 26).
4. The operation should be definitive and the deformity permanently corrected. For example, when a nail or portion of a nail needs to be removed, the corresponding

by good podiatric treatment and follow-up (see Chapters 20 and 33). The physician should take into consideration the intelligence and educability of the patient, opportunity for observation, general condition and associated systemic diseases, age, occupation, activity, and evaluation of circulation, and neuropathy and should definitively treat many more of the nail, toe, and distal foot abnormalities while the opportunity exists. Treatment after entry of infection and beginning local spread is often unavailing.

The nail, toe, and distal foot abnormalities in the diabetic foot are numerically so overwhelming that not all of them can be attended to, but certainly lesions that have already given rise to minor infections should be corrected. With the passage of time, ingrown nails, incurving nails, bunions, calluses, and hammer toes only become worse. After a minor infection arising in a friction ulcer has been contained and the ulcer has healed, the scar is more vulnerable to later friction and is likely to ulcerate again. The scar epithelium is less durable than the originally intact skin. The capillaries and arterioles beneath this epithelium have been thrombosed, and on healing they only partly recanalize and reform.

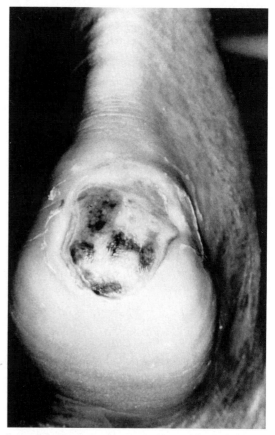

Figure 23–28 ■ Heel ulcer began as blister after one episode of excessive walking in patient with severe neuropathy.

generative area of the nail should also be removed.

5. Simple operations should be used. Osteoplastic operations and tendon transfers require more tissue handling than do the more simple amputations, osteotomies, ostectomies, and removal of exostoses.

6. Scar on weight-bearing sites should be avoided. In distal toe amputations the plantar flap should be longer than the dorsal flap. Incisions for removal of metatarsal heads should be made in the dorsum of the foot.

7. Muscle imbalances should be avoided. An amputation through the middle phalanx of a toe will often result in the toe being pulled into extension unless an extensor tenotomy is also done.

Major Infections

Mead and Mueller[17] recognize three basic anatomic types of major foot infection. These three types, which represent different problems and require different treatments, are (1) abscess occurring in the deep spaces of the foot, chiefly in the central plantar space; (2) nonsuppurative phlegmon of the dorsum of the foot; and (3) mal perforans ulcer of the plantar surface of the foot. In a prospective study of major foot infections in 300 diabetic patients, Isakov et al.[12] found that the initial anatomic site of the lesions resulting in amputations in diabetics was as follows: digits, 62.2%; distal foot under metatarsal heads, 8.0%; midfoot and heel, 8.5%; dorsum of foot, 3.3%; and ankle or lower leg, 5.7%.

Central Plantar Space Abscess

Central plantar space abscess can be the most devastating infection in the foot. Infection may enter the deep plantar space in several ways. Direct penetration by foreign bodies in the insensitive foot may not be recognized until the abscess is well established and has produced swelling so pronounced that it can be seen or can prevent putting on shoes.

Web space infections may begin with superficial breaks in the skin caused by fungus infections or by maceration associated with poor hygiene. Infection in the web space extends to the bursa of the lumbrical muscle then into the central plantar space. Infec-

tions anywhere in the toes may spread into the central plantar space by means of suppurative tenosynovitis of the flexor tendon sheath.

Of Bose's[3] 240 cases of plantar abscess, 70 began as initial lesions near the nail or nail bed, 140 began as web space infections, and 30 were caused by direct penetration of the soles.

Once the infection is established in the plantar space, the characteristic signs of plantar abscess appear. The longitudinal arch and the skin creases disappear, and the area of the longitudinal arch may bulge. The sole of the foot becomes edematous. Frequently in the diabetic patient, pain and tenderness are absent and ambulation may continue, adding dependency and the milking action of motion to other factors influencing spread of the infection. In a few days edema of the dorsum of the foot appears. The usual systemic signs of severe infection such as fever and malaise occur. Loss of diabetic control and ketoacidosis are often present. The appearance of glucosuria is sometimes the first abnormality noted by the patient and even sometimes is the feature that precipitates a visit to the physician.

At the proximal end of the central plantar space, the long flexor tendons of the toes are again surrounded by bursa sheaths. After exiting from the plantar space, the tendons lie posterior to the medial malleolus. Through this route infection may be carried to the leg.

Thrombotic obliteration of small- and medium-sized vessels may occur in established plantar abscess, resulting in progressive necrosis of the plantar fascia, tendon, and tendon sheath. If extensive, this necrosis may prohibit salvage of the foot. The plantar digital arteries of the second, third, and fourth toes arise from the plantar arch; with nearby infection, trombotic occlusion of the plantar arch can appear and lead to necrosis of all or portions of those toes, particularly the middle toe.

The *lateral* and *medial plantar spaces* contain the abductor and short flexor muscles of the first and fifth toes. In addition to infection by direct penetrating trauma, infection may enter these spaces from infected bunions. Frequently these difficulties start with new shoes, which abrade the skin in the first and fifth metatarsophalangeal areas. Penetration through the subcutaneous tissue and erosion of the joint capsule with septic arthri-

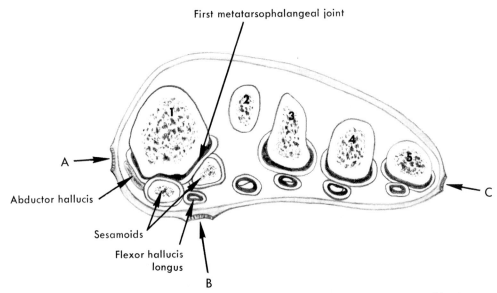

First metatarsophalangeal joint

A →

Abductor hallucis

Sesamoids

Flexor hallucis
longus

B

→ C

Figure 23-29 ■ Common modes of spread of infection in distal foot. *A,* Infection from ulcerated bunion may enter lateral plantar space or first metatarsophalangeal joint fairly readily. Joint infection then can penetrate into central plantar space. *B,* Mal perforans fixes flexor tendons. With progression of infection, plantar space or joint may be entered. *C,* Ulcerated tailor's bunion finds meager tissue barrier to entry into fifth metatarsophalangeal joint.

tis may follow (Fig. 23–29). Medial and lateral plantar space abscesses seldom spread into the central plantar space.

Dorsal Foot Phlegmon

The extensor tendons are not encased in sheaths but lie in loose areolar tissue on the dorsum of the foot. Deep to the extensor tendons, a dense fascia overlies the interossei and metatarsal muscles. The extensor tendons are covered by a thin superficial fascia, which is continuous with the extensor retinaculum of the anterior ankle. This fascia serves to contain the tendons and prevent bowstringing.

Spread in the dorsum of the foot is by the lymphatics. At first, the soft tissues of the dorsum become red and edematous. Again, as in the diabetic foot in general, pain and tenderness depend on the degree of neuropathy. The edema may be of impressive proportions in diabetics with neuropathy, whose lack of pain permits dependency and motion. The dorsal phlegmon of the diabetic foot does not differ from cellulitis in nondiabetics except that the infection is perpetuated and spread by continuing use of the foot in diabetics with neuropathy, whereas persons with normal sensation elevate and rest the foot of their own volition. With infective occlusions

of small vessels in the skin and lack of opportunity to develop collateral flow, the result may be necrosis of the skin overlying the phlegmonous area. Infections that may be controlled in nondiabetics lead in the diabetic, with microangiopathy, to death of tissue.

Mal Perforans

Mal perforans is a chronic, indolent ulcer of the sole of the foot, usually over the head of the first, second, or fifth metatarsal (Fig. 23–30). Ordinarily it is caused by ulceration of a preexisting callus. After the ulceration occurs, the hard, thickened area of hyperkeratinization continues to surround the crater. When seen, mal perforans is uniformly associated with neuropathy and probably is a direct consequence of it. Most of the patients with mal perforans do not have ischemia.[7] Characteristically the mal perforans implies severe neuropathy in the presence of good blood flow.

The initial calluses are the result of concentrated weight bearing, chronic friction, and minor irritation in the insensitive foot. The high incidence of calluses in the diabetic foot is associated with a combination of sensory deficit and neurogenic small-muscle atrophy. The small-muscle atrophy produces

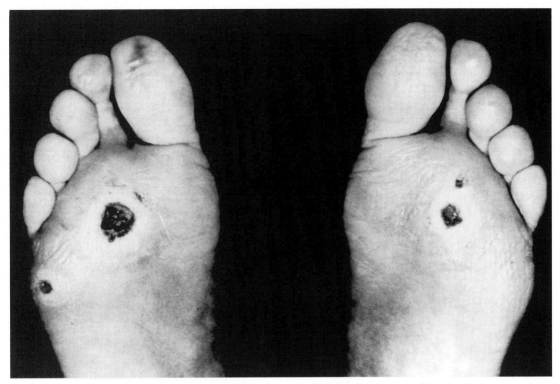

Figure 23–30 ■ Mal perforans ulcers of both feet over metatarsal heads.

abnormal foot alignment, which forces the body weight to be borne on surfaces poorly designed, anatomically, for that purpose. Fissuring and cracking in the calluses allow a variety of organisms to enter. The subsequent minor infection is ignored, and continued walking results in central excavation of the callus.

Penetration of the subcutaneous tissue in the sole of the foot is limited from lateral spread by the dense fibrous septa that partition the subcutaneous fat into lobules, giving resiliency to the walking surface. For a long time deep penetration may be limited to skin and subcutaneous tissue. The plantar fascia is partly deficient over the metatarsal heads, because the fibers of the plantar aponeurosis split and pass between the metatarsal heads. The flexor tendon may then form the base of the ulcer. The flexor tendon becomes fixed to its sheath and to the underlying metatarsophalangeal joint capsule and periosteum. Ultimately, the tendon is eroded and the joint entered, with subsequent septic arthritis and osteomyelitis. The depth of penetration of the plantar ulcer is often underestimated on clinical examination. More of them penetrate to deeper structures than is ordinarily sus-

pected.[11] Newman et al.,[20] by bone biopsy and bone culture, found osteomyelitis in 68% of diabetic foot ulcers. Only 32% of those with osteomyelitis had been diagnosed clinically by the referring physician.

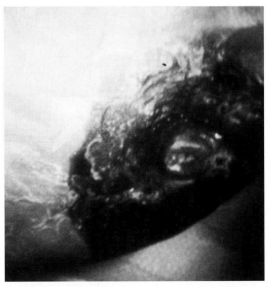

Figure 23–31 ■ Gangrene spreading radially from mal perforans after superficial femoral artery thrombosis.

When bone is identified by probing, specialized radiography and radionuclide studies to identify osteomyelitis may be unnecessary.[11]

Episodes of quiescence alternate with flareups of infection. The arterial circulation is usually good; otherwise, this infection would not be tolerated. Gangrene of the skin spreading radially from the mal perforans center often means that occlusion of a major vessel (superficial femoral, popliteal) higher in the leg has occurred and is an indication for angiography (Fig. 23–31).

REFERENCES

1. Armstrong DG, Lavery LA, Stern S, Harkless LB: Is prophylactic diabetic foot surgery dangerous? J Foot Ankle Surg 35:585, 1996.
2. Beach KW, Bedford GR, Bergelin RO, et al: Progression of lower extremity arterial occlusive disease in type II diabetes mellitus. Diabetes Care 11(Suppl):464, 1988.
3. Bose K: A surgical approach for the diabetic foot. Int Orthop 3:177, 1979.
4. Bresäter L-E, Welin L, Romanus B: Foot pathology and risk factors for diabetic foot disease in elderly men. Diabetes Res Clin Pract 32:103, 1996.
5. Delbridge L, Cterecteko G, Gowler C, et al: The aetiology of diabetic neuropathic ulceration of the foot. Br J Surg 72:1, 1985.
6. Edelson GW, Armstrong DG, Lavery LA, Caicco G: The acutely infected diabetic foot is not adequately evaluated in an inpatient setting. J Am Podiatr Med Assoc 87:260, 1997.
7. Fernando DJ, et al: Risk factors for nonischemic foot ulceration in diabetic neuropathy. Diabet Med 8:223, 1990.
8. Frykberg RG: Neuropathic orthopathy: The diabetic Charcot's foot. Diabetes Educ 9:17, 1984.
9. Gooding GAW, Stess RM, Graf PM, et al: Sonography of the sole of the foot: Evidence for loss of foot pad thickness in diabetes and its relationship to ulceration of the foot. Invest Radiol 21:45, 1986.
10. Grant JBC: An Atlas of Anatomy, 6th ed. Baltimore: Williams & Wilkins, 1972.
11. Grayson ML, Gibbons GW, Balogh K, et al: Probing to bone in infected pedal ulcers: A clinical sign of underlying osteomyelitis in diabetic patients. JAMA 273:721, 1995.
12. Isakov E, Budoragin N, Shenhav S, et al: Anatomical sites of foot lesions resulting in amputation among diabetics and nondiabetics. Am J Phys Med Rehabil 74:130, 1995.
13. Kastrup J, Lassen NA, Parving H-H: Diabetic microangiopathy: A factor enhancing the functional significance of peripheral occlusive arteriosclerotic disease. Clin Physiol 4:367, 1984.
14. Kumar S, Ashe HA, Darnell LN, et al: The prevalence of foot ulceration and its correlation in type 2 diabetic patients: A population-based study. Diabetic Med 11:480, 1994.
15. Lee BY, Guerra J, Civelek B: Compartment syndrome in the diabetic foot. Adv Wound Care 8:36, 1995.
16. Lewis BL: Microscopic studies of fetal and mature nail and surrounding soft tissue. Arch Dermatol Syph 70:752, 1954.
17. Meade JW, Mueller CB: Major infections of the foot. Med Times 96:154, 1968.
18. Meyerson MS: Management of compartment syndrome of the foot. Clin Orthop 271:239, 1991.
19. Murray HV, Young MJ, Hollis S, Boulton AJ: The association between callus formation, high pressures, and neuropathy in diabetic foot ulceration. Diabet Med 13:979, 1996.
20. Newman LG, Waller J, Palestro CJ, et al: Unsuspected osteomyelitis in diabetic foot ulcers, diagnosis and monitoring by leukocyte scanning with indium oxyquinoline. JAMA 266:1246, 1991.
21. Plummer ES, Albert SG: Foot care assessment in patients with diabetes: A screening algorithm for patient education and referral. Diabetes Educ 21:47, 1995.
22. Spencer F, Sage R, Graner J: The incidence of foot pathology in a diabetic population. J Am Podiatr Assoc 75:590, 1985.
23. Tooke JE, Brash PD: Microvascular aspects of the diabetic foot disease. Diabet Med 13:526, 1996.
24. Walsh CH, Soler NG, Fitzgerald MG, et al: Association of foot lesions with retinopathy in patients with newly diagnosed diabetes. Lancet 1:878, 1975.
25. Worth CT, McEwen JA: A follow-up study of diabetic patients with foot problems in Nottingham, 1971–1978. Practitioner 226:2085, 1982.
26. Valente LA, Nelson MS: Patient education for diabetic patients. An integral part of quality health care. J Am Podiatr Med Assoc 85:177, 1995.

Chapter 24

MEDICAL MANAGEMENT OF DIABETIC PATIENTS DURING THE PERIOPERATIVE PERIOD

■ Molly C. Carr and Irl B. Hirsch

Recent surveys estimate that as many as 15.7 million Americans have diabetes, while older estimates suggest that diabetic patients have a 50% chance of undergoing surgery at least sometime during their life.[32, 39] We suspect that this risk of surgery has increased as mortality rates for diabetes-related deaths have decreased over the past 20 years allowing diabetic patients longer life spans.[35] If one considers all of the operations a patient with diabetes may need over the course of a lifetime related to one of the microvascular or macrovascular complications (in addition to non–diabetes-related surgery), the chance for surgery in a diabetic individual is likely much higher than 50%.

The prevalence of peripheral vascular disease (PVD) and distal symmetric polyneuropathy with diabetes is important to appreciate. Diabetic patients, who account for more than 50% of all nontraumatic lower limb amputations in the United States, represent only 3% of the population.[33] Lower limb surgery is responsible for more than one half of all types of surgery in diabetic patients. From 1993 to 1995, about 67,000 amputations were performed each year among people with diabetes,[32] and greater than 75% of total hospital bed days used for patients with diabetes were for either "chronic ulcer of the skin or other peripheral vascular disease" compared to 30% in nondiabetic patients.[7] Neuropathy is present in 8% of diabetic patients at diagnosis, but after 25 years one half of the patients with diabetes have developed symptoms of neuropathy.[3] Therefore, if only one half of the 15.7 million people in the United States with diabetes live 20 years (a conservative estimate), there would be approximately 4 million diabetic individuals with PVD and neuropathy. This is consistent with the estimate that 25% of diabetic patients will eventually develop foot or leg problems.

Most diabetic patients requiring lower extremity surgery will have type 2 diabetes (previously termed non–insulin-dependent diabetes), albeit many will be insulin requiring. It is important for the health care provider to make the distinction between type 1 diabetes (previously called insulin-dependent) and type 2 diabetes. Without insulin, patients with the former condition will develop ketosis and severe hyperglycemia, whereas patients with the latter will usually have more significant hyperglycemia without significant ketosis. A position statement was recently published by the American Diabetes Association that set forth a new diabetes classification system.[38] The terms insulin-dependent and non–insulin-dependent have been eliminated in favor of type 1 and type 2 diabetes, respectively. The serum glucose criteria for the diagnosis of diabetes has been changed to a fasting glucose greater than or equal to 126 mg/dL (7.0 mmol/L) or a nonfasting serum glucose greater than or equal to 200 mg/dL (11.1 mmol/L) on two occasions. Unfortunately, this system of diabetic classification is sometimes difficult phenotypically if individuals do not fit into a single class, such as in a thin, adult-onset, insulin-requiring patient. The disease label is less important than understanding the pathogenesis and treating the patient effectively, which in most cases means treating perioperatively with insulin.

Thus it is important for all health care professionals to be familiar with the medical management of the diabetic patient having surgery. There is still controversy regarding both the degree of metabolic control required during the perioperative period and the medical regimen that would be best suited for a specific situation. Laxity of blood glucose control has been viewed as acceptable by many because it avoids the risks of hypoglycemia, the most feared metabolic complication of surgery. A 1995 survey of 172 anesthesiologists in the United Kingdom[14] revealed that attitudes toward the perioperative management of diabetes have changed significantly since 1985. The study found that a greater percentage of anesthesiologists are attempting to maintain bedside glucose levels below 180 mg/dL and that there is a major trend away from the use of combined glucose, insulin, and potassium (GIK) infusions[24] in favor of separate glucose and insulin infusions.[14]

Because of a lack of controlled studies, there is no consensus on the optimum manner in which to manage the metabolic changes in patients with diabetes that occur during the perioperative period. However, if certain fundamental principles (e.g., the metabolic effects of anesthesia, the pharmacokinetics and dynamics of subcutaneous and intravenous insulin, and glucose re-

quirements during the perioperative period) are better understood, a more rational approach to the perioperative management of patients with diabetes could be developed.

Pathophysiology of Hyperglycemia

High glucose levels (>250 mg/dL) allow for increased rates of postoperative infection and decreased rates of wound healing. Poor wound healing is a well-established problem in diabetic patients and hyperglycemia contributes in several ways. Hyperglycemia has been shown to both inhibit polymorphonuclear leukocyte phagocytic activity and decrease the antibody response to *Staphylococcus* toxin.[20] A large study of 1,042 patients undergoing total hip replacement found a significant increase in the postoperative wound infection rate in diabetic versus nondiabetic patients (11% vs. 2%).[42] Elevated glucose levels act to decrease wound tensile strength as well as decrease phagocytosis by macrophages.[45] Hyperglycemia has also been shown to slow the influx of fibroblasts, new vessels, and nutrients into the healing wound.[17] Furthermore, high glucose levels that exceed the renal threshold (160 to 180 mg/dL) cause spillage of glucose into the urine leading to an osmotic diuresis. This causes loss of intra- and extracellular water as well as electrolytes. However, there are no controlled clinical studies to show that uncontrolled diabetes results in an inferior outcome in terms of these end points or prolonged hospital stay. Few would argue that acute complications of uncontrolled diabetes might be avoided by providing adequate attention to the various metabolic parameters.

Metabolic Response to Surgery and Anesthesia

Hyperglycemia is not uncommon in the nondiabetic inpatient population.[29] Elevated blood glucose levels are caused by both (relative) insulin deficiency and insulin resistance.[20] Insulin secretion has consistently been found to be blunted with general anesthesia, and the increase in insulin resistance is presumed to be secondary to elevated counterregulatory hormone levels. The exact stress response is a function of the degree of trauma and can be modified by anesthesia. Therefore, declaring that surgery causes an increase in the four principal counterregulatory hormones (glucagon, the catecholamines epinephrine and norepinephrine, growth hormone, and cortisol) is an oversimplification of a complex metabolic process. Studies to date have shown remarkable variations in the individual counterregulatory hormone response to surgery,[20, 30] and this is likely the result of variations in surgical procedure, surgical technique, and type of anesthesia used.

The individual effects of the counterregulatory hormones include the following: (1) glucagon and epinephrine both stimulate gluconeogenesis (because epinephrine also inhibits pancreatic insulin secretion, there is decreased peripheral glucose uptake with catecholamine hypersecretion); (2) cortisol increases both gluconeogenesis and the resistance to glucose uptake by muscle; and (3) growth hormone secretion is somewhat more complicated, because it exerts both insulin-like and insulin-antagonistic effects. The former effect is weak and of minor importance, whereas the latter becomes evident after a lag period of 2 to 3 hours and induces insulin resistance in both the liver and peripheral tissues.[10, 28]

Another important aspect of the counterregulatory hormones is their effect on fat metabolism. Epinephrine, cortisol, and growth hormone all stimulate lipolysis, whereas glucagon has little, if any, effect on fat catabolism.[25] Insulin is the only antilipolytic hormone. The combination of absolute insulin deficiency, as seen in type 1 diabetes, and generalized counterregulatory hormone excess can potentially lead to metabolic decompensation with unrestrained lipolysis and ketoacidosis. It is therefore not surprising that if sufficient fluids are administered to the patient with type 1 diabetes (with normal renal function), significant ketoacidosis may occur without the typical elevations in plasma glucose concentrations. A condition known as "euglycemic diabetic ketoacidosis"[31] may account for up to 17% of all episodes of diabetic ketoacidosis.

Preoperative Evaluation

Preoperative issues may be separated into two categories: (1) the assessment of the acute metabolic status and (2) the evaluation of the chronic complications of diabetes that may affect the surgical outcome. With regard to the former issue, because of the potential deleterious metabolic effects of surgery, significant preoperative hyperglycemia and electrolyte abnormalities should be corrected. Therefore, preoperative plasma glucose level and electrolyte concentrations, in addition to urinary ketone levels, should be assessed, as significant ketosis may occur without the typical elevations in plasma glucose concentrations. Significant metabolic instability (e.g., ketosis, blood glucose levels >400 mg/dL, hypokalemia) will require admission before elective surgery, although most patients may be treated successfully with admission on the day of the procedure.

The complete assessment of the various chronic complications should ideally be completed before admission. Cardiovascular disease is the most common cause of perioperative mortality among patients with diabetes. Patients with diabetes are two to five times as likely to report having heart disease than their nondiabetic counterparts, and about two thirds of deaths in people with diabetes are caused by cardiovascular disease.[44] Although extremely common, heart disease in patients with diabetes can be difficult to diagnose because frequently these patients do not manifest classic cardiac symptoms.

The optimum preoperative cardiovascular assessment is controversial,[12, 16] in part because of the high frequency of asymptomatic myocardial ischemia in this population,[27] but also because of the relatively low predictive value of routine cardiovascular evaluation, especially in patients with renal disease. The American Heart Association recently set forth 1997–1998 guidelines[12] that recommend that all patients with diabetes be considered "intermediate cardiovascular risk" even without cardiac symptoms and "high cardiovascular risk" if diabetic patients have symptoms of angina, arrhythmias, or decompensated congestive heart failure. Cardiac evaluation for diabetic patients prior to a low-risk procedure (i.e., cataract surgery or superficial procedures) is usually not necessary. With intermediate risk (orthopedic, head and neck, intraperitoneal, and intrathoracic surgery) and high-risk procedures (peripheral vascular, aortic, and other major vascular surgery) the American Heart Association guidelines recommend a more thorough cardiac evaluation. This topic is too extensive to be covered in greater detail but excellent reviews are available.[11–13]

Preoperative evaluation also requires the assessment of diabetic nephropathy. A serum creatinine concentration is not a sufficient indicator for renal disease in diabetic patients because its level usually remains normal until the nephropathy is advanced.[37] Because the first harbinger of diabetic nephropathy is proteinuria, dipstick for urinary protein should be included in the minimum assessment of renal disease. It is now well established that persistent proteinuria with as little as 30 mg/24 hr is a strong predictor of nephropathy in patients with types 1 and 2 diabetes.[8] Albumin excretion rates between 30 and 300 mg/24 hr are called "microalbuminuria." Unfortunately, dipstick-positive proteinuria does not usually occur until urinary albumin excretion exceeds 250 to 300 mg/24 hr. Therefore, the American Diabetes Association now recommends yearly assessments for microalbuminuria for all patients with diabetes.[4] The preoperative assessment of proteinuria is important for two reasons. First, any potential nephrotic agent should be avoided for the patient with proteinuria. In addition, proteinuria is a predictor of mortality (mainly cardiovascular) in patients with type 2 diabetes.

Autonomic neuropathy should also be assessed before surgery. One report showed that diabetic patients with autonomic dysfunction had increased risk of perioperative hypotension.[6] Therefore, routine preoperative history should include questioning about the typical symptoms of autonomic dysfunction (resting tachycardia, early satiety, abdominal bloating and pain, gustatory sweating, diarrhea [often nocturnal] alternating with constipation and orthostatic hypotension). Autonomic dysfunction may be measured with much greater sensitivity by measuring variation in RR interval (between QRS complexes on electrocardiogram) during deep breathing, heart rate response to Valsalva maneuver, as well as the blood pressure and heart rate response to standing.[15]

The need for medical consultation will vary depending on the surgeon's comfort with the various preoperative issues. Because of the complexity of medical problems, many of these patients should be followed by their family practitioner, internist, or endocrinologist during the perioperative period. Surgery in patients with diabetes is another situation that requires a team approach for the optimum care. Indeed, more hospitals are now using a diabetes clinical nurse specialist to consult with all patients admitted with diabetes.

Anesthesia and Hypoglycemia

Selection of the anesthetic modality is the prerogative of the anesthesiologist and is based on the type of surgery, the medical and surgical risks, and individual preferences without primary consideration of the presence of diabetes. Modern inhalation anesthesia has relatively little effect on metabolic regulation; spinal, epidural, and peripheral nerve blocks produce the least disturbance in glycemic control.[20] Ankle block is preferred for most patients requiring foot surgery. The prudent use of preoperative medication, including sedation and muscle relaxants, facilitates the anesthetic induction. These agents should be carefully titrated in elderly patients.

Any type of sedation may also impair symptom recognition of hypoglycemia. It is well documented that asymptomatic hypoglycemia is a common event in diabetic patients who are not receiving central nervous system depressants. One study documented a 29% incidence (each night) of asymptomatic nocturnal hypoglycemia (defined as plasma glucose concentration <55 mg/dL).[36] The Diabetes Control and Complications Trial (DCCT) has described their experience with 1,441 subjects spanning 6½ years screening for severe hypoglycemia (an event with symptoms consistent with hypoglycemia in which the patient required the assistance of another person).[40] These authors reported that 35% of conventionally treated (standard community care) diabetic patients have had a hypoglycemic event requiring assistance. There are few published data regarding perioperative hypoglycemia. One review[22] has found a 13% incidence of perioperative hypoglycemia (blood glucose level <60 mg/dL) in a group of 85 patients with type 1 diabetes. Therefore, any patient receiving a glucose-lowering agent and any sedation requires regular blood glucose monitoring.

Type 1 Diabetes

There is general agreement that patients with type 1 diabetes receiving general anesthesia should receive their insulin as a continuous intravenous (IV) infusion.[1, 21] Insulin availability after subcutaneous insulin injections is unpredictable in the usual outpatient setting[19]; in the perioperative setting, with fluid shifts and hemodynamic changes, insulin absorption is even more erratic. A study comparing subcutaneous and intravenous insulin use in the perioperative period in type 1 patients showed significantly higher mean glucose levels and wide swings in glucose levels with subcutaneous insulin even with aggressive monitoring.[26] Intravenous insulin infusions have been shown to be safe and provide improved metabolic control compared with perioperative subcutaneous insulin injections.[34, 43] Hypoglycemia also tends to be less of a problem with the use of an IV infusion because the more predictable and instantaneous insulin availability diminishes the risk of delivering an excessive amount of hormone.

Despite the agreement that patients with type 1 diabetes receiving general anesthesia should be administered insulin by IV infusion, subcutaneous insulin is often used.[22] Probably the primary reason for this is simply custom. Anesthesiologists frequently administer large IV boluses of insulin during the intraoperative period. Because the half-life of IV insulin is only 4 to 5 minutes, and the biologic half-life is less than 20 minutes,[41] this practice is not recommended. Besides wide swings in glucose levels another risk with IV insulin boluses is severe electrolyte shifts that could potentially cause iatrogenic complications. Our experience with short procedures (<1 hour) that require general anesthesia is that subcutaneous insulin is probably reasonable. There are few data to support this practice, but with the short duration of the procedure, it is reasonable to treat with a fraction of the NPH dose, all of the ultralente dose, or continuing with the basal rate with continuous subcutaneous insulin infusion (insulin pump).

The IV insulin infusion for an elective procedure with the patient under general anesthesia may be started on the morning of surgery. It is inappropriate to withhold insulin in the patient with type 1 diabetes. When serum insulin levels decline below a critical level, unrestrained hepatic lipolysis and ketogenesis may quickly develop into ketoacidosis. Basal insulin administration is required for patients with type 1 diabetes that are not eating. Because of its relatively short duration, subcutaneous regular insulin or in-

sulin lispro (see below) is best suited for anticipatory mealtime glycemic excursions. Therefore, if the operation is scheduled for late morning or during the afternoon, it is less cumbersome to initiate the basal insulin with an IV insulin infusion than to administer subcutaneous insulin. If the blood glucose concentration is less than 120 mg/dL, the insulin infusion should be delayed until it rises above this level.

Variable rate insulin infusions are considered by most to be the most simple and easily adaptable to patients with widely ranging insulin requirements (see Table 24–1). Regular insulin is diluted in normal saline at a concentration of 1 U/10 mL and dispensed by infusion pump. Most authors suggest initiating the infusion at 1.0 U/hr; however, we recommend beginning at 0.5 U/hr in thin women with type 1 diabetes, who tend to be more insulin sensitive. The infusion rate is adjusted in incremental steps of 0.3 U/hr based on bedside glucose measurements (see Table 24–2). A glucose infusion must be given in a separate infusion pump at a rate of 5 to 10 gm dextrose per hour (D5 1/2 NS or D10 1/2 NS at 100 mL/hr). The algorithm in Table 24–2 is a guide that we have found to be quite effective, but extremely high or low blood glucose levels will require adjustments. Table 24–3 is an option to consider when there are large changes in blood glucose. To avoid any problems with insulin adsorption to the plastic, 50 mL of the infusion mixture should be flushed through the tubing before it is connected to the patient.

Table 24–1 ■ VARIABLE RATE INTRAVENOUS INSULIN INFUSION PREPARATION

1. Mix 25 U regular human insulin into 250 mL normal saline solution (0.1 U/mL).
2. Flush 50 mL of the infusion mixture through the tubing.
3. Do not start insulin infusion until the blood glucose level is >120 mg/dL.
4. General guidelines for initial dose in patients with Type 1 diabetes: men, 1.0 U/hr; women, 0.5 U/hr Type 2 diabetes: 1.0 U/hr for all patients
5. Blood glucose levels should be measured hourly during and immediately after surgery.
6. Adjust insulin infusion using standard insulin algorithm (Table 24–2).
7. Do not stop insulin infusion until patient is able to tolerate food orally; at that time, give usual dose of premeal regular insulin (may give 4–8 U SC regular insulin before lunch if insulin is not usually given then).

Table 24-2 ■ STANDARD INSULIN ALGORITHM*

BLOOD GLUCOSE (mg/dL)	
<70	Turn off infusion for 15 min. Administer 10 gm glucose[†]
70–120	Decrease infusion by 3 mL/hr (0.3 U/hr)
121–180	No change in infusion rate
181–240	Increase infusion by 3 mL/hr (0.3 U/hr)
241–300	Increase infusion by 6 mL/hr (0.6 U/hr)
>300	Increase infusion by 10 mL/hr (1.0 U/hr)

* If patient's blood glucose is changing rapidly, use alternate insulin algorithm (Table 24–3) for large glycemic fluctuations. When blood glucose is no longer fluctuating by 60 mg/dL per hour then revert back to standard insulin algorithm.
[†] Restart infusion at 3 mL/hr (0.3 U/hr) after the blood glucose level is >100 (should be remeasured 15 min after turning off insulin infusion); if blood glucose is still <100 mg/dL, may wait another 15 min.

Sufficient glucose is required during the perioperative period both for basal energy requirements and for the prevention of hypoglycemia. Again, there are no data regarding the optimum quantity of glucose in diabetic patients. Most authors give 5 or 10 gm of glucose each hour. The larger glucose infusion rate is preferred by some because of the greater energy provided in addition to a more anabolic quantity of insulin required. If 5 gm of glucose is administered each hour in the presence of ketonuria and blood glucose levels are near target values, the glucose infusion should be increased to 10 gm/hr. The ketonuria in this situation is likely caused by a lack of glucose.

Bedside fingerstick measurements must be made every 1 to 2 hours, and the aim is for blood glucose levels between 120 and 180 mg/dL, but slightly higher targets (e.g., 150

to 200 mg/dL) are also acceptable. These values are chosen to minimize the risk of hypoglycemia and also to decrease the risk of excessive catabolism from insulin deficiency and hyperglycemia. Maintaining blood glucose levels less than 200 mg/dL will also diminish the deleterious effects of hyperglycemia, namely, impaired wound healing and strength, impaired phagocyte function, exacerbation of ischemic brain damage, and hyperosmolarity.

As a general guideline, most patients will require between 0.3 and 0.4 units of insulin per gram of glucose per hour to achieve targeted glucose goals.[2] Patients with foot infections often require 0.6 to 0.8 units of insulin per gram of glucose per hour. Insulin requirements will vary greatly depending on patient weight and degree of insulin resistance. Patients with severe liver or renal dysfunction may require a significantly lower insulin dose because the half-life of insulin is increased with the delayed metabolism of insulin. With a variable-rate insulin infusion, the rate may be increased or decreased, and targeted blood glucose levels can rapidly be achieved.

Another virtue of the variable-rate insulin infusion is the ease of managing the diabetes with postoperative vomiting. Vomiting may be related to anesthesia and surgery alone or to gastroparesis from the diabetes. If food is not tolerated, blood glucose levels may be easily managed without the guesswork involved with subcutaneous insulin. Because metoclopramide is the only antiemetic approved in the United States for the treatment of gastroparesis, it should be considered the drug of choice of the treatment of postoperative vomiting in diabetic patients.

The insulin analog lispro (Humalog; Eli Lilly, Indianapolis, IN) was introduced to the

Table 24-3 ■ ALTERNATE INSULIN ALGORITHM*

BLOOD GLUCOSE (mg/dL)	IF BG INCREASED >60 mg/dL/hr	IF BG DECREASED <60 mg/dL/hr
<70	N/A	Stop infusion[†]
71–120	No change	Decrease rate by 0.6 U/hr
121–180	Increase rate by 0.3 U/hr	Decrease rate by 0.3 U/hr
181–240	Increase rate by 0.6 U/hr	No change
241–300	Increase rate by 1.0 U/hr	No change
>300	Increase rate by 1.5 U/hr	No change

* When blood glucose is no longer fluctuating by 60 mg/dL per hour then revert back to standard insulin algorithm (Table 24–2).
[†] Stop infusion for 30 min. Administer 10 gm glucose. Recheck BG in 20 min and restart when BG >100 mg/dL. Restart infusion at 3 mL/hr (0.3 U/hr) after the blood glucose level is >100 (should be remeasured 15 min after turning off insulin infusion); if blood glucose is still <100 mg/dL, may wait another 15 min.

United States market in 1996. This new insulin analog is absorbed more quickly than the regular insulin now available. This allows for physiologic control because insulin lispro is absorbed in a similar rate as food absorption and better controls postprandial glucose excursions. Its onset of action is approximately 15 minutes when given subcutaneously and peaks in 1 hour, with an average duration of action of 3 to 4 hours as opposed to 6 to 8 hours with regular insulin. Studies using insulin lispro during the perioperative period are not available, but the more physiologic rapid absorption may lead to fewer hypoglycemic events, as observed in the ambulatory setting.[23] Insulin lispro may be particularly useful for correcting premeal hyperglycemia by administering additional insulin to the usual insulin dose.[19] In the perioperative period, this advantage could be particularly useful.

Another controversial issue regards the required frequency of metabolic monitoring. Most authors agree that with general anesthesia blood glucose and electrolyte levels should be measured just before and after surgery. While the patient is receiving the IV insulin infusion, we prefer to obtain bedside glucose determinations every hour during and immediately after surgery, and every 2 hours after that if there are no problems. Others believe it is safe to monitor less frequently.[1] There are no data investigating the optimum frequency of perioperative blood glucose monitoring. Urinary ketone levels should also be routinely measured in patients with type 1 diabetes. For patients who are not eating, urinary ketones should be measured daily until food is tolerated. This will identify any patient with early ketosis that may be exacerbated by starvation.

Recommendations for the perioperative management for the patient with type 1 diabetes having local anesthesia are less clear. For patients receiving ultralente insulin as their basal insulin or those using subcutaneous insulin infusion pumps, we find it easiest to continue with the home regimen during procedures requiring local anesthesia. For those using NPH or Lente at home, a fraction of the usual morning dose may be given at the usual time (e.g., one-half the usual dose of intermediate and short-acting insulin), a glucose infusion should be initiated, and bedside glucose levels should be monitored every hour during and immediately after the procedure. Variable-rate insulin infusion is also

acceptable although probably not necessary in this situation. As noted above, subcutaneous insulin for short (<1 hour) procedures using regular insulin can be done safely.

Type 2 Diabetes

Patients with type 2 diabetes comprise the majority of individuals requiring lower limb surgery. However, many patients with type 2 diabetes are insulin requiring and so metabolic control is achieved with the same principles of management as type 1 patients.

For procedures requiring general anesthesia, most authors agree that special treatment other than close blood glucose monitoring (hourly during surgery) is not required for patients whose diabetes is well controlled by diet therapy alone.[1, 2, 5, 20] Because of the overall hyperglycemic response to the surgery, the presence of a preexisting lower limb infection will contribute to insulin resistance, and therefore, many of these patients will require insulin to control their hyperglycemia. As mentioned previously, the insulin should be administered with a variable-rate IV insulin infusion. Targeted blood glucose concentrations are identical to those for patients with type 1 diabetes, and thus we suggest initiating insulin when the blood glucose level exceeds 200 mg/dL. This value is also chosen because fasting blood glucose levels greater than this manifest absolute deficiency with respect to insulin secretion.[9]

There is some disagreement regarding management strategies for patients requiring general anesthesia whose diabetes is well controlled with sulfonylureas. We agree with Alberti,[1] who recommends withholding all oral agents on the morning of surgery for procedures requiring either general or local anesthesia, because with the former, an insulin infusion will likely be required to control the hyperglycemia. If insulin is not instituted at the beginning of the procedure, it should be initiated when the blood glucose level exceeds 200 mg/dL. Although as a general rule, subcutaneous insulin should not be used for any patient receiving general anesthesia[1, 20] subcutaneous insulin appears safe for short procedures.

There have been extraordinary advances made in oral antihyperglycemic agents used to treat type 2 diabetes in the last decade. There are many more options now than the sulfonylureas and some have special considerations in the perioperative period.

The biguanide metformin (Glucophage; Bristol-Myers Squibb, Princeton, NJ) is an antihyperglycemic agent introduced onto the American market in 1994 (see Table 24–4). This class of drugs has a rare but serious side effect of lactic acidosis when used in patients with preexisting renal or hepatic dysfunction, with an average incidence of 0.03 per 1,000 patient years. Metformin should be discontinued immediately prior to and restarted 48 hours after the surgical procedure and reinitiated only when renal function has been assessed and found to be normal (metformin package insert). In 1998, the prescribing information was changed with regard to radiologic procedures using iodinated contrast media. Metformin should be discontinued at the time of radiologic studies and withheld for 48 hours after the procedures and reinstituted only after renal function has been found normal. In the case of emergent procedures, although there are no data available, it would be reasonable to discontinue metformin, hydrate the patient for as long as possible prior to surgery, and continue for at least 12 hours afterward.[18] Again, metformin should only be restarted a minimum of 48 hours postoperatively and the serum creatinine measured.

The first thiazolidinedione (Troglitazone; Parke-Davis, Parsippany, NJ) was released onto the U.S. market in 1997 as a unique class of oral hypoglycemics that increases peripheral tissue sensitivity to insulin. It acts to improve sensitivity to insulin in muscle and adipose tissue and inhibits hepatic gluconeogenesis. The thiazolidinediones are metabolized and excreted exclusively by the liver and so should not be used in patients with hepatic dysfunction. It is recommended

that the drug be discontinued before the surgical procedure and then restarted once the patient is eating.

The α-glucosidase inhibitor acarbose (Precose; Bayer, West Haven, CT) is an oral antihyperglycemic that binds to gut brush border enzymes and interferes with carbohydrate absorption. This action delays carbohydrate digestion and absorption and blunts postprandial rises in plasma glucose and insulin. The predominant side effects are flatulence, diarrhea, and abdominal discomfort. It has no benefit if patients are not eating and should be discontinued perioperatively if patients are NPO and restarted once patients are eating (acarbose package insert).

Repaglinide (Prandin; Novo Nordisk, Princeton, NJ) is the first agent in a new class of oral antihyperglycemic drugs called benzoic acid analogs. Although it is structurally unrelated to sulfonylurea drugs, it has a similar mechanism of stimulating insulin release from the pancreas. There is a similar risk of hypoglycemia with repaglinide as with the sulfonylurea drugs except with a short half-life of 1 hour and so must be taken before each meal. It is recommended that repaglinide be used cautiously in patients with impaired liver function (repaglinide package insert). Preoperatively, repaglinide should be withheld on the day of surgery in a manner similar to sulfonylureas.

Treatment decisions for patients with type 2 diabetes receiving local anesthesia are similar, except that patients with well-controlled diabetes who are treated with diet alone or diet with oral agents likely will not require additional insulin. One study showed that 93% of patients with type 2 diabetes (mean fasting blood glucose levels 133 mg/dL) can achieve acceptable blood glucose control without insulin.[24] Therefore, unless blood

Table 24–4 ■ ORAL ANTIHYPERGLYCEMIC DRUGS

DRUG CLASS	DURATION OF ACTION	TRADE NAME	GENERIC NAME	HYPOGLYCEMIA RISK WITH MONOTHERAPY
Sulfonylureas	24 hours	Diabeta	Glyburide	Present
	12–24 hours	Glynase Glucotrol	Glipizide	Present
Benzoic acid analogs	1–2 hours	Prandin	Repaglinide	Present
Biguanides	6 hours	Glucophage	Metformin	Absent
Thiazolidinediones	16–34 hours	Rezulin	Troglitazone	Absent
α-Glucosidase inhibitors	2–4 hours	Avandia	Rosiglitazone	Absent
		Actos	Pioglitazone	Absent
		Precose	Acarbose	Absent

glucose levels rise above the targeted values, no further specific therapy will be required, and the sulfonylureas may be safely omitted for that day. If insulin is required, there is no particular advantage of IV insulin over subcutaneous insulin in this population. If subcutaneous insulin is used, we suggest starting with 4 to 6 U of regular insulin every 4 hours.

Patients whose diabetes is poorly controlled before their admission using oral agents will require insulin to maintain targeted blood glucose goals. Furthermore, administering these agents could be potentially dangerous in the patients with well-controlled diabetes if enough calories were not provided.

Insulin-requiring patients with type 2 diabetes receiving local anesthesia should be managed similarly to patients with type 1 diabetes. Many of these patients are insulin-openic and thus behave metabolically like those with type 1 diabetes. Most clinicians prefer subcutaneous insulin for this situation.

Postoperative Treatment

Because any patient with diabetes requiring general anesthesia for more than an hour should be receiving a variable-rate insulin infusion (except the patient with type 2 diabetes whose blood glucose concentrations do not exceed 200 mg/dL), postoperative management is simple. If the patient cannot tolerate food and blood glucose levels remain in the targeted range after 12 hours, the frequency of blood glucose monitoring often can be decreased to every 2 to 4 hours, although if any changes in the insulin dose are required, blood glucose measurements must be made more frequently. We measure urinary ketone levels daily because the presence of ketonuria in the presence of well-controlled glycemia indicates the need for greater quantities of glucose (starvation ketosis). Alternatively, ketonuria with unexplained hyperglycemia could represent one of a variety of problems, including sepsis, myocardial infarction, or possibly a pharmacy error with the insulin mixture. Finally, serum electrolyte levels should be measured immediately after surgery for all diabetic patients and on a daily basis for those receiving an insulin infusion.

We have found it easiest to continue the insulin infusion until solid food is tolerated.

Thus, if nausea and vomiting are present, there will be no interruption of glucose and insulin therapy. If solid food is permitted for the lunch or supper meal on the day of the surgery, the regular home dose of insulin may be administered 20 to 30 minutes before the meal and the insulin (and glucose) infusion stopped just before the meal. If regular insulin is not usually given before the lunch meal, 4 to 6 U of regular insulin (subcutaneous) may be given. If the patient will be spending the night in the hospital, it is sometimes easier to continue with the insulin infusion until the next morning to ensure that the morning meal is well tolerated.

With local anesthesia, patients using ultralente insulin or an insulin pump at home should continue with their usual doses of "basal" insulin, and supplemental regular insulin (or lispro) may be administered subcutaneously as needed every 4 hours. Because of the guesswork involved when NPH and lente preparations are administered, recommendations are difficult if one decides to administer these insulins to patients with type 1 diabetes or those with type 2 diabetes who require insulin. If food is tolerated immediately after surgery, regular insulin may or may not be required, depending on the time of the day in relation to the "peaking" intermediate insulin. This problem is eliminated if an insulin infusion is used.

With the increasing emphasis on outpatient procedures, it is imperative that patients with diabetes are instructed how to manage their diabetes after discharge. Blood glucose monitoring should be continued every 1 to 2 hours after the patient returns home. For patients receiving insulin, a predetermined plan for insulin supplements should be created before discharge from the hospital. For those diet controlled or receiving a sulfonylurea, the patient should be instructed to contact the health care provider should the blood glucose concentration exceed a certain level. We would not encourage sending patients home if there are any problems with postoperative nausea and vomiting. However, should this develop after discharge, the patient should call the provider for further instructions. Patients with type 1 diabetes should always have the ability to measure urinary ketone levels at home, and any diabetic patient with nausea and vomiting should be screened for ketonuria. Most important, all patients should have specific guidelines as to when their providers should be contacted.

Summary

Lower limb surgery is a common occurrence for patients with diabetes, but large trials examining the optimal medical management and its relationship to surgical outcome of these patients are lacking. Although there is some disagreement about the perioperative management of these patients, there is general consensus about how these patients should be managed. Blood glucose levels should be maintained at less than 200 mg/dL while avoiding hypoglycemia. All insulin-requiring patients (both type 1 and type 2) who are receiving general anesthesia for more than 1 hour should be administered a variable-rate insulin infusion. Patients with type 1 diabetes who are administered local anesthesia generally do well with subcutaneous insulin, although the few studies suggest that they may do even better with a variable-rate insulin infusion during and after surgery.

However, there is the least amount of information about the most common situation, the poorly controlled patient with type 2 diabetes receiving local anesthesia. For these patients, there is probably no advantage in using IV insulin compared with subcutaneous insulin if the patient will resume normal eating within the day. Well-controlled type 2 patients on sulfonylureas, acarbose, Troglitazone, or repaglinide should omit their tablets on the day of surgery until their first meal. Consideration should be given to metformin, which should be withheld on the day of surgery and then restarted 48 hours after the procedure only after the renal function has been assessed

REFERENCES

1. Alberti KGMM: Diabetes and surgery [editorial]. Anesthesiology 74:209–211, 1991.
2. Alberti KGMM, Gill GV, Elliot MJ: Insulin delivery during surgery in the diabetic patient. Diabetes Care 5:65–77, 1982.
3. American Diabetes Association: 1991 Vital Statistics. Alexandria, VA: American Diabetes Association, 1991.
4. American Diabetes Association: Diabetic nephropathy. Diabetes Care 21:S50–S53, 1998.
5. Arauz-Pacheco C, Raskin P: Surgery and anesthesia. Therapy for Diabetes Mellitus and Related Disorders, 2nd ed. Alexandria, VA: American Diabetes Association, 1994.
6. Burgos LG, Ebert TJ, Asiddao C, et al: Increased intraoperative cardiovascular morbidity in diabetics with autonomic neuropathy. Anesthesiology 70:591–597, 1989.
7. Currie CJ, Morgan CL, Peters JR: The epidemiology and cost of inpatient care for peripheral vascular disease, infection, neuropathy, and ulceration in diabetes. Diabetes Care 21:42–48, 1998.
8. DeFronzo RA: Diabetic nephropathy: Etiologic and therapeutic considerations. Diabetes Rev 3:510–565, 1995.
9. DeFronzo RA, Ferrannini E, Kovisto V: New concepts in the pathogenesis and treatment of non-insulin-dependent diabetes mellitus. Am J Med 74:52–81, 1983.
10. Domalik LJ, Feldman JM: Carbohydrate metabolism and surgery. Surgical Management of the Diabetic Patient. New York: Raven Press, 1991.
11. Eagle KA: Surgical patients with heart disease: Summary of the ACC/AHA guidelines. Am Fam Physician 56:811–818, 1997.
12. Eagle KA, Brundage BH, Chaitman BR, et al: Guidelines for perioperative cardiovascular evaluation for noncardiac surgery. Report of the American college of Cardiology/American Heart Association Task Force on Practice Guidelines (Committee on Perioperative Cardiovascular Evaluation for Noncardiac Surgery). J Am Coll Cardiol 27:910–948, 1996.
13. Eagle KA, Brundage BH, Chaitman BR, et al: Guidelines for perioperative cardiovascular evaluation for noncardiac surgery: An abridged version of the report of the American College of Cardiology/American Heart Association Task Force on Practice Guidelines. Mayo Clin Proc 72:524–531, 1997.
14. Eldridge AJ, Sear JW: Peri-operative management of diabetic patients: Any changes for the better since 1985? Anaesthesia 51:45–51, 1996.
15. Ewing DJ, Clarke BF: Diagnosis and management of diabetic autonomic neuropathy. Br Med J 285:916–918, 1982.
16. Freeman WK, Gibbons RJ, Shub C: Preoperative assessment of the cardiac patients undergoing noncardiac surgical procedures. Mayo Clin Proc 64:1105–1117, 1989.
17. Hansis M: Pathophysiology of infection—a theoretical approach. Injury 27:SC5–SC8, 1996.
18. Hirsch IB: Approach to the patient with diabetes undergoing a vascular or interventional procedure. J Vasc Interv Radiol 8:329–336, 1997.
19. Hirsch IB: Current strategies for the treatment of type I diabetes. Med Clin North Am 82:689–719, 1998.
20. Hirsch IB, McGill JB, Cryer PE, et al: Perioperative management of surgical patients with diabetes mellitus. Anesthesiology 74:346–359, 1991.
21. Hirsch IB, Paauw DS: Diabetes management in special situations. Endocrinol Metab Clin North Am 26:631–645, 1997.
22. Hirsch IB, White PF: A retrospective review of the perioperative management of IDDM during surgery. Anesth Rev 21:53–59, 1994.
23. Holleman F, Schmitt H, Rottiers R, et al: Reduced frequency of severe hypoglycemia and coma in well-controlled IDDM patients treated with insulin lispro. The Benelux-UK Insulin Lispro Study Group. Diabetes Care 20:1827–1832, 1997.
24. Husband DJ, Thai AC, Alberti KG: Management of diabetes during surgery with glucose-insulin-potassium infusion. Diabet Med 3:69–74, 1986.

25. Jensen MD, Heiling VJ, Miles JM: Effects of glucagon on free fatty acid metabolism in humans. J Clin Endocrinol Metab 72:308–315, 1991.
26. Kaufman FR, Devgan S, Roe TF, et al: Perioperative management with prolonged intravenous insulin infusion versus subcutaneous insulin in children with type I diabetes mellitus. J Diabetes Complications 10:6–11, 1996.
27. Koistinen MJ: Prevalence of asymptomatic myocardial ischaemia in diabetic subjects. BMJ 301:92–95, 1990.
28. Lager I: The insulin-antagonistic effect of the counterregulatory hormones. J Intern Med 229:41–47, 1991.
29. Levetan CS, Passaro M, Jablonski K, et al: Unrecognized diabetes among hospitalized patients. Diabetes Care 21:246–249, 1998.
30. Monk TG, Mueller M, White PF: Treatment of stress response during balanced anesthesia. Anesthesiology 76:39–45, 1992.
31. Munro JF, Campbell IW, McCuish AC, et al: Euglycaemic diabetic ketoacidosis. Br Med J 2:578–580, 1973.
32. National Institutes of Health (U.S.), National Institute of Diabetes and Digestive and Kidney Disease (U.S.): Diabetes Statistics. Bethesda, MD: National Institutes of Health, 1995.
33. Palumbo PJ, Melton LJ III: Peripheral Vascular Disease and Diabetes. Diabetes in America, 2nd ed. Bethesda, MD: National Institutes of Health, 1995.
34. Pezzarossa A, Taddei F, Cimicchi MC, et al: Perioperative management of diabetic subjects. Subcutaneous versus intravenous insulin administration during glucose-potassium infusion. Diabetes Care 11:52–58, 1988.
35. Portuese E, Orchard T: Mortality in Insulin-Dependent Diabetes. Diabetes in America, 2nd ed. Bethesda, MD: National Institutes of Health, 1995.
36. Pramming S, Thorsteinsson B, Bendtson I, et al: Nocturnal hypoglycaemia in patients receiving conventional treatment with insulin. Br Med J Clin Res Ed 291:376–379, 1985.
37. Reddi AS, Camerini-Davalos RA: Diabetic nephropathy: An update. Arch Intern Med 150:31–43, 1990.
38. Report of the Expert Committee on the Diagnosis and Classification of Diabetes Mellitus. Diabetes Care 20:1183–1197, 1997.
39. Root HF: Pre-operative care of the diabetic patient. Postgrad Med 40:439, 1989.
40. The Diabetes Control and Complications Trial Research Group: Hypoglycemia in the Diabetes Control and Complications Trial. Diabetes 46:271–286, 1997.
41. Turner RC, Grayburn JA, Newman GB, et al: Measurement of the insulin delivery rate in man. J Clin Endocrinol Metab 33:279–286, 1971.
42. Vannini P, Ciavarella A, Olmi R, et al: Diabetes as pro-infective risk factor in total hip replacement. Acta Diabetica Lat 21:275–280, 1984.
43. Watts NB, Gebhart SS, Clark RV, et al: Postoperative management of diabetes mellitus: Steady-state glucose control with bedside algorithm for insulin adjustment. Diabetes Care 10:722–728, 1987.
44. Wingard DL, Barrett-Connor E: Heart Disease and Diabetes, Diabetes in America, 2nd ed. Bethesda, MD: National Institutes of Health, 1995.
45. Yue DK, McLennan S, Marsh M, et al: Effects of experimental diabetes, uremia, and malnutrition on wound healing. Diabetes 36:295–299, 1987.

Chapter 25

THE ROLE OF VASCULAR SURGERY IN THE DIABETIC PATIENT

■ Michael Y. Hu and Brent T. Allen

Diffuse vascular disease is the most important factor leading to the increased mortality and morbidity in patients with diabetes mellitus. Diabetes is the seventh leading cause of death in the United States and is the most frequent cause of nontraumatic amputations.[153] The vascular complications of diabetes mellitus can occur in multiple locations including the coronary, cerebral, retinal, renal, and peripheral circulation. Patients with diabetes mellitus are two to four times more likely to die from heart diesease and two to six times more likely to suffer a stroke. Diabetes is the leading cause of blindness between the ages of 25 and 74 years and accounts for 40% of the new cases of end-stage renal disease each year.[153] Patients with diabetes are 15 times more likely to have peripheral vascular disease and 22 times more likely to have foot ulceration or gangrene than nondiabetics.[99]

Vascular disease in diabetics is a tremendous burden to the health care system. The total health care cost of diabetes mellitus in the United States in 1992 was estimated to be $92 billion. Direct medical costs were estimated at $45 billion with an addition $47 billion attributed to indirect costs of disability, work loss, and premature mortality.[153]

Diabetes accounted for 1.6% of all hospital discharges in 1994,[78] and the total cost of in-hospital treatment for late complications of diabetes was estimated at $5.1 billion by the 1987 National Hospital Discharge Survey.[100] Peripheral arterial diabetic complications accounted for $873 million (17%) of this total and ranked second only to heart disease as the most costly of diabetic complications requiring hospitalization. Peripheral vascular disease accounted for more in-hospital days (14.4) than any other complication of diabetes.[100]

Incidence

Diabetes affects as many as 15.7 million people in the United States, approximately 5 to 6% of the American population. More than 798,000 new cases are diagnosed each year and the incidence has increased during the 1980s.[153] The prevalence tends to be slightly higher in women than in men, especially in black Americans.[153]

Melton[147] found that the incidence of symptomatic occlusive arterial disease in 1,073 diabetic patients was 21.3 and 17.6 per 1,000 persons per year for men and women, respectively. The incidence of peripheral vascular disease increased with age and duration of the diabetes. Furthermore, approximately 20% of diabetics with occlusive arterial disease had experienced gangrene. The cumulative incidence of vascular disease in diabetics has been estimated to be 15% at 10 years after the initial diagnosis of the disease and 45% at 20 years.[153] Uusitupu[223] reported that the age-adjusted incidence of claudication was significantly higher among middle-aged diabetic males and diabetic females (males, 20.3% vs. 8.0%; females, 21.8% vs. 4.2%, respectively). Janka et al.[101] estimated a 16% prevalence of peripheral vascular disease in 623 diabetic patients when patients with symptoms were screened with Doppler measurements of limb perfusion. There was a marked increase in peripheral vascular disease with age from 3.2% of those patients under 50, to 55% of those over 80 years of age. Duration of diabetes and degree of hyperglycemia correlated with distal peripheral vascular disease but did not correlate with proximal arterial disease.

Diabetes appears to augment atherosclerosis and it has its greatest impact in populations with other risk factors such as smoking and hypertension. Sternby[208] showed that diabetes is a strong risk factor for peripheral vascular disease involving the aorta, cerebral, femoral, and coronary arteries. The atherogenic effect of diabetes seems to be clinically more pronounced in the peripheral and coronary arteries than in the aorta or cerebral circulation, which may explain the absence of diabetes-aggravated atherosclerosis in some animal models in which the aorta has been the vessel studied.

Pathogenesis

Three factors combine to promote tissue necrosis in diabetic feet: trauma, neuropathy, and ischemia. The relative contribution of each of these factors varies among patients. Trauma and neuropathy are interrelated, as patients with severe neuropathy are prone to traumatic ulceration because of alterations in weight-bearing forces producing pressure points and because of loss of protective sensation. If the traumatized tissue has adequate blood supply, then patients often develop a chronic ulcer surrounded by hypertrophic callus that bleeds easily when debrided. Traumatized tissue in patients with

arterial insufficiency lacks the blood supply to support healing mechanisms or resist infection. In this setting ischemic ulcerated tissue is likely to become septic and progressively enlarge, thus jeopardizing the foot. The initial and most important step in managing diabetic foot ulceration is to control sepsis in the foot with antibiotics and debridement of necrotic tissue. This is performed during the patient's initial management while the degree of arterial insufficiency is being assessed.

A common misconception is that diabetic ulceration is primarily due to "microvascular" disease. This mechanism was first suggested by Goldenberg[77] after retrospectively studying diabetic and nondiabetic amputation specimens with light microscopy. Histologic examination reportedly revealed a material that was positive on periodic acid–Schiff staining in the arterioles of diabetics. This material was thought to be the obstructing pathogenic lesion in diabetic vascular disease. However, subsequent prospective investigations have failed to confirm the presence of an obstructive arteriolar lesion in diabetics.[12, 98] Diabetic patients do have muscle capillary basement membrane thickening that may not involve all capillaries in all patients to the same degree. The thickened capillary basement membrane apparently does not represent a barrier to gas exchange in studies documenting no difference in transcutaneous oxygen tension in diabetic or nondiabetic patients with vascular disease of similar severity.[240]

While diffusion of oxygen through diabetic capillaries does not appear impaired, an alteration in capillary blood and serum viscosity as well as flow abnormalities in leukocytes, erythrocytes, platelet, and plasma proteins has been reported.[61, 105, 146, 200] The hyperviscosity seen in diabetic patients stems from hyperglycemic glycosylation of the red cell membrane leading to membrane stiffening and subsequent decreased red cell deformability and increased erythrocyte aggregation. Red cell membrane glycosylation is directly proportional to serum glucose levels. The hemoglobin molecule is also susceptible to glycosylation, a reaction that increases hemoglobin's affinity for oxygen and therefore may contribute to ischemia in affected tissues.[193]

Diabetics are unique in their propensity toward calcific obstructive atherosclerosis that is most prominent in the tibial arteries between the knee and ankle. The arterial lesions in this location are the most important reason for the increased risk of tissue necrosis and limb loss in the diabetic population. Commonly, the lower extremity vessels proximal to the knee and in the foot are less diseased. The basis for the distribution of diabetic lower extremity vascular disease is unknown. Fortunately, the frequent sparing of the proximal femoral and pedal arteries allows for femoral-pedal artery bypass and limb salvage in many cases.

Finally, diabetics are susceptible to the atherogenic factors common to nondiabetic patients such as smoking, family history, hypertension, and hyperlipidemia. Diabetes in patients with such risk factors seems to potentiate the chance of cardiovascular complications from atherosclerosis.

Clinical Presentation

History

Patients consulting a vascular surgeon for evaluation of lower extremity ischemia typically complain of muscle pain with ambulation (claudication), constant foot pain (rest pain), or tissue necrosis (ulceration or gangrene).

Lower extremity claudication, the most common presenting symptom of patients with peripheral vascular disease, is a weakness, cramping, or fatigue of exercised muscle groups associated with prompt relief by rest. Although usually very specific in its presentation, occasionally it can be difficult to differentiate from "pseudoclaudication syndromes" such as degenerative arthritis of the spine, hips, or feet; neuritis; and venous claudication. In arterial claudication, the prompt relief by rest, the reproducibility of the symptoms during exercise, and the absence of symptoms at rest differentiates it from the pseudoclaudication syndromes. Patients with pseudoclaudication usually must sit or lie down to obtain relief, while in arterial claudication, cessation of the exercise is usually sufficient. The length of time for resolution of the pain is longer in pseudoclaudication than in arterial claudication, often requiring 20 to 30 minutes in the former and 2 to 3 minutes in the latter.

Generally the level of the vascular obstruction can be estimated by the muscle groups producing the symptoms of claudication.

Claudication in the buttocks indicates a blockage in the terminal aorta. Thigh claudication indicates disease in the iliac arteries, and calf claudication suggests obstruction in the superficial femoral arteries. Fatigue or paresthesias in the foot is an uncommon symptom of claudication but may indicate obstructive disease of the vessels of the calf. Claudication alone, as will be discussed later, is typically not associated with limb-threatening ischemia but may be severely disabling.

Claudication often slowly worsens and is accompanied by other symptoms of arterial insufficiency. As claudication progresses from walking three blocks to walking only one block, to walking from the bedroom to the bathroom, the patient may begin to complain of numbness of the foot, night pain, and later, rest pain, ischemic ulcers, or gangrene.

Nighttime numbness and pain in the foot, termed "rest pain," are frequently located on the forefoot and are prominent complaints in patients with limb-threatening ischemia. Sleeping supine eliminates gravity's contribution to arterial perfusion and the blood pressure normally drops during sleep, hence the foot becomes more ischemic as the flow through the collateral vessels decreases. Ischemic pain arouses the patient from sleep, who gets relief by walking a few steps. This presumably elevates the blood pressure, restores gravity's effect, and improves perfusion of the feet. Frequently patients with severe rest pain sleep in chairs with their feet in a dependent position to minimize discomfort. Rest pain, persistent numbness, painful ulcers, and frank gangrene are symptoms of limb-threatening ischemia and require prompt investigation.

Diabetic Neuropathy

The symptoms of lower extremity arterial insufficiency in diabetics are sometimes difficult to distinguish from neuropathy. Diabetic patients frequently are referred for vascular evaluation because of a constant burning pain or tingling sensation in the foot. These symptoms are typical of neuropathic pain; they are most severe at night and generally not relieved by position change. The pain usually circumferentially involves the entire foot or lower leg in a "stocking-and-glove" distribution, and commonly is bilateral. This type of neuropathic pain is not caused by macrovascular disease and often is found in diabetic patients with normal limb perfusion. It may be present in patients with other symptoms of arterial insufficiency (i.e., claudication) but is not improved with revascularization.

Ulceration of the diabetic foot is another common stimulus for a vascular evaluation. Diabetic neuropathy may compromise protective sensation and predispose diabetics to ulceration. This may occur in spite of normal perfusion and lead to a chronic draining wound that won't heal until the source of trauma is eliminated. The classic example of this is the mal perforans ulcer that heals rapidly once traumatic ambulation is avoided.

Neuropathic ulceration may be the inciting event leading to severe sepsis or gangrene in an ischemic diabetic foot. Once traumatic ulcers have developed in ischemic limbs, the blood flow may be insufficient to promote healing or resist infection. Septic necrosis (gangrene) may progress quickly, involving previously viable tissue and producing limb- or life-threatening complications.

Diabetic neuropathy may delay the presentation of patients with critical limb ischemia. Patients with severe neuropathy frequently do not experience classic ischemic rest pain as a warning sign of impending tissue necrosis. Hence, they seek medical attention only after a nonhealing ulcer or a gangrenous toe develops. Thomas et al.[222] noted the absence of preoperative ischemic pain in diabetic versus nondiabetic patients with limb-threatening arterial insufficiency (44% vs. 68%). The prevalence of tissue necrosis in diabetics compared to nondiabetic patients with peripheral vascular disease is illustrated by our experience at Barnes Hospital with 228 patients who required amputations in the foot (toe and transmetatarsal) for tissue necrosis. Diabetics accounted for 70% (160 patients) of this group.

Physical Examination

Physical examination yields important clues to the degree of vascular impairment in the diabetic patient. Funduscopic examination can sometimes provide important information regarding the severity and duration of the vascular involvement. Palpation and auscultation of the extracranial carotid artery may detect a thrill or bruit, which sug-

gests the possibility of atherosclerotic narrowing at the carotid bifurcation and should be further evaluated with duplex sonography. Cardiac evaluation may detect arrhythmias or abnormal heart sounds indicative of ischemic heart disease. Examination of the abdomen may detect an asymptomatic abdominal aortic aneurysm or identify bruits associated with visceral, renal, or iliac artery occlusive disease.

Evaluation of the extremities in the diabetic patient is extremely important and can often pinpoint the level of arterial obstruction. An audible bruit or the absence of pulses in the groin indicates aortoiliofemoral occlusive disease, which is less common than distal disease in diabetics. The palpation of popliteal, posterior tibial, and dorsalis pedis pulses helps to localize the site of infrainguinal occlusive disease. Although uncommon, occasionally a weak pedal pulse may be palpable in spite of an occluded superficial femoral artery, indicating extensive collateral blood flow from the deep femoral artery to the popliteal artery. Diminished hair growth, reduced perspiration, and decreased temperature in the lower leg are all suggestive of inadequate circulation.

In diabetics, careful inspection of the feet is important (see Chapter 9). Sensory changes (pain, light touch, position sense) should be noted. The presence of erythematous pressure points, ischemic ulcers, neuropathic ulcers ("mal perforans" ulcers), gangrenous toes, calluses, and hypertrophic nails may provide important information regarding the degree of vascular or neuropathic involvement of the extremity. Dependent cyanosis and rubor of the feet suggests arterial insufficiency, especially in patients who note relief of rest pain with foot dependency. Dependent rubor results from vasodilation secondary to ischemia and is more indicative of distal arterial obstruction. Cyanosis may be present because of venous insufficiency in patients with little or no arterial disease.

Diagnosis

Noninvasive Vascular Diagnostic Techniques

The noninvasive vascular laboratory is a cornerstone in the objective evaluation of patients with vascular disease (see Chapter 16).

The vascular laboratory can provide accurate information regarding the location and severity of occlusive disease, the need for angiography, and the establishment of a baseline for serial follow-up. These studies are well accepted by patients, as they are noninvasive and inexpensive, and can be performed on an outpatient basis. The noninvasive vascular studies can help clarify the contribution of vascular disease to lower extremity symptoms in diabetic patients with neuropathy.

Lower extremity systolic Doppler arterial pressures and waveform analysis obtained at the proximal thigh, above-knee, below-knee, ankle, and toe levels have become the "gold standard" in the noninvasive evaluation of patients with peripheral vascular disease. This technique utilizes pneumatic cuffs to occlude vessels and depends on the compressibility of vessels. The blood pressure at the ankle in one of the pedal arteries is compared to the brachial artery pressure and an ankle-brachial index (ABI) is calculated. However, peripheral arteries may be relatively incompressible secondary to marked medial calcification common in diabetics (Fig. 25–1).[81, 156] Tenembaum et al.[218] demonstrated that the average foot pressure in the diabetic was 20 mm Hg greater than the pressure in nondiabetic controls. This complicates the use of segmental pressures alone for assessing lower extremity perfusion. In extreme cases of arterial calcification, occlusive compression is not possible even at 300 mm Hg; thus, segmental pressures in such situations cannot assess arterial perfusion.

Since ABI may not be reliable in some diabetic patients due to vessel incompressibility, a technique for the measurement of *digital* systolic pressures has been reported as being more informative regarding degree of distal macrovascular disease.[82, 130] This technique, expressed as a toe-brachial index (TBI) or in certain cases as a toe-ankle index

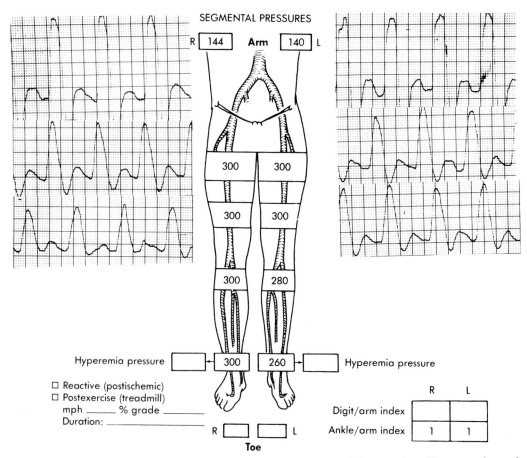

Figure 25–1 ■ Lower extremity segmental pressures and waveforms in a diabetic patient. Note normal waveforms but falsely elevated segmental pressures from vessel incompressibility.

(TAI), permits the evaluation of pressure proximal to the toes as well as changes distal to the ankle. Some studies[129, 156] have demonstrated excellent correlation of TBI with angiographic findings. No differences in the TBIs of diabetic and nondiabetic groups among patients with claudication was reported by Vincent and collaborators.[229] The use of toe pressures and toe-brachial indices for assessing healing potential has been previously described by various investigators. Barnes et al.[13] reported the healing of all foot amputations in diabetics if the toe pressures were greater than 10 mm Hg and greater than 25 mm Hg in nondiabetics. Ramsey et al.[179] reported healing of foot ulcers in diabetics if they had toe pressure of 30 mm Hg or higher. Conversely, Bone and Pomajzl[28] reported that a minimal toe pressure of 45 mm Hg was required to ensure healing of forefoot amputations. These data indicate that toe blood pressure in the range of 25 to 45 mm Hg is a good indicator of healing potential of ulcers and amputations in the diabetic foot.

Arterial waveform analysis is an important component of the lower extremity Doppler blood pressure evaluations, especially in diabetics with noncompressible vessels (Fig. 25–2). This technique becomes especially useful for evaluation of disease in the femoral, popliteal, and tibial regions, where blunted monophasic waveforms suggest occlusive arterial disease even in the presence of normal Doppler pressures secondary to incompressible vessels. The routine evaluation of waveforms in conjunction with the segmental pressures and segmental indices increases the accuracy of Doppler testing.

The use of radioisotope clearance has been reported as a valuable technique in the evaluation of ischemic limbs and specifically for determining the proximal amputation site.[124, 131, 135] Malone et al.[135] demonstrated that 70 of 74 (95%) amputations with xenon-133 clearance of over 2.2 mL/100 gm tissue/min healed primarily. The presence of diabetes mellitus did not affect the incidence of primary healing when compared to nondiabetics. However, the isotope is not widely commercially available and requires both a subcutaneous injection and radiation exposure. As a result, other noninvasive diagnostic techniques have been developed.

Another noninvasive technique is the transcutaneous Po_2 (TcPo_2) measurement of ischemic extremities. The technique seems to be equally applicable in diabetics and nondiabetics,[107, 239] and reports have cited predictive accuracies of 90% or greater.[45, 107] Kram

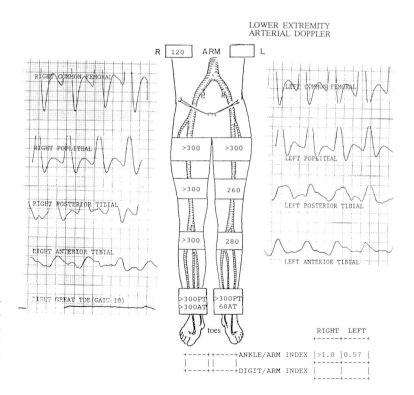

Figure 25–2 ■ Lower extremity segmental pressures and waveforms in a diabetic patient with severe infrapopliteal occlusive disease. Note falsely elevated ankle pressures with abnormal waveforms.

and associates[120] found that preoperative anterior and posterior calf transcutaneous oxygen tension was significantly lower in patients that failed to heal a below-knee amputation when compared to patients who healed their amputation. Successful amputation healing occurred in only 50% of patients with calf oxygen tensions less than 20 mm Hg, but healing occurred in 96% of patients with calf oxygen tensions greater than 20 mm Hg.

However, a wide variation in the threshold value of $TcPo_2$ needed for adequate lower extremity wound healing has been reported, ranging from 10 to 40 mm Hg.[45, 107, 165] In addition, a higher level of $TcPo_2$ may also be needed in the presence of infection.[45] A well-defined threshold may not exist, and the role of $TcPo_2$ may be to furnish the surgeon with a quantitative ischemic risk to help guide medical and surgical therapy.

Laser Doppler velocimetry is another noninvasive technique that has been developed to aid in evaluating the ischemic lower extremity. The laser provides a light source that penetrates the skin to a maximum depth of 1.5 mm. The light is reflected from the moving red blood cells within the surface capillaries and the Doppler-shifted reflected light is measured. The Doppler shift is directly proportional to the velocity of blood flow and is expressed in units of millivolts (mV). Like $TcPo_2$, the threshold wound healing value for laser Doppler velocimetry to achieve predictive accuracies of 90% has also varied, ranging from 40 to 125 mV.[107, 165] Other variations in the use of laser Doppler have included combining laser Doppler perfusion imaging with digital photography[29] and using laser Doppler to measure skin perfusion pressure.[2]

Radiographic Evaluation of Vascular Disease

A variety of radiographic techniques have been developed over the last six decades to visualize large- and small-caliber vessels. Important modifications in the contrast materials and the techniques of arteriography have occurred since the original description by Brooks for lower extremity arteriography in 1924[37] and later for aortic visualization by Dos Santos in 1929.[63]

Soft tissue x-rays are helpful in determining the extent of vascular calcifications (Figs. 25–3, 25–4, and 25–5). Twenty to 25% of

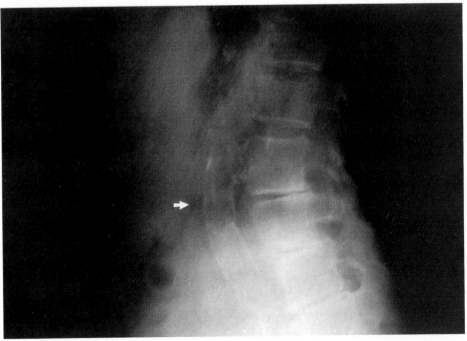

Figure 25–3 ■ Marked aortic calcification in a diabetic patient ("egg shell aorta").

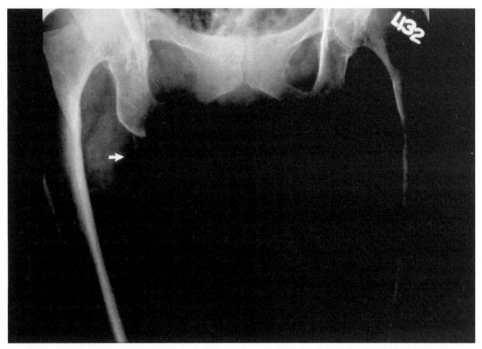

Figure 25–4 ■ Diffuse femoral artery calcification in a diabetic patient.

patients with adult-onset diabetes have radiographic evidence of arterial calcification.[5, 75, 221] Interestingly, calcification of the media that is typically seen in diabetics is *not* commonly associated with complete vascular occlusion. Correlation between sites of vascular calcifications and patent vessels on the arteriogram can provide important information regarding the appropriate surgical procedure.

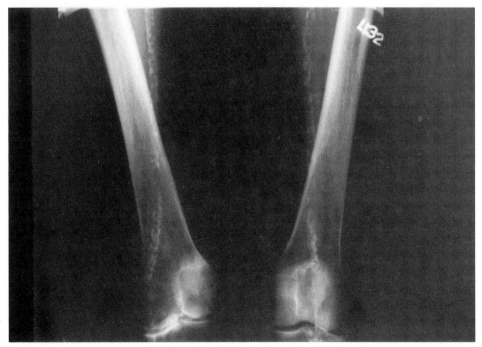

Figure 25–5 ■ Extensive superficial femoral and popliteal calcification in a diabetic patient.

Transfemoral arteriography has become the routine approach for radiologic evaluation of the aortoiliac and leg vessels. This technique has been previously described by various authors.[113, 194, 235] Due to the increased incidence of renal impairment in the diabetic population, minimal radiographic contrast administration combined with adequate hydration prior to and after the procedure is mandatory. Although in most patients the renal impairment is reversible, a high incidence of chronic renal failure is found especially if the patients have serum creatinine levels higher than 5 mg/dL. Dehydration and a large contrast load seem to be aggravating factors. Eisenberg et al.[67] reported no acute renal failure in 537 patients who underwent adequate hydration prior to major angiography. In a study evaluating renal dysfunction after arteriography, Mason et al.[140] found no clinically significant renal failure and a 25% decrease in glomerular filtration rates in only 18% of diabetics who were appropriately hydrated. Harkonen and Kjellstrand[84] reported significant renal impairment following intravenous pyelography in 76% of diabetics with serum creatinine levels of 2 mg/dL or higher.

Besides saline hydration, the administration of mannitol or furosemide has also been proposed as a prophylactic measure prior to angiography. In uncontrolled trials, the addition of either mannitol or furosemide seems to decrease the incidence of contrast dye–induced renal dysfunction.[6, 26, 159] However, a prospective randomized study by Solomon et al.[202] showed no benefit to the addition of mannitol or furosemide versus saline hydration alone in a group of patients at high risk for contrast-induced renal dysfunction. In this study, patients scheduled for angiography who had serum creatinine concentrations exceeding 1.6 mg/dL or creatinine clearance rates below 60 mL/min were randomized to either saline hydration alone or saline hydration plus either mannitol or furosemide. There were statistically significant increases in mean serum creatinine at 24 hours in both the mannitol- and furosemide-treated groups compared to saline alone. In addition, the percentage of patients suffering an increase in serum creatinine by at least 0.5 mg/dL was higher in the patients who received mannitol (28%) and furosemide (40%) versus saline alone (11%; $p = 0.02$). Thus, saline hydration alone was associated with the lowest incidence of contrast-induced renal dysfunction in this study, with no protective effect associated with the addition of mannitol or furosemide in the periprocedure period.

An important potential hazard in using iodinated contrast agents in diabetics taking the drug metformin hydrochloride (Glucophage; Bristol-Myers Squibb, Princeton, NJ) has recently been reported.[52, 94, 157, 173, 180] Metformin is an oral hyperglycemic drug used in the treatment of non–insulin-dependent diabetes mellitus. Excreted almost entirely by the kidney, metformin is associated with a rare incidence of lactic acidosis of 0.03 cases per 1,000 patients per year, with approximately 50% of the cases resulting in death.[52] A small number of published, reported cases of metformin-associated lactic acidosis have been specific to patients who had also received parenteral contrast materials.[186] As a result, iodinated contrast material is specifically listed as a contraindication during metformin use. Recommendations included with the medication advise the avoidance of metformin 48 hours prior to and 48 hours subsequent to the use of parenteral contrast agents, with reevaluation of renal function prior to reinstitution of metformin. This is the only drug of which we are aware that lists iodinated contrast material as a contraindication to its use.

Contrast-induced nephrotoxicity is believed to be mediated primarily by adenosine phosphodiesterase, which causes vasoconstriction of the afferent arterioles and vasodilation of the efferent arterioles. In concert, these actions decrease the glomerular perfusion pressure.[111] Blocking renal vascular adenosine receptors with theophylline has also been proposed as a method to reduce contrast-induced renal dysfunction. In preliminary studies in patients undergoing angiography with ionic, high-osmolality contrast media, patients receiving hydration and oral theophylline just prior to and for 2 days after angiography had less of a decrease in creatinine clearance compared to those patients receiving hydration alone.[110] Additional trials are warranted to confirm these results.

The use of less nephrotoxic contrast agents is another strategy to lower adverse side effects of contrast angiography. Several prospective randomized trials have shown a better safety profile for lower osmolar, nonionic contrast agents compared to standard higher osmolar, ionic contrast media.[15, 92, 112, 150, 205] In a multicenter trial reported by Hill et al.,[92] the incidence of all contrast media adverse effects were 31.6% with the higher osmolar agent diatrizoate compared to 10.2% with the lower osmolar agent iohexol. In a study by Katholi et al.[112] of patients receiving low-osmolality agents, creatinine clearance decreased by 19% at 24 hours and recovered by 48 hours. In patients receiving high-osmolality agents, creatinine clearance decreased by 40% at 24 hours and remained depressed by 47% at 48 hours. Although lower osmotic, nonionic contrast agents have a better safety profile, their higher cost, up to 20 times that of ionic contrast agents,[205] prohibits their standard use. Various risk factors of those patients who might benefit from the use of nonionic contrast agents have included age over 60,[205] unstable angina,[205] New York Heart Association classification III or IV,[92] serum creatinine greater than 1.5 mg/dL,[92] and diabetes.[125]

Most diabetics with peripheral vascular disease have significant occlusive disease in the distal popliteal artery or below the trifurcation; yet the aortoiliac and femoral vessels can be relatively disease free (Fig. 25–6). In patients with unilateral leg ischemia and adequate femoral arterial inflow (determined by physical exam and noninvasive techniques), isolated angiography of the symptomatic limb should be considered to decrease the contrast load. Adequate preangiography information to the radiologist regarding the presence or absence of a popliteal pulse, along with the noninvasive results, may avoid the excessive use of dye in an attempt to maximize visualization of the distal tibial and foot vessels. Close attention to postangiography urine output and serum creatinine levels is important. Because of its potential complications, arteriography should only be considered in patients who are potential candidates for angioplasty and/or surgical revascularization.

The importance of visualizing the arterial anatomy of the foot and its direct correlation with patency of arterial bypass procedures has been described by O'Mara and collaborators.[158] Similarly, Imparato et al.[97] also demonstrated the importance of visualizing the pedal arch and its relationship to graft patency. In their series of extended distal bypasses, 35 of 40 (87.5%) limbs with an intact

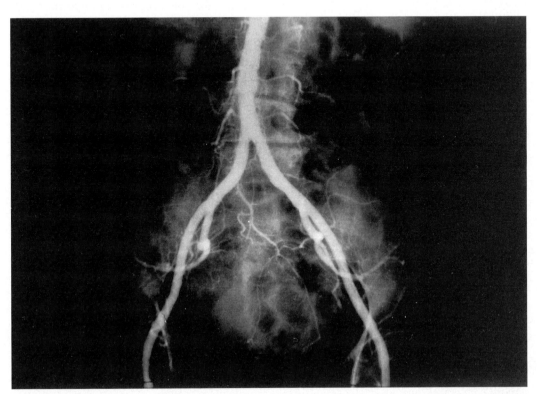

Figure 25–6 ■ Arteriogram in a diabetic patient with significant femoropopliteal occlusive disease but minimal aortic and iliac artery vascular disease.

primary or secondary arch demonstrated early graft patency, while only 2 of 16 limbs (12.5%) without a patent primary or secondary arch underwent successful revascularization.

Occasionally, inadequate visualization of the subtrifurcation circulation by routine arteriography may lead to unnecessary amputation. If the Doppler examination suggests patent vessels in the distal leg, the use of preoperative or intraoperative downstream (antegrade) arteriography may enhance distal vessel visualization that could lead to a limb salvage procedure rather than amputation. The technique of intraoperative arteriography prior to the bypass as an antegrade injection with proximal inflow occlusion, as described by Flanigan et al.,[72] provides excellent visualization of the distal circulation in most patients.

Recent advances in computerized radiology have opened new avenues in the field of arterial dye visualization. Digital vascular imaging (DVI) using an intravenous or intraarterial bolus of contrast is an old concept[24, 206] that had to await the development of image-intensified television fluoroscopy systems, which offer electronic subtraction. Venous injections were hoped to be an effective method of evaluating the arterial system.[183] However, they require relatively large contrast loads and produce poor-quality images. Digital imaging with intra-arterial injection requires only small volumes of contrast and produces high-quality images. Intra-arterial digital subtraction angiography is now the state of the art and is able to produce excellent angiograms even in the distal pedal circulation with a minimal amount of contrast.

Magnetic resonance angiography (MRA) is another available method that can replace contrast angiography in certain settings. MRA can be used as an alternative to angiography in patients allergic to iodinated contrast material, have renal insufficiency, or in whom long-term follow-up would otherwise require repeated angiography. Further discussion of MRA can be found in Chapter 15.

Management of Symptomatic Peripheral Vascular Disease

Medical Management

Intermittent calf claudication is not a mandatory indication for operative intervention unless it becomes incapacitating. Boyd[30] in 1962 followed 1,440 patients with intermittent claudication and found an amputation rate of 7.2% at 5 years. Imparato et al.[96] followed 104 patients with intermittent claudication and found that 82 of 104 (79%) improved or remained with stable claudication and only 6 of 104 (5.8%) required amputation at 2.5 years' follow-up. Therefore, claudication is not limb threatening and in most patients has a benign natural history. Diabetics, however, are a unique subset of patients with a prevalence of claudication four to six times higher than the nondiabetic population.[207] The natural history of claudication in diabetics appears less favorable in a study by Jonason et al.,[104] who noted the 6-year amputation rate in diabetic claudicants to be 12.8% versus 0.5% in nondiabetics. McAllister[142] followed 100 consecutive claudicants for 1 to 18 years and noted progressive ischemia in 16 of the 87 nondiabetics (18%) and 6 of the 13 diabetics (46%), with an average follow-up of 6 years. Only one of the nondiabetics (1%) required amputation, whereas six of the diabetics (46%) underwent amputation during the study period. Thus, diabetics with moderate claudication and a history of significant disease progression in a short period of time should undergo prompt and aggressive evaluation and possible revascularization.[19]

Most patients with one or more block claudication or symptoms of mild coolness in the feet usually do not require reconstructive arterial surgery and are best treated by conservative means. Sometimes when claudication first appears it is severe (less than one block), and is usually related to progression of stenosis to complete occlusion or occlusion of an important collateral. These symptoms typically will improve with conservative therapy as collateral circulation increases. Recommendations for conservative therapy are as follows:

1. Discuss the problem with the patient, including advance notice that action must be taken if the symptoms should worsen.
2. Advise the patient to stop smoking.
3. Recommend leg exercises, especially walking, which can be useful in extending pain-free ambulation.
4. Emphasize the importance of foot care; the treatment of any mycotic infections, prevention of dryness and cracking of the

feet, wearing comfortable shoes, good foot hygiene, and nail care.

5. Normalize the cholesterol and lipid levels to prevent progression of the disease.

6. Maintain diabetic control to help reduce neuropathy.

7. Consider pharmacologic therapy (see below).

8. Repeat vascular laboratory arterial studies in 6 months and every 12 months thereafter to better assess improvement, stabilization, or progression of disease.

Pharmacologic Treatment

A variety of drugs have been used to treat symptomatic peripheral vascular disease including vasodilators, antiplatelet or anticoagulant drugs, hemorheologic drugs, and metabolic agents. The rationale for pharmacologic intervention in lower extremity ischemia is to increase oxygen delivery or improve utilization of oxygen in ischemic tissues.

The use of vasodilators in patients with lower extremity ischemia has been advocated to improve blood flow by reducing vascular resistance. But in patients with obstructive vascular disease, the main determinant of blood flow is the vascular stenosis, not vascular tone. Additionally, hypoxia has a potent vasodilator effect and thus patients with lower extremity ischemia are already maximally vasodilated.[226] The calcium channel blockers produce vasodilatation by preventing the influx of calcium into smooth muscle cells. Recent studies using the calcium channel blocker nifedipine as a vasodilator failed to improve walking ability in patients with claudication.[203] However, the calcium channel blocker verapamil has shown clinical benefits in patients with moderate intermittent claudication in a short-term study by Bagger et al.[10] In this randomized, double-blind, placebo-controlled, crossover study of 44 patients, verapamil did show increased mean pain-free walking distance by 29% from 44.9 m to 57.8 m and maximal walking distance by 49% from 100.7 m to 149.8 m compared with placebo.

Antiplatelet agents including aspirin, prostacylin (PGI$_2$), ticlopidine, and thromboxane synthetase inhibitors have been extensively studied because of the platelet's key role in arterial thrombosis and atherosclerosis. Aspirin, a cyclooxygenase inhibitor, when used in combination with dipyridamole has been shown to reduce the risk of cardiac death in patients with atherosclerotic disease and reduce the incidence of combined stroke and transient ischemic attacks in patients with carotid artery stenosis.[71, 219] Importantly, aspirin and dipyridamole may prolong prosthetic graft patency in lower extremity revascularization when started preoperatively,[46, 47] but aspirin with or without dipyridamole has not been shown to improve claudication.

PGI$_2$ is a potent inhibitor of platelet aggregation and a vasodilator. It has been effective in relieving ischemic rest pain, healing ischemic ulcers, and improving claudication in some studies, but its use is limited by the requirement for intravenous administration, short duration of action, and side effects of nausea and hypotension.[17, 95, 132] Although newer prostaglandin preparations have been developed and have shown efficacy in randomized trials,[16, 60] the continued need for intravenous administration may prevent their widespread clinical use.

Ticlopidine, an inhibitor of adenosine diphosphate (ADP)-induced platelet aggregation, has been evaluated in multicenter trials to demonstrate small improvements in ambulatory distance in patients with claudication.[7, 11] The modest improvement with ticlopidine in patients with claudication may be in part related to its anticoagulant effect and its ability to reduce blood viscosity and red cell deformability.[174] Added benefits to the use of ticlopidine are its beneficial vascular effects throughout the body. Randomized trials have shown a benefit in morbidity and mortality from vascular events with the use of ticlopidine.[27, 102] In summary, antiplatelet agents may slow the progression of atherosclerotic disease but do not seem to offer meaningful symptomatic improvement in claudication.

Anticoagulation may improve ambulatory walking distance in claudicants as demonstrated by Dettori et al.[58] in a controlled study of 30 patients who demonstrated a 236% increase in pain-free walking over a 12-month period when treated with acenocoumarol and pentoxifylline compared to a 149% increase in controls. Two (6.7%) major bleeding complications occurred, however, suggesting that the risk of anticoagulation does not justify its use in claudication.

Pentoxifylline, a hemorheologic drug derived from methylxanthine, decreases erythrocyte membrane rigidity, plasma fibrinogen levels, blood viscosity, and platelet aggregation.[4, 190, 211] It enjoys distinction as being the only medication approved by the Food and Drug Administration (FDA) in the United States for the treatment of ischemic claudication. Pentoxifylline has undergone extensive evaluation regarding its efficacy in the treatment of intermittent claudication.[117] Most investigations have concluded that it is moderately effective in increasing initial and absolute claudication distances as measured by the exercise treadmill test. Additionally, patients with ischemic rest pain or paresthesias may benefit from its use.[117] While claudication does not usually resolve completely, pentoxifylline may improve ambulatory distance in claudication enough to be of practical benefit. In a review of two multicenter, randomized, placebo-controlled studies, improvement in treadmill distances were converted to comparable distances on flat ground. Improvements on pentoxifylline therapy translated to walking distances that enabled greater daily function and added to the quality of life of the patients.[76] Maximal therapeutic benefit of pentoxifylline requires several weeks of drug administration. The drug has approximately a 5% incidence of significant gastrointestinal side effects (nausea) that may require cessation of therapy.

Carnitine and naftidrofuryl are two agents that appear to increase the metabolic efficiency of ischemic muscle. Naftidrofuryl increases delivery of carbohydrate and fatty acids to muscle mitochondria, while carnitine is an important cofactor for skeletal muscle metabolism promoting pyruvate uptake into the Krebs cycle and transport of long-chain fatty acids into mitochondria, thus increasing the production of adenosine triphosphate (ATP) and reducing the loss of pyruvate into the muscle.[31] Both agents have been shown to increase ambulatory distances in patients with claudication.[32, 33, 109, 149] In a double-blind study of propionyl-L-carnitine in intermittent claudication, patients able to walk less than 250 m had significantly improved physical function compared with placebo. In patients with baseline maximal walking capacity greater than or equal to 250 m, propionyl-L-carnitine did not improve walking performance, indicating that propionyl-L-carnitine may be only beneficial in patients with more severely limited walking capacity.[33]

Newer drugs undergoing trials for claudication include indobufen,[166] sulodexide,[198] and buflomedil.[43]

Perhaps one of the most effective nonoperative treatments for ischemic claudication is supervised treadmill exercise. Many studies have demonstrated an increase in treadmill exercise performance and a reduction in claudication symptoms with an exercise conditioning program.[49, 53, 54, 68, 69, 90, 123, 133, 134, 137, 138] In addition, there is essentially no morbidity or mortality from this mode of treatment. A recent study[91] in controlled exercise conditioning at the University of Colorado demonstrated an increase in maximal walking time on a graded treadmill by 123% and in pain-free walking time by 165%. Peak systemic oxygen consumption improved by 30%, confirming that the exercise tolerance was increased. It appears that a dedicated supervised program of progressive walking exercise can improve exercise performance and reduce claudication pain in patients with lower extremity ischemia.

Interventional Radiology

Traditionally, surgical therapy in the form of bypass or endarterectomy was the only treatment option available in severe lower extremity ischemia. The last three decades have witnessed an explosion in percutaneous radiographically monitored catheter techniques, collectively referred to as endovascular procedures, to treat vascular stenoses or, in some cases, occlusions. The most common of these catheter-based procedures is balloon dilatation angioplasty, a concept first introduced by Dotter and Judkins in 1964[64] and later modified by Gruntzig,[80] who brought it to its present level of technology. In addition to balloon angioplasty, a variety of other endovascular procedures are available including laser angioplasty, mechanical atherectomy, and intravascular stents. Endovascular techniques are attractive as minimally invasive procedures that are well tolerated and well received by patients. Ohki, Marin, and Veith recently summarized the literature concerning the use of endovascular grafts in nonaneurysmal arterial disease.[160] Their review of a largely uncontrolled and preliminary experience with this technology indicate a technical success rate of over 90%, an operative mortality of less than 2%, a major complication rate of 2 to 8%, and a primary patency rate of over 80% with generally short follow-up. However, the long-term durability of endovascular treatments for occlusive disease is unknown. Therefore, the indications for these new procedures are not well defined and patients being treated with catheter-based interventions should be carefully selected and followed. The radiologist's role in the treatment of diabetic vascular disease is discussed further in Chapter 19.

Surgical Management of Lower Extremity Arterial Insufficiency in the Diabetic Patient

Lower extremity ischemia is classified according to the location of the arterial obstruction. Since ischemic symptoms can result from intra-abdominal vascular disease (aortic, common, or external iliac arteries) or vascular lesions in the leg (common femoral artery, superficial femoral artery, popliteal artery, or subtrifurcation arteries), the inguinal ligament serves as a convenient landmark to stratify patients on initial examination. Patients with obstructive intra-abdominal aortoiliac arterial pathology (inflow disease) complain of claudication that progresses proximally to involve the thigh and buttocks and have poor femoral pulses often associated with a thrill or bruit. Ischemic rest pain in patients with such proximal disease is relatively uncommon because of the extensive collateral network that develops.

Obstructive infrainguinal arterial lesions are further divided into femoral popliteal and more distal infrapopliteal (subtrifurcation) disease. These lesions typically produce calf claudication or, in more extensive cases, rest pain or tissue necrosis in the foot and have nonpalpable popliteal or pedal pulses. Combinations of abdominal inflow and infrainguinal pathology (multilevel disease) frequently occur and require careful investigation and judgment to determine if one or both levels of occlusive disease need to be corrected to alleviate ischemic symptoms.

Diabetics are unique in their propensity to develop severe infrainguinal disease with relative sparing of the aortoiliac inflow segment (Figs. 25–6 and 25–7). The most severely affected vessels are often the subtri-

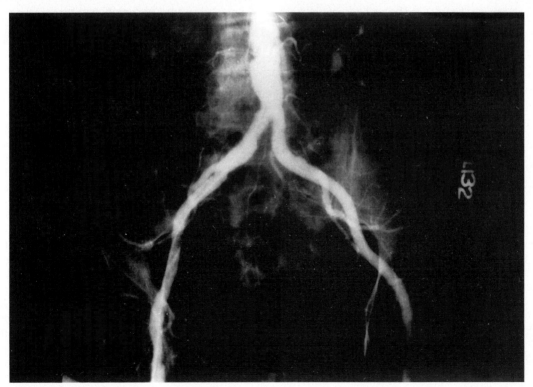

Figure 25–7 ■ Arteriogram in a diabetic patient showing moderate aortoiliac and right femoral artery vascular disease. This patient had marked distal disease.

furcation arteries: the anterior tibial, posterior tibial, and peroneal vessels (Figs. 25–8 and 25–9). The increased incidence of distal lower extremity vascular disease in diabetics is demonstrated by our experience at Barnes Hospital in patients undergoing vascular reconstruction for various levels of arterial disease (Fig. 25–10). Interestingly, no significant difference of atherosclerotic renal artery stenosis has been found between diabetics and nondiabetics.[152]

Aortoiliac Occlusive Disease

Although most diabetics do not have isolated aortoiliac occlusive disease, occasionally patients with occlusions below the inguinal ligament will also present with concomitant aortoiliac obstructive disease (Fig. 25–11). As mentioned, patients with aortoiliac occlusive disease usually do not have rest pain or

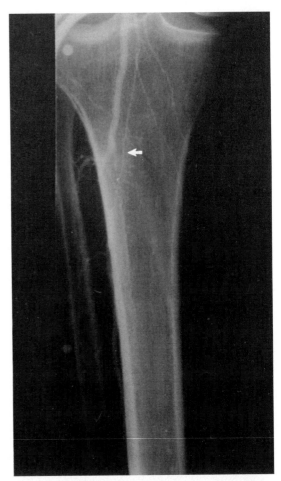

Figure 25–9 ■ Arteriogram in same patient shows marked anterior tibial and common tibioperoneal trunk occlusive disease (*arrow*).

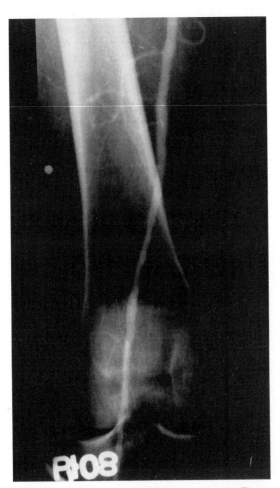

Figure 25–8 ■ Arteriogram of same patient in Figure 25–7 demonstrates minimal popliteal vascular disease.

distal gangrene unless there are ulcerated atherosclerotic plaques that embolize to the foot or there is associated obstructive lesions in the femoropopliteal or infrapopliteal arterial segments. Restoring adequate aortoiliac inflow usually relieves claudication symptoms in both patients with isolated aortoiliac lesions and those with multilevel disease. However, in patients with multilevel occlusive disease and distal tissue necrosis or rest pain, a limb salvage rate of only 70 to 85% should be expected with an inflow procedure *alone*. Brewster et al.[35] reviewed the results of aortofemoral reconstruction of 181 patients with multilevel occlusive disease. In their series, a limb salvage rate of 85% (80 of 94) was achieved in patients with limb-threatening ischemia, but 29% of these patients required both an inflow and infrainguinal bypass to adequately revascularize the

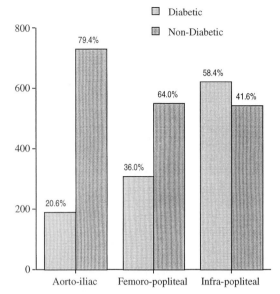

Figure 25–10 ■ Incidence of diabetes mellitus and the location of symptomatic arterial obstruction in 2,844 patients undergoing vascular reconstruction at Barnes Hospital, 1985–1997.

lower extremities. In patients with multilevel disease who were operated on for claudication, both an inflow and infrainguinal bypass were required in 12 of 87 (10%) patients. More recently, Dalman and associates[55] re-

ported 62 patients undergoing simultaneous multilevel repair of lower extremity occlusive disease. Tissue necrosis or rest pain was present in 80%, and 48% were diabetic. The mortality rate (1.8%), morbidity rate, and operative time in this group were not significantly different than in a nonrandomized concurrent group of patients undergoing isolated inflow procedures. All patients with claudication were completely relieved of symptoms, and the cumulative limb salvage at 36-month follow-up was 90.9%. Although numerous noninvasive techniques have been described in an attempt to predict which patients will need a distal bypass combined with inflow procedure, the reliability of these tests has not been convincing.[25, 119]

The options in surgical revascularization in aortoiliac occlusive disease has remained an area of controversy among vascular surgeons. Aortoiliac endarterectomy, bypass grafting (aortoiliac or aortofemoral), and extra-anatomic reconstructions (i.e., axillofemoral, femorofemoral) have all been reported to be effective. Most surgeons agree that aortic reconstruction is best performed with bypass grafts, although some cases (i.e., localized aortoiliac disease, unilateral iliac occlusive disease) can benefit from aortoiliac endarterectomy. The long-term success of

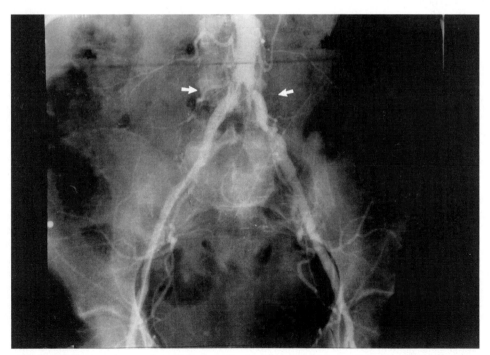

Figure 25–11 ■ The arteriogram in a diabetic patient with marked bilateral common iliac artery stenoses.

unilateral iliofemoral endarterectomy was emphasized in a report from Van den Dungen,[225] who noted no deaths in 94 patients undergoing iliofemoral endarterectomy with patency rates of 94%, 83%, and 65% at 1 year, 5 years, and 10 years, respectively. In selected cases, a familiarity with endarterectomy adds an important tool to the armamentarium of the vascular surgeon. A common technique of aortoiliac endarterectomy is depicted in Figure 25–12. An alternate novel technique of closed aortoiliac surgical endarterectomy using a "plaque cracker" instrument was originally described by LeVeen[128] and is gaining popularity.[20, 237] This instrument permits separation of the atherosclerotic plaque from the vessel wall without opening the vessel and subsequent extraction with a minimal number of arteriotomies (Fig. 25–13). We have found this technique helpful, especially in unilateral iliac occlusive disease. Butcher and Jaffe[41] reported their experience with aortoiliac endarterectomy in 94 patients from 1959 to 1970 at Barnes Hospital. The 5-year patency rate

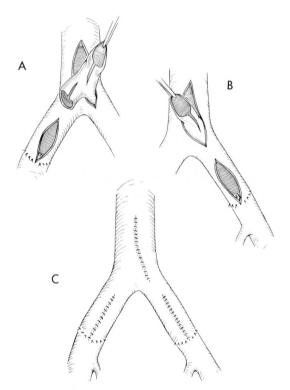

Figure 25–12 ■ Technique of aortoiliac endarterectomy. Note the importance of suturing down distal intima to avoid elevation of flap and thrombosis.

was 84% and 70% for nondiabetic and diabetic patients, respectively (Table 25–1).

The frequent presence of extensive disease involving both the aortoiliac and bilateral iliofemoral segments and the availability of durable and flexible synthetic grafts has made aortobifemoral grafting the procedure of choice for most patients with abdominal inflow arterial obstruction. Although some authors[171] prefer end-to-end aorta to graft proximal anastomosis, we have found the end-to-side graft to aorta anastomosis as effective. End-to-side anastomosis may be potentially advantageous in certain anatomic patterns of disease, most notably when the occlusive disease involves the external iliac arteries.[36] In such an example, end-to-end anastomosis with bypass to the femoral level may effectively devascularize the pelvic region due to the lack of retrograde flow up the iliac arteries to supply the hypogastric vascular beds. The most common techniques are depicted in Figure 25–14. Most series indicate an early (30 days) graft patency rate of 95 to 99% and a 5-year patency from 74 to 92% (Table 25–2). Progression of atherosclerotic disease in the distal vessels accounts for the decrease in the 10-year patency rate to 62 to 77% in most series. Improvement in graft material, surgical techniques, and perioperative management have made this procedure successful and safe, with mortality rates less than 5% commonly reported.

The retroperitoneal approach to aortoiliac reconstruction may be better tolerated than the classic transperitoneal route by patients operated on for both aortoiliac occlusive and aneurysmal disease. Two prospective randomized studies have been published comparing transabdominal and retroperitoneal approaches for aortic reconstruction.[42, 199] Cambria et al. randomized 113 patients between the two approaches and found no difference in intraoperative details, respiratory complications, return of gastrointestinal function, narcotic requirements, incidence of major and minor complications, and hospital stay.[42] A larger prospective randomized trial of 145 patients by our group at Washington University[199] did find shorter intensive care unit stays, lower hospital charges, as well as a decreased incidence of overall complications, postoperative ileus, and small bowel obstruction in the retroperitoneal group. Overall, both techniques can be considered comparable, with choice of approach individ-

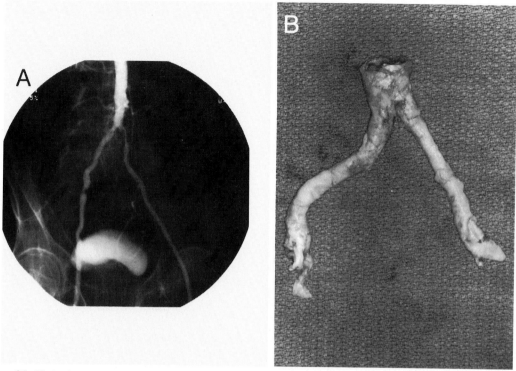

Figure 25–13 ■ Aortoiliac angiogram (*A*) and atherosclerotic plaque (*B*) from a patient undergoing a bilateral aortoiliac endarterectomy using the "plaque cracker" technique.

ualized to the patient. The retroperitoneal exposure is clearly advantageous in some patients (i.e., previous abdominal surgery, obesity, cases requiring left renal artery reconstruction, horseshoe kidney, significant juxtarenal or pararenal disease) and should be a consideration in these types of cases. Our experience with these two approaches using endarterectomy or bypass in occlusive aortoiliac disease is shown in Table 25–3.

In patients with less severe aortoiliac occlusive disease, percutaneous angioplasty with the selective use of stenting has become a first-line treatment at some centers. In a multicenter trial of stenting versus angioplasty in the iliac and femoral arteries reported by Martin et al.,[139] the primary clinical patency in the iliac system was 81% at 1 year and 71% at 2 years. The secondary clinical patency was 91% and 86%, respectively.

Table 25–1 ■ AORTOILIAC ENDARTERECTOMY (BARNES HOSPITAL, 1959–1970)*

	NUMBER OF PATIENTS	5-YEAR PATENCY (%)	P VALUE
Diabetes			
Nondiabetic	84	84	NS
Diabetic	16	70	
Degree of ischemia			
Claudication alone	73	83	<0.02
Rest pain, ulcer, gangrene	26	70	
Femoral pulse			
Palpable femoral pulse	53	92	<0.02
Absent femoral pulse	108	78	

* From Butcher H, Jaffe B: Treatment of aortoiliac arterial occlusive disease by endarterectomy. Ann Surg 173:925–932, 1971, with permission.

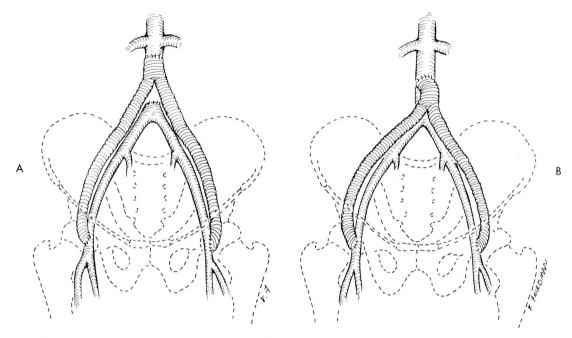

Figure 25–14 ■ Technique commonly used for aortofemoral bypass. *A*, End-to-end graft to aortic anastomosis. *B*, End-to-side graft to aortic anastomosis.

In the femoral arteries the primary clinical patency was 61% at 1 year and 49% at 2 years. The secondary patency was 84% and 72%, respectively. These results were similar to earlier reports for stents in the iliac arteries and with angioplasty alone in the iliac and femoral regions.

Some patients have aortoiliac disease that is not amenable to direct reconstruction. Such patients include those with cardiac disease that would not tolerate intraoperative aortic occlusion or those with previously failed aortic reconstruction. Lower extremity revascularization in these cases can usually be achieved with an extra-anatomic bypass (a prosthetic bypass between a donor and recipient artery that is tunneled through a nonanatomic route). An example is a bypass from the axillary artery (donor vessel) to the femoral artery (recipient vessel) tunneled through the subcutaneous tissues along the lateral chest and abdominal wall to unilaterally revascularize the leg in a patient with an obstructed iliac artery. In the past this technique has had poor patency rates when used unilaterally in comparison to other

Table 25–2 ■ AORTOFEMORAL GRAFT PATENCY RATES OF SELECTED SERIES

AUTHORS	YEAR	NUMBER OF PATIENTS	PATENCY		OPERATIVE MORTALITY (%)
			5 Years	10 Years	
Duncan, Linton, and Darling[66]	1971	87	74	—	2.3
Malone et al.[136]	1975	180	82	66	2.5
Brewster and Darling[34]	1978	406	88	74	1.1
Nevelsteen et al.[154]	1980	352	80	62	5.1
King et al.[115]	1983	79	79	—	4.8
Sladen et al.[201]	1986	100	84	78	—
Szilagyi et al.[213]	1986	1,647	77	77	5.0
Poulias et al.[175]	1992	1,000	82	76	3.3
Passman et al.[170]	1996	139	80		<1.0
McDaniel et al.[145]	1997	~4,160 (meta-analysis)	82–92	74–78	3.1 ± 2.2

Table 25-3 ■ ELECTIVE REPAIR AORTOILIAC OCCLUSIVE DISEASE (BARNES HOSPITAL, 1985-1997)

PROCEDURE	RETROPERITONEAL	TRANSPERITONEAL	LEG/GROIN	TOTAL
Aortobi-iliac bypass	13	25	—	38
Aortobifemoral bypass	87	145	1	233
Endarterectomy	13	26	8	47
Total	113(35.6%)	196(61.6%)	9(2.8%)	318
Mortality	3 (2.7%)	3 (1.5%)	—	6 (1.9%)

forms of aortoiliac reconstruction. Recently, better results have been noted when this type of bypass has been used for bilateral lower extremity revascularization (axillobifemoral bypass). The addition of reinforcing plastic rings to these grafts prevents external compression in their subcutaneous location and has been another favorable modification. Harris et al.[85] noted a life table primary patency of 85% in 76 axillobifemoral bypass grafts performed with externally supported grafts and followed for an average of 28 months.

It has generally been agreed that extra-anatomic axillobifemoral bypass has been a compromise choice for aortoiliac occlusive disease, trading inferior long-term durability and less comprehensive hemodynamic improvement for lower morbidity and mortality in high-risk patients.[36, 188, 189] However, a recent report by Passman et al.[170] has challenged this view. In their retrospective review, they compared the results of 117 axillobifemoral bypasses with 139 aortobifemoral bypasses over a 6-year period. Patients undergoing axillobifemoral bypasses were older, had more comorbid diseases, and were operated for limb salvage indications more often. Not unexpectedly, 5-year patient survival was less for patients undergoing axillobifemoral bypasses versus aortobifemoral bypasses (45% vs. 72%). However, 5-year patency (74% vs. 80%), limb salvage (89% vs. 79%), and operative mortality rate (3.4% vs. < 1.0%) were comparable between the axillobifemoral and aortobifemoral bypass groups, respectively. Although this was a nonrandomized group of patients and a retrospective review, if these results are confirmed, this would indicate that the axillobifemoral bypass may be an operation that can be selected with confidence in older high-risk patients that are high operative risks for aortic cross-clamping or have aortoiliac disease not amenable to direct reconstruction without concern of inferior patency or compromise of limb salvage rates.

Femoral Popliteal Occlusive Disease

Arterial occlusive lesions in the femoropopliteal region can compromise the distal circulation of the lower extremity, resulting in claudication, rest pain, and/or tissue necrosis. Since mild claudication is associated with a low incidence of amputation as described by Boyd[30] and Imparato,[96] most surgeons agree that the only absolute indications for femoral popliteal reconstruction should be disabling claudication or limb-threatening ischemia (rest pain, ischemic ulceration, and gangrene). Most series involving femoropopliteal reconstruction report an incidence of diabetes that ranges between 15 and 40% (Fig. 25-10). Unfortunately, most diabetics with arterial disease of the lower extremity will have not only femoropopliteal lesions but concomitant trifurcation disease, which complicates revascularization procedures.

In patients with simple occlusion of the superficial femoral artery, the procedure of choice is a bypass from the common femoral artery to the popliteal artery (Fig. 25-15). The distal anastomosis can be performed to the above-knee (AK) or below-knee (BK) segment of the popliteal artery depending on which portion of the vessel is most suitable. An important consideration in femoropopliteal reconstruction is the type of vascular graft used in the bypass. Most prospective and retrospective studies have demonstrated the superiority of autogenous saphenous vein over synthetics as a conduit for bypass surgery.[228, 236] However, a number of patients will have had the vein used in a previous revascularization (i.e., coronary artery bypass) or, less frequently, it is inadequate for use as an arterial conduit. A variety of synthetic grafts are available in the absence of saphenous vein, but most vascular surgeons have used a graft constructed of polytetrafluoroethylene (PTFE), knitted Dacron, or less frequently a glutaraldehyde tanned umbilical vein wrapped with a supporting Dacron mesh. We have preferred PTFE in this instance be-

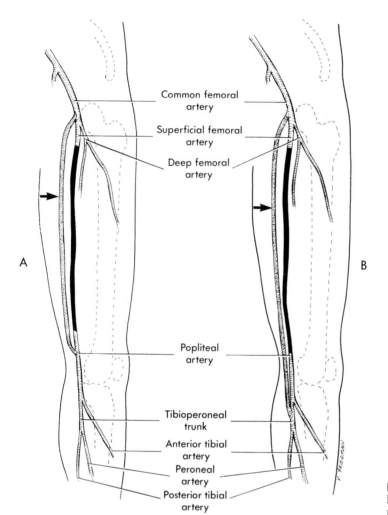

Figure 25–15 ▪ Technique of above-knee (*A*) and below-knee (*B*) femoro-popliteal bypass (*arrows*).

cause of its attractive handling characteristics and performance.

The saphenous vein can be harvested for use as a "reversed" saphenous vein graft similar to the technique used in coronary artery bypass or it can be prepared for use "in situ" by dividing the venous valves with an intraluminal valvulotome to permit proximal to distal flow and ligating the venous tributaries to prevent arteriovenous fistula formation. The proximal and distal ends of the vein are then anastomosed to the donor and recipient arteries, respectively. Both of these techniques yield 5-year secondary patency rates (includes graft revisions) of 75 to 80% (Table 25–4). Many surgeons prefer the in situ method because of the better size match between the proximal and distal portions of the vein to the femoral and popliteal arteries, but both methods

can yield satisfactory results in well-trained hands.

When autogenous vein is not available, a synthetic graft bypass to the popliteal artery is an acceptable alternative. A comparison between PTFE and Dacron synthetic grafts was recently reported in a prospective, randomized, multicenter trial.[1] Two hundred forty-four patients were randomized to above-knee PTFE or collagen-impregnated knitted Dacron. At 1 and 3 years, primary and secondary patency as well as limb salvage rates were equivalent between the two groups.[1] Interestingly, although no graft size was specified in the study protocol, small graft size proved to be the most powerful risk factor for graft occlusion. Three-year patency was approximately 79% for 7- to 8-mm-diameter grafts and 60% for 5- to 6-mm-diameter grafts. Again, in the smaller or larger graft

Table 25-4 ■ RECENT REPORTS CONTAINING 5-YEAR PATENCY FOR INFRAINGUINAL AUTOGENOUS VEIN BYPASS*

STUDY	YEAR	CHARACTERISTICS OF VEIN	NO. OF CASES	DISTAL ANASTOMOSIS	PATENCY		% FOR CLAUDICATION
					Primary	Secondary	
Hobson et al.[93]	1985	Reversed saphenous	75	BK popliteal	74	—	<14
			50	Infrapopliteal	42	—	
Veith et al.[227]	1986	Reversed saphenous	98	AK popliteal	68	—	18
			49	BK popliteal		—	
Berkowitz et al.[23]	1987	Reversed saphenous	102	Infrapopliteal	47	70	14
Leather et al.[126]	1988	In situ	304	BK popliteal	59	76	3
			608	Infrapopliteal			
Kent et al.[114]	1988	Reversed 80%	87	AK popliteal	78	—	100
		In situ 20%	80	BK popliteal		—	
Barnes et al.[14]	1989	In situ 74%	150	AK popliteal	66	—	31†
		Nonreversed		BK popliteal			
		Translocated 15%		Infrapopliteal			
		Reversed 11%					
Taylor et al.[217]	1990	Reversed saphenous or alternative vein	76	AK popliteal	76	76	20
Harris et al.[86]	1993	Reversed saphenous (82%)	199	BK popliteal	80	86	
			241	Infrapopliteal	69	77	
			451 men	Infrainguinal	71	—	22
				BK popliteal	71	—	
				Infrapopliteal	70	—	
			341 women	Infrainguinal	67	—	15
				BK popliteal	73	—	
				Infrapopliteal	59	—	
Shah et al.[197]	1995	In situ	2058	Infrainguinal	72	81	6
			48	AK popliteal	71	76	
			587	BK popliteal	72	83	
			1,423	Infrainguinal	71	81	
Belkin et al.[18]	1996	In situ	568	Infrainguinal	72	82	32
				Infrapopliteal	64	75	
		Nonreversed saphenous	168	Infrainguinal	65	74	11
				Infrapopliteal	69	77	

* Adapted from Porter JM, Mayberry JC, Taylor LM Jr, et al: Chronic lower-extremity ischemia. Part 2. Curr Probl Surg 28:132, 1991, with permission.
† %from series including 52 polytetrafluoroethylene grafts.
AK, above-knee; BK, below-knee.

sizes, there was no difference found between PTFE and Dacron.[1]

Table 25–5 contains the primary patency rates for selected series of femoral popliteal bypass using PTFE to the above-knee or below-knee popliteal artery. The best patency rates are generally found when bypasses can be performed to the AK popliteal artery and in patients operated on for claudication. These patients typically have less severe vascular disease than patients with limb-threatening ischemia and therefore have better graft patency. The influence of disease distal to the popliteal artery (runoff) on patency was demonstrated by Prendiville,[176] who noted in a series of 59 AK PTFE grafts with two or three patent runoff vessels from the popliteal artery a 4-year patency rate of 70% compared to 28% in grafts with poor runoff. Both cigarette smoking and diabetes adversely affected prosthetic graft patency. In contrast, Szilagyi[214] found no difference in cumulative patency rates at 5 and 10 years between the diabetics and nondiabetics who underwent femoropopliteal and femoroinfrapopliteal bypass grafts. Similarly, Bergan et al.[22] could not demonstrate any difference in patency for all femoropopliteal grafts in diabetics compared to nondiabetics at 12 and 24 months, respectively. Cutler et al.[51] reported a 5-year patency rate of 70% in patients with diabetes mellitus compared to 75% in patients without diabetes mellitus.

An important consideration in selecting an autogenous vein graft or synthetic graft for a femoral popliteal bypass is the patient's general health and the estimated chance that progressive vascular disease distal to the bypass will require further reconstruction in the future. Bergan and associates[22] demonstrated in a randomized prospective study that the patency rate at 2½ years was not significantly different between saphenous vein and PTFE grafts to the popliteal artery. At our institution, a retrospective review of our femoral popliteal bypass grafts for claudication revealed no statistically significant difference in primary or secondary patency rates between autogenous saphenous vein and PTFE at 5 years.[3] Saphenous vein graft bypasses (reversed or in situ) generally require larger incisions and longer anesthesia times that may not be well tolerated by medically fragile patients. Therefore, a PTFE

Table 25–5 ■ RECENT REPORTS CONTAINING 5-YEAR PATENCY FOR INFRAINGUINAL POLYTETRAFLUOROETHYLENE BYPASS*

STUDY	YEAR	NO. OF CASES	DISTAL ANASTOMOSIS	PRIMARY PATENCY	% OF CASES DONE FOR CLAUDICATION
McAuley et al.[143]	1984	90	AK popliteal	40	30%
		37	BK popliteal		
Sterpetti et al.[209]	1985	90	AK popliteal	58	46%
Ascer et al.[8]	1985	228	AK popliteal	55	Limb salvage cases
		199	BK popliteal		
Hobson et al.[93]	1985	80	BK popliteal	22	<14%
		41	Infrapopliteal	12	
Veith et al.[227]	1986	118	AK popliteal	38	11%
		53	BK popliteal		
Quinones-Baldrich et al.[178]	1988	101	AK popliteal	63	42%
		45	BK popliteal	44	
Kent et al.[114]	1988	63	AK popliteal	52	100%
		19	BK popliteal		
Barnes et al.[14]	1989	52	AK popliteal	46	31%†
			BK popliteal		
			Infrapopliteal		
Whittemore et al.[236]	1989	182	AK popliteal	42	28%
		97	BK popliteal	28	
		21	Infrapopliteal	12	
Prendiville et al.[176]	1990	114	AK popliteal	42	39%
Allen et al.[3]	1996	128	AK popliteal	58	100%
		45	BK popliteal	55	
Parsons et al.[169]	1996	66	Infrapopliteal	28	Limb salvage cases

* Adapted from Porter JM, Mayberry JC, Taylor LM Jr, et al: Chronic lower-extremity ischemia. Part 2. Curr Probl Surg 28:135, 1991, with permission.
† % from series also including 150 vein grafts.
AK, above-knee; BK, below-knee.

graft may be preferred over a saphenous vein graft in elderly patients with a limited life expectancy (<2 years) who have a popliteal artery with good runoff.

Catheter-based procedures have not been very helpful in managing arterial lesions in the femoral popliteal segment. Jeans and associates[103] recently reported a 7-year prospective study of 370 patients undergoing 500 percutaneous transluminal angioplasties. The 5-year cumulative patency rate in patients with femoropopliteal lesions was 41%. As was found in the surgical treatment of this problem, the 3-year patency rate in patients with two- or three-vessel runoff was better (78%) than in those patients with one-vessel runoff (25%). The potential for improved results with the addition of laser-assisted balloon angioplasty has been much publicized. A 3-year prospective trial of 28 patients (27 with advanced disease) undergoing laser thermal-assisted angioplasty was recently reported by White and associates.[234] They noted successful recanalization in 18 patients (67%). However, the cumulative patency for successful procedures by life table analysis was 55.5%, 38.8%, and 11.1% at 3, 6, and 12 months, respectively. Hence, laser-assisted angioplasty at the present level of development seems to be of limited use in patients with severe femoropopliteal disease. In general, the addition of laser energy to balloon angioplasty in the treatment of femoropopliteal lesions does not improve the results of balloon angioplasty alone and is associated with an increased complication rate.

We recommend an aggressive surgical approach to diabetic patients, especially those with significant lower extremity vascular insufficiency with less than one-block calf claudication. When obstructive lesions in the superficial femoral artery are found in a diabetic with *progressive* symptoms and an ankle-arm index by Doppler pressures of less than 0.30, revascularization (bypass or rarely angioplasty; see Chapter 19) should be considered based on the arteriographic findings. Although saphenous vein remains the conduit of choice for femoropopliteal bypass, PTFE grafts can provide an adequate alternative, especially at the above-knee level when autogenous vein is not available.

Infrapopliteal Vascular Occlusive Disease

The incidence of infrapopliteal vascular occlusive disease in the diabetic patient is higher than in the nondiabetic population and is the most important vascular factor in the propensity for diabetic patients to develop ischemic symptoms in the foot. The peroneal artery is a frequent site of distal bypass, as seen in a series by Dardik et al.[56] Other studies have reported the incidence of diabetes mellitus in patients presenting with infrapopliteal vascular disease to range from 47% to 88% (Fig. 25–10).[9] Occlusive vascular disease in the smaller muscular arteries of the leg in diabetic patients frequently requires an arterial bypass from the femoral artery in the groin to the tibial, peroneal, or dorsalis pedis arteries of the lower leg or foot for limb salvage. Preoperative angiography, often with digital subtraction techniques, is critical to determine which of these distal vessels are patent and in communication with the plantar arcades. The size of the vessel, the amount of disease, and the runoff into the foot usually determine the site of the distal anastomosis. Saphenous vein bypass using the in situ technique currently is the most common method of revascularization for infrapopliteal disease at our institution. This technique minimizes trauma and warm ischemia to the vein graft. Additionally, the vasa vasorum, which supply nutrients to the vessel, are preserved over the majority of the vein's length. Meticulous technique, including careful dissection of the vessel, preservation of arterial tributaries, and use of magnifying loops to ensure a properly constructed anastomosis, is important in the success of these distal procedures. The propensity for diabetic vessels to develop medial calcification can make these procedures especially challenging. Most vascular surgeons advise an intraoperative completion arteriogram to ascertain the lack of technical errors, the absence of clot formation at the distal anastomosis, and the integrity of the distal vessels communicating with the plantar arterial arch.

A common misconception is that the results of distal vascular reconstruction are worse in diabetics than in nondiabetics. It is important to emphasize that distal vascular reconstruction is at least as successful if not more successful in the diabetic population when compared to nondiabetics. The findings of Rosenblatt and coauthors[184] support this observation (Fig. 25–16). They noted in diabetics undergoing distal arterial reconstruction cumulative 1- and 4-year patency rates of 95% and 89%, respectively, while the rates in nondiabetics were 85% and 80%, respec-

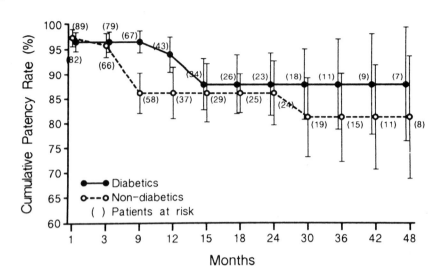

Figure 25-16 ■ The 48-month cumulative patency in diabetics and nondiabetics undergoing distal arterial reconstruction. (From Rosenblatt MS, Quist WC, Sidway AN, et al: Results of vein graft reconstruction of the lower extremity in diabetic and nondiabetic patients. J Am Coll Surg (formerly Surg Gynecol Obstet) 171:331–335, 1990, with permission from the American College of Surgeons.)

tively. The 1-year patency rate in diabetic versus nondiabetic patients undergoing revascularization for threatened limb loss approached statistical significance ($p = 0.056$) in favor of diabetics. In a review of 2,058 in situ venous bypasses reported by Shah et al.,[197] no differences in primary and secondary patency between diabetics and nondiabetics at 1, 5, and 10 years were found. Therefore, distal vascular reconstruction should not be categorically withheld from diabetic patients because of anticipated poor results.

An important element in the long-term success of infrapopliteal bypass is the availability and quality of an autogenous vein graft. Prospective randomized trials comparing in situ and reversed vein grafts in infrapopliteal bypasses have shown equivalent results in patency and limb salvage rates.[86, 233] The patency rates for PTFE placed to the infrapopliteal vessels has been disappointing; approximately 40% at 1 year and 10% at 5 years. Bergan et al.[22] reported 2-year patency rates of 77% and 34% for infrapopliteal bypass grafts for autogenous vein and PTFE grafts, respectively. Similarly, Ricco et al.[181] demonstrated a 20% 2-year patency rate in PTFE grafts compared to a 62% 2-year patency rate for autogenous grafts when used in the infrapopliteal position. Flinn et al.[73] have noted modest improvement in infrapopliteal prosthetic graft patency through the use of long-term anticoagulation. The 2- and 4-year cumulative patency rates were 45% and 37%, respectively, in a series of 75 infrapopliteal PTFE

grafts maintained initially on heparin and then long-term warfarin. A slight increase in bleeding complications (17%) was noted.

In patients without the option of autogenous vein as a bypass graft conduit, improvements in infrapopliteal prosthetic graft patency have also been noted with the addition of vein cuffs or patches to the distal anastomosis.[151, 155, 238] In a prospective randomized trial, Stonebridge et al.[210] did find that the addition of a vein cuff at the distal anastomosis improved patency in PTFE grafts to the below-knee popliteal artery but not the above-knee popliteal artery. In this study, the 12-month patency rates for cuffed and uncuffed above-knee popliteal artery PTFE bypass grafts were 80% and 84%, and the 2-year patency rates were 72% and 70%, respectively. The patency rates for bypass grafts to the below-knee popliteal artery at 12 months were 80% and 65% and at 2 years 52% and 29%, respectively ($p = 0.03$). At the below-knee site, this was reflected in a 24-month difference in limb salvage rates of 84% and 62%, respectively ($p = 0.08$). Thus, the addition of a vein cuff seems to provide a patency advantage in prosthetic grafts as the anastomotic site becomes more distal on the extremity. This is borne out in a retrospective series by Pappas et al.,[168] who reported a cumulative 2-year life-table patency for infrapopliteal PTFE bypasses with vein cuffs of 62% compared to previous primary patency for PTFE bypasses without vein cuffs of 12% at the same level. In patients with critical ischemia, PTFE with a vein cuff interposed at the distal anastomosis may be a reasonable substitute when vein is not available.

The lesser saphenous vein or arm veins are important alternate sources of autogenous vein grafts when the ipsilateral or contralateral greater saphenous vein is unavailable. Although the harvesting of these grafts requires multiple incisions and frequently short segments of vein must be anastomosed to achieve adequate lengths, the long-term patency is clearly better than prosthetic material when bypassing to the infrapopliteal arteries, as demonstrated by Harris and co-authors.[87] They reported patency rates at 1, 3, and 5 years in 67 patients undergoing 70 cephalic vein bypasses of 85%, 72%, and 68%, respectively. Overall limb salvage was 85% at 5 years in these patients, 90% of whom required construction of the distal anastomosis at the infrapopliteal level.

Although most reports dealing with infrapopliteal bypass grafts describe the common femoral artery as the donor site for the inflow, various reports have documented the suitability of the popliteal artery as an adequate inflow site in those patients without significant superficial femoral artery disease, as commonly found in diabetics.[70] In diabetic patients with good inflow to the popliteal artery, a popliteal-to-distal bypass allows the use of a shorter saphenous vein or other autogenous vein and can be extended to pedal arteries with good results.[38, 39] In a series supported by Schuler et al.,[191] 23 of 29 (79%) patients with popliteal-to-infrapopliteal bypass for limb salvage were diabetics. They reported an 84% graft patency rate at 31 months. The limb salvage rate in this study was lower (70% vs. 84%) than the cumulative graft patency rate, which differs from the report of DeWeese et al.[59] and more recently Bergan,[22] which demonstrate that limb salvage exceeds long-term graft patency by as much as 20%.

The fact that the rate of limb salvage is typically higher than patency rate after lower extremity vascular bypass is an important concept to emphasize. Many diabetic patients have marginal perfusion in an otherwise normal appearing foot. Minor trauma can damage the skin and lead to nonhealing ulcers or infection because of the minimal blood supply. These injuries may progress and ultimately destroy the foot, resulting in an amputation. Revascularization of the leg can promote healing of the ulcer and restore

foot viability. Once the ulcer is healed, graft thrombosis most frequently causes the limb to revert to its prebypass level of marginal but adequate perfusion; hence limb salvage is greater than graft patency.

Although the limb salvage rate seems to be higher for the femorotibial than the femoral peroneal bypass graft, the results with a peroneal bypass in the presence of a patent pedal arch are acceptable. Furthermore, the use of the in situ technique has provided excellent results for peroneal artery bypass.[108] Dardik et al.[56] demonstrated a cumulative patency rate of 50% at 12 months in diabetics who underwent femoral peroneal bypass graft. In this report, the cumulative limb salvage rate of 79% at 30 months for the peroneal groups makes this reconstruction worthwhile, especially in selected cases with a patent pedal arch (Fig. 25–17). Occasion-

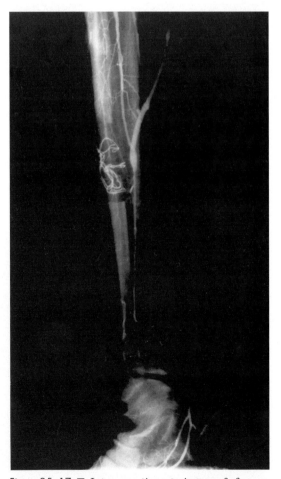

Figure 25–17 ■ Intraoperative arteriogram of a femoroperoneal in situ saphenous vein bypass in a diabetic patient. Note posterior perforating branch from peroneal artery filling posterior tibial artery and plantar arch.

ally, there is not a suitable artery to bypass to above the ankle, but a dorsalis pedis artery, posterior tibial artery, or plantar artery reconstitutes in the foot. In other cases, none of the distal vessels are seen at angiography but a Doppler signal is audible in the dorsalis pedis or posterior tibial areas. In this group of patients, if amputation is inevitable, an exploration of the pedal vessels is indicated and can lead to successful revascularization (Fig. 25–18). Auer et al.[9] demonstrated a 62% 5-year patency in dorsalis pedis bypass grafts in 29 patients. Common procedures done to the infrapopliteal and pedal vessels are shown in Figure 25–19. Routine use of intraoperative postbypass arteriography, especially in distal tibial, peroneal, or pedal bypass, provides information regarding the presence or absence of technical errors (Fig. 25–20) or thrombi (Fig. 25–21), and a better visualization of the vasculature distal to the bypass.

Limb Salvage with Tissue Transfer

The application of tissue transfer procedures to diabetic foot ulcers has enhanced our ability to avoid amputation in patients with extensive tissue loss. This technique is frequently performed by vascular and plastic surgeons working together. Patients undergoing these type of procedures generally have more critically threatened limbs with significant bone, tendon, and joint exposure.[195] In addition, these patients often have contralateral amputations or other factors that would prevent ambulation if a primary amputation were performed, resulting in compromise of independent activity and nursing home placement.[196]

Areas of tissue loss requiring coverage are often on the hindfoot or the ankle that have developed in association with peripheral neuropathy.[50] Patients who develop forefoot ulcers may best be treated with local plastic procedures or distal amputations and may not need free tissue transfer after revascularization. Healthy muscle with or without overlying skin is harvested from distant sites (latissimus dorsi, serratus anterior, rectus abdominus, or forearm muscle flaps based on the radial artery) with preservation of the artery and vein supplying the tissue. The flap is placed in the wound and locally revascu-

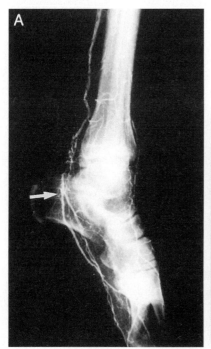
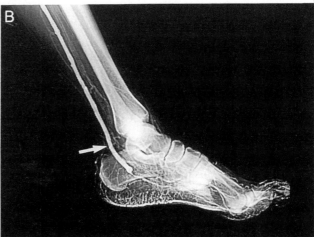

Figure 25–18 ■ *A,* Preoperative arteriogram in a diabetic patient with gangrene of the fourth and fifth toes showing no suitable recipient vessel for distal bypass above ankle. Plantar arteries (*arrow*) reconstitute in foot and are minimally diseased. *B,* Intraoperative angiogram demonstrating revascularization of common plantar artery with a saphenous vein graft (*arrow*) originating from the popliteal artery.

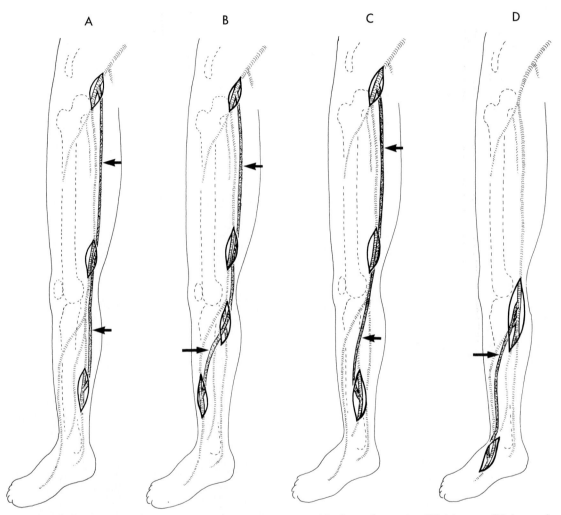

Figure 25–19 ■ Technique for femoral posterior tibial bypass (*A*), femoral anterior tibial bypass (*B*) (*arrows*), femoral peroneal bypass (*C*), and popliteal to dorsalis pedis bypass (*arrows*).

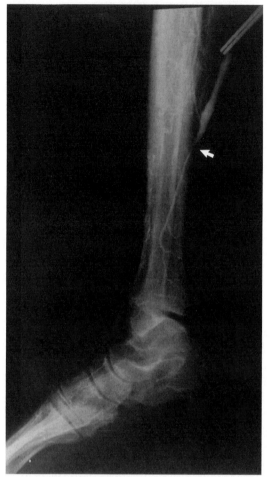

Figure 25–20 ■ Intraoperative arteriogram of a femoral posterior tibial bypass in a diabetic patient. Note obstruction in anastomotic area (*arrow*) secondary to thrombus that required postangiography embolectomy.

larized, oftentimes from a femoropedal vessel saphenous vein graft (Fig. 25–22). Application of a well-vascularized free flap can promote healing in the presence of local infection, including osteomyelitis.[141, 195] Limb salvage rates of 75 to 80% can be expected as well as ambulation in the majority of patients.[44, 79] Additional information on the role of the plastic surgeon in limb salvage is discussed in Chapter 26.

Lumbar Sympathectomy

The benefit of lumbar sympathectomy in the treatment of occlusive arterial disease remains controversial.[127, 215] In diabetic patients, the benefit of this procedure is more disputed due to the common occurrence of

autosympathectomy as a result of the associated neuropathy.[118, 177] Our opinion is that sympathectomy in the diabetic patient is of little benefit and its use not warranted.

Postoperative Follow-up

Atherosclerotic vascular disease is a progressive systemic condition especially in patients with associated risk factors (diabetes, smoking, hypertension, hyperlipidemia). The most common cause of death postoperatively or in the long run death in the patient with reconstructive vascular surgery is myocardial infarction and/or stroke. Moreover, patients with reconstructive vascular surgery tend to develop progression of vascular disease in the bypass graft or the distal arteries.

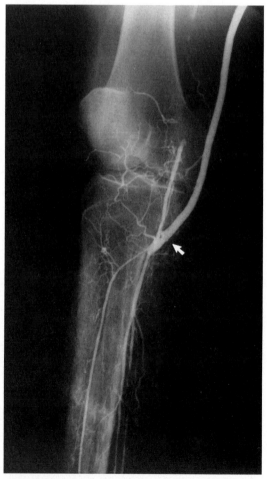

Figure 25–21 ■ Intraoperative arteriogram after thrombectomy of PTFE femoropopliteal bypass. Note irregularity in distal PTFE graft (*arrow*) secondary to intimal hyperplasia. This was resolved by endarterectomy and patch angioplasty.

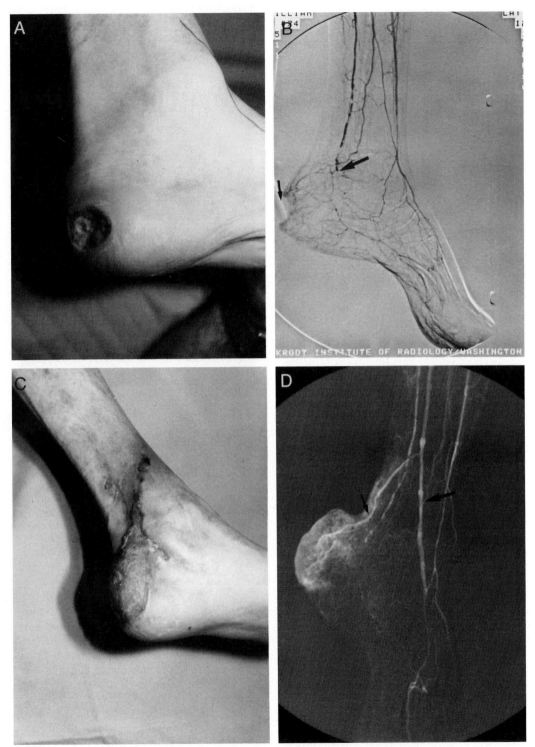

Figure 25–22 ■ *A*, Chronic left heel ulcer in diabetic patient at prolonged bed rest for hip fracture. *B*, Preoperative angiogram demonstrating poor perfusion to ulcer (*small arrow*) secondary to occlusion of posterior tibial artery (*large arrow*). *C*, Ulcer healed 6 weeks after serratus anterior muscle free flap and skin graft revascularized from popliteal to dorsalis pedis reversed saphenous vein bypass. *D*, Postoperative angiogram demonstrating revascularization of free flap. Popliteal to dorsalis pedis reversed saphenous vein graft (*large arrow*). Artery to free flap (*small arrow*).

Cessation of smoking, tight control of hypertension and hyperglycemia, as well as weight control, are important components of the follow-up of diabetics with reconstructive vascular procedures. Furthermore, frequent (every 6 to 12 months) evaluation in the noninvasive vascular laboratory may detect stenosis in the vascular graft or progression of disease distal to the graft. In a study by Sanchez et al., most failing grafts (79%) were detected in the first 2 years.[187] Although there is no consensus on the duration of follow-up needed for bypass grafts, with detailed follow-up every 6 months and surgical revision as needed, Shah et al. reported an outstanding secondary patency of vein bypasses of 70% at 10 years.[197]

Up to 25% of patients with failing grafts may be asymptomatic.[212] Early detection of a stenosis in the bypass graft (Fig. 25–23) or distal to the graft may allow for salvage of the conduit prior to thrombosis either by percutaneous angioplasty or by reoperation. Secondary graft patency in failing stenotic grafts revised before thrombosis is superior to secondary patency of thrombosed then revised grafts. In a study by Bergamini et al., 3-year secondary graft patency of in situ grafts revised prior to thrombosis was 93% compared to 47% if revised after thrombosis.[21]

Occasionally, acute occlusion of chronically implanted grafts will result in recurrence of prebypass symptoms or more severe limb ischemia. Limb-threatening ischemia should be evaluated by angiography to define the anatomy and assess progression of disease since the revascularization procedure. Further options in reconstruction will depend on the arteriographic findings.

Thrombolytic therapy has gained popularity in the nonoperative management of thrombosed vascular grafts or thrombosis proximal to a stenosis in a native vessel. Although systemic heparinization can be of help in acute arterial thrombosis, it will only benefit those patients with adequate collateral flow distal to the acute occlusion.[57, 83] Most radiologists and vascular surgeons agree that systemic thrombolytic therapy administered intravenously for graft thrombolysis is contraindicated because of the significant hemorrhagic complications associated with a systemic lytic state. The best method of thrombolytic therapy for arterial or graft thrombosis is that of high-dose local therapy administered directly into the thrombus, since it is associated with less systemic com-

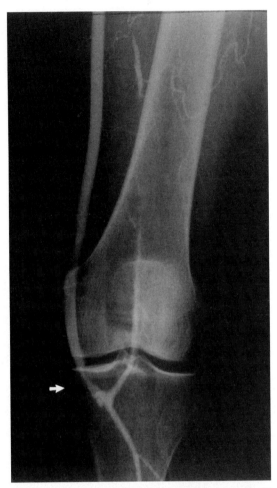

Figure 25–23 ■ Femoral arteriogram obtained 20 months after a PTFE femoropopliteal bypass. Note marked stenosis in distal graft (*arrow*). Arterial noninvasive studies demonstrated a diminished ankle-arm index, which suggested a stenosis despite a patent graft. Patient underwent successful endarterectomy and patch angioplasty.

plications.[224] The basic technique requires percutaneous placement of an intra-arterial catheter directly into the clot or just proximal to it. Patients are started on a thrombolytic agent (urokinase, streptokinase, or tissue plasminogen activator) administered through the catheter into the thrombus. Preinfusion and every-4-hour coagulation studies are performed to avoid systemic thrombolysis. Distal perfusion and potential bleeding sites are monitored carefully and progress is monitored angiographically every 4 to 12 hours. If ischemic symptoms progress or bleeding complications occur, the thrombolytic agent is discontinued and surgical thrombectomy performed. A favorable experience with thrombolytic salvage of 30 thrombosed lower extremity vascular grafts was reported by Seabrook.[192] Patency was initially restored to all bypasses. However, adjunctive surgical thrombectomy was necessary to remove persistent thrombus after thrombolytic infusion in six cases. Underlying morphologic defects (intimal hyperplasia) were noted in 15 grafts; seven connected with balloon angioplasty and eight with surgery. Five (33%) significant hemorrhagic complications occurred, one of which resulted in a lethal myocardial infarction.

Three recent prospective randomized trials comparing thrombolysis and surgery have provided significant insight into the management of acute lower limb ischemia. The first is the Rochester Trial, a single-institution study[162]; the second is the STILE trial (Surgery Versus Thrombolysis for Lower Extremity Ischemia), a 31-center trial[48, 220, 231]; and the third is the TOPAS trial (Study of Thrombolysis or Peripheral Arterial Surgery), a 79-center trial.[163, 164] The three trials collectively randomized 720 patients between lytic agents and surgical therapy, allowing a number of different and clinically important conclusions to be made.[232] First, the technical success of lytic therapy can be highly variable. Successful catheter placement with delivery of thrombolytic therapy occurred in 61% of the patients in STILE compared to 96% in the Rochester Trial and 92% in TOPAS. This difference was most likely due to the greater chronicity (up to 6 months) in STILE versus 7 days and 14 days in the Rochester Trial and TOPAS, respectively. However, this also underscores the need to consider locally available technical expertise when managing lower extremity ischemia. Second, the type of lytic agent does not seem to be a significant factor between urokinase (UK), recombinant urokinase (r-UK), or recombinant tissue plasminogen activator (rt-PA). Bleeding complications ranged from 5 to 20%, with the majority of complications being minor. Third, all three studies showed a reduction in the magnitude of procedure after successful thrombolysis, although the impact on limb salvage was variable. Equivalent amputation rates in both thrombolytic and surgery groups were found in the Rochester Trial and TOPAS, while a benefit for thrombolysis was found in subgroup analysis of patients with acute bypass graft occlusion in STILE.

In the STILE trial, when patients with native artery occlusion were stratified by location, limb salvage for iliac common femoral occlusions were equivalent for surgery or thrombolysis. However, limb salvage was improved when superficial-femoral occlusions were surgically treated compared to thrombolysis.[231] In patients with bypass grafts, prosthetic grafts randomized to both surgical and thrombolysis groups tended to have statistically significant increased major morbidity compared with autogenous grafts. Although patients with autogenous graft occlusion tended to do better than patients with prosthetic occlusion, once patency was restored either by thrombolysis or surgery, there were no outcome differences at 30 days or 1 year.[231]

An investigation of the costs associated with two treatment options for acute peripheral arterial occlusions, thrombolysis and surgical intervention was reported by Ouriel et al.[161] One hundred fourteen patients were randomly assigned to receive urokinase ($n = 57$) or to undergo an operation ($n = 57$) as the initial therapeutic intervention. The total treatment costs did not differ significantly between the two treatment groups ($22,171 ± $4,959 in the thrombolytic group and $19,775 ± $5,253 in the operative group). The total hospital charges were similar between the two groups. Overall, the total charges were remarkably similar between the two treatment groups, averaging $40,823 ± $8,764 in the thrombolytic group and $41,930 ± $10,398 in the operative group. An economic analysis of the data confirmed that the total economic impact of thrombolysis approximated that of initial operative therapy.

Thrombolytic therapy is an important consideration in the initial management of acute vascular graft thrombosis. Caution must be exercised, however, in choosing thrombolytic treatment, which often takes several hours or days to complete. Thrombolysis should be avoided in favor of surgical thrombectomy in critically ischemic limbs that are immediately threatened.

Nonreconstructible Disease

Despite the ability of modern surgical techniques to bypass to distal tibial or even pedal vessels, there is a small population of patients who will be nonreconstructible. These patients may include those in whom prior bypasses have failed or are not technically feasible, those who refuse surgery, or those that are at too high risk for the reconstruction necessary for limb salvage. In these patients, nonhealing gangrenous ulcers or intractable pain may be the symptoms that push the patient and surgeon toward lower extremity amputation (see Chapters 28, 29, and 36). The options other than amputation are limited in these cases and not universally accepted as standard therapy.

Hyperbaric Oxygen

Oxygen plays a key role in healing, and the absence of oxygen is a cause of chronic nonhealing wounds. If tissue oxygenation cannot be improved by improving tissue perfusion with bypass techniques, in theory, increasing the oxygen content of the blood that can be delivered may be helpful for wound healing. Hyperbaric oxygen therapy consists of breathing 100% oxygen while the entire body is surrounded by pressure greater than atmospheric. This treatment can only be given in a hyperbaric chamber. Prospective studies supporting the use of hyperbaric oxygen in diabetics with gangrenous foot ulcers are few, contain small numbers of patients, and are nonrandomized.[62, 241] Studies that are available have shown only modest improvements in wound healing or control of distal infection. With the lack of data from prospective randomized trials showing efficacy of hyperbaric oxygen therapy, this modality cannot be recommended with confidence in the treatment of nonhealing diabetic foot ulcers.

Topical Growth Factors

A variety of endogenous polypeptide growth factors have been identified that play central roles in the stimulation of cell proliferation, differentiation, and maintenance of viability. Growth factors have emerged as potential agents that may facilitate and accelerate healing, particularly in hard-to-heal wounds in diabetic patients.[121] Although a number of industry-sponsored clinical trials of various growth factors have been approved by the FDA, the most widely studied agent for facilitating the healing of chronic wounds is a mixture of growth factors and other platelet-derived factors called platelet-derived wound-healing factors (PDWHFs). Randomized trials have shown mixed results with

regard to efficacy,[116, 122] but even proponents of these topical growth factors recommend their use only in the setting of a comprehensive clinical wound care protocol including strict glucose regulation, meticulous wound care, arterial revascularization, control of infection, and careful follow-up.[65] Another randomized trial testing recombinant human platelet-derived growth factor (rh-PDGF) has also shown efficacy in healing chronic diabetic neurotrophic ulcers.[204] Again, in this study, patients were treated with comprehensive wound care and had transcutaneous oxygen tensions of 30 mm Hg or greater.[204] Although these topical agents may hold great promise as future therapeutic agents, in the setting of nonreconstructible disease with chronic limb ischemia, their use should be limited to highly selected patients and only as an adjunct to comprehensive wound care.

Intractable Pain

In patients with intensely painful ischemic ulcers and/or rest pain, but who have no reasonable chance of revascularization, there are few alternatives to amputation. One alternative is multisensory peripheral nerve severing in the affected limb.[167] Considerable pain relief may be obtained, but only a third of the patients may retain a functional lower extremity over 6 months. Epidural spinal stimulation with a permanently implantable pulse generator is another reported technique in this highly selected group of end-stage vascular patients. Symptomatic relief has been reported in approximately 80% of patients with ischemic rest pain in preliminary studies both in the United States and in Europe.[40, 74, 230] Despite these encouraging results, the role of epidural spinal stimulation in the treatment of intractable ischemic pain is yet to be clearly determined, and we have not used it in our practice.

Upper Extremity Complications in Diabetics

Occlusive arterial lesions of the upper extremity are much less common than in the lower extremity and may be associated with thoracic outlet syndrome or collagen vascular disorders. It has been estimated that two thirds of patients with localized finger gangrene have large artery proximal obstruction and the remaining one third have systemic diseases associated with diffuse occlusions of palmar and digital arteries.[216] In the latter group, collagen vascular disorders like hypersensitivity angiitis, scleroderma, systemic lupus erythematosus, and others are the main causative factor.

Diabetes mellitus, although not commonly associated with upper extremity gangrene, can occasionally lead to severe finger ischemia, especially in the dialysis or post–renal transplant patient. The decreased blood flow to the digits secondary to vascular access procedures, along with the digital arterial occlusive disease and the common practice of glucose monitoring with blood obtained from fingersticks, makes the uremic patient at risk for hand ischemia and gangrene (Fig. 25–24). These factors are responsible for the increased incidence of upper or lower limb loss. In the series reported by Mitchell[148] of 16 diabetic patients with successful renal allografts, eight (50%) required one or more amputations and four had amputations of two or more extremities including the upper extremity. Careful selection of vascular access sites, good hand care, and intentional

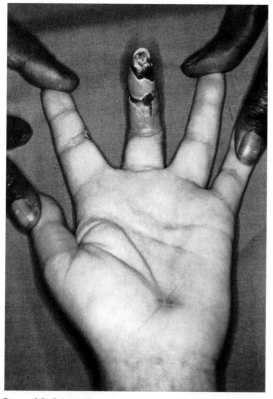

Figure 25–24 ■ Gangrene in the middle finger in a diabetic patient on steroids following renal transplant.

interruption of the vascular access after successful allograft may decrease this complication.

Venous Stasis Ulcers

Chronic venous insufficiency is associated with clinical severity ranging from superficial varicosities to cutaneous ulceration. Mild chronic venous insufficiency may manifest as superficial varicosities or mild ankle edema. Moderate chronic venous insufficiency is manifest by brawny edema, hyperpigmentation of the skin, and subcutaneous fibrosis without ulceration. Severe chronic venous insufficiency is associated with ulceration, eczematous changes, and severe edema. As with arterial insufficiency, patients with venous insufficiency should undergo noninvasive vascular studies to evaluate the underlying level of venous incompetence, which can be either the superficial or deep venous systems, or a combination of the two. The cornerstone of treatment for chronic venous insufficiency has been nonoperative, consisting of skin care, elimination of local cellulitis, limb elevation, leg exercise, and compressive therapy.[185] Skin care includes keeping the skin well hydrated and moist to prevent drying and fissuring. Neutral soaps for washing as well as topical corticosteroids for dermatitis and pruritis are also useful. Although venous stasis ulcers are often chronically contaminated, antibiotics are reserved for the treatment of cellulitis and not recommended for chronic use. Patients should avoid prolonged standing or sitting with their legs in a dependent position, since exposure to a hydrostatic column of blood is an important etiology of cutaneous venous stasis manifestations. Since the calf muscle pump is an important factor in returning blood to the heart in the lower limb, a program of exercise while wearing a gradient fitted elastic stocking should also be instituted. Compressive therapy is recommended in all patients with skin changes, ulceration, and leg edema. Therapy often consists of Unna's boot or graduated pressure elastic stockings. Other nonoperative treatment options include the use of sequential gradient pneumatic compression systems.[144]

Surgical treatment of chronic venous insufficiency is reserved for those patients that fail nonoperative therapy, and is tailored to the underlying venous abnormality. For patients with superficial venous insufficiency, ligation and stripping of the greater or lesser saphenous venous system, with ligation of incompetent perforating veins between the superficial and deep venous systems, may be indicated. Patients with deep venous insufficiency may benefit from surgical ligation of incompetent perforating veins. This can be accomplished transcutaneously for perforators localized around an ulcer bed; or in patients with severe lipodermatosclerosis, it can be accomplished subfascially by open or endoscopic techniques.[88, 89, 106, 172] Other less commonly employed surgical modalities include operative valvuloplasty, venous transposition, and venous bypass.[182]

REFERENCES

1. Abbott WM, Green RM, Matsumoto T, et al: Prosthetic above-knee femoropopliteal bypass grafting: Results of a multicenter randomized prospective trial. Above-Knee Femoropopliteal Study Group. J Vasc Surg 25:19–28, 1997.
2. Adera HM, James K, Castronuovo JJ Jr, et al: Prediction of amputation wound healing with skin perfusion pressure. J Vasc Surg 21:823–829, 1995.
3. Allen BT, Reilly JM, Rubin BG, et al: Femoropopliteal bypass for claudication: Vein vs. PTFE. Ann Vasc Surg 10:178–185, 1996.
4. Ambrus J, Ambrus CM, Taheri S, et al: Red cell flexibility and platelet aggregation in patients with chronic obstructive vascular disease (CAOD) and study of therapeutic approaches. Angiology 35:418–426, 1984.
5. Ansell G, Tweedie M, West C, et al: The current status of reactions to intravenous contrast media. Invest Radiol 15(Suppl):S32–S39, 1980.
6. Anto HR, Chou S-Y, Porush JG, Shapiro WB: Infusion intravenous pyelography and renal function: Effects of hypertonic mannitol in patients with chronic renal insufficiency. Arch Intern Med 141:1652–1656, 1981.
7. Arcan J, Blanchard J, Boissel J, et al: Multicenter double-blind trial of ticlopidine in the treatment of intermittent claudication and the prevention of its complications. Angiology 39:802–811, 1988.
8. Ascer E, Veith F, Gupta S, et al: Six year experience with expanded polytetrafluoroethylene arterial grafts for limb salvage. J Cardiovasc Surg 26:468–472, 1985.
9. Auer A, Hurley J, Binnington H, et al: Distal tibial vein grafts for limb salvage. Arch Surg 118:597–602, 1983.
10. Bagger JP, Helligsoe P, Randsbaek F, et al: Effect of verapamil in intermittent claudication. A randomized, double-blind, placebo-controlled, crossover study after individual dose-response assessment. Circulation 95:411–414, 1997.
11. Balsano F, Coicheri S, Libretti A, et al: Ticlopidine in the treatment of intermittent claudication: A 21 month double-blind trial. J Lab Clin Med 114:84–91, 1989.
12. Barner H, Kaiser G, Willman V: Blood flow in the diabetic leg. Circulation 43:391–394, 1971.
13. Barnes R, Shanik G, Slaymaker E: An index of healing in below-knee amputation: Leg blood pressure by Doppler ultrasound. Surgery 79:13–20, 1976.
14. Barnes R, Thompson B, MacDonald C, et al: Serial noninvasive studies do not herald postoperative failure of femoropopliteal or femorotibial bypass grafts. Ann Surg 210:486–493, 1989.
15. Barrett BJ, Parfrey PS, Vavasour HM, et al: A comparison of nonionic, low-osmolality radiocontrast agents with ionic, high-osmolality agents during cardiac catheterization. N Engl J Med 326:431–436, 1992.
16. Belch JJ, Bell PR, Creissen D, et al: Randomized, double-blind, placebo-controlled study evaluating the efficacy and safety of AS-013, a prostaglandin E1 prodrug, in patients with intermittent claudication. Circulation 95:2298–2302, 1997.
17. Belch JJ, Newman P, Drury JK, et al: Intermittent epoprostenol (prostacyclin) infusion in patients with Raynaud's syndrome: A double-blind controlled trial. Lancet 1:313–315, 1983.
18. Belkin M, Knox J, Donaldson MC, et al: Infrainguinal arterial reconstruction with nonreversed greater saphenous vein. J Vasc Surg 24:957–962, 1996.
19. Bendick P, Glover J, Kuebler T, Dilley R: Progression of atherosclerosis in diabetics. Surgery 93:834–838, 1983.
20. Bengoechea E, Cuesta M, Doblas M: Extensive endarterectomy of the aorta, common and external iliac arteries and common femoral arteries by a modified LeVeen method. Surgery 99:537–548, 1986.
21. Bergamini TM, Towne JB, Bandyk DF, et al: Experience with in situ saphenous vein bypass during 1981 to 1989: Determinant factors of long-term patency. J Vasc Surg 13:137–149, 1996.
22. Bergan J, Veith F, Banhard V, et al: Randomization of autogenous vein and polytetrafluoroethylene grafts in femoral-distal reconstruction. Surgery 92:921–930, 1982.
23. Berkowitz H, Greenstein S: Improved patency in reversed femoral-infrapopliteal autogenous vein grafts by early detection and treatment of the failing graft. J Vasc Surg 5:755–761, 1987.
24. Bernstein E, Greenspan R, Loken M: Intravenous abdominal aortography: A preliminary report. Surgery 44:529, 1958.
25. Bernstein E, Rhodes G, Stuart S, et al: Toe pulse reappearance time in prediction of aortofemoral bypass success. Ann Surg 193:201, 1981.
26. Beroniade VC: Prevention of acute renal failure secondary to radiocontrast agents [abstract]. Abstracts of the 8th International Congress of Nephrology. Athens. Basel, Switzerland: Karger, 1981, p 380.
27. Blanchard J, Carreras LO, Kindermans M: Results of EMATAP: A double-blind placebo-controlled multicentre trial of ticlopidine in patients with peripheral arterial disease. Nouv Rev Fran Hematol 35:523–528, 1994.
28. Bone G, Pomajzl M: Toe blood pressure by photoplethysmography: An index of healing in forefoot amputation. Surgery 89:569–574, 1981.
29. Bornmyr S, Martensson A, Svensson H, et al: A new device combining laser Doppler perfusion imaging and digital photography. Clin Physiol 16:535–541, 1996.

30. Boyd A: The natural course of arteriosclerosis of the lower extremities. Proc R Soc Med 55:591, 1962.

31. Bremer J: Carnitine metabolism and functions [review]. Physiol Rev 63:1420–1480, 1983.

32. Brevetti G, Chiariello M, Ferulano G, et al: Increases in walking distance in patients with peripheral vascular disease treated with L-carnitine: A double-blind, cross-over study. Circulation 77:767–773, 1988.

33. Brevetti G, Perna S, Sabba C, et al: Effect of propionyl-L-carnitine on quality of life in intermittent claudication. Am J Cardiol 79:777–780, 1997.

34. Brewster D, Darling R: Optimal methods of aortoiliac reconstruction. Surgery 84:739–748, 1978.

35. Brewster D, Perler B, Robinson J, Darling R: Aortofemoral graft for multilevel occlusive disease. Predictors of success and need for distal bypass. Arch Surg 117:1593–1600, 1982.

36. Brewster DC: Current controversies in the management of aortoiliac occlusive disease. J Vasc Surg 25:365–379, 1997.

37. Brooks B: Intra-arterial injection of sodium iodide. JAMA 82:1016, 1924.

38. Buchbinder D, Pasch A, Rollins D, et al: Results of arterial reconstruction of the foot. Arch Surg 121:673–677, 1986.

39. Buchbinder D, Pasch A, Verta M, et al: Ankle bypass: Should we go the distance? Am J Surg 150:216–219, 1985.

40. Bunt TJ, Holloway GA, Lawrence P, et al: Experience with epidural spinal stimulation in the treatment of end-stage peripheral vascular disease. Semin Vasc Surg 4:216–220, 1991.

41. Butcher HR Jr, Jaffe B: Treatment of aortoiliac arterial occlusive disease by endarterectomy. Ann Surg 173:925–932, 1971.

42. Cambria R, Brewster D, Abbott W, et al: Transperitoneal versus retroperitoneal approach for aortic reconstruction: A randomized prospective study. J Vasc Surg 11:314–324, 1990.

43. Chacon-Quevedo A, Eguaras MG, Calleja F, et al: Comparative evaluation of pentoxifylline, buflomedil, and nifedipine in the treatment of intermittent claudication of the lower limbs. Angiology 45:647–653, 1994.

44. Chowdary R, Celani V, Goodreau J, et al: Free-tissue transfers for limb salvage utilizing in situ saphenous vein bypass conduit as the inflow. Plast Reconstr Surg 87:529–535, 1991.

45. Cina C, Katsamouris A, Megerman J, et al: Utility of transcutaneous oxygen tension measurements in peripheral arterial occlusive disease. J Vasc Surg 1:362–371, 1984.

46. Clagett G, Genton E, Salzman E: Antithrombotic therapy in peripheral vascular disease [review]. Chest 95(Suppl):128S–139S, 1989.

47. Clyne CA, Archer TJ, Atuhaire LK, et al: Random control trial of a short course of aspirin and dipyridamole (Persantin) for femorodistal grafts. Br J Surg 74:246–248, 1987.

48. Comerota AJ, Weaver FA, Hosking JD, et al: Results of a prospective, randomized trial of surgery versus thrombolysis for occluded lower extremity bypass grafts. Am J Surg 172:105–112, 1996.

49. Creasy TS, McMillan PJ, Fletcher EW, et al: Is percutaneous transluminal angioplasty better than exercise for claudication? Preliminary results from a prospective randomised trial. Eur J Vasc Surg 4:135–140, 1990.

50. Cronenwett JL, McDaniel MD, Zwolak RM, et al: Limb salvage despite extensive tissue loss. Free tissue transfer combined with distal revascularization. Arch Surg 124:609–615, 1989.

51. Cutler BS, Thompson JE, Kleinsasser LJ, Hempel GK: Autologous saphenous vein femoropopliteal bypass: Analysis of 298 cases. Surgery 79:325–331, 1976.

52. Dachman AH: New contraindication to intravascular iodinated contrast material [letter]. Radiology 197:545, 1995.

53. Dahllof A, Bjorntorp P, Holm J, Schersten T: Metabolic activity of skeletal muscle in patients with peripheral arterial insufficiency. Effect of physical training. Eur J Clin Invest 4:9–15, 1974.

54. Dahllof AG, Holm J, Schersten T, Sivertsson R: Peripheral arterial insufficiency, effect of physical training on walking tolerance, calf blood flow, and blood flow resistance. Scand J Rehabil Med 8:19–26, 1976.

55. Dalman RL, Taylor LM Jr, Moneta GL, et al: Simultaneous operative repair of multilevel lower extremity occlusive disease. J Vasc Surg 13:211–219, 1991.

56. Dardik H, Ibrahim IM, Dardik II: The role of the peroneal artery for limb salvage. Ann Surg 189:189–198, 1979.

57. Dardik H, Sussman BC, Kahn M, et al: Lysis of arterial clot by intravenous or intra-arterial administration of streptokinase. Surg Gynecol Obstet 158:137–140, 1984.

58. Dettori AG, Pini M, Moratti A, et al: Acenocoumarol and pentoxifylline in intermittent claudication. A controlled clinical study. The APIC Study Group. Angiology 40:237–248, 1989.

59. DeWeese JA, Rob CG: Autogenous venous grafts ten years later. Surgery 82:755–784, 1977.

60. Diehm C, Balzer K, Bisler H, et al: Efficacy of a new prostaglandin E1 regimen in outpatients with severe intermittent claudication: Results of a multicenter placebo-controlled double-blind trial. J Vasc Surg 25:537–544, 1997.

61. Dintenfass L: Blood viscosity factors in severe nondiabetic and diabetic retinopathy. Biorheology 14:151–157, 1977.

62. Doctor N, Pandya S, Supe A: Hyperbaric oxygen therapy in diabetic foot. J Postgrad Med 38:112–114, 1992.

63. Dos Santos R, Lamas A, Pereira C: Arteriografia da aorta e dos vasos abdominas. Med Contemp 47:93, 1929.

64. Dotter CT, Judkins MP: Transluminal treatment of arteriosclerotic obstruction. Description of a new technic and a preliminary report of its application. 1964 [classical article]. Radiology 172:904–920, 1989.

65. Doucette MM, Fylling C, Knighton DR: Amputation prevention in a high-risk population through comprehensive wound-healing protocol. Arch Phys Med Rehabil 70:780–785, 1989.

66. Duncan WC, Linton RR, Darling RC: Aortoiliofemoral atherosclerotic occlusive disease: Comparative results of endarterectomy and Dacron bypass grafts. Surgery 70:974–984, 1971.

67. Eisenberg RL, Bank WO, Hedgcock MW: Renal failure after major angiography. Am J Med 68:43–46, 1980.

68. Ericsson B, Haeger K, Lindell SE: Effect of physical training of intermittent claudication. Angiology 21:188–192, 1970.

69. Ernst EE, Matrai A: Intermittent claudication, exercise, and blood rheology. Circulation 76:1110–1114, 1987.

70. Feldman AJ, Nevonen M, Berguer R: Experience with popliteal-infrapopliteal bypass grafting. Surg Gynecol Obstet 154:238–240, 1982.

71. Fields WS, Lemak NA, Frankowski RF, Hardy RJ: Controlled trial of aspirin in cerebral ischemia. Stroke 8:301–314, 1977.

72. Flanigan DP, Williams LR, Keifer T, et al: Prebypass operative arteriography. Surgery 92:627–633, 1982.

73. Flinn WR, Rohrer MJ, Yao JS, et al: Improved long-term patency of infragenicular polytetrafluoroethylene grafts. J Vasc Surg 7:685–690, 1988.

74. Galley D, Rettori R, Boccalon H, et al: Electric stimulation of the spinal cord in arterial diseases of the legs. A multicenter study of 244 patients. J Mal Vasc 17:208–213, 1992.

75. Geoffroy J, Hoeffel JC, Pointel JP, et al: Osteoarticular lesions of the foot in diabetic patients. A systematic review of 1,501 radiological reports [author's translation]. J Radiol 59:557–562, 1978.

76. Gillings DB: Pentoxifylline and intermittent claudication: Review of clinical trials and cost-effectiveness analyses. J Cardiovasc Pharmacol 25 (Suppl 2):S44–S50, 1995.

77. Goldenberg SG, Alex M, Joshi RA, Blumenthal HT: Nonatheromatous peripheral vascular disease of the lower extremity in diabetes mellitus. Diabetes 8:261–273, 1959.

78. Graves EJ, Gillum BS: National Hospital Discharge Survey: Annual Summary, 1994. Vital Health Stat 13:128, 1997.

79. Greenwald LL, Comerota AJ, Mitra A, et al: Free vascularized tissue transfer for limb salvage in peripheral vascular disease. Ann Vasc Surg 4:244–254, 1990.

80. Gruntzig A, Hopff H: Percutaneous recanalization after chronic arterial occlusion with a new dilator-catheter (modification of the Dotter technique) [author's translation]. Dtsch Med Wochenschr 99:2502–2511, 1974.

81. Guggenheim W, Koch G, Adams AP, et al: Femoral and popliteal occlusive vascular disease. A report on 143 diabetic patients. Diabetes 18:428–433, 1969.

82. Gundersen J: Segmental measurements of systolic blood pressure in the extremities including the thumb and the great toe. Acta Chir Scand Suppl 426:1–90, 1972.

83. Hargrove WC, Berkowitz HD, Freiman DB, et al: Recanalization of totally occluded femoropopliteal vein grafts with low-dose streptokinase infusion. Surgery 92:890–895, 1982.

84. Harkonen S, Kjellstrand CM: Exacerbation of diabetic renal failure following intravenous pyelography. Am J Med 63:939–946, 1977.

85. Harris EJ Jr, Taylor LM Jr, McConnell DB, et al: Clinical results of axillobifemoral bypass using externally supported polytetrafluoroethylene. J Vasc Surg 12:416–421, 1990.

86. Harris PL, Veith FJ, Shanik GD, et al: Prospective randomized comparison of in situ and reversed infrapopliteal vein grafts. Br J Surg 80:173–176, 1993.

87. Harris RW, Andros G, Dulawa LB, et al: Successful long-term limb salvage using cephalic vein bypass grafts. Ann Surg 200:785–792, 1984.

88. Hauer G, Barkun J, Wisser I, Deiler S: Endoscopic subfascial discission of perforating veins. Surg Endosc 2:5–12, 1988.

89. Healey PJ, Healey EH, Wong R, Schaberg FJ Jr: Surgical management of the chronic venous ulcer: The Rob procedure. Am J Surg 137:556–559, 1979.

90. Hedberg B, Langstrom M, Angquist KA, Fugl-Meyer AR: Isokinetic plantar flexor performance and fatigability in peripheral arterial insufficiency. Effects of training vs. vascular surgery. Acta Chir Scand 154:363–369, 1988.

91. Hiatt WR, Regensteiner JG, Hargarten ME, et al: Benefit of exercise conditioning for patients with peripheral arterial disease. Circulation 81:602–609, 1990.

92. Hill JA, Winniford M, Cohen MB, et al: Multicenter trial of ionic versus nonionic contrast media for cardiac angiography. The Iohexol Cooperative Study. Am J Cardiol 72:770–775, 1993.

93. Hobson RWD, Lynch TG, Jamil Z, et al: Results of revascularization and amputation in severe lower extremity ischemia: A five-year clinical experience. J Vasc Surg 2:174–185, 1985.

94. Hornsby VP: Intravascular injection of iodinated contrast media [letter]. Clin Radiol 51:820, 1996.

95. Hossmann V, Auel H, Rucker W, Schror K: Prolonged infusion of prostacyclin in patients with advanced stages of peripheral vascular disease: A placebo-controlled cross-over study. Klin Wochenschr 62:1108–1114, 1984.

96. Imparato AM, Kim GE, Davidson T, Crowley JG: Intermittent claudication: Its natural course. Surgery 78:795–799, 1975.

97. Imparato AM, Kim GE, Madayag M, Haveson S: Angiographic criteria for successful tibial arterial reconstructions. Surgery 74:830–838, 1973.

98. Irwin ST, Gilmore J, McGrann S, et al: Blood flow in diabetics with foot lesions due to 'small vessel disease'. Br J Surg 75:1201–1206, 1988.

99. Jacobs J, Sena M, Fox N: The cost of hospitalization for the late complications of diabetes in the United States. Diabet Med 8:S23–S29, 1991.

100. Jacobs J, Sena M, Fox N: The cost of hospitalization for the late complications of diabetes in the United States. Diabet Med, 8:S23–S29, 1991.

101. Janka HU, Standl E, Mehnert H: Peripheral vascular disease in diabetes mellitus and its relation to cardiovascular risk factors: Screening with the Doppler ultrasonic technique. Diabetes Care 3:207–213, 1980.

102. Janzon L: The STIMS trial: The ticlopidine experience and its clinical applications. Swedish Ticlopidine Multicenter Study. Vasc Med 1:141–143, 1996.

103. Jeans WD, Armstrong S, Cole SE, et al: Fate of patients undergoing transluminal angioplasty for lower-limb ischemia. Radiology 177:559–564, 1990.

104. Jonason T, Ringqvist I: Diabetes mellitus and intermittent claudication. Relation between peripheral vascular complications and location of the occlusive atherosclerosis in the legs. Acta Med Scand 218:217–221, 1985.

105. Jones RL, Peterson CM: Hematologic alterations in diabetes mellitus. Am J Med 70:339–352, 1981.
106. Jugenheimer M, Junginger T: Endoscopic subfascial sectioning of incompetent perforating veins in treatment of primary varicosis. World J Surg 16:971–975, 1992.
107. Karanfilian RG, Lynch TG, Zirul VT, et al: The value of laser Doppler velocimetry and transcutaneous oxygen tension determination in predicting healing of ischemic forefoot ulcerations and amputations in diabetic and nondiabetic patients. J Vasc Surg 4:511–516, 1986.
108. Karmody AM, Leather RP, Shah DM, et al: Peroneal artery bypass: A reappraisal of its value in limb salvage. J Vasc Surg 1:809–816, 1984.
109. Karnik R, Valentin A, Stollberger C, Slany J: Effects of naftidrofuryl in patients with intermittent claudication. Angiology 39:234–240, 1988.
110. Katholi RE, Taylor GJ, McCann WP, et al: Nephrotoxicity from contrast media: Attenuation with theophylline. Radiology 195:17–22, 1995.
111. Katholi RE, Taylor GJ, Woods WT, et al: Contrast medium nephrotoxicity in humans is mediated by intrarenal adenosine and related to osmotic load [abstract]. Radiology 181(P):285, 1991.
112. Katholi RE, Taylor GJ, Woods WT, et al: Nephrotoxicity of nonionic low-osmolality versus ionic high-osmolality contrast media: A prospective double-blind randomized comparison in human beings. Radiology 186:183–187, 1993.
113. Katzen BT: Angiography of the abdominal aorta and its branches. Interventional Diagnostic and Therapeutic Procedures. New York: Springer Verlag, 1980.
114. Kent KC, Donaldson MC, Attinger CE, et al: Femoropopliteal reconstruction for claudication. The risk to life and limb. Arch Surg 123:1196–1198, 1988.
115. King RB, Myers KA, Scott DF, Devine TJ: The choice of operation in aortoiliac reconstructions for intermittent claudication. World J Surg 7:334–339, 1983.
116. Knighton DR, Ciresi K, Fiegel VD, et al: Stimulation of repair in chronic, nonhealing, cutaneous ulcers using platelet-derived wound healing formula. Surg Gynecol Obstet 170:56–60, 1990.
117. Kokesh J, Kazmers A, Zierler RE: Pentoxifylline in the nonoperative management of intermittent claudication. Ann Vasc Surg 5:66–70, 1991.
118. Kott I, Urca I, Sandbank U: Lumbar sympathetic ganglia in atherosclerotic patients, diabetic and nondiabetic. A comparative morphological and ultrastructural study. Arch Surg 109:787–792, 1974.
119. Kozloff L, Collins GJ Jr, Rich NM, et al: Fallibility of postoperative Doppler ankle pressures in determining the adequacy of proximal arterial revascularization. Am J Surg 139:326–329, 1980.
120. Kram HB, Appel PL, Shoemaker WC: Multisensor transcutaneous oximetric mapping to predict below-knee amputation wound healing: Use of a critical Po2. J Vasc Surg 9:796–800, 1989.
121. Krupski WC: Growth factors and wound healing. Semin Vasc Surg 5:249–256, 1992.
122. Krupski WC, Reilly LM, Perez S, et al: A prospective randomized trial of autologous platelet-derived wound healing factors for treatment of chronic nonhealing wounds: A preliminary report. J Vasc Surg 14:526–632. 1991.
123. Larsen OA, Lassen NA: Effect of daily muscular exercise in patients with intermittent claudication. Lancet 2:1093–1096, 1966.
124. Lassen NA, Holstein P: Use of radioisotopes in assessment of distal blood flow and distal blood pressure in arterial insufficiency. Surg Clin North Am 54:39–55, 1974.
125. Lautin EM, Freeman NJ, Schoenfeld AH, et al: Radiocontrast-associated renal dysfunction: Incidence and risk factors. AJR Am J Roentgenol 157:49–58, 1991.
126. Leather RP, Shah DM, Chang BB, Kaufman JL: Resurrection of the in situ saphenous vein bypass. 1000 cases later. Ann Surg 208:435–442, 1988.
127. Lee BY, LaPointe DG, Madden JL: Evaluation of lumbar sympathectomy by quantification of arterial pulsatile waveform. Vasc Surg 5:61–87, 1971.
128. LeVeen HH, Diaz C, Ip WM: Extraperitoneal aortoiliac disobliteration with plaque cracker. Am J Surg 136:221–224, 1978.
129. Lezack JD, Carter SA: The relationship of distal systolic pressures to the clinical and angiographic findings in limbs with arterial occlusive disease. Scand J Clin Lab Invest Suppl 128:97–101, 1973.
130. Lezack JD, Carter SA: Systolic pressures in the extremities of man with special reference to the toes. Can J Physiol Pharmacol 48:469–474, 1970.
131. Lindbjerg IF: Diagnostic application of the 133xenon method in peripheral arterial disease. Scand J Clin Lab Invest 17:589–599, 1965.
132. Linet OI, Mohberg NR, Sinzinger H, et al: Cycloprostin (epoprostenol) is effective in peripheral vascular disease. Cardiovascular Pharmacotherapy International Symposium 1985. Geneva, Switzerland, 1985.
133. Lundgren F, Dahllof AG, Lundholm K, et al: Intermittent claudication—surgical reconstruction or physical training? A prospective randomized trial of treatment efficacy. Ann Surg 209:346–355, 1989.
134. Lundgren F, Dahllof AG, Schersten T, Bylund-Fellenius AC: Muscle enzyme adaptation in patients with peripheral arterial insufficiency: Spontaneous adaptation, effect of different treatments and consequences on walking performance. Clin Sci 77:485–493, 1989.
135. Malone JM, Leal JM, Moore WS, et al: The "gold standard" for amputation level selection xenon-133 clearance. J Surg Res 30:449–455, 1981.
136. Malone JM, Moore WS, Goldstone J: The natural history of bilateral aortofemoral bypass grafts for ischemia of the lower extremities. Arch Surg 110:1300–1306, 1975.
137. Mannarino E, Pasqualini L, Innocente S, et al: Physical training and antiplatelet treatment in stage II peripheral arterial occlusive disease: Alone or combined? Angiology 42:513–521, 1991.
138. Mannarino E, Pasqualini L, Menna M, et al: Effects of physical training on peripheral vascular disease: A controlled study. Angiology 40:5–10, 1989.
139. Martin EC, Katzen BT, Benenati JF, et al: Multicenter trial of the Wallstent in the iliac and femoral arteries. J Vasc Intervent Radiol 6:843–849, 1995.
140. Mason RA, Arbeit LA, Giron F: Renal dysfunction after arteriography. JAMA 253:1001–1004, 1985.
141. Mathes SJ, Alpert BS, Chang N: Use of the muscle flap in chronic osteomyelitis: Experimental and

clinical correlation. Plast Reconstr Surg 69:815–829, 1982.

142. McAllister FF: The fate of patients with intermittent claudication managed nonoperatively. Am J Surg 132:593–595, 1976.

143. McAuley CE, Steed DL, Webster MW: Seven-year follow-up of expanded polytetrafluoroethylene (PTFE) femoropopliteal bypass grafts. Ann Surg 199:57–60, 1984.

144. McCulloch JM, Marler KC, Neal MB, Phifer TJ: Intermittent pneumatic compression improves venous ulcer healing. Adv Wound Care 7:22–26, 1994.

145. McDaniel MD, Macdonald PD, Haver RA, Littenberg B: Published results of surgery for aortoiliac occlusive disease. Ann Vasc Surg 11:425–441, 1997.

146. McMillan DE, Gion KM: Glucosylated hemoglobin and reduced erythrocyte deformability in diabetes. Horm Metab Res Suppl 11:108–112, 1981.

147. Melton LJD, Macken KM, Palumbo PJ, Elveback LR: Incidence and prevalence of clinical peripheral vascular disease in a population-based cohort of diabetic patients. Diabetes Care 3:650–654, 1980.

148. Mitchell JC: End-stage renal failure in juvenile diabetes mellitus: A 5-year follow-up of treatment. Mayo Clin Proc 52:281–288, 1977.

149. Moody AP, al-Khaffaf HS, Lehert P, et al: An evaluation of patients with severe intermittent claudication and the effect of treatment with naftidrofuryl. Cardiovasc Pharmacol 23(Suppl 3):S44–S47, 1994.

150. Moore RD, Steinberg EP, Powe NR, et al: Nephrotoxicity of high-osmolality versus low-osmolality contrast media: Randomized clinical trial. Radiology 182:649–655, 1992.

151. Morasch MD, Couse NF, Colgan MP, et al: Lower extremity bypass for critical ischemia using synthetic conduit and adjuvant vein cuff. Ann Vasc Surg 11:242–246, 1997.

152. Munichoodappa C, D'Elia JA, Libertino JA, et al: Renal artery stenosis in hypertensive diabetics. J Urol 121:555–558, 1979.

153. National Diabetes Fact Sheet: National estimates and general information on diabetes in the United States. Atlanta, GA: U.S. Department of Health and Human Services, Centers for Disease Control and Prevention, 1997.

154. Nevelsteen A, Suy R, Daenen W, et al: Aortofemoral grafting: Factors influencing late results. Surgery 88:642–653, 1980.

155. Neville RF, Attinger C, Sidaway AN: Prosthetic bypass with a distal vein patch for limb salvage. Am J Surg 174:173–176, 1997.

156. Nielsen PE, Rasmussen SM: Indirect measurement of systolic blood pressure by strain gauge technique at finger, ankle and toe in diabetic patients without symptoms of occlusive arterial disease. Diabetologia 9:25–29, 1973.

157. Nugent RA, Flak B: Contrast-enhanced imaging studies contraindicated in patients receiving Glucophage [letter]. Can Assoc Radiol J 47:225, 1996.

158. O'Mara CS, Flinn WR, Neiman HL, et al: Correlation of foot arterial anatomy with early tibial bypass patency. Surgery 89:743–752, 1981.

159. Oguagha C, Porush JG, Chou SY, et al: Prevention of acute renal failure (ARF) following infusion intravenous pyelography (IVP) in patients with chronic renal insufficiency (CRI) by furosemide (F) [abstract]. Abstracts of the 8th International Congress of Nephrology. Athens. Basel, Switzerland: Karger, 1981, p 290.

160. Ohki T, Marin ML, Veith FJ: Use of endovascular grafts to treat nonaneurysmal arterial disease. Ann Vasc Surg 11:200–205, 1997.

161. Ouriel K, Kolassa M, DeWeese JA, Green RM: Economic implications of thrombolysis or operation as the initial treatment modality in acute peripheral arterial occlusion. Surgery 118:810–814, 1995.

162. Ouriel K, Shortell CK, DeWeese JA, et al: A comparison of thrombolytic therapy with operative revascularization in the initial treatment of acute peripheral arterial ischemia. J Vasc Surg 19:1021–1030, 1994.

163. Ouriel K, Veith FJ, Sasahara AA: A comparison of recombinant urokinase with vascular surgery as initial treatment for acute arterial occlusion of the legs. Thrombolysis or Peripheral Arterial Surgery (TOPAS) Investigators. N Engl J Med 338:1105–1111, 1998.

164. Ouriel K, Veith FJ, Sasahara AA: Thrombolysis or peripheral arterial surgery: Phase I results. TOPAS Investigators. J Vasc Surg 23:64–75, 1996.

165. Padberg FT Jr, Back TL, Hart LC, Franco CD: Comparison of heated-probe laser Doppler and transcutaneous oxygen measurements for predicting outcome of ischemic wounds. J Cardiovasc Surg 33:715–722, 1992.

166. Panchenko E, Eshkeeva A, Dobrovolsky A, et al: Effects of indobufen and pentoxifylline on walking capacity and hemostasis in patients with intermittent claudication: Results of six months of treatment. Angiology 48:247–254, 1997.

167. Papa MZ, Amsalem Y, Bass A, et al: Peripheral nerve section as palliation for severe ischemic foot pain. J Cardiovasc Surg 25:115–117, 1984.

168. Pappas PJ, Hobson RWN, Meyers MG, et al: Patency of infrainguinal polytetrafluoroethylene bypass grafts with distal interposition vein cuffs. Cardiovasc Surg 6:19–26, 1998.

169. Parsons RE, Suggs WD, Veith FJ, et al: Polytetrafluoroethylene bypasses to infrapopliteal arteries without cuffs or patches: A better option than amputation in patients without autologous vein. J Vasc Surg 23:347–356, 1996.

170. Passman MA, Taylor LM, Moneta GL, et al: Comparison of axillofemoral and aortofemoral bypass for aortoiliac occlusive disease. J Vasc Surg 23:263–271, 1996.

171. Pierce GE, Turrentine M, Stringfield S, et al: Evaluation of end-to-side v end-to-end proximal anastomosis in aortobifemoral bypass. Arch Surg 117:1580–1588, 1982.

172. Pierik EG, van Urk H, Wittens CH: Efficacy of subfascial endoscopy in eradicating perforating veins of the lower leg and its relation with venous ulcer healing. J Vasc Surg 26:255–259, 1997.

173. Pond GD, Smyth SH, Roach DJ, Hunter G: Metformin and contrast media: Genuine risk or witch hunt? [letter; comment]. Radiology 201:879–880, 1996.

174. Porter JM, Mayberry JC, Taylor LM Jr, et al: Chronic lower-extremity ischemia. Part I. Curr Probl Surg 28:1–92, 1991.

175. Poulias GE, Doundoulakis N, Prombonas E, et al: Aorto–femoral bypass and determinants of early success and late favourable outcome. Experience with 1000 consecutive cases. J Cardiovasc Surg 33:664–678, 1992.

176. Prendiville EJ, Yeager A, O'Donnell TF Jr, et al: Long-term results with the above-knee popliteal expanded polytetrafluoroethylene graft. J Vasc Surg 11:517–524, 1990.

177. Quayle JB: Diabetic autonomic neuropathy in patients with vascular disease. Br J Surg 65:305–307, 1978.

178. Quinones-Baldrich WJ, Busuttil RW, Baker JD, et al: Is the preferential use of polytetrafluoroethylene grafts for femoropopliteal bypass justified? J Vasc Surg 8:219–228, 1988.

179. Ramsey DE, Manke DA, Sumner DS: Toe blood pressure. A valuable adjunct to ankle pressure measurement for assessing peripheral arterial disease. J Cardiovasc Surg 24:43–48, 1983.

180. Rasuli P, French G, Hammond DI: New contraindication to intravascular contrast material [letter; comment]. Radiology 201:289–290, 1996.

181. Ricco JB, Flinn WR, McDaniel MD, et al: Objective analysis of factors contributing to failure of tibial bypass grafts. World J Surg 7:347–352, 1983.

182. Rodriguez AA, O'Donnell TFJ: Surgical management of chronic venous insufficiency. In Stanley J, Ernst C (eds): Current Therapy in Vascular Surgery, 3rd ed. St. Louis: Mosby-Year-Book, 1995, pp 914–919.

183. Rosen RJ, Roven SJ, Taylor RF, et al: Evaluation of aorto-iliac occlusive disease by intravenous digital subtraction angiography. Radiology 148:7–8, 1983.

184. Rosenblatt MS, Quist WC, Sidawy AN, et al: Results of vein graft reconstruction of the lower extremity in diabetic and nondiabetic patients. Surg Gynecol Obstet 171:331–335, 1990.

185. Rummel MC, Kernstein MD: Nonoperative management of chronic venous insufficiency. In Stanley J, Ernst C (eds): Current Therapy in Vascular Surgery, 3rd ed. St. Louis: Mosby-Year-Book, 1995, pp 910–913.

186. Safadi R, Dranitzki-Elhalel M, Popovtzer M, Ben-Yehuda A: Metformin-induced lactic acidosis associated with acute renal failure. Am J Nephrol 16:520–522, 1996.

187. Sanchez LA, Gupta SK, Veith FJ, et al: A ten-year experience with one hundred fifty failing or threatened vein and polytetrafluoroethylene arterial bypass grafts. J Vasc Surg 14:729–738, 1991.

188. Schneider JR, Golan JF: The role of extraanatomic bypass in the management of bilateral aortoiliac occlusive disease. Semin Vasc Surg 7:35–44, 1994.

189. Schneider JR, McDaniel MD, Walsh DB, et al: Axillofemoral bypass: Outcome and hemodynamic results in high-risk patients. J Vasc Surg 15:952–963, 1992.

190. Schroer RH: Antithrombotic potential of pentoxifylline. A hemorheologically active drug. Angiology 36:387–398, 1985.

191. Schuler JJ, Flanigan DP, Williams LR, et al: Early experience with popliteal to infrapopliteal bypass for limb salvage. Arch Surg 118:472–476, 1983.

192. Seabrook GR, Mewissen MW, Schmitt DD, et al: Percutaneous intraarterial thrombolysis in the treatment of thrombosis of lower extremity arterial reconstructions. J Vasc Surg 13:646–651, 1991.

193. Searles JM Jr, Colen LB: Foot reconstruction in diabetes mellitus and peripheral vascular insufficiency. Clin Plast Surg 18:467–483, 1996.

194. Seldinger SI: AIF techniques. Catheter replacement of needle in percutaneous arteriography: New technique. Acta Radiol 39:368, 1953.

195. Serletti JM, Deuber MA, Guidera PM, et al: Atherosclerosis of the lower extremity and free-tissue reconstruction for limb salvage. Plast Reconstr Surg 96:1136–1144, 1995.

196. Serletti JM, Hurwitz SR, Jones JA, et al: Extension of limb salvage by combined vascular reconstruction and adjunctive free-tissue transfer. J Vasc Surg 18:972–980, 1993.

197. Shah DM, Darling RCR, Chang BB, et al: Long-term results of in situ saphenous vein bypass. Analysis of 2058 cases. Ann Surg 222:438–448, 1995.

198. Shustov SB: Controlled clinical trial on the efficacy and safety of oral sulodexide in patients with peripheral occlusive arterial disease. Curr Med Res Opin 13:573–582, 1997.

199. Sicard GA, Reilly JM, Rubin BG, et al: Transabdominal versus retroperitoneal incision for abdominal aortic surgery: Report of a prospective randomized trial. J Vasc Surg 21:174–183, 1995.

200. Skovborg F, Nielsen AV, Schlichtkrull J, Ditzel J: Blood-viscosity in diabetic patients. Lancet 1:129–131, 1966.

201. Sladen JG, Gilmour JL, Wong RW: Cumulative patency and actual palliation in patients with claudication after aortofemoral bypass. Prospective long-term follow-up of 100 patients. Am J Surg 152:190–195, 1986.

202. Solomon R, Werner C, Mann D, et al: Effects of saline, mannitol, and furosemide to prevent acute decreases in renal function induced by radiocontrast agents. N Engl J Med 331:1416–1420, 1994.

203. Solomon SA, Ramsay LE, Yeo WW, et al: Beta blockade and intermittent claudication: Placebo controlled trial of atenolol and nifedipine and their combination. BMJ 303:1100–1104, 1991.

204. Steed DL: Clinical evaluation of recombinant human platelet-derived growth factor for the treatment of lower extremity diabetic ulcers. Diabetic Ulcer Study Group. J Vasc Surg 21:71–81, 1995.

205. Steinberg EP, Moore RD, Powe NR, et al: Safety and cost effectiveness of high-osmolality as compared with low-osmolality contrast material in patients undergoing cardiac angiography. N Engl J Med 326:425–430, 1992.

206. Steinberg I, Finby N, Evans JA: A safe and practical intravenous method for abdominal aortography, peripheral arteriography and cerebral angiography. AJR Am J Roentgenol 82:758, 1959.

207. Stemmer EA: Influence of diabetes on patterns of peripheral vascular disease. Surg Rounds 13:43–53, 1990.

208. Sternby NH: Atherosclerosis in a defined population. An autopsy survey in Malmo, Sweden. Acta Pathol Microbiol Scand Suppl 194:5, 1968.

209. Sterpetti AV, Schultz RD, Feldhaus RJ, Peetz DJ Jr: Seven-year experience with polytetrafluoroethylene as above-knee femoropopliteal bypass graft. Is it worthwhile to preserve the autologous saphenous vein? J Vasc Surg 2:907–912, 1985.

210. Stonebridge PA, Prescott RJ, Ruckley CV: Randomized trial comparing infrainguinal polytetrafluoroethylene bypass grafting with and without vein interposition cuff at the distal anastomosis. The Joint Vascular Research Group. J Vasc Surg 26:543–550, 1997.

211. Strano A, Davi G, Avellone G, et al: Double-blind, crossover study of the clinical efficacy and the hemorheological effects of pentoxifylline in patients

with occlusive arterial disease of the lower limbs. Angiology 35:459–466, 1984.

212. Sullivan TR Jr, Welch HJ, Iafrati MD, et al: Clinical results of common strategies used to revise infrainguinal vein grafts. J Vasc Surg 24:909–919, 1996.

213. Szilagyi DE, Elliott JP Jr, Smith RF, et al: A thirty-year survey of the reconstructive surgical treatment of aortoiliac occlusive disease. J Vasc Surg 3:421–436, 1986.

214. Szilagyi DE, Hageman JH, Smith RF, et al: Autogenous vein grafting in femoropopliteal atherosclerosis: The limits of its effectiveness. Surgery 86:836–851, 1979.

215. Szilagyi DE, Smith RF, Scerpella JR, Hoffman K: Lumbar sympathectomy. Current role in the treatment of arteriosclerotic occlusive disease. Arch Surg 95:753–761, 1967.

216. Taylor LM Jr, Baur GM, Porter JM: Finger gangrene caused by small artery occlusive disease. Ann Surg 193:453–461, 1981.

217. Taylor LM Jr, Edwards JM, Porter JM: Present status of reversed vein bypass grafting: Five-year results of a modern series. J Vasc Surg 11:193–206, 1990.

218. Tenembaum MM, Rayfield E, Junior J, et al: Altered pressure flow relationship in the diabetic foot. J Surg Res 31:307–313, 1981.

219. The Canadian Cooperative Study Group: A randomized trial of aspirin and sulfinpyrazone in threatened stroke. N Engl J Med 299:53–59, 1978.

220. The STILE Investigators: Results of a prospective randomized trial evaluating surgery versus thrombolysis for ischemia of the lower extremity. The STILE trial. Ann Surg 220:251–268, 1994.

221. The University Group Diabetes Program: A study of the effects of hypoglycemic agents on vascular complications in patients with adult-onset diabetes. I: Design, methods, and baseline characteristics. Diabetes 19(Suppl 2):747–783, 1970.

222. Thomas JH, Steers JL, Keushkerian SM, et al: A comparison of diabetics and nondiabetics with threatened limb loss. Am J Surg 156:481–483, 1988.

223. Uusitupa MI, Niskanen LK, Siitonen O, et al: 5-year incidence of atherosclerotic vascular disease in relation to general risk factors, insulin level, and abnormalities in lipoprotein composition in non-insulin-dependent diabetic and nondiabetic subjects. Circulation 82:27–36, 1990.

224. van Breda A, Katzen BT: Radiologic aspects of intra-arterial thrombolytic therapy. In Comerata AJ (ed): Thrombolytic Therapy. Orlando, FL: Grune & Stratton, 1988.

225. van den Dungen JJ, Boontje AH, Kropveld A: Unilateral iliofemoral occlusive disease: Long-term results of the semiclosed endarterectomy with the ring-stripper. J Vasc Surg 14:673–677, 1991.

226. Vanhoutte PM: Endothelium and control of vascular function. State of the art lecture. Hypertension 13:658–667, 1989.

227. Veith FJ, Gupta SK, Ascer E, et al: Six-year prospective multicenter randomized comparison of autologous saphenous vein and expanded polytetrafluoroethylene grafts in infrainguinal arterial reconstructions. J Vasc Surg 3:104–114, 1986.

228. Veith FJ, Gupta SK, Wengerter KR, et al: Changing arteriosclerotic disease patterns and management strategies in lower-limb-threatening ischemia. Ann Surg 212:402–414, 1990.

229. Vincent DG, Salles-Cunha SX, Bernhard VM, Towne JB: Noninvasive assessment of toe systolic pressures with special reference to diabetes mellitus. J Cardiovasc Surg 24:22–28, 1983.

230. Visconti W, Fontana P, Buonocore P, et al: Spinal electrostimulation in the treatment of advanced chronic obliterating arteriopathies. Minerva Cardioangiol 44:19–27, 1996.

231. Weaver FA, Comerota AJ, Youngblood M, et al: Surgical revascularization versus thrombolysis for nonembolic lower extremity native artery occlusions: Results of a prospective randomized trial. The STILE Investigators. Surgery versus Thrombolysis for Ischemia of the Lower Extremity. J Vasc Surg 24:513–523, 1996.

232. Weaver FA, Toms C: The practical implications of recent trials comparing thrombolytic therapy with surgery for lower extremity ischemia. Semin Vasc Surg 10:49–54, 1997.

233. Wengerter KR, Veith FJ, Gupta SK, et al: Prospective randomized multicenter comparison of in situ and reversed vein infrapopliteal bypasses. J Vasc Surg 13:189–199, 1991.

234. White RA, White GH, Mehringer MC, et al: A clinical trial of laser thermal angioplasty in patients with advanced peripheral vascular disease. Ann Surg 212:257–265, 1990.

235. White RI Jr: Principles of percutaneous catheterization. In Fundamentals of Vascular Radiology. Philadelphia: Lea & Febiger, 1976.

236. Whittemore AD, Kent KC, Donaldson MC, et al: What is the proper role of polytetrafluoroethylene grafts in infrainguinal reconstruction? J Vasc Surg 10:299–305, 1989.

237. Widdershoven RM, LeVeen HH: Closed endarterectomy. Preferred operation for aortoiliac occlusive disease. Arch Surg 124:986–990, 1989.

238. Wolfe JH, Tyrrell MR: Improving the patency of prosthetic grafts with vein cuffs. Semin Vasc Surg 8:246–252, 1995.

239. Wyss CR, Harrington RM, Burgess EM, Matsen FAD: Transcutaneous oxygen tension as a predictor of success after an amputation. J Bone Joint Surg Am 70:203–207, 1988.

240. Wyss CR, Matsen FAD, Simmons CW, Burgess EM: Transcutaneous oxygen tension measurements on limbs of diabetic and nondiabetic patients with peripheral vascular disease. Surgery 95:339–346, 1984.

241. Zamboni WA, Wong HP, Stephenson LL, Pfeifer MA: Evaluation of hyperbaric oxygen for diabetic wounds: A prospective study. Undersea Hyperb Med 24:175–179, 1997.

Chapter 26

PLASTIC SURGICAL RECONSTRUCTION OF THE DIABETIC FOOT

■ Janice F. Lalikos, William A. Wooden, and Joseph C. Benacci

The field of plastic and reconstructive surgery emphasizes the restoration of form and function as its primary goal. The diabetic patient represents a significant challenge to the medical profession due to the progressive unrelenting impact that diabetes mellitus has on the body as a whole. When specifically addressing the impact of diabetes mellitus on the lower limb, the fight is certainly one of limb salvage. The plastic surgeon is often faced with difficult wound healing challenges requiring intricate reconstructive solutions. As a result, the field has developed an extensive understanding of wound healing from a metabolic and surgical standpoint and can provide significant support in the team management of the diabetic patient.

The human foot is comprised of a very complex and interdependent array of structures that function to support the body during standing, climbing, and ambulation. The feet are exposed to significant forces, yet an intricate interaction exists between the soft tissue envelope, the musculotendinous structures, and the bony support of the foot. The unique weight-bearing properties of the foot as well as its necessary sensibility enables ambula-

tion. When there is a breakdown or destruction of any of these structures, significant disability results. Approximately 20% of all diabetic patients who are hospitalized are admitted with foot-related problems.[1] Similarly, between 50 and 80% of lower limb amputations are performed in the diabetic population.[2] Obviously, the most efficacious and cost-effective long-term management of diabetic foot should involve prevention of foot ulceration. Evidence indicates that there are four significant factors responsible for diabetic foot ulceration: (1) poor blood supply to the foot secondary to the infrapopliteal vascular disease present within the lower limb, (2) pressure points on the plantar foot secondary to orthopedic deformities (e.g., Charcot joint deformity) with or without concomitant hyperkeratosis at points of chronic trauma (Fig. 26–1), (3) neuropathic conditions that result in decreased sensibility also leading to repeated unrecognized foot trauma (Fig. 26–2A), and (4) poor serum glucose control, which may allow rapid progression of cellulitis or soft tissue infection (Fig. 26–3A).

Prevention of foot ulceration accordingly may be addressed in four specific categories:

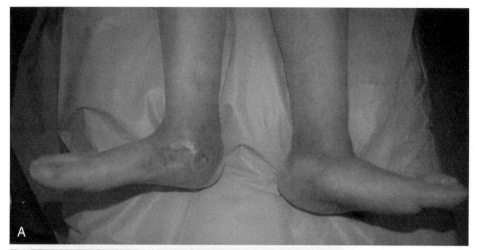

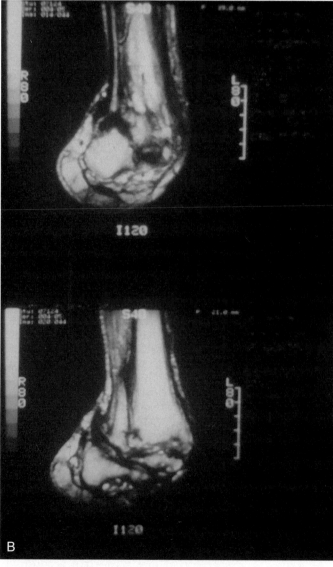

Figure 26–1 ■ *A,* Example of Charcot deformity of the right and left ankle as a result of severe and progressive neuropathic changes, repetitive trauma. *B,* Magnetic resonance imaging (MRI) scan of patient's right foot and ankle showing advanced radiographic changes.

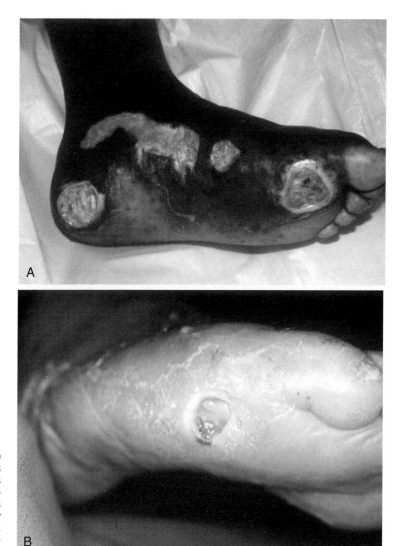

Figure 26–2 ■ *A,* Classic example of neurotrophic ulcer formation at the heel, medial arch, and first metatarsal with hammer-toe deformity and early Charcot changes. *B,* Neurotrophic ulcer overlying the fifth metatarsal head with chronic epidermal and dermal changes and necrotic base.

(1) prevention and vigilant attention to early signs of skin breakdown, pressure, or hyperkeratosis, particularly on the plantar and lateral aspects of the foot; (2) absolute glucose control; (3) optimization of the macrovascular blood flow in the infrapopliteal region with appropriate medical (i.e., alteration of red cell fluidity with pentoxyphylline) and perhaps surgical treatment of the atherosclerotic occlusive disease; and (4) decompression of pedal sensory nerves in the properly selected candidate to improve sensibility to the plantar foot. To be maximally effective and ensure patient compliance, prevention also mandates education of both patients and physicians involved to the importance of the multidisciplinary strategy.

Despite the most comprehensive and aggressive modes of prevention, either primary or secondary ulceration of the foot will be encountered. In these instances, plastic surgical reconstruction of the skin surface may be necessary and can be divided into discrete categories of treatment. First, the basics of wound care, which are not particularly different for the diabetic foot ulcer than for the nondiabetic patient, need to be instituted (Table 26–1). Thereafter, skin grafts, limited amputation, or local flaps can be used for discrete areas that do not heal primarily. For

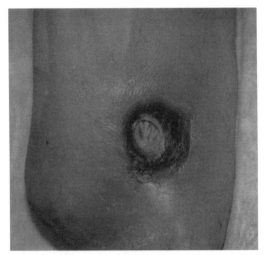

Figure 26–3 ■ Necrotic dorsal foot wound in insulin-dependent diabetic with surrounding necrosis, cellulitis, and necrotic wound base. Tissue cultures revealed both a polymicrobial floral as well as *Aspergillus*.

larger or more difficult locations, free tissue transfer may be necessary to provide adequate coverage. Ultimately, the goal of all reconstruction is to provide the opportunity for a painless bipedal ambulation.

When faced with a new ulceration in the diabetic foot, several questions need to be initially addressed, such as: What is the vascularity of the foot? This requires evaluation of both the arterial and the venous system, as compromise in either system may be partially or solely responsible for foot ulceration. An arterial pulse examination is necessary, but by itself is notoriously unpredictable for predicting wound healing. Ankle-brachial indices are also frequently misleading, as 30% of diabetics have noncompressible arterial walls, which falsely elevates the results.[8] Therefore, Doppler noninvasive duplex scanning of the arterial system or angiography is often needed to elucidate specific flow abnormalities and anatomic lesions in the lower limb. Both of these studies are more reliable in predicting the likelihood of wound healing than pulse examination, but are not absolute indicators of success or failure. Transcutaneous oxygen mapping has also been used as a parameter of healing. $TcPo_2$ readings of 25 mm Hg or less are much less likely to heal[10] (<10 mm Hg = frank ischemia[1]). Duplex evaluation of the venous drainage of the foot may be useful in identifying those patients with concomitant venous hypertension but provides no absolute predictors for outcome. Early assessment of vascularity should be made prior to wide debridement of the wound in order to assess the likelihood of healing. If the vascularity to the foot is poor, amputation need not be the only treatment alternative; vascular reconstructive efforts should be exhausted first. Since expeditious return to ambulation is the goal, only evidence of failed arterial reconstruction, nonreconstructible bypasses, gangrenous lesions, or significant soft tissue necrosis from infection should overwhelmingly prohibit salvage of the foot or any portion thereof. Revascularization should also be considered to ensure survival of a foot reconstructed with skin grafts, local flaps, or free tissue transfer. It is important to understand and monitor for segmental ischemia. In diabetic patients with disease distal to the infrapopliteal region, lower extremity revascularization may not ensure the survival of the leg or the entirety of the foot.

Table 26-1 ■ MINIMAL CLINICAL ASSESSMENT

General
  Complete history
  Complete physical
Wound specific
  Infection
    Tissue culture–specific treatment
  Vascularity
    Need for revascularization
  Oxygenation
    Need for revascularization
    Need for hyperbaric oxygen therapy
  Metabolic assessment
    Glucose control
    Nutritional assessment
    Other factors (e.g., hypothyroidism)
  Need for surgical treatment
    Debridement
    Revascularization
    Flap reconstruction
    Amputation
  Orthotic or orthopedic
    Unloading of the wound
  Dressing
    Wound specific

■ CASE STUDY 1

Figure 26–4A and B demonstrates the difficulty of wound management and the importance of revascularization. The patient is a middle-aged female insulin-dependent diabetic who presented with a dorsal lateral foot wound. On initial assessment she was felt to have reasonable vascularity to the foot and

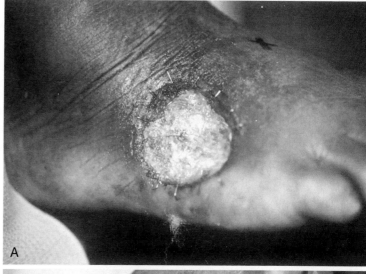

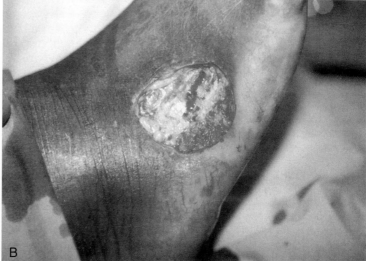

Figure 26–4 ■ *A,* Failed initial skin graft prior to revascularization. *B,* Same wound following debridement at time of revascularization. Note well-perfused wound base.

leg. The wound was treated with debridement, culture-specific antibiotics, and local wound care. The wound improved and was felt to be suitable for split-thickness skin grafting; this was done and failed. The patient was then referred to plastic surgery for reassessment. More detailed investigation revealed that the patient's arterial inflow was inadequate and the patient subsequently underwent revascularization per the vascular surgical service. This procedure restored flow to her foot, but note in Figure 26–4 that she still exhibited poor healing of her bypass incisions. Ultimately, the patient did well, but the scenario demonstrates the importance of a complete vascular evaluation in all diabetic patients, even if their wound seems minor.

Wound Management

The basic principles of wound management in the diabetic foot are not dissimilar to that of the nondiabetic foot. These include detailed wound evaluation of not only the skin and soft tissue structures but also the bony structures. Both the neurologic function and the vascular status of the foot need to be thoroughly catalogued. Then, the full wound evaluation is put in the context of the patient's overall condition and performance status. All of these factors determine not only the patient's initial wound healing perfor-

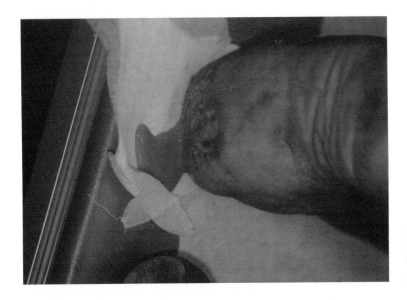

Figure 26–5 ■ Small heel ulcer in insulin-dependent diabetic with minimal clinical symptomatology but advanced plantar abscess and gross purulent drainage.

mance but also his or her ultimate outcome, and thereby dictate treatment planning.

For those individuals with obvious cellulitis, elevation of the foot and appropriate tissue culture–directed antibiotic therapy is mandatory. In patients with suspected loculated cavities of infected materials, aggressive exploration, drainage, and requisite debridement of all necrotic debris is performed (Fig. 26–5). Oftentimes, the diabetic patient may masquerade gross purulence and necrosis within the deeper spaces of the foot; therefore, a high index of suspicion should be present in the early evaluation to prevent significant and often rapid progression of an infectious process. Sometimes, aspiration with an 18-gauge needle can unveil a subfascial space abscess.[8] Following drainage of purulent material and the debridement of necrotic tissue, open wound packing with possible whirlpool or pulse irrigation lavage may facilitate clearing of the infection. Multiple debridements as well as amputations may be necessary prior to entertaining wound coverage options (Fig. 26–6). Of particular note, bony debridement of dead devitalized osteomyelitic bone segments may also be necessary. Accurate diagnosis of true osteomyelitis is oftentimes difficult in these situations because surrounding soft tissues are so contaminated.

Soft Tissue Reconstruction

Within the plastic surgical literature, foot reconstruction has been classified according to a number of criteria. One of the more prevalent schemas is to divide the foot into anatomic areas for reconstruction.[5] The four regions most commonly described are (1) the heel and the midplantar region (Fig. 26–7), (2) the distal plantar region (Fig. 26–8), (3) The malleolar, Achilles tendon and non–weight-bearing posterior heel area (Fig. 26–9), and (4) the dorsum (Fig. 26–10). The needs of each region will vary and therefore dictate specific solutions to satisfy its coverage needs.

The weight-bearing plantar surface is without question the most challenging area, as it ideally requires a sensate surface that will tolerate the trauma of weight bearing as well as provide a stable surface for the sheer forces related to ambulation. Ideally, that stable surface should be glabrous skin, which is difficult to recruit barring the plantar surface of the foot or palm of the hand. Conversely, the dorsal foot does not require the durability of the plantar foot and coverage need not require sensation to allow for safe ambulation. Therefore, skin grafts, either full thickness or split thickness, can work well in this location (Figs. 26–11 and 26–12).

Local Flaps

A number of local skin and muscle flaps are available within the foot itself. Many of these flaps are ideal for small defects. Local flaps, while providing like tissue for a foot defect, are limited by their arch of

Text continued on page 577

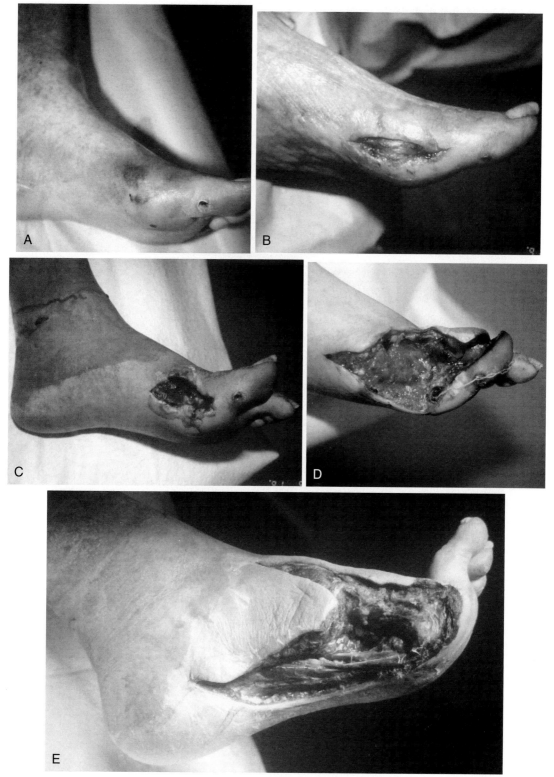

Figure 26–6 ■ *A*, Middle-aged white male with longstanding insulin-dependent diabetes mellitus presenting with small trophic ulcer over the first metatarsal head and signs of early infection surrounding the metatarsal head presenting for incision and drainage. *B*, Initial incision and drainage identifying involvement of the first metatarsal phalangeal joint and surrounding soft tissues. *C*, Progressive necrosis despite aggressive antibiotic therapy and debridement. *D*, Continued necrosis despite bony resection and systemic antibiotic therapy and serial debridement. *E*, Continued necrosis as a result of poor perfusion and hypovascularity.

Illustration continued on opposite page

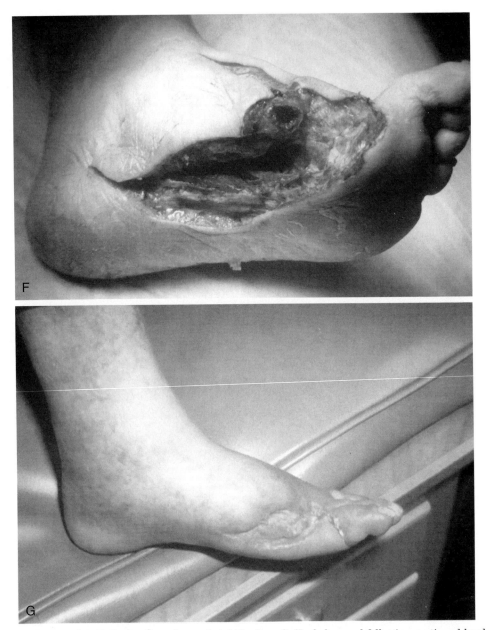

Figure 26–6 *Continued* ■ *F*, Early signs of wound stabilization. *G*, Healed wound following continued local wound care and subsequent split-thickness skin graft.

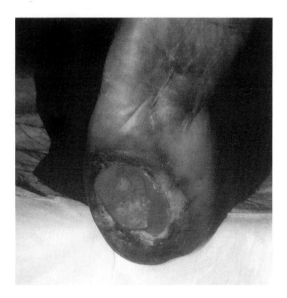

Figure 26–7 ■ Classic longstanding trophic heel ulcer with neuropathic, Charcot changes.

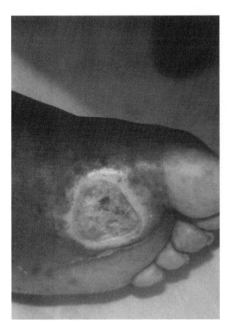

Figure 26–8 ■ Classic neuropathic changes and first metatarsal head ulceration.

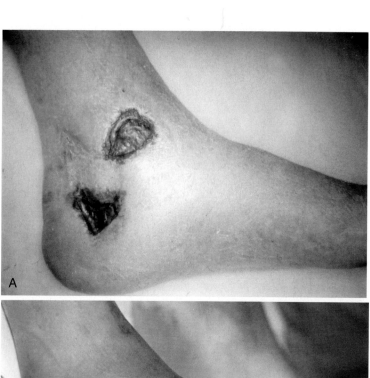

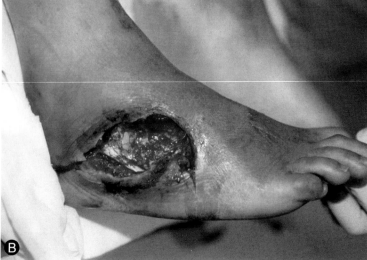

Figure 26–9 ■ *A,* Subacute medial malleolus and ankle wounds of longstanding duration. *B,* Acute lateral malleolus and dorsal foot wound secondary to minor trauma and secondary infection.

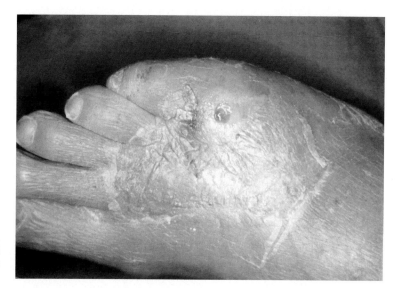

Figure 26–10 ■ Dorsal foot ulceration secondary to and associated with deep infection of the fifth toe and metatarsophalangeal joint.

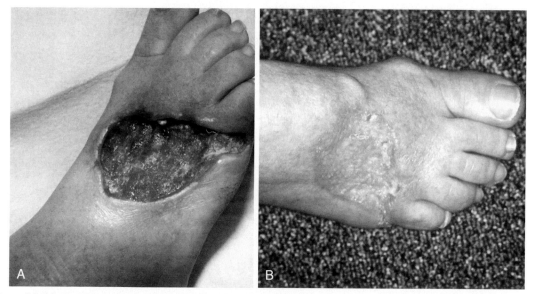

Figure 26–11 ■ A, Complex dorsal foot wound following serial debridement, antibiotic therapy, and local wound care. B, Healed wound following split-thickness skin graft.

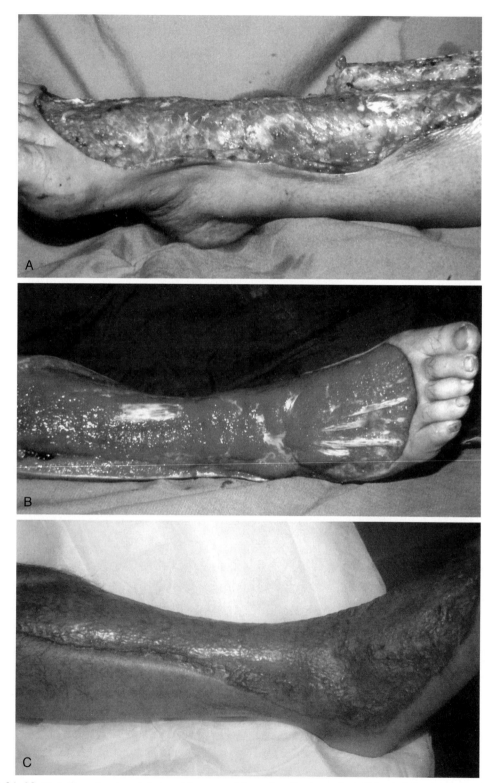

Figure 26–12 ■ *A*, Complex dorsal foot and leg wound in an insulin-dependent diabetic following a local trauma and soft tissue infection. *B*, Same wound following antibiotics and aggressive local wound management. *C*, Wound following successful split-thickness skin grafting.

rotation and sometimes by the vascular anatomy of the foot. Consequently, poor arterial inflow or collateral circulation between the anterior tibial, posterior tibial, and peroneal arteries may compromise the surgeon's ability to perform any of the local flaps. In addition, for larger defects they are often inadequate. Despite the above-mentioned limitations, the following local flaps have been successfully used to close foot wounds.[4, 8, 11]

1. Local random flaps such as the V-Y flap or rotational skin flap.
2. The medial plantar artery flap (Fig. 26–13).
3. The lateral calcaneal artery flap (Fig. 26–14).

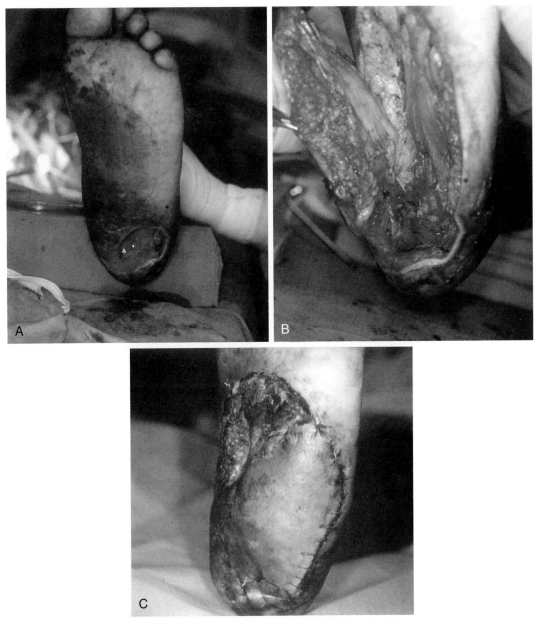

Figure 26–13 ▪ *A,* Stable but chronic heel ulcer in a longstanding insulin-dependent diabetic with prior first metatarsal head ulcer now healed and epithelialized for reconstruction using medial plantar artery flap and split-thickness skin grafting to the instep of foot. *B,* Medial plantar flap elevated. *C,* Flap insert with split-thickness graft to instep.

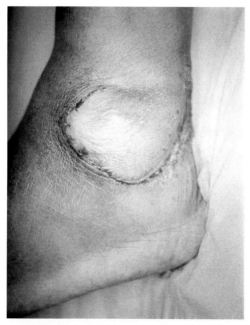

Figure 26–14 ■ Lateral malleolar ulcer closed with rotation flap and skin graft to cover defect.

4. The superior malleolar artery flap.
5. The medial calcaneal artery flap (Fig. 26–15).
6. The extensor digitorum brevis muscle flaps off of the lateral tarsal artery (Fig. 26–16).
7. The abductor hallucis muscle flap.
8. The abductor digiti minimi muscle flaps (lateral malleolar defects) (Fig. 26–17).
9. The flexor digiti minimi/flexor digitorum brevis muscle flaps (proximal small toe metatarsal defects) (Fig. 26–18).
10. The toe fillet flap (particularly useful in plantar defects on the weight-bearing heads of the metatarsophalangeal joints).

Free Tissue Transfer

For those patients in whom adequate debridement of the wounds has been accomplished and a clean wound with no evidence of infection is present, free tissue transfer may be necessary for wounds with adequate arterial inflow but which have defects too large for skin graft or local flap coverage. Also, free tissue may be indicated for wounds with exposed tendons or bony structures or in which a durable yet pliable skin surface is otherwise not available. The free tissue transfer allows one the ability to resurface essentially any size defect in the foot. This freedom allows for aggressive resection of scarred cicatricial skin as well as infected or necrotic soft tissue when appropriate. However, free tissue transfer should still be reserved for those patients in whom lesser local plantar flaps or skin grafts are not suitable, as the expenditure of patient and physician time as well as the delay in ultimate unaided ambulation is greater in the free tissue transfer reconstruction than in local flap reconstruction.[6]

There are basically two types of free flap options for the foot: the fasciocutaneous flap (free radial forearm flap, free lateral arm flap, free tensor fascia latae flap) and the muscle flap with overlying skin graft (free rectus abdominus muscle flap, free gracilis muscle flap, free latissimus dorsi flap, free serratus anterior flap). Many variables are analyzed before choosing the type of free tissue transfer. The size of the defect, of course, is one major factor. The need for muscle bulk or fill versus the need for thin pliable resurfacing is contemplated. Also, the recipient blood vessels and the length of the donor vessels determine the mechanical feasibility of the microvascular anastamosis. Lastly, the impact or functional loss of the donor tissue is also taken into account. Table 26–2 outlines the most commonly used free flaps for lower extremity reconstruction and their specifications.[3] It should be noted that the free tissue transfer, although often the only viable reconstructive solution, is a difficult and costly option requiring a dedicated patient and surgical team. It often requires an extensive hospitalization for recovery and rehabilitation. Therefore, strict patient selection and screening is warranted.

■ CASE STUDY 2

This case demonstrates the clinical complexity often encountered in the diabetic patient. This gentleman is a middle-aged insulin-dependent diabetic who had a long history of poor control and prior foot ulcers. He suffered an acute silent myocardial infarction requiring an emergent cardiac bypass. The postoperative period was quite complicated, accentuated by early mediastinitis requiring serial debridements and flap reconstruction. During this period he developed a limb-threatening heel ulcer exposing his calcaneus and Achilles tendons. After stabilization from cardiac, metabolic, nutritional, and wound standpoints, he underwent complete vascular assessment, which

Text continued on page 583

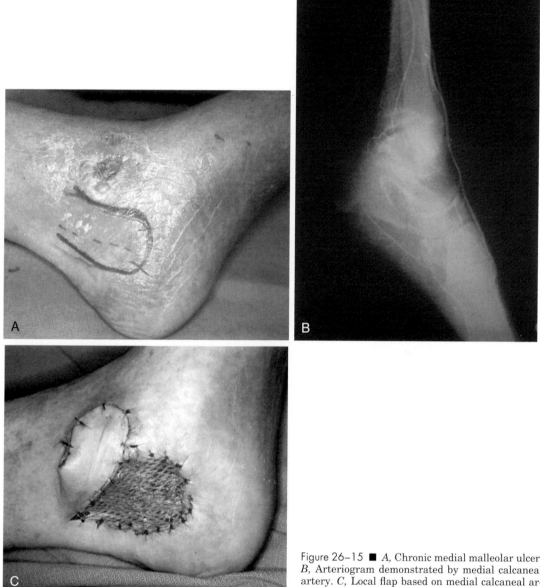

Figure 26–15 ■ *A*, Chronic medial malleolar ulcer. *B*, Arteriogram demonstrated by medial calcaneal artery. *C*, Local flap based on medial calcaneal artery and split-thickness skin graft to donor site.

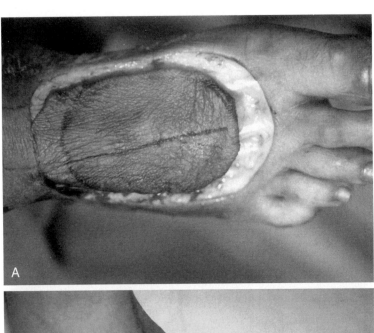

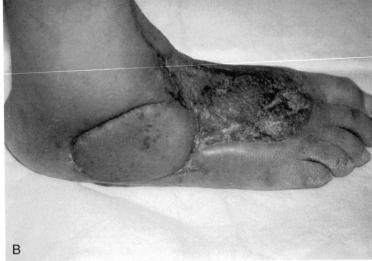

Figure 26–16 ■ *A*, Dorsalis pedis artery flap for coverage of a complex lateral ankle with open ankle joint secondary to *Cryptosporidium* infection. *B*, Healed flap and donor site skin graft.

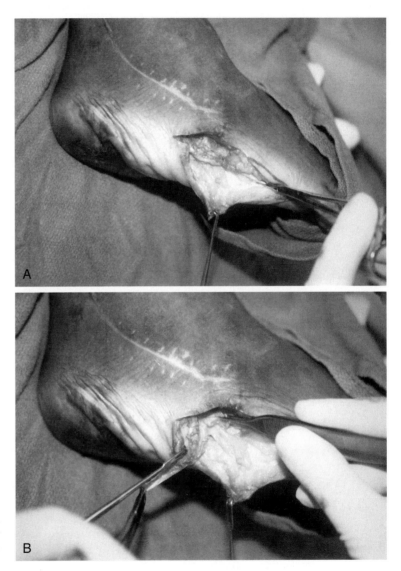

Figure 26–17 ■ *A* and *B*, Elevation and dissection of an adductor digiti minimi muscular flap being elevated for reconstruction of a proximal lateral foot ulcer.

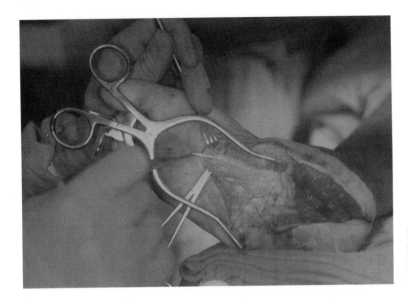

Figure 26–18 ■ Elevation and demonstration of a flexor digiti brevis muscular flap for reconstruction of a proximal heel ulceration.

Table 26-2 ■ ADVANTAGES AND DISADVANTAGES OF VARIOUS TYPES OF PRETISSUE TRANSFER

FLAP TYPE	ADVANTAGES	DISADVANTAGES
Fasciocutaneous Flaps		
Radial forearm	Easily accessible, long vascular pedicle. Potential for providing sensation using dorsal sensory branch of radial nerve. Relatively thin and pliable.	Potential arm morbidity, may require radial artery reconstruction. Limited by prior radial artery cannulation or injury.
Scapular/parascapular	Relatively large flap(s) potentially for multiple components including muscle and/or bone on a single large vascular pedicle.	Potential need to reposition during operative procedure. Donor site morbidity, shoulder stiffness, wide scars. Potential requirement for secondary skin grafting.
Lateral arm flap	Relatively accessible with reasonable pedicle length. Potential for providing sensation.	Potentially bulky—creates relatively large visible donor site.
Muscle Flaps		
Serratus muscular flap	Can be harvested in multiple segments depending on size of defect. Pedicle is consistent, relatively reliable, and large.	Creates a degree of shoulder and scapular weakness. Dissection can be difficult at times along the thoracodorsal nerve.
Latissimus dorsi flap	Large relatively straightforward dissection. Good vascular pedicle length.	Potentially bulky, creates relatively large donor site with degree of shoulder girdle weakness.
Rectus abdominus flap	Easily accessible, reliable vascular pedicle and anatomy.	Potential abdominal wall weakness and secondary hernia formation. Potential for atherosclerotic involvement of vascular pedicle.
Gracilis muscle flap	Generally accessible minimal donor site morbidity. Fairly reliable vascular pedicle.	Short vascular pedicle that can sometimes be affected by atherosclerotic disease.

demonstrated good arterial inflow and venous outflow. Plastic surgery was consulted and it was decided that no local options were available for durable wound coverage; hence a free tissue transfer. The potential flap selections included the radial forearm, scapular fasciocutaneous, rectus abdominus, and latissimus dorsi free flaps. Due to the superior quality of muscle in general to cover bony prominences and clear bacteria, the rectus abdominus muscle free flap was chosen with an overlying skin graft. Arteriography was performed and the posterior tibial vessels were chosen as recipient sites. The anastomosis was carried out in end-to-side fashion allowing for continued foot perfusion. The case is outlined in Figure 26–19.

Other Adjuncts

Other important adjuncts in the fight to heal diabetic wounds come into play either preoperatively or postoperatively. A rather new modality for wound healing is subatmospheric, negative-pressure treatment for wounds with impaired healing. Now widely available is the Vacuum Assisted Wound closure device, currently marketed by KCI Corporation. The VAC therapy concept was pioneered at Bowman Gray University and applies a vacuum (negative pressure) to a wound. This system has been shown to augment the formation of healthy granulation

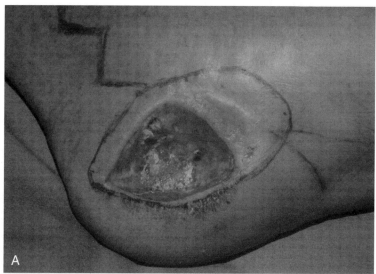

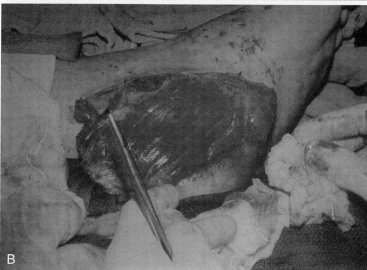

Figure 26–19 ■ *A,* Complex heel wound following revascularization and local wound care. *B,* Flap following vascular repair prior to skin graft.

tissue in an open wound bed in a carefully selected group of patients.[7] Orthotic devices also provide valuable support and protection to the healing wound. In some patients, a total non–weight-bearing patellar tibial brace with contralateral custom orthotic shoe lift allows patients to maintain a moderate degree of mobility while still providing non–weight-bearing status to the limb (Fig. 26–20).

Summary

Although there are a great many adjuncts to wound healing the critical factors remain as follows:

1. The control of infection both locally and systemically.
2. The control of metabolic factors such as glucose control, nutrition, concurrent illnesses, and medications such as steroids.
3. An educated, compliant, cooperative patient with the ability to participate in his or her assessment and care.

4. A care team including the full spectrum of medical and nonmedical support.
5. Mechanical unloading of the extremity.
6. Appropriate and complete debridement, drainage.
7. Vascular perfusion or reperfusion of the extremity.

Without perfusion, the tissues cannot be oxygenated or nourished, infections will not be cleared, and tissues will not heal and thus will not be eligible for reconstruction. A consistent, thorough vascular assessment is critical to salvage of a limb in the diabetic patient. Any plastic surgical reconstructive efforts, be they flaps or grafts, can provide an important adjunct to the salvage and maintenance of an extremity; however, without perfusion the limb is ultimately lost. Figure 26–21 provides a broad conceptual algorithm through which lower limb salvage can be considered. The threatened extremity (i.e., one that demonstrates severe claudication, rest pain, significant tissue loss, dependent rubor, or deep infection) requires intervention from a medical as well as a surgical

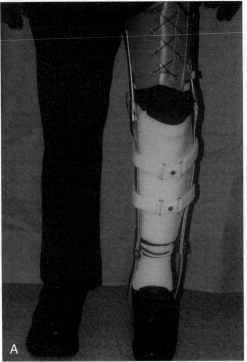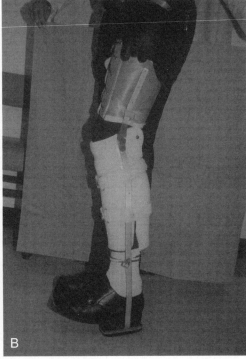

Figure 26–20 ■ *A* and *B*, Anterior and lateral photograph of the full non–weight-bearing patellar tibial brace with contralateral orthotic shoe with sole lift, allowing secondary healing of weight-bearing foot ulcers in the postoperative period following reconstruction.

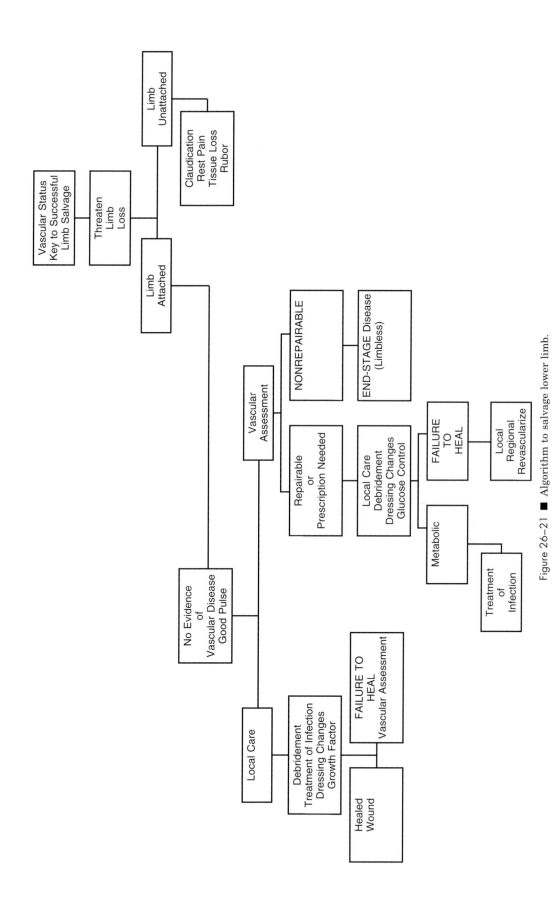

Figure 26–21 ■ Algorithm to salvage lower limb.

standpoint. Revascularization alone does not take the place of local adjuncts, medical management, and metabolic correction but proceeds rapidly in concert with the other interventions. Unfortunately, despite all our efforts, some wounds often still fail to heal due to factors as yet unknown to us. Thus continues the great challenge within the art and practice of medicine.

REFERENCES

1. Attinger CE: Foot and ankle preservation. *In* Aston SJ, Beasley RW, Thorne CMH (eds): Grabb and Smith's Plastic Surgery, 5th ed. Philadelphia: Lippincott-Raven Publishers, 1997, pp 1059–1075.
2. Banis JC, Derr JW, Richardson JD: A rational approach to ischemia and ischemic-diabetic foot reconstruction. *In* Jurkiewicz MJ, Culbertson JH (eds): Operative Techniques in Plastic and Reconstructive Surgery-Foot Reconstruction, Vol. 4, Philadelphia: WB Saunders, 1997, pp 217–235.
3. Germann G, Erdmann D: Foot reconstruction with microvascular flaps. *In* Jurkiewicz MJ, Culbertson JH (eds): Operative Techniques in Plastic and Reconstructive Surgery-Foot Reconstruction, Vol. 4, Philadelphia: WB Saunders, 1997, pp 172–182.
4. Heinz TR: Local flaps for hind foot reconstruction. *In* Jurkiewicz MJ, Culbertson JH (eds): Operative Techniques in Plastic and Reconstructive Surgery-Foot Reconstruction, Vol. 4, Philadelphia: WB Saunders, 1997, pp 157–164.
5. Hidalgo DA, Shaw WW: Reconstruction of foot injuries. Clin Plast Surg 13:663–680, 1986.
6. Levin LS: The reconstructive ladder—an orthoplastic approach. Orthop Clin Am 24:393–409, 1993.
7. Morykwas MJ, Argenta LC: Use of negative pressure to increase the rate of granulation tissue formation in chronic open wounds presented at the annual meeting. Federation of American Society for Experimental Biology—March 28–April 1, 1993, New Orleans.
8. Parker JA, Searles JM: Local flaps for forefoot and midfoot reconstruction. *In* Jurkiewicz MJ, Culbertson JH (eds): Operative Techniques in Plastic and Reconstructive Surgery-Foot Reconstruction, Vol. 4, Philadelphia: WB Saunders, 1997, pp 148–157.
9. Reiber GE, Lipsky BA, Gibbons GW: The burden of diabetic foot ulcers. Am J Surg 176:5S–10S, 1998.
10. Rhodes G, Skudder P: Salvage of ischemic diabetic feet: Roles of transcutaneous O_2 mapping and multiple configurations of in situ bypass. Am J Surg 152:165–169, 1986.
11. Saltz R, Hochberg J, Given KS: Muscle and musculocutaneous flaps of the foot. Clin Plast Surg 18:627–638, 1991.

Chapter 27

CHARCOT NEUROPATHY OF THE FOOT: SURGICAL ASPECTS

■ Jeffrey E. Johnson

Nonsurgical treatment utilizing total-contact casting followed by appropriate bracing and footwear is the "gold standard" for treatment of the majority of foot and ankle neuropathic (Charcot) fractures and dislocations. However, surgical treatment is indicated for chronic recurrent ulceration, joint instability or, in some cases, pain that has failed nonoperative treatment. Selected acute fractures may also have operative indications. The goals of operative treatment are to preserve functional activity with the aid of appropriate footwear or bracing and to prevent amputation. These goals are achieved through restoration of the contour or alignment of the affected foot and ankle segment. Despite the potential for significant operative complications, the overall success rate of limb salvage reconstruction is approximately 80 to 90%.[9, 15, 20, 22, 25, 30]

Neuropathic (Charcot) osteoarthropathy is a noninfective, destructive bone and joint fracture and/or dislocation associated with a peripheral neuropathy. Diabetes is the most common cause for these deformity-causing fractures in the United States, and neuropathic arthropathy has been estimated to occur in 0.1 to 0.5% of patients with diabetes mellitus.[16, 17] There are an estimated 16 mil-

lion diabetic patients in the United States.[2] Because of improvements in diabetes care, diabetic patients are living longer. Therefore, neuropathic arthropathy, a late effect of peripheral neuropathy of the foot and ankle, continues to be a major clinical problem.

The etiology and pathophysiology of neuropathic bone and joint destruction is still poorly understood. However, the stages of bone and joint destruction followed by fracture healing and remodeling were described by Eichenholtz.[10] The Eichenholtz classification is based on the characteristic clinical and radiographic changes that occur with neuropathic joint destruction or fracture over time and is therefore a temporally based classification.[12] These changes progress from the acute phase (dissolution), through the healing phase (coalescence), to the resolution phase. The timing and selection of a surgical procedure in a neuropathic patient should be made with a thorough understanding of the natural history and the temporal stage of the patient's neuropathic process.

Several authors have described classifications for the characteristic patterns of neuropathic bone and joint destruction.[5, 8, 11, 26] An understanding of these patterns is helpful in making the diagnosis of a Charcot foot in cases of occult neuropathy and in planning operative or nonoperative treatment.

Foot and ankle deformities from a neuropathic fracture or dislocation cause difficulty with shoe fit and marked alteration in weight-bearing loads, all leading to an increased propensity for ulceration in high-pressure areas (Fig. 27–1). These ulcers may become a portal of entry for bacteria, resulting in superficial or deep infection. Deformity may also be associated with joint instability, which is accentuated by weight-bearing, especially with hindfoot or ankle involvement. These changes result in loss of a plantigrade foot position and development of progressive varus, valgus, equinus, or calcaneus deformity.

Surgical Treatment

Nonoperative management is indicated for the vast majority of Charcot foot and ankle deformities. However, surgical treatment is

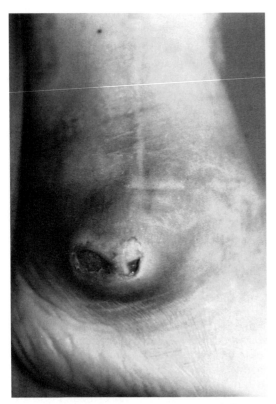

Figure 27–1 ■ Right Charcot ankle fracture dislocation following open reduction and internal fixation of a bimalleolar ankle fraction. The resulting varus deformity caused recurrent ulceration over the distal fibula despite bracing.

indicated for severe foot and ankle deformities (which are not amenable to custom bracing or custom footwear); significant instability (usually involving the hindfoot and ankle); recurrent ulceration; and selected acute fractures. A markedly unstable Charcot joint may be associated with pain; however, unlike painful osteoarthritis, a painful Charcot joint is rarely the sole reason for operative treatment.

Goals of Surgical Treatment

The goals of surgical treatment of the Charcot foot and ankle are to restore the stability and alignment of the foot and ankle so that footwear and bracing is possible. For most patients with a deformity severe enough to require operative treatment, a partial foot or transtibial amputation is usually the only alternative treatment option. Therefore, an additional goal of operative intervention is to prevent inevitable amputation of a limb that is destined to develop recurrent ulceration.

Patients with a significant deformity from neuropathic arthropathy will require specialized footwear with custom total-contact inserts and in some cases custom bracing to prevent recurrent ulceration and progressive deformity, whether or not they have surgery. Therefore, the treatment decision is not between operative treatment *or* prescription footwear and bracing, but rather between operative treatment followed by prescription footwear and bracing *or* prescription footwear and bracing alone. Operative treatment is primarily indicated to make these patients better candidates for shoe and brace wear. Although some patients with a solid realignment arthrodesis may eventually be weaned from their ankle-foot orthosis (AFO), it is an unrealistic goal for many patients and may lead to recurrent ulcerations or stress fractures of the tibia.[15, 18]

Timing of Operative Treatment

Operative treatment of the Charcot foot is usually done in the quiescent, resolution phase of the fracture pattern (Eichenholtz stage III), after casting, footwear, and bracing have failed. Acute fractures in neuropathic patients may be openly reduced and fixed if treatment is performed early before significant neuropathic fracture inflammation occurs, while bone stock is still sufficient for rigid fixation. However, most patients do not present for treatment early enough for this approach to be utilized. Once the acute dissolution phase (Eichenholtz stage I) has begun, regional bone demineralization (which hinders rigid internal fixation) and swelling make surgical management of the fracture difficult, leading to a higher rate of fixation failure, recurrent deformity, and infection.

Foot ulcers in association with significant neuropathic deformity are treated until healed (if possible) with total-contact casting so that the incision for the reconstructive procedure may be made through intact skin to reduce the possibility of postoperative infection. If underlying osteomyelitis is suspected in association with the neuropathic fracture, nuclear imaging with a combined technetium-99m (^{99m}Tc) bone scan and indium-111 (^{111}In) white blood cell (WBC) scan utilizing the dual-window technique is helpful to make this determination.[13, 14, 27] If osteomyelitis is present, appropriate debridement and antibiotic treatment is administered until wound healing and resolution of the infection occur. At this time, the decision regarding operative versus nonoperative treatment for the remaining deformity can be made.

Reconstructive Procedures for Neuropathic Deformity

There are two types of procedures for treatment of severe neuropathic deformities. For the patient with a stable forefoot or midfoot deformity from a bony prominence, an ostectomy (bumpectomy) is often satisfactory to prevent recurrent ulceration and relieve severe shoe fitting problems. Severe deformities associated with instability, especially in the hindfoot and ankle, require realignment and stabilization by arthrodesis to provide long-term correction of deformity.

Ostectomy

The midfoot is the most common location for neuropathic destruction.[4] The apex of the rocker bottom foot deformity that results is a frequent source of recurrent ulceration. The most common operative procedure for a neu-

ropathic deformity is removal of a bony prominence on the medial, lateral, or plantar aspect of the foot that is creating recurrent ulceration and difficulty with footwear.

The first step in the operative treatment of any neuropathic deformity is to obtain closure of the overlying ulcer, if possible, so that the incision to remove the bony prominence can be made through intact skin. An alternative technique is to ellipse the ulcer through a plantar longitudinal incision made directly over the prominence.[20] However, this technique exposes a significant amount of underlying cancellous bone to the open ulcer with a potential for bacterial colonization of the underlying bone.

The author's preferred method (Fig. 27–2) is to obtain ulcer closure with total-contact casting and make an incision through intact skin on the medial or lateral border of the foot closest to the bony prominence.[5] The skin incision is made as a full-thickness flap down to the bony prominence. A periosteal elevator is used to separate the overlying soft tissue from the protuberant bone. A small power saw or an osteotome is used to resect the bone surface, which is then rasped, to provide a smooth broad surface in the weight-bearing area. Major tendon attachments such as the peroneus brevis, anterior tibial tendon, posterior tibial tendon, and Achilles tendon should be respected and reattached to bone if they are detached. Resection of a large medial midfoot prominence (especially if it involves the medial cuneiform) should include reattachment of the anterior tibial tendon through drill holes into the remaining bone. Many patients have a coexistent tendo Achilles contracture and percutaneous tendo Achilles lengthening is frequently performed at the time of plantar ostectomy.[21]

The skin is closed over a suction drain, which is left in place for 24 hours with a compression splint. The following day, a total-contact cast is applied to stabilize the soft tissues, promote wound healing, and allow the patient limited weight-bearing. It is important to avoid excessive bone resection, especially in the midfoot, where removal of the plantar ligaments may cause progression of the rocker bottom deformity. Plantar midfoot ostectomy is more successful when the neuropathic deformity is stable, without sagittal or transverse plane instability.[20]

The sutures are removed once the incision has healed, usually 2 to 3 weeks after the

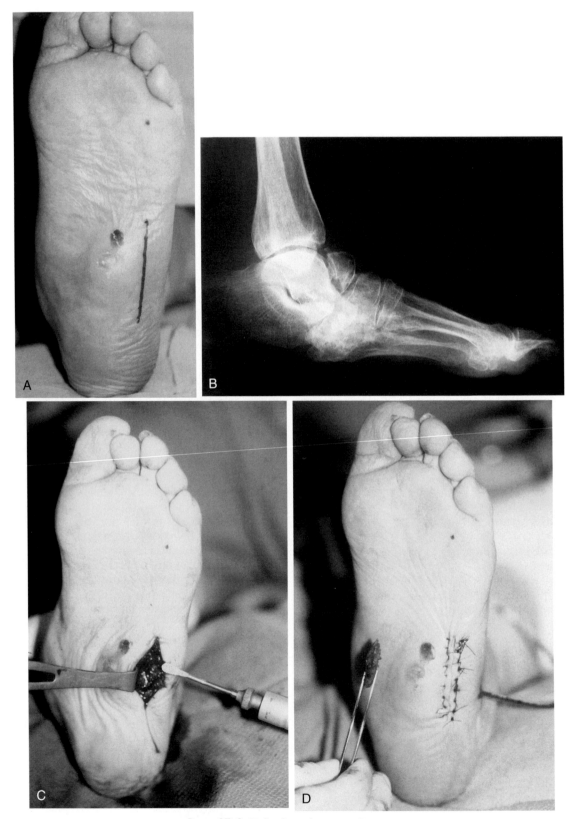

Figure 27–2 ■ *See legend on opposite page*

procedure. A mold for a total-contact insert is made of the foot at one of the cast changes so that once healing has occurred, the appropriate footwear and custom insert will be ready for dispensing at the time of cast removal.

Realignment and Arthrodesis

Severe Charcot foot and ankle deformity or instability is treated with realignment of the involved joint and stabilization by arthrodesis. For most patients considering this treatment, bracing and footwear have failed and amputation is the only other reasonable option for treatment (Fig. 27–3). The goal of operative treatment is to restore the alignment and stability of the foot to allow bracing and footwear. An operation is not intended to substitute for appropriate footwear or bracing.

Contraindications to arthrodesis include the following:

1. Soft tissue or bone infection (unless arthrodesis is performed as a staged procedure after the infection has been treated, all osteomyelitic bone has been resected, and the soft tissues have healed).
2. Acute dissolution phase of neuropathic fracture disease process (Eichenholtz stage I).
3. Uncontrolled diabetes or malnutrition.
4. Significant peripheral vascular disease.
5. Insufficient bone stock to obtain rigid fixation.
6. Inability to comply with the postoperative regimen (psychosocial problems).

Realignment and Arthrodesis Technique

Preoperatively, total-contact casting is performed until the acute phase of the Charcot fracture process has subsided and the skin is intact. Extensile longitudinal incisions are utilized with full-thickness skin flaps to bone. If deformity is limited to the ankle and subtalar joints, a posterior approach to the tibiotalocalcaneal fusion may be used if there is mild to moderate deformity.[24] For correction of a severe deformity, exposure is enhanced by medial and lateral ankle incisions (Fig. 27–3). Bone is resected to allow correction of the deformity and opposition of stable bleeding bone surfaces to promote successful fusion. Achilles tendon contractures are addressed with percutaneous lengthening, especially when performing a midfoot or hindfoot arthrodesis. Autologous bone graft is utilized to fill any defects and to provide both an intra- and extra-articular arthrodesis when possible. Morselized pieces of resected tibia and fibula may also be used when bone graft is primarily needed for extra-articular application. Rigid internal fixation with screws, large threaded Steinmann pins, compression blade plates, or custom intramedullary rods are used in whatever combination will provide adequate rigid internal fixation (Figs. 27–3 through 27–6). Plating of the plantar aspect of the medial column of the midfoot has been advocated to enhance the rigidity of midfoot arthrodeses.[28] External fixation provides adequate stability, but positioning the foot and ankle is more difficult with an external fixator and is reserved for open wounds requiring bony stabilization. Pin site problems may also force early removal of the fixator, leading to nonunion or malunion.

Long-term immobilization is critical in obtaining bony union. In general, the immobilization period for an arthrodesis in a neuropathic patient is doubled in comparison to the postoperative regimen for nonneuropathic patients. The postoperative regimen includes 3 months of non–weight-bearing in a total-contact cast followed by 1 to 2 months in a weight-bearing total-contact cast. The

Text continued on page 600

Figure 27–2 ■ *A*, Plantar view demonstrating chronic recurrent plantar ulcer beneath rocker bottom deformity. The ulcer was healed with total-contact casting prior to exostectomy. Note incision for resection of plantar prominence is on plantar-lateral border of foot. *B*, Lateral radiograph demonstrating neuropathic midfoot rocker bottom deformity with large plantar prominence. Note equinus position of hindfoot secondary to Achilles contracture. *C*, Intraoperative photograph demonstrating incision lateral to healed ulcer for resection of plantar prominence. A power reciprocating rasp is used to smooth the bone surface after the prominence has been osteotomized. Percutaneous tendo Achilles lengthening also performed. *D*, Postoperative photograph following plantar ostectomy demonstrating amount of bone resected. Patient has remained healed in a double-upright calf lacer ankle-foot orthosis attached to an in-depth shoe with a custom total-contact insert.

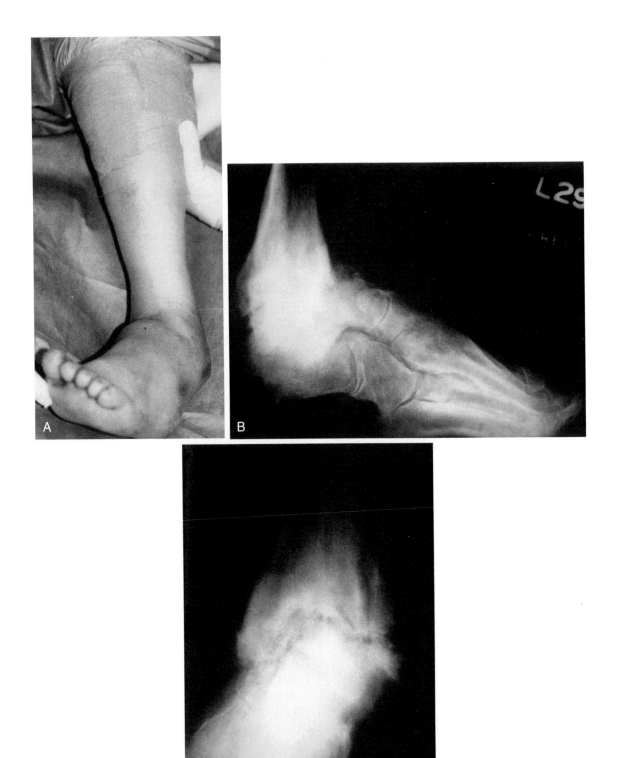

Figure 27–3 ■ *A,* Preoperative photograph of neuropathic arthropathy of the ankle and hindfoot with marked varus deformity. Note prominence of lateral malleolus with impending skin breakdown. *B,* Lateral radiograph of same patient demonstrating neuropathic fracture dislocation of the hindfoot with dissolution of the body of the talus. *C,* Anteroposterior (AP) radiograph demonstrating varus angulation of the tibiotalocalcaneal joints.

Illustration continued on opposite page

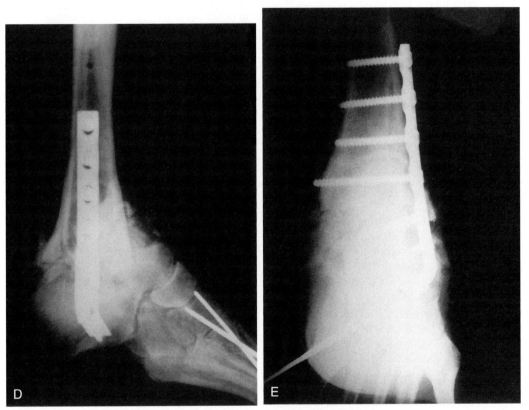

Figure 27–3 *Continued* ■ *D,* Lateral radiograph following open reduction, realignment, and tibiotalocalcaneal arthrodesis through lateral and medial incisions. Note the Steinmann pin fixation of the first metatarsal dorsiflexion osteotomy for correction of fixed forefoot valgus. *E,* AP radiograph demonstrating 4.5-mm titanium blade plate fixation of tibiotalocalcaneal fusion.

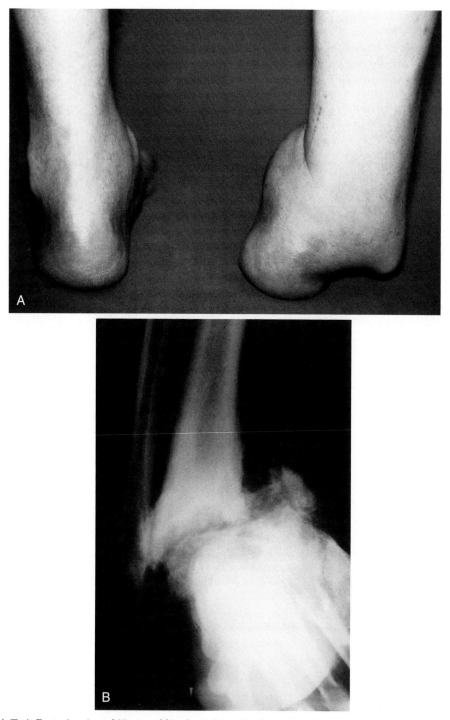

Figure 27–4 ■ *A*, Posterior view of 65-year-old male with insulin-dependent diabetes mellitus and severe peripheral neuropathy with progressive right hindfoot varus following ankle injury. *B*, AP radiograph of same patient demonstrating old fracture dislocation of tibiotalar joint and marked varus angulation.

Illustration continued on opposite page

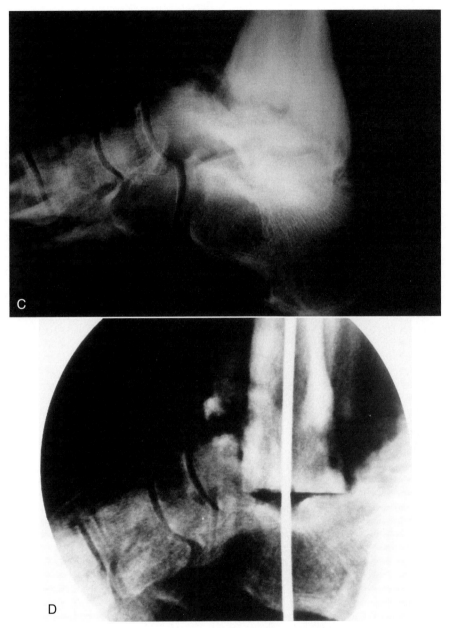

Figure 27–4 Continued ■ C, Lateral radiograph of ankle demonstrating collapse of talar body and destruction of ankle and subtalar joints. D, Intraoperative lateral fluoroscopic image of same patient demonstrating removal of the talar neck and body with retention of talar head to maintain length of the medial column of the foot. Note the distal tibia has been osteotomized and "mortised" into the anterior portion of the calcaneus. A guide pin has been placed from the plantar aspect of the calcaneus up the medullary canal of the distal tibia in preparation for insertion of the interlocking intramedullary rod.

Illustration continued on following page

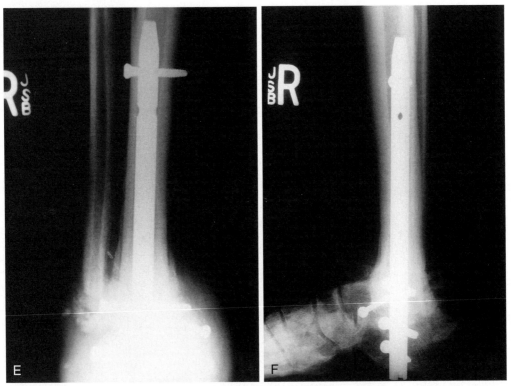

Figure 27–4 *Continued* ■ *E,* Postoperative AP radiograph demonstrating corrected alignment of the ankle joint with the interlocking screws placed lateral to medial. *F,* Lateral radiograph at 6 months postoperatively. Note the plantigrade position of the foot with the appropriate calcaneal pitch angle. The talar neck has fused to the anterior tibia.

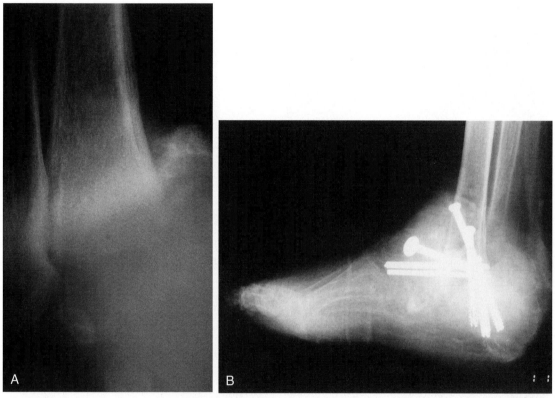

Figure 27–5 ■ *A*, AP radiograph of 72-year-old female with kidney-pancreas transplant and progressive hindfoot varus deformity from neuropathic arthropathy of the hindfoot. *B*, Postoperative lateral radiograph demonstrating realignment and arthrodesis utilizing multiple cannulated cancellous screws augmented with threaded Steinmann pins.

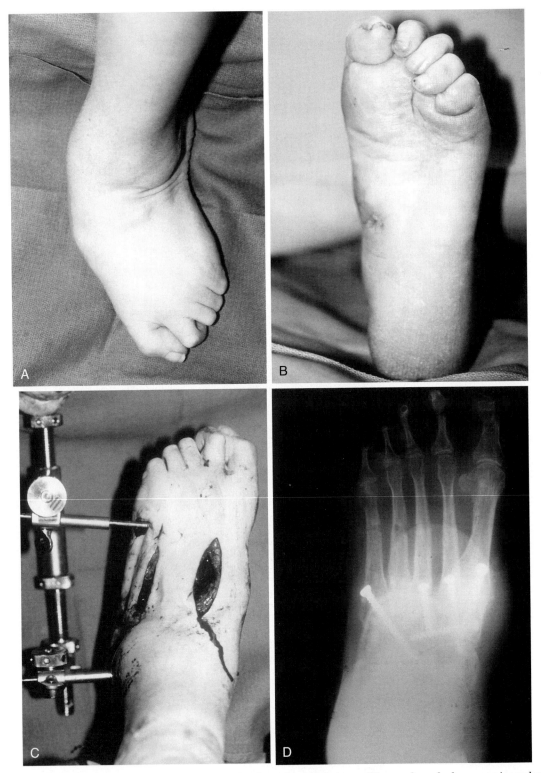

Figure 27–6 ■ *A,* Fifty-year-old female with insulin-dependent diabetes mellitus and marked progressive valgus deformity left foot with recurrent plantar medial midfoot ulceration despite custom footwear. *B,* Plantar view demonstrating pressure area beneath medial midfoot and severe clawtoe deformities. *C,* Intraoperative photograph of the same patient demonstrating the use of the femoral distractor to assist in correction of the deformity. After the tarsometatarsal joints were denuded of their cartilage, a Schanz pin was placed in the calcaneus and the fourth metatarsal. Distraction on the lateral side of the foot corrected the severe forefoot abduction until the internal fixation was placed. *D,* AP radiograph demonstrating screw fixation of the arthrodesis across all five tarsometatarsal joints.

Illustration continued on opposite page

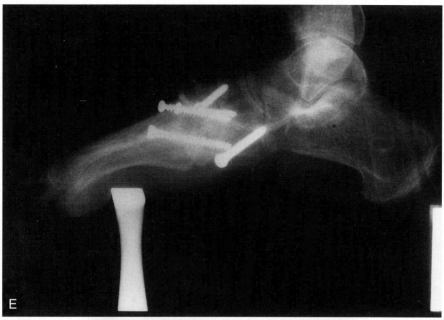

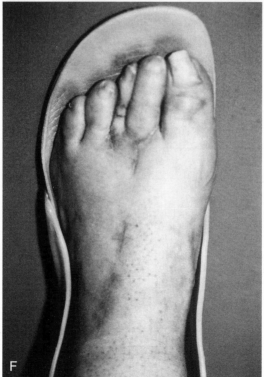

Figure 27–6 Continued ■ E, Lateral radiograph demonstrating restoration of the medial longitudinal arch following arthrodesis. F, Six months postoperatively, demonstrating correction of midfoot and forefoot deformity. Note the posterior shell ankle-foot orthosis is used for 12 to 18 months postoperatively.

limb is then placed into a bivalved ankle foot orthosis with a rocker sole added to the foot plate until footwear and definitive bracing is possible. Bracing is continued for 12 to 18 months postoperatively, similar to the treatment of a neuropathic fracture. For midfoot fusions, if swelling is minimal and the arthrodesis is solid, an in-depth shoe with an extended steel shank and a rocker sole may be used. For hindfoot and ankle involvement, this type of shoe is attached to either a double upright calf lacer or patellar tendon-bearing ankle-foot orthosis (Fig. 27–7). A custom molded polypropylene ankle-foot orthosis may be utilized inside a shoe with a rocker sole if the foot deformity is not severe (Figs. 27–6F and 27–8).

When there is significant deformity in the foot, it is preferable to use whatever customized shoe and foot orthosis combination is necessary to accommodate the foot deformity and then have this shoe attached to a double-upright brace (Fig. 27–7). A custom molded

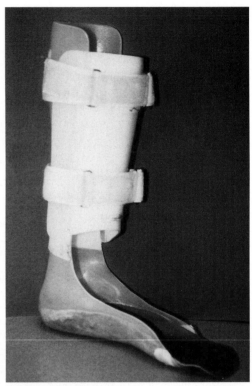

Figure 27–8 ■ Two-piece polypropylene clamshell type ankle-foot orthosis used for immobilization of an Eichenholtz stage II or III neuropathic fracture or following hindfoot arthrodesis of a neuropathic deformity.

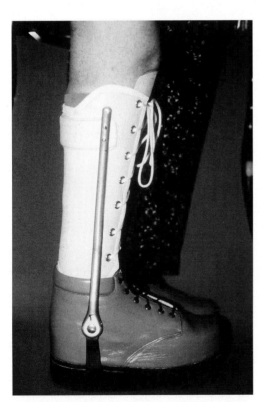

Figure 27–7 ■ Double-upright modified calf lacer ankle-foot orthosis (AFO) attached to an in-depth shoe with an extended steel shank and a rocker sole. This style of AFO is utilized when there is significant foot deformity that requires specialized footwear for accommodation.

polypropylene ankle-foot orthosis that extends into the foot region takes up space in the shoe and may not allow as much accommodation for severe deformities of the foot, thereby causing a recurrent ulceration.

Bracing is required following midfoot, hindfoot, and ankle fusions for at least the first 12 to 18 months postoperatively to allow complete healing and return to weight-bearing. Ankle, hindfoot, and midfoot fusions at the talonavicular joint level are prone to either recurrent Charcot changes at adjacent joints or stress fractures[12, 15, 26] and should be protected by bracing indefinitely. Midfoot fusions distal to the talonavicular joint level may remain stable in an in-depth shoe with a total-contact insert, an extended steel shank, and rocker soles.

The choice of whether to wean a patient from their ankle-foot orthosis at 12 to 18 months following arthrodesis depends on multiple factors including union and stability at the arthrodesis site, reliability of the patient, activity level, and location of the arthrodesis. Hindfoot arthrodeses involving the tibiotalocalcaneal joints in active patients are prone to distal tibial stress fractures (Fig. 27–9). These fractures are usually minimally displaced and will heal with 6 to 12 weeks of total-contact casting. Bracing is utilized for strenuous weight-bearing activities to prevent stress fractures due to the stresses placed on the tibia from the foot acting as a long, rigid lever arm.[12, 15, 26]

Results of Charcot Reconstruction

The reported bony union rates of foot and ankle fusions for neuropathic deformity range from 66 to 100%.[1, 15, 20, 22, 25, 30] However, the goal of achieving a stable, braceable, and shoeable foot is obtainable in 80% of patients following the initial operative procedure regardless of whether a solid arthrodesis or a stable nonunion is obtained.[9, 15] Complications that may lead to failure of the procedure requiring a repeat procedure include deep wound infection, unstable nonunion, and malunion.

Although earlier reports expressed caution in performing arthrodeses for neuropathic arthropathy,[7, 29] modern techniques of internal fixation and prolonged immobilization have significantly improved the union rate and decreased complications. The satisfaction rate for these procedures is high, in large part because pain is not a major factor.[1, 3, 9, 15, 20, 22, 25, 30] Most patients are grateful if they can be restored to walking status in an appropriate shoe or brace and avoid amputation.

In a recent study, 32 procedures for arthrodesis of neuropathic deformities of the foot and ankle were performed on 27 feet in 25 patients.[15] Five of these procedures were repeat procedures following an initial attempt at realignment arthrodesis by the authors and included two rearthrodesis procedures and three plantar ostectomies. Including these reoperations, 26 of the 27 feet were eventually rendered stable and braceable (96%). The goals of surgery were not met in one patient who developed a deep infection requiring transtibial amputation.[15]

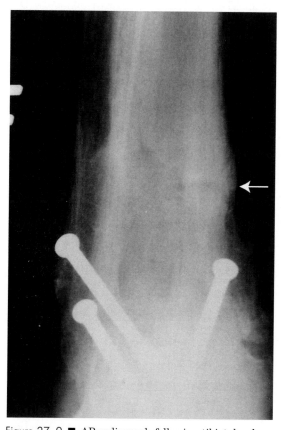

Figure 27–9 ■ AP radiograph following tibiotalocalcaneal arthrodesis with cannulated screws. Note the cortical lucency proximal to the arthrodesis site indicating a tibial stress fracture. The fracture occurred while the patient was walking without her brace or in-depth shoe with rocker soles. The fracture was treated with 8 weeks of total-contact casting followed by resumption of brace use.

Charcot Reconstruction: Technical Triumph Over Reason?

Because of the technical difficulty in managing these patients, the potential complications, and the prolonged treatment time required, some practitioners favor amputation rather than reconstruction for the unbraceable neuropathic deformity. Previous studies on energy expenditure and amputation level demonstrate that walking requires less energy expenditure the more distal the level of amputation.[23] Therefore, it would seem logical that the Charcot reconstruction arthrodesis patient would have less energy expenditure with walking and have a higher functional level than an amputee, especially in patients with limited cardiovascular reserve.

Perhaps the most compelling reason for limb salvage is the long-term uncertainty about the status of the other foot. Peripheral vascular disease or an ulcer leading to a deep wound infection may occur on the contralateral foot, necessitating an amputation in the future. Reconstruction instead of amputation for the "salvageable" neuropathic deformity may avoid creating a future bilateral amputee.

Prevention of Charcot Deformity and Acute Fracture Management in Patients with Neuropathic Arthropathy

The most important factor in successful management of an acute fracture and prevention of late deformity in a neuropathic patient is to recognize the fact that the patient has a significant peripheral neuropathy. A series of small monofilament nylon "hairs" (Semmes-Weinstein monofilaments) may be used to determine the severity and location of the sensory neuropathy.[19] If Semmes-Weinstein monofilament sensory testing shows loss of protective sensation (level 5.07/10 gm or greater), it is important to alter the typical treatment regimen to help prevent subsequent Charcot joint destruction. It is also important to warn the patient about the potential risk of Charcot joint involvement whether operative or nonoperative treatment of the fracture is undertaken.

The first step in acute fracture management is to differentiate an acute neuropathic fracture (i.e., Eichenholtz stage I) from an acute fracture in a patient who has a significant peripheral neuropathy. This differentiation can often be made by the patient's history. For example, the patient who suffers a relatively minor injury such as an ankle or foot "sprain," followed by several days or weeks of erythema and swelling and presents with a displaced fracture would usually be treated as an Eichenholtz stage I injury in a total-contact cast. However, the patient with a significant diabetic peripheral neuropathy who sustains an acute displaced fracture may be treated with the same operative or nonoperative fracture management principles as the nonneuropathic patient if seen acutely. The caveat is that a higher rate of complications should be anticipated and a prolonged postoperative period of non–weight-bearing and total-contact cast immobilization followed by bracing is therefore indicated. Routine postoperative fracture management with early range of motion, limited weight-bearing, and removable prefabricated walking braces may result in failure of fixation prior to fracture healing (Fig. 27–10).

Acute fractures of the ankle, talus, and midfoot may be treated with the established indications for open reduction and internal fixation assuming that the patient is medically fit, vascular status is adequate, and there is minimal swelling and the skin is intact and in good condition. Patients that have already entered Eichenholtz stage I with early demineralization and soft tissue inflammation are poorer candidates for operative treatment of their acute fracture.

Traditional ankle fracture internal fixation is augmented by the addition of one or two Steinmann pins across the ankle and subtalar joints[6] to prevent hardware failure, mortise displacement, and joint deformity (Fig. 27–11). The pins are cut off below the level of the plantar skin and removed in 6 to 10 weeks at a cast change.

It is important to extend the length of immobilization for a given fracture in neuropathic patients to approximately double the normal length of time that the patient would otherwise be non–weight-bearing. Therefore, the typical ankle fracture would be kept non–weight-bearing for approximately 3 months (as opposed to 6 weeks) and casting would continue until approximately 4 to 5 months following injury when the patient is able to be fully ambulatory in a cast and the fracture demonstrates radiographic union. Bracing the foot and ankle for hindfoot and ankle fractures is then utilized for 1 year following the injury to prevent the late development of a Charcot joint. If the patient has a stable, well-aligned ankle and hindfoot following acute fracture management and bracing at 12 to 18 months following injury, the patient may be weaned from their brace into appropriate footwear. During this period they are carefully monitored for the development of a Charcot joint.

This protocol for prolonged immobilization may be over-treatment for some patients who are not destined to progress to a Charcot joint. However, there are no known predictors of which fracture in a given neuropathic patient will progress to a Charcot joint. Therefore, it seems prudent to treat every patient with loss of protective sensation as if a Charcot joint will develop in hopes of preventing severe deformity.

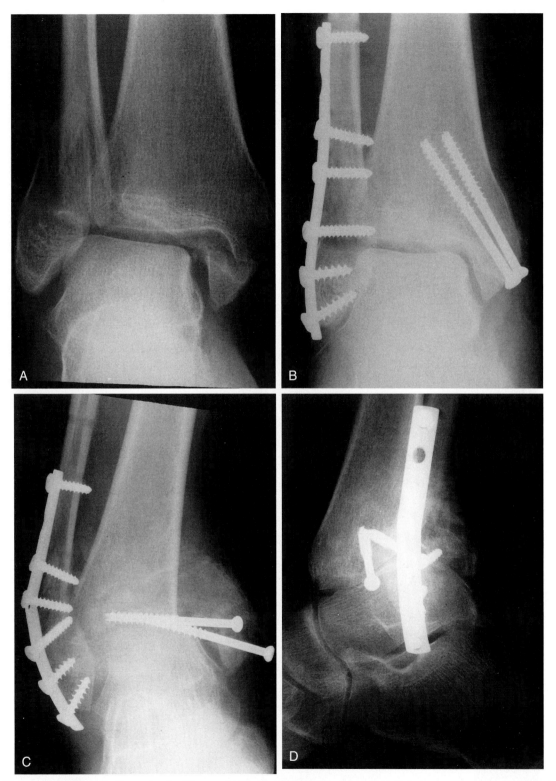

Figure 27–10 ■ *A*, Radiograph of a 33-year-old female with insulin-dependent diabetes mellitus and peripheral neuropathy with loss of protective sensation and a bimalleolar right ankle fracture. *B*, AP radiograph of the same patient following open reduction and rigid internal fixation of bimalleolar ankle fracture. The patient was placed in a prefabricated removable brace for postoperative immobilization. *C*, Touch weight-bearing was allowed and this varus deformity was noted within 4 weeks postoperatively. Note the displacement of the medial malleolus and the bending of the fibular plate with varus angulation at the ankle joint. *D*, Lateral radiograph at 4 weeks postoperatively demonstrating posterior subluxation of the talar body and collapse of the posterior malleolus, which was not present on the initial injury radiographs.

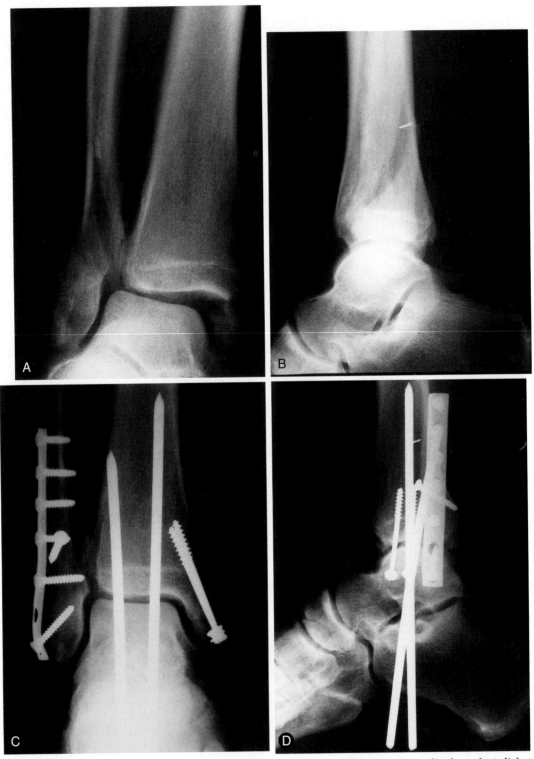

Figure 27–11 ■ *A* and *B*, Mortise and lateral radiographs of a 58-year-old male with insulin-dependent diabetes mellitus and severe peripheral neuropathy with displaced bimalleolar right ankle fracture. *C*, Postoperative mortise view radiograph following open reduction and internal fixation of the bimalleolar ankle fracture and insertion of two smooth Steinmann pins across subtalar and ankle joints to enhance stability. *D*, Lateral radiograph following open reduction and internal fixation. Note that one of the pins engages the posterior cortex of the tibia, significantly improving pin fixation.

Illustration continued on opposite page

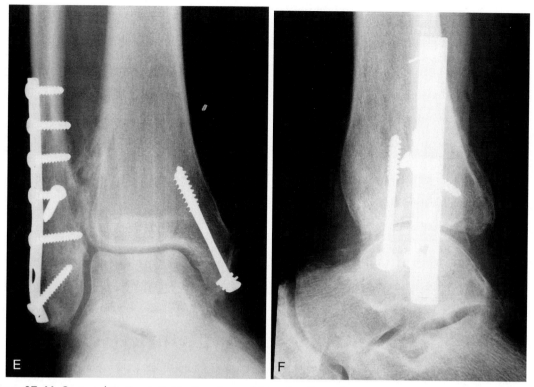

Figure 27–11 *Continued* ■ *E* and *F,* Mortise view and lateral radiographs at 5 months postoperatively. Note the healing of the fracture without displacement or destruction of the ankle joint. Ankle range of motion on this patient immediately after cast removal was 5 degrees of ankle dorsiflexion and 40 degrees of ankle plantar flexion without pain.

Conclusion

Reconstruction of the Charcot foot and ankle is a valuable technique for the patient with a severe deformity who cannot be managed by appropriate footwear and bracing. Goals of surgery are to render the patient shoeable and braceable and to prevent amputation. Despite complications, the overall success rate is approximately 80%. Stability and appropriate alignment are more important than bony union in obtaining a successful result. Important operative techniques include meticulous handling of the soft tissues and rigid internal fixation with bone grafting. Prolonged immobilization is necessary with doubling of the standard periods for non–weight-bearing and weight-bearing casting followed by bracing. Limb salvage with realignment and arthrodesis of the severely deformed foot and ankle will in most cases prevent amputation and likely provide a more functional limb. Using these operative indications and techniques, patient satisfaction following these procedures is high.

REFERENCES

1. Alvarez RG, Perkins TD, Barbour TM: Tibiocalcaneal arthrodesis for nonbraceable neurotrophic ankle deformity. Presented at the American Orthopaedic Foot and Ankle Society, 8th Annual Summer Meeting, Napa, CA, July 15–19, 1992.
2. American Diabetes Association: Diabetes: 1996 Vital Statistics. Alexandria, VA, 1996.
3. Bono JV, Roger DJ, Jacobs RL: Surgical arthrodesis of the neuropathic foot. A salvage procedure. Clin Orthop 296:14–20, 1993.
4. Brodsky JW: The diabetic foot. *In* Mann RA, Coughlin MJ (eds): Surgery of the Foot and Ankle, St. Louis: CV Mosby Co, 1993.
5. Brodsky JW, Rouse AM: Exostectomy for symptomatic bony prominences in diabetic Charcot feet. Clin Orthop 296:21–26, 1993.
6. Childress HM: Vertical transarticular-pin fixation for unstable ankle fractures. J Bone Joint Surg 47-A:1323–1334, 1965.
7. Cleveland M: Surgical fusion of unstable joints due to neuropathic disturbance. Am J Surg 43:580, 1939.
8. Cofield RH, Morrison RC, Beabout JW: Diabetic neuroarthropathy in the foot. Patient characteristics and patterns of radiographic change. Foot Ankle Int 4:15, 1983.
9. Early JS, Hansen ST: Surgical reconstruction of the diabetic foot: A salvage approach to midfoot collapse. Foot Ankle Int 17:325–330, 1996.
10. Eichenholtz SN: Charcot Joints. Springfield, IL: Charles C Thomas, 1966.

11. Harris JR, Brand PW: Patterns of disentegration of the tarsus in the anesthetic foot. J Bone Joint Surg 48B:4–16, 1966.

12. Johnson JE: Surgical reconstruction of the diabetic Charcot foot and ankle. Foot Ankle Clin 2:37–55, 1997.

13. Johnson JE, et al: Prospective study of bone, indium-111-labeled white blood cells, and gallium-67 scanning for the evaluation of osteomyelitis in the diabetic foot. Foot Ankle Int 17:10–16, 1996.

14. Johnson JE, Mitchell JR, Lipman BT, et al: MRI, nuclear medicine, and x-ray imaging of the neuropathic foot for suspected osteomyelitis. American Orthopaedic Foot and Ankle Society Annual Summer Meeting, Asheville, NC, July 25, 1993.

15. Johnson JE, O'Brien TS, Hart TS, et al: Reconstruction of the Charcot foot and ankle: An outcome study of long-term results. American Orthopaedic Foot and Ankle Society 12th Annual Summer Meeting, Hilton Head, SC, June 27–30, 1996.

16. Johnson JTH: Neuropathic fractures and joint injuries. J Bone Joint Surg 49-A:1–30, 1967.

17. Kristiansen B: Ankle and foot fractures in diabetics provoking neuropathic joint changes. Acta Orthop Scand 51:975–979, 1980.

18. Mitchell JR, Johnson JE, Collier DB, Gould JS: Stress fracture of the tibia following extensive hindfoot and ankle arthrodesis: A report of three cases. Foot Ankle Int 16:445–448, 1995.

19. Mueller MJ: Identifying patients with diabetes mellitus who are at risk for lower-extremity complications: Use of Semmes-Weinstein monofilaments. Phys Ther 76:68–71, 1996.

20. Myerson MS, et al: Symposium: Neuroarthopathy of the foot. Contemp Orthop 26:43–64, 1993.

21. Myerson MS, et al: Management of midfoot diabetic neuroarthropathy. Foot Ankle Int 15:233–241, 1994.

22. Papa J, Myerson M, Girard P: Salvage, with arthrodesis, in intractable diabetic neuropathic arthropathy of the foot and ankle. J Bone Joint Surg 75-A:1056–1066, 1993.

23. Pinzur MS, et al: Energy demands for walking in dysvascular amputees as related to the level of amputation. Orthopedics 15:1033–1037, 1992.

24. Russotti GM, Johnson KA, Cass JR: Tibiotalocalcaneal arthrodesis for arthritis and deformity of the hind part of the foot. J Bone Joint Surg 70-A:1304–1307, 1988.

25. Sammarco GJ, Conti SF: Reconstruction of neuropathic (Charcot) foot deformity. Presented at the American Orthopaedic Foot and Ankle Society 8th Annual Summer Meeting, Napa, CA, July 15–19, 1992.

26. Sanders LJ, Frykberg RG: Diabetic neuropathic osteoarthropathy: The Charcot foot. In Frykberg RG (ed): The High Risk Foot in Diabetes Mellitus. New York: Churchill Livingstone, 1991.

27. Schauwecker DS, et al: Combined bone scintigraphy and indium-111 leukocyte scans in neuropathic foot disease. J Nucl Med 29:1651–1655, 1988.

28. Schon LC, Marks RM: The management of neuroarthropathic fracture-dislocations in the diabetic patient. Orthop Clin Am 26:375–392, 1995.

29. Stuart MJ, Morrey BF: Arthrodesis of the diabetic neuropathic ankle joint. Clin Orthop 253:209–211, 1990.

30. Tisdel CL, Marcus RE, Heiple KG: Triple arthrodesis for diabetic peritalar neuropathy. Foot Ankle Int 16:332–338, 1995.

Chapter 28

MINOR AND MAJOR LOWER LIMB AMPUTATION IN PERSONS WITH DIABETES MELLITUS

■ John H. Bowker and Thomas P. San Giovanni

The surgeon who is consulted regarding disorders of the foot and ankle in diabetic patients will inevitably face the need for amputation of part or all of the foot. Most often this situation arises emergently as a result of infection with or without ischemia and, on occasion, as a failure of nonsurgical or surgical treatment of Charcot neuroarthropathy. The real challenge to the attitude of the surgeon is to regard amputations and disarticulations as reconstructive procedures, not as failures of medical science or personal skills. Indeed, an ablation should be regarded as the first step in returning patients to their former functional status. This chapter serves as an introduction to this much-underrated area of care, which has been dynamized over the past few years by significant advances in material science, resulting in continual improvement in partial foot prostheses, foot orthoses, and shoewear. Descriptions of the most commonly utilized procedures are given, along with their expected functional outcomes. Evaluation and management of limb-threatening emergencies, with emphasis on decision making, are thoroughly discussed.

It should be noted that there are several important advantages of partial foot ablations over transtibial or higher amputations. These include preservation of end-weight-bearing along normal proprioceptive pathways as well as limited disruption of body image, which is easily masked with an orthosis, a limited prosthesis, or simply with shoe modifications. These devices can restore near-normal walking function, relative to the loss of forefoot lever length and the associated musculature at the level selected.

Until the last half of the 20th century, partial foot amputations and disarticulations were rarely done except for trauma. When wet gangrene related to infection or dry gangrene due to peripheral vascular disease occurred, the customary treatment was a major lower limb amputation. More often than not, the transfemoral level was chosen, since the rationale was to amputate where primary healing could safely be anticipated. Failure of primary healing due to wound ischemia or infection posed a very real danger of death in the preantibiotic era, when the emphasis was not on functional rehabilitation, but on survival.

In many geographic areas, however, the choice of level was often dictated by local prejudice on the part of surgeons and/or prosthetists. This premise was borne out by a statistical survey of 12,000 new amputations done in the early 1960s in nine major cities across the United States. At that time, an average of 56% of major lower limb amputations were transfemoral except in Baltimore, where only 42% were at that level.[15] A similar study of 6,000 new amputations was done a decade later to assess the effect on surgical practice of findings regarding the superior functional results of transtibial amputations. During that interval, the average percent of transfemoral amputations had happily fallen from 56% to 38%. In Baltimore, however, the percent had *risen* from 42% to 50%, while in nearby Philadelphia the percent of transfemoral amputations had decreased from 67% to 50%. Further emphasizing regional variations, two western U.S. cities had reduced transfemoral amputations from an average of 60% to 28%.[26]

With the convergence of advances in diverse but interrelated fields, such as nutrition, wound healing, tissue oxygenation, antibiotic drugs as well as vascular reconstruction, amputation surgery, and prosthetics, the surgeon now has the opportunity to consider the foot rather than the femur or tibia as the level of choice for amputation in selected cases of diabetic infection with or without peripheral vascular disease.[6]

A remaining question is how to best utilize these advances in order to conserve all tissue commensurate with the diagnosis and good future ambulatory function. Unfortunately, many surgeons still consider a transverse ablation, such as a transmetatarsal amputation, to be the best solution for forefoot infection, even if only a ray (toe and metatarsal) is involved, analogous to the automatic selection of a transfemoral over a transtibial level in the past.

The most common cause for partial foot ablations in persons with diabetes mellitus is infection (wet gangrene). The initiating etiology is most often a normal bony prominence combined with sensory neuropathy and inappropriate shoewear. Infection follows ulcerative penetration of the full thickness of the skin into the bones and joints of the foot. Thermal injuries from hot foot soaks or baths, automobile floor boards or transmission tunnels, solar radiation, fireplaces, or floor-furnace grids are also common. Dry gangrene, in contrast, is most often seen in diabetics as a result of dysvascularity associated with sensory neuropathy. Smoking can be an aggravating factor in all of these situations.

As stated above, an amputation or disarticulation should be regarded as the first major step in restoring the diabetic's quality of life to an acceptable level. It should be considered on a par with any other major limb reconstructive procedure, such as a hip replacement. Amputation is not to be treated offhandedly as a failure of salvage attempts, exemplified by assigning it to the most junior surgical trainee to do without close intraoperative supervision. In addition, there is no longer any excuse for a poorly fashioned residual limb. Instead, modern amputation surgery should result in the creation of a modified locomotor end-organ that will interface comfortably with a prosthesis, orthosis, or modified shoewear and provide the most efficient, energy-conserving gait possible.

To achieve these goals, a well-planned amputation or disarticulation will conserve all tissue commensurate with the diagnosis and with good function. Although, as a basic requirement, amputation must be done proximal to gangrenous tissue or an otherwise irreparably damaged body part, a determined effort should be made to save maximum length to enhance ambulatory function.

The next consideration is the creation of a mobile soft-tissue envelope for the residual skeleton, which will absorb direct (normal) and shear forces during prosthetic usage. In most foot ablations, the soft tissue envelope is formed of plantar skin, subcutaneous tissue, and fascia alone, unlike more proximal amputations, where muscle tissue forms an integral part of the soft tissue envelope.

It is essential to properly contour cut bones, with removal of sharp edges and corners, to prevent damage of the soft tissue envelope from within as the soft tissues are compressed between the bones and the prosthesis, orthosis, or shoe. Above all else, adherence of skin directly to bone must be minimized to prevent ulceration from shear forces during walking. This is best accomplished by avoiding, insofar as possible, coverage with split skin grafts on the distal, lateral, and weight-bearing plantar surfaces of the residual foot because split graft in these areas often ulcerates. In contrast, split graft placed dorsally, even on bony surfaces covered only with granulation tissue, can last indefinitely with reasonable care (Fig. 28–1). To prevent further damage to already compromised skin, flaps should never be handled with forceps during surgery.

In all transverse ablations proximal to the metatarsophalangeal joints, close attention must be directed to prevention of equinus contracture of the ankle joint. This is most easily accomplished by casting the foot for several weeks in slight dorsiflexion to encourage triceps surae atrophy. A more muscle-balanced residual foot will result by thus weakening the ankle plantar flexors relative to the dorsiflexors. Once full weight-bearing is resumed, full dorsiflexion should be easily retained.

Determining the Level of Amputation

There are a number of factors that influence the level of amputation or disarticulation. Some are reversible and/or controllable by the efforts of the surgeon and some are not. As noted above, amputation must be done proximal to the level of gangrenous tissue or

an irreparably damaged body part. Here, the location of necrosis can be critical. For example, it is difficult to recommend an ablation distal to the transtibial level in cases of gangrenous changes of the heel pad. In contrast, while tissue oxygen perfusion levels are often a major determinant of level, they can sometimes be improved by the vascular surgeon. Before attempting the distal procedures described in this chapter, therefore, thorough evaluation of arterial blood flow is essential. (see Chapters 16 and 25). In the case of foot abscesses, prompt incision and drainage in the emergency department will, by controlling proximal spread of infection, tend to allow preservation of the greatest limb length at the time of definitive debridement. Several other factors that are reversible and/ or controllable come to mind, some with strong behavioral overtones, both on the part of the patient and the physician. Although these factors alone should not dictate level selection, they do deserve adequate preoperative evaluation and appropriate correction. The most obvious examples are patients with uncontrolled psychosis or a history of major

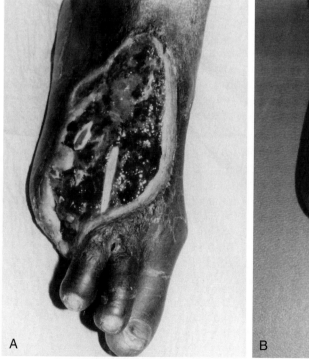
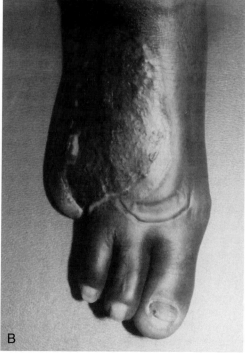

Figure 28–1 ■ *A,* Right foot of 52-year-old diabetic woman following disarticulation of fourth and fifth toes and necrotic dorsal skin. The wound is well covered with granulation tissue and ready for a split skin graft. *B,* The same foot 3 months after grafting. The graft has now tolerated shoe wear for many years. (From Bowker JH: Partial foot amputations and disarticulations. Foot Ankle Clin 2:153, 1997, with permission.)

noncompliance with foot care programs. In these situations, the surgeon may be deterred from performing a procedure that requires a high degree of patient compliance both in the immediate postoperative period and long term for success to be ensured, such as a Syme ankle disarticulation. Lack of protective sensation, by itself, should not be considered a criterion for more proximal amputation through sensate skin, since the decrease in sensation can be compensated for by the skillful use of protective interface materials in prostheses, orthoses, and shoewear.

Factors Affecting Wound Healing

Tissue oxygen perfusion may be profoundly decreased by the chronic use of vasoconstrictors. The use of nicotine and caffeine should, therefore, be actively discouraged. Smoking is a risk factor of real significance, due not only to the short-term effects of vessel constriction, but over time due to enhanced development of atherosclerosis. In smokers, healing is also retarded by the decreased ability of the blood to deliver oxygen to tissues because of carbon monoxide binding to sites on hemoglobin that normally carry oxygen. This is clearly seen in decreased baseline percutaneous oxygen levels in the hands and feet of smokers as compared to nonsmokers. Ricci et al. found that oxygen levels fell significantly within 10 minutes after smoking one cigarette, reached their lowest point in 30 minutes, and were still below baseline for 60 minutes. Use of nicotine gum or patches resulted in levels intermediate between those of smokers and nonsmokers and were recommended as aids to achieve smoking cessation in those with acute or chronic wounds.[42] A study by Lind et al. showed a marked increase in complications after primary amputations of the lower limb in those patients who continued to smoke cigarettes postoperatively. This group's rate of infection and reamputation was 2.5 times higher than in cigar smokers and nonsmokers. The authors concluded that smoking should cease at least 1 week preoperatively to allow platelet function and fibrinogen levels to normalize.[30]

Another reversible and/or controllable factor influencing wound healing is nutritional status. This is reflected in serum albumin levels below 3.0 gm/dL, which can be indicative of starvation, severe renal disease with loss of protein in the urine, acute stress, or a combination of these factors. Wound-healing potential is also diminished in patients who are immunosuppressed, as indicated by a total lymphocyte count below 1,500/mm³. In a retrospective study, Dickhaut and associates reviewed the healing rate of Syme ankle disarticulation in 23 diabetic patients who met Wagner's criteria for that level. Serum albumin levels and total lymphocyte counts that had been obtained on admission were evaluated as possible additional screening criteria of wound-healing potential. Eighty-six percent of patients with a serum albumin level of at least 3.5 gm/dL and a total lymphocyte count of at least 1,500/mm³ healed, in contrast to 43% of those who failed to meet these additional criteria. Of the two criteria, serum albumin appeared to be the more significant.[10] A similar study by Pinzur et al. showed an 82% healing rate when all criteria were met. They concluded that a minimum serum albumin level of 3.0 gm/dL was sufficient.[41] In this regard, it must be remembered that, in attempting to improve the nutrition of diabetics by increasing their caloric intake, a matching increase in hypoglycemic agents will be required to avert iatrogenic hyperglycemia.

Diffuse tissue glycation, which results from prolonged uncontrolled hyperglycemia, can be inferred from high levels of glycohemoglobin. Levels of seven or more tend to indicate poor adherence to blood glucose control on the part of patients and may impair wound healing. Although direct evidence of poor wound healing in humans secondary to poor blood glucose control is lacking, several studies implicating uncontrolled glucose levels in poor wound healing in rats have been published. The wounds exhibited decreased numbers of leukocytes and impaired neovascularization as well as decreased nitric acid (NO) synthesis, wound strength, collagen content, and granulation tissue mass.[13, 44, 51, 52] Additionally, the dramatic decrease in complications affecting the eyes, kidneys, and nerves in diabetic humans, thoroughly documented by the Diabetes Control and Complications Trial (DCCT) is sufficient to recommend tight blood glucose control.[9]

Cosmesis and Function

Partial foot amputations result in the least disruption of body image of all lower limb ablations and may require only shoe modifications or a limited prosthesis or orthosis. The degree to which normal walking function is prosthetically restored is relative to the loss of forefoot/midfoot lever length and associated muscles.

The partial foot amputee or Syme ankle disarticulate continues to bear weight on the residual foot in a manner that approximates the normal in regard to proprioceptive feedback, in contrast to the transtibial level, in which an entirely new feedback pattern must be interpreted. Many adult-onset diabetics with peripheral neuropathy also retain some protective sensation in the arch and heel areas. In the case of partial foot amputees, the heel lever is intact while variable portions of the forefoot/midfoot lever remain, ranging from full length, in the case of single ray (toe and metatarsal) amputation to virtually none in the case of midtarsal (Chopart) disarticulation.

Postoperative Management

The most important aspect of postoperative management is compliance with the program on the part of the patient. This includes avoidance of body weight transfer through the foot until the wound is sound enough for suture removal (usually 3 to 4 weeks). This is virtually impossible for the average diabetic to achieve due to poor balance secondary to decreased lower limb proprioception, often associated with truncal obesity. By permitting just touch-down weight-bearing of the involved foot while using a walker, body balance is retained with only the weight of the limb transferred through the foot to the floor. Other vital elements of postoperative management include nutritional support, continued avoidance of vasoconstrictors such as nicotine and caffeine, and tight control of blood glucose levels. The foot should be kept elevated to reduce the negative effect of wound edema on healing whenever the patient is not doing the minimal walking essential for activities of daily living. For the first few weeks, the wound should be evaluated weekly. If the wound has been closed primarily, the last partial weight-bearing cast can be removed at 3 weeks with resumption of active ankle and subtalar motion at that time. In the case of open ablations of the forefoot, it is often possible to allow protected weight-bearing using a heel-bearing weight-relief shoe.

Once sound healing has been achieved, the emphasis must shift to prevention of future skin ulceration and infection. In recent years, great advances in the long-term protection of feet following toe, ray, and transmetatarsal amputations have been provided through organized pedorthic care (see Chapter 34). At more proximal levels in the foot (tarsometatarsal and midtarsal), however, the residual foot becomes progressively more difficult to capture for successful late stance phase gait activity. Here, successful fitting may require the multiple skills of an orthotist, prosthetist, and pedorthist. (See Chapter 34.)

Management of Limb-Threatening Emergencies

Ischemia (Dry Gangrene)

Ischemia of the foot often results from peripheral vascular disease associated with diabetes mellitus. Since this often presents as *dry* gangrene, it is extremely important to avoid the use of soaks, wet dressings, and debriding agents. These "treatments" often result in conversion of a localized, fairly benign condition to limb-threatening wet gangrene. Conversely, as long as the necrotic areas remain dry, there is ample time to allow completion of the demarcation between viable and dead tissue and a thorough evaluation of vascular perfusion. If arterial circulation proximal to the necrotic tissue is found to be significantly impaired, consultation with a vascular surgeon is advised regarding the feasibility of arterial bypass or recanalization with concomitant limited distal amputation. If blood flow cannot be restored, amputation at the appropriate more proximal level should be done at the same time to minimize deconditioning due to immobility. In selected cases, maximum tissue preservation can be achieved by allowing autoamputation of the necrotic parts. This is especially true if gangrene is limited to the digits. The entire process may take many months (Fig. 28–2).

Infection (Wet Gangrene)

As soon as the patient is seen, all further weight-bearing should be prohibited to avoid

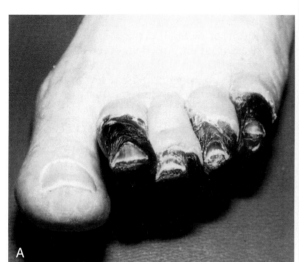
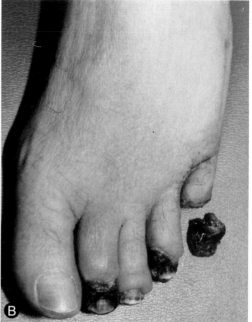
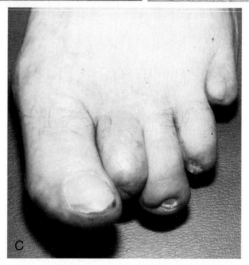

Figure 28-2 ■ *A,* Left foot of a 77-year-old diabetic male with a 30-year-history of smoking. Note dry gangrene of four lateral toes. Vascular reconstruction was not feasible due to cardiac status. *B,* Three months later, the apparent gangrene had receded in all toes and the fifth toe had partially sloughed. *C,* The final result at 6 months, showing considerable salvage of toe tissue by allowing completion of autoamputation without surgical interference. (*A* and *C* from Bowker JH, Poonekar PD: Amputation. Oxford: Butterworth-Heinemann, 1996, with permission.)

the proximal spread of pus along tissue planes. The inciting skin wound is then probed with a sterile cotton-tipped applicator. If bone is contacted, a presumptive diagnosis of osteomyelitis may be confidently made with easy confirmation by coned-down radiographs.[19] In the authors' experience, the expense of bone scans is rarely justified. Aerobic and anaerobic cultures should be taken at this time, allowing initial selection of anti-

biotics, pending the result of cultures and antibiotic sensitivities. Due to the polymicrobial nature of most diabetic foot infections, broad-spectrum antibiotics should be given intravenously.[43] These should be effective against staphylococci and streptococci as well as the commonly encountered gram-negative bacilli and anaerobes.[18] This criterion can be largely met by a variety of regimens, including ticarcillin-clavulanate, ampicillin-sulbactam, or clindamycin combined with either ciprofloxacin or a third-generation cephalosporin.[25]

To control further spread of infection along tissue planes from internal pressure of the abscess, initial abscess drainage should be done promptly in the emergency department. Drainage can be done under ankle block anesthesia or without any anesthesia if profound loss of pain sensation from diabetic neuropathy exists. Any decompressive incision(s) must respect normal weight-bearing surfaces such as the heel pad and lateral sole as well as all skin directly plantar to the metatarsal heads, although incisions may pass between the heads. Incisions should be longitudinally oriented to avoid as many vascular and neural structures as possible. By inadvertently extending a midsole incision into the heel pad or proximal to the ankle joint, a later procedure, such as a Syme ankle disarticulation, may be severely compromised. Control of blood glucose should be initiated, although this is somewhat compromised in the presence of infection. Treatment with antibiotics alone, without controlling blood glucose levels, will be only partially effective because of the inhibitory effect of hyperglycemia on leukocyte functions and the thrombosis of blood vessels in an abscessed area.[1] The interdependence of these factors reinforces the need for prompt surgical debridement of all necrotic and infected tissue, including bone. Iatrogenic hypoglycemia in these often very ill patients is to be avoided.

Prior to definitive debridement under ankle block anesthesia in the operating room, it is important to get a thorough preoperative noninvasive evaluation of the arterial circulation. This and plain radiographs will quickly determine the available options for foot salvage. Nonetheless, at the beginning of debridement, the surgeon cannot be absolutely certain of the full proximal extent of an infective process nor of the viability of all tissues remaining at the conclusion of surgery. The patient and family must understand that the exploration is somewhat tentative in nature and, based upon the preoperative studies and the findings at exploration, the surgeon will be as conservative as possible in removal of tissue, even to the extent of leaving some skin with marginal perfusion in hopes that it may recover. If blood flow is found to be less than adequate,

consultation with a vascular surgeon following initial debridement is advised.

Both plantar and dorsal incisions may be required to permit fully open drainage of all abscess pockets. The guidelines for incision placement discussed above should be carefully followed. The central plantar spaces described by Grodinsky and later confirmed by Loeffler and Ballard can be opened by a single extensile plantar incision. This starts posterior to the medial malleolus and ends distally between the first and second metatarsal heads. The incision may be extended deeply into the first web space as well. Either part or all of this incision may be used, depending on the extent of the infection.[20, 34] Distal infections involving the metatarsal fat pad may track across the entire distal foot, requiring a transverse plantar incision at the base of the toes, its length depending on the extent of spread of the infection. If two dorsal longitudinal incisions are required for full exposure of infection, they should be as widely separated as possible. Even with this precaution, the intervening skin bridge may necrose because of septic thrombosis of its small skin vessels. First and foremost, however, the disease process must be controlled by excision of all involved tissues. Following removal of patently necrotic tissue, the dorsal and plantar surfaces of the foot should be firmly stroked from proximal to distal along tendon sheaths and fascial planes to empty and thus discover pockets of pus. These recesses are then probed to their proximal end, widely opened and thoroughly debrided. If the infection involves the midfoot extensively, but spares the heel pad, an open Syme ankle disarticulation may be done. Spread of infection into the heel pad or ankle joint or along tendon sheaths proximal to the ankle joint generally precludes anything but an open ankle disarticulation as a prelude to transtibial amputation. Although exploration should be aggressively pursued to fully determine the extent of involvement, it can be done efficiently as well as conservatively by application of basic anatomic knowledge, rarely adding significantly to the overall operative time.

In addition to obviously infected and necrotic tissue, all poorly vascularized tissues, such as articular cartilage, joint capsules, volar plates, and tendons should be removed as part of a thorough debridement. Otherwise, the wound may remain open, often for months, with these tissues fostering residual, progressive infection. All visually uninvolved, well-vascularized tissue should be saved for secondary reconstruction. Since gangrenous areas vary so much in their extent, however, the skin flaps preserved for immediate or delayed closure will frequently be "nonstandard." The "guillotine" approach to amputation, in contrast, will preclude creative use of otherwise salvageable tissues in preserving limb length. All wounds should be *lightly* packed with saline-moistened gauze to allow free wicking of infective fluids to the surface. Thrice-daily damp saline gauze dressings, as described below, start on the first postoperative day.

If the infective process is acute and purulent, the surgeon must be willing to redebride the foot. This may become necessary for several reasons. First, it is sometimes difficult to be certain that all involved tissue has been removed. Second, some areas of skin, optimistically left at the initial debridement, may now be frankly necrotic. Third, the infection may have persisted. Secondary debridements can be done either at the bedside or more formally in the operating room, if the patient has sufficient retained sensation to require ankle block anesthesia or if the procedure will be extensive.

Conversely, if the wound had little or no initial purulence and is visually clean following debridement with no residual pus or compromised tissue, a primary loose closure can generally be done. When the wound has sufficient volume (ray or transmetatarsal ablations, for example), it can be closed over a Kritter flow-through irrigation system to remove residual detritus.[28] The author's version of this is as follows: a 14-gauge polyethylene venous catheter is passed into the depths of the wound from an adjacent site by means of its integral needle. The needle is then discarded and the catheter is sutured to the skin and then connected to a bag of normal saline solution. The fluid exits the wound between the widely spaced simple skin sutures at the rate of 1 L/24 hr for 3 days (Fig. 28–3). The fluid is collected in an absorbent dressing consisting of three rolls of bulky cotton gauze (Fig. 28–4). The outer layers only of the dressing are changed every 4 to 5 hours.[4] On the third day, the edges of the wound are gently compressed by the surgeon. If there is any purulence seen, the sutures are removed and the wound packed. This should be an uncommon occurrence if patients have been carefully selected. Advantages of this method include primary healing, usually within 3 weeks, thus avoiding the need for secondary closure or the several months required for healing by secondary intention. In addition, skin grafting is avoided, resulting in better cosmesis.

Postoperative Management of Open Amputations

Damp saline gauze dressings, gently packed into all areas of the wound, work well for most open amputations. This method possesses the advantages of easy execution and

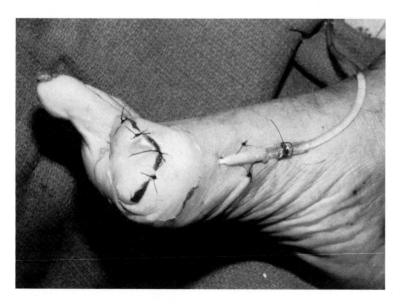

Figure 28–3 ■ Disarticulation of right great toe for diabetic gangrene with closure using flaps salvaged from lateral aspect of toe. Note Kritter flow-through irrigation system. Sutures are widely spaced to permit egress of irrigation fluid. (From Bowker JH: The choice between limb salvage and amputation: Infection. *In* Bowker JH, Michael JW [eds]: Atlas of Limb Prosthetics, 2nd ed. St. Louis: Mosby Year Book, 1992, with permission.)

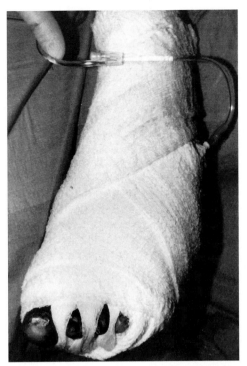

Figure 28–4 ■ Kritter irrigation system installed in left second ray amputation wound. Note the bulky bandage used to absorb irrigation fluid. The outer of three rolls is replaced every three hours. (From Bowker JH: The choice between limb salvage and amputation: Infection. *In* Bowker JH, Michael JW [eds]: Atlas of Limb Prosthetics, 2nd ed. St. Louis: Mosby Year Book, 1992, with permission.)

low cost. Since it requires only "clean" technique, it is easily taught to the patient and family prior to discharge.

A dressing change is done every 8 hours. This allows the drying gauze to adhere to the wound surface and debride detritus with each change. If the wound is producing an excess of fluid, the gauze may be used dry until this stops. Conversely, if the wound is too dry, or if a vital tendon or joint capsule is exposed, the dressing is rewetted exteriorly with saline 4 hours after each dressing change to prevent critical tissues from ever drying. Povidone-iodine or hydrogen peroxide should not be used because repeated exposure of the wound surface to these substances can be cytotoxic to granulation tissue.[40, 43] If a greenish tinge to the dressings occurs, indicating *Pseudomonas* colonization, a 0.25% acetic acid solution can be used for a few days to suppress it. Because its antibacterial activity is exceeded by its fibroblast toxicity, use must be limited.[31]

Every 24 to 48 hours, the surgeon should manually compress the infected areas from proximal to distal in order to locate pockets of infection that escaped initial detection and require redebridement. Adequate pre- and postoperative nutritional support must be provided, including sufficient caloric intake to compensate for the catabolic effects of infection and bedrest as well as for a low initial serum albumin level. Supplemental iron, zinc and vitamin C, as well as multivitamins, provide essential elements for collagen formation in wound healing.[45, 47] Oral hyperalimentation in diabetics will require concomitant adjustment in hypoglycemic medication to prevent iatrogenic hyperglycemia.

The surgeon should await formation of granulation tissue throughout the depths of the wound before discharging the patient to outpatient status. The diabetologist will have been consulted at the time of admission not only to assist in preoperative control of blood glucose levels but to provide a management program that will continue after discharge to assist in wound healing by decreasing tissue glycation. The infectious disease specialist will have been involved in cases of unusual infection. All possible factors that will likely delay healing should be evaluated and corrected, such as malnutrition and the use of vasoconstrictors, such as nicotine and caffeine. Weight-bearing should be limited to the absolutely essential and then only with a weight-relief shoe. The patient is taught to prevent continual wound-site edema by avoiding dependency of the foot.

Partial Foot Amputations and Disarticulations

There are two important advantages of partial foot ablations over the transtibial and higher levels. These include preservation of end-weight-bearing along normal proprioceptive pathways and a limited disruption of body image, which is easily masked with an orthosis or limited prosthesis or simply with a modified shoe. These devices can restore near-normal walking function, relative to the loss of forefoot lever length and associated musculature.

If the criteria for level selection are met and the factors required for wound healing are correctly assessed, no amputation level in the foot need be excluded on the basis of associated diabetes mellitus. Longitudinal rather than transverse amputation should be the goal whenever possible. By only narrowing rather than shortening the foot, postoperative fitting of shoewear is greatly enhanced. Conversely, the surgeon should also consider the possibility that a forefoot or midfoot ablation, too close to extensive infection, may forfeit the chance for a Syme ankle disarticulation; therefore, he or she must be reasonably sure that a partial foot amputation is the logical initial procedure. Specific levels of amputation or disarticulation, starting with the great toe, will now be considered.

Toe Disarticulations

Method

In cases of osteomyelitis of the distal phalanx of the great toe, sufficient viable skin can often be salvaged to permit closure of an interphalangeal disarticulation. To close the wound without tension, it may be necessary to trim the prominent condylar portions of the proximal phalanx as well as to shorten it slightly by removing the articular cartilage. The sesamoid bone within the flexor hallucis longus tendon at the level of the interphalangeal joint is removed by shortening the tendon. The proximal phalanx will continue to

aid with standing balance due to preservation of the windlass mechanism in this procedure, in contrast to disarticulation at the metatarsophalangeal joint where it is lost with removal of the flexor hallucis brevis/sesamoid complex (Fig. 28–5).

Osteomyelitis of the distal phalanx of an insensate lesser toe often follows ulceration of a fixed mallet toe deformity. It is most commonly noted in the second toe in association with a long second metatarsal bone, especially following disarticulation of the great toe (Fig. 28–6). Removal of the infected distal phalanx shortens the toe so that it no longer projects beyond the adjacent toes, reducing the risk of future ulceration.

In regard to the great toe, the metatarsophalangeal joint is the next site of election if a major portion of the proximal phalanx is infected. After release of the flexor hallucis brevis tendon insertions on the proximal phalanx, the sesamoid bones will displace proximally. This maneuver exposes the prominent crista on the plantar surface of the first metatarsal head. The medial sesamoid, especially, may produce a bony prominence of its own just proximal to the metatarsal head. For these reasons, the sesamoids and their fibrocartilaginous plate should be excised and the crista removed with a rongeur. The articular cartilage should also be re-

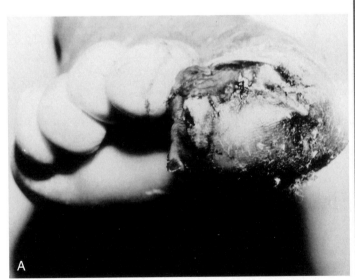
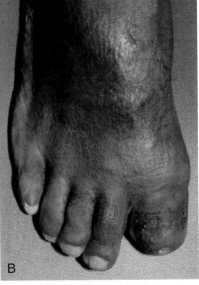

Figure 28–5 ■ *A,* Right foot of 49-year-old diabetic male with necrosis of the great toe and adequate perfusion proximally. *B,* Same case following interphalangeal disarticulation made possible by conservative debridement and primary closure over a Kritter flow-through irrigation system. (From Bowker JH: AAOS Instructional Course Lectures 39:355, 1990, with permission.)

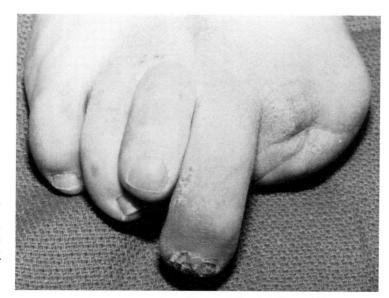

Figure 28–6 ■ Right foot of a 46-year-old diabetic male with osteomyelitis of distal phalanx of insensate second mallet toe. Disarticulation at distal interphalangeal joint was curative. Previous metatarsophalangeal joint disarticulation of the great toe left the second toe exposed to trauma.

moved and the metatarsal head smoothly rounded with a file.

Disarticulation of the second toe at the metatarsophalangeal joint often creates a secondary problem by removing the lateral support it provides to the great toe. A hallux valgus (bunion) deformity is likely to follow (Fig. 28–7). To avoid this iatrogenic bony prominence in an insensate foot, which invites future ulceration, it is better to remove the second metatarsal through its proximal metaphysis along with the toe. Following this second ray amputation, the forefoot can then narrow as the first and third metatar-

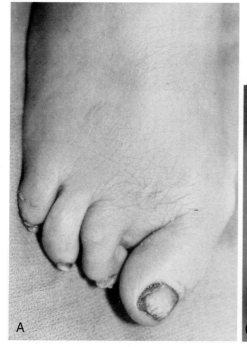

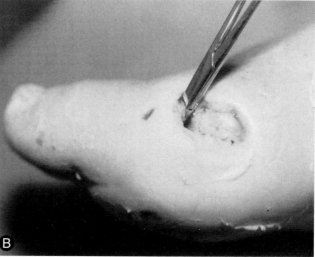

Figure 28–7 ■ Result following disarticulation of right second toe in an 87-year-old diabetic male. *A,* Note hallux valgus deformity secondary to loss of lateral support of second toe. *B,* Note ulcer penetrating metatarsophalangeal joint.

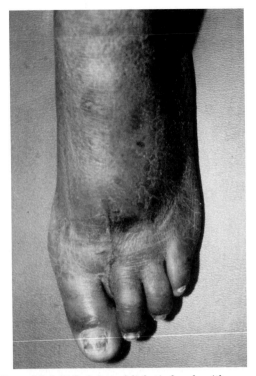

Figure 28–8 ■ Left foot of diabetic female with second ray resection for osteomyelitis shows no significant hallux valgus because of lateral support provided by third toe after postoperative forefoot narrowing. (From Bowker JH: The choice between limb salvage and amputation: Infection. *In* Bowker JH, Michael JW [eds]: Atlas of Limb Prosthetics, 2nd ed. St. Louis: Mosby Year Book, 1992, with permission.)

sals approximate each other, resulting in a good cosmetic and functional result (Fig. 28–8). If the third or fourth toes alone are disarticulated, the adjacent ones will tend to close the intervening space, thus restoring a smooth contour to the distal forefoot. Amputation of the fifth toe alone leaves its metatarsal head prominent laterally. If the head is excessively wide, it can be narrowed by trimming its lateral condyle sagittally. Leaving a lesser toe isolated by removing the toes on either side should be avoided because of the increased susceptibility to injury of the isolated and functionless toe (Fig. 28–9).

Expected Functional Outcome

Following toe disarticulations, walking function should approach normal, provided that a shoe with a firm sole and soft molded insert with any required filler has been fitted. Function will be most affected by disarticulation of the great toe at the metatarsophalangeal joint. This is because the specialized function of the first ray in the final transfer of weight during late stance phase is lost. Mann et al. found that following removal of the great toe, the end-point of progression of the moving center of plantar pressure during stance had shifted from the second metatarsal head to the third. This occurred despite a dropping of the first metatarsal head, due to loss of the great toe's stabilizing windlass mechanism

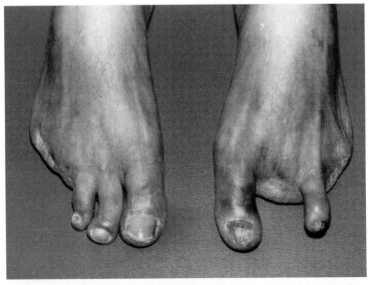

Figure 28–9 ■ Note striking difference in distal forefoot contours of right and left feet. On the right, the remaining lesser toes are protected by the great toe. On the left, the fourth toe is constantly exposed to minor trauma and does not contribute to propulsion or foot length like the great toe. It should have been removed with the other lesser toes.

associated with the flexor hallucis brevis complex.[36] Removal of lesser toes, in contrast, appears to cause little clinical difficulty.

Ray Amputations

Methods

A ray amputation consists of excision of a toe and its metatarsal. In regard to the first (medial) ray, shortening of the metatarsal shaft should be as limited as possible to allow effective orthotic support of the medial arch by means of a custom-molded insert fitted into a shoe with a rigid rocker bottom (Fig. 28–10). Preservation of first metatarsal shaft length is relatively easy because the usual source of infection is a penetrating ulcer plantar to the first metatarsal head/sesamoids, resulting in septic arthritis of the metatarsophalangeal joint. Only a portion of the head may need to be removed to eradicate the infection, preserving all uninvolved portions of the shaft. The extent of osteomyelitis in a metatarsal can generally be determined

visually. If in doubt, the marrow cavity contents can be curetted and cultured. The shaft should be beveled on its plantar aspect to avoid a high-pressure area during rollover at the end of the stance phase of gait.

Single lesser ray amputations will affect only the width of the forefoot, giving a nice cosmetic result. The bone is divided through the proximal metaphysis where the involved ray intersects with the adjacent metatarsals (Fig. 28–11). The fifth metatarsal is best transected obliquely with an inferolateral-facing facet. The uninvolved half to two thirds of the shaft is left to retain the insertion of the peroneus brevis muscle (Fig. 28–12).

On occasion, multiple lateral ray resections are required in cases of massive forefoot infection. In this situation, the lateral metatarsals can be divided obliquely with an inferolateral-facing facet. Each affected metatarsal is cut somewhat longer as one progresses toward the first ray (Fig. 28–13). If all but the first ray are involved, it can be left as the only complete one (Fig. 28–14). This strategy retains both

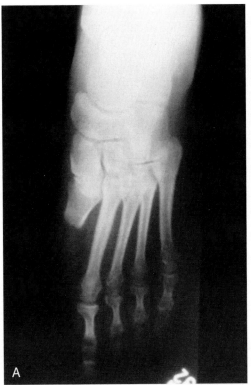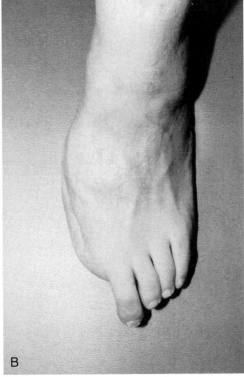

Figure 28–10 ■ *A*, Radiograph of left foot after radical first ray amputation for diabetic infection. There is insufficient metatarsal shaft remaining to allow effective medial orthotic support. *B*, Note planovalgus position of foot secondary to loss of medial column support. (From Bowker JH: J Prosthet Orthot 4:23, 1991, with permission.)

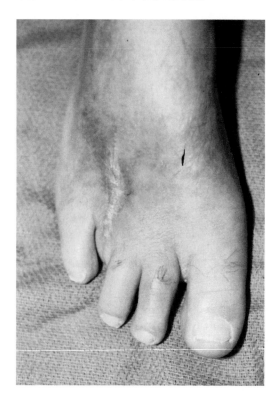

Figure 28–11 ■ Right foot of diabetic male with fourth ray amputation that healed by secondary intention. Note narrowing of forefoot and excellent distal forefoot contour. (From Bowker JH, San Giovanni TP: Amputations and disarticulations. *In* Myerson M [ed]: Foot and Ankle Disorders. Philadelphia: WB Saunders Company, 2000, with permission.)

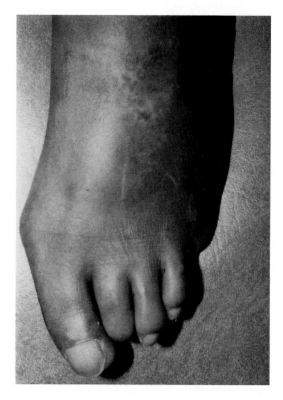

Figure 28–12 ■ Left foot of diabetic female with healed fifth ray amputation. Proximal half of shaft was left to retain insertion of peroneus brevis tendon.

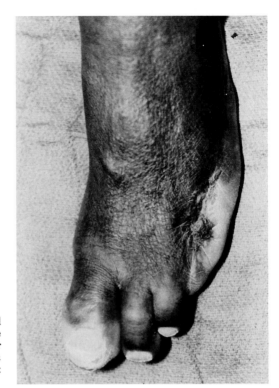

Figure 28–13 ■ Left foot of diabetic male with fourth and fifth ray amputations. He functions well in a depth shoe with custom-molded inlay with lateral filler. (From Bowker JH, San Giovanni TP: Amputations and disarticulations. *In* Myerson M [ed]: Foot and Ankle Disorders. Philadelphia: WB Saunders Company, 2000, with permission.)

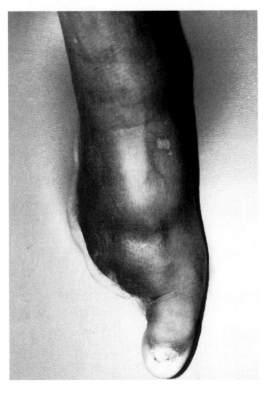

Figure 28–14 ■ Right foot of a diabetic male with the lateral four rays excised in an oblique fashion for a severe diabetic foot abscess. The first ray was left intact. Good function was present with customized footwear.

rollover function at the end of stance and full foot length in the shoe. With proper pedorthic fitting, this is far preferable to a transmetatarsal amputation. Removal of two or more central rays is to be avoided; here it is better to include the uninvolved lateral ray(s) in the resection to obviate a poor functional and cosmetic result (Fig. 28–15). In all ray amputations, the full thickness of the inciting ulcer can be easily cored out with a #11 blade down to the underlying bone. Even when it is feasible to close the primary wound over a Kritter flow-through irrigation system, the ulcer wound can be left open to contract and heal secondarily from depth to surface.

This is greatly assisted by twice-daily *gentle* packing of the wound with normal saline-moistened gauze dressings or other absorbent material, provided it is nontoxic to granulation tissue.

Expected Functional Outcome

First ray amputation involving major removal of the first metatarsal is devastating to stance and gait because an intact medial column is essential to proper foot function during both stance and forward progression. The effectiveness of orthotic restoration of the medial arch is directly related to the length of the first metatarsal shaft preserved. Single lesser ray amputation, in contrast, will provide an excellent result from both the functional and cosmetic points of view. In these cases, only the width of the forefoot is affected, while rollover function during terminal stance appears to remain essentially normal. Removal of several lateral rays, if done as conservatively as possible, can be adequately compensated by good pedorthic fitting. Barefoot walking appears to be markedly impaired in all but the single lesser ray amputations.

There are occasional cases in which a penetrating ulcer has destroyed the first metatarsophalangeal joint, leaving the great toe viable. In this instance, in lieu of a first ray amputation, the joint alone can be removed. This is done through a medial longitudinal in-

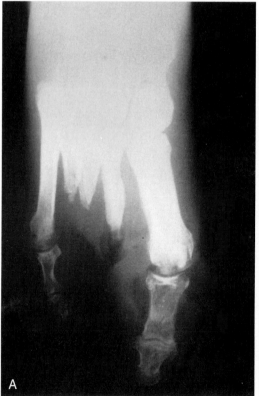 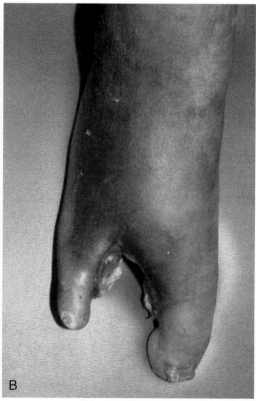

Figure 28–15 ■ *A*, Radiograph of right foot of diabetic male after excision of three central rays for abscess. *B*, Poor cosmetic and functional result. A transmetatarsal amputation was required to correct chronic plantar ulceration. An initial oblique removal of all lateral rays might have averted this outcome (*B* From Bowker JH: Medical and surgical considerations in the care of patients with insensitive dysvascular feet. J Prosthet Orthot 4:23, 1991, with permission.)

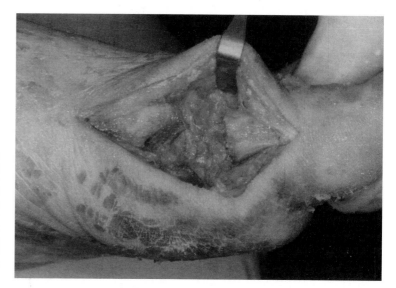

Figure 28–16 ■ Intraoperative medial view of the left forefoot showing excision of chronically infected first metatarsophalangeal joint. Note plantar bevel of the metatarsal metaphysis. Joint infection had followed penetration from plantar ulcer. (From Bowker JH: Partial foot amputations and disarticulations. Foot Ankle Clin 2:153, 1997, with permission.)

cision over the joint. The inciting ulcer should be excised as described above. All relatively avascular tissues should be removed, including the sesamoid complex, articular cartilage, joint capsule, and flexor tendons as well as infected cancellous bone (Fig. 28–16). If the wound is sufficiently clean at the conclusion of the procedure, it can be closed loosely over a Kritter flow-through irrigation system as described above.[28] The cosmetic and shoe-fitting result is much better than following great toe amputation, although the stabilizing windlass mechanism is lost with the excision of the flexor hallucis brevis complex. Active dorsiflexion of the great toe is retained if the usually uninvolved extensor hallucis longus tendon is preserved (Fig. 28–17).

Transmetatarsal Amputation

Method

This should be considered whenever control of infection requires that most or all of the first metatarsal bone or two or more medial rays must be removed. To ensure maximum function, it is important to save all metatarsal shaft length that can be covered distally with good plantar skin, avoiding the use of split skin grafts in this area as well as plantarly (Fig. 28–18). In contrast, residual dorsal defects can be easily closed with split skin grafts. With avoidance of shear forces and with properly fitted footwear, these dorsal grafts rarely ulcerate. To assist in preserving

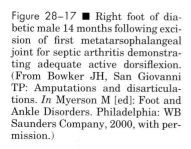

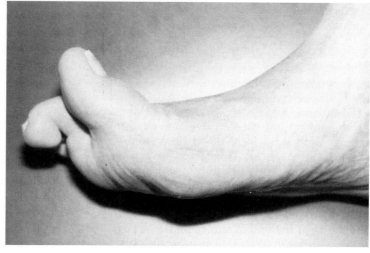

Figure 28–17 ■ Right foot of diabetic male 14 months following excision of first metatarsophalangeal joint for septic arthritis demonstrating adequate active dorsiflexion. (From Bowker JH, San Giovanni TP: Amputations and disarticulations. In Myerson M [ed]: Foot and Ankle Disorders. Philadelphia: WB Saunders Company, 2000, with permission.)

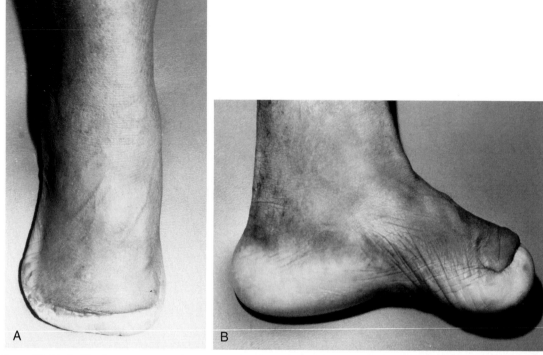

Figure 28–18 ■ Ideal transmetatarsal amputation. *A,* Dorsal view. *B,* Medial view. Note placement of distal plantar flap, overall length of residual forefoot, maintenance of medial arch, and absence of equinus deformity.

forefoot skeletal length and in ensuring distal coverage of the metatarsal shafts with a durable soft tissue envelope, the transverse plantar and dorsal incisions are made at the base of the toes. To further assist in preserving length, the shaft cuts should begin medially with the first metatarsal, taking off as little as possible while removing all involved bone. The surgeon should reproduce the 15-degree transverse angle parallel to the metatarsophalangeal joint, which parallels the normal "toe break" of the shoe. The metatarsal shafts should also be beveled plantarly to reduce distal plantar peak pressures during rollover. If a large necrotic plantar forefoot ulcer is present, it can be excised in a longitudinal elliptic manner with closure done in a "T" fashion (Fig. 28–19). At closure, all flaps are trimmed to fit without tension or redundancy. With good local blood flow, healing should be uneventful. If no active *or* passive ankle dorsiflexion is present, a concomitant percutaneous fractional lengthening of the Achilles tendon is indicated to effectively reduce distal peak pressures over the metatarsal shafts at the end of stance phase. A Kritter flow-through irrigation system, described

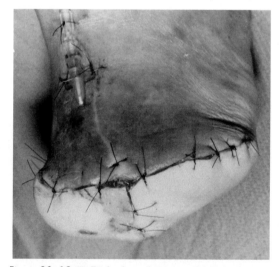

Figure 28–19 ■ Right foot of 62-year-old diabetic male following transmetatarsal amputation. The infection was initiated by a large penetrating ulcer beneath the second metatarsal head. Wide excision of the ulcer required a "T"-shaped closure. Note the Kritter flow-through irrigation system. (From Bowker JH, San Giovanni TP: Amputations and disarticulations. *In* Myerson M [ed]: Foot and Ankle Disorders. Philadelphia: WB Saunders Company, 2000, with permission.)

above under "Management of Limb-Threatening Emergencies," is useful in removing wound detritus. Before discharge, a well-padded total-contact cast is applied with the foot in a slightly dorsiflexed position to protect the wound and prevent equinus contracture. The cast is changed weekly until the wound is sound, usually at 6 weeks, when a shoe with a stiff rocker sole and custom-molded insert with filler, previously measured, is fitted. In the case of associated tibialis anterior weakness (drop foot), common in diabetics, a well-padded ankle-foot orthosis will be necessary.

Expected Functional Outcome

Published healing rates of transmetatarsal amputations have varied widely. In a mixed group of diabetics with arterial gangrene, Gerolakos and May noted healing in 68%. No follow-up information regarding function was given.[14] Hobson et al. noted a 50% healing rate in 30 amputees with preoperative gangrene, rest pain, or infection; again without functional data.[22] In both groups, patient selection was on clinical grounds alone, including skin appearance and extent of gangrene, without studies of tissue perfusion. Durham and associates reported on a series of 43 open transmetatarsal amputations. Fifty-three percent healed by wound contraction or split skin grafting at a mean time of 7.1 ± 5.6 months. Ninety-one percent of those that healed (21 of 23 patients) became independent walkers, but no long-term data regarding durability of the scarred or grafted wounds were provided.[11]

In 1949, prior to the availability of any laboratory methods of determining tissue perfusion, McKittrick obtained transmetatarsal healing in 91% of 215 diabetic patients with a 78% satisfactory functional outcome in walking.[38] This clearly demonstrates what a high level of clinical acumen can achieve.

Following transmetatarsal amputation, a steel shank or carbon fiber stiffener and rocker should be added to the shoe sole to avoid distal stump ulcers from the shoe curling around the end of the residual foot. A distal filler will also be needed to prevent crushing of the toebox. Some patients, for simplicity, will elect a custom-made short shoe, but this will cause an unequal "drop-off" gait due to the shortened forefoot lever arm.

Tarsometatarsal (Lisfranc) Disarticulation

Method

This disarticulation, at the junction of the tarsus and metatarsus, was described for trauma cases by Lisfranc in 1815, at the conclusion of the Napoleonic Wars.[32] It can also be used in cases of foot infection in diabetics if one is very selective, since failure to control the infection at this level will risk the failure of a Syme ankle disarticulation. The Lisfranc procedure results in a major loss of forefoot lever length; therefore, it is important to preserve the tendon insertions of the peroneus brevis, peroneus longus, and tibialis anterior muscles in order to maintain a muscle-balanced residual foot. These muscles will help to counteract the massive triceps surae complex and prevent equinus contracture as well as provide eversion and inversion of the residual foot. Careful dissection will spare the proximal insertions of the peroneus longus and tibialis anterior tendons on the medial cuneiform bone. The distal insertions of these tendons on the first metatarsal can also be carefully skived off and reattached for reinforcement. While the first, third, and fourth metatarsals can be disarticulated, the "keystone" base of the second metatarsal should be left in place to preserve the proximal transverse arch. Leaving a portion of the base of the fifth metatarsal will preserve the insertion of the peroneus brevis tendon. Prevention of equinus contracture can also be enhanced by doing a primary percutaneous fractional heel cord lengthening followed by application of a rigid cast with the foot in a slightly dorsiflexed position.[33] Another method that the author now uses in lieu of heel cord lengthening is cast immobilization of the residual foot in ankle dorsiflexion for 3 to 4 weeks to weaken the triceps surae relative to the ankle dorsiflexors (Fig. 28–20).

Expected Functional Outcome

This level represents a significant loss of forefoot length with a corresponding decrease in barefoot walking function. To restore fairly effective late stance phase walking function, an intimately fitting fixed-ankle prosthesis or orthosis is required, which is then placed into a shoe with a rigid rocker bottom.

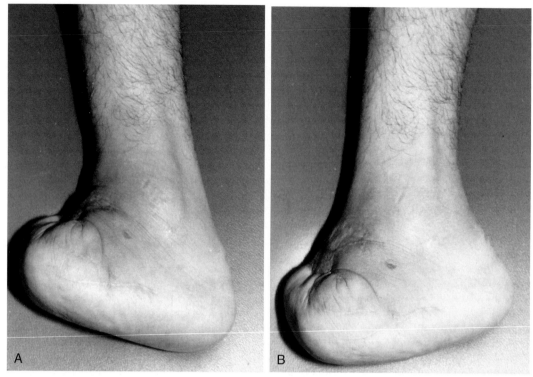

Figure 28–20 ■ Lateral views of right foot of male with Lisfranc disarticulation, demonstrating range of ankle motion available with preservation of midfoot insertions of extrinsic muscles. *A,* Maximum active dorsiflexion. *B,* Maximum active plantar flexion. (From Bowker JH, San Giovanni TP: Amputations and disarticulations. *In* Myerson M [ed]: Foot and Ankle Disorders. Philadelphia: WB Saunders Company, 2000, with permission.)

Midtarsal (Chopart) Disarticulation

Method

This disarticulation is through the talonavicular and calcaneocuboid joints, leaving only the hindfoot (talus and calcaneus). It can be used only occasionally in diabetic foot infections because of its proximity to the heel pad as discussed under tarsometatarsal disarticulation. Since no muscles insert on the talus, all active dorsiflexion function is lost at the time of disarticulation. Dorsiflexion can be restored, however, to this extremely short residual foot by reattachment of the anterior tibialis tendon to the anterolateral talus by a variety of methods, either through a drill hole in the talar head or with sutures to a groove in the head.[29] Rather than lengthen the Achilles tendon to maintain functional balance between dorsiflexors and plantar flexors, the author has found it more effective to remove 2 to 3 cm of the tendon just proximal to the calcaneus. This is easily done through a separate longitudinal incision just medial to the tendon, leaving the sheath of the tendon in place to allow rapid reconstitution at its new length. A well-padded total-contact cast is applied with the ankle in slight dorsiflexion. This is worn for about 6 weeks with changes as necessary for wound evaluation. In addition to preventing equinus contracture of the hindfoot, this method allows secure healing of the tibialis anterior tendon to the talus.

The author has treated several cases of equinus contracture following Chopart disarticulation in which the anterior tibial tendon had not been surgically attached to the talus. Active dorsiflexion with restoration of comfortable heel pad weight-bearing was obtained by partial Achilles tendon excision and cast immobilization as described above. This simple salvage procedure, recommended by Burgess, avoids revision to a Syme or higher level[8] (Fig. 28–21).

Expected Functional Outcome

Although this disarticulation does allow direct end-bearing, it provides no inherent rollover function. Due to preservation of stabil-

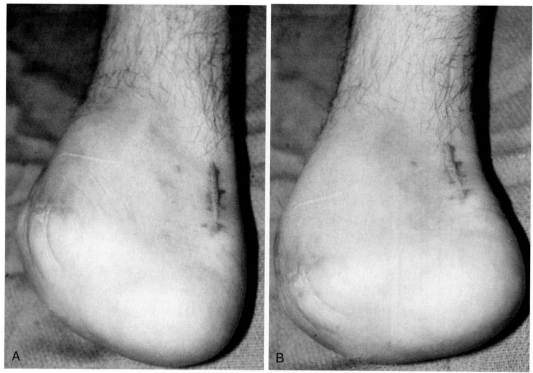

Figure 28–21 ■ Medial views of right foot of 17-year-old male with Chopart disarticulation. He presented with distal stump pain while walking in prosthesis secondary to severe equinus deformity. Photographs taken 3 weeks after excision of 2 cm of the Achilles tendon to restore the heel pad to a plantigrade position. Note the short medial incision. *A*, Maximum active dorsiflexion. *B*, Maximum active plantar flexion. (From Bowker JH, San Giovanni TP: Amputations and disarticulations. *In* Myerson M [ed]: Foot and Ankle Disorders. Philadelphia: WB Saunders Company, 2000, with permission.)

ity of the heel-pad and full leg length, the amputee may do limited walking without a prosthesis, in contrast to the Syme level, where the prosthesis is essential to heel-pad stability and leg-length equality. Nonetheless, the Chopart prosthesis is required for reasonable walking function. As with the Lisfranc disarticulation, this level also requires a very intimately fitted rigid ankle prosthesis or orthosis which then slips into a shoe with a rigid rocker sole to permit adequate late stance phase gait.

Syme Ankle Disarticulation

Methods

In 1843, James Syme, Professor of Surgery at the University of Edinburgh, succinctly described his operation as "disarticulation through the ankle joint with preservation of the heel flap to permit weight-bearing on the end of the stump."[48] Because the heel pad is salvaged, it may be considered a type of partial-foot ablation. Its main indication is the inability to salvage a more distal functional level in an infected or traumatized foot with an adequate posterior tibial artery, the main source of blood supply to the heel pad. As noted above, it is also indicated if an infection is too close to the heel pad to risk failure of a Lisfranc or Chopart disarticulation. Syme ankle disarticulation can also be a reasonable choice in certain cases of severe neuroarthropathic destruction of the ankle joint. It offers these patients a much more rapid return to weight-bearing status than ankle arthrodesis because it requires no fusion or fibrous ankylosis of bones (Fig. 28–22).

Contraindications include inadequate blood flow to the heel pad, infection of the heel pad, or ascending lymphangitis uncontrolled by systemic antibiotics.[49] A low serum albumin due to diabetic nephropathy or malnutrition as well as decreased immunocompetence reflected in a low total lymphocyte count can also seriously impede healing.[2, 10, 41] Uncompensated congestive heart

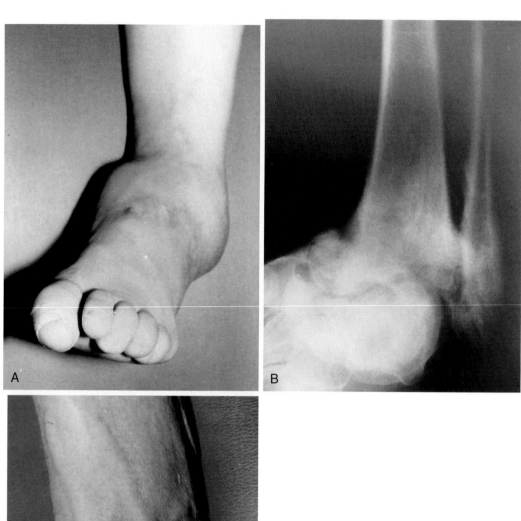

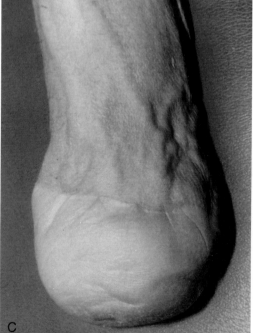

Figure 28–22 ■ Feet of 32-year-old female with type 1 diabetes 1 year after undisplaced bimalleolar fracture of left ankle treated in cast for 6 weeks. She was insensate to just below the knees. *A,* Anterior view showing severe medial displacement of left foot. Pressure ulcer was present over lateral malleolus from misguided use of ankle-foot orthosis to control this irreducible, increasing deformity. *B,* Anteroposterior radiograph showing foot displacement with ankle joint and hindfoot dissolution. *C,* Stump appearance 8 years after surgery. She actively wears her prosthesis 14 to 16 hours daily.

failure will also prevent healing by keeping wound tissues edematous.[2] A past history of poor compliance or overt psychosis should alert the surgeon to the likelihood of failure of this procedure.

This operation must be meticulously done in order to preserve the posterior tibial neurovascular structures and the integrity of the vertically oriented fat-filled fibrous chambers of the heel pad, which provide shock absorption on heel strike. These points are thoroughly discussed and well-illustrated in the classic article by R.I. Harris.[21] Wagner modified Harris' traditional method of removing 1 cm of the distal tibia by simply cutting the malleoli flush with the tibial plafond and also narrowing the malleoli to match the width of the metaphyseal flare. He recommended that the procedure be done in two stages to reduce the chance of recurrent infection.[49] In the absence of infection directly adjacent to the heel pad, however, both stages can be safely combined.[2, 41] If infection is close to the heel pad, the wound should be left open for 7 to 10 days before closure to determine if drainage and antibiotics have controlled it. If closure is then clearly indicated, the tibia will need to be shortened as described by Harris to accommodate interval shrinkage of the heel pad flap.[21] If infection has not been controlled, a long transtibial amputation is done without further delay.

Closure must be snug, but not tight, with the heel pad perfectly centered under the leg (Fig. 28–23). The heel pad flap can be accurately centered under the tibia by suturing the plantar fascia to the anterior tibial cortex through drill holes. Closed wound irrigation, using a modified Foley catheter or Shirley drain, inserted through a lateral stab wound, is continued for 3 days (Fig. 28–24).

Postoperative Management

Immediately after removal of the catheter, a carefully molded cast is applied, holding the heel pad centered and slightly forward. The cast is changed weekly for 4 to 5 weeks to accommodate volume reduction, at which time a temporary prosthesis is applied, consisting of a cast with a walking heel. This is changed whenever it becomes loose, but at least every 2 weeks, until limb volume has stabilized (Fig. 28–25). A definitive prosthesis is then fabricated and applied by the prosthetist.

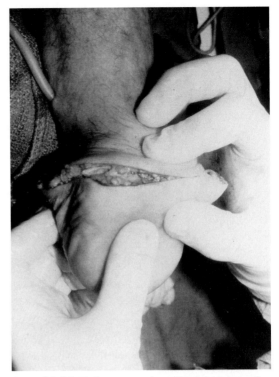

Figure 28–23 ■ Syme procedure. Prior to closure, flap length is carefully checked. If redundant, skin can be removed from the proximal flap. If too snug, the tibia will need to be appropriately shortened, most accurately with a broad hand saw. (From Bowker JH, San Giovanni TP: Amputations and disarticulations. *In* Myerson M [ed]: Foot and Ankle Disorders. Philadelphia: WB Saunders Company, 2000, with permission.)

Expected Functional Outcome

Because the Syme ankle disarticulation preserves heel-pad bearing along normal proprioceptive pathways, minimal prosthetic gait training is required. This level is also more energy efficient than the transtibial level.[50] The stump is remarkably activity tolerant, even if insensate, provided an intimately fitted socket firmly holds the thick fat-filled heel pad directly under the tibia (Fig. 28–26). This position must then be maintained by timely replacement of the prosthesis, as the inevitable calf atrophy occurs over time. Although the prosthesis is more difficult to contour cosmetically in its distal half as compared to its transtibial counterpart, the patient's ability to comfortably engage in a wide variety of activities should lead to much wider use of this procedure than at present.

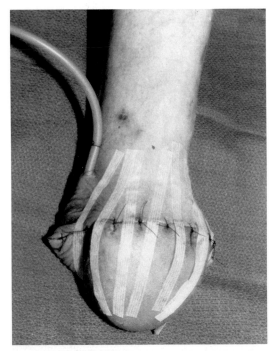

Figure 28–24 ■ Syme procedure. Note modified Foley catheter exiting through lateral stab wound. Also note that "dog-ears" have not been trimmed. This avoids any narrowing of the heel pad pedicle. (From Bowker JH, San Giovanni TP: Amputations and disarticulations. *In* Myerson M [ed]: Foot and Ankle Disorders. Philadelphia: WB Saunders Company, 2000, with permission.)

Transtibial Amputation

Methods

Despite the obvious functional advantages of partial foot ablations and notwithstanding the desire of the progressive amputation surgeon to conserve all possible length, at times it is impossible to salvage any portion of the foot. Once this has been strongly suspected by the primary physician, a thorough review of the problem should be done by a surgical consultant with a definite bias toward preservation of locomotor function. If the consultant also finds the foot unsalvageable, a prompt transtibial amputation should be done. As much length as possible should be preserved and early prosthetic fitting should be a priority. The patient and family should fully participate in the decision and follow-up to provide the best chance of optimum rehabilitation.

After determining that the foot cannot be saved and that the knee joint is usable, a choice must be made regarding the length to be retained. The shortest useful transtibial

amputation must include the tibial tubercle to preserve knee extension by the quadriceps with flexion provided by the semimembranosus and the biceps femoris. Stable prosthetic socket fitting at this level is markedly enhanced by removal of the fibular head and neck and high transection of the peroneal nerve[46] (Fig. 28–27). To ensure that the inevitable peroneal neuroma will be proximal to the knee, gentle traction is applied to the nerve with the knee flexed and the hip extended, allowing maximum length to be excised.

Beyond universal acceptance of this shortest possible functional transtibial level, no agreement has been reached regarding the best length for optimum prosthetic function. Several amputation surgeons have strongly endorsed as distal a site as possible compatible with healing and good prosthetic func-

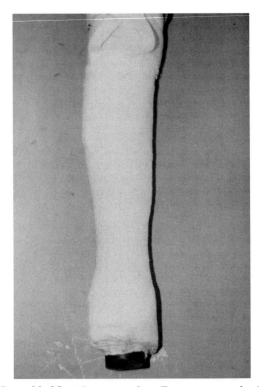

Figure 28–25 ■ Syme procedure. Temporary prosthesis applied by the surgeon after 4 to 5 weeks of non–weight-bearing casts, changed weekly. This weight-bearing cast is changed every 10 to 14 days until no further atrophy occurs. A definitive prosthesis is fitted at that time. It is important that the patient is never without external support for the heel pad until the definitive prosthesis is fitted. (From Bowker JH, San Giovanni TP: Amputations and disarticulations. *In* Myerson M [ed]: Foot and Ankle Disorders. Philadelphia: WB Saunders Company, 2000, with permission.)

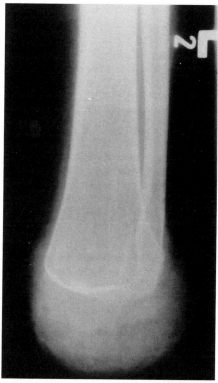

Figure 28–26 ■ Syme procedure. Radiograph of Syme stump. Note the thickness of the heel pad, which provides excellent end-weight-bearing within the prosthetic socket.

abscess has spread proximally along tissue planes under pressure into the crural compartments. Although involvement may extend to the proximal leg, it may not yet involve the knee joint. If this is so, and sufficient vascularity can be demonstrated, there is no need to amputate above the infection (i.e., at the transfemoral level). Instead, an emergent ankle disarticulation is done. If the distal tibial cancellous bone has been affected, a very low supramalleolar transection is indicated. Each crural compartment, in turn, is then manually stripped from proximal to distal while closely observing the cross-section at the ankle for expressed pus. Involved compartments are then incised longitudinally, beginning distally and extending proximally to the limit of involvement. These may include the anterior and lateral as well as the deep and superficial posterior compartments. If all compartments must be opened, the required anterolateral and pos-

tion.[12, 37, 39] This conservative position is supported by a study showing that transtibial amputees with longer stumps require less energy to walk.[16] In addition, most patients with diabetic wet gangrene who have good perfusion will heal at the junction of the proximal two thirds and distal one third of the leg. Even in dysvascular cases, healing can usually be achieved at the midleg level.

In a patient with dry gangrene of the entire foot, however, there may be no palpable pulses even at the groin. If the limb below the knee is warm, transcutaneous oxygen mapping of the skin will help assess healing potential. If skin perfusion is found to be poor, even with an oxygen challenge, an *interested* vascular surgeon should determine if proximal bypass or recanalization is feasible. Even when patches of gangrenous tissue are present distal to the knee at the time of a successful bypass, a short transtibial amputation can often be fashioned using nonstandard flaps.

Another major challenge to preservation of the knee joint occurs when a massive foot

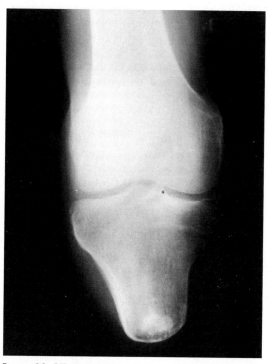

Figure 28–27 ■ Anteroposterior radiograph of a very short right transtibial amputation. Note the excellent contour achieved by removal of the nonfunctional fibular head. The prosthetic socket can now be intimately molded to the lateral tibia for greater stability. (From Bowker JH, Goldberg B, Poonekar PD: Transtibial amputation: Surgical procedures and immediate postsurgical management. *In* Bowker JH, Michael JW [eds]: Atlas of Limb Prosthetics, 2nd ed. St. Louis: Mosby Year Book, 1992, with permission.)

teromedial incisions must be spaced sufficiently apart to avoid too narrow an anterior flap. *All* infected and necrotic tissue is thoroughly excised.

The thigh tourniquet is then deflated, hemostasis achieved, and the wounds firmly packed after final inspection for residual necrotic tissue. Beginning the next day, the wounds are then lightly packed thrice daily with wet-to-dry saline gauze dressings. After 10 to 14 days, the wounds should be well granulated and ready for reexcision and myodesis closure at the long transtibial level with a posterior myofasciocutaneous flap[5] (Fig. 28–28).

Expected Functional Outcome

From a rehabilitation point of view, preservation of the knee joint cannot be stressed enough. Analysis of several studies evaluating the prosthetic rehabilitation of persons with transtibial versus transfemoral amputations revealed that 75% of transtibial versus 25% of transfemoral amputees successfully achieved prosthetic rehabilitation.[3]

A modern, well-fitted transtibial prosthesis can restore a surprising amount of function, provided that good comfort is achieved. A dynamic response foot provides good shock absorption at heel contact as well as giving a sense of propulsion in late stance phase. A rotator unit can be added to reduce torsional loads at the stump-socket interface. For a detailed discussion of all aspects of transtibial amputation, including surgical technique, the reader is referred to Chapter 18A of the *AAOS Atlas of Limb Prosthetics,* 2nd ed.[5]

Knee Disarticulation

Whenever the knee joint cannot be salvaged, knee disarticulation should be strongly considered as the next best level, rather than transfemoral amputation. It is a simpler, less shocking procedure with minimal blood loss

and rapid postoperative recovery because virtually no muscle tissue is transected. The prosthetic advantages include end-weight-bearing along normal proprioceptive pathways as well as a strong, muscle-balanced lever arm with the thigh in a normally adducted position. Prosthetic suspension is enhanced by the metaphyseal flare. Even if the patient is permanently bed and chair bound, there are advantages over the transfemoral level including greater bed mobility due to retention of good kneeling and turning abilities as well as better sitting balance and easier transfers between various sitting surfaces. To provide a superior soft tissue envelope, the authors advocate the use of a long posterior myofasciocutaneous flap, which includes the gastrocnemius bellies. This method, first reported by Klaes and Eigler, allows comfortable direct end-weight-bearing.[7, 27] Strong hip extension is restored by reattaching the biceps femoris and semimembranosus tendons and the iliotibial band to the capsular structures.[24] The patellar tendon is sewn to the cruciate stumps to restore proper quadriceps muscle tension.

Transfemoral Amputation

Following transfemoral amputation, only about 25% of patients become functional prosthesis users, because the excess energy expenditure is 65% or more, far beyond what many patients can safely generate due to cardiovascular disease.[3, 16] If a transfemoral amputation is unavoidable, however, all length that can be adequately covered with muscle and skin should be saved to minimize this excess energy expenditure and to provide a more symmetric gait.[23]

On the basis of cadaver studies, Gottschalk calculated that up to 70% of hip adductor power and considerable hip extensor power are lost with the division of the adductor magnus muscle. This is related to its large cross-sectional area and distal attachment at

---

Figure 28–28 ■ *A,* Severely abscessed right foot of 43-year-old type 1 diabetic prior to supramalleolar amputation and wide debridement of ascending infection of all crural compartments. *B,* The anterior compartment wound at 17 days demonstrates granulation. It is ready for excision and distal closure. *C,* Lateral view of distal closure. The proximal portion at the wound healed by secondary intention. Only enough bone was removed to effect myodesis closure. *D,* Lateral view 3 months following initial open amputation; the limb is ready for prosthetic fitting. (From Bowker JH, Goldberg B, Poonekar PD: Transtibial amputation: Surgical procedures and immediate postsurgical management. *In* Bowker JH, Michael JW [eds]: Atlas of Limb Prosthetics, 2nd ed. St. Louis: Mosby Year Book, 1992, with permission.)

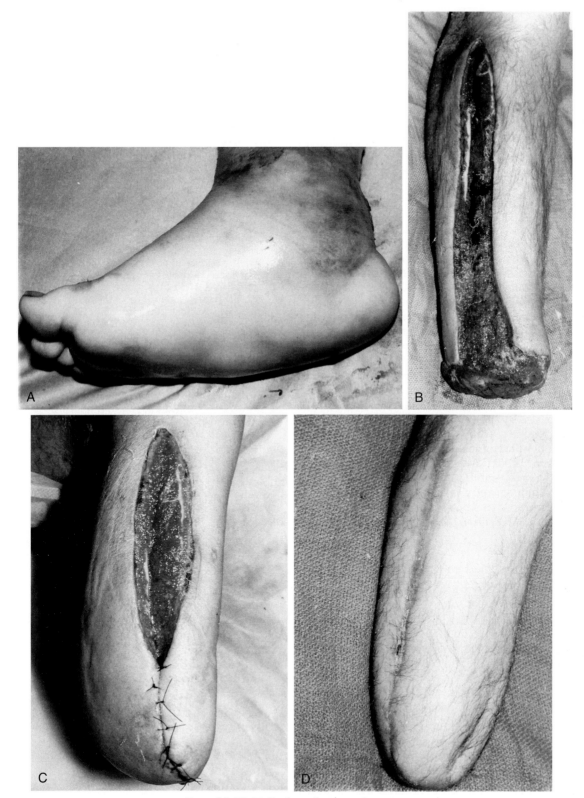

Figure 28–28 ■ *See legend on opposite page*

the abductor tubercle. The resulting muscular imbalance between hip abductors and adductors leads to a lurching prosthetic gait due to a relatively abducted position of the stump in the prosthetic socket. This increase of lateral translation of the body's center of gravity during gait is one of the major causes of excess energy expenditure at this level. Based on these findings, Gottschalk developed a vastly improved technique for transfemoral amputation that preserves adductor magnus power.[17]

Following division of the femur 10 to 12 cm above the knee joint line, the sterile tourniquet is removed prior to setting muscle tensions. With the femur held in maximum adduction and extension, the adductor magnus tendon is reattached to the distal-lateral cortex of the femur. The quadriceps muscle, which had been detached from the superior pole of the patella, is centered over the end of the femur and attached to posterior femoral drill holes, thus providing an excellent distal end pad.[17] The hamstrings and the iliotibial band are firmly reattached to assist in hip extension.[24]

In summary, this chapter may act as a reliable guide to both beginning and experienced team members as they face the daunting task of providing the most conservative treatment possible to diabetic patients facing minor or major loss of tissue of the lower limb due to infection, dysvascularity, or trauma and various combinations thereof. The extensive bibliography is meant to stimulate exploration of this challenging and rewarding, but often-neglected, area of care.

ACKNOWLEDGMENT

The authors wish to express their thanks to Ms. Patsy Bain for her expert preparation of this manuscript.

REFERENCES

1. Bagdade JD, Nielsen K, Root R, et al: Host defense in diabetes mellitus: The feckless phagocyte during poor control and ketoacidosis. Diabetes 19:364, 1970.
2. Bowker JH, Bui VT, Redman S, et al: Syme amputation in diabetic dysvascular patients. Orthop Trans 12:767, 1988.
3. Bowker JH: Transtibial (below-knee) amputation. Report of ISPO Consensus Conference on Amputation Surgery. Copenhagen: International Society for Prosthetics and Orthotics, 1992, p 10.
4. Bowker JH: The choice between limb salvage and amputation: Infection. *In* Bowker JH, Michael JW (eds): Atlas of Limb Prosthetics, 2nd ed. St. Louis: Mosby Year Book, 1992, p 39.
5. Bowker JH, Goldberg B, Poonekar PD: Transtibial amputation: Surgical procedures and immediate postsurgical management. *In* Bowker JH, Michael JW (eds): Atlas of Limb Prosthetics, 2nd ed. St. Louis: Mosby Year Book, 1992, p 429.
6. Bowker JH: Partial foot amputations and disarticulations. Foot Ankle Clin 2:153, 1997.
7. Bowker JH, San Giovanni TP, Pinzur, MS: An improved technique for knee disarticulation utilizing a posterior myofasciocutaneous flap [abstract]. *In* Conference Book of the Ninth World Congress of the International Society for Prosthetics and Orthotics. Amsterdam, 1998, p 373.
8. Burgess EM: Prevention and correction of fixed equinus deformity in mid-foot amputations. Bull Prosthet Res 10:45, 1966.
9. Diabetes Control and Complications Trial Research Group: The effect of intensive treatment of diabetes on the development and progression of long-term complications in insulin-dependent diabetes mellitus. N Engl J Med 329:977, 1993.
10. Dickhaut SC, DeLee JC, Page CP: Nutritional status: Importance in predicting wound healing after amputation. J Bone Joint Surg 66A:71, 1984.
11. Durham JR, McCoy DM, Sawchuk AP, et al: Open transmetatarsal amputation in the treatment of severe foot infections. Am J Surg 158:127, 1989.
12. Epps CH Jr: Amputation of the lower limb. *In* Evarts MC (ed): Surgery of the Musculoskeletal System, 2nd ed. New York: Churchill Livingstone, 1990, p 5121.
13. Fahey TJ III, Sadaty A, Jones WG II, et al: Diabetes impairs the late inflammatory response to wound healing. J Surg Res 50:308, 1991.
14. Geroulakos G, May ARL: Transmetatarsal amputation in patients with peripheral vascular disease. Eur J Vasc Surg 5:655, 1991.
15. Glattly HW: A statistical study of 12,000 new amputees. S Med J 57:1373, 1964.
16. Gonzalez EG, Corcoran PJ, Reyes RL: Energy expenditure in below-knee amputees: Correlation with stump length. Arch Phys Med Rehabil 55:111, 1974.
17. Gottschalk F: Transfemoral amputation: Surgical procedures. *In* Bowker JH, Michael JW (eds): Atlas of Limb Prosthetics, 2nd ed. St. Louis: Mosby Year Book, 1992, p 501.
18. Grayson ML: Diabetic foot infections. Antimicrobial therapy. Infect Dis Clin North Am 9:143, 1995.
19. Grayson JL, Gibbons GW, Balogh K, et al: Probing to bone in infected pedal ulcers. A clinical sign of underlying osteomyelitis in diabetic patients. JAMA 273:721, 1995.
20. Grodinsky M: A study of fascial spaces of the feet. Surg Gynecol Obstet 49:737, 1929.
21. Harris RI: Syme's amputation: The technical details essential for success. J Bone Joint Surg 38B:614, 1956.
22. Hobson MI, Stonebridge PA, Clason AE: Place of transmetatarsal amputations: A 5-year experience and review of the literature. J R Coll Surg Edinb 35:113, 1990.
23. Jaegers SM, Arendzen JH, deJongh HJ: Prosthetic gait of unilateral transfemoral amputees: A kinematic study. Arch Phys Med Rehabil 76:736, 1995.
24. Jaegers SM, Arendzen JH, deJongh HJ: An electromyographic study of the hip muscles of transfemoral amputees in walking. Clin Orthop 328:119, 1996.

25. Karchmer AW, Gibbons GW: Foot infections in diabetes: Evaluation and management. *In* Remington JS, Swartz MN (eds): Current Clinical Topics in Infectious Diseases, Vol XIV. Boston: Blackwell Scientific, 1994, p 7.

26. Kay HW, Newman JD: Relative incidence of new amputations: Statistical comparison of 6,000 new amputees. Orthot Prosthet 29:3, 1975.

27. Klaes W, Eigler F: Eine neue Technik der transgenikulären Amputation. Chirurg 56:735, 1985.

28. Kritter AE: A technique for salvage of the infected diabetic foot. Orthop Clin North Am 4:21, 1973.

29. Letts M, Pyper A: The modified Chopart's amputation: Clin Orthop 256:44, 1990.

30. Lind J, Kramhoff M, Bodker S: The influence of smoking on complications after primary amputations of the lower extremity. Clin Orthop 267:211, 1991.

31. Lineaweaver W, Howard R, Soucy D, et al: Topical antimicrobial toxicity. Arch Surg 120:267, 1985.

32. Lisfranc J: Nouvelle Methode Operatoire pour l'Amputation du Pied dans son Articulation Tarsometatarsienne: Methode Precedee des Nombreuses Modifications qu'a Subies celle de Chopart. Paris: Gabon, 1815.

33. Livingston R, Jacobs RL, Karmody A: Plantar abscess in the diabetic patient. Foot Ankle 5:205, 1985.

34. Loeffler RD Jr, Ballard A: Plantar fascial spaces of the foot and a proposed surgical approach. Foot Ankle 1:11, 1980.

35. Louie TJ, Bartlett JG, Tally FP, et al: Aerobic and anaerobic bacteria in diabetic foot ulcers. Ann Intern Med 85:461, 1976.

36. Mann RA, Poppen NK, O'Kinski M: Amputation of the great toe. A clinical and biomechanical study. Clin Orthop 226:192, 1988.

37. McCullough NC III, Harris AR, Hampton FL: Below-knee amputation. *In* Atlas of Limb Prosthetics. St. Louis: Mosby Year Book, 1981, p 341.

38. McKittrick LS, McKittrick JB, Risley TS: Transmetatarsal amputation for infection or gangrene in patients with diabetes mellitus. Ann Surg 130:826, 1949.

39. Moore TJ: Amputations of the lower extremities. *In* Chapman MW (ed): Operative Orthopaedics, 2nd ed. Philadelphia: JB Lippincott, 1993, p 2443.

40. Oberg MS, Lindsey D: Do not put hydrogen peroxide or povidone-iodine into wounds! [editorial]. Am J Dis Child 141:27, 1987.

41. Pinzur MS, Smith D, Osterman H: Syme ankle disarticulation in peripheral vascular disease and diabetic infection: The one-stage versus two-stage procedure. Foot Ankle Int 16:124, 1993.

42. Ricci MA, Fleishman C, Gerstein N: The effects of cigarette smoking and smoking cessation aids on transcutaneous oxygen levels. J Vasc Med Biol 4:256, 1993.

43. Rodeheaver G, Bellamy W, Kody M, et al: Bactericidal activity and toxicity of iodine-containing solutions in wounds. Arch Surg 117:181, 1982.

44. Schaffer MR, Tantry U, Efron PA, et al: Diabetes-impaired healing and reduced wound nitric oxide synthesis, a possible pathophysiologic correlation. Surgery 121:513, 1997.

45. Sieggreen MY: Healing of physical wounds. Nurs Clin North Am 22:439, 1987.

46. Spira A, Steinbach T: Fibulectomy and resection of the peroneal nerve for "short tibial stumps". Acta Orthop Scand 44:589, 1973.

47. Stotts NA, Washington DF: Nutrition: A critical component of wound healing. AACN Clin Issues 1:585, 1990.

48. Syme J: On amputation at the ankle joint. London Edinb Month J Med Sci 2:93, 1843.

49. Wagner FW Jr: The Syme ankle disarticulation: Surgical procedures. *In* Bowker JH, Michael JW (eds): Atlas of Limb Prosthetics, 2nd ed. St. Louis: Mosby Year Book, 1992, p 413.

50. Waters RL: The energy expenditure of amputee gait. *In* Bowker JH, Michael JW (eds): Atlas of Limb Prosthetics, 2nd ed. St. Louis: Mosby Year Book, 1992, p 381.

51. Yue DK, McLellan S, Marsh M, et al: Effects of experimental diabetes, uremia and malnutrition on wound healing. Diabetes 36:295, 1987.

52. Yue DK, Swanson B, McLennan S, et al: Abnormalities of granulation tissue and collagen formation in experimental diabetes, uraemia and malnutrition. Diabet Med 3:221, 1986.

Chapter 29

REHABILITATION OF THE DIABETIC AMPUTEE

■ Robert S. Gailey, Jr., and Curtis R. Clark

There are approximately 115,000 to 135,000 lower limb amputations performed in the United States annually.[72] An estimated 70 to 90% are the result of peripheral vascular disease (PVD) with the greater percentage (45 to 83%) of PVD amputations being related to diabetes mellitus.[3, 35] The American Diabetes Association estimates that annually there are 40,000 to 60,000 amputations performed on diabetics.[2, 64] Patients with diabetes are 15 times more likely to undergo a second amputation than the general population,[43, 45, 52] at an annual medical cost in 1992 dollars of greater than $2 billion.[66] The rate of new amputation after 1, 3, and 5 years has been suggested to be 14%, 30%, and 49%, respectively.[42] The mortality rate 1, 3, and 5 years after the first amputation was found to be 15%, 38%, and 68%, respectively.[42]

Metabolic Cost of Amputee Ambulation

The conservation of effort is one of the most important concerns of the amputee and as a result can have a tremendous impact on the successful return to premorbid lifestyle. If the labor of ambulation is too great, there is a good chance the person will become sedentary or even reluctant to complete their course of rehabilitation. For this reason, an overview of the physiologic energy requirements for prosthetic ambulation becomes worthwhile.

For amputees in general, the metabolic cost of ambulation is increased, while overall walking velocity is deceased.[64] This issue becomes of concern for the diabetic amputee, who typically will experience decreased cardiopulmonary capacity and additional comorbid conditions that frequently further impact their overall physical health. Other declining abilities such as memory, attention, concentration, and organizational and cognitive skills for successful prosthetic management create additional concerns.[63]

Summarizing the past two decades of relevant publications provides the following generalizations concerning the metabolic cost of ambulation for the amputee. The greater the loss of limb, the greater the energy expenditure the amputee will have to exert while walking at a substantially lower velocity.[61, 75] Two exceptions to this principle should be noted, the first involving the knee disarticulation amputee (KD). The KD amputee has a significantly higher O_2 cost (mL/kg·m) than both the transtibial amputee (TTA) and transfemoral amputee (TFA); however, the speed of walking does fall between the two, being slightly faster than the TFA while still slower than the TTA.[75]

The relationship between the ankle disarticulation (AD) and the TTA is the second exception to the generalization concerning ambulation efficiency. Ankle disarticulation amputees do appear to walk faster than TTAs; however, both groups expend the same relative energy cost.[4] Interestingly, there does appear to be a significant reduction in rate of oxygen consumption (ml/kg·min) between short TTA (<20% of total tibial length) and standard TTA length (20 to 40% of tibial length).[28] The long TTA (>40% of tibial length) currently does not appear to have been investigated with respect to the standard TTA or AD amputation. In general, these findings appear to emphasize the longstanding philosophy first noted by Nathan Smith in 1825 that "as a general rule, you should save all the stump you can."[67] In effect, it appears that the greater the residual limb length the more likely that there will be a decrease in relative energy expenditure and/or the potential for improved ambulation velocity.

Aside from length of the residual limb, the cause of amputation, vascular or nonvascular, is directly related to the oxygen cost and speed of ambulation (Table 29–1). Vascular amputees will adopt a comfortable walking speed (CWS) that will enable them to reach their desired destination without undue exertion. Keeping in mind that most diabetic amputees suffer from significant deconditioning from inactivity, ambulation is often reserved for short distances or areas that are difficult to access with a wheelchair.

Because approximately one third of diabetic amputees will lose the contralateral limb within 3 years after the primary limb amputation, it is important to note the escalating metabolic effort that is required by the bilateral amputee over the unilateral amputee. Unfortunately, most data available are from studies performed on relatively small sample size (Table 29–1). The key to ambulation success for the diabetic bilateral amputee is the preservation of at least one anatomic knee.[73] The likelihood of ambulation as a bilateral TFA is very remote with this population, not only because of the physiologic expectations[32] but also because the time required for the process of prosthetic fitting and gait rehabilitation becomes overwhelming. For the bilateral vascular amputee, use of a wheelchair becomes a considerably more efficient form of mobility, reducing energy cost and increasing velocity.[16, 48]

It is important to note that for nonamputees using crutches, either underarm or forearm with a three-point gait, the energy cost compared to normal walking was approximately twice as great.[21] Likewise, Pagliarulo et al. demonstrated that for TTAs having no vascular disease, the energy rate rose significantly from a mean of 15.5 mL O_2/kg/min with a prosthesis to 22.3 mL O_2/kg/min when ambulating with crutches only.[59] This suggests that the amputee should be encouraged to use the prosthesis even if an assistive device is required.

It should be mentioned that particular components of the prosthesis itself have not been shown to reduce the energy cost of ambulation. Numerous authors have demonstrated that there is no metabolic cost differ-

Table 29–1 ■ ENERGY EXPENDITURE OF UNILATERAL AND BILATERAL VASCULAR AMPUTEES*

VASCULAR AMPUTEE	SPEED (m/min)	O_2 RATE (ml/kg·min)	O_2 COST (ml/kg·m)	PULSE (bpm)
Unilateral				
TF	36	10.8	0.28	126
TT	45	9.4	0.20	105
AD	54	9.2	0.17	108
Bilateral				
TT/TT	40	11.6	0.31	113
AD/AD	62	12.8	0.21	99
Nonamputee				
Adults (20–59 yr)	80	12.1	0.15	99

* Data from Bowker JH, Michael JW: Atlas of Limb Prosthetics, 2nd ed. St Louis: Mosby-Year Book, 1992; and Waters RL, Perry J, Antonelli D, Hislop H: The energy cost of walking of amputees—influence of level amputation. J Bone Joint Surg 58(A): 42–46, 1976. TF, transfemoral; TT, transtibial; AD, ankle disarticulation.

ence between dynamic and nondynamic response foot-ankle assemblies.[28, 46, 62] Although the ability to vary cadence with fluid-controlled prosthetic knee units is a possibility, conservation of energy has yet to be established. Even though there may exist a possibility for socket designs to influence energy cost, this has only been demonstrated at a higher walking speed (2.5 mph) with traumatic TFAs, and not at slower speed (1.75 mph) with vascular amputees.[22] It had long been perceived that any reduction in the weight of the prosthesis would have a direct effect on the energy cost to the wearer. However, when additional weight of up to 2 lbs with TTAs[23] and 3 lbs with TFAs[13, 29, 30] was applied to the shanks of the average prosthesis, there was no appreciable influence on the metabolic cost during ambulation. Therefore, the addition of components that will improve the overall function and durability of the prosthesis might be of more importance than the overall mass of the prosthesis.

No one entity may be responsible for reducing the metabolic cost of ambulation for the amputee. The diabetic and vascular amputee, in most instances, will walk more slowly while exerting a greater effort to cover the same distances as their nonamputee counterparts. Collectively, the surgery, prosthetic fitting, and therapy may make a difference. Surgery should be skillfully designed to preserve limb length and anatomic joints whenever possible. A satisfactory overall prosthetic fitting will help ensure that the amputee will accept and wear the limb regularly. Finally, the proper strength, endurance, and prosthetic gait training program should lead to maximal use of the prosthesis by reducing the amputee's efforts with daily activities.

The importance of being a physically fit prosthetic ambulator cannot be minimized. A properly fitting prosthesis that is worn daily will permit the opportunity for greater mobility and probably increase the activity level over that of amputees who do not wear a prosthesis. Several authors have suggested that an amputee's level of activity is not dictated by the level of amputation, cause of amputation, number of limbs amputated, or age.[6, 24, 51] More importantly, the level of activity prior to the amputation appears to be the most important predictor of postamputation activity. If the amputee was involved and motivated before amputation, chances are they will continue to remain so after amputation. If they were sedentary and noncompliant before the loss of limb, unfortunately the prospects for change are not strong.

Immediate Postsurgical Treatment

Bedside Management

Generally, the goals of postoperative treatment for the new amputee are to reduce edema, promote healing, prevent loss of motion, increase cardiovascular endurance, and improve strength. Functional skills must also be introduced as early as possible to promote independence in bed mobility, transfers, and ambulation techniques. Prevention of further adversity may be addressed with education in the self-care of the residual and sound limbs. Moreover, each member of the rehabilitation team should be aware of the need to assist the patient with the psychological adjustment to limb loss.

Acute Bedside Amputee Assessment

The initial assessment of the amputee postsurgically has many significant components. The obvious responsibility is to obtain the baseline information necessary to determine the goals of rehabilitation and to formulate a treatment plan. However, the rehabilitation team must view the amputation surgery as a constructive procedure, not a destructive one. Therefore, action must be taken to restore the amputee to a premorbid lifestyle and prevent further adversity. This requires that the amputee be immediately taught how to care for the healing residual limb, and instructed in functional skills, protection of the sound limb, and avoidance of physical deconditioning, all in preparation for prosthetic training.

Throughout the short time the amputee is seen on an inpatient basis, the rehabilitation team must focus on endorsing the total rehabilitation process from the acute stages to completion of prosthetic training. Educating the person may reduce the anxiety of not knowing what lies ahead and enhance compliance as the amputee is made aware of the whole process and the value of each step. The inclusion of amputee support groups or peer visitation can be a tremendous asset when the support personnel involved are well informed and hold views consistent with those of the rehabilitation team.

Postoperative Dressing

Postoperative dressing selection will vary according to the level of amputation, surgical technique, healing requirements, patient compliance, and physician's preference. The four major types are soft dressings, semi-rigid/rigid dressings, immediate postoperative prostheses (IPOP), and removable rigid dressings. Soft dressings are most often used for vascular patients where regular dressing changes may be performed and alternative wound environments may be used. The disadvantage to soft dressings is that patients frequently decrease their bed mobility, as they are more hesitant to move the painful operated limb.[7] Semirigid and rigid dressings, in addition to controlling edema and providing protection and support, will assist in preventing knee flexion contractures with TTAs while offering the amputee greater confidence with bed mobility.

IPOP dressings, besides offering the aforementioned benefits, allow the amputee the ability to ambulate with an assistive device with limited weight-bearing status. Furthermore, they afford the amputee the physiological and psychological advantage of walking with a limb. To date there has been no evidence that IPOPs lead to an increased number of falls or injury to the healing residual limb. In fact, additional support to the amputated limb, in the case of the amputee with a neuropathic sound limb, can potentially reduce foot pressures, improve balance, and reduce the effort of ambulation with an assistive device.

Removable rigid dressings originally were fabricated from plaster and suspended with a variety of supracondylar cuff systems. They may now consist of a prefabricated copolymer plastic shell with a soft lining and, in some instances, the ability to attach a pylon and foot to create an IPOP. The removable rigid dressing provides the protection and other benefits of the classic rigid dressing with the option of removal for wound inspection or bathing. Additionally, socks may be added or the system tightened for progressive shrinkage of the residuum and has been shown to shorten the time to ambulatory discharge from hospital with a temporary prosthesis.[77]

Positioning

The transfemoral amputee should place a pillow laterally along the residual limb to maintain neutral rotation with no abduction, when in a supine position. If the prone position is tolerable during the day or evening, then a pillow is placed under the residual limb to maintain hip extension. Transtibial amputees should avoid knee flexion for prolonged periods of time. A residual limb board will help maintain knee extension when using a wheelchair. All amputees must be made aware that continual sitting in a wheelchair without any effort to promote hip extension may lead to limited motion during prosthetic ambulation.

Bed Mobility

The importance of good bed mobility extends beyond simple positional adjustments for comfort, or to get in and out of bed. The patient must acquire bed mobility skills to maintain correct bed positioning in order to prevent contractures and to avoid excessive friction of the sheets against the suture line or frail skin. Regardless of age, each patient should be taught a safe and efficient manner in which to roll, come to sitting, or adjust his or her position. If the patient is unable to perform the skills necessary to maintain proper positioning, a family member or caregiver must be taught how to provide assistance.

Transfers

Once bed mobility is mastered, the patient must learn to transfer from the bed to a chair or a wheelchair and then progress to more advanced transfer skills such as toilet, tub, and car transfers. In cases where an immediate postoperative or temporary prosthesis is utilized, weight-bearing through the prosthesis can assist the patient in the transfer and provide additional safety. For transtibial amputees who are not ambulatory candidates, a lightweight transfer prosthesis may allow more independent transfers. This prosthesis is typically fit when the residual limb is healed and the patient is ready for training. Bilateral amputees who are not fitted with an initial prosthesis transfer in a "head-on" manner where the patient slides forward from the wheelchair onto the desired surface by lifting the body and pushing forward with both hands.

Wheelchair Propulsion

The primary means of mobility for a large majority of vascular amputees, either temporarily or permanently, will be the wheelchair. The energy conservation of the wheelchair over prosthetic ambulation is considerable with some levels of amputation.[16, 48] Therefore, wheelchair skills should be taught to most amputees as a part of their rehabilitation program. Bilateral and older amputees may require greater use of the wheelchair, while unilateral and younger amputees will be more likely to utilize other assistive devices when not ambulating with their prosthesis. Because of the loss of body weight anteriorly, the amputee will be prone to tipping backwards while in the standard wheelchair. Amputee adapters set the wheels back approximately 2 inches, thus moving the center of mass anteriorly to prevent tipping, especially when ascending ramps or curbs. An alternative method to prevent tipping would be the addition of anti-tippers in place of, or in addition to, the amputee wheel adapters. Transtibial amputees will also require an elevating leg rest or residual limb board designed to maintain the knee in extension, thus preventing prolonged knee flexion and reducing the dependent position of the limb in order to control edema. Finally, it is recommended that the wheelchair be fitted with removable armrests to enable ease of transfer to or from either side of the chair.

Ambulation with Assistive Devices without a Prosthesis

A traditional evaluation of the patient's potential for ambulation is performed, including strength of the sound lower limb and both upper limbs, single limb balance, coordination, and mental status. The selection of an assistive device should meet with the amputee's level of skill, keeping in mind that with time the assistive device may need to be changed. Some patients who have difficulty ambulating on one limb secondary to obesity, blindness, poor balance, or generalized weakness can still be successful prosthetic ambulators when additional support is provided by the prosthesis.

Ambulation with Assistive Devices

All amputees will need an assistive device for times when they may choose not to wear their prosthesis, or on occasions when they are unable to wear their prosthesis secondary to edema, skin irritation, or a poor prosthetic fit. Other amputees will require an assistive device while ambulating with the prosthesis. Safety is the primary factor when selecting the appropriate assistive device; however, mobility is a secondary consideration that cannot be overlooked. The criteria for selection should include: (1) the ability for unsupported standing balance, (2) the degree of upper limb strength, (3) coordination and skill with the assistive device, and (4) cognition. A walker is chosen when an amputee has fair to poor balance, strength, and coordination. If balance and strength are good to normal, Lofstrand (Canadian) crutches may be used for ambulation with or without a prosthesis. A cane may be selected to ensure safety when balance is questionable while ambulating with a prosthesis.

Residual Limb Care

Phantom Sensation, Pain, and Residual Limb Pain

Some of the most common and least understood phenomena experienced by amputees are phantom pain, phantom sensation, and residual limb pain.[14] It is estimated that 85% of amputees will experience one or all three forms of pain or sensation at one time or another. During the first year after amputation, the majority of amputees will have the greatest number of episodes, with a significant decrease in intensity and duration as time after amputation increases. The amputee eventually becomes familiar with the unique manner in which the phantom sensation or pain will present to them with respect to onset, type of sensation, duration, intensity, and effective treatment.

Prior to the 1960s, many amputees were reluctant to describe their phantom pain or sensation for fear that they would lose their physician's confidence. However, current literature suggests that these phenomena and their symptoms are independent of age, sex, race, cause of amputation, health status, or psychological profile.[14] As a result, the suggestion that particular personalities or "types" of patients are more prone to complain of phantom sensation or pain is not an accepted theory today. Moreover, many practitioners are now adopting the regular practice of discussing this occurrence prior to or immediately after amputation to reassure the amputee that these feelings are totally normal and to be expected.

Unfortunately, there still is not a universally accepted explanation of the cause of phantom sensation or pain. Multiple theories exist; however, a review of these theories is beyond the scope of this chapter. Clinically, the ability to compare and contrast the three forms of adverse sensation is presumably of more importance and will be briefly presented.

Phantom Sensation

Phantom sensation is defined as a nonpainful sensation or awareness that gives form to a body part with specific dimensions, weight, or range of motion. Phantom sensation is more frequently described than phantom pain. Jensen et al. identified three categories of phantom sensation: (1) kinesthetic sensation that gives rise to the impression of postural changes, length and volume of the limb; (2) kinetic sensation described as the perception of willed, spontaneous or associated movements, and (3) extroceptive sensations such as touch, temperature, pressure, and other more commonly experienced sensations that are not painful in nature (wetness, itching, fatigue, and generalized discomfort).[38]

Phantom Pain

Phantom pain is a painful sensation experienced within the nonexisting amputated limb. It is unpredictable with regard to predisposing factors, severity, frequency, duration, character, and initiating stimuli. The more common provoking stimuli are emotional stress, exposure to cold, and local irritation. Phantom pain differs from phantom sensation in that perceived sensations are indeed painful in nature and that most postural experiences place the limb in unnatural positions such as a foot backwards or a twisted leg. Other painful sensations include dull aching, burning, knife-like stabbing, sticking, squeezing, electrical shocks or the feeling that the leg is being pulled off.[69] Traumatic amputees may complain of pain that replicates the painful sensation experienced during the trauma. Longstanding pain from limb pathology prior to amputation may persist in the form of phantom pain after amputation.

Residual Limb Pain

Residual limb pain arises from a specific anatomic structure that can be identified within the residual limb. Some of the more common causes include improperly fitting prosthesis, entrapped neuromata, abnormal tissue (bone, joint, or soft tissue), sympathetic pain, referred pain (radiculopathy, joint pain, myofascial pain), and residual limb changes (skin thinning, muscle atrophy, changes in blood flow, and insufficient nutrition).[14]

A wide variety of treatments for amputees who experience phantom sensation or pain have been administered with relatively little consistent success. Sherman's survey of 8,000 amputees found that only 7% benefited from their treatments and that there was no consistency in the type of treatment.[69]

It is important for the clinician to assure the amputee that phantom pain and sensation are very common and are experienced by most amputees some time after amputation. The clinician must accurately assess the nature of pain or sensation and then be open to administering a variety of therapies. Unfortunately, most treatments are unsuccessful for any length of time. The most effective treatment is the use of the prosthesis and should always be encouraged by the rehabilitation team.

Desensitization

Postsurgically, many amputees experience hypersensitive skin sensation as a result of the disruption of the neuromuscular system and associated edema. As wound compression techniques reduce the edema, progressive desensitization of the residual limb frequently becomes necessary to assist in restoring normal sensation. The primary concept of this technique is to gradually introduce stimuli that reduce the hyperirritability of the limb. For example, a soft material such as cotton cloth or lamb's wool is rubbed around the residual limb followed by gradually coarser materials such as corduroy. The amputee should progress as quickly as possible to tapping with the hand, massage and, eventually, when the suture line is healed, applying pressure through the residual limb as with transfers, mobility skills, and exercise. These measures will help expedite the ability to wear the prosthesis.

Education

Educating the amputee about self-care and a home exercise program are critical to the ultimate outcome of the rehabilitation process. The most difficult task is ensuring retention and compliance. The use of a checklist that the amputee may take home can assist in achieving a positive outcome. The value of an itemized list not only aids the amputee at home but also provides the clinician with a format that will help avoid the possibility that important items are being overlooked. An itemized checklist designed for the diabetic amputee provides the clinician with a systematic method of educating the amputee and should be offered as a home guide to the patient (Fig. 29–1).

Residual Limb Compression Dressing

Early rigid, semirigid dressings, compression wrapping, or the use of shrinker garments for the residual limb can (1) decrease edema, (2) increase circulation, (3) assist in shaping, (4) provide skin protection, (5) reduce redundant tissue problems; (6) reduce phantom limb pain/sensation, and (7) desensitize the residual limb. Rigid dressings with TTAs casted in extension will prevent knee flexion contractures and aid in greater confidence with early bed mobility.[7] In the case of transfemoral residual limbs, there may be some value in counteracting contracture forces with specific compression wrapping techniques.

Controversy does exist around the use of traditional compression wrapping versus the use of residual limb shrinker socks. Currently, many institutions prefer commercial shrinkers for their ease of donning. Advocates of compression wrapping state that they provide more control over pressure gradients and tissue shaping.[49] Condie et al. found that both TTAs and TFAs using a shrinker sock within 10 days after amputation demonstrated a significantly reduced time from amputation to prosthetic casting from those amputees using wrapping methods.[11] Moreover, even shorter time to prosthetic casting has been observed with TTAs receiving semirigid and rigid dressings.[11, 49]

Many programs prefer to wait until after the sutures or staples have been removed before using a shrinker sock. In the case of diabetic amputees, this time period may often be as long as 21 days. However, compression therapy can begin with wraps or rigid dressings and progress to shrinkers after the suture line has healed. This is a controversial area, and each rehabilitation team should determine the best course for their respective clients.

All compression techniques must be performed correctly and in a consistent manner to prevent (1) circulation constriction, (2) poor residual limb shaping, and (3) edema. Likewise, compliance is considered to be an intricate part of the compression program. All methods of wrapping or shrinker sock use should be routinely checked or reapplied several times per day. Furthermore, the application of a nylon sheath over the residual limb prior to wrapping or donning the shrinker sock may reduce shearing forces to skin and provide additional comfort.

Limb Management

Sound Limb Issues

When planning treatment for the diabetic amputee, management of the sound limb plays an important role. Preservation of the sound limb in many cases permits continued bipedal ambulation and delays further medical complications that can reduce the quality of life. One reason for this concern is that the sound limb routinely compensates for the amputee's inability to maintain equal weight distribution between limbs, resulting in altered gait mechanics. Two effects on the non-amputated limb raise concern: the first is force being placed on the weight-bearing surfaces of the foot and the second is the change in ground reaction forces (GRF) throughout the skeletal structures of the limb.

Increased forces placed on the intact limb can be of considerable concern during ambulation, since the foot often presents with neuropathic symptoms and is vulnerable to soft

Physical Therapy Diabetic Amputee Limb Care Check List

Topic Item	Date Completed
Skin Inspection Education	
Daily inspection of skin with mirror for difficult to see areas	
Attention to bony prominences, between toes and scars	
Attention to problem areas	
Skin Care	
Daily cleansing techniques mild unscented soap	
Application of moisturizer	
Avoid hot water	
Minimize exposure to perspiration and wet weather	
Minimize exposure extreme heat and cold	
Foot Care	
Toe deformity care (lamb wool between toes)	
Clean, dry socks without elastic bands	
Extra depth shoes with custom molded inserts	
Appropriate house slipper or shoes worn at all times in the home	
Never walk barefoot especially on beaches, hot surfaces or at night in the home	
Assistance with nail and callus trimming (if patient is independent use nail file for nails and pumice stone for corns & calluses, **No Sharp Implements**)	
Friction Reduction	
Bed mobility avoid excessive sound limb use	
Posture and positioning	
Transfer techniques	
Equal weight-bearing during standing and ambulation	
Ambulation turning techniques, avoid pivoting on sound foot	
Appropriate shoe wear with socks	
Residual Limb	
Skin inspection (same as above)	
Skin care (same as above)	
Positioning	
Prosthetic Care	
Sock regulation (correct plys, sock application & main dry sock wear)	
Prosthetic wear schedule (discuss procedure if skin lesions appear)	
Daily socket cleansing	
Compression Therapy	
Wrapping or shrinker application techniques	
Precautionary signs (pain and swelling)	
Phantom Sensation and Pain	
Awareness and desensitization	
Support Group Participation	
Contact person and phone number	
Shoe Wear	
Suggest purchase of 2-3 pairs of proper shoes for daily rotation of shoes	
Change shoes with perspiration or when wet and soiled. Methods of assessment to insure proper fit of shoes	
Inspect the inside of shoes daily for foreign objects	
Inspect for excessive wear (sole wear, split in leather, holes etc.)	
Wear dry cotton or wool socks without elastic bands	
Wound Care	
Always follow prescribed treatment from your healthcare professional	
Insure that dressing always remain dry and clean	
Check for drainage of the wound into the sock or shoe; if this occurs, have dressing changed	
Take all prescribed medication and never alter the dosage without consulting your physician	

Date item understood or mastered by amputee is signified in the "Date Completed" column.

Figure 29–1 ■ Checklist for diabetic amputee limb care. For use in the clinical or home setting. (Adapted from Clark CR, Gailey RS: From One Step Ahead: An Integrated Approach to Lower Extremity Prosthetics and Amputee Rehabilitation. Course workbook. Advanced Rehabilitation Therapy Inc, 1998, with permission.)

tissue injury brought about by altered biomechanics. The overall gait pattern of the neuropathic diabetic is tentative as a result of feeling unsafe during standing and walking.[9] This conservative walking style is characteristically the product of poor proprioception, diminished sensory information, and an overall lack of stability resulting in a reduction of velocity and stride length with an altered displacement of forces.[55] Nonamputee diabetic subjects with peripheral neuropathy demonstrate alterations in foot biomechanics that could increase peak foot pressures, and facilitate foot injuries or ulceration.[39] In some cases, a shuffling gait is adopted that, while reducing peak foot pressures by distributing applied forces over a greater area, will cause increased fatigue from the inefficient gait pattern.[33]

Nonamputee diabetics with peripheral neuropathy have a high risk for developing plantar ulcers, and it is believed that most of these ulcers develop during walking.[5, 53] Fifty percent of diabetic nonamputees will also develop contralateral foot infections and possible amputation within 2 years.[17, 31] Therefore, the clinican working with a diabetic amputee must be alerted to the potential of complications that may arise with the nonamputated foot. The term "sound" limb can be very misleading. In fact, it is probably just a twist of fate that one foot became infected before the other and thus only a matter of time before problems begin to arise with the contralateral limb if the patient does not take extreme care. The odds are certainly working against them, especially if any other deformity is present as the amputee learns to use the prosthesis.

Because the diabetic amputee with neuropathy will often avoid full weight-bearing through the prosthesis, the contralateral limb must accept a greater proportion of body weight. Specifically, there is an increase of GRF at anatomic heel contact, comparatively decreased midstance time, with a rapid and significantly increased GRF during terminal stance as the foot rolls over the metatarsal heads.[36, 54] In the case where the great toe is amputated, as with so many diabetics, peak foot pressures become significantly higher under the first metatarsal head, lesser metatarsal heads, and toes.[44] Unfortunately, if not closely monitored, this can lead to ulceration and infection and possible amputation.

Serroussi demonstrated that the amputee's intact ankle at terminal stance works about 33% more than a normal ankle during terminal stance.[68] The increased work of the intact limb during terminal stance may be a compensatory mechanism for the lack of push-off by the prosthetic foot or might provide additional stability needed during double support as the prosthetic limb enters stance phase. Additionally, the intact limb has a significantly longer period of stance phase support than the prosthetic limb,[37] with greater hip extensor work during early stance,[36, 68] further compounding the forces placed on the plantar surface of the "sound" foot. Moreover, it has been shown that the loss of subtalar joint motion in the intact ankle can result in higher foot pressures and has the potential to lead to ulceration with the nonamputee diabetic.[15, 20] Consequently, it is important for clinicians to be aware that the increased work at the hip and ankle coupled with potentially limited ankle joint mobility of the sound limb can have a tremendous impact on the ground forces exerted on the plantar surface of the intact forefoot during the stance phase of gait.

Alterations in ambulation not only affect the soft tissues of the foot but also have an influence on the forces inherent to the sound limb joint articulations. Amputees experience a significantly greater incidence of osteoarthritis in the knee of the nonamputated leg.[34] Hungerford and Cockin compared the incidence of hip osteoporosis and joint space narrowing in addition to patellofemoral osteoarthritis in the nonamputated limb of three age-matched groups of World War II veterans.[34] He found an increased incidence of hip osteoporosis and joint space narrowing and that 63% of the TFAs, 41% of the TTAs, and 22% of the control group demonstrated positive findings for patellofemoral osteoarthritis on radiographs. Burke et al. reported that 52% of nonvascular TTAs had symptoms resulting from bony changes seen on radiographs from the nonamputated limb.[8]

Mussman et al. described the chief complaint in 55% of their subjects, primarily traumatic amputees, as a painful contralateral knee joint. Other complaints were fewer: foot pain (30%), ankle pain (28%), and hip pain (23%).[57] Separating TTA from TFA, the following percentages of subjects reporting joint pain in the contralateral limb were: TTA subjects: 29% hip, 46% knee, 29% ankle, and 29% foot; and TFA subjects: 19% hip, 75% knee, 38% ankle, and 38% foot.[57]

Lemaire attributed the significant increase in sound side knee osteoarthritis to the significant increase in horizontal and vertical forces being placed on the TTA knee during gait.[47] Even though the amputee subjects walked considerably slower than the control group, the joint reaction forces were markedly higher during weight acceptance. The combination of slower gait and increased forces may contribute to the early sound limb joint degeneration in lower limb amputees. In contrast, lower gait velocities in nonamputees result in reduced joint reaction forces.

The transfemoral amputee demonstrates additional variations in gait that, individually, may not have a critical impact, but collectively may influence the arthrokinematics of the sound limb. Jaegers supported Murray's work that double-limb support is longer when the intact limb is initiating stance phase.[36, 56] This asymmetry was reduced as walking speed increased, reaching what would be considered normal gait velocity.[36] In addition, the intact knee remained in a flexed position throughout the entire stance phase, never reaching the knee extension observed in nonamputee ambulators.[36] Also, Engsberg found that TTA children tended to cross midline with the sound limb.[19] Clinical observation with TTA and TFA adults finds that there is also a tendency for placement of the sound limb more towards midline during stance, rather than observing the typical 5- to 10-cm width of walking base. By maintaining the center of mass over the intact limb, the amputee may feel more confident, but consequently may be placing greater torsional forces on the joint surfaces from the excessive limb adduction.

The combination of additional vertical forces and shear stresses placed on the intact foot and the increased possibility of disproportionate weight-bearing can result in increased skin lesions, ulcers, and/or joint degeneration. Therefore, the goal of rehabilitation must include education and instructional measures designed to reduce risk of skin lesions or ulceration and the risk of additional degeneration of the sound limb.

The loss of a limb and the addition of a prosthetic device clearly have an impact on gait biomechanics in most diabetic amputees. There are substitutions from normal gait kinematics that increase vertical and shear forces in combination with preexisting abnormal sensation, devascularization, scar tissue, and any preexisting foot and/or ankle deformity. Collectively, this represents a dire situation not only for the limb but also for the patient's general health. This is apparent by the 50% increased incidence of amputation in the same or contralateral limb within 4 years after the primary amputation.[17, 40, 50, 76] Without hesitation, the patient should be made aware of the impending dangers from the onset of rehabilitation. Accordingly, foot care becomes even more critical after amputation for the diabetic amputee, especially since a high percentage will lose their contralateral limb within a few years and their chances of achieving functional ambulation as a bilateral amputee will decline.

Prosthetic Management

Prescription of prosthetic componentry has become a very complex and subjective topic. There are literally hundreds of combinations of components when considering suspension devices, socket designs, knee systems, and foot-ankle assemblies. Suspension methods have grown considerably from straps, cuffs, and simple suction to include pin-and-lock mechanisms, more complex suction approaches, and a wide variety of liner/suspension combinations. Socket designs have expanded tremendously over the past two decades to improve muscular function, suspension methods, and comfort. Knee units have become lighter, with improved durability and performance. Improved foot-ankle assemblies and lighter weight and more dynamic foot keels have permitted amputees greater mobility on varied terrain and improved performance during higher level activities. The addition of rotators, shock absorbers, and more versatile coupling systems have given more options and improved overall comfort and function to the finished prosthesis. The majority of these advances have been the result of incorporating a wider variety of materials into prosthetics. The ongoing prosthetic technology revolution was spawned by the demand of amputee clients who are no longer complacent in their acceptance of outdated technology and by the concerted effort of prosthetists and manufacturers worldwide.

To adequately cover the subject of prosthetic componentry with any kind of depth in this chapter would be almost impossible, while reducing the information to a general or most basic level would be an injustice to the developments within the profession. Currently, there are some excellent resources that explain in detail specific components, their design, and their function.[4] For this reason, the information presented will be directed toward those components that interface with the protection of the skin, the management of the residual limb, and prosthetic gait training designed to prevent further adversity of the residual and intact limb. The information discussed will be directed toward the diabetic/dysvascular amputee.

Some might argue that even though many advances have been made in prosthetics, the latest technology is focused on the younger, more active amputee and not the older diabetic/dysvascular amputee. However, the geriatric population has benefited tremendously from advancements first utilized by the younger traumatic amputee and as a result now enjoys more comfortable and better functioning prosthetic devices. Therefore, the prescription of newer prosthetic designs is, in many cases, just as appropriate for the older amputee as for their younger counterparts. The selection of more sophisticated components for senior amputees, however, must be solely on the basis of improved function.

Problem Detection/Skin Care

The socket should be cleaned daily to promote good hygiene and prevent deterioration of prosthetic materials. As a rule, laminate plastic, copolymer plastic, and silicone materials are cleaned with a mild soap on a damp cloth and foam materials are cleansed with rubbing alcohol. After using the cleaning agent, a clean damp cloth should be used to wipe away any residue. To ensure maximum life and safety of the prosthesis, patients are reminded that routine maintenance of their prosthesis should be performed by the prosthetist.

Every patient should be instructed to visually inspect the residual limb as well as the sound limb foot on a daily basis or after any strenuous activity. The residual limb is inspected to determine whether there are any abnormal pressures from the socket. Inspection of the sound limb has greater importance after amputation, since addition axial and shear forces, as described earlier, will be experienced by the foot in compensation for prosthetic weight-bearing adjustment. More frequent inspection of both limbs should be performed in the initial months of prosthetic training. A hand mirror may be used to view the posterior residual limb and plantar foot. Reddened areas should be monitored very closely as potential sites for abrasions. Amputees with visual impairment should seek the assistance of a family member for daily inspections. If a skin abrasion occurs, the amputee must understand that, in most cases, the prosthesis should not be worn until healing occurs. In some cases, a protective barrier may be used to avert further insult to the integrity of the tissue while permitting continued use of the prosthesis. In all cases, any lesion to the skin should be reported and followed clinically to avoid further complications.

With regard to the residual limb, the amputee must understand that the care of skin and scar tissue is extremely important to prevent breakdown during prosthetic rehabilitation. This practice becomes significant as the healing time is usually increased for the diabetic population and that the inability to wear the prosthesis secondary to skin healing will delay prosthetic rehabilitation and lead to further deconditioning. Therefore, the patient must be orientated to the proper fit of the socket and taught the difference between weight-bearing and pressure-sensitive areas.

Sock Regulation and Suspension Sleeve Use

Sock regulation is of extreme importance to prevent "pistoning" in the socket from occurring. The patient should carry extra socks at all times to add if pistoning occurs or for a change in case of extreme perspiration. A thin nylon sheath covering the residual limb will assist in reducing friction at the stump/socket interface. Stump socks are available in assorted plys or thickness, permitting the patient to obtain the desired fit within the socket. Socks should be applied wrinkle free with the seam horizontal and on the outside to prevent additional irritation to the skin. Many suppliers now offer seamless socks to eliminate this problem.

Recently, the use of silicone suspension sleeves and gel liners has gained widespread acceptance and use. Some of the benefits of suspension sleeves include reduced pistoning, better management of unstable limb volume, improved cosmesis and, in some cases, easier donning with impaired hand function.

Frequently, gel liners can be used as suspension devices in addition to reducing shear forces over scar areas and bony prominences.

Suspension sleeves and liners have not received universal acceptance, although the benefits appear to outweigh the negatives. A few reservations have surfaced concerning skin reaction and other unfavorable effects. Most of these concerns have been directed toward the types of materials used, since not all silicones and gels are medical grade, resulting in adverse reactions in some amputees. Fortunately, there are so many product lines available today that if problems do arise, the clinician is left with a wide variety of alternative materials to use. Another option is the use of a nylon sheath as a protective layer beneath the sleeve or liner.

Lake and Supan found through a survey of suspension sleeve users that the low to moderately active amputee and the older diabetic/dysvascular amputee reported a lower incidence of perspiration, heat rash, and folliculitis, with the latter also having less trouble with contact dermatitis and residual limb soreness. Although these results were not statistically significant, the differences were worth noting. One other interesting finding was that the longer the amputee used a silicone suspension sleeve, the greater the likelihood of dermatologic problems. In light of this study, silicone suction sleeves do offer the diabetic/dysvascular amputee a viable alternative to traditional suspension with less risk of problems than the younger traumatic amputee with longer prosthetic wear times.[41]

Physical Conditioning and Prosthetic Preparation

General Conditioning

Encouraging activity as soon as possible after amputation surgery helps speed recovery in several ways. First, it will offset the negative effects of immobility by promoting movement through the joints, muscle activity, and increased circulation. Second, the patient will begin to reestablish his or her independence, which may have been perceived as threatened due to the loss of limb. Finally, the psychological advantage derived from activity and independence will impact the motivational status of the patient throughout the rehabilitation process.

Often, decreased general conditioning and cardiovascular endurance are contributory factors leading to difficulties in learning functional activities, and prosthetic gait training. Regardless of age or present physical condition, a progressive general exercise prescription can be written for every patient beginning immediately after surgery, through the preprosthetic period to be continued as part of the daily routine.

The list of possible general strengthening/endurance exercise activities is vast: cuff weights in bed, dynamic stump exercises, wheelchair propulsion for a predetermined distance, ambulation with assistive device prior to the prosthesis, lower or upper limb ergometry, wheelchair aerobics, swimming, aquatic therapy, lower and upper body strengthening at the local fitness center, and any sport or recreational activity of interest. The amputee should select one or more of these activities and begin participation to tolerance, progressing to a minimum of 20 minutes to 60 minutes or more a day. The advantages of participation extend well beyond improving the chances of ambulating well with a prosthesis. The individual has the opportunity to experience and enjoy activities probably not thought possible. If difficulties are experienced, the amputee is still within an environment where assistance may be readily obtained either from the therapist or from a fellow amputee who has mastered a particular activity.

Prevention of decreased range of motion (ROM) and contractures is a major concern to all involved. Limited ROM can often result in difficulties with prosthetic fit, gait deviations, or the inability to ambulate with a prosthesis altogether. The best way to prevent loss of ROM is to remain active and ensure full ROM of affected joints. A daily stretching program can be of substantial benefit in preparation for prosthesis as well as general fitness.

Eisert first described dynamic stump exercises in 1954.[18] Since then, his antigravity exercises have been the most favorable method of strengthening the residual limb. Dynamic stump exercises require little in the way of equipment. A towel roll and step stool are all that are required. These exercises offer additional benefits aside from strengthening, such as desensitization, bed mobility, and joint ROM. Incorporating isometric contractions at the peak of the isotonic movement will help to maximize strength increases.[26]

All amputees should consider performing the abdominal and back extensor strengthening exercises with the intent to maintain trunk strength, decrease the possible risk of back pain, and assist in the reduction of gait deviations associated with the trunk. The strengthening of the trunk and pelvic musculature can best be achieved by stabilization or dynamic closed kinetic chain exercises performed with a Swiss ball or some other compliant surface in conjunction with other strengthening exercises.[27]

Amputees who have access to a health care or health club setting with isotonic equipment can take advantage of the benefits derived from these forms of strengthening with few modifications in patient positioning on the weight machines. The major advantage to participating at a supervised exercise facility is that the amputee is creating a healthy exercise habit. If introduced to the benefits of regular exercise during rehabilitation and continuation is integrated into lifelong practice, the secondary rewards achieved can reduce a variety of complications associated with inactivity.

Prosthetic Gait Training

The need to know the specific gait training protocol or treatments is probably not necessary for the majority of clinicians with the exception of the physical therapist. There is a need nonetheless for those on the rehabilitation team, primarily the physician and prosthetist, who are involved in assessing gait, to understand specific limitations or deviations that could have an adverse effect on the residual and sound limb. The following are selected alterations in gait commonly observed in amputees and their effect on the determinants of gait. If not attended to, there exists a greater opportunity for the amputee to fall short of reaching their full ambulatory potential, regardless of age, and potential experienced additional problems.

Standing Balance

After the loss of a limb, the decrease in body weight will alter the body's center of mass (COM). In order to maintain the single-limb balance necessary during stance without the prosthesis, ambulating with an assistive de-

vice or single-limb hopping, the amputee will shift the COM over the base of support (BOS), which will be the foot of the sound limb. However, the amputee must learn to maintain the COM and thus their body's weight equally over the prosthesis and sound limb to maintain the COM midline during bipedal standing and ambulation activities. Various methods of proprioceptive and visual feedback may be employed to promote the amputee's ability to optimize the displacement of the COM over the BOS. The amputee must learn to displace the COM in all directions in order to maintain balance during dynamic activities such as walking.

Furthermore, with the nonamputee neuropathic diabetic, Courtemanche illustrated nicely that a deterioration of the peripheral sensory system could produce gait and balance problems because of increasing attentional demands for the postural tasks.[12] The diabetic neuropathic patient feels less safe during standing and walking and as a result, fear of falling and the attendant lack of confidence alters postural control and gait behavior.[1, 71] The neuropathic amputee must be permitted early on in gait training to reorganize their postural strategies and to adapt to the prosthetic limb in a pseudostatic environment of standing prior to accepting the overwhelming dynamic act of walking. If prematurely forced into an insecure walking setting, the amputee's fear will frequently terminate progress and their true potential will never be reached.

Single-Limb Standing Balance

Weight acceptance onto the prosthesis is one of the most difficult challenges facing the amputee. Without the ability to maintain full single-limb weight-bearing and balance on the prosthesis for an adequate amount of time (0.5 second minimum) the amputee will exhibit a number of gait deviations, including (1) decreased stance time on the prosthetic side resulting in a faster step with intact limb that will strike the floor at an accelerated speed, thus increasing shear forces; (2) a shortened stride length on the sound side; or (3) lateral trunk bending over the prosthetic limb. More importantly for the vascular amputee, if their confidence increases in balancing over the prosthetic limb, the forces placed on the sound limb will decrease as the weight is shared between both limbs.

The amputee's ability to control sound limb advancement during walking is directly related to the ability to control prosthetic limb stance. The following are three contributing factors that may help the amputee achieve adequate balance over the prosthetic limb. The first is control of the musculature of the residual limb to maintain balance over the prosthesis. Second, the patient must learn to utilize the available sensation within the stump/socket interface, such as proprioception, in order to control the prosthesis. Likewise, the amputee must also begin to appreciate the amount of force or pressure that must be experienced at the residual limb/socket interface. For most the pressure is far greater than could ever be imagined. Third, the amputee must visualize the prosthetic foot and its relationship to the ground and therefore develop a sense of where their body weight is in relationship to the prosthetic foot.[26]

Gait Training Skills

Prosthetic developments in the last two decades have provided limbs that closely replicate the mechanics of the human leg. Therefore, the goal of gait training should be the restoration of function to the remaining joints of the amputated limb. Prosthetic gait training should not alter the amputee's gait mechanics for the prosthesis, but instead, the mechanics of the prosthesis should be designed around the amputee's individual gait.

For the majority of amputees, if pelvic and trunk movements can be returned to their premorbid level of function, the ability of the prosthetic limb to accomplish stability during the stance phase and advance naturally during the swing phase of gait should require very little effort. However, understanding the role of the pelvis and trunk in controlling COM over BOS and thus providing balance with functional movement patterns is essential.

The pelvis and the body's COM move as a unit in four directional manners: (1) vertical displacement, (2) lateral shift, (3) horizontal tilt, and (4) transverse rotation. Each of these motions can directly affect the amputee's gait; resulting in gait deviation with a concomitant rise in energy consumption during ambulation. If restoration of function to the remaining joints of the amputated limb is the goal of gait training, then the pelvic motions

play a decisive role in determining the final outcome of an individual's gait pattern.

Vertical Displacement

Vertical displacement is simply the rhythmic up-and-downward motion of the body's COM. The knee must flex 10 to 15 degrees during loading response,[61] and extension must be obtained during midstance. The TTA has the ability to flex and extend the knee during the stance phase of gait. The TFA unfortunately, is at a disadvantage, as the knee must remain in extension throughout the entire stance phase in order to avoid buckling or collapsing of the prosthetic knee.

Lateral Shift

Lateral shift occurs when the pelvis shifts from side to side approximately 5 cm. The amount of lateral shift is determined by the width of the BOS, which is 5 to 10 cm, depending on the height of the individual.[61] Because amputees have to spend an inordinate amount of time single-limb standing on the sound limb, such as when they are on crutches, hopping without the prosthesis, or during relaxed standing, amputees are adept at maintaining COM over the sound limb and therefore have a habit of crossing midline with the sound foot. Often, adequate space for the prosthetic limb to follow a natural line of progression is not available. The result is an abducted or circumducted gait with greater lateral displacement of the pelvis toward the prosthetic side. More frequently, this is observed in TFAs; however, this altered BOS may also be seen with TTAs.

The consequence of this deviation was discussed earlier; however, the importance of reducing the torsional forces to the joints of the limb must not be ignored. By simply reestablishing the position of the sound limb during initial contact and throughout the stance phase, improved balance with less stress to the limb can be achieved.

Horizontal Tilt

Horizontal tilt of the pelvis is normal up to 5 degrees. Typically, weak hip abductor musculature, specifically the gluteus medius, has been identified as the primary cause of excessive pelvic tilt. Maintenance of the residual femur in adduction via the socket theoretically places the gluteus medius at the optimal length-tension ratio. However, if the limb is in an abducted position in the socket, the muscle is placed in a compromised position, and is unable to function properly. The result is a compensatory Duchenne's gait, where the trunk leans laterally over the prosthetic limb in an attempt to maintain the body's center of mass over the base of support.

Some amputees, however, have long residual limbs and very strong abductor muscles, yet display the same gait pattern. As a result, an argument can be made that the bone length and loss of muscle may not be entirely responsible. In fact, another very significant deficit is the loss of mechanoreceptors or proprioceptors of the distal joints being the ankle and possibly the knee. The ankle strategies or the mechanism of continual movements of the neuromuscular system about the ankle that accommodates for sway assists in maintaining single-limb balance. The loss of the ankle and possibly the knee contribute to the additional loss of not only muscle but also joint proprioception, which is responsible for providing the necessary somatosensory feedback at a reflexive level. This phenomenon becomes apparent when comparing acquired to congenital amputees. Congenital amputees, especially bilateral amputees, have extremely good balance as compared to acquired amputees. This difference may not be the result of strength differences, but instead may be due to the superior somatosensory system of the congenital amputee as their joint proprioceptors gain this awareness throughout the neurodevelopmental process.

This is also evident through the observation that many TFAs walk with a slightly abducted gait with the prosthetic limb, using the prosthesis as a strut and thus decreasing the need for muscular effort to control the pelvis. Because the gluteus medius and minimus are intact, greater pelvic stability should be possible, since only the tensor fascia latae is lost in TFAs. However, many amputees of all levels have difficulty maintaining horizontal pelvic control. Therefore, effective gait training should include educating the hip musculature to function at a more rapid rate to control for sway. Moreover, for the neuropathic diabetic amputee who already has a significant loss of sensory feedback with the intact limb, this form of training undoubtedly has even greater significance.

Transverse Rotation

Transverse rotation of the pelvis occurs around the longitudinal axis approximately 5 to 10 degrees to either side.[61] This rotation assists in shifting the body's COM from one stance limb to the other, as well as providing adequate step length. In addition, it also helps to initiate the 30 degrees of knee flexion during toe-off, which is necessary to achieve 60 degrees of knee flexion during the acceleration phase of swing. Knee flexion during toe-off is created by other influences as well, including plantar flexion of the foot, horizontal tilt of the pelvis, and gravity. No prosthetic foot permits active plantar flexion, and since horizontal tilt greater than 5 degrees is abnormal, restoration of transverse rotation of the pelvis becomes of great importance in order to obtain sufficient knee flexion.

Another benefit to the restoration of pelvic rotation is the chance that the work and peak pressures produced by the contralateral ankle-foot could be reduced. For the insensate foot, prone to ulceration, this could be of great value not only in reducing pressures, but also in reducing the effort required to walk.

There are a wide variety of training techniques that may be utilized by the physical therapist to restore normal pelvic and lower limb biomechanics. Resistive gait training methods assist in facilitating appropriate movements, strength, and timing. Normalization of trunk, pelvic, and limb biomechanics should, however, be taught to the amputee in a systematic way. First, independent movements of the various joint and muscle groups are developed. Second, the independent movements are incorporated into functional movement patterns of the gait cycle. Finally, all component movement patterns are integrated to produce a smooth normalized gait.

Maintenance of equal stride length may not be immediately forthcoming, as many amputees have a tendency to take a longer step with the prosthetic limb than the sound limb.[36] When adequate weight-bearing through the prosthetic limb has been achieved, the amputee does have the ability to maintain equal stride length. One technique to promote equality in stride length is to have the amputee take longer steps with the sound limb and slightly shorter steps with the prosthetic limb. This principle also applies when increasing the cadence.

Normal cadence is considered to be 90 to 120 steps per minute, or 2.5 to 3.0 mph.[70] Arm swing, which is the result of trunk rotation in opposition to pelvic rotation, provides balance, momentum, and symmetry of gait, and is directly influenced by the speed of ambulation.[60] As speed of walking is increased, arm swing increases, thus permitting a more efficient gait. Amputees who walk at slower speeds will demonstrate a diminished arm swing, especially on the prosthetic side. Returning trunk rotation and arm swing is easily accomplished by utilizing a variety of gait training techniques such as manually guiding the trunk as the amputee ambulates.

Both amputees who will be independent ambulators and those who will require an assistive device can benefit to varying degrees from the above systematic rehabilitation program. Most patients can be progressed to the point of ambulating out of the parallel bars. At that time, the amputee must practice ambulating with the chosen assistive device, maintaining pelvic rotation, adequate BOS, equal stance time, and equal stride length, all of which can have a direct influence on the energy cost of walking. Trunk rotation will be absent with amputees utilizing a walker as an assistive device; however, those ambulating with crutches or a cane should be able to incorporate trunk rotation into their gait.

Considering the special needs of each individual patient, the therapist can design a customized program to meet the needs of each amputee. In many cases, the amputation may be only one of many comorbidities for which the patient is being treated. The clinician or patient must not internalize frustration for the delays in prosthetic rehabilitation as adequate time for treatment of the other more serious conditions is allowed. The amount of physical deconditioning that can occur during these times may be devastating. For this reason, the clinician must keep focused on the overall progress of the amputee and realize that the amputation may be a lifesaving procedure because of other anatomic system failures. Once the health status of the patient improves, then and only then can a successful prosthetic rehabilitation program begin.

Conclusion

It is important for the clinician to remember that age can influence the amputee's ability to ambulate with a prosthesis, just as age influences the gait of nonamputee ambulators. This is not to say that age alone dictates the amputee's capabilities. On the contrary, level of activity prior to amputation has a greater influence on the rehabilitation outcome than age, level of amputation, or number of limbs involved.[6, 10, 51, 58, 65, 74] Therefore, it is wrong to predetermine the outcome of the amputee based on the information presented in a chart. Motivation, character, and personality prior to amputation play a far greater role in determining the final result.

Since the diabetic/dysvascular amputee may have the same rehabilitation potential as the traumatic amputee of the same age, preconceived bias must be eliminated prior to the clinician's initial assessment. The key to improving quality of life and preventing further adversity is protecting the intact foot and limb by teaching the amputee to become reliant on the prosthetic limb. The rehabilitation team must stress the need for rehabilitation compliance and further emphasize the need for participation in follow-up foot and postamputation clinics and health care appointments. The process of prosthetic gait training must include the same gait principles taught to other amputees, recognizing that comorbidities associated with the diabetic patient may result in some delays during convalescence and will require additional variations in the treatment progression. The key to success with the diabetic amputee is teamwork, which includes a meaningful educational program for the patient and family. For, if diabetic amputees are willing to participate fully in their own rehabilitation program, the potential of once again being productive members of society will increase tremendously.

REFERENCES

1. Alexander NB: Postural control in older adults. J Am Geriatr Soc 42:93–108, 1994.
2. American Diabetes Association: 1991 fact sheet on diabetes. Alexandria, VA, 1991.
3. Armstrong DG, Lavery LA, Harkless LB, Van Houtum WH: Amputation and re-amputation of the diabetic foot. J Am Podiatr Med Assoc 87:255–259, 1997.
4. Bowker JH, Michael JW: Atlas of Limb Prosthetics, 2nd ed. St Louis: Mosby-Year Book, 1992.
5. Brand PW: The diabetic foot. In Ellenberg M, Rifkin H (eds): Diabetes Mellitus: Theory and Practice, 3rd ed. Hyde Park, NY: Medical Examination Publishing Co Inc, 1983, pp 829–849.
6. Brodzka WK, Thornhill HL, Zarapkar SE, et al: Long term function of persons with atherosclerotic

bilateral below-knee amputation living in the inner city. Arch Phys Med Rehabil 71:898–900, 1990.

7. Burgess EM: Immediate postsurgical prosthetic fitting: A system of amputee management. Phys Ther 51:139–143, 1971.

8. Burke MJ, Roman V, Wright V: Bone and joint changes in lower limb amputees. Ann Rheum Dis 37:252–254, 1978.

9. Cavanagh PR, Derr JA, Ulbrecht JS, et al: Problems with gait and posture in neuropathic patients with insulin dependent diabetes mellitus. Diabet Med 9:469–474, 1992.

10. Chan KM, Tan ES: Use of lower limb prosthesis among elderly amputees. Ann Acad Med 19:811–816, 1990.

11. Condie E, Jones D, Treweek S, Scott H: A one-year national survey of patients having a lower limb amputation. Physiotherapy 82:14–20, 1996.

12. Courtemanche R, Teasdale N, Boucher P, et al: Gait problems in diabetic neuropathic patients. Arch Phys Med Rehabil 77:849–855, 1996.

13. Czerniecki JM, Gitter A, Weaver K: Effect of alterations in prosthetic shank mass on the metabolic costs of ambulation in above-knee amputees. Am J Phys Med Rehabil 73:348–352, 1994.

14. Davis RW: Phantom sensation, phantom pain, and stump pain. Arch Phys Med Rehabil 74:79–91, 1993.

15. Delbridge L, Perry P, Marr S, et al: Limited joint mobility in the diabetic foot: Relationship to neuropathic ulceration. Diabet Med 5:333–337, 1988.

16. DuBow LL, Witt PL, Kadaba MP, et al: Oxygen consumption of elderly persons with bilateral below knee amputations: Ambulation vs. wheelchair propulsion. Arch Phys Med Rehabil 64:255–259, 1983.

17. Ecker ML, Jacobs BS: Lower extremity amputations in diabetic patients. Diabetes 19:189–195, 1970.

18. Eisert O, Tester OW: Dynamic stump for lower extremity amputees. Arch Phys Med Rehabil 33:695–704, 1954.

19. Engsberg JR, Lee AG, Patterson JL, Harder JA: External loading comparisons between able-bodied and below-knee amputee children during walking. Arch Phys Med Rehabil 72:657–661, 1991.

20. Fernando DJS, Masson EA, Veves A, Boulton AJM: Relationship of limited joint mobility to abnormal foot pressures and diabetic foot ulceration. Diabetes Care 14:8–11, 1991.

21. Fisher SV, Patterson RP: Energy cost of ambulation with crutches. Arch Phys Med Rehabil 62:250–256, 1981.

22. Gailey R, Lawrence D, Burditt C, et al: Comparison of metabolic cost during ambulation between the contoured adducted trochanteric-controlled alignment method and the quadrilateral socket. Prosthet Orthot Int 17:95–106, 1993.

23. Gailey R, Nash M, Atchley T, et al: The effects of prosthesis weight on metabolic cost of ambulation in nonvascular transtibial amputees. Prosthet Orthot Int 21:9–15, 1997.

24. Gailey RS: Recreational pursuits of elders with amputation. Top Geriatr Rehabil 8:39–58, 1992.

25. Gailey RS: One Step Ahead: An Integrated Approach to Lower Extremity Prosthetics and Amputee Rehabilitation. Miami: Advanced Rehabilitation Therapy, 1996.

26. Gailey RS, Gailey AM: Prosthetic Gait Training for Lower Extremity Amputees. Miami: Advanced Rehabilitation Therapy Inc, 1989.

27. Gailey RS, Gailey AM, Sandelbach SJ: Home Exercise Guide for Lower Extremity Amputees. Miami: Advanced Rehabilitation Therapy Inc, 1995.

28. Gailey RS, Wenger MA, Raya M, et al: Energy expenditure of transtibial amputees during ambulation at self-selected pace. Prosthet Orthot Int 18:84–91, 1994.

29. Gitter A, Czerniecki J, Meinders M: Effect of prosthetic mass on swing phase work during above-knee amputee ambulation. Am J Phys Med Rehabil 76:114–121, 1997.

30. Gitter A, Czerniecki J, Weaver K: A reassessment of center-of-mass dynamics as a determinate of the metabolic inefficiency of above-knee amputee ambulation. Am J Phys Med Rehabil 74:332–338, 1995.

31. Goldner MG: The fate of the second leg in the diabetic amputee. Diabetes 9:100, 1960.

32. Hoffman MD, Sheldahl LM, Buley KJ, Sandford PR: Physiological comparison of walking among bilateral above-knee amputee and able-bodied subjects, and a model to account for the differences in metabolic cost. Arch Phys Med Rehabil 78:385–392, 1997.

33. Hongshen Z, Wertsch JJ, Harris GF, et al: Foot pressure distribution during walking and shuffling. Arch Phys Med Rehabil 72:390–397, 1991.

34. Hungerford DS, Cockin J: Fate of the retained lower limb joints in Second World War amputees. Proceedings and Reports Univ Colleges, Council Associations 57-B:111, 1975.

35. Isakov E, Burdoragin N, Shenhav S, et al: Anatomic sites of foot lesions resulting in amputation among diabetics and non-diabetics. Am J Phys Med Rehabil 74:130–133, 1995.

36. Jaegers SMHJ, Arendzen JH, de Jongh HJ: Prosthetic gait of unilateral transfemoral amputees: A kinematic study. Arch Phys Med Rehabil 76:736–743, 1995.

37. Jaegers SMHJ, Arendzen JH, de Jongh HJ: An electromyographic study of the hip muscles of transfemoral amputees in walking. Clin Orthop 328:119–128, 1996.

38. Jensen TS, Krebs B, Nielsen J, Rasmussen P: Nonpainful phantom limb phenomena in amputees: Incidence, clinical characteristics and temporal course. Acta Neurol Scand 70:407–414, 1984.

39. Katoulis EC, Ebdon-Parry H, Vileikyte L, et al: Gait abnormalities in diabetic neuropathy. Diabetes Care 20:1904–1907, 1997.

40. Kucan JO, Robson MC: Diabetic foot infections: Fate of the contralateral foot. Plast Reconstr Surg 77:439–441, 1986.

41. Lake C, Supan TJ: The incidence of dermatological problems in the silicone suspension sleeve user. J Prosthet Orthot 9:97–104, 1997.

42. Larsson J, Agadh CD, Apelqvist J, Stenström A: Long term prognosis after healed amputation in patients with diabetes. Clin Orthop 350:149–157, 1998.

43. Lavery LA: Epidemiology and prevention of diabetic foot disease. In The High Risk Foot in Diabetes Mellitus. New York: Churchill Livingstone, 1991.

44. Lavery LA, Ashry HR, Van Houtum W: Variation in the incidence and proportion of diabetes-related amputations in minorities. Diabetes Care 19:48, 1996.

45. Lavery LA, Lavery DC, Quebedeax TL: Increased foot pressures after great toe amputation in diabetes. Diabetes Care 18:1460–1462, 1995.

46. Lehmann JF, Price R, Boswell-Bessette S, et al: Comprehensive analysis of energy storing prosthetic feet: Flex foot and Seattle foot versus standard SACH foot. Arch Phys Med Rehabil 74:1225–1231, 1993.

47. Lemaire ED, Fisher FR: Osteoarthritis and elderly amputee gait. Arch Phys Med Rehabil 75:1094–1099, 1994.

48. Malone JM, Snyder M, Anderson G, et al: Prevention of amputation by diabetic education. Am J Surg 158:520–523, 1989.

49. May BJ: Stump bandaging of the lower extremity amputee. Phys Ther 44:808, 1964.

50. McCollough NC, Jennings JJ, Sarmiento A: Bilateral below-the-knee amputation in patients over fifty years of age. J Bone Joint Surg 54:1217–1223, 1972.

51. Medhat A, Huber PM, Medhat MA: Factors that influence the level of activities in persons with lower extremity amputation. Rehabil Nurs 13:13–18, 1990.

52. Most RS, Sinnock P: The epidemiology of lower extremity amputations in diabetic individuals. Diabetes Care 6:87–91, 1983.

53. Mueller MJ, Diamond JE, Delitto A, Sinacore DR: Insensitivity, limited joint mobility, and plantar ulcers in patients with diabetes mellitus. Phys Ther 69:453–462, 1989.

54. Mueller MJ, Minor SD, Sahrmann SA, et al: Differences in gait characteristics of patients with diabetes and peripheral neuropathy compared with age-matched controls. Phys Ther 74:299–313, 1994.

55. Mueller MJ, Sinacore DR, Hoogstrate S, Daly L: Hip and ankle walking strategies: Effect on peak plantar pressures and implications for neuropathic ulceration. Arch Phys Med Rehabil 75:1196–1200, 1994.

56. Murray MP, Sepic SB, Gardner GM, Mollinger LA: Gait patterns of above-knee amputees using constant friction knee components. Bull Prosthet Res 17:35–45, 1980.

57. Mussman M, Twerger WA, Eisenstein J, et al: Contralateral lower extremity evaluation with a lower limb prosthesis. J Am Podiatr Assoc 73:344–346, 1983.

58. Nissen SJ, Newman WP: Factors influencing reintegration to normal living after amputation. Arch Phys Med Rehabil 73:548–551, 1992.

59. Pagliarulo MA, Waters R, Hislop HJ: Energy cost of walking of below-knee amputees having no vascular disease. Phys Ther 59:538–543, 1979.

60. Peizer E, Wright DW, Mason C: Human locomotion. Bull Prosthet Res 10:48–105, 1969.

61. Perry J: Gait Analysis: Normal and Pathological Function. Thorofare, NJ: Slack Inc., 1992.

62. Perry J, Shanfield S: Efficiency of dynamic elastic response prosthetic feet. J Rehabil Res Dev 30:137–143, 1993.

63. Pinzur MS, Gold J, Schwartz D, et al: Energy demands for walking in dysvascular amputees as a result of the level of amputation. Orthopedics 15:1033–1036, 1992.

64. Pinzur MS, Gottschalk F, Smith D, et al: Functional outcome of below-knee amputation in peripheral vascular insufficiency. A multi-center review. Clin Orthop 286:170–172, 1993.

65. Pinzur MS, Littooy F, Daniels J, et al: Multidisciplinary assessment and late function in dysvascular amputees. Clin Orthop 281:239–243, 1992.

66. Reiber GE: Diabetic foot care: Financial implications and practice guidelines. Diabetes Care 15(Suppl 1):29–31, 1992.

67. Sanders GT: Lower Limb Amputation: A Guide to Rehabilitation. Philadelphia: FA Davis, 1986.

68. Seroussi RE, Gitter A, Czerniecki JM, Weaver K: Mechanical work adaptations of above-knee amputee ambulation. Arch Phys Med Rehabil 77:1209–1214, 1996.

69. Sherman RA: Stump and phantom limb pain. Neurol Clin 7:249–264, 1989.

70. Smidt G (ed): Clinics in Physical Therapy: Gait in Rehabilitation. New York: Churchill Livingstone, 1990, p 312.

71. Tinetti ME, Powell L: Fear of falling and low self-efficacy: A case of dependence in elderly persons. J Gerontol 48(special issue):35–48, 1993.

72. U.S. Department of Health and Human Services. Vital and health statistics: Detail diagnosis and procedures. Hyattsville, MD: Public Health Service, Centers for Disease Control, National Center for Health Statistics, 1993.

73. Volpicelli LJ, Chambers RB, Wagner FW Jr: Ambulation levels of bilateral lower-extremity amputees. Analysis of one hundred and three cases. J Bone Joint Surg Am 65:599–605, 1983.

74. Walker CRC, Ingram MG, Hullen MG, et al: Lower limb amputation following injury: A survey of long-term functional outcome. Injury 25:387–392, 1994.

75. Waters RL, Perry J, Antonelli D, Hislop H: The energy cost of walking of amputees—influence of level amputation. J Bone Joint Surg 58(A):42–46, 1976.

76. Whitehouse FW, Jurgensen C, Block MA: The later life of the diabetic amputee: Another look at fate of the second leg. Diabetes 17:520–521, 1968.

77. Wu Y, Keagy RD, Krick HJ, et al: An innovative removable rigid dressing technique for below-the-knee amputation. J Bone Joint Surg 61:724–729, 1979.

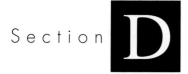

Section **D**

TEAM APPROACH

Chapter 30

ORGANIZING AN EDUCATION-BASED DIABETIC FOOT CLINIC

■ John H. Bowker and Nancy P. Wade

The number of diabetic persons is inexorably increasing. It is estimated that by 2025, there will be 250 million diabetics worldwide, compared to 120 million in 1996. With the onset of sensory neuropathy, the feet of many of these people will be at risk of ulceration. It has been found that foot ulcer precedes 85% of nontraumatic amputations in diabetics.[6, 9] Most significantly, it has been estimated that 75% of these amputations would have been prevented by early identification and education of those at risk of ulceration. Such a service can only be effectively supplied by a group of caregivers with complementary skills who can work in an interdisciplinary, proactive manner with "preventive rehabilitation" as their common goal. This approach is necessary if the current deplorable number of major lower limb amputations is to be reduced.

It is clear from the preceding that the need exists for education-based diabetic foot clinics in every community where diabetics reside. Unfortunately, even in the most developed areas, despite the presence of the personnel required to staff such clinics, diabetic foot care remains a fragmented process with little coordination and communication among caregivers. The standard "medical model," in which patients are seen at separate times and venues by various physicians, surgeons, podiatrists, nurses, and other caregivers, perpetuates this fragmented, ineffective, and costly care of the foot in diabetic patients. An education-based diabetic foot clinic, in contrast, can be designed to provide an integrated, thus inherently more cost-effective, approach to the management of these needy patients, by recognizing the fact that no one specialist possesses all the skills needed to prevent lower limb amputation. Funding for these clinics will vary among locales and countries (see Chapter 10).

The clinic does *not* have to be associated with a large regional or university hospital; successful programs can be organized in any community by a local group of interested health professionals. All that is necessary is recognition of the need and a willingness to apply well-known principles of care to these patients. Next, the team members should visit a well-established diabetic foot-care clinic as a group to see how it operates on a day-to-day basis.[1] If this is not feasible, one or more consultants from that clinic could be brought in to meet with the team members for formal and informal lectures and discussions. An excellent handbook for diabetic foot care, recently published by the International Working Group on the Diabetic Foot, is highly recommended for review prior to organizing a clinic.[5]*

Exactly how the clinic is organized and who staffs it can vary widely, as is amply demonstrated by the differing combinations of specialists who successfully run such programs throughout the world (see Chapter 10). What is important is that the clinic have certain basic programmatic elements and that the specialists most often required be in attendance at the clinic. Those needed less frequently should be available at short notice to provide their expertise as required. The clinic should meet regularly and frequently with provision for prompt, effective self-referral both during and after regular clinic hours. In short, for such a program to be effective, its services must be readily accessible.

Clinic Organization

The Team

The central figure on the team *must* be the patient together with responsible family members, domestic partners, or friends. Without their full cooperation in treatment, the team's work will be an exercise in futility. In most cases, an internist or surgeon will head the clinic team, with the choice often based on which person has the most interest and time available for this task. Inclusive of the team leader, a complete physician roster should include a diabetes physician, a foot-ankle surgeon, a vascular surgeon, a plastic surgeon, a rehabilitation physician, and a dermatologist. As noted above, not all physician members need to be present at all clinic meetings, but should be readily available for consultation. The nurse-educator, by virtue of possessing a complete overview of clinic function, can perform as an effective team coordinator in addition to her or his more traditional roles. Other essential nonphysician team members include the dietitian, podiatrist, pedorthist, orthotist, prosthetist, physical therapist, social worker, psychologist, and health administrator.

---

* Available from International Working Group on the Diabetic Foot. P. O. Box 9533, 1006 GA Amsterdam, The Netherlands.

Basic Organization

There are many possible ways to organize the day-to-day operations of an interdisciplinary diabetic foot clinic. One format that has worked well in a large inner-city county hospital for the authors will be described as *one* approach to managing a large number of patients. From its beginnings as a unified clinic in 1982, the program rapidly evolved into a two-tiered system, based on the acuity of the patient's foot condition. Our first-tier "full-team" clinic is held once each week for patients who, for a wide variety of social and economic reasons, present late with foot problems of high acuity. Patients with problems of lower acuity are seen initially and for follow-up in two clinics each week staffed by a miniteam consisting of a surgeon and nurse-educator with additional team members available as needed. Patients with acute events such as wet gangrene or sudden ischemic episodes are, of course, seen promptly in either clinic. Chronic ulcerative wounds are also seen as well as all postoperative wounds, usually by the operating surgeon.

The second-tier clinic, termed the patient-family education clinic (PFEC), provides long-term care for all stable patients and is managed by the same nurse-educator who attends the first-tier clinic. Patients are usually seen at bimonthly intervals in one of two meetings each week. The goal of this clinic is foot health maintenance by the provision of basic foot care and the prevention of initial or recurrent foot lesions through comprehensive education in self-care.[7, 11] The teaching involves both the patient and "family" members. The term "family" is used in its broadest sense and includes family members, domestic partners, and friends. In fact, the PFEC becomes an integral part of the diabetic patient's support network. We will now expand on the essential programmatic elements of a diabetic foot care program.

Essential Elements of the Acute Care (First-Tier) Program

Intake Evaluation

History

As in managing any other disease entity, a thorough, pertinent history will serve to enhance the subsequent examination and more effectively guide the care of the individual diabetic patient. While obtaining facts regarding other disease processes is essential to holistic management, the majority of the questions will be specific to diabetes mellitus. The replies given will allow the historian to assess both the patient's knowledge of diabetes and their level of involvement in self-care. The answers obtained to the following basic questions will often lead to further lines of questioning:

1. Time since onset of diabetes symptoms
2. Time since diagnosis of diabetes (often significantly less than time since onset of symptoms)
3. Type of medical practitioner seen
   Diabetes specialist
   General internist
   Family physician
   Surgeon
   Podiatrist
   Other
   None
4. Method of serum glucose management
   Diet only
   Oral agents only
   Oral agents and insulin
   Insulin only
   None
5. Schedule of serum glucose measurements
   Home (how often, what meter, meter average)
   Doctor's office
   None
6. Frequency and results of follow-up care for diabetes mellitus
   Glycohemoglobin measurements
   Eye examinations
   Kidney function tests
   Foot examinations
   Dietetic reviews
   Cholesterol
   Blood pressure
   Cardiac evaluations
7. Complications to date
   Eyes
   Kidneys
   Feet
   Cardiac problems
   Vascular problems
   Neuropathy
      Pain
      Numbness
      Sexual dysfunction
      Gastrointestinal/Bladder dysfunction
      Sudomotor disturbances
      Postural dizziness
8. Smoking history
   Current consumption
   Time of cessation
   Pack-years
9. Vocation/avocations
   Hours on feet/passive versus active
10. Type of footwear commonly used
   High-fashion shoes
   Walking shoes
   Sport shoes
   Work boots
   Sandals
   Slippers
   None
11. Footwear use
   At all times
   Outside house only
   Work only
   Rarely
12. Details of presenting foot complaint
   Time since onset
   Cause of problem
   Care to present

Foot Examination

It is essential that *both* feet be examined at *every* visit. Patients with profound neuropathy will frequently fail to note obvious abnormalities of one foot if the other foot happens to be of more immediate concern to them. To avoid missing any significant findings, the feet should be at a level readily accessible to the eyes and hands of the examiner. First, observe the overall conformation of the feet and ankles and note common deformities such as clawed toes with secondarily depressed metatarsal heads, bunions, bunionettes, and plantar, medial, or malleolar masses secondary to Charcot neuroarthropathy. Second, look for signs of acute and chronic shoe pressure over bony prominences, such as localized redness, hard corns or web-space soft corns, and ulcers, the latter two often associated with maceration and ulcer formation.

Third, check for signs of abnormal plantar weight distribution including calluses and/or ulcers under prominent metatarsal heads or midfoot and other bony masses secondary to Charcot neuroarthropathy. Areas of clinically significant callus formation will not be missed if the examiner lightly passes his or her hands over all foot surfaces. Because an ulcer may be partially or fully developed beneath a visually intact callus or corn, but not yet elevated by underlying fluid, corns and calluses should always be carefully shaved to assess this possibility. Ulcers can be visually deceiving in regard to their actual depth; therefore, they should always be probed to determine if they penetrate to the bone and/or joint beneath. This is most easily done with a sterile cotton-tipped applicator. If bone is felt, one may safely assume that osteitis or osteomyelitis is present.[4]

Fourth, one should look for signs of neuropathic changes specific to the feet. *Sensory* neuropathy results in the loss of protective sensation and is detected by application of the 10-gm Semmes-Weinstein filament to multiple sites on the foot (see Chapters 3 and 20). Vibratory sensation can be assessed with a 128-Hz tuning fork or a Biothesiometer. Joint proprioception can be tested at the level of the great toe, ankle, and knee. *Motor* neuropathy should also be sought, especially weakness of the ankle dorsiflexors as noted by manual resistance testing. *Autonomic* neuropathy results in dryness and fissuring of the skin and evidence of arteriovenous shunting in the feet. The latter can be deduced from the presence of dorsal vein engorgement persisting on elevation of the foot. We will now turn to the evaluation of a late but serious result of neuropathy. When a diabetic patient presents with a swollen, warm ankle or foot and shows no signs of systemic illness, the diagnosis of *Charcot neuroarthropathy* should always be seriously considered (see Chapter 21). Even if the initial radiographs are negative for fracture and/or dislocation, it is still the most likely diagnosis until disproved by serial radiographs. If the process appears to involve the foot, obtain initial anteroposterior, lateral, and oblique views of the foot, weight-bearing. Alternatively, if the ankle is affected, anteroposterior, lateral, and mortise views of the ankle, also weight-bearing, are appropriate. Management is discussed below.

Fifth, the examiner should check for loss of functional range of motion of the toe and ankle joints secondary to glycation of their capsules. Sixth, the arterial inflow to the feet should be evaluated. Lack of hair growth, coolness to touch, and dependent rubor of the feet followed by blanching on elevation should alert the examiner to the probability of arterial insufficiency. Although this can

often be confirmed quite easily by palpation for the dorsalis pedis, posterior tibial, popliteal, and femoral pulses, more quantitative testing may be required (see Chapter 16). Seventh, the feet should next be examined with the patient in the standing position, since their conformation can change remarkably on weight-bearing. The position of the toes should be observed for persistence of apparent clawing as well as height of the medial arch noting whether there is a very high arch (cavus), a normal arch, an absence of arch (planovalgus), or a reversed arch (rocker bottom). Plantar bony prominences can be easily documented in a semiquantitative manner for the patient record with a Harris mat imprint. Lastly, observe the patient walking away from, towards, and then back and forth in front of the examiner. Carefully note signs of ataxia related to poor proprioceptive function or a drop-foot or steppage gait secondary to weakness of the foot dorsiflexors. Careful correlation of the historical and examination data will allow the risk level for foot lesions to be estimated (see Chapter 20).

Shoe Examination

Evaluation of the patient's shoes is as much an integral part of the intake evaluation as examination of the foot, because of their intimate interrelation. By correlating the findings on foot examination with those of shoe evaluation, the causation of skin lesions is often made quite apparent. To begin, evaluate the design and fit, then note the materials (leather or plastic) from which the upper and counter are formed. Shake out the shoes to remove any foreign objects and then insert the hand into the toe box of the shoe to find any irregularities such as internally projecting seams, creases, or a torn or worn lining. The inserts should be removed and examined for impressions from plantar bony prominences. The wear patterns of the shoe can also be quite helpful. As examples, severe wear of the sole at the toe indicates a drop foot gait, while lateral shifting of the shoe upper and/or counter to the medial or lateral side, associated with abnormal wear of the sole may indicate major malalignment of the foot. It is essential to attempt correlation of any abnormalities of the shoes with deformities of the feet in order to correct stance and gait mechanisms leading to callus formation and ulceration.

Table 30–1 ■ BASIC EQUIPMENT NEEDED FOR A DIABETIC FOOT CLINIC

1. 1-, 10-, and 75-gm Semmes-Weinstein filaments
2. 128-Hz tuning fork
3. Glucometer
4. Nonsterile latex gloves
5. Nail clipper
6. #15 scalpels
7. Rongeurs
8. Thumb forceps
9. Surgical scissors
10. Small straight or curved hemostats
11. Orange sticks
12. Cotton-tipped applicators
13. 15-cm rule
14. Clear radiographic film and marker
15. Camera
16. Dressing materials
17. Bandage scissors
18. Weight-relief shoes
19. Casting materials
20. Brannock shoe-measuring device
21. Radiographic equipment (readily accessible)

If any skin breakdown has been noted during the examination, this should be carefully classified in regard to its depth and any signs of peripheral ischemia. Brodsky's classification (see Chapter 11) is quite complete and easy to use for this purpose. If a penetrating lesion is confined to the distal forefoot or to a specific toe, coned-down anteroposterior, lateral, and oblique radiographs of those areas will be the most useful. In determining a plan of treatment, bone scans are rarely needed. If the lesion is associated with significant ischemia, however, further testing may be deemed necessary by the team's vascular surgeon (see Chapter 16).

Clinic Management of Acute Foot Problems

As noted previously, care of wounds is an essential service provided by the acute care clinic. These include ulcers, debridement wounds, and partial foot amputations left open because of the severity of the infection. Treatment for ulcers which demonstrate adequate perfusion, are not infected, and do not involve bone consists of regular sharp debridement of overhanging callus and the use of total-contact casts or various other weight-relief devices or shoes (see Chapters 13 and 14 and Table 30–1). If accessible (i.e., not casted), the ulcers are dressed with moist

saline gauze changed two times daily. If the patient cannot comply with this program for any reason, a series of total-contact casts is recommended but only if the ulcer is Brodsky classification 1A. The cast is changed every 7 to 10 days for ulcer care and observation. If localized superficial infection is present, cultures should be taken and broad-spectrum antibiotics prescribed.

Wounds from major debridements or partial foot amputations are usually treated with twice-daily moist-to-dry normal saline gauze dressings to assist in wound debridement. If a joint capsule is exposed in the wound, however, a saline wet-to-wet technique is taught in which the intact outer bandage is moistened every 2 to 3 hours to prevent any drying of the wound between dressing changes. For home preparation of normal saline solution, see Table 30–2A. If the dressings show a greenish tinge, indicating *Pseudomonas* colonization, a ¼% acetic acid solution can be used for a few days only to suppress it. Use must be limited because its fibroblast toxicity exceeds its bactericidal activity.[8] For home preparation of ¼% acetic acid solution, see Table 30–2B. At times, a copiously draining wound may benefit from a few days of dry gauze dressings. As soon as the drainage is less copious, normal saline dressings can be started. The patient and/or family members are taught to change these dressings with clean, not sterile technique,

Table 30–2 ■ HOME PREPARATION OF WOUND DRESSING SOLUTIONS

A. Normal saline solution
1. Wash teaspoon, measuring cup, glass jar, and lid in warm, soapy water. Rinse well in hot water.
2. Boil a pot of water for 20 minutes and allow to cool.
3. Pour four cups of boiled water into jar.
4. Add two teaspoons of salt, cap, and store in refrigerator.
5. Make a new solution each week.

B. One-quarter percent (1/4%) acetic acid solution
1. Wash tablespoon, measuring cup, glass jar and lid in warm, soapy water. Rinse well in hot water.
2. Boil a pot of water for 20 minutes and allow to cool.
3. Pour five cups of boiled water into jar.
4. Add four tablespoons of white vinegar, cap and store in refrigerator.
5. Make a new solution each week.

thus keeping the cost reasonable without compromising the result. Patients are warned to avoid the use of hydrogen peroxide and iodine solutions, alcohol, or other home remedies, which have been shown to inhibit wound healing.[8] As in the case of ulcers, these wounds are also relieved of weight-bearing by the use of weight-relief orthoses or shoes, sometimes augmented with the external support of a walking frame. The progress of wound closure can be followed by photographs, measurements, or tracings on clear radiographic film from which the ulcer area can be measured, if desired. Reviewing the progress of healing with the patient can be helpful in securing compliance with wound care.

If healing is not proceeding as expected with regular reductions in wound volume, the reasons are sought. They may be physiologic, related to poor tissue oxygen perfusion secondary to peripheral vascular disease or anemia, poor nutrition, renal disease, chronic hyperglycemia, and/or persistent infection, possibly requiring surgical intervention. Behavioral factors affecting wound healing include failure to use weight-relief devices, chronic use of vasoconstrictors such as nicotine and caffeine, and noncompliance with overall diabetic management, based on denial, depression, or displaced locus of control or a combination of these.[2]

In managing acute Charcot neuroarthropathy, a total-contact cast is applied immediately after satisfactory radiography. Minimal weight-bearing with a walking frame to assist balance is allowed for essential walking with constant elevation of the foot while sitting. The initial cast will need to be changed in 1 week or less due to reduction in edema. Thereafter, cast changes are done every 3 weeks or whenever the cast loosens, becomes wet, or is otherwise damaged. Radiographs are taken every 6 weeks until the foot structure is deemed to be stable and clinical signs of inflammation such as localized excessive heat and swelling are totally gone. This interval may last up to 6 months, after which full weight-bearing in a cast is permitted. If there is no recurrence of inflammation over the next few weeks, a Charcot restraint orthotic walker (CROW) is fitted and used for up to 4 months. Thereafter, ready-made in-depth shoes with custom inserts and soles are fitted, unless the foot is grossly deformed. In this case, both shoes and inserts should be custom made. In regard to Charcot neuroarthropathy of the ankle, the authors have often seen patients with unstable ankle fracture-dislocations placed in an ankle-foot orthosis (AFO) and told to bear full weight. It should be noted that an AFO, no matter how well-fitted, cannot prevent an unstable ankle deformity from increasing with full weight-bearing nor can it reduce a fixed deformity. Since an ankle-foot orthosis utilizes a three-point pressure system, ulcers will inevitably occur. The end result is often amputation of the foot. For a discussion of the *surgical* management of Charcot neuroarthropathy, see Chapter 27.

The frequency of visits to the acute care clinic is determined by the progress of wound healing and can range from weekly to monthly. Once healing is complete, the patient is referred to the patient-family education clinic for long-term foot health maintenance. If a new lesion develops or an old one recurs, the patient is referred back to the acute clinic for management.

Essential Elements of the Chronic Care Program

There are several groups of patients who are referred to the patient-family education clinic for long-term care. The first consists of patients *without* foot lesions who have completed intake evaluation and have been fitted with protective shoes. Those with sensory neuropathy, bony deformities, and evidence of peripheral vascular disease are seen every 3 months. Patients with sensory neuropathy but no foot deformities are seen every 6 months, while those patients without sensory neuropathy, that is, essentially normal feet, will be seen yearly following thorough counseling on foot care and shoe wear. The second group are those whose wounds have either healed completely or to the point where they are expected to heal without further active intervention on the part of the surgeon. These patients are seen every 1 to 3 months, partially depending on their demonstrated level of compliance. The third group consists of diabetic amputees, many of whom have had a major unilateral amputation, but continue to be active walkers with a prosthesis. The remaining foot is often intact, but is at increased risk of amputation, thus requiring regular preventive care. In addition, patients can be referred directly from general medical clinics or from the emergency department for triage on days when the acute care clinics are not meeting.

The main goal of foot health maintenance is met in our patient-family education clinic by providing several specific services in addition to education. These include monitoring of foot condition by visual inspection and palpation, regular nail and callus trimming, careful shoe and insert inspection, and referral to the pedorthist for shoe repair or replacement as needed. Shoes and inserts are replaced on an annual basis for all patients who are legal residents regardless of funding status. Compliance with instruction from the doctors managing their diabetes and eyecare is also closely monitored with assistance provided for patients in obtaining referrals to the appropriate clinics.

One of the most important functions of the patient-family education clinic is the instruction of patients in specific preventive foot care measures. The style of instruction, including the terminology used, is tailored to the patient's ability to understand their disease. It is also very important that instruction given by all team members be consistent and repeated as often as necessary to ensure comprehension. Most importantly, patients are taught to *never* walk barefoot and to remove their shoes for visual examination of the feet twice daily, if necessary with a mirror. If retinopathy has reduced vision, family members are shown how to perform this essential task. At these times, the feet should also be palpated for areas of increased warmth, which may indicate inflammation from chronic trauma. Patients are encouraged to use their protective shoes at all times, changing them at midday if possible and alternating shoes daily. They are also taught to shake foreign bodies, such as small stones, out of their shoes before putting them on. Patients are also told to avoid thermal injury from home-heating sources such as floor furnace grids and fireplaces as well as from hot water bottles, heating pads, and hot baths. They are also informed of the dangers of direct exposure to solar radiation (sunburn) and to avoid walking directly on hot sand or paving at the beach or pool by wearing commercially available "water shoes." Contact with car heaters or transmission tunnels in older automobiles is also dangerous to the unwary on long motor trips. They are warned to limit outdoor exposure in cold climates to avoid frostbite to an insensate part. The de-

structive effect of salicylic acid–based callus removers is emphasized. Patients are encouraged to avoid any form of "home surgery" and instead to come in on a regular basis for nail and callus trimming. They are encouraged to take shorter, slower steps and avoid excessive walking to decrease chronic foot trauma, which can lead to tissue breakdown. The use of emollients to compensate for skin dryness is recommended, except between the toes. Vegetable shortening is recommended as an inexpensive, effective substance for this purpose. Many very helpful education booklets on diabetic foot care are provided free of charge by manufacturers of insulin and oral hypoglycemic agents for distribution to diabetic patients. They are very useful in reinforcing the team member's instructions and as a rapid home reference for the patient and family.

Among the chief reasons for poor patient compliance with even the most comprehensive clinic programs are the three "Ds": denial, depression, and displaced locus of control. The patient-family education clinic is the ideal place to address these issues in a gently repetitive, nonconfrontational manner. The result of this informal counseling should be the empowerment of the patient to assume responsibility for care of the feet as well as other aspects of his or her diabetic management. If the patient proves resistant, referral to the team psychologist may be appropriate. In the event a new or recurrent acute problem should arise, the patient is referred to the appropriate caregiver, most often the full clinic team, or if they will not be available in the near future, to the emergency department.

An additional feature of great value is the telephone "hotline." For assistance or advice outside of regular clinic hours, the patient is given a specific number to report foot problems. If the person receiving the call judges the situation to be urgent, the patient is referred immediately to the emergency department. Otherwise, the patient is given some simple instructions regarding care and told to come in the very next morning for further evaluation in whichever clinic is meeting that day. This method encourages the early reporting of foot problems and essentially avoids the dangerous delay in treatment that is common whenever patients without the benefit of pain use their own judgment in regard to when they will appear for treatment.

In summary, a well-organized diabetic foot clinic, providing consistent patient education as well as preventive and acute care for diabetic foot problems, can be expected to bring about a marked reduction in major lower limb amputation rates.[3, 10]

REFERENCES

1. Blair VP III, Drury DA: Starting the diabetic foot center. *In* Levin ME, O'Neal LW (eds): The Diabetic Foot, 4th ed. St. Louis: Mosby Year Book, 1988.
2. Bowker JH: An holistic approach to foot wound healing in diabetic persons with or without dysvascularity. Wounds 12(Suppl A):2000 (in press).
3. Edmonds M, Foster AVM: Diabetic foot clinic. *In* Levin ME, O'Neal LW, Bowker JH, (eds). The Diabetic Foot, 5th ed. St. Louis: Mosby Year Book, 1993.
4. Grayson JL, Gibbons GW, Balogh K et al: Probing to bone in infected pedal ulcers. A clinical sign of underlying osteomyelitis in diabetic patients. JAMA 273:721–723, 1995.
5. International Consensus on the Diabetic foot: International Working Group on the Diabetic Foot. Amsterdam, 1999.
6. Larsson J, Agardh C, Apelquist J, Stenstrom A: Long-term prognosis after healed amputations in patients with diabetes. Clin Orthop 350:149–158, 1998.
7. Lemerman RD, Wade NP: A rehabilitation clinic for the client and family. Rehabil Nurs 9:21–23, 1984.
8. Lineaweaver W, Howard R, Soucy D, et al: Topical antimicrobial toxicity. Arch Surg 120:267–270, 1985.
9. Pecoraro RE, Reiber GE, Burgess EM: Pathways to diabetic foot amputation: Basis for prevention. Diabetes Care 13:513–521, 1990.
10. Spraul M, Chamberlain E, Schmid M: Education of the patient, the diabetic foot clinic: A team approach. *In* Bakker K, Nieuwenhvijzen Kruseman AC (eds). The Diabetic Foot. Amsterdam: Excerpta Medica, 1991, pp 150–161.
11. Wade NP, Lemerman RD, Mastrionni EJ: Rehabilitation care and education: Practical guidelines for preparing the patient to function at home. Rehabil Nurs 5:32–34, 1983.

Chapter 31

LOWER LIMB SELF-MANAGEMENT EDUCATION

■ Linda B. Haas and Jessie H. Ahroni

The education of patients and health care professionals to reduce risk factors for lower limb morbidity and prevent limb loss is an important strategy in diabetes management. Appropriate diabetes self-management education and preventive care are believed to be able to reduce lower limb complications.[41, 43, 47, 49] This important knowledge must be transferred to patients with diabetes, since they are the only ones who can incorporate this knowledge into self-care behaviors. Clinicians who are convinced that foot care is a critical component of diabetes regimens can help patients change their attitudes, and ultimately their foot self-care behaviors.

Diabetes Education Effectiveness

Does diabetes self-management education improve outcomes? The Diabetes Control and Complications Trial (DCCT) showed that the experimental subjects, who had intensive diabetes education and treatment, were able to improve their glycemic control, and decrease the development of eye, kidney, and nerve complications by 50 to 75%, while maintaining a high quality of life.[56] This landmark study showed that intensive self-management education and management could change behavior and reduce morbidity. In addition, other studies have demonstrated the effectiveness of self-management education in diabetes management.[13, 16, 20, 28–30, 32]

Foot Care Education Effectiveness

Does diabetic foot care education lead to behavior changes that alter risk factors? Despite the longstanding role of foot care education in diabetes management, randomized controlled trials evaluating its effects are sparse. Barth et al. compared the results of a comprehensive program of foot care education with a conventional program.[8] This study found that an intensive foot care education program resulted in greater knowledge and compliance, and a lower frequency of foot problems in the experimental group compared to the conventional group.

Del Aguila et al.[18] documented that clinicians, when aware of patients' elevated risk for lower limb amputation, as evidenced by a history of a foot ulcer, were more likely to prescribe preventive foot care behaviors. The authors recommended that physicians, in addition to patients, receive periodic education and reinforcement to modify care delivered to individuals at high risk for lower limb complications.

In a randomized controlled trial, Litzelman et al.[43] showed that by educating a group of patients and a group of clinicians in proper foot care, there were reduced foot problems when compared with a group of patients and providers who were not equally educated. This research is remarkable in that patient, clinician, and systems interventions were examined in a 12-month multifaceted study.[43] The patient educational intervention was effective in increasing self-care activities such as bathing, and foot and shoe inspection, and eliminating soaking. The clinician educational intervention led to providers who were more likely to document pulses, dry or cracked skin, calluses, and ulcers. There were fewer minor and serious foot lesions in the intervention group, and these patients were three times more likely to report appropriate foot care behaviors and have foot exams during office visits.

Assal et al.[7] showed that education and training of patients with diabetes markedly decreased lower limb amputations: 12 times fewer above-knee amputations, reduction by half of below-knee amputations, and a four-fold decrease in toe amputations.

One study found a 78% long-term decrease in the incidence of major amputations following implementation of a multidisciplinary program for prevention, education, and treatment of diabetic foot ulcers.[42] A prospective, randomized, controlled trial[47] evaluated the influence of education on the incidence of lower limb complications in diabetes patients. Although there were no significant differences in medical management or risk factors between the two groups, the ulceration and amputation rates were three times higher in the group that did not receive the educational intervention.

Thus, it appears that diabetic foot care self-management education activities and programs can, and do, improve foot care behaviors and decrease lower limb morbidities.

Diabetes Foot Care Education

Foot care education is more than imparting information; the ultimate goal is behavior change.[38] For many patients, simply acquiring the appropriate knowledge will be enough for them to practice good foot care hygiene and select appropriate footwear. However, for others, the educational process will have to include assistance so patients can see and reach their feet, or identifying resources, such as family members, support systems, or community resources to assist in lower limb care.

Diabetes self-management foot care education must involve the person with diabetes in all phases of the education process.[5, 24] Doing so may alleviate some of the well-known difficulties with compliance.[24, 40] With mutual planning, the individual with diabetes is at least partially responsible for goal determination. Mutual goal determination is important because patients are ultimately responsible for implementing the indicated behavior changes. For persons with diabetes to assume the therapeutic role, they must have the knowledge they need and want. Clinicians can help patients see the need for this knowledge, promote motivation to learn about lower limb self-care, teach foot care self-management principles, and assist in identification of resources. Clinicians can also demonstrate the importance of foot care by examining patients' feet frequently and asking about self-care behaviors and problems.

Adult Education

Before delineating the aspects of foot care self-management education, it may be appropriate to review the principles of adult learning, as the majority of persons with diabetes are adults, particularly those with current or potential foot problems. These principles, which should be utilized in development of educational plans are that adults[4, 21]:

- *Assume responsibility for lifelong learning and continually learn and apply new concepts and skills.* The clinician can point out how new knowledge and skills can be applied and incorporated into patients' activities of daily living.
- *Build on previously acquired experience and knowledge.* Pointing out how adults have learned previous skills is helpful, and encourages them to apply prior successes to current challenges.
- *Have already formulated major life and learning goals.* An educational assessment can identify these goals. Then, family,

work, and leisure goals can be incorporated into the self-care management plan to create a "win/win" situation.

- *Translate new information into practical applications.* Adults are problem oriented, rather than theory oriented. Adult learners, for the most part, want to know how to use information. If an adult patient with diabetes is supposed to select shoes based on particular criteria, they want to know exactly what the criteria are, and how the task is best accomplished within their frame of reference.

- *Want to see a need for learning.* Adults want to know why they should make changes and how health care interventions will affect their everyday lives, and how to make the interventions work. Therefore, the educational focus should be on necessary knowledge, rather than academic facts that may be interesting but not necessary.

- *Critique new knowledge.* Adults will continually evaluate new knowledge in terms of who is making the recommendation, what they already know (or think they know), what others say (including friends and relatives), and what they are willing to do. This principle causes adults to pose the same question to several health care providers. Thus, to establish credibility, clinicians should be consistent in their information. When scientific evidence is not established, it is helpful to tell patients there is no one right answer to their question, but that several approaches may be acceptable. Then providers can help patients select the intervention that best fits their needs and lifestyles.

The Diabetes Self-Management Educational Process

Diabetes foot care education is an individualized, planned process that includes assessment, planning, the actual teaching, and evaluation.[4, 48, 52] It is more than handing out a preprinted foot care pamphlet.[21] It is a continuous process, determined by the physical, emotional, and social status of the patient, which is, in turn, determined by the educational assessment.[37]

Assessment

The principles of an educational assessment are similar to those of a physical assessment.

Determining educational readiness and the most efficacious educational approaches are the primary goals of educational assessment for a particular patient or group of patients.[4, 52] Areas to explore when doing an educational assessment of an adult include[37]:

- *Usual health practices.* Specifically for diabetes foot care, by asking questions such as, how, and how often they examine their feet, what types of footwear they use, where and how they buy their shoes, the amount and type of exercise they do, and type of shoes worn during exercise, clinicians can identify educational areas on which to focus.

- *Health beliefs.* It is important to assess whether patients believe they can make a difference in their health status and who they believe is responsible for their health (e.g., health care providers, their spouses [external control], a higher power, fate [chance control], or themselves [internal control]).[54] Knowing patients' health beliefs can help clinicians determine whether to use collaborative or authoritarian educational approaches.

- *Present knowledge level and abilities (especially problem-solving abilities).* Assessment for foot care self-management education should include patients' current knowledge of diabetes and its effect on the lower limbs, current foot care behaviors, beliefs, attitudes, and ability to solve problems.[57]

- *Attitudes toward health in general, and diabetes specifically.* Patients' feelings and concerns about their susceptibility to the consequences of diabetes should be explored, as well as any negative impacts of diabetes on their lives. Assessment should include whether patients believe that following recommendations can make a difference, and whether the benefits of self-care offset the personal and financial costs. Affirmative answers to these questions indicate that the patient will most likely be receptive to education. Negative answers, on the other hand, indicate that work that is more preliminary needs to be done. Often, clinicians will have to develop rapport with patients, to assist them to believe they can make a difference, and that what they do for their own self-care will be beneficial.

- *Functional status.* Employment status; independence in activities of daily living; visual, auditory, mobility, hand-eye coordination abilities; and tremors are important functional areas to assess. If there are difficulties in any of these areas, resources such as family, friends, or visiting nurses may need to be identified.

- *Cognitive ability.* Assessment should include patients' ability to understand and remember directions and any short-term memory loss or confusion.
- *Educational level.* Although educational level is not a surrogate measure for intelligence,[21] it often indicates the types of educational materials and approaches that might be most appropriate, and may be an indicator of reading level.
- *Literacy level.* Whether patients spend their time watching TV or videos, or reading and what types of material they read, and familiarity with computers can help determine if educational interventions should include video, written materials, or computer-assisted materials.

Identification of the Foot at Risk

Not all patients with diabetes need the same foot care self-management education. To be efficient with providers' and patients' time, it is reasonable to identify patients' risk for lower extremity morbidity. Self-management education for those at low risk can focus on preventive measures, whereas education for those at high risk will be more intensive. Screening refers to the application of a test, procedure, or examination to people who are asymptomatic in order to classify them regarding their likelihood of having a particular disease or outcome. The screening procedure itself does not diagnose the outcome, but indicates those who are at high risk. Thus, in addition to an educational assessment, patients should be screened to determine their risk for lower limb morbidity.

History

A study at the Veterans Affairs Puget Sound Health Care System, Seattle Division used two step-wise logistic regression models to identify risk factors to predict (1) lower limb ulceration and (2) amputation.[2] The five variables that predicted foot ulceration were:

- Sensory neuropathy (inability to perceive the 5.07 monofilament)

- History of amputation
- Absent toe vibration (128-Hz tuning fork)
- Insulin treatment
- History of ulceration

When all five variables are absent, the probability of foot ulceration was 0.05%. When all five of the variables are present, the probability of foot ulceration was 68% with a likelihood ratio of 11. This same study also identified five variables that predicted amputation, which were:

- History of foot ulceration or amputation
- Charcot foot
- Diabetes duration greater than 10 years
- Hammer or claw toes
- Self-reported nephropathy

When all five variables were absent, the probability of a lower limb amputation was 0.05%. When all five variables were present, the probability of an amputation was 84% with a likelihood ratio of 164.

Three predictors of foot ulceration (history of ulceration, amputation, and insulin treatment) and possibly all five of the above predictors for amputation can be obtained by questioning patients. Patients who have had a foot ulceration or amputation can be categorized as "high risk" and no further screening questions or examinations are necessary.

Physical Examination of the Foot

Patients understand the importance of diabetic foot care better when it is demonstrated by a provider who examines the feet carefully at least annually, and asks about foot problems at every visit. A standardized assessment form that lists the specific screening activities to be done, foot risk categories, and the recommended interventions facilitates implementation and documentation of this activity.

Along with questions about a history of foot ulceration, peripheral vascular disease, or amputation, a foot risk-screening visit includes questions about limb changes since the last visit, such as intermittent claudication and symptoms of neuropathy. The presence or absence of current foot ulceration should be recorded.

Since a foot inspection includes the tops, bottoms, and sides of each foot and between the toes, patients' abilities to do this self-care behavior should be assessed. A vision examination with a handheld or wall-mounted Snellen chart will give clues whether patients can see their feet well enough for a visual inspection. Vision worse than 20/40 in both eyes may be inadequate. If vision is poor, manual inspections may substitute for visual inspections. If visual or mobility impairment makes it difficult for patients to reach their feet, a mirror, magnifying glass, or magnifying mirror may be used. Alternatively, family members, neighbors, or other caregivers may need to assist with daily limb inspection.

Patients should demonstrate ability to reach their feet for foot care and manual inspection. Thomson showed that in three groups of elderly patients (mean age 76 years), two groups of whom had diabetes, only 14% could remove 0.5-cm red dots that had been placed on their plantar surfaces, over the first and fifth metatarsal heads.[56a]

Limited joint mobility has been shown to be associated with development of foot ulcers.[17] This lack of joint mobility may significantly limit patients' abilities to perform lower limb self-care. Other barriers can be obesity, with inability to see or reach feet, neuropathy (autonomic, motor, and sensory), peripheral vascular disease, homelessness, and presence of alcohol and drug abuse.

Environmental factors, such as occupation, financial resources, physical surroundings, and social support should be assessed, as these may impact patients' abilities to perform adequate lower limb hygiene.

Sensory Examination

In the clinical setting, sensory examination with a 5.07 monofilament is the single most practical measure of neuropathy.[33, 53, 55] After demonstrating the procedure in an area of intact sensation, such as the arm, the examiner should use the modified two alternative forced choice method[33] to test the most common sites of potential ulceration, the plantar surface of the great toe, and the first, third, and fifth metatarsal heads.[23] When the plastic wire bends to a C shape, 10 gm of pressure is being applied. Insensitivity is the inability to feel this monofilament at any site on either foot. The 5.07 monofilament is the best discriminator between those with protective sensation and those without.[19, 33, 53]

Peripheral Vascular Disease

A recent study showed that the probability of peripheral vascular disease (PVD) can be obtained from knowledge of patients' age, history of vascular disease, venous filling time, and palpation of lower limb pulses.[11] Palpation of the dorsalis pedis (DP) and posterior tibialis (PT) pulses should be recorded as present or absent. Determination of the ankle-arm index (AAI) should be made in patients without palpable pulses, or those otherwise suspected of having PVD.

Venous filling time is determined after identification of a prominent pedal vein. Examiners assist patients to elevate their legs to 45 degrees for 1 minute. Patients are then asked to sit up and hang their legs over the side of the examining table. The time in seconds until the veins bulge above the skin level is recorded. The time to reappearance of the veins can be recorded, or results can be classified as normal (≤20 seconds) or abnormal (>20 seconds).

Structural Deformities

Structural deformities include the presence or absence of prominent metatarsal heads; hammer or claw toes; Charcot foot deformity (collapse of the foot arch); bony prominences (exostosis); hallux valgus (bunion); hallux limitus (also called hallux rigidus, stiff great toe joint with limited range of motion); and corns and calluses. Corns and callused areas are signs of increased pressure.

Footwear

Shoes and socks should be examined to determine fit and condition.

Skin Abnormalities

Skin abnormalities include excessive dryness and macerated intertriginous areas indicating severe tinea pedis (athlete's foot fungus). Nail deformities such as fungal dystrophy (thickened and deformed toenails) or ingrown toenails should be noted. In addition, the way the nails are trimmed should be noted.

After the examination, the foot risk category is determined, and a plan for foot care education and annual foot exams is made for low-risk patients. High-risk patients will require more frequent foot exams by clinicians, and more detailed self-management education emphasizing daily inspection, protective footwear, and the need to report foot problems promptly.

Planning

Educational plans for adults are most effective when there is patient participation in the planning process.[24] The elements of an effective teaching plan for knowledge and skills acquisition include measurable behavioral objectives; selection of appropriate content; teaching materials and instructional methods; and a plan to evaluate learning and skills. The actual educational process should take place in a comfortable, well-lit, relaxed environment. When feasible, several short sessions, with each session focused on a specific topic, are more effective than one long session during which everything is covered.

The educational plan is developed with the principles of adult education in mind. Patients should be asked what they want to learn about diabetic foot care. It is reasonable for clinicians to set educational goals and objectives, but patients should be asked if the goals and objectives are acceptable. Providers need to be flexible and open to change. If the clinician's goal is to teach foot self-care according to guidelines, and the patient wants to learn how to select shoes for hiking, the session may be ineffective and lead to frustration for both teacher and learner.

Once goals are set, measurable objectives should be delineated, with the patient's input. Objectives can be related to any aspect of the management plan, but they must be specific, measurable, and time limited.[12, 44] For example, a goal may be to ensure that a patient with insensate feet who plans to start a walking program protects his/her feet. Objectives under that goal might be:

- The patient describes how to purchase and break in the appropriate shoes.
- The patient states the appropriate type of socks to wear.
- The patient identifies appropriate surfaces for a walking program.
- The patient demonstrates how to examine his/her feet after exercise and describes what reddened areas or blisters indicate.

- The patient has the name and telephone number of whom to call at the earliest sign of foot problems.

The plan must be feasible and achievable within a reasonable time. Although prevention of amputation is the ultimate goal of foot care self-management education, the educational session focuses on behaviors that lead to short term goals and objectives. The focus should be on keeping skin soft by application of emollients, or daily foot inspections, rather than never having a lower limb amputation. Written contracts may help patients adhere to the self-care process.[52]

When the behavioral objectives have been determined, the appropriate presentation methods are identified, since people learn in different ways.[48] Most people are visual learners; they learn best by seeing. These people will say "I see what you are saying." However, some people learn better by hearing and others by touching. People who learn best audibly may say things such as "I hear what you are saying," while kinesthetic learners use the word "feel" frequently. Thus, in a group situation, it is advisable to use different methods, such as lecture, slides, videos, demonstrations, return demonstrations, problem solving, handouts, repetition, and feedback.

Teaching Methodology

Teaching involves imparting information and ensuring that learners have acquired the required knowledge or skills and are able to apply these concepts. The teaching content is based on the identified objectives. Principles involved in teaching a skill, such as toenail trimming, involve determining and facilitating readiness to learn, modeling (demonstrating) the desired task, having active participation by patients (return demonstration), and giving feedback as to the appropriateness of the learners' techniques. When learning new psychomotor skills, people have better retention if the procedural steps are verbalized as they are performed. This can be evaluated in a return demonstration. The return demonstration should be repeated until safe behavior is demonstrated. Feedback enables patients to know how they are doing and is often motivating.

Repetition facilitates learning. Therefore, material should be repeated, preferably in different ways, or using different analogies or examples, to make the same point. Material should be presented in a positive manner, stressing what patients can do to protect their feet, rather than with a threatening attitude, stressing that if they do not do these things, they will lose a limb. It is important to repeat the most critical facts learners need to know at the end of the session.

Written Educational Materials

Written educational materials give patients tangible reminders of what to do to prevent lower limb problems, when to do it, and what to do if problems occur. The written educational materials should be appropriate in terms of ethnicity, age, and reading level for each patient.[9, 21, 22, 34, 61] Twenty percent of adults in the United States have reading skills below the fifth-grade level, and the average reading level in the United States is about eighth grade,[21, 22] although it may be even lower in the elderly.[48] Unfortunately, the majority of health education materials are written at higher than a ninth grade reading level.[22, 27] Therefore, a selection of patient education materials should be available for different patient groups. Illustrations in handouts or take-home materials should be of the type to which patients can relate. For example, written materials for patients with type 2 diabetes starting an exercise program should not use a picture of children playing at school recess as an illustration. To personalize the information, providers should review all handouts with patients and highlight principles to emphasize, or cross out irrelevant items. Patients need practical and realistic information provided with a "can do" attitude.

Teaching Content

There are several essentials of foot care self-management education for people with diabetes.

Inspection

Patients with neuropathy should be instructed how to perform daily visual or manual foot inspection. Patients without neuropathy will be likely to perceive injuries to their feet, but daily foot inspection is a good habit

for everyone with diabetes. It does not have to be a burden, but can consist of a brief examination of the feet in good light, when drying them after a shower or bath, when putting on socks or skin lotion, or before going to bed.

The feet and interdigital areas should be inspected daily. Patients should be instructed to look for cuts, blisters, bruises, and anything unusual. A magnifying glass, mirror, or magnifying mirror may be helpful. After the daily foot inspection has been explained and demonstrated, patients, families, or other care givers should perform a return demonstration, and verbalize what they will look for.

Daily Hygiene

Patients should be instructed to wash and dry their feet thoroughly, especially between the toes. Patients should be instructed to check the bath water temperature with their forearms, elbows, or a bath thermometer to prevent burns. Routine soaking is not recommended, as it may cause dry skin. Emollients such as lanolin or hand lotion should be applied to dry skin, but not between their toes, where the excess moisture may cause maceration. A strand of lamb's wool may be wound between the toes to separate overlapping or contacting toes and help prevent maceration.

Toenails. Patients should be instructed to cut or file their toenails keeping to the contour of the toe. All sharp or jagged edges should be smoothed with a file or emery board. If patients have poor vision or difficulty reaching their feet, other resources such as family members, nurses, or podiatrists should be identified to trim patients' toenails.

Self-Treatment of Abnormal Conditions

Patients should be instructed to never use chemicals, sharp instruments, or razor blades on their feet. Flaky fungal debris can be loosened with a soft nailbrush during regular bathing. Patients or family members should be instructed to gently buff corns or calluses with a pumice stone or towel after bathing, and to apply a moisturizer while the skin is damp, to help soften corns or calluses.

Foot Wear

Patients should be instructed to wear socks that do not have seams or holes, and should be instructed that socks with holes should be discarded, rather than mended. Patients with sweaty feet should be instructed to wear well-fitting soft cotton or wool socks that will absorb moisture and to avoid a warm, moist environment, in which fungus can thrive. Socks with extra padding may provide comfort and added protection for high-risk patients.[58]

Since the most common cause of foot trauma has been shown to be related to shoes,[10, 15, 35, 36, 49, 51] shoe selection and maintenance is a critical component of foot care self-management education. Patients should be instructed to purchase shoes in the middle of the day. Patients with sensory neuropathy should be instructed to have shoes fitted by a professional, if possible. If these patients must buy shoes "off the rack," the shapes of their feet can be traced on a piece of paper. Then, when buying shoes, patients can be sure that these shapes fit the shoes being purchased.

Patients should be instructed to wear athletic shoes[50] or oxford type shoes with adjustable vamps, made from leather or canvas. Instruction should also include that new shoes should fit well around the heel so the heel does not move around in the shoe, which can cause blisters. Patients should also be instructed that when purchasing new shoes, they should stand upright in them to be sure that the heel counter is firm and the ball width, the widest part of the shoe, corresponds to the metatarsal heads. Since manufacturers' sizes are only guidelines, and variable, patients with insensate feet should be instructed not to buy shoes by size alone.

Shoes must provide adequate toe room. Therefore, patients should learn that the adequacy of the toe box is related to the style of the shoe, rather than the size. They should wear shoes that have an adequate toe box, to accommodate their forefeet and toes, and yet fit well at the heel. Shoes with extra depth may be needed. The shoe length should be approximately $\frac{1}{2}$ inch longer than the longest toe. If claw or hammer toes are present, extra depth or custom shoes may be indicated. In addition, people with severe foot deformities may need custom molded footwear.[14, 15, 26, 60]

Energy-absorbing insoles can distribute weight-bearing forces equally over the plantar surfaces. Since Medicare will cover 80% of the cost of therapeutic shoes and orthotics for enrollees with Medicare Part B, the educational process may need to include assisting patients to access this benefit.[36]

Shoes should be broken in gradually, worn only 1 or 2 hours a day for the first week. Patients should be instructed to examine their feet after removing the shoes and to look for reddened areas, which may indicate increased pressure. Patients should also be instructed to alternate shoes during the day for pressure relief. If alternating shoes is not possible, they should remove their shoes for 10 to 15 minutes every 2 to 3 hours to limit repetitive local pressures.

Patients with any limb insensitivity should be instructed to examine their shoes before putting them on, and to feel inside the shoes for torn or loose linings, cracks, pebbles, nails or other objects, or irregularities that may irritate the skin. Patients should be instructed to develop the habit of shaking out their shoes before putting them on to find "lost" objects.

Patients with insensate feet should be instructed to never go barefoot (except in the shower or bed), in order to avoid trauma, puncture wounds, and burns from hot sand or pavement. Patients with diabetes and neuropathy should not apply external heat to their feet. If their feet are cold, socks can be worn to bed.

When to Seek Assistance

It is important that patients know, and can state, when, how, and whom to contact regarding limb problems. Patients should be instructed to report the following: any breaks in the skin or discoloration that does not begin healing after 2 to 3 days; swelling of the limbs; abnormal shapes; burns; frostbite; or obvious infection. Patients should be given a specific name and telephone number, or the telephone number of the emergency room or contact. They should be encouraged to call with any problems or concerns they have regarding their lower limbs.

Exercise

Exercise is an important modality in the management of diabetes. However, before beginning an exercise program, the patient with diabetes should undergo a medical evaluation to screen for the presence of conditions that may be worsened by exercise.[31] The medical history and physical examination should focus on the signs and symptoms of cardiovascular, cerebrovascular, and peripheral vascular disease, and peripheral sensory neuropathy. For patients planning to participate in low-intensity forms of exercise, such as walking, the clinician may use judgment in deciding whether diagnostic studies are necessary. The vast majority of people with diabetes in good metabolic control and without complications can participate in exercise if they are careful to avoid hypoglycemia during periods of increased activity.

A standard recommendation for all exercise sessions is to include proper warm-up and cool-down periods. A warm-up consists of 5 to 10 minutes of aerobic activity at a low-intensity level, followed by gently stretching for another 5 to 10 minutes. A cool-down period of another 5 to 10 minutes of low-intensity activity should follow the high-activity exercise period.[6]

Patients starting moderate to high-intensity exercise programs may need graded exercise testing, especially if they are elderly, have a long history of diabetes, have additional risk factors for cardiovascular disease, or have established complications of diabetes. Patients with known coronary artery disease should undergo a supervised evaluation of the ischemic response to exercise, ischemic threshold, and the propensity to arrhythmia during exercise.

Autonomic neuropathy may limit patients' exercise capacity and increase the risk of adverse cardiovascular events during exercise. Hypotension and hypertension after vigorous exercise are more likely to develop in patients with autonomic neuropathy, particularly when starting a new exercise program. Because these individuals may have difficulty with thermoregulation, they should avoid exercise in hot or cold environments and be vigilant about adequate hydration.[59]

When patients have active proliferative diabetic retinopathy, strenuous activity may precipitate vitreous hemorrhage or retinal detachment. These individuals should avoid anaerobic exercise and exercise that involves straining, jarring, or Valsalva-like maneuvers.[3]

Patients with peripheral arterial disease may self-limit their walking due to intermittent claudication. After an evaluation for lower limb blood flow, a supervised walking program may be recommended as a treatment for intermittent claudication.

Patients with peripheral neuropathy and loss of protective sensation to their feet should limit or avoid repetitive weight-bearing exercises such as jogging, prolonged walking, treadmills, and stair step exercises. Patients with sensory peripheral neuropathy must be cautioned to avoid hot sand and pavement around pools and sport courts. These surfaces can be too hot for neuropathic feet even when shoes are worn, if the shoes are thin soled like many sandals and moccasins.

The presence of an active foot ulcer is an absolute contraindication for weight-bearing exercise. Even patients who have a healed ulcer must take special precautions when exercising to prevent a recurrence. Special shoes and padded socks appropriate to the particular activity are important for injury prevention. Patients with healed ulcers or with severe foot deformities can participate in non–weight-bearing exercising such as swimming, bicycling, rowing, and upper body exercises.

In spite of these cautions, exercise programs are beneficial for patients with diabetes. Several long-term studies have demonstrated the positive effects of regular exercise on carbohydrate metabolism and insulin sensitivity. Exercise also has the potential to decrease cardiovascular risk factors and is associated with improvements in dyslipidemia, hypertension, and obesity.[1, 39, 45, 46]

Evaluation

Evaluation of the educational process is necessary to ensure that the goals and objectives were met. Providers and patients evaluate the education session and process by referring back to the goals and objectives.[4, 12, 37, 44] If met, praise and feedback are very encouraging for patients, and may encourage them to set and achieve further-reaching goals and objectives. If goals were not met, the feasibility of the objectives should be reassessed and another educational plan developed. Occasionally posttests are used to evaluate knowledge. If used, posttest questions should relate to the learning objectives. The most important evaluation relates to behavior change. These behaviors include that patients incorporate foot care management into their daily lives, practice good lower limb hygiene, and obtain and wear adequate footwear. Clinicians can question patients at subsequent visits to determine if they are changing their behaviors.

Another evaluation method is problem-solving questions. Patients can be asked what they would do in particular situations. For example, "What would you do if you notice a blister after your exercise?" or "What foot problems would you call me about?"

Conclusions

Most patients with diabetes are fearful of lower limb amputations, and sensitivity must be used to present accurate information to encourage behavior changes, but that avoid scaring the patient. The most important lower limb self-care concepts for patients to understand and incorporate into their diabetes self-management regimens are: proper foot inspection and care; selection and safe use of footwear; and when and how to contact a health care provider.

Teaching and learning about lower limb self-care are not easy tasks. Foot care self-management education is a complex, ongoing process. Every office visit should be an opportunity for self-management education. Families and support systems should be included whenever possible, since family and social support has been shown to increase adherence.[25, 62] Lower limb self-management education involves giving persons with diabetes the knowledge to make intelligent choices about their behavior, and the changes they can and will make to improve their chances of delaying or avoiding the devastating lower limb complications of diabetes.

REFERENCES

1. Agurs-Collins TA, Kumanyika SK, Ten Have TR, Adams-Campbell LL: A randomized controlled trial of weight reduction and exercise for diabetes management in older African-American subjects. Diabetes Care 20:1503, 1997.
2. Ahroni JH: The evaluation and development of diabetic foot risk stratification tools. In Health Services. Minneapolis, MN: Walden University, 1997, p 206.
3. Aiello L, Cavallerano J, Aiello LP, et al: Retinopathy. In Ruderman N, Devlin JT (eds): The Health Professional's Guide to Diabetes and Exercise. Alexandria, VA: American Diabetes Association, Inc, 1995, pp 143–151.
4. Anderson RM: Educational principles and strategies. In Peragallo-Dittko V (ed): A Core Curriculum for Diabetes Education. Chicago: The American Association of Diabetes Educators and the AADE Education and Research Foundation, 1993, pp 1–26.

5. Anderson RM, Genthner RW: A guide for assessing a patient's level of personal responsibility for diabetes management. Patient Educ Couns 16:269, 1990.
6. Armstrong JJ: A brief overview of diabetes mellitus and exercise. Diabetes Educ 17:175, 1991.
7. Assal JP, Peter-Riesch B, Vaucher J: The cost of training a diabetic patient: Effects on prevention of amputation. Diabetes Metab 19:491, 1993.
8. Barth R, Campbell L, Allen S, et al: Intensive education improves knowledge, compliance, and foot problems in type 2 diabetes. Diabet Med 8:111, 1991.
9. Bernier MJ, Yasko J: Designing and evaluating printed education materials: Model and instrument development. Patient Educ Couns 18:251, 1991.
10. Boulton AJM: Why bother educating the multidisciplinary team and the patient—the example of prevention of lower extremity amputation in diabetes. Patient Educ Couns 26:183, 1995.
11. Boyko EJ, Ahroni JH, Davignon D, et al: Diagnostic utility of the history and physical examination for peripheral vascular disease among patients with diabetes mellitus. J Clin Epidemiol 50:659, 1997.
12. Brink S, Siminerio L, Hinnen-Hentzen D, et al: Diabetes Education Goals. Alexandria, VA: American Diabetes Association, Inc, 1995.
13. Brown SA: Effects of educational interventions and outcomes in diabetic adults: A meta-analysis revisited. Patient Educ Couns 16:189, 1990.
14. Chantelau E, Haage P: An audit of cushioned diabetic footwear: Relation to patient compliance. Diabet Med 11:114, 1993.
15. Chantelau E, Kushner T, Spraul M: How effective is cushioned therapeutic footwear in protecting diabetic feet? A clinical study. Diabet Med 7:335, 1990.
16. Clement S: Diabetes self-management education: Technical review. Diabetes Care 18:1204, 1995.
17. Crausaz FM, Clavel S, Liniger C, et al: Additional factors associated with plantar ulcers in diabetic neuropathy. Diabet Med 5:771, 1988.
18. Del Aguila MA, Reiber GE, Koepsell TD: How does provider and patient awareness of high-risk status for lower-extremity amputation influence foot care practice? Diabetes Care 17:1050, 1994.
19. de Sonnaville JJ, Colly LP, Wijkel D, Heine RJ: The prevalence and determinants of foot ulceration in type II diabetic patients in a primary health care setting. Diabetes Res Clin Pract 35:149, 1997.
20. DeWeerdt I, Visser, Adriaan PH, et al: Determinants of active self-care behavior of insulin treated patients with diabetes: Implications for diabetes education. Soc Sci Med 30:605, 1990.
21. Doak CC, Doak LG, Root JH: Teaching Patients with Low Literacy Skills. Philadelphia: JB Lippincott, 1996.
22. Dollahite J, Thompson C, McNew R: Readability of printed sources of diet and health information. Patient Educ Couns 27:123, 1996.
23. Dorgan MB, Birke JA, Moretto JA, et al: Performing foot screening for diabetic patients. Am J Nurs 95:32, 1995.
24. Duchin S, Brown SA: Patients should participate in designing diabetes educational content. Patient Educ Couns 16:255, 1990.
25. Dunbar-Joseph J, Dwyer K, Dunning EJ: Compliance with antihypertensive regimen: A review of the research in the 1980s. Ann Behav Med 13:31, 1991.
26. Edmonds ME, Blundell MP, Morris ME, et al: Improved survival of the diabetic foot: The role of a

specialized foot clinic. Q J Med New Series 60:763, 1986.

27. Farrell-Miller P, Gentry P: How effective are your patient education materials? Guidelines for developing and evaluating written education materials. Diabetes Educ 15:418, 1989.

28. Franz MJ, Monk A, Barry B, et al: Effectiveness of medical nutrition therapy provided by dietitians in the management of non-insulin-dependent diabetes mellitus: A randomized, controlled clinical trial. J Am Dietet Assoc 95:1009, 1995.

29. Funnell MM, Haas LB: National standards for diabetes self-management education programs: Technical review. Diabetes Care 18:100, 1995.

30. Glasgow RE, Toobert DJ, Hampson SE, et al: Improving self-care among older patients with type II diabetes: The "Sixty something. . ." Study. Patient Educ Couns 19:61, 1992.

31. Gordon NF: The exercise prescription. In Ruderman N, Devlin JT (eds): The Health Professional's Guide to Diabetes and Exercise. Alexandria, VA: American Diabetes Association, Inc, 1995, pp 70–82.

32. Gruesser M, Bott U, Ellerman P, et al: Evaluation of a structured treatment and teaching program for non-insulin-treated type II diabetic outpatients in Germany after the nation-wide introduction of reimbursement policy for physicians. Diabetes Care 16:1268, 1993.

33. Holewski JJ, Stess RM, Graf PM, Grunfeld C: Aesthesiometry: Quantification of cutaneous pressure sensation in diabetic peripheral neuropathy. J Rehabil Res Dev 25:1, 1988.

34. Hosey GM, Freeman WL, Stracqualursi F, Gohdes D: Designing and evaluating diabetes education material for American Indians. Diabetes Educ 16:407, 1990.

35. Isakov E, Susak Z, Budoragin N, Mendelevich I: Self-injury resulting in amputation among vascular patients: A retrospective epidemiological study. Disabil Rehabil 14:78, 1992.

36. Janisse DJ: Commentary: Accessing the Therapeutic Shoe Bill. Diabetes Spectrum 8:214, 1995.

37. Joint Commission on the Accreditation of Healthcare Organizations: Educating Hospital Patients and Their Families: Examples of Compliance. Oakbrook Terrace, IL: Joint Commission on the Accreditation of Healthcare Organizations, 1996.

38. Kaplan RM: Behavior as the central outcome in health care. Am Psychol 45:1211, 1990.

39. Kaplan RM, Hartwell SL, Wilson DK, Wallace JP: Effects of diet and exercise interventions on control and quality of life in non-insulin-dependent diabetes mellitus. J Gen Intern Med 2:222, 1987.

40. Kaplan RM, Simon HJ: Compliance in medical care: Reconsideration of self-predictions. Ann Behav Med 12:66, 1990.

41. Kruger S, Guthrie D: Foot care: Knowledge retention and self-care practices. Diabetes Educ 18:487, 1992.

42. Larson J, Apelqvist J, Agardh CD, Stenstrom A: Decreasing incidence of major amputation in diabetic patients: A consequence of a multidisciplinary foot care team approach? Diabet Med 12:770, 1995.

43. Litzelman DK, Slemenda CW, Langefeld CD, et al: Reduction of lower extremity clinical abnormalities in patients with non-insulin-dependent diabetes mellitus: A randomized, controlled trial. Ann Intern Med 119:36, 1993.

44. Lorig K: Patient Education: A Practical Approach. Thousand Oaks, CA: Sage Publishers, Inc, 1996.

45. Manson JE, Spelsberg A: Reduction in risk of coronary heart disease and diabetes. In Ruderman N, Devlin JT (eds): The Health Professional's Guide to Diabetes and Exercise. Alexandria, VA: American Diabetes Association, Inc, 1995, pp 51–58.

46. McCargar LJ, Tauton J, Pare S: Benefits of exercise training for men with insulin-dependent diabetes mellitus. Diabetes Educ 17:179, 1991.

47. Malone JM, Snyder M, Anderson G, et al: Prevention of amputation by diabetic education. Am J Surg 158:520, 1989.

48. Moss VA: Assessing learning abilities, readiness for education. Semin Perioperative Nurs 3:113, 1994.

49. Pecoraro RE, Reiber GE, Burgess EM: Pathways to diabetic limb amputation: Basis for prevention, Diabetes Care 13:513, 1990.

50. Perry JE, Ulbrecht JS, Derr JA, Cavanagh PR: The use of running shoes to reduce plantar pressures in patients who have diabetes. J Bone Joint Surg 77A:1819, 1995.

51. Rausher H, Rausher SR, Friedman EA: Preserving feet in the uremic diabetic: The physician's role. J Diabetes Complications 1:145, 1988.

52. Redman BK: The Process of Patient Education. St. Louis: Mosby-Year Book, 1993.

53. Rith-Najarian SJ, Stolusky T, Gohdes DM: Identifying diabetic patients at high risk for lower-extremity amputation in a primary health care setting: A prospective evaluation of simple screening criteria. Diabetes Care 15:1386, 1992.

54. Ruzicki DA: Relationship of participation preference and health locus of control in diabetes education. Diabetes Care 7:372, 1984.

55. Skolnick AA: Foot care program for patients with leprosy also may prevent amputations in persons with diabetes. JAMA 267:2288, 1992.

56. The Diabetes Control and Complications Research Group: The effect of intensive treatment of diabetes on the development and progression of long-term complications in insulin-dependent diabetes mellitus. N Engl J Med 329:977, 1993.

56a. Thomson FJ, Masson EA: Can elderly diabetic patients co-operate with routine foot care? Age Ageing 21:333–337, 1992.

57. Toobert DJ, Glasgow RE: Problem solving and diabetes self-care. J Behav Med 14:71, 1991.

58. Veves A, Masson EA, Fernando DJS, Boulton AJM: Studies of experimental hosiery in diabetic neuropathic patients with high foot pressures. Diabet Med 7:324, 1990.

59. Vinik AI: Neuropathy. In Ruderman N, Devlin JT (eds): The Health Professional's Guide to Diabetes and Exercise. Alexandria, VA: American Diabetes Association, Inc, 1995, pp 182–197.

60. Ward AB: Footwear and orthoses for diabetic patients. Diabet Med 10:497, 1993.

61. Weinrich SP, Boyd M: Education in the elderly: Adapting and evaluating teaching tools. J Gerontol Nurs 18:15, 1992.

62. Zink MR, Gadomski M, O'Connell PB, Nizzi-Herzog M: Collaborative project to examine social support in elder homebound diabetics. J Home Health Care Pract 4:52, 1992.

Chapter 32

ROLE OF THE WOUND CARE NURSE

■ Dorothy B. Doughty

It is clear that optimal management of the diabetic foot is a complex challenge, involving preventive, interventional, and follow-up care; it is equally evident that the best approach to this multifaceted problem is a team approach that utilizes each member's unique knowledge, skills, and frame of reference. The benefits of the team approach and the specific roles and expertise of other health care professionals are addressed in separate chapters within this text; in this chapter, I will address the qualifications, skills, and role of the wound care nurse.

Qualifications of the Wound Care Nurse

The term "wound care nurse" is not an "official" (i.e., trademarked) title and can therefore be used by any nurse who "sees" herself or himself as a "wound specialist." The issue is further clouded by the fact that the title "nurse" is used to refer to professionals with significantly different educational backgrounds—including the licensed practical or licensed vocational nurse (LPN/LVN), who has graduated from a 12- to 18-month training program, the registered nurse (RN) (who may have graduated from a two-year associate degree nursing program, a 3-year di-

ploma program, or a 4-year baccalaureate program), and the "advanced practice" nurse (nurse practitioner). While all nursing education programs include *some* content related to wound care, it is typically procedurally focused, limited in both depth and scope, and sometimes out-of-date. This means that the title "nurse" does not signify preparation for complex wound care, though it does signify basic knowledge regarding the various disease processes that predispose to skin and tissue breakdown as well as skill in clean versus sterile technique, and in basic wound care procedures such as dressing changes and wound irrigations. All RN programs also include significant content related to holistic health care, factors impacting on patient and family compliance with established management plans, issues and strategies for effective patient and family education, and basic research principles.

While the title "nurse" is an "umbrella" term for practitioners with varied educational backgrounds, and the title "wound care nurse" can be self-assumed, there *are* titles and certifications that speak to knowledge and skill in the area of wound care. Formal education is available through certificate programs accredited by the Wound Ostomy Continence Nurses Society[9]; these programs provide intense theoretical instruction as well as clinical preceptorship, and graduation signifies demonstration of acceptable knowledge and skill in the area of wound care. These programs are available in a variety of formats; some are "wound care only" programs, while others provide wound care as a component of a program that also includes instruction in ostomy care and continence care. Programs are available in traditional, "split-option," and distance-learning formats. The traditional program is a 3- or 4-week-long program that involves at least 120 hours of classroom and clinical instruction. The split-option program is a variant of the traditional program in which the student comes to campus for the didactic instruction, and then completes the clinical preceptorship in her/his own area with approved qualified preceptors. The distance-learning program provides self-study modules for completion of the didactic component; testing is completed via proctored examinations. Following completion of the didactic portion, students complete the clinical requirement with a qualified preceptor. The core curriculum for these programs is guided by accreditation requirements[9]: all programs must demonstrate adequate scope and depth in the areas of anatomy and physiology; etiologic factors for skin breakdown (with a focus on elimination or amelioration of these etiologic factors); pathophysiology of chronic wounds (to include lower limb ulcerations and pressure ulcers); critical assessment factors and techniques (to include primary vascular and sensorimotor assessment for the individual with a lower limb ulceration); systemic factors affecting wound repair, with a strong emphasis on nutritional requirements for repair; principles and products for topical therapy; indications for adjunctive therapies (e.g., growth factors, electrical stimulation, hyperbaric oxygen therapy, and surgery); and current regulatory and reimbursement issues related to wound care. Many programs also include primary foot and nail care for the individual with a compromised lower extremity (e.g., patient with lower extremity arterial disease or diabetes mellitus). Some of these programs award graduate credits (the program is equivalent to a 2- or 3-semester-hour course), but all award certificates signifying successful completion of the program. Upon graduation, these nurses have earned the title "wound care nurse"; they are then eligible for the national certification examination provided by the Wound Ostomy

Continence Nursing Certification Board (WOCNCB).

In addition to these accredited certificate programs, there are a number of continuing education programs in the area of wound care; these programs are usually open to any nurse, regardless of educational background. The objectives and content vary, but all CE-approved programs have been reviewed and determined to be valid educational offerings. Many nurses who become interested in wound care attend multiple CE programs in wound care, and also subscribe to wound care journals, in order to strengthen their knowledge base regarding wound care.

For the nurse who has not completed a formal certificate program, certification programs provide the opportunity for documenting and validating their knowledge base. There are several pathways and two options for certification. One option for certification is the national certification exam administered and governed by the WOCNCB[11]; there are three pathways by which a nurse can attain eligibility for this examination. The first is by graduation from an accredited certificate program, the second is by satisfactory completion of graduate coursework in the area of wound care (documented by transcript), and the third is by documentation of at least 1 year of full-time experience in wound care, verified by a supervisor.[11] It must be emphasized that *eligibility* for certification can be acquired by any of these pathways; however, certification itself is dependent upon satisfactory completion of the certification exam. Upon satisfactory completion of the certification exam, the nurse has earned the credential of Certified Wound Care Nurse (CWCN) or Certified Wound Ostomy Continence Nurse (CWOCN); the title CWOCN is limited to nurses who have satisfied requirements for certification in all three of these areas. (Prior to June 1998, satisfactory completion of the certification exam in wound ostomy continence nursing earned the credential of CETN, i.e., certified in ET nursing. This title was changed to CWOCN in 1998 to more clearly reflect the areas of ET nursing expertise.) Certification obtained through the WOCNCB is valid for 5 years; at that time the certificant must recertify to maintain the credential. Recertification can be obtained by retesting or by documenting professional activities related to wound care that are indicative of current knowledge and practice.[11] There is a specific format to be followed and criteria to be addressed when recertifying by the "Professional Growth Points" program, and each portfolio is reviewed against the established criteria.

The second option for certification is through the American Academy of Wound Management (AAWM).[1] At this time, the AAWM offers three levels of certification: the diplomate level, the fellow level, and the clinical associates level. The diplomate certification is available to physicians, nurses, physical therapists, and other health care providers who are doctorally prepared and who have at least 2 years of experience in wound care, and the fellow level of certification is open to health care professionals who are master's-prepared and who have at least 2 years of experience in wound care. The third level of certification is the clinical associates level, which is open to registered nurses, certified physicians assistants, individuals with a baccalaureate degree, or other health care providers with extensive training and background in wound care; certificants must have 5 years of clinical or research experience in the field of wound care. Currently, certification is obtained through portfolio submission and review; AAWM plans to initiate testing as a requirement for certification in 1999. Professionals attaining board certification through the AAWM earn the title of certified wound specialist, or CSW. Contact information for the WOCNCB and AAWM is listed in Table 32–1.

In summary, a wound care nurse typically has at least a baccalaureate degree and has

Table 32–1 ■ ORGANIZATIONS OFFERING CERTIFICATION

America Academy of Wound Management
1720 Kennedy Causeway, Suite 109
North Bay Village, FL 33141
305-866-9592
fax: 305-868-0905
e-mail: woundnet@aol.com

Wound Ostomy Continence Nursing Certification
    Board
1550 S. Coast Highway, Suite 201
Laguna Beach, CA 92651
888-4-WOCNCB (496-2622)
fax: 714-376-3456
e-mail: www.\\.wocncb.org

validated her/his knowledge regarding wound care through satisfactory completion of an accredited certificate program and/or through satisfactory completion of the certification process.[10] The prospective employer would therefore be well advised to look for the specific titles that bespeak completion of formal training and/or validation of knowledge and skills through a certification process; if the individual being considered has completed no formal training and is not certified in wound care, the employer should certainly look beyond the individual's self-assumed title and ask for explanations regarding preparation and education for the role of wound care nurse.

Services Provided by the Wound Care Nurse

The wound care nurse can contribute significantly to the prevention and management of diabetic foot wounds; in some settings the wound care nurse has primary responsibility for screening assessment, preventive care, wound management, and initiation of referrals, while in other settings the role of wound care nurse is defined by the needs of the multidisciplinary team in addition to the knowledge and skills of the nurse.

Whatever the setting, the wound care nurse is prepared to provide the following services[5, 6, 9, 11]:

I. Comprehensive nursing assessment, to include:
   a. Vascular status (i.e., presence and quality of pulses; capillary refill; measurement of ankle-brachial index; inspection of skin, hair, and nails for ischemic changes)
   b. Sensorimotor status (i.e., response to monofilament testing; vibratory sense; position sense; range of motion; reflexes; gait; presence/absence of deformities; wear patterns in shoes and Harris mat testing)
   c. Autonomic function (i.e., hyperhidrosis or anhidrosis; Charcot deformity)
   d. Status of skin and nails (i.e., skin turgor and skin condition; hygiene status and hygiene routine; presence/absence of skin lesions, rashes, ulcers, corns, calluses; length, thickness, and color of nails; presence/absence

of hypertrophic or excessively long nails, deformed nails, encurvated nails, "ingrown" nails, infected nails)

e. Self-care status (i.e., understanding of diabetes, management plan, and preventive foot care; visual acuity; manual dexterity; ability to perform own foot care safely)

f. For patient with ulcer/lesion: etiologic factors (e.g., painless trauma, abnormal weight bearing, ischemia, prolonged pressure); ulcer characteristics (i.e., dimensions, depth, undermined or tunneled areas, status of wound bed/stage in wound healing process, status of surrounding tissue, status of wound edges, volume and character of exudate, indicators of infection); systemic factors impacting on healing process (e.g., perfusion, nutritional status, glucose control); behavioral factors impacting on healing process (e.g., patient and family understanding of etiologic factors for ulcer, potential seriousness of ulcer, potential for adverse outcomes/amputation, principles and specifics of management plan, ability to access and afford needed care; willingness and ability to comply with treatment plan); risk factors for further/recurrent injury.

II. Preventive foot and nail care, to include:
   a. Instruction in proper hygienic care
   b. Assessment of skin and nail status and risk for injury (as outlined above)
   c. Clipping of nails and debridement of hypertrophic nails with electric grinder
   d. Paring of corns and calluses
   e. Instruction in preventive foot care and proper footwear
   f. Referrals as indicated for complex foot conditions

III. Holistic management of patient with foot ulceration, to include:
   a. Correction of etiologic factors (i.e., instruction in principles and strategies for "offloading," with referrals as indicated for orthotics, contact casting or aircast application, or temporary wheelchair use; patient education re: strategies to prevent painless trauma; referrals as indicated for vascular assessment/revascularization; patient instruction regarding measures to maximize perfusion, to include smoking cessation)
   b. Systemic support measures (i.e., instruction in dietary modifications to maintain normoglycemia and provide the protein, calories, vitamins, and minerals required for healing; nutritionist referral as indicated)
   c. Appropriate topical therapy (i.e., selection of appropriate wound cleansing techniques and dressings/topical agents based on assessment of wound status and principles of moist wound healing; conservative sharp wound debridement when indicated and ordered by physician; $AgNO_3$ cauterization of hypertrophic granulation tissue or closed nonproliferative wound edges when indicated and ordered by physician)
   d. Initiation of referrals for adjunctive therapies when indicated (i.e., hyperbaric oxygen therapy, topical application of growth factors, electrical stimulation)
   e. Patient and family education regarding principles and procedures for wound care, expected outcomes, indications of adverse outcomes and appropriate response (prompt reporting), and follow-up care to prevent recurrence.

In addition to providing clinical services, the wound care nurse is prepared to educate other caregivers regarding etiologic/risk factors for breakdown, preventive strategies, and the principles and procedures involved in comprehensive wound management; education is provided through inservice programs, one-on-one interactions, and updated policies, procedures, protocols, and algorithms for care.[8] In order to promote optimal care, the wound care nurse must remain abreast of current research findings and product development in the area of wound care. In addition to serving as a research consumer and disseminator, the wound care nurse is prepared to contribute to the body of research by participating in clinical research studies.

The wound care nurse is also prepared to coordinate the various services needed to optimize wound healing and to prevent recurrence, and to interface with third-party payors to obtain appropriate reimbursement.

Role of the Wound Care Nurse

As noted above, the specific role of the wound care nurse varies according to the setting, as well as the availability and involvement of other health care professionals.[8, 10] In the acute care setting, the wound care nurse frequently has primary responsibility for topical therapy, and shared responsibility for correction of etiologic factors and provision of systemic support for wound healing. In the home health setting, the wound care nurse may function either as the primary nurse, or as a consultant to the primary nurse; in either case, the wound care nurse is responsible for providing or directing comprehensive assessment and holistic management, to include correction of etiologic factors, systemic support measures, appropriate topical therapy, and initiation of indicated referrals. In the outpatient setting, the wound care nurse typically functions as a member of a multidisciplinary team, with specific functions determined by the team member mix and needs.[7] Alternatively, the wound care nurse may function as the primary caregiver/coordinator in a nurse-managed clinic with medical oversight; in this case, the role of the wound care nurse is to provide primary care and to initiate and coordinate appropriate referrals.

In many settings, the wound care nurse is assuming the role of the case manager.[3] The wound care nurse is well equipped to assume this role, since she/he has a broad understanding of the care issues involved in both prevention and management of foot ulcers, is skilled in patient/family education and counseling, is familiar with the services provided by other team members, and is usually able to follow the patient through the various care settings (assuming compatibility with employment contract and demands). In addition, nurses have traditionally been responsible for coordinating the various services needed by patients and are therefore skilled in this role.

Benefits Provided by the Wound Care Nurse

The ability to improve outcomes and reduce costs is of critical importance in today's managed care environment; the wound care nurse is prepared to contribute significantly to each of these goals, and to assist with the development of "care maps" or "critical pathways" that standardize this outcomes-oriented approach to care. Specific ways in which wound care nurses impact on outcomes and costs include the following[3, 4, 7]:

1. Immediate establishment of a comprehensive management plan based on thorough assessment of the patient's care needs. Prompt establishment of a comprehensive management plan minimizes the time to healing (or reduces the risk of ulceration) and thus minimizes the associated costs.

2. Ongoing monitoring of progress in healing (or in maintenance of intact skin status), and prompt intervention whenever there is a lack of progress or a regression in wound status, or an increased risk of ulceration. This approach again minimizes the time to healing (or the risk of acute ulceration), which reduces the cost of care in addition to improving outcomes.

3. Appropriate referrals for further evaluation or adjunctive therapies. The wound care nurse can identify patients who require additional services and/or evaluation, which serves to maximize outcomes while ensuring appropriate resource utilization.

4. Cost-effective use of supplies. The wound care nurse is extremely knowledgeable with regard to the many products available for wound management; this permits her/him to select products for topical therapy that are therapeutically appropriate yet cost effective, taking into consideration the cost of the dressing, the frequency of dressing change, additional supplies required, and potential impact on time to healing.

5. Improved patient compliance resulting from a "team" approach in which the patient and family are recognized as team members who are integral to success of the management plan, and a strong emphasis on patient education and counseling. Wound care nurses are prepared to address psychosocial issues that interfere with patient compliance, and to initiate "patient-provider" contracts when indicated to promote compliance.

6. Communication with third-party payors to explain rationale for recommended therapies from both an outcomes and cost perspective, thus promoting reimbursement for appropriate care.

Studies in the home care setting have supported the value of the wound care nurse in management of chronic wounds; patients who were managed by wound care nurses had a significantly greater healing rate and a significantly lower cost of care, despite use of "more expensive" products.[2]

Summary

Management of the diabetic foot is a complex challenge that is most effectively handled by a multidisciplinary team. The wound care nurse is a critical component of this team; she/he is prepared to assist with preventive care as well as the effective management of the ulcerated foot. Specific services provided by the wound care nurse include comprehensive patient assessment; establishment of a holistic management plan; patient and caregiver education; dissemination of current research; coordination of needed services; and communication with third-party payors to optimize reimbursement. The importance of these services is underscored by studies documenting significantly higher healing rates and reduced care costs when a wound care nurse is involved in the care of patients with chronic wounds.

REFERENCES

1. American Academy of Wound Management: Certification and Membership Information. North Bay Village, FL: AAWM, 1997.
2. Arnold N, Weir R: Retrospective analysis of healing in wounds cared for by ET nurses versus staff nurses in a home setting. J Wound Ostomy Continence Nurs 21:156–160, 1994.
3. Blaylock B, Murray M: Case management: A new practice model for ET nurses. J Wound Ostomy Continence Nursing 23:66–72, 1996.
4. Gartner M, Twardon C: Care guidelines: Journey through the managed care maze. J Wound Ostomy Continence Nursing 22:118–121, 1995.
5. Gordon B: Conservative sharp wound debridement: State Boards of Nursing positions. J Wound Ostomy Continence Nurs 23:137–143, 1996.
6. Kelechi T, Lukacs K: Foot Care Course Syllabus. Charleston, SC: Medical University of South Carolina, 1995.
7. Ratliff C, Rodeheaver G: The chronic wound care clinic: "One-stop shopping." J Wound Ostomy Continence Nurs 22:77–80, 1995.
8. Robinson SM: Advancing home care nursing practice with an ET clinical nurse specialist. Home Healthcare Nurse 14:269–274, 1996.
9. Wound Ostomy Continence Nurses Society: Accreditation Policy and Procedure Manual. Laguna Beach, CA: ADI, 1997.
10. Wound Ostomy Continence Nurses Society: Position statement: Wound care nurse specialist. Laguna Beach, CA: ADI, 1997.
11. Wound Ostomy Continence Nursing Certification Board. Candidate Handbook. Laguna Beach, CA: ADI, 1997.

Chapter 33

ROLE OF THE PODIATRIST

■ Lawrence B. Harkless, V. Kathleen Satterfield, and Kenrick J. Dennis

Just as the endocrinologist orchestrates a symphony of metabolic and systemic interactions, the podiatrist serves a similar role for mechanical and metabolic conditions affecting the foot. Periodic professional foot care serves a fundamental role in diabetic preventive care (Fig. 33–1). Today, it is not enough to simply educate the diabetic patient and their family. Routine evaluation and management is the key to success.

Diabetes is a complex disease process involving much more than the metabolism of glucose. As evidenced by this text, it involves many organ systems including dermatologic, renal, neurologic, cardiovascular, ocular, gastrointestinal, urinary, musculoskeletal, and immunologic systems. This complex process requires the attention of various medical specialties and is often manifested as pathology of the lower extremity. Ongoing education, aggressive follow-up, and thorough evaluation are all vital elements in reducing the morbidity and mortality from diabetic lower extremity limb infections.[18]

There are an estimated 200 million diabetics worldwide, and diabetes affects 2.4 to 5% of the American population. Diabetes in all forms is the leading cause of new blindness and the third leading cause of death in the United States.[18, 28] Diabetes remains the leading cause of atraumatic amputations in the United States.[26, 31] In 1991, 54,000 people had at least one amputation during the year at an average cost of \$33,444 and an average hospital stay of 23 days.[10] The number of hospital days as well as the costs to the health care system are well documented.[24] Boulton in 1988 noted that 50% of atraumatic amputations in the United States are on diabetic patients.[8] It is obvious that diabetic limb infections have both a monetary and human cost. As members of the health care team, we have significantly impacted these statistics. In recent studies utilizing vascular surgery and foot care specialists, these joint clinical efforts resulted in an 85% limb salvage rate.[3, 12, 33, 34] However, as a team, we will continue to strive for increased quality of life.

Since the initial publication of this text, the importance of foot care has become a major issue in diabetic care. In fact, position statements have now been issued by the American Diabetes Association (ADA) which include, "Patients with a history of foot lesions, especially those with prior amputation, require preventive foot care and lifelong surveillance, preferably by a foot care specialist."[2] This is an incredibly strong statement; these patients "require" professional care. It is not fair to the patient, their family, or to the other members of the health care team to teach foot care and then send the

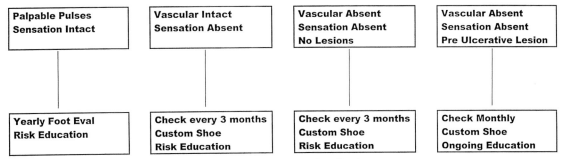

Palpable Pulses Sensation Intact	Vascular Intact Sensation Absent	Vascular Absent Sensation Absent No Lesions	Vascular Absent Sensation Absent Pre Ulcerative Lesion
Yearly Foot Eval Risk Education	Check every 3 months Custom Shoe Risk Education	Check every 3 months Custom Shoe Risk Education	Check Monthly Custom Shoe Ongoing Education

Figure 33–1 ■ Frequency of podiatric care.

patient home only to return when the inevitable tissue breakdown occurs. Today we must partner with our patients to provide those things that loss of sensation, poor vision, and immunocompromise have robbed them of. The second half of the position statement implores lifelong surveillance. This pathology will not go away by looking the other way, but with open eyes and a realistic vision of the job at hand, outcomes may be improved.

This is not meant to imply that the podiatrist is the only member of the health care team capable of providing such service. On the contrary, orthopedists, wound care specialists, and physicians all have the facility and expertise to provide comprehensive care. But the podiatric visit continues to represent an optimum time to focus on the pedal manifestations of disease. As patients are referred for these encounters it is hoped that the patient's experience will be one of regular preventative care rather than of emergency interventional care. Harrington in an analysis of diabetic foot ulcers using Medicare claims data for 1995–96 found that 70% of patients had treatment with little or no follow-up.[15]

More and more multidisciplinary centers have developed in order to provide comprehensive service for the patient with diabetes. There is no doubt that this approach provides impact on major foot complications.[12, 19, 25, 33] The team approach has been in place for many years. It continues to develop and mature, becoming more sophisticated and sensitive to the needs of the patient. There are obviously many factors that play a role in diminishing amputation rate, but patient education and responsibility play a significant role. Armstrong et al.[4] encouraged a positive approach for referrals to multidisciplinary

foot-care teams for a more multifactorial, long-term treatment and management plan for the patient.

History

When evaluating the patient with diabetes, specific questions about vascular disease should be asked:

1. Where is the patient along the risk spectrum of vascular disease?
2. Do they have mild, moderate or severe disease?
3. What evidence is there to support the disease spectrum by history and examination?

Specific questions will help to assess the patient's risk spectrum.

1. Macrovascular disease: Is there a history of coronary artery disease or stroke?
2. Microvascular disease: Is there a history of retinopathy, nephropathy or neuropathy? Has the patient been followed for these conditions? Also, has the patient had laser surgery? A history of laser surgery is indicative of proliferative retinopathy. This indicates development of advanced microcirculation disease. If they have disease in the eyes, they will have the same disease evident in their lower extremity. It is not imperative that they have symptoms.
3. Functional microcirculation: Does the patient have a history of gastroparesis or impotence? The autonomic nervous system controls the body's blood flow and these symptoms are related to autonomic

neuropathy. A depletion of nitric oxide, a condition prevalent in patients with long-standing diabetes, causes impairment of the smooth muscle vasodilation. This, in turn, leads to endothelial cell damage along with capillary leakage with resultant difficulty in wound healing.[27]

4. Insulin resistance syndrome: Does the patient have a history of dyslipidemia (i.e., elevated lipids and cholesterol)? Is there a history of glucose intolerance or insulin resistance? A history of obesity, central adiposity, hypertension, or smoking is also an indicator.

5. Family history: Is there a familial history of diabetes? Did any of the family members have renal dysfunction or lower extremity amputations? In the family with a history of diabetes with microvascular complications there is the likelihood of the patient having similar problems due to a genetic predisposition.

6. Duration of diabetes: Vascular complications are directly related to the duration of diabetes with poor control.

We have found that when patients with a history of diabetes over 10 years have eight of these particular questions positive, they usually have moderate disease along the vascular risk spectrum. Moreover, if they have signs and symptoms of vascular disease in the foot and leg, this denotes a more severe risk spectrum.

Examination

The intimate relationship of neuropathy and vascular disease[7] forms the foundation for future diabetic foot complications (Fig. 33–2). By recognizing early signs of diabetic peripheral neuropathy, such as plantar xerosis, contracture of the toes with associated corns and calluses, and then understanding the predictive nature of these clinical findings, simple education and home care may be implemented. From Figure 33–2, it is easy to see how early neurotrophic changes might easily participate with vascular changes yielding catastrophic results.

The ability to notice subtle pathology and correlate these pathologic changes with long-term prognosis is critical to reducing the morbidity associated with longstanding diabetes.[16] Various clinical factors along with the clinical presentation help identify increased risk for disease (Fig. 33–3). The history should include the patient's last physical exam and relevant findings, duration of diabetes, medication and allergic history, surgical history, and any history of slow healing or recovery. Additional risk factors to assess are smoking, subjective cold, burning or numb feet, previous infection or amputation, and average blood sugar monitoring at home. Asking the patient how they take care of their feet can also give clues to future prob-

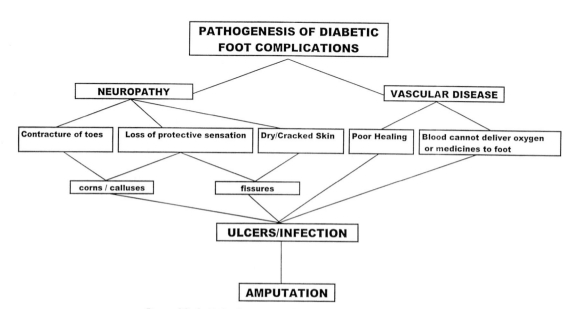

Figure 33–2 ▪ Pathogenesis of diabetic foot complications.

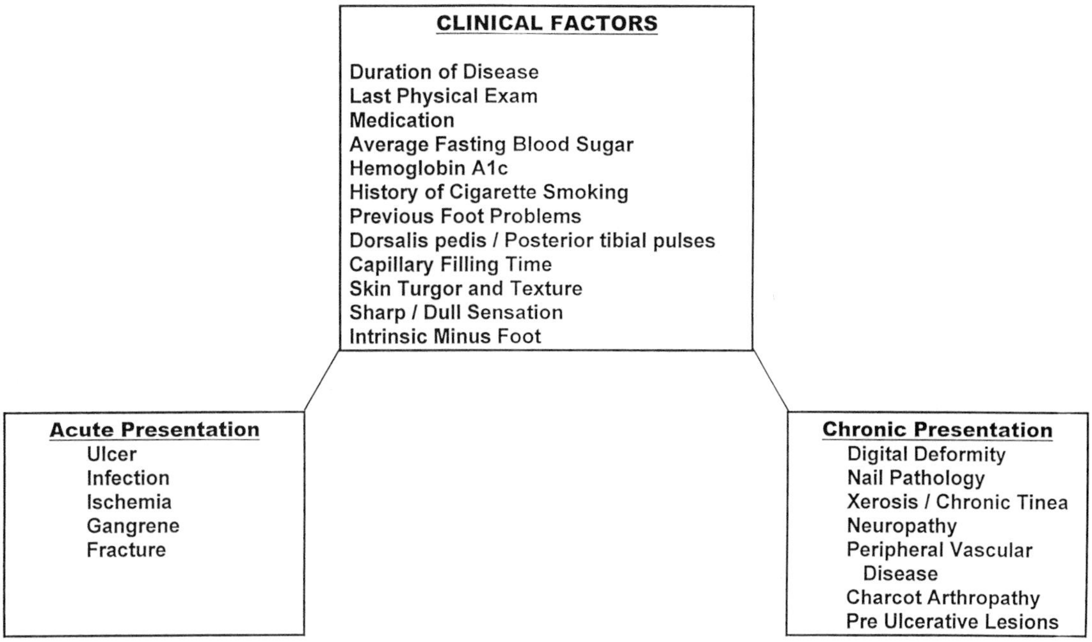

CLINICAL FACTORS

Duration of Disease
Last Physical Exam
Medication
Average Fasting Blood Sugar
Hemoglobin A1c
History of Cigarette Smoking
Previous Foot Problems
Dorsalis pedis / Posterior tibial pulses
Capillary Filling Time
Skin Turgor and Texture
Sharp / Dull Sensation
Intrinsic Minus Foot

Acute Presentation
Ulcer
Infection
Ischemia
Gangrene
Fracture

Chronic Presentation
Digital Deformity
Nail Pathology
Xerosis / Chronic Tinea
Neuropathy
Peripheral Vascular
  Disease
Charcot Arthropathy
Pre Ulcerative Lesions

Figure 33–3 ■ Diabetic foot problems.

lems. The patient with retinopathy who shaves their calluses with a razor, trims their nails with tin snips, or soaks their feet in a pot of hot water (Fig. 33–4 and 33–5) needs to be counseled immediately of the inherent dangers of "bathroom surgery."

Physical examination of the diabetic limb should be approached from a systems perspective: vascular, dermatologic, neurologic, and musculoskeletal/biomechanical. A thorough lower extremity examination should take no more than 5 minutes and requires little instrumentation (Fig. 33–6).

Vascular Exam

The ability to ascertain the patient's risk spectrum by history will provide an index of

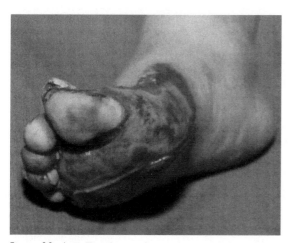

Figure 33–4 ■ Foot burn, plantar aspect of the sulcus of second and third toes.

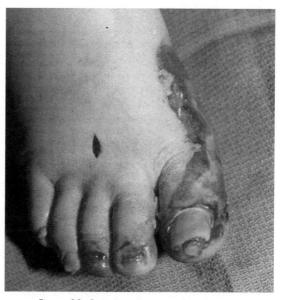

Figure 33–5 ■ Foot burn on dorsal feet.

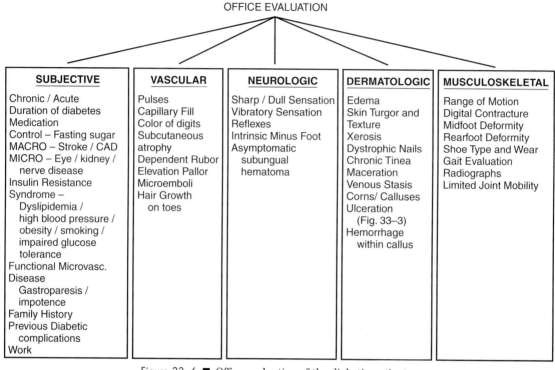

OFFICE EVALUATION

SUBJECTIVE	VASCULAR	NEUROLOGIC	DERMATOLOGIC	MUSCULOSKELETAL

Chronic / Acute
Duration of diabetes
Medication
Control – Fasting sugar
MACRO – Stroke / CAD
MICRO – Eye / kidney /
  nerve disease
Insulin Resistance
Syndrome –
  Dyslipidemia /
  high blood pressure /
  obesity / smoking /
  impaired glucose
  tolerance
Functional Microvasc.
Disease
  Gastroparesis /
  impotence
Family History
Previous Diabetic
  complications
Work
	Pulses
	Capillary Fill
	Color of digits
	Subcutaneous
	atrophy
	Dependent Rubor
	Elevation Pallor
	Microemboli
	Hair Growth
	  on toes
		Sharp / Dull Sensation
		Vibratory Sensation
		Reflexes
		Intrinsic Minus Foot
		Asymptomatic
		  subungual
		  hematoma
			Edema
			Skin Turgor and
			Texture
			Xerosis
			Dystrophic Nails
			Chronic Tinea
			Maceration
			Venous Stasis
			Corns/ Calluses
			Ulceration
			  (Fig. 33–3)
			Hemorrhage
			  within callus
				Range of Motion
				Digital Contracture
				Midfoot Deformity
				Rearfoot Deformity
				Shoe Type and Wear
				Gait Evaluation
				Radiographs
				Limited Joint Mobility

Figure 33–6 ■ Office evaluation of the diabetic patient.

suspicion for vascular disease. An index of suspicion for vascular disease will be found in the patient's history prior to the physical exam. Symptoms of vascular disease are cold feet, edema, blue toes, muscle cramps with activity or at rest, and pain at night. Patients with intermittent claudication complain of pain or cramping in the legs with activity that is usually reproducible. A patient may relate muscle cramps after walking a certain distance and only obtains relief after resting or sitting for 10 to 15 minutes. The symptoms are usually unilateral, and may include the musculature of the foot, calf, thigh, and gluteal group. Night cramps are also of clinical importance, as arterial flow, which requires the assistance of gravity, indicates significant compromise.

The vascular exam should include palpation of the femoral, popliteal, dorsalis pedis, and posterior tibial pulses in both extremities and noting any differences. Capillary fill time should be assessed with the foot raised above the level of the heart. Pallor on elevation and rubor on dependent position of the limb should also be assessed. Subcutaneous atrophy indicates poor functional vascular status to the distal tuft of the toe. This is easily visualized as the physician squeezes

the end of the toe; the poorly vascularized toe feels quite similar to a "baked potato," a poor prognostic sign (Fig. 33–7). This is indicative of poor arterial flow to the limb, and the patient may be at an increased risk for ulceration and infection. The presence of small focal areas of gangrene may be present from embolic phenomena distally. Sparse hair growth of the foot and skin atrophy are

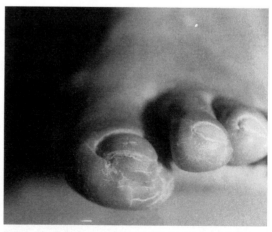

Figure 33–7 ■ Loss of subcutaneous tissue with lack of resiliency in distal soft tissue in hallux: "baked potato toe."

DIABETIC PERIPHERAL NEUROPATHY

AUTONOMIC	MOTOR	SENSORY
Eccrine Sweat Pores Decreased Lubrication to skin Generalized Dryness Heel Fissures Pallor Bounding Pulse	Atrophy of Intrinsic Muscles Leads to digital contractures Apropulsive (Steppage) Gait	Loss of Protective Sensation Blisters do not hurt Ingrown nails do not hurt

Figure 33–8 ■ Diabetic peripheral neuropathy.

a clue to vascular disease of the foot and leg. Nonpalpable pulses may be found using a hand held Doppler flow unit. In severely compromised patients, or patients with symptoms of arterial insufficiency, a vascular work-up including Doppler exam and an arteriogram may be indicated.[29, 32]

Neurologic Exam

Diabetic neuropathy affects much more than the feet. In fact, diabetic neuropathy affects every major organ system of the body.[7, 36] The differential diagnosis for peripheral neuropathy should always include alcoholism, malignancy, malnutrition, vitamin deficiencies, lead poisoning, spinal cord lesions, syphilis, and medications. Diabetic peripheral neuropathy affects motor, sensory, and autonomic nerves of the foot and leg (Fig. 33–8). These specific types of neuropathy may cause the patient to complain of burning, tingling,

heavy feet, socks rolled under the toes, cold feet, numbness, muscle weakness, or very dry xerotic skin. Sweat glands on the plantar aspect of the foot are controlled by the autonomic nervous system. Neuropathic patients lose eccrine gland function, resulting in decreased skin moisture, dryness, and fissuring of tissues, which creates an infection portal (Fig. 33–9). Motor neuropathy leads to changes in foot structure and gait patterns. Initially, the small intrinsic musculature of the foot begins to atrophy due to a loss of motor innervation. The end result of this loss of these intrinsic muscles is the loss of the stabilizing effect they provide and an overpowering of the long flexors and extensors, which in turn leads to contracted digits with retrograde forces being placed on the metatarsal heads (Fig. 33–10).

Diabetic patients may present with one or more of the following types of neuropathies: distal symmetric sensorimotor polyneuropathy, autonomic neuropathy, mononeuropa-

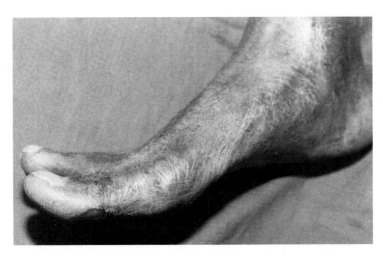

Figure 33–9 ■ Xerosis and scaling, intrinsic atrophy, with hallux extensus.

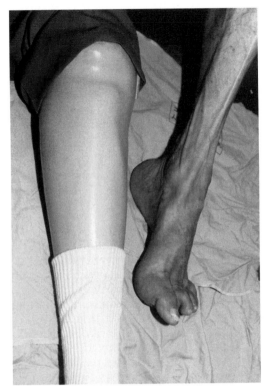

Figure 33–10 ■ Diabetic patient status post below-the-knee amputation with contracted toes, prominent extensor tendons, anterior cavus, and prominent metatarsal heads. This is a classic high-risk intrinsic minus foot.

thy multiplex, cranial neuropathy, radiculopathy, and plexopathy. Neurologic testing (Fig. 33–3) of the diabetic limb should include Achilles and patellar reflexes, sharp dull sensation, sensation threshold, vibratory and proprioceptive sensation, and temperature. These tests are easily performed in the exam room with a pin, swab, percussion hammer, and tuning fork. Have the patient recline and close their eyes as these are performed. A sensory testing nylon filament may be used to monitor or grade the level of neuropathy. The standard filament used is the Semmes-Weinstein 5.07/10-gm filament. This 10-gm filament probably represents the pressure threshold required to protect against ulceration.[36] The patient that cannot feel the filament on the skin is at increased risk for skin ulceration or injury. All areas of the dorsal and plantar nerve distributions must be tested to rule out specific nerve pathology. However, this examination needs to be coupled with a subjective history of neuropathic symptoms (i.e., numbness, burning, tingling sensations).

If more quantitative nylon monofilament wires are not available, an easy sharp-dull test can be performed by breaking a wooden/cotton swab and using the point of a broken end for sharp and the cotton for dull sensation; again, test all areas. Tubes of warm and cold water or ice can be placed against the skin to determine sensitivity to temperature. These tests are important to determine a level of risk for the patient and as a baseline to follow progression of neuropathy.

For the clinical exam, the tuning fork provides an easy but crude evaluation of the patient's peripheral large afferent fiber function. The patient's ability to detect the vibration in his or her foot is compared to the examiner's ability to feel the vibration in his or her hand. Therefore, one must assume that the examiner has "normal" sensation. The vibration perception threshold (VPT) can be measured using a handheld tactor, such as a Biothesiometer (Biomedical Instrument Corporation, Newbury, OH) (Fig. 33–11). The tactor is balanced vertically on the pulp of the toe. Voltage is increased on the base unit until the patient perceives a

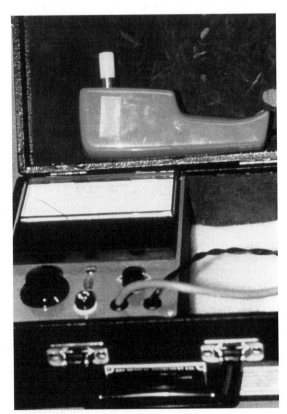

Figure 33–11 ■ Biothesiometer used to measure the vibration perception threshold.

vibration, which is documented as the VPT. The ability to quantitate the VPT is a major advantage for documentation or comparison of the progression of neuropathy since vibratory sensation is lost first in diabetic patients. Young et al. reported that a VPT greater than 25 V carried a sevenfold risk of foot ulceration compared with VPT of less than 15 V.[35] Abbott et al. also demonstrated in a multicenter study of the incidence and predictive risk factors for diabetic neuropathic foot ulcerations that VPT and Michigan DPN scores for muscle strength and reflexes were significant predictors of foot ulceration.[1, 35]

A recent study by Armstrong et al.,[20] which attempted to identify a practical neurologic screening test, reported that a positive Semmes-Weinstein test in which patients lacked perception of four out of ten sites on the foot was 97% sensitive and 83% specific for positively identifying loss of protective sensation. The Biothesiometer was 90% sensitive and 84% specific at a cutoff of 25 V. However, when combined with either or both being positive, there was 100% sensitivity and 77% specificity. Overall, the best modality for evaluating loss of protective threshold was a combination of modalities, which with a positive monofilament test and focused neuropathy symptom score yielded a 97% sensitivity and 86% specificity. Therefore, a thorough, multifactorial examination should be elicited to accurately assess the patient's neurologic status.

Dermatologic

The skin is the largest body organ and the first barrier against infection. In the diabetic, the skin is compromised by arterial, neurologic, and musculoskeletal disease. Assessment of the skin should include skin quality, turgor/texture, and hair growth. Diabetic patients with arterial disease commonly have shiny atrophic skin of the dorsum of the foot. The nails are also a skin appendage that must be evaluated. Koilonychia (or spoon-shaped nails), pitting of the nail plate, onycholysis, subungual hemorrhages, and nail color changes are associated wth diabetes mellitus.[17] The importance of nail care cannot be stressed enough as seen with subungual ulcerations secondary to onychomycosis as well as infected ingrown nails (Fig. 33–12). With immunologic compromise, diabetic patients are susceptible to both bacterial and fungal infections. Areas of interdigital maceration, venous stasis, corns, and calluses are all potential portals of infection in the lower extremity. Chronic tinea pedis with its "moccasin" distribution and slightly erythematous superficial scaling and xerosis are common presentations.

Autonomic neuropathy has been indicated in several of the cutaneous findings in diabetics. With an extensive patient history, one will usually find the patient complaining of cold feet, pruritus associated with xerotic skin, and occasional burning, all of which result from such neuropathy. However, the most common manifestation of loss of autonomic control is decreased or lost vasomotor activity resulting in the inability to adequately hydrate the pedal skin, although most patients may complain of increased sweating in other areas of the body. A resultant thickening of the stratum corneum is

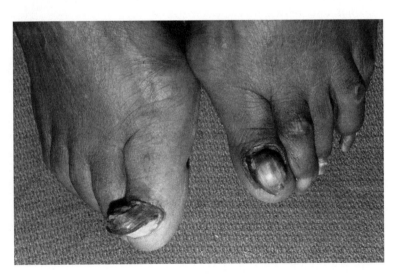

Figure 33–12 ■ Mycotic, hypertrophic hallux nails.

then observed with the formation of brittle callosities on the feet which, when coupled with peripheral neuropathy, become high-pressure areas for ulceration. The key to control is to stress the importance of adequate hygiene in these patients and the use of moisturizing emollients. Another consequence of autonomic neuropathy is loss of sympathetic control, which will result in vasodilation, arteriovenous shunting, and edema. These findings are witnessed by prominent vessels and varicosities of the feet and should be considered an impairment in the peripheral circulation of the patient.

Calluses are usually located in areas of high pressure, and their presence in the diabetic foot is considered pathologic. Simply put, a callus is the body's protective mechanism for an area of chronic irritation, but they are the most destructive skin lesion in the diabetic patient. The etiology is structural deformity with abnormal biomechanical function. Repetitive pressure in the neuropathic foot has been consistently described within the literature as a compounding factor in callus formation along with neuropathy. It has also been stated that nonenzymatic glycosylation results in alterations of the structural stability of the skin, predisposing the diabetic to increased callus formation. Although witnessed in patients with good glycemic control, keratin and collagen disturbances have been most commonly related to elevated blood glucose levels making the tissue rigid, inflexible, and more resistant to collagenase digestion. According to Delbridge,[11] such glycosylated keratin will build up secondary to repetitive pressure and not be removed from the superficial layers of the foot and result in hyperkeratoses and ultimately neuropathic ulceration. He also describes several steps in the development of a neuropathic ulceration in the diabetic foot. First, there is an initial hyperkeratotic lesion, which with continued repetitive pressure will result in breakdown of deeper tissue. Eventually a cavity will form, fill with blood, and enlarge to the point where it ruptures and forms an ulceration.

Pedal ulceration is probably of the greatest concern in diagnosing and treating the diabetic patient.

The most destructive lesion of the skin is the diabetic ulceration. These lesions are most commonly a continuum of a callus that went unrecognized and untreated. A callus is simply the body's protective mechanism for an area of chronic irritation. Callus sets up increased shear and ultimately will blister and ulcerate.

The importance of identification of the diabetic foot ulcer and then ensuring proper follow-up was identified even more clearly in a recent study that revealed that Medicare expenditures for patients with diabetic foot ulcers were three times higher than for Medicare patients in general—$15,309 versus $4,226. Care for ulcers represented 24% of spending for that patient population. The fact that the majority of patients had little or no follow-up on a regular basis was the reason attributed for the discrepancy.[15]

Seven simple questions should be asked for a thorough evaluation of an ulceration and its classification. They are as follows:

1. *Where is the ulcer located?* There is an intimate relationship between the location of an ulcer and its etiology. For example, ulcers located along the lateral or medial foot margins are secondary to constant low pressures (i.e., tight shoe irritation), and wounds found on the plantar aspect of the foot are caused by repetitive moderate pressures (i.e., prominent metatarsal head) (Fig. 33–13).

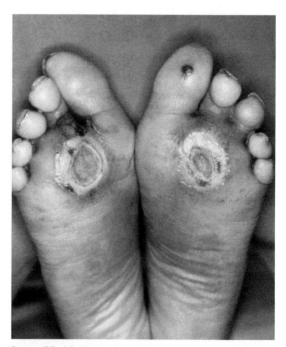

Figure 33–13 ■ Neuropathic ulcer sub–second metatarsal, bilateral, due to hammer toes with lack of motion of the second metatarsals.

2. *How large is the ulcer?* This will be a key factor in determining the duration for wound healing with wound size recorded at each visit to gauge healing progression.
3. *What do the wound margins look like?* The margins can tell a lot about a wound. If adequate debridement and off-loading have been implemented, the margins should be well adhered to the surface of the underlying subcuticular structures with a gentle slope toward normal epithelium. However, if a wound has been inadequately debrided and off-loaded, undermining of the leading edge will predominate (Fig. 33–14). This phenomenon is due to the "edge-effect" which dictates that an interruption in any matrix (in this case, the dermal matrix) magnifies both vertical and shear stress on the edges of that interruption. This subsequently causes shearing from underlying epithelium (making the wound larger by undermining) and increased vertical pressure, which makes the wound progressively deeper. This effect can be mitigated with regular, adequate debridement and off-loading techniques. Based on this concept, wound margins should be described as undermined, adherent, macerated, and/or viable versus nonviable.
4. *What does the wound base look like?* The commonly descriptive terms used to describe the base of a wound include granular, fibrotic, or necrotic. Also, one should note the absence or presence of any serous or purulent drainage from the wound as well as the odor.
5. *How deep is the ulcer and which underlying structures are involved?* Wound depth is by far the most commonly utilized descriptor in wound classification.

In order to effectively treat ulcerations, it is helpful to have an established classification and risk system. Besides the advantage of being a proven protocol, it also allows the medical and research communities to speak a common language.

The University of Texas Wound Classification System fulfills these requirements. In addition, it allows the practitioner to predict expected outcomes based on ulcer qualities and the patient's comorbidities. It was developed based on treatment of 360 patients evaluated over a 6-month period for complications (Fig. 33–15).[6, 27]

The University of Texas Health Sciences Center at San Antonio wound classification system is a simple system that has been validated by the ADA. This system provides a proven treatment protocol and allows the practitioner to predict expected outcomes based on ulcer qualities and patient comorbidities. The depth of the ulceration is categorized according to the anatomic level that is involved:

Grade 0: Pre-/postulcerative lesion— completely epithelialized
Grade 1: Full-thickness skin—superficial lesion
Grade 2: Deep to tendon and/or capsule
Grade 3: Deep to exposed bone

Practitioners have felt that wounds that penetrate to bone frequently have osteomyelitis. Grayson and colleagues indicated that probing to bone is up to 66% sensitive and 85% specific in diagnosing osteomyelitis.[14]

6. *Is the ulcer infected?* The diabetic, in light of an infection, may be unable to mount an adequate immune response. Therefore, white blood cell (WBC) counts may be normal over half of the time in these patients.[23] Similarly, fever and other subjective signs of infection are absent approximately 86% of the time.[2] This makes diagnosis of infection a difficult one; however, one must watch for the five cardinal signs of infection: rubor, calor, tumor, do-

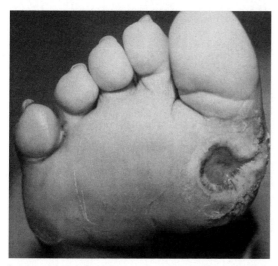

Figure 33–14 ■ Neuropathic ulceration sub–first metatarsal.

		GRADE / DEPTH "How deep is the wound?"			
		0	**I**	**II**	**III**
STAGE / COMORBIDITIES "Is the wound infected, ischemic, or both"?	**A**	Pre- or postulcerative lesion, completely epithelialized	Superficial wound, not involving tendon, capsule, or bone	Wound penetrating to tendon or capsule	Wound penetrating to bone or joint
	B	Pre- or postulcerative lesion completely epithelialized with infection	Superficial wound, not involving lesion, capsule, or bone, with infection	Wound penetrating to tendon or capsule, with infection	Wound penetrating to bone
	C	Pre- or postulcerative lesion, completely epithelialized with infection and ischemia	Superficial wound, not involving tendon, capsule, or bone, with ischemia	Wound penetrating to tendon or capsule, with ischemia	Wound penetrating to bone or joint, with ischemia
	D	Pre- or postulcerative lesion, completely epithelized with infection and ischemia	Superficial wound, not involving tendon, capsule, or bone, with infection and ischemia	Wound penetrating to tendon or capsule, with infection and ischemia	Wound penetrating to bone or joint, with infection and ischemia

Figure 33–15 ▪ The University of Texas Classification System for Diabetic Foot Wounds

lor, and loss of function. Infection is loosely defined as the presence of cellulitis, the presence of purulence, or more than two of the cardinal signs (Fig. 33–16).

7. *Is the ulcer ischemic?* The determination of an ischemic ulcer can be based upon its appearance, which is usually necrotic (Fig. 33–17) and lacking a good, red granular base or if the wound is slow healing in the face of adequate local wound care and off-loading techniques. Findings such as these warrant the evaluation of noninvasive vascular studies and possibly a vascular consult for possible surgical in-

tervention to optimize perfusion of the area and ultimately wound healing once these questions are answered (Figs. 33–18 and 33–19).

Several other dermatologic findings have been observed in the diabetic patient including paronychia, yellow nails, fungal nails,

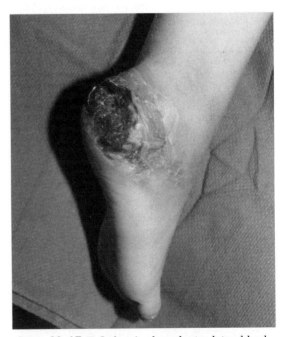

Figure 33–17 ▪ Ischemic ulcer plantar lateral heel.

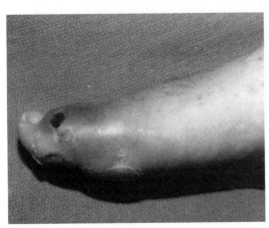

Figure 33–16 ▪ Cellulitis secondary to neuropathic ulceration.

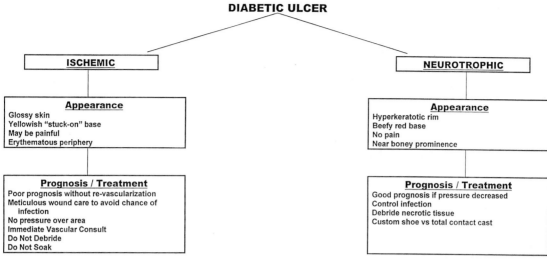

Figure 33–18 ■ Diabetic ulcer.

pigmented purpura, periungual telangiectasias, and necrobiosis lipoidica diabeticorum (NLD). Some of these conditions have been attributed to the level of glucose control, nonenzymatic glycosylation, and/or the degree of vascular compromise of the patient. Yellowing of the skin, though once thought to be due to carotenemia, is now thought to be due to glycosylation end-products, which become yellow and give such a hue to the skin. Pigmented purpura, on the other hand, is attributed to the extravasation of red blood cells

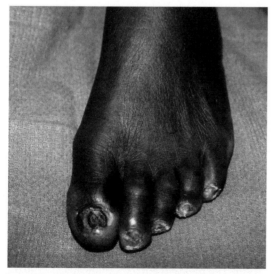

Figure 33–19 ■ Patient exhibits all the signs of vascular disease in the foot and leg; shiny atrophic skin, no hair, and ischemic ulcer of hallux nail bed, dystrophic nails.

from the superficial vascular plexus. These lesions are commonly referred to as "cayenne pepper spots" and consist of tan/orange patches, notably on the shins. The purpura is commonly found in conjunction with diabetic dermopathy and precipitated by lower extremity edema.

Found in up to 65% of diabetic patients, shin spots or diabetic dermopathy is considered the most common dermatologic manifestation in this population. Lesions are usually bilateral, asymmetric, circumscribed, atrophic, hyperpigmented macules on the shins of affected individuals. The etiology of such lesions is unknown, though they have been closely associated with posttraumatic atrophy and postinflammatory hyperpigmentation in poorly vascularized skin. These lesions have, however, been observed in nondiabetics, and it has been postulated that the presence of four or more lesions is more definitive of diabetic dermopathy. One study found 14% of diabetics and none of the nondiabetics to be affected by such multilesional dermopathy. Regardless, the lesions continue to be a consistent finding in the diabetic population and, although not fully understood, they may be another indicator of vascular disease.

Paronychia has been attributed to several factors including trauma, nail dystrophy, tight shoegear, nail morphology, and improper nail debridement. Trauma and nail morphology being the only uncontrollable factors, one should be aware of the remaining factors and work toward preventing their progression. However, should the diabetic patient present with a paronychia, the degree of the infection, noted by purulence and erythema, should be noted as well as the duration of symptoms. In light of adequate pedal pulses and capillary fill time, the offending border may usually be removed by performing a partial matrixectomy. If vascular status is of concern, antibiotic therapy as well as adequate conservative debridement of the offending border should be implemented with close continued follow-up of the patient.

Onychomycosis, which is common in the general population, is also highly prevalent and a greater risk in the diabetic patient. Though its etiology is unclear, it has been proposed that undetected subungual hemorrhage secondary to neuropathy acts as a nidus for fungal infection and results in thickened, hypertrophic nails. Other factors of concern are immunopathy and vasculopathy, which decrease the ability to fight off such infections. Invasion of the nail bed results in increased subungual debris causing dorsal lifting of the nail and, coupled with the thickened, dystrophic nature of the nail, can result in pressure from shoegear and future subungual ulceration. For these reasons, adequate regular debridement is important in the pedal care of the diabetic patient.

Also, with the high incidence of fungally infected toenails, tinea pedis as well as interdigital tinea become associated risk factors. Common findings with such infection include vesicular lesions, areas of skin breakdown, and interdigital macerations, all of which may cause invasion of the subcutaneous layers by the skin's normal flora. The consequence of such events may lead to a superimposed bacterial infection.

Musculoskeletal/Biomechanical Evaluation

The musculoskeletal anatomy of the foot is dynamic and complex and cannot be thoroughly appreciated by a solely non–weight-bearing exam. One mandatory aspect of a complete lower extremity exam is the evaluation of the foot in its weight-bearing attitude (Fig. 33–6). The foot must be able to handle many times the body's weight while converting rapidly from a mobile adapter at heel contact to a rigid lever for propulsion in gait.

When functioning properly, the foot is efficient at dispersing loads, shear, and friction. During this phase of the clinical examination, one must identify areas of pressure, shear, and increased friction. Subtle changes in color, skin lines, bony prominences, hyperkeratosis, erythema, and pain are good indicators of problem areas. No matter the foot type, potential complications may result. The cavus foot, with its contracted toes and high arch, may have digital and metatarsal pressure areas, just as the pathologically flat (or planus) foot may show the changes of Charcot arthropathy and midfoot ulceration.

Range of motion, both qualitative and quantitative, should be assessed, including the metatarsophalangeal joints, the midtarsal joint, and the subtalar and ankle joints. Manual muscle testing of all muscle groups should be performed.

Weight-bearing radiographic studies of both feet should be considered as a baseline if the neurologic exam is positive for peripheral neuropathy. Remember, the foot functions significantly differently in a weight-bearing versus non–weight-bearing attitude. Early collapse of the midtarsal and subtalar joints, which is effectively treated with orthotic devices, would only be evident on a weight-bearing study.

During gait, bony prominences or shoe pressure may cause blood to be displaced from the tissue, creating a transient local area of ischemia. In the neurologically intact foot, this would normally cause pain, but in the neuropathic patient, the protective reflex is absent. Shear and pressure forces combine over these areas of ischemia to produce hyperkeratosis initially, and continued stress eventually leads to tissue breakdown and ulceration. Pressure points may be created by long or plantarflexed metatarsals, prominent sesamoid bones, exostoses, contracted digits, and shoegear (Figs. 33–20 and 33–21).

Of great concern in the final, overall assessment of the musculoskeletal function of the diabetic patient is the degree of joint mobility and the rigidity versus flexibility of any deformities encountered. These findings have been extensively discussed by several authors including Fernando,[13] Delbridge,[11] and Lavery et al.[21] It has also been attributed to joint stiffening secondary to glycosylation of soft tissue structures. Lavery et al. discuss that limited joint mobility can best be appreciated by assessing the range of motion of the first metatarsophalangeal joint. Findings

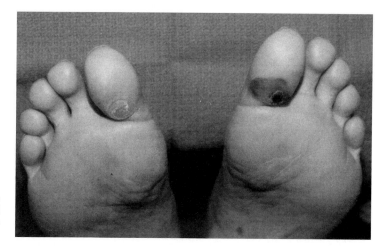

Figure 33–20 ■ Callus of plantar aspect of the hallux interphalangeal joint bilateral due to hallux interphalangeal sesamoid.

of less than 50 degrees of non–weight-bearing passive dorsiflexion have been accepted as an increased risk for ulceration. One must also take into consideration the amount of motion at the metatarsophalangeal joint, subtalar joint, and the ankle, since any limitation in these areas may result in increased pressures.

Off-loading

One of the areas where the podiatrist can be most effective in preventing initial presentation or return of ulcerations is in off-loading. The podiatrist has a keen understanding of materials, foot function, and the interaction with ulcerations.

Again, questioning the patient about footwear specifics is the foundation of proper treatment. The practitioner needs to know:

- What did the patient wear to the appointment?
- Is this typical of what they wear at home?
- Do they go barefoot at home? Examine the feet for debris that may reveal the answer.
- Has the patient been provided with prescription footwear and is it being worn? Examine the shoes for wear patterns. Too often the patient will report that the prescription footwear is being saved for "special occasions." The patient must be educated about the fact that the shoes are similar to medication and must be used exactly as prescribed.

At the same time, the podiatrist cannot be rigid and inflexible in dealing with the patient. The practitioner must take into consideration the patient's social, work, and personal needs when prescribing footwear. For instance, a patient who works in the con-

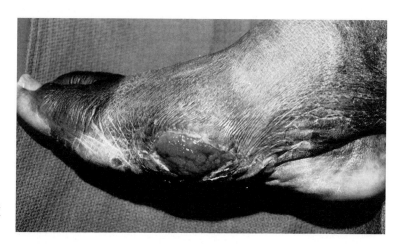

Figure 33–21 ■ Ulceration in a patient with Charcot arthropathy with collapsed medial column.

struction industry is not likely to wear a prescription shoe in a fashionable wing-tip style for the workday.

Besides appropriateness of style, care must be taken to utilize those materials and features that will best benefit the patient. While these are specific to the patient, certain features are universally important: a deep toe box to accommodate digital deformities, a sturdy heel counter to stabilize the foot, and accommodation through insoles to protect pressure points.

The same philosophy of protection is used in off-loading principles used during the treatment phase. An example is the use of the total-contact cast (TCC). The biomechanics of the TCC are better understood now because of determination of plantar pressure and ground reaction forces in the device,[30] and with that knowledge comes the ability to best use this modality.

Shaw et al. determined that the TCC is successful in treating forefoot ulcers on a dependable basis but that treatment of rearfoot ulcers is dependent upon appropriate foam padding.[30]

Following a detailed diabetic foot examination, a clear description of risk that expresses the salient findings from the history and physical examination is of paramount importance when structuring any treatment plan designed to reduce lower extremity amputation. The University of Texas Foot Classification System was devised by Armstrong et al.[5] (Figs. 33–22 and 33–23) to adequately communicate where a patient lies on the

---

Category 0: No Pathology

- Patient diagnosed with Diabetes Mellitus
- Protective sensation intact
- Ankle Brachial Index (ABI) >0.80 and toe systolic pressure >45 mmHg
- Foot deformity may be present
- No history of ulceration

POSSIBLE TREATMENT FOR CATEGORY 0
- Two to three visits a year to assess neurovascular status, dermal thermometry and foci of stress
- Possible shoe accommodations
- Patient education

Category 1: Neuropathy, No Deformity

- Protective sensation absent
- Ankle Brachial Index (ABI) >0.80 and toe systolic pressure >45 mmHg
- No history of ulceration
- No history of diabetic neuropathic osteoarthropathy (Charcot's joint)
- No foot deformity

POSSIBLE TREATMENT FOR CATEGORY 1
Same as category 0 plus:
- Possible shoe gear accommodation (pedorthic/orthotist consultation)
- Quarterly visits to assess shoe gear and monitor for signs of irritation

---

Category 2: Neuropathy with Deformity

- Protective sensation absent
- Ankle Brachial Index (ABI) >0.80 and toe systolic pressure >44 mmHg
- No history of neuropathic ulceration
- No history of Charcot's joint
- Foot deformity present (focus of stress)

POSSIBLE TREATMENT FOR CATEGORY 2
Same as Category 1 plus:
- Pedorthic/orthotist consultation for possible custom molded/extra depth shoe accommodation
- Possible prophylactic surgery to alleviate focus of stress (e.g., correction of hammertoe or bunion deformity)

Category 3: History of Pathology

- Protective sensation absent
- Ankle Brachial Index (ABI) >0.80 and toe systolic pressure >45 mmHg
- History of neuropathic ulceration
- History of Charcot's joint
- Foot deformity present (focus of stress)

POSSIBLE TREATMENT FOR CATEGORY 3
Same as Category 2 plus:
- Pedorthic/orthotist consultation for custom molded/extra depth shoe accommodation
- Possible prophylactic surgery to alleviate focus of stress (e.g., correction of bunion or hammertoe)
- More frequent visits may be indicated for monitoring

Figure 33–22 ■ The University of Texas Diabetic Foot Classification System: Categories 0–3: Risk Factors for Ulceration

---

Category 4A: Neuropathic Ulceration

- Patient diagnosed with Diabetes Mellitus
- Sensorium may or may not be intact
- Ankle Brachial Index (ABI) >0.80 mmHg and toe systolic pressure of >45 mmHg
- Foot deformity normally present
- No infected neuropathic ulceration
- No acute diabetic neuropathic osteoarthropathy (Charcot's joint) present

POSSIBLE TREATMENT FOR CATEGORY 4A
Same as category 3 plus:
- Offweighting program instituted
- Dressing change program instituted
- Debridement program instituted
- Dermal thermometric monitoring
- Weekly to biweekly visits as needed
- Possible prophylactic surgery

Category 4B: Acute Charcot's Joint

- Patient diagnosed with Diabetes Mellitus
- Sensorium absent
- Ankle Brachial Index (ABI) >0.80 mmHg and toe systolic pressure of >45 mmHg
- Noninfected neuropathic ulceration may be present
- Diabetic neuropathic osteoarthropathy (Charcot's joint) present

POSSIBLE TREATMENT FOR CATEGORY 4B
Same as category 3 plus:
- Offweighting program instituted; possible total contact cast
- Weekly to biweekly visits (as per contact casting regimen)
- Dermal thermometric and radiographic monitoring
- If ulcer is present, treatment same as for category 4A

Category 5: Infected Diabetic Foot

- Patient diagnosed with Diabetes Mellitus
- Sensorium may or may not be intact
- Infected wound
- Charcot's joint may be present

POSSIBLE TREATMENT FOR CATEGORY 2
Same as Category 4 plus:
- Debridement of infected necrotic tissue and bone
- Possible hospitalization
- Antibiotic therapy
- Medical management
- Contact casting generally contraindicated until diabetic category drops to 4

Category 6: Dysvascular Foot

- Patient diagnosed with Diabetes Mellitus
- Sensorium may or may not be intact
- Ankle brachial index of <0.80 mmHg or toe systolic pressure of <45 mmHg or pedal transcutaneous oxygen tension of <40 mmHg
- Ulceration may be present

POSSIBLE TREATMENT FOR CATEGORY 3
- Vascular consult, possible revascularization
- If infection present, treatment same as for category 5
- Vascular consultation concomitant with control of sepsis
- Contact casting generally contraindicated

Figure 33–23 ■ The University of Texas Diabetic Foot Classification system: Categories 4A–6: Risk Factors for Amputation.

spectrum of risk throughout the entire course of care. Moreover, generalized treatment guidelines are designed to bring the patient from a high-risk category into the lowest possible category for that patient. Categories 0 to 3 are risk factors for ulceration and 4 to 6 are risk factors for amputation. Risk factors for development of ulceration include neuropathy, deformity or limited joint mobility, and a previous history of ulceration or amputation. Lavery et al.[20] evaluated 255 subjects in a case comparison study and found that those falling into category 1 neuropathy (loss of protective sensation) were at 1.7 times greater risk of ulceration. Patients in foot category 2 neuropathy plus deformity were

at 12 times greater risk for ulceration. Those patients in category 3 neuropathy plus deformity plus a history of ulceration Charcot arthropathy or amputation were at 36 times greater risk for ulceration. Clearly, all diabetic patients should be screened and placed in the appropriate risk category and followed appropriately. This system will allow practitioners to communicate and classify cumulative risk and help predict outcomes.

Conclusions

The pedal manifestations of diabetes may be quite complex, with multiple etiologic factors combining to complicate the clinical presentation. A thorough understanding of the pathogenesis of foot disease provides the basis for effective treatment. As stated by Cavanagh,[9] the key is linking all of the associated risk factors of structure, function, footwear, and lifestyle or activity level. These risk factors are dynamic, not static, and therefore constant evaluation and assessment are essential to prevention. This understanding must be followed by a systematic implementation in order to also provide efficient and effective treatment. When knowledge and implementation meet, the physician is afforded an exceptional opportunity to truly make a difference in the quality of life for the diabetic patient.

REFERENCES

1. Abbott CA, Vileikyte L, et al: Multicenter study of the incidence of and predictive risk factors for diabetic neuropathic foot ulceration. Diabetes Care 21:1071–1075, 1998.
2. American Diabetes Association: Foot care in patients with diabetes mellitus [position statement]. Diabetes Care 21(Suppl 1):554–555, 1998.
3. Apelqvist J, Larsson J, Agardh CD: Long-term prognosis for diabetic patients with foot ulcers: J Intern Med 233:485–491, 1993.
4. Armstrong DG, Harkless LB: Outcomes of preventative care in a diabetic foot specialty clinic. J Foot Ankle Surg 37:460–466, 1998.
5. Armstrong DG, Lavery LA, Harkless LB: Treatment based classification system for assessment and care of diabetic feet. J Am Podiatr Med Assoc 86:311–316, 1996.
6. Armstrong DG, Lavery L, Harkless LB: Validation of a diabetic wound classification system. Diabetes Care 23:855–859, 1998.
7. Boulton AJM: The pathogenesis of diabetic foot problems: An overview. Diabet Med 13:S12–S16, 1996.
8. Boulton AJM: The diabetic foot. Med Clin North Am 72:1513–1530, 1988.
9. Cavanagh PE: In Boulton AM (ed): The Foot in Diabetes, 2nd ed. New York: John Wiley & Sons, 1994.
10. Del Aguila M, Reiber G, Koepseli T: How does provider and patient awareness of high risk status for lower extremity amputation influence foot-care practices? Diabetes Care 17:9, 1994.
11. Delbridge L, Ellis CS, Robertson K, et al: Non-enzymatic glycosylation of keratin from the stratum cornea of the diabetic foot. Br J Dermatol 112:547–554, 1985.
12. Edmonds ME, Blundell MP, Morris ME, et al: Improved survival of the diabetic foot: The role of a specialized foot clinic. Q J Med 232:763–771, 1986.
13. Fernando DJS, Masson EA, Veves A, Boulton AJM: Relationship of limited joint mobility to abnormal foot pressure and diabetic foot ulceration. Diabetes Care 14:8–11, 1991.
14. Grayson ML, Balaugh K, et al: Probing to bone in infected pedal ulcers: A clinical sign of underlying osteomyelities in diabetic patients. J Am Podiatr Med Assoc 273:721–723, 1995.
15. Harrington CA, The Lewin Group, et al: An analysis of Diabetic Foot Ulcers Using Medicare Claims Data [abstract] ADA Annual Meeting, 1999.
16. Heus-vann Putten MA, Schaper NC, Bakker K: The clinical examination of the diabetic foot in daily practice. Diabet Med 13:S55–S57, 1996.
17. Herzberg A: Nail manifestations of systemic disease. Clinics in Podiatric Medicine and Surgery. Philadelphia: WB Saunders Company, 1995, pp 314–317.
18. Kozak G, Hoar C, Rowbatham J, et al: Management of the Diabetic Foot Problems. Philadelphia: WB Saunders Company, 1984, pp 1–8.
19. Larsson J, Apelquist J, Agardh DD, Stenstron A: Decreasing the incidence of major amputation in diabetic patients: A consequence of a multidisciplinary foot care team approach. Diabet Med 12:770–776, 1995.
20. Lavery LA, Armstrong DG, et al: Choosing a practical screening instrument to identify patients at risk for diabetic foot ulceration. Arch Intern Med 158:157–162, 1998.
21. Lavery LA, Armstrong DG, et al: Practical screening criteria for patient at high risk for diabetic foot ulceration. Arch Intern Med 158:157–162, 1998.
22. Lavery LA, Armstrong DG, Harkless LB: Classification of diabetic foot wounds. J Foot Ankle Surg 35:528–531, 1996.
23. Lavery LA, Armstrong DG, Quebedeaux TL, et al: Puncture wounds: The frequency of normal laboratory values in the face of severe foot infections of the diabetic foot in diabetic and non-diabetic adults. Am J Med 101:521–525, 1998.
24. Levin ME: Preventing amputation in the patient with diabetes. Diabetes Care 18:1383–1394, 1995.
25. Litzelman DK, Slemenda CW, Langefeld CD, et al: Reduction in lower extremity clinical abnormalities in patients with non-insulin dependent diabetes mellitus. Ann Intern Med 119:36–41, 1993.
26. Moss R, Klein R, Klein BEK: The prevalence and incidence of lower extremity amputation in a diabetic population. Arch Intern Med 152:610–616, 1999.
27. Pham H, et al: The role of endothelial function on the foot. Clin Podiatr Med Surg 15:85–94, 1998.
28. Reiber GE: The epidemiology of diabetic foot problems. Diabet Med 13:S6–S11, 1996.
29. Schaper NC: Early atherogenesis in diabetes mellitus. Diabet Med 13:S17, 1996.
30. Shaw JE, Van Schie CHM, Carrington AL, et al: An analysis of dynamic forces transmitted through the foot in diabetic neuropathy. Diabetes Care 21:1955–1959, 1998.
31. Shenaq SM, Klebuc MJA, Vargo D: How to help diabetic patients avoid amputations. Postgrad Med 96:177–192, 1994.
32. Takolander R, Rauweda JA: The use of non-invasive vascular assessment in diabetic patients with foot lesions. Diabet Med 24:S39–S42, 1996.

33. Thomson FJ, Veves A, Ashe H, et al: A team approach to diabetic foot care: The Manchester experience. Foot 2:75–82, 1991.
34. Van Gils CC, Wheeler LA, Mellstrom M, et al: Amputation prevention by vascular surgery and podiatry collaboration in high-risk diabetic and nondiabetic patients. Diabet Care 22:678–683, 1999.
35. Young MJ: The prediction of diabetic neuropathic foot ulceration using vibration perception thresholds: A prospective study. Diabetes Care 17:557–560, 1999.
36. Ziegler D: Diagnosis and management of diabetic peripheral neuropathy. Diabet Med 13:S34–S38, 1996.

34

PEDORTHIC CARE OF THE DIABETIC FOOT

■ Dennis J. Janisse

Role of Board-Certified Pedorthist

Pedorthics is the design, manufacture, fit, and modification of shoes and foot orthoses to alleviate foot problems caused by disease, overuse, or injury.[23] Pedorthists fit and dispense footwear according to a physician's prescription. A board-certified pedorthist (CPed) is trained in foot anatomy and construction of shoes and foot orthotic devices. In order to achieve certification, a candidate's qualifications have been tested and accepted by the Board for Certification in Pedorthics (BCP). Certified pedorthists are required to participate in a continuing education program under BCP auspices.[23] The CPed designation is intended to provide the prescribing physician and consumer with the assurance of competence in dispensing prescription footwear. Both the BCP and the Pedorthic Footwear Association (PFA) work to establish standards and provide educational opportunities for individuals involved in the practice of pedorthics.

As a member of the team involved in the long-term treatment of the patient with diabetes, the certified pedorthist plays an important role in the care of the insensate foot.[3, 12, 19] First, the pedorthist can provide the necessary prescription footwear by main-taining the required inventory to ensure that the patient receives the type of shoes prescribed and that they fit properly. He or she can also take foot impressions and provide any needed external shoe modifications and total-contact orthoses (TCOs). When necessary, the pedorthist can also construct custom-made shoes.

The second part of the pedorthist's role is in the area of patient education. Levin[19] has stated, "Of all the approaches to saving the diabetic foot, the most important is patient education"; the importance of patient education has also been noted by Boulton[3] and others.[7, 9, 20, 30] The pedorthist is a valuable resource for instructing patients in all aspects of footwear: the purpose and proper use of the prescribed footwear, criteria of a good fit, and appropriate shoe materials and styles for the diabetic foot. The pedorthist can reinforce information given by other team members, such as foot inspection and hygiene procedures and injury prevention. The need for follow-up is emphasized, including any necessary minor adjustments to the current footwear, as well as future changes in the prescription itself as the patient experiences changes in his or her feet.

Finally, the certified pedorthist plays an important role in monitoring patient progress. Ideally the pedorthist should meet in a clinic setting with both the physician and the patient to determine the patient's footwear needs and formulate an effective prescription. (The role of specialized foot clinics in reducing amputation and other diabetic foot complications has been documented.[8, 20, 30]) However, because pedorthists may work with a large number of referring physicians, seeing every patient in a clinic setting is often not practical, with the result that most patients come to the pedorthist with a written prescription from their physician. In these cases, the pedorthist must serve as the link between the physician and the patient. In return visits to the pedorthist the patient can report success or any problems experienced with the prescription footwear. The pedorthist should inspect both the footwear and the patient's feet, looking for signs of undue skin pressure. The overall effectiveness of the prescription footwear should be noted and reported to the prescribing physician with recommendations for additional modifications or adjustments. The pedorthist should see patients several times, until it is certain the prescription is filled correctly and functioning properly.

As patient progress is monitored, additional opportunities are created for patient education and reinforcement of important foot care concepts. The pedorthist will often be able to prevent a foot problem through early detection; for example, in a routine foot inspection the pedorthist might notice a red spot or a developing ulcer that the patient has overlooked, especially if he or she has any loss of sensation. (The importance of regular foot inspection has been noted by Levin[19] and others.[3, 7, 20, 30]) In addition, detailed footwear records should be maintained for all patients, facilitating effective follow-up and long-term management of diabetic foot problems.

Objectives in the Pedorthic Care of the Diabetic Foot

Before the specific types of prescription footwear that a pedorthist can provide are discussed, it is first necessary to identify the objectives in the pedorthic care of the diabetic foot. These can be stated as follows[11, 12]:

1. *Relief of areas of excessive plantar pressure.* Repetitive application of high pressures during the walking and standing activities of daily life can lead to ulceration on the plantar surface of the insensitive foot. Specific high-pressure areas, such as the metatarsal heads, are particularly susceptible to neuropathic ulceration. By relieving high-pressure areas and more evenly spreading forces over the plantar surface, one can attempt to reduce the incidence and recurrence of ulceration.[4, 26, 29]

2. *Reduction of shock.* Even moderate amounts of pressure, when repetitive, can lead to ulceration in the insensitive foot; therefore, in addition to relieving specific high-pressure areas, a reduction in the overall amount of vertical pressure, or shock, on the plantar surface is desirable.[3, 9, 29] This is especially important for a foot with undue bony prominences or with the abnormal bone structure associated with Charcot neuroarthropathy.

3. *Reduction of shear.* The reduction of horizontal and vertical movement of the foot within the shoe, leading to skin shear, is also an important consideration in minimizing ulceration, callus buildup, and excessive heat because of friction.[5, 6, 9]

4. *Accommodation of deformities.* Deformities resulting from conditions such as Charcot neuroarthropathy, loss of fatty tissue, and amputations must be accommodated. It is also vital to minimize pressure from shoe uppers on hammer toes or claw toes.[3, 4, 28]

5. *Stabilization and support of deformities.* Many deformities need to be stabilized to relieve pain and avoid further destruction, whereas flexible deformities may need to be controlled or supported in a more normal or neutral position to decrease progression of the deformity.[7, 28]

6. *Limitation of joint motion.* Limiting the motion of involved joints can often reduce inflammation, relieve pain, and result in a more stable and functional foot.[28] For example, supporting the heel and arch to limit pronation can decrease pain and inflammation of the midfoot and subtalar joints.

It is important to note that pedorthic care for ulcers is intended strictly as a long-term management technique for maintaining healed ulcers and preventing further ulceration; it is not generally considered an appropriate treatment or healing measure for open ulcers.[6, 19, 26] Therefore, in this chapter, when referring to ulcers, it is always with the understanding that pedorthic care for ulcers is limited to maintenance and prevention after healing.

Achieving Proper Shoe Fit

To meet the objectives in the pedorthic care of the diabetic foot, one must begin with a properly fitting shoe. The excessive pressure and friction from poorly fitting shoes can lead to blisters, calluses, and ulcers in the insensitive foot.[3, 7, 8, 19] In this section, the two basic components of shoe fit, that is, shape and size, as well as guidelines for proper shoe fit are discussed.

Shoe Shape

Proper shoe fit is attained when shoe shape is matched to foot shape.[10, 25] The shape of a shoe, including the shape of both the sole and the upper, is dependent on the *last,* the mold over which the shoe is made. The standard last is the single, basic shoe shape from which most mass-produced shoes are made. Prescription footwear, on the other hand, are made over a variety of last shapes: examples include the combination last, which has a narrower heel than the standard last; the inflare last, which provides more medial fore- foot surface area; and the in-depth last, which is shaped to allow extra volume for the foot inside the shoe and provides enough room for a generic insole or a custom orthosis.

Specific parts of the shoe upper also affect shoe fit. Terms useful in describing the shoe upper are (1) *counter,* the part of the shoe extending around the heel; (2) *toe box,* the part that covers the toe area; (3) *vamp,* the part that covers the instep; and (4) *throat,* the part at the bottom of the laces. These, along with other important parts of a shoe, are illustrated in Figure 34–1.

The counter controls the heel and determines heel fit. Strong counters are necessary to adequately control the foot inside the shoe.[7, 10] A shoe that has a high toe box and a rounded, or oblique, toe provides the best fit by allowing the toes to fit comfortably inside the shoe. A shoe with a tapered toe box or a pointed toe is therefore inappropriate for the diabetic foot, because it applies pressure to the toes and forces them into an unnatural shape, leading to calluses, ulcers, and eventual deformity.[7, 8] As with the toe box, the vamp should be high enough to prevent pressure on the instep. A shoe with laces is best for the diabetic foot because laces provide the adjustability needed for any edema or other deformities and allow the shoe to be fit properly without any danger of it slipping off. Pumps and slip-ons often have virtually no vamp, so that they must be fitted

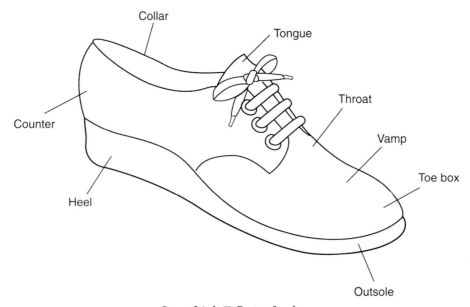

Figure 34–1 ■ Parts of a shoe.

too snugly or they will fall off. Of the two types of throat openings, the blucher is preferred over the balmoral because it allows for greater adjustability, easier entry, and is more compliant to foot shape (Fig. 34–2).[10, 14, 25]

Shoe Size

Once the properly shaped shoe has been found, the next step is to determine the proper size. There are three essential measurements in determining shoe size: overall foot length (heel to toe), arch length (heel to arch, or first metatarsal), and width. The proper shoe size is the one that accommodates the first metatarsophalangeal joint (i.e., the widest part of the foot) in the widest part of the shoe; it is for this reason that shoes must be fit by arch length rather than by overall foot length.[10, 14, 25] The feet in Figure 34–3 have the same overall foot length but require different size shoes because of the difference in arch length.

Guidelines for Proper Shoe Fit

The following is a set of guidelines that can be used to achieve proper shoe fit.[1, 10, 14, 25]

1. Measure both feet with an appropriate measuring device; the Brannock measuring device is recommended. Measure both length and width.
2. Remember that shoe sizes are not standard; they vary among brands and styles. Look in a size range, based on the results of measuring.
3. Fit shoes on both feet while weight-bearing.
4. Check for the proper position of the first metatarsophalangeal joint. It should be in the widest part of the shoe.
5. Check for the correct toe length. Allow ⅜ to ½ inch between the end of the shoe and the longest toe.
6. Check for the proper width, allowing adequate room across the ball of the foot.
7. Look for a snug fit around the heel.
8. Determine that proper fit over the instep has been achieved by an appropriately high vamp, preferably with laces to allow adjustability.

A properly fitting shoe is absolutely essential for the diabetic foot, especially if there has been any loss of sensation or previous instances of callusing, ulceration, or deformity, to prevent recurrence or further damage.[3, 7, 8] The patient with a loss of sensation

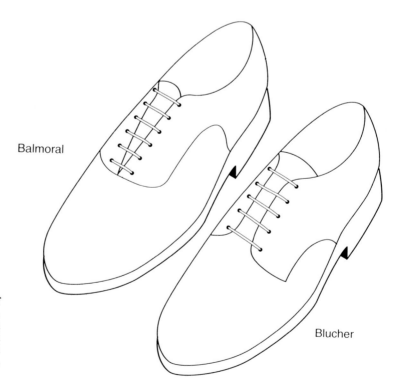

Figure 34–2 ■ The two types of throat openings. *Left,* Balmoral. *Right,* Blucher. (Redrawn from Rossi WA, Tennant R: Professional Shoe Fitting. New York: National Shoe Retailers Association, 1984, with permission.)

Balmoral

Blucher

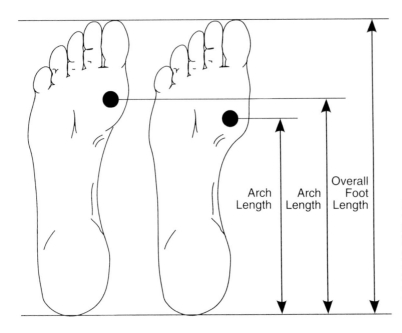

Figure 34–3 ■ Overall foot length versus arch length. These feet have the same overall foot length, but the foot on the left would require a larger size shoe because it has a longer arch length. (Redrawn from Rossi WA, Tennant R: Professional Shoe Fitting. New York: National Shoe Retailers Association, 1984, with permission.)

will tend to purchase a shoe that is too tight; the size that feels right is often too small because of the loss of sensation.[3, 12, 19, 28] It is highly recommended that shoe fitting for these patients be done by a certified pedorthist or professionally trained shoe fitter.

Prescription Footwear for the Diabetic Foot

For patients in the early stages of diabetes who have no history of foot problems and no signs of neuropathy, a properly fitted shoe made of soft materials with a shock-absorbing sole may be all that is necessary. However, for many patients the objectives listed previously can be achieved only with the use of prescription footwear. The following modalities are discussed in this section: (1) healing shoes and appliances, (2) in-depth shoes, (3) external shoe modifications, (4) TCOs, and (5) custom-made shoes.

Healing Shoes and Appliances

Immediately following surgery or other trauma, or in the case of healing ulcers, the presence of swelling, edema, or bulky dressings may necessitate the use of some type of healing shoe or appliance before a regular in-depth or custom-made shoe can be worn.

In this section, five types of healing shoes and appliances are covered.[14] (See Chapter 14.)

Heat-Moldable Healing Shoe

Made from a nylon-covered moldable polyethylene foam, this closed-toe, soft, extra-wide healing shoe can be molded directly to the patient's foot (Fig. 34–4). It also has a

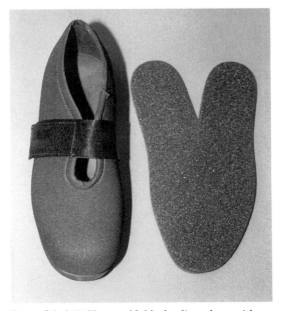

Figure 34–4 ■ Heat-moldable healing shoe, with removable Plastazote insoles.

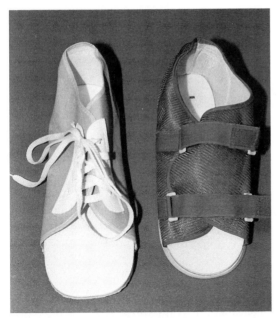

Figure 34–5 ■ Postoperative shoes. *Left,* Canvas upper with lace closure. *Right,* Nylon mesh upper with Velcro closure.

removable Plastazote insole, a Velcro strap or lace closure, and a crepe sole. It is commonly used following amputation or skin grafting but can be used whenever a soft, flexible, accommodative healing shoe is needed. These healing shoes are also available with leather covers for a more durable, permanent shoe.

Postoperative Shoe

This shoe is generally open-toed, with uppers made of canvas or nylon mesh; the upper may be padded for additional comfort (Fig. 34–5). It has a wide forefoot opening with either Velcro straps or lace closures and can accommodate extreme swelling and the bulkiest dressings. The postoperative shoe can be made with a flexible crepe sole, but is most often found with a more rigid sole made of firm crepe or lightweight wood. This is particularly helpful for allowing ambulation while limiting motion.

Negative Heel Shoe

Designed to provide extreme forefoot relief by transferring the patient's weight to the heel area, the negative heel shoe (Fig. 34–6) can be used for wound healing of metatarsal and distal toe ulcers. The padded insole lies on top of a hard polyurethane sole, and this type of healing shoe may or may not have a foot bed under the forefoot. It has Velcro closures to allow for adjustability and is available in multiple sizes.

Heel Relief Shoe

Similar in construction to the negative heel shoe, the heel relief shoe (Fig. 34–7) is designed instead to provide extreme heel relief by suspending the heel and eliminating all weight-bearing from the heel area. It can be used for wound healing of calcaneal ulcers.

Controlled Ankle Motion Device

For the patient who can be mobile but must maintain a fixed ankle position or limited ankle motion, the controlled ankle motion device can provide the necessary stability and support while allowing a comfortable, natural gait pattern. This appliance is essentially a postoperative shoe to which medial-lateral uprights and a posterior Achilles plate have been added (Fig. 34–8). The foot

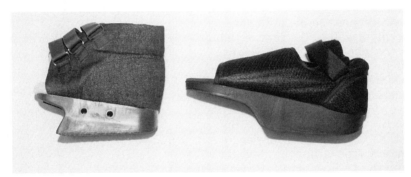

Figure 34–6 ■ Negative heel shoes. *Left,* Without foot bed under the forefoot. *Right,* With foot bed under the forefoot.

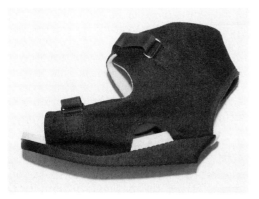

Figure 34–7 ■ Heel relief shoe.

and ankle are held in place with wide Velcro straps, and the ankle joint may be held in a fixed position or allowed to move within a limited range of motion. A cushioned liner provides pressure relief, and a rocker sole allows a natural walking gait. The use of a total-contact orthosis inside a controlled ankle motion device can be used for wound healing as an alternative to total-contact casting, allowing the patient easier access to view, dress, and bathe the wound.[2]

In-Depth Shoes

The majority of diabetic footwear prescriptions begin with the in-depth shoe. It is generally a blucher-style oxford or athletic shoe with an additional ¼ to ½ inch of depth throughout the shoe. This provides the extra volume needed to accommodate both the foot and a TCO, a special insole custom made to fit the exact contours of the individual foot. The additional depth is also useful in accommodating deformities associated with the diabetic foot, such as hammer toes and claw toes, as well as moderate medial and lateral bony prominences resulting from Charcot deformities.[3, 12]

Other features common to in-depth shoes that are especially useful in the care of the diabetic foot include their light-weight, shock-absorbing soles and strong counters. In-depth shoes are made with a variety of upper materials, including deerskin and cowhide; some have a heat-moldable lining material that allows the upper to be molded to the individual foot, especially useful for severe deformities. A new type of in-depth shoe is shaped wider in the midfoot area to accommodate a Charcot deformity. In-depth shoes

also come in a wide range of shapes and sizes to accommodate almost any foot except those with severe skeletal distortion, and as a greater number of manufacturers become involved, their appearance has steadily improved.

External Shoe Modifications

The outside of the shoe can be modified in a variety of ways.[12] The following external shoe modifications are covered in this section: rocker sole, stabilization, extended steel shank, cushion heel, wedge, and customized upper.

Rocker Sole

The rocker sole is one of the most commonly prescribed shoe modifications. As its name suggests, the basic function of a rocker sole is to literally rock the foot from heel-strike to toe-off without bending the shoe or foot. However, the actual shape of a rocker sole varies according to (1) the patient's specific foot problems and (2) the desired effect of the rocker sole. In general the biomechanical

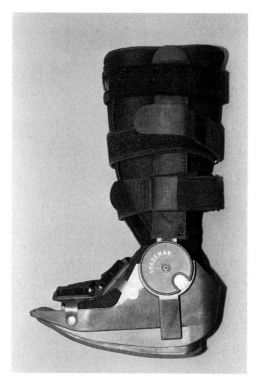

Figure 34–8 ■ Controlled ankle motion device.

effects of a rocker sole are (1) restoring lost motion in the foot, ankle, or both related to pain, deformity, or stiffness, resulting in an overall improvement in gait[12, 28]; and (2) relieving pressure on a specific area of the plantar surface.[12, 22]

There are two terms relevant to a discussion of rocker soles: (1) the *midstance,* or the portion of the rocker sole that is in contact with the floor when in a standing position: and (2) the *apex,* or high point, of the rocker sole, located at the distal end of the midstance. These terms are illustrated in Figure 34–9. It is important to note that the apex must be placed behind any area for which pressure relief is desired. For example, a rocker sole designed to relieve pressure on the metatarsal heads must be made with the apex behind the metatarsal heads.

In general, rocker soles are custom made for each patient; however, the following basic types of rocker soles can be identified:

Mild Rocker Sole. The most widely used and most basic of the rocker soles has a mild rocker angle at both the heel and the toe (Fig. 34–10A). This type of rocker sole can relieve metatarsal pressure and may assist gait by increasing propulsion and reducing the amount of energy expended in walking. It is appropriate for the foot that is not at risk and is typically found on athletic walking shoes. The other types of rocker soles are essentially variations of this basic, mild rocker sole.

Heel-to-Toe Rocker Sole. This type of rocker sole is shaped with a more severe angle at both the heel and the toe (Fig. 34–10B). It is intended to aid propulsion at toe-off, decrease heel-strike forces on the cal-

caneus, and reduce the need for ankle motion. The heel-to-toe rocker sole may be indicated for patients with a fixed claw toe or rigid hammer toe, midfoot amputation, or calcaneal ulcers.

Toe-Only Rocker Sole. As the name suggests, the toe-only rocker sole has a rocker angle only at the toe, with the midstance extending to the back end of the sole (Fig. 34–10C). The purpose of this type of rocker sole is to increase weight-bearing proximal to the metatarsal heads, to provide a stable midstance, and to reduce the need for toe dorsiflexion on toe-off. Indications for the toe-only rocker sole include hallux rigidus, callus, or ulcer on the distal portion of a claw, hammer, or mallet toe and metatarsal ulcers.

Severe Angle Rocker Sole. This type of rocker sole also has a rocker angle only at the toe, but it is a much more severe angle than that found on the toe-only rocker sole (Fig. 34–10D). The purpose of the severe rocker angle at the toe is to eliminate the weight-bearing forces anterior to the metatarsal heads. It is indicated for extreme relief of ulcerated metatarsal heads.

Negative Heel Rocker Sole. Shaped with a rocker angle at the toe and a negative heel, this type of rocker sole results in the patient's heel being at the same height or lower than the ball of the foot when in a standing position (Fig. 34–10E). The purpose of the negative heel rocker sole is to accommodate a foot that is fixed in dorsiflexion or to relieve forefoot pressure by shifting it to the hindfoot and midfoot. Its indications include an ankle that is fixed in dorsiflexion, prominent metatarsal heads with extreme ulcers or callus-

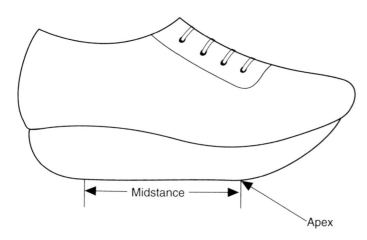

Figure 34–9 ■ Rocker sole, illustrating midstance and apex.

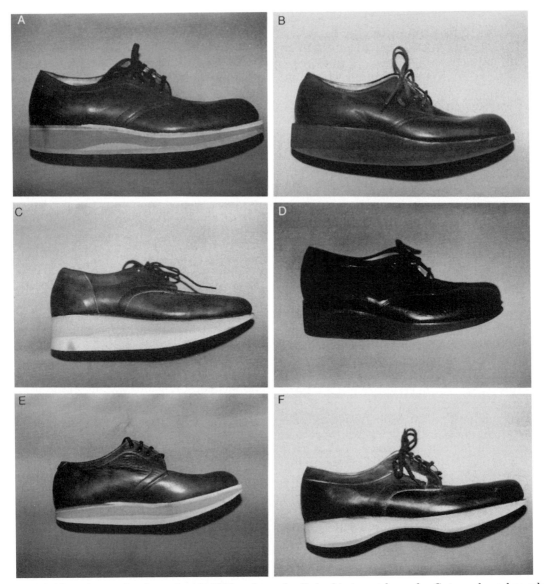

Figure 34–10 ■ Types of rocker soles. *A,* Mild rocker sole; *B,* heel-to-toe rocker sole; *C,* toe-only rocker sole; *D,* severe angle rocker sole; *E,* negative heel rocker sole; *F,* double rocker sole.

ing, and distal toe ulcers. Also, because forefoot pressure relief is accomplished through the use of a negative heel, the depth or height of the sole itself can be minimized, thereby increasing overall stability of the shoe. It is therefore indicated for patients who feel unstable with the normal height of a rocker sole. The negative heel rocker sole is to be used with caution, however, because inability to attain the necessary ankle dorsiflexion will cause discomfort and may increase pressure on the problem area.

Double Rocker Sole. This type of rocker sole is a mild rocker sole with a section of the sole removed in the midfoot area, thereby giving the appearance of two rocker soles—one at the hindfoot and one at the forefoot—and two areas of midstance (Fig. 34–10*F*). Because the thinnest area of the double rocker sole is at the midfoot, it is used to relieve a specific midfoot problem area, such as a midfoot prominence associated with a rocker bottom foot or a Charcot foot deformity.

Clearly, there are many types of rocker soles, and each must be individualized for a given patient's foot condition and the desired effect. A poorly or improperly designed rocker sole can actually worsen the problem it was supposed to help correct. When a rocker sole is prescribed, it is essential that the physician clearly specify the desired effect or purpose of the rocker sole. A certified pedorthist is trained to know which type of rocker sole will best achieve that purpose. The pedorthist will also take measurements, obtain floor reaction imprints, and provide follow-up care to make sure that the rocker sole is performing properly for the individual patient.

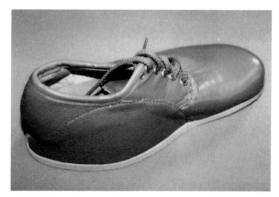

Figure 34–12 ■ Medial stabilizer.

Stabilization

A second type of external shoe modification involves the addition of material to the medial or lateral portion of the shoe to stabilize some part of the foot.

Flare. A flare is an extension to the heel of the shoe, the sole, or both (Fig. 34–11). Flares can be medial or lateral, and their purpose is to stabilize a hindfoot, midfoot, or forefoot instability. For example, a medial heel flare might be used to support a foot with a fixed valgus heel deformity.

Stabilizer. A stabilizer is an extension added to the side of the shoe, including both the

sole and upper (Fig. 34–12). Made from rigid foam or crepe, a stabilizer provides more extensive stabilization than a flare and is used for more severe medial or lateral instability of the hindfoot or midfoot, for example, with a medially collapsed Charcot foot. Before a stabilizer is added, the patient must wear the shoe for a few weeks until it is "broken in" (i.e., has taken on the shape of the deformed foot). Adding a stabilizer to a new shoe can lead to serious skin breakdown in the diabetic foot.

Extended Steel Shank

An extended steel shank is a strip of spring steel inserted between the layers of the sole, extending from the heel to the toe of the shoe (Fig. 34–13). New, lighter weight carbon fiber materials are also available for this modi-

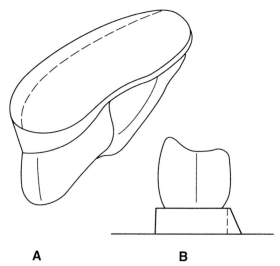

A   **B**

Figure 34–11 ■ Lateral flare. A, Plantar view, B, Posterior view.

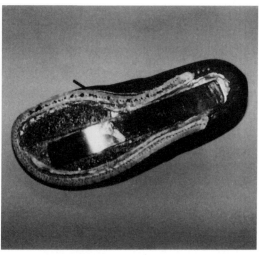

Figure 34–13 ■ Extended steel shank.

fication. It is most commonly used in combination with a rocker sole and helps maintain the shape and effectiveness of the rocker sole. An extended steel shank can also prevent the shoe from bending, limit toe and midfoot motion, aid propulsion on toe-off, and strengthen the entire shoe and sole. It is indicated for hallux limitus or rigidus, limited ankle motion, and more proximal partial foot amputations.

Cushion Heel

A cushion heel consists of a wedge of shock-absorbing material layered into the heel area of the shoe (Fig. 34–14). Its purpose is to provide a maximum amount of shock absorption under the heel (in addition to that provided by a total-contact orthosis) while maintaining a stable stance. It is indicated for calcaneal ulcers or for a rigid ankle and hindfoot as a result of Charcot deformity.

Wedge

A wedge of sole material is sometimes added medially or laterally to the heel of the sole or to both the heel and sole (Fig. 34–15). It can be inserted between the upper and the sole or added directly to the bottom of the shoe to redirect the weight-bearing position of the foot. A wedge is also useful in stabilizing a flexible deformity in a corrected position or in accommodating a fixed deformity (by essentially bringing the ground to the foot). A medial wedge is indicated in cases of extreme pronation, whereas a lateral wedge can be used for ankle instability or a varus heel deformity.

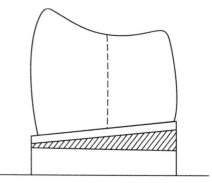

Figure 34–15 ■ Lateral wedge, inserted between the upper and the sole.

Customized Upper

Occasionally, to accommodate a severe or unusual (but often localized) foot deformity, it becomes necessary to make a shoe modification that does not fit into any of the previous categories. By use of a customized shoe upper, the patient whose foot will otherwise fit into a stock in-depth shoe can avoid the expense and delay associated with a custom-made shoe. A Charcot foot deformity is a good example of the type that might require a customized upper. For example, Figure 34–16 shows a shoe with a custom-molded lateral "pocket" designed to accommodate a severe Charcot deformity. Another type of customized upper, for patients who have difficulty tying their shoes, is the addition of a Velcro opening that maintains the appearance of shoelaces (Fig. 34–17).

Total-Contact Orthosis

The TCO is a special insole that is custom made over a model of the patient's foot, thereby achieving "total contact" with the plantar surface of the foot, using the same total contact concept as the total-contact cast (see Chapter 13). The TCO is composed of a *shell,* the layer of material next to the foot and in total contact with the foot, and the *posting,* the material that fills in the space between the shell and the shoe (Fig. 34–18). A properly designed TCO can achieve the objectives for pedorthic care of the diabetic foot in the following ways[11]:

1. Relieve areas of excessive plantar pressure by evenly distributing pressure over the entire plantar surface.

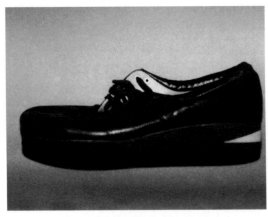

Figure 34–14 ■ Cushion heel.

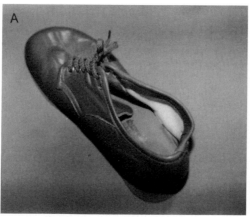
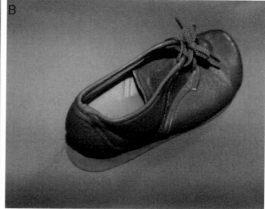

Figure 34–16 ■ Two views of custom-molded lateral "pocket" designed to accommodate a severe Charcot deformity. Notice that this shoe has also been stretched for a hammer toe deformity.

2. Reduce shock through the use of shock-absorbing materials in the TCO.
3. Reduce shear, because the total contact minimizes horizontal and vertical foot movement.
4. Accommodate deformities with the use of soft, moldable materials in the TCO's shell.
5. Stabilize and support deformities with the use of more rigid, supportive materials in the posting.
6. Limit the motion of joints, also through the use of supportive materials.

Recent studies report the effectiveness of custom-molded TCOs in relieving plantar pressure.[17, 21] It is important to note that even though premade insoles may provide some degree of shock absorption, they cannot fulfill the other objectives because of the absence of total contact.

Design and Fabrication

For a TCO to accomplish the desired objectives, it should be designed and fabricated by an experienced professional who can:

1. Understand and evaluate the biomechanics of the lower limb.
2. Identify areas of excessive plantar pressure.
3. Utilize the appropriate impression techniques.
4. Select the appropriate TCO materials.

A certified pedorthist is an ideal choice, having been trained in all of these areas. In addition, a detailed diagnosis and explanation of the desired function of the TCO from the prescribing physician are essential.

Evaluation of Lower Limb Biomechanics. The position and relationship of the hindfoot,

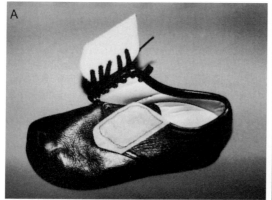
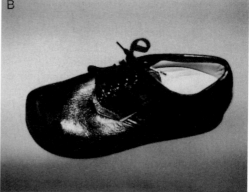

Figure 34–17 ■ A, Customized Velcro opening addition. B, When closed, the shoe maintains the appearance of shoelaces.

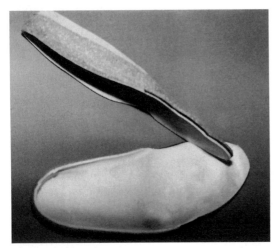

Figure 34–18 ▪ Multiple-layer total-contact orthosis. This TCO has a polyethylene foam shell, a middle layer of micropore rubber, and cork posting.

midfoot, and forefoot is simple yet critical information to be obtained. For example, a patient with valgus heels may have compensatory deformities on weight-bearing, such as varus forefeet; this must be taken into consideration when the TCO is designed.[11]

The range of motion in the joints of the lower limb must also be evaluated. Ankle dorsiflexion and plantar flexion, as well as limited or fixed inversion or eversion, are important to observe. The midtarsal joints must be evaluated in terms of dorsiflexion and plantar flexion and pronation and supination. Range of motion in the metatarsophalangeal and phalangeal joints also needs to be noted, including clawed toes, hammer toes, mallet toes, and dropped metatarsal heads. Limited range of motion in any of these joints will have an impact on TCO design. For example, a fixed forefoot varus deformity that is not properly accommodated will result in excessive pressure being exerted on the lateral border of the foot with resultant strain in the midfoot area.

Finally, it is important that any examination of lower limb biomechanics be done in both static and dynamic states.[16] Because the TCO must accommodate the foot while sitting, standing, and walking, the changes that these activities produce in the foot must be determined.

Identification of Areas of Excessive Plantar Pressure. Areas of excessive plantar pressure need to be defined so that they can be relieved by proper TCO design. This evaluation should begin with a physical examination of the plantar surface of the foot, looking for calluses, blisters, ulcers, red spots, or any other indications of excessive pressure or shear. The examination should also identify bony prominences, such as depressed metatarsal heads, or bony deformity, such as a varus heel, associated with areas of soft tissue breakdown.

In addition to a physical examination of the foot, areas of excessive plantar pressure can be identified through more objective means, such as the Harris mat floor reaction system.[11, 28] It consists of a rubber grid with ridges at three different heights. Ink is applied to the mat, and as the patient stands or walks over it, the ridges collapse under varying amounts of weight, thereby identifying areas of high pressure by the intensity of the ink impression on the underlying paper. Newer, more costly methods for evaluating plantar pressure use computerized force plate systems that provide detailed maps of the plantar surface, with quantitative measurements of plantar pressure. Either of these methods provides valuable information in determining the areas of high pressure that the TCO design must relieve.

Foot Impression Techniques. As noted earlier, the TCO is made from a model of the patient's foot. There are five principal techniques used to take a foot impression, with the choice of technique determined by (1) the results of the biomechanical and pressure evaluations described earlier and (2) the desired function of the TCO. In terms of function, two basic types can be identified[11, 16]: (1) *accommodative,* whose primary function is to accommodate a fixed deformity or one that places the foot particularly at risk; and (2) *functional,* which is designed to control a flexible deformity by providing support and stability. The function of the TCO depends on the specific foot condition. Many TCOs for the diabetic foot are both accommodative and functional to some degree. Foot impression techniques include the following[11, 16]:

Plaster Cast. A traditional plaster cast is applied to the foot, similar to the process of total-contact casting. This technique, when the foot is maintained in a neutral position, is useful when the purpose of the TCO is primarily functional. It is also especially useful for a very complicated foot, such as an amputation or severe deformity, because the moldability of the plaster provides greater detail.

Wax. A thin sheet of wax is heated in warm water and then molded to the foot. This procedure gives a good, clean impression and is a general purpose technique that can be used for both functional and accommodative TCOs.

Sand and Wax. This technique is similar to the wax procedure, but as the sheet of wax is being molded to the foot, the patient stands in a tray of fine silica sand. As a consequence, the soft tissue is compressed, and the resulting TCO will be especially effective in relieving bony prominences.

Foam Box. The patient's foot is pushed into a box of crushable rigid foam, or the impression can be taken with the patient weight-bearing. This technique is best used when the TCO is to be completely accommodative and results in a TCO with passive support and maximum accommodation.

Computerized Scanning. This technique bypasses the process of taking a foot impression and making a model of the foot. Instead the foot itself is electronically scanned. The TCO provider is therefore required to have a computerized foot scanning system in his or her office. The foot is electronically scanned, and the digital model created by the computer is sent to a computerized milling device that fabricates the TCO. This milling device may or may not be at the provider's office; the digital model of the foot can be sent via computer modem to any orthotics laboratory that has a compatible milling device. The advantages of using this technology are numerous: elimination of the impression process, faster turnaround time, and increased accuracy. However, the scanning systems can be cost prohibitive for many providers.

Selection of Appropriate TCO Materials. As with impression techniques, the selection of materials for the TCO is determined by its desired function. Total-contact orthosis materials can be described in terms of their function and can be divided into three types[11, 16]:

Soft. Cross-linked polyethylene foams are the most common soft materials currently in use. They are made by a large number of manufacturers and are rapidly being developed and improved. Generally they are moldable with application of heat (120° to 150°C)

and come in a variety of densities. Their function is accommodative, and they are used close to the foot (i.e., in the shell). Studies show, however, that they decrease in thickness quickly, a phenomenon referred to as "bottoming out."[5] Soft, nonmoldable materials such as closed-cell expanded rubber and polyurethane foam are accommodative but do not bottom out so quickly as moldable polyethylene. They often are used in conjunction with a moldable foam to provide an additional soft layer of shock absorption with minimal bottoming out.

Semiflexible. Leather and cork fall into this category. Many of the cork materials are being combined with plastic compounds to make them moldable when heated. Semiflexible materials are somewhat accommodative but provide more functional support than the soft type and do not bottom out as quickly.

Rigid. Acrylic plastics and thermoplastic polymers are considered rigid materials. They are moldable at very high temperatures and are primarily functional. They are the most durable and most supportive of the three types.

To provide maximum moldability (essential for total contact) along with the necessary shock absorption and control, a TCO for the diabetic foot should generally be made from a combination of materials.[5, 11, 28] A triple-layer molded TCO can offer the needed combination of accommodative and functional properties. This type of TCO would consist of the following:

1. Top layer (shell): soft, moldable polyethylene foam.
2. Middle layer: closed cell neoprene rubber or a urethane polymer for long-lasting shock absorption.
3. Bottom layer (posting): cork, or possibly a denser polyethylene foam, for control.

The specific materials used for each layer can vary according to the needs of the individual patient.

Custom-Made Shoes

When extremely severe deformities are present, it may be that the foot cannot be fit with an in-depth shoe, even with extensive modifications. In these instances, a custom-made shoe, constructed from a cast or model of the patient's foot, is required. These cases are rare, but can include severe Charcot foot deformities and partial foot amputations.

Another type of custom-made shoe used more commonly for patients with diabetes is the custom-made sandal (Fig. 34–19). Made from multiple layers of polyethylene foam, with nylon straps and Velcro closures, the custom-made sandal has multiple uses: as a slipper, a shower or pool shoe, or as an interim shoe to be worn after wound healing and before a regular shoe can be worn. The custom-made sandal can even be dressed up with leather and worn as a regular sandal for casual wear.

Applications

In this section, pedorthic care for the following problems associated with the diabetic foot are considered: ulcers, amputations, and Charcot joints and deformities. After the treatment objectives are identified, appropriate prescription footwear recommendations are made, including shoes, external shoe modifications, and TCOs. Most patients will not require all of the prescription footwear modalities described. Depending on the individual foot, the severity of the problems, and the degree of deformity, any or all of the footwear recommendations may be used. The use of in-depth shoes is recommended for all of the following unless otherwise indicated.

Ulcers

As noted earlier in the chapter, pedorthic care for ulcers is intended strictly as a long-term management technique for maintaining healed areas and preventing further ulceration. Appropriate prescription footwear is considered an important factor in this effort, particularly in the insensate foot.[3, 8, 19] Two recent studies demonstrate the effectiveness of in-depth shoes with orthoses in preventing reulceration.[24, 27]

Plantar Ulcers

Objectives. The objectives in the pedorthic management of plantar ulcers are (1) even distribution of plantar pressure by transfer from areas of high pressure, such as the metatarsal heads, to areas of lower pressure; (2) shock absorption; (3) reduction of friction and shear; (4) limiting of joint motion; and (5) accommodation of deformities.

Shoes. Proper shoe fit is essential in maintaining healed plantar areas and preventing further ulceration. It is crucial that the shape of the shoe match the shape of the foot to limit overall pressure on the foot, to eliminate any particular high-pressure areas, and to accommodate any deformities. A shoe with a heat-moldable upper may be required for more severe deformities or in cases of mismated feet.

Other important characteristics for a shoe used in the pedorthic management of plantar ulcers include (1) a long medial counter to control the heel and medial arch and to decrease shear forces; (2) a blucher opening to allow easy entry into the shoe; (3) a shock-absorbing sole to reduce impact shock; and (4) a low heel to decrease pressure on the metatarsal heads and the toes.

External Shoe Modifications. Addition of an appropriate rocker sole will aid in reducing overall pressure and impact shock; it will also limit motion of the joints and improve the weight-bearing transfer. Adding an extended steel shank will enhance the effects of the rocker sole. A negative heel rocker sole may be used for additional reduction of pressure and impact shock on the forefoot.

TCOs. The use of a TCO can be quite effective in the distribution and transfer of plantar pressure and in reduction or elimination of weight-bearing in problem areas. A TCO is also useful in stabilizing or restricting joint motion. To provide the maximum moldability essential for achieving total contact, along with the necessary shock absorption and con-

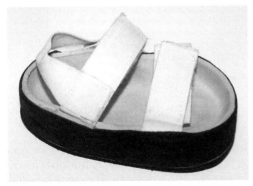

Figure 34–19 ▪ Custom-made sandal.

trol, a multiple-layer TCO is generally preferred.

Dorsal Ulcers

Objectives. Prescription footwear for dorsal ulcers should reduce friction and shear, accommodate any deformities and, most important, reduce pressure from the shoe upper.

Shoes. With dorsal ulcers, proper fit of the shoe upper is especially important. It should be made of a soft, pliable material such as deerskin; heat-moldable uppers may be necessary for more severe deformities. The upper should also be free of unnecessary seams or designs in the toe area to minimize the possibility of skin irritation. A blucher opening allows easier entry, especially if a hammer toe deformity is present, and a low heel will prevent the foot from sliding forward in the shoe.

External Shoe Modifications. The primary modification for dorsal ulcers is the stretching or molding of the shoe upper to accommodate deformities and reduce pressure in specific problem areas. For particularly severe deformities, a part of the shoe upper can be cut out and replaced with a moldable "pocket" (see Fig. 34–16).

TCOs. A TCO with a metatarsal pad can be especially helpful for dorsal ulcers on flexible hammer toes. The metatarsal pad aids in relaxing the hammer toe deformity, allowing the toes to extend slightly and reduce the possibility of pressure from the shoe upper.

Partial Foot Amputations

Prescription footwear for several types of amputations are covered in this section: toe, ray, transmetatarsal, tarsometatarsal (Lisfranc), and midtarsal (Chopart). Although the pedorthic care for each type of amputation is different, several objectives are common to all amputations:

1. *Provide shoe filler.* Unless the amputation is extensive and a custom-made or shortened shoe is used, some type of shoe filler is needed for the portion of the foot that has been amputated. In most cases, the filler can be incorporated into the TCO.
2. *Equalize weight-bearing.* Amputation of a portion of the foot will often result in uneven patterns of weight-bearing on the remaining foot. Just as with the intact diabetic foot, any areas of excessive pressure must be eliminated and even distribution of weight-bearing maintained.
3. *Protect and accommodate remaining portion of the foot.* Because the occurrence of an amputation implies severe foot problems, special care must be taken to protect and accommodate the remaining portion of an at-risk foot. The presence of skin grafts, scar tissue, or other postsurgical complications must also be taken into consideration when one is providing prescription footwear for a foot that has undergone partial amputation.
4. *Improve gait.* When part of the foot has been amputated, a natural gait pattern is no longer possible. The addition of an appropriate type of rocker sole can often improve the gait pattern after an amputation.

The proper shoe for a partially amputated foot is determined by the extent of the amputation. If the metatarsal heads remain intact, shoe size does not change. Only when one or more metatarsal heads have been removed can the patient be fit with a shorter (i.e., smaller size) shoe.

Toe and Ray Amputations

Objectives. The first three of the objectives stated earlier are the most relevant to toe and ray amputations; depending on the extent of the amputation, gait may not be significantly affected. A shoe filler can help to minimize drifting of the remaining toes, which is particularly important after a great toe amputation. In the case of a ray amputation, especially the first ray, the removal of one or more metatarsal heads results in increased pressure on the remaining heads; it is therefore important to maintain even distribution of weight-bearing to protect the remaining metatarsal heads.[18]

Shoes. As indicated earlier, shoe size after a toe amputation does not change because the metatarsal heads remain intact. Even after a ray amputation, where one or more metatarsals have been removed, a well-constructed shoe filler can usually allow the patient to wear a full shoe. Other important shoe features include a strong medial counter for stability, especially if the first ray has been removed, and a soft, moldable upper to protect and accommodate the remaining foot.

External Shoe Modifications. Many shoes for toe and ray amputations do not require external modifications; however, possible modifications include a rocker sole with an extended steel shank (to improve gait and protect remaining metatarsal heads) and a flare (for additional stability, especially if more than one ray has been removed).

TCOs. After removal of one or more toes, those remaining have a tendency to drift out of position. The use of a TCO with a filler will help to maintain the position of the remaining toes; it can also equalize weight-bearing, thereby eliminating excessive pressure on the remaining toes and metatarsals.

Transmetatarsal Amputation

Objectives. The shoe filler provided for the amputated portion of the forefoot will help prevent creasing of the shoe at the point of amputation, avoiding breakdown and eventual collapse of the shoe. A filler can also help control the remaining foot inside the shoe, decrease soft tissue shear at its distal end, and often eliminate the need for a costly, less cosmetically appealing custom-made shoe. Equalizing weight-bearing is especially important after a transmetatarsal amputation.

Shoes. A shoe with a blucher opening and a long medial counter can best control the remaining foot and help decrease soft tissue shear. The upper should be made of a soft, moldable leather to accommodate and protect the remaining foot. A custom-made shoe is generally not necessary with a transmetatarsal amputation because enough of the foot remains to keep a shoe on with the aid of a filler; however, a smaller size shoe may be appropriate if the patient finds it cosmetically acceptable.

External Shoe Modifications. An extended steel shank in conjunction with an appropriate rocker sole can reduce pressure and impact shock while aiding propulsion and reducing the amount of shoe distortion. The use of a cushion heel will further minimize impact shock. Medial and lateral flares may be added to stabilize and control the amputated foot and decrease shear.

TCOs. A TCO with a filler will help to stabilize or restrict joint motion, accommodate bony prominences and deformities, decrease shear and shoe distortion, and equalize weight-bearing. Socks are now available that are especially made for use following a transmetatarsal amputation, which may also be helpful in protecting and accommodating the remaining foot.

Tarsometatarsal and Midtarsal Amputations

Objectives. In addition to the objectives already listed, pedorthic care for a tarsometatarsal or midtarsal amputation should also be concerned with containing the remaining foot inside the shoe and preventing equinus contracture.

Shoes. A high-top shoe is best after this type of amputation because it can most effectively contain the foot in the shoe and provide the control necessary to prevent equinus contracture. A strong counter can also aid in providing control while improving medial and lateral stability. A wedge sole will provide a broader base of support, and a shorter shoe size will decrease the resistance to roll-over on toe-off and aid in propulsion. For the smaller remaining foot, a custom-made shoe will best meet the treatment objectives by providing total accommodation of the foot.

External Shoe Modifications. An extended steel shank and appropriate rocker sole are needed to decrease shock impact, decrease shoe distortion, and aid in propulsion. A medial or lateral flare can improve stability and weight bearing. Because a smaller area must assume the weight that would normally be spread out over the entire foot, the use of a cushion heel will reduce shock at heel strike and further improve gait.

TCOs. A TCO with any necessary filler will give maximum accommodation and protection of the remaining foot while stabilizing or restricting joint motion. A TCO will also decrease shear, decrease shoe distortion, and equalize weight-bearing. Further protection of the remaining foot is made possible with the use of a custom-made sock.

As an alternative to incorporating the shoe filler into the TCO, a Chopart filler boot with a built-in shoe filler may be used. This orthotic device is made of leather, laces up the ankle, and resembles a high-top boot without a sole. Made to fit inside the patient's shoe, it offers additional control and helps maintain medial and lateral stability without the need for a high-top shoe.

Charcot Joints and Deformities

Objectives. The objectives in pedorthic care of Charcot joints and deformities are (1) to accommodate fixed or flexible deformities, (2) to restrict or control unstable or painful joint motions, (3) to relieve or transfer pressure, and (4) to improve gait patterns.

Shoes. The proper shoe for midfoot Charcot joint deformities will be wide in the midfoot region to accommodate the collapsed midfoot. The extra width will also reduce or eliminate pressure on any bony prominences and provide a good base of support for the foot. A heat-moldable upper may be necessary to accommodate deformities and relieve pressure. A blucher opening allows for easy entry of the foot into the shoe and will help control the foot, decrease shear, and accommodate edema. Further control and reduction of shear are accomplished with a long medial counter while a shock-absorbing sole will reduce plantar pressure and shock. For severe deformities, such as a rocker bottom foot or extreme angulation or displacement of any part of the foot, a custom-made shoe will be necessary.

External Shoe Modifications. A sole and heel flare (medial or lateral as appropriate) can help to stabilize the Charcot deformity by providing a broader base of support, by reducing medial or lateral tilt, and by minimizing ligament strain. For the more severe deformity, such as a collapsed foot, a stabilizer can provide additional support and improve weight-bearing. A properly designed rocker sole can assist in immobilizing unstable, damaged joints; it can also decrease midfoot pressure and strain, decrease impact shock, and improve gait.

Modifications to the counter of the shoe can accommodate some of the more severe deformities. A custom-molded addition to the medial or lateral counter, or counter "pocket" (see Fig. 34–16), can be used for extreme medial and lateral deformities in the midfoot and hindfoot regions. For the rocker bottom foot, extending the height of the counter in the rear of the shoe may be necessary to help hold the heel inside the shoe.

TCOs. A TCO with any necessary modifications to accommodate prominences and relieve pressure is an essential component of the pedorthic management of Charcot joints and deformities.

Writing Footwear Prescriptions

A complete written prescription from the physician is necessary to ensure that the certified pedorthist will be able to achieve the desired treatment results. It is often the only communication between the physician and the pedorthist. Even if a patient's footwear needs have been ideally determined in consultation with the physician in a clinic setting, a written prescription becomes a permanent part of the pedorthist's patient records, serving as a valuable resource for providing follow-up care, monitoring patient progress, and obtaining insurance reimbursement.

The written footwear prescription should include the following[15]:

1. *Complete diagnosis.* It is important to provide the patient's complete diagnosis, including both primary and secondary diagnoses. The physician should never rely on the patient to communicate diagnoses to the pedorthist. It is also important that the diagnosis be as specific as possible; for example, a diagnosis of "foot sores" should more appropriately read, "diabetes, peripheral neuropathy, plantar ulcer under third metatarsal head."

2. *Desired effect.* The prescription should include a precise description of the desired effect or function of the footwear. For the previously mentioned diagnosis, this might say, "to relieve pressure on metatarsal heads."

3. *Specific footwear required to produce desired effect.* The physician should give the pedorthist some direction on how to accomplish the desired effect, such as in-depth shoes, external shoe modifications, and TCOs. Because the physician may not be familiar with the specific materials, shoes, construction techniques, or potential modifications, he or she may find it desirable to give the pedorthist some latitude in this area.

Case Studies

The following case studies illustrate the broad range of pedorthic care for the diabetic foot.

Case 1: Plantar Ulcer

A 45-year-old man 6 feet tall and 225 lb, with size 14 feet and a 20-year history of insulin-dependent diabetes, had pes cavus feet with very little remaining fatty tissue, impaired sensation, and a history of numerous ulcers associated with severe callusing under the metatarsal heads (Fig. 34–20A). (The pes cavus foot does not absorb shock well; it puts extreme weight-bearing on the metatarsal heads, which are already at risk because of the lack of fatty tissue and impaired sensation.)

His original prescription was for in-depth shoes and TCOs with a viscoelastic polymer added under the metatarsal heads to provide metatarsal pressure relief. Callus build-up improved somewhat but remained problematic under the first and fourth metatarsal heads. Addition of toe-only rocker soles provided further relief, but hemorrhaging under the first metatarsal calluses continued.

After consultation with the prescribing physician, it was decided that the TCO should be modified by adding posting material to transfer the excessive plantar pressure on the first and fourth metatarsal heads to the second and third. As seen in Figure 34–20B, the new TCO has extreme posting proximal to the metatarsal heads, with plantar pressure transferred to the second and third metatarsal heads. The callus has virtually disappeared since the patient began wearing the new TCO.

Case 2: Complex Plantar Ulcer

This 55-year-old, overweight man (5 feet 6½ inches, 225 lb) had a 15-year history of insulin-dependent diabetes. His vascular insufficiency had been improved with a vein bypass, but peripheral neuropathy had resulted in a completely insensate foot.

Visual examination revealed a severe calcaneal ulcer stretching from the plantar to the posterior part of the heel (Fig. 34–21A). Radiologic examination revealed soft tissue involvement only; no osteomyelitis was present (Fig. 35–21B). The ulcer was treated with total-contact casting, which successfully closed the ulcer, except for a small area that subsequently healed while using a custom Plastazote sandal. Maintaining this healed area was especially challenging because due to a very large deficit and a considerable amount of scar tissue, the heel remained extremely susceptible to breakdown.

The prescription called for a heat-moldable shoe to provide maximum accommodation for this at-risk foot. The shoe was modified with a heel-to-toe rocker sole and, very importantly, a cushion heel to absorb additional shock on heel strike (Fig. 34–21C). With the cushion heel and rocker sole, there was virtually no weight-bearing on the postulcer heel area; significant weight-bearing began at a position that was distal to the heel.

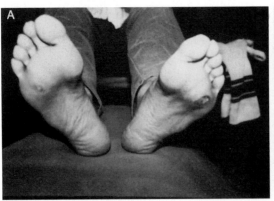 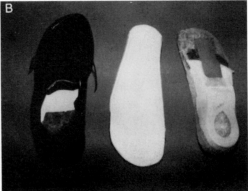

Figure 34–20 ■ Case 1. A, Pes cavus feet with plantar ulcer under left fourth metatarsal head. B, In-depth shoe and TCI with posting to relieve pressure on first and fourth metatarsal heads.

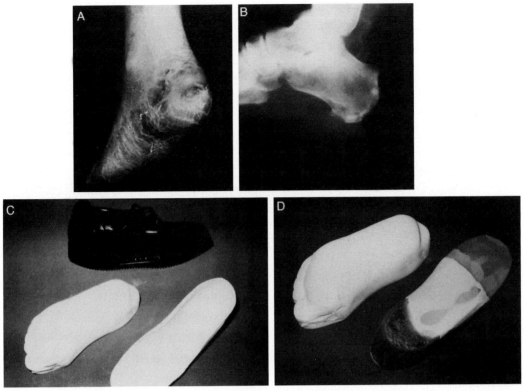

Figure 34–21 ■ Case 2. *A,* Healed calcaneal ulcer. *B,* Radiograph showing absence of osteomyelitis. *C,* Heat-moldable shoe with rocker sole. (TCO and plaster foot model are also shown.) *D,* Plantar view of TCO. Notice the heel deficit in the plaster model used to make the TCO.

A triple-layer TCO served to further protect and accommodate the heel deficit as well as other minor plantar prominences. The shell was made of soft Plastazote, and the deficit area of the heel was filled and supported with a low-density viscoelastic polymer (Fig. 34–21*D*). After 2 years, the patient has no recurrence of ulceration or tissue breakdown.

Case 3: Dorsal Ulcer

A 66-year-old woman with a 19-year history of insulin-dependent diabetes had a chronic dorsal ulcer on her second toe (Fig. 34–22*A*). Her insensate foot had collapsed medially, and she had a dynamic hammer toe deformity (i.e., the deformity worsened while walking).

Her first prescription was for a heat-moldable shoe and TCO. The shoe was stretched as much as possible over the second toe in an attempt to eliminate pressure from the shoe upper, but even after repeated attempts to further stretch the upper, reulceration of the toe occurred. The patient was treated in between shoe-stretching attempts with a custom Plastazote sandal with no pressure on the toes, resulting in rapid healing.

The final solution was to remove all of the moldable lining material from the shoe in the area over the hammer toe. The remaining deerskin was extremely soft and even more stretchable without the lining material (Fig. 34–22*B*). For the past 4 years, there has been no recurrence of the ulcer.

This case illustrates the importance of evaluating the foot dynamically. In most cases the initial stretching of the shoe would probably have been successful, but this patient's toe position changed so dramatically while walking that normal stretching was ineffective in relieving dorsal pressure.

Case 4: Ray Amputation

This 51-year-old man with a 32-year history of insulin-dependent diabetes had periph-

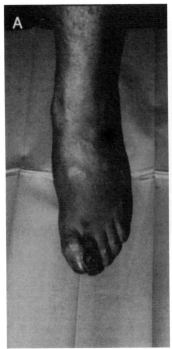
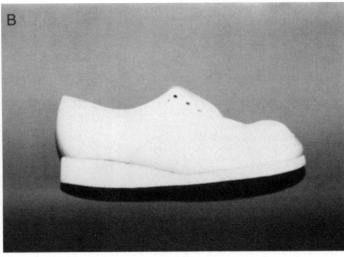

Figure 34–22 ■ Case 3. *A,* Dorsal ulcer on second toe. *B,* Shoe with stretched upper to reduce pressure on dynamic hammer toe.

eral neuropathy resulting in completely insensate feet and a history of metatarsal ulcers.

He had a persistent plantar ulcer under the first metatarsal head of his left foot. His physician requested that we try to close the ulcer in-shoe so that the man could continue to work. This was done using in-depth steel-toed boots, rocker soles, and a triple-layer TCO with extensive relief of the first metatarsal head. The ulcer had nearly closed when a sudden infection occurred. The bone infection was so severe that the first toe and a portion of the first metatarsal had to be amputated (Fig. 34–23A). The foot was closed dorsally and medially with a skin graft, but the skin on the plantar surface remained intact and was therefore not especially difficult to maintain (Fig. 34–23B).

The new prescription made use of the patient's previous oblique-toed in-depth shoes (Fig. 34–23C). The rocker sole was modified to provide a small amount of heel rock but considerably more rock on the toe. An extended steel shank was also added. The new triple-layer TCO had a mild toe filler added to maintain the position of the lesser toes. Supportive material was added under the re-maining first metatarsal so that it would bear some weight and therefore balance over-all weight-bearing on the foot. This also served to eliminate excessive plantar pressure on the second through fifth metatarsal heads, thereby minimizing the chances of future callusing and ulceration (Fig. 34–23D).

Case 5: Transmetatarsal Amputation

This 37-year-old man with a 15-year history of insulin-dependent diabetes was a heavy user of alcohol and was otherwise noncompliant. He had twice frozen his insensate feet, resulting in bilateral transmetatarsal amputations (Fig. 34–24A). His plantar skin was in good condition.

The choice of prescription footwear was made easy by the patient's desire to return to work. High-top work shoes with added rocker soles controlled his remaining feet well. (A smaller size was used because of the lack of metatarsal heads.) A TCO made with a combination of medium and firm density materials served to protect and balance the remaining foot and provide the necessary toe filler (Fig. 34–24B).

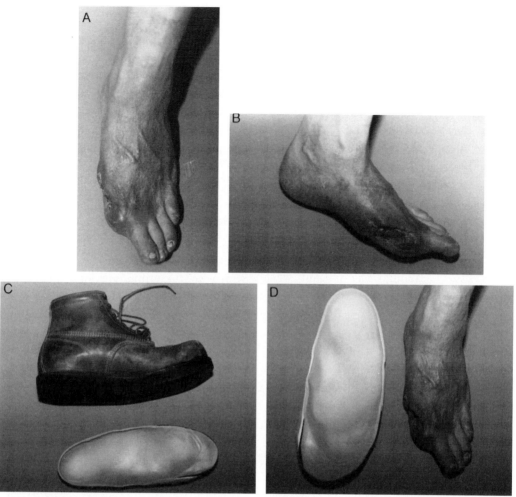

Figure 34–23 ■ Case 4. *A,* First ray amputation, dorsal view. *B,* Medial view, showing skin graft. *C,* Oblique-toed in-depth boots with rocker sole; dorsal view of TCO. *D,* TCO with toe filler; dorsal view of foot.

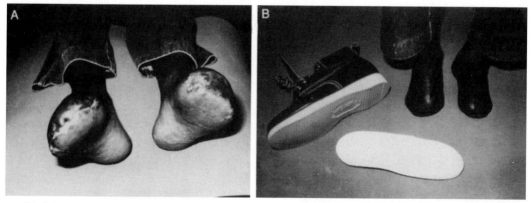

Figure 34–24 ■ Case 5. *A,* Bilateral transmetatarsal amputations. *B,* High-top work shoe and TCO; dorsal view of amputated feet.

Case 6: Midtarsal Amputation

This 70-year-old man had a 25-year history of insulin-dependent diabetes. An infection occurred 2 years previously in his right foot, resulting in a midtarsal amputation (Fig. 34–25A). The original prescription after the amputation called for in-depth shoes (of the same size on both feet) and TCOs. The use of the same-size shoe on the amputated foot caused gait problems due to its length, creating the potential for breakdown in the distal portion of the amputated foot.

The prescription was reevaluated, and the decision was made to use a custom-made shoe with a triple-layer TCO and a rocker sole (Fig. 34–25B). A custom-made sock was also fabricated for the amputated foot (Fig. 34–25C). Although the patient was initially concerned with the appearance of different-sized shoes, he was willing to give the shorter custom-made shoe a try. He found the comfort, protection, and ease of gait so much improved that acceptance came easily. He is now wearing his second pair.

Case 7: Charcot Foot (Conventional In-Depth Shoe)

A 66-year-old woman with a 20-year history of insulin-dependent diabetes had impaired sensation and a history of ulceration on the medial plantar aspects of her feet. She had bilateral medially collapsed Charcot foot deformities (Fig. 34–26A). The patient had been wearing standard cowhide in-depth shoes, which were hard to break-in and caused callusing and discomfort until "deformed" enough to conform to the shape of her feet.

Her prescription included a triple-layer TCO (with a Plastazote shell) that molded well to the entire plantar surface of her foot; the TCO therefore had an increased midfoot width to accommodate her medially collapsed midfoot. A viscoelastic polymer was added to the TCO under the bony prominences (Fig. 34–26B).

A thermal moldable shoe was used because of its soft, accommodating upper, which was molded for some hammer toe deformities also present. As shown in Figure 34–26C, the sole

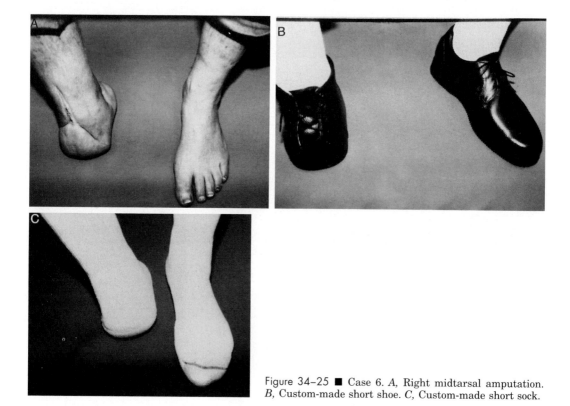

Figure 34–25 ■ Case 6. *A,* Right midtarsal amputation. *B,* Custom-made short shoe. *C,* Custom-made short sock.

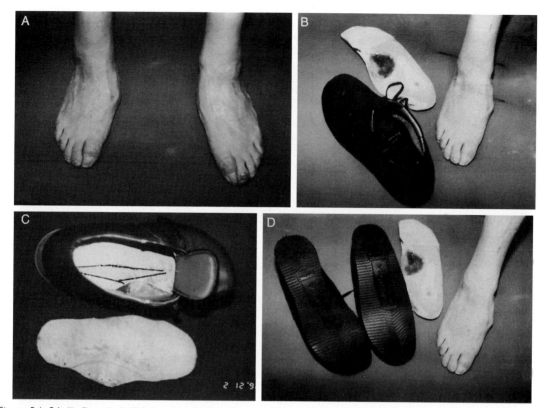

Figure 34–26 ■ Case 7. *A*, Bilateral medially collapsed Charcot foot deformities. *B*, Plantar view of TCO, showing addition of viscoelastic polymer. (Shoe and foot are also shown.) *C*, Split sole modification. *D*, Plantar view of shoe, before split sole modification (*left*) and after (*right*). (TCO and foot are also shown.)

of the shoe was cut lengthwise (through both the outsole and insole) and split apart to accommodate her deformed foot (i.e., making shoe shape match foot shape). Figure 34–26D shows a plantar view of the patient's shoe both before and after the modification. A double rocker sole with an extended steel shank was also added.

This patient was extremely satisfied with the "split sole" modification, because her entire foot was contained within the shoe. Previously she had always felt that the medial aspect was either falling out of the shoe or off the side of the shoe.

Case 8: Charcot Foot (Custom-Made Shoe)

This 66-year-old man, 5 feet 9 inches tall, weighing 280 lb, had insulin-dependent diabetes for 18 years. He had a severely deformed left foot and ankle because of Charcot destruction. The foot was very large, with extremely prominent medial displacement and hallux varus (Fig. 34–27A and B).

In the past he had experienced plantar ulceration on the medial prominences. A plastic patella-tendon-bearing (PTB) orthosis had apparently contributed to the ulceration problem, because the foot was quite mobile and moved within the orthosis. The Charcot foot was stabilized with the use of total-contact casting. The physician followed this with the use of a PTB orthosis attached to a shoe for 6 months. The brace was then removed, and the patient now needs only a custom-made shoe.

As the photographs illustrate, a conventional shoe would simply not be possible for this foot, even with extensive modifications. A custom-made shoe was therefore prescribed (Fig. 34–27C). It was able to accommodate the extensive deformities and was made with a padded collar because of the large size of the patient's legs. The TCO was

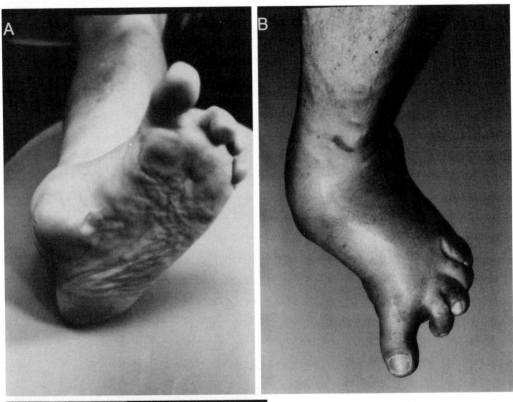

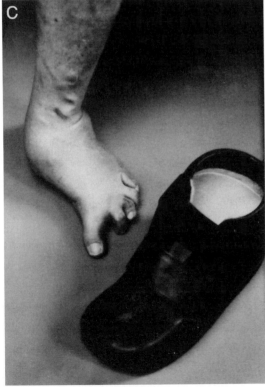

Figure 34–27 ■ Case 8. *A*, Severe Charcot foot deformity with prominent medial displacement, plantar view. *B*, Dorsal view, showing hallux varus. *C*, High-top custom-made shoe with Velcro closures and padded collar. Notice the medial extension of the TCO.

extended quite high on the medial aspect of the foot for maximum protection. Velcro closures were added, because the patient cannot reach his feet to tie laces. The shoe was made as a high-top to offer added ankle support. This prescription has been highly successful for the past three years.

Summary

Current research in the care of the diabetic foot emphasizes (1) a team approach, (2) patient education, and (3) prevention. The certified pedorthist can make an important contribution in each of these areas. Whether on the staff of a diabetic foot clinic or in a private pedorthic practice, the pedorthist's specialized knowledge of prescription footwear for the diabetic foot and ability to provide properly fitting shoes, shoe modifications, and foot orthoses make the pedorthist a valuable member of the treatment team. In addition, the pedorthist can educate patients not only in footwear but also in complete foot care. Foot and footwear inspections performed during follow-up visits and monitoring of prescription footwear effectiveness offer the opportunity for early detection and prevention of serious complications. Studies showing the importance of prescription footwear in preventing both ulcer recurrence and amputation point to their significance in the long-term management of the diabetic foot. Medicare has also recently acknowledged the effectiveness of prescription footwear for patients with diabetes by adding coverage for therapeutic shoes and orthoses.[13, 23]

REFERENCES

1. American Orthopaedic Foot and Ankle Society, National shoe Retailers Association, Pedorthic Footwear Association: Shoe Fit: What You to Know. Columbia, MD: Pedorthic Footwear Association, 1997.
2. Baumhauer JF, et al: A comparison study of plantar foot pressure in a standardized shoe, total contact cast, and prefabricated pneumatic walking brace. Foot Ankle Int 18:26–33, 1997.
3. Boulton AJM: The diabetic foot. Med Clin North Am 72:1513–1530, 1988.
4. Boulton AJM, Veves A, Young MJ: Etiopathogenesis and management of abnormal foot pressures. In Levin ME, O'Neal LW, Bowker JH (eds): The Diabetic Foot, 5th ed. St. Louis: Mosby-Year Book, 1993, pp 233–246.
5. Brodsky JW, et al: Objective evaluation of insert material for diabetic and athletic footwear. Foot Ankle 9:111–116, 1998.
6. Cavanagh PR, Ulbrecht JS: Biomechanics of the foot in diabetes mellitus. In Levin ME, O' Neal LW, Bowker JH (eds): The Diabetic Foot, 5th ed. St. Louis: Mosby-Year Book, 1993, pp 199–232.
7. Coleman WC: Footwear in a management program for injury prevention. In Levin ME, O'Neal LW, Bowker JH (eds): The Diabetic Foot, 5th ed. St. Louis: Mosby-Year Book, 1993, pp 531–547.
8. Edmonds ME, et al: Improved survival of the diabetic foot: The role of a specialised foot clinic. Q J Med 60:763–771, 1986.
9. Edmonds ME, Watkins PJ: Management of the diabetic foot. In Dyck PJ, et al (eds): Diabetic Neuropathy. Philadelphia: WB Saunders Company, 1987.
10. Janisse DJ: The art and science of fitting shoes. Foot Ankle 13:257–262, 1992.
11. Janisse DJ: A scientific approach to insole design for the diabetic foot. Foot 3:105–108, 1993.
12. Janisse DJ: The role of the pedorthist in the prevention and management of diabetic foot ulcers. Ostomy Wound Management 40:54–65, 1994.
13. Janisse DJ: Accessing the therapeutic shoe bill. Diabetes Spect 8:214–215, 1995.
14. Janisse DJ: The shoe in rehabilitation of the foot and ankle. In Sammarco GJ (ed): Rehabilitation of the Foot and Ankle. St. Louis: Mosby-Year Book, 1995.
15. Janisse DJ: Footwear prescriptions. Foot Ankle Int 18:526–527, 1997.
16. Janisse DJ, Wertsch JJ, Del Toro DR: Foot orthoses and prescription shoes. In Redford JB, Basmajian JV, Trautman P (eds): Orthotics: Clinical Practice and Rehabilitation Technology. New York: Churchill Livingstone, 1995.
17. Kogler GF, Solomonidis SE, Paul JP: Biomechanics of longitudinal arch support mechanisms in foot orthoses and their effect on plantar aponeurosis strain. Clin Biomech 11:243–252, 1996.
18. Lavery LA, Lavery DC, Quebedeax-Farnham TL: Increased foot pressures after great toe amputation in diabetes. Diabetes Care 18:1460–1462, 1995.
19. Levin ME: Pathogenesis and management of the diabetic foot. In Levin ME, O'Neal LW, Bowker JH (eds): The Diabetic Foot, 5th ed. St. Louis: Mosby-Year Book, 1993, pp 17–60.
20. Litzelman DK, et al: Reduction of lower extremity clinical abnormalities in patients with non-insulin-dependent diabetes mellitus. Ann Intern Med 119:36–41, 1993.
21. Lord M, Hosein R: Pressure redistribution by molded inserts in diabetic footwear: A pilot study. J Rehabil Res Dev 31:214–221, 1994.
22. Nawoczenski DA, Birke JA, Coleman WC: Effect of rocker sole design on plantar forefoot pressures. J Am Podiatr Med Assoc 78:455–460, 1998.
23. Pedorthic Footwear Association: Pedorthic Reference Guide. Columbia, MD: Pedorthic Footwear Association, 1996.
24. Reiber GE, et al: Design and pilot testing of the DVA/Seattle Footwear System for diabetic patients with foot insensitivity. J Rehabil Res Dev 34:1–8, 1997.

25. Rossi WA, Tennant R: Professional Shoe Fitting. New York: National Shoe Retailers Association, 1984.

26. Sinacore DR, Mueller MJ: Total-contact casting in the treatment of neuropathic ulcers. *In* Levin ME, O'Neal LW, Bowker JH (eds): The Diabetic Foot, 5th ed. St. Louis: Mosby-Year Book, 1993, pp 283–304.

27. Uccioli L, et al: Manufactured shoes in the prevention of diabetic foot ulcers. Diabetes Care 18:1376–1378, 1995.

28. Ullman BC, Brncick M: Orthotic and pedorthic management of the diabetic foot. *In* Sammarco GJ (ed): The Foot in Diabetes. Philadelphia: Lea & Febiger, 1991.

29. Veves A, et al: The risk of foot ulceration in diabetic patients with high foot pressure: A prospective study. Diabetologia 35:660–663, 1992.

30. Weaver FM, Burdi MD, Pinzur MS: Outpatient foot care: Correlation to amputation level. Foot Ankle Int 15:498–501, 1994.

Chapter 35

PSYCHOSOCIAL AND PSYCHOLOGICAL ASPECTS OF DIABETIC FOOT COMPLICATIONS

■ James E. Aikens and Patrick J. Lustman

Although two of the top five predictors of mortality in diabetes are psychosocial or behavioral in nature (social effects of illness and smoking history),[20] these factors receive little clinical attention compared to physiologic factors such as glycosylated hemoglobin (HbA_{1c}). An impressive array of psychosocial, psychological, and behavioral problems have been empirically documented in patients with both type 1 and type 2 diabetes mellitus. These include poor adherence to diabetes self-care regimen,[3,74] elevated rates of depression and anxiety,[26,47] fear of hypoglycemia,[34] psychological stress,[2–4] compromised quality of life,[21] sexual dysfunction, eating disorders, and numerous additional difficulties.[71]

Psychosocial problems may contribute to foot complications, result from them, or both. For example, effort and diligence are required to prevent and/or manage complications such as those affecting the foot. The quality of self-care behavior probably deteriorates in response to declines in psychological functioning. On the other hand, psychosocial difficulties may be exacerbated by the presence of foot ulceration, amputation, or related foot complications. For example, even a "medically optimal" lower extremity amputation is widely acknowledged as a severe stressor, one which frequently limits function and quality of life.[41,86] Even for patients who manage to avoid amputation, the presence of pain, disability, or reduced access to meaningful activities may drastically reduce quality of life. Over time, such stressors may also increase the risk for developing serious psychiatric problems such as major depression.

Psychosocial and Psychological Problems in Diabetes

Psychosocial Problems and Complications of the Diabetic Foot

Only a handful of studies have directly focused on adaptational difficulties specifically associated with complications of the diabetic foot. Reiber et al.[68] compared male diabetic patients prior to lower extremity amputation to diabetic controls undergoing surgeries other than amputation. Those undergoing

727

amputation demonstrated less acknowledgment of the importance of diabetes self-care, lower levels of social support, and fewer social connections. Pre-amputees were about twice as likely to be unmarried (i.e., single, separated, divorced, or widowed), have no visits in the past month from friends or relatives, and not belong to any club or organization. Pre-amputees were roughly four times as likely to not attend religious services and to be dissatisfied with their personal life, and they were more socially isolated and socially disconnected.

Other studies raise the possibility that such psychosocial disruption also affects diabetic patients who have other foot complications. In comparison to controls without foot disease, elderly male diabetic patients with a history of any type of foot disease were over three times as likely to be divorced or have significant alcohol abuse history.[11] Carrington et al.'s study[16] indicated that diabetic patients with either unilateral lower extremity amputations or chronic foot ulceration alone were significantly more depressed, had a more negative attitude towards the foot and its care, showed poorer overall psychosocial adjustment to illness, and had more illness-related disruption in domestic and social environments than diabetic controls with no ulceration or amputation history. However, only patients with chronic ulceration exceeded controls in vocational problems and psychological stressors, whereas only those with lower extremity amputation exceeded controls in psychosocial difficulties with health care. In another study, diabetic patients with neuropathy rated their health more negatively than did those with vascular disease or no foot complications, despite a lack of group differences in glycosylated hemoglobin and body mass index.[90] Finally, elderly individuals with diabetic foot ulcers report strikingly low levels of social support,[37] although this level does not differ significantly from the support levels of nondiabetic patients with leg ulcers. Thus, both chronic foot ulceration and lower extremity amputation are associated with a broad set of psychosocial problems, poor quality of life, and negative attitudes towards foot care.

Psychosocial Problems and Other Diabetes Complications

The broader literature concerning diabetes complications contains further data relevant to foot complications. Of numerous medical factors studied, complication rate was the only variable associated with increased risk for anxiety and depression.[64] Associations have also been demonstrated between depressive symptoms and neuropathy,[84] retinopathy,[35, 38] macrovascular disease,[13, 45] and visual impairment.[8] Visual impairment has furthermore been associated with poor self-esteem and high divorce rate.[8] Such associations are not surprising, particularly because depression has been associated with various medical risk factors for diabetes complications, such as (1) obesity,[70] (2) poor diabetes regimen adherence,[42, 57] and (3) poor glycemic control.[22, 25, 52, 54, 56, 58]

Diabetic patients with complications have been shown to be more likely than those without to report problems in vocation, leisure activity, family life, nonfamily social life, and relationship with partner, whereas they were less likely to be worried about developing new complications.[27] The emergence of complications was rated as more psychologically difficult than diabetes onset. Patients with HbA_{1c} exceeding 9.3% rate their physical and emotional functioning as significantly worse than patients with lower HbA_{1c}.[89] The presence of retinopathy, albuminuria, and/or neuropathy was associated with worse perceived health, pain, sexual dysfunction, and functional limitations. A remarkably high rate of separation and divorce is reported among patients with diabetes-related visual complications.[8]

Mechanism Underlying Associations Between Complications and Psychosocial Problems

The psychosocial problems associated with diabetes complications are summarized in Table 35–1. The precise mechanism underlying these associations is uncertain. Psychological problems may increase complication risk by interfering with dietary and medication compliance.[42, 57] Depression in particular would be expected to be associated with reduced physical activity level and eating disorders with extreme dietary nonadherence, whereas dysfunctional family relationships, low socioeconomic status, and severe psychological stressors might broadly interfere with numerous aspects of diabetes self-care. Depression could also interfere with both the

Table 35-1 ■ PSYCHOSOCIAL FACTORS
ASSOCIATED WITH DIABETES COMPLICATIONS

FACTORS ASSOCIATED WITH FOOT COMPLICATIONS

Increased

Depression
Divorce rate
Alcohol abuse
Disruption in social, domestic, health care, and
   vocational environments
Negative attitude towards foot and foot care

Decreased

Acknowledgment of importance of general
   diabetes self-care
Psychosocial adjustment to illness
Social support and family support, social
   connections (marriage, friends, clubs)

OTHER FACTORS ASSOCIATED WITH COMPLICATIONS

Increased

Anxiety
Pain

Decreased

Self-esteem
Worry about developing new complications
Perceived quality of health
Satisfaction with health

learning and performance of necessary foot self-care behaviors.

Alternatively, complications such as pain, decreased mobility, or altered body image may increase the risk of depression and other psychosocial problems. This prevalent view is expressed in the colloquialism, "You'd be depressed, too, if you were that sick" (or disabled, limited, disfigured, etc.). While popular, this view of psychosocial problems as exclusively secondary to diabetes complications seems overly simplistic. For example, in comorbid depression and type 2 diabetes, depression onset precedes diabetes onset by 5 to 10 years.[53]

A third possibility is framed in stress-diathesis models of depression, which assert that underlying psychological and biologic vulnerabilities interact with life stressors to trigger depressive episodes. It is also possible that the same biologic factors contribute to both diabetes complications and psychiatric difficulties. For example, there is evidence that chronic glucocorticoid abnormalities similar to those seen in diabetes may result in hippocampal shrinkage, possibly leading to both cerebrovascular disease and depression.[77] More generally, chronic hyperglycemia may alter autonomic tone, which in turn may contribute to depression and/or cardio-

vascular disease.[14, 73] Finally, because none of these hypothetical causal mechanisms are mutually exclusive, it is possible that the association is multidimensional or bidirectional.

Factors Associated with Poor Diabetes Self-Care

A host of factors may need to be considered in order to understand why a patient does or does not perform adequate foot self-care behaviors. These factors may include regimen characteristics, patient knowledge, past reinforcement for self-care behavior, patient beliefs about their ability to perform the necessary behaviors, concern over potential amputation, and concern over quality versus length of life. A patient's willingness to wear specialized protective footwear is affected by many of these factors as well as the cosmetic acceptability, cost, and availability of modified shoes.[12, 17]

Because the overall diabetes regimen is one of the most complex, intrusive, and burdensome of all the prevalent chronic illnesses, general regimen adherence (or "compliance") is a prevalent and serious clinical problem.[3, 74] In fact, regimen nonadherence is probably the statistical norm, rather than the exception. Although most diabetic patients are aware that intensive diabetes management effectively controls glucose and reduces long-term complications,[82] estimates suggest that between 58 and 80% of diabetic patients fail to adhere adequately to their diet and insulin administration recommendations.[74] The Pittsburgh Epidemiology of Diabetes Complications Study[45] reported that chronically poor glycemic control was associated with adherence difficulties and low social support. Paralleling the foot self-care data reviewed above, male patients demonstrate poorer self-care behavior[45] and reported less worry about developing long-term complications or acute hypoglycemia than diabetic females.[27] As noted above, poor diabetes adherence has also been associated with depression and anxiety (reviewed above), as well as maladaptive personality traits[50] and poor coping skills.[24]

A host of additional psychological and cognitive factors could hypothetically predict the quality and consistency of self-care behavior.[3, 19, 71] These include patient beliefs about whether they can influence their diabetes (e.g., locus of control),[63] perceived ability to self-manage diabetes,[36] environmental barriers to adherence,[33] and perceived immediate costs versus long-term benefits of treatment adherence. Social and family factors also appear to be relevant, such as familial dysfunction in children and adolescents with type 1 diabetes[5] and diabetes-specific family support for adults with type 2 diabetes.[28]

Therapeutic Interventions

A list of therapeutic interventions for psychosocial problems that commonly accompany foot complications is presented in Table 35–2.

Biofeedback

Biofeedback is one of the few psychological interventions that directly targets physiological processes. In biofeedback, physiologic activity is electronically monitored, amplified, and "fed back" to the patient. With appropriate repetition and reinforcement, the patient can gain voluntary control over these physiologic responses.[3] Typically, the target parameter falls below the patient's sensory threshold, either due to normal sensory limitations or disease factors such as neuropathy. In most nondiabetes applications, the target function is autonomically mediated and stress-responsive, such as: blood flow,

pulse, respiration, skin temperature, galvanic skin response (or electrodermal response), and frontalis muscle activity.

By decreasing peripheral sympathetic nervous system activity, distal temperature biofeedback increases peripheral blood flow,[65] raising the possibility of prophylactic or therapeutic use for certain diabetic foot problems. In a sample of diabetic patients without peripheral vascular disease or neuropathy, 1 hour of temperature biofeedback followed by 4 weeks of daily audiotaped foot-warming instructions produced increases in blood volume pulse and skin temperature in the toe, with decreases in arm diastolic blood pressure.[69] Two controlled biofeedback studies on nondiabetic patients with peripheral vascular disease and intermittent claudication[30, 31] report similar improvements. Compared to physical therapy, temperature biofeedback produced a tenfold increase in walking distance, and reduced resting systolic blood pressure. A related technique incorporating hypnotic suggestion (autogenic training) decreased foot and leg symptoms in 65% of diabetic patients with angiopathy accompanied by intermittent claudication or toe coldness.[29] Saunders et al.[76] reported increased foot temperature, normalized blood pressure, and complete remission of severe claudication in a 48-year-old type 2 diabetes patient with peripheral vascular disease who underwent temperature biofeedback-assisted relaxation training. Finally, a potential role in diabetes wound healing is suggested by a case study of biofeedback applied to the pre-

Table 35–2 ■ PSYCHOSOCIAL PROBLEMS IN DIABETES, WITH POTENTIAL INTERVENTIONS AND USUAL PROVIDERS

PROBLEM	TREATMENT	PROVIDER
Intermittent claudication, toe coldness, foot pain	Temperature biofeedback	Psychologist trained in biofeedback
Stress and anxiety	Behavior therapy, relaxation training	Psychologist, psychiatrist, or social worker trained in behavior therapy
	EMG biofeedback	Psychologist trained in biofeedback
Poor self-care	Improved cues and reinforcement	Physician, dietitian, nurse educator
	Behavior therapy	Medical psychologist
Obesity and cigarette smoking	Behavior therapy	Health care professional trained in behavior therapy
Alcohol abuse	Cognitive behavioral therapy	Psychologist
	Alcoholics Anonymous (AA)	AA group
	Medication	Physician
Depression	Antidepressant medication	Primary physician or psychiatrist
	Cognitive-behavioral therapy or interpersonal therapy	Psychologist, psychiatrist, social worker, or counselor with specialized training
Poor social support	Individual and family therapy, diabetes support groups	Various mental health providers and paraprofessionals

gangrenous hand of a 39-year-old male with type 1 diabetes complicated by double amputation and severe visual impairment.[62] The patient showed rapid increase in hand temperature (~3°F), reduced pain and depression, and eventual hand healing. Although these preliminary temperature results are promising, controlled studies are needed to determine the appropriate role of biofeedback in preventing and managing complications.

Frontalis electromyographic (EMG) biofeedback-assisted relaxation training, the most prevalent biofeedback modality, has been evaluated as a method for improving glucose control in both type 1 and type 2 diabetes. The rationale for this application is that stress-related neurohormonal activity might directly induce hyperglycemia via sympathetic inhibition of insulin production and action, and stimulation of hepatic glucose release.[79] While some studies show glycemic improvement with the intervention, others show no effect.[19, 79] To the extent that relaxation training possibly might reduce glycemia, benefits are probably most likely for type 2 patients who are chronically hyperglycemic[39] or psychologically stressed.[10] High trait anxiety and improved glucose tolerance with alprazolam (an anxiolytic agent) predict reduced glycemia following biofeedback-assisted relaxation training,[40] whereas low trait anxiety predicts reduced glycemia following group-delivered nonbiofeedback relaxation training.[1]

Possible Psychological Effects of Foot Examination

Routine foot examinations by the physician[23] may yield psychological benefits beyond the obvious functions of lesion screening or monitoring. The ritual of having the physician meticulously inspect the feet reinforces to the patient the concept that foot tissue integrity is critical and deserves constant vigilance.[85] Each foot examination is an opportunity to behaviorally model the attitude of foot concern as well as the actual procedures of skin inspection and footwear selection. It is also a chance to reinforce patient awareness of tactile-sensory deficits via actual demonstration of areas of reduced sensation. Exams also represent a potent opportunity to reward or redirect patient efforts. Patient foot self-care might improve merely as a simple

function of expecting an exam, and there is always the possibility that short-term improvements is self-care will maintain and become enduring habits. In sum, patient acquisition and performance of foot self-care will probably be enhanced as a direct function of the quality and number of physician-conducted foot exams.

Behavioral Interventions to Improve Self-Care

In the past two decades, increased emphasis has been placed upon preventative education in general diabetes management. Foot care education has received attention in both clinical texts[9, 18] and, increasingly, in the research literature as well. Although the multidisciplinary foot clinic typically has a strong educational component, behavioral methods to optimize health behavior adoption are not always systematically applied.

Foot care education is thoroughly covered elsewhere in this volume (see Chapter 31). These programs often integrate behavior therapy principles, such as those described in the controlled trial by Litzelman et al.[43] Individualized behavioral contracts for the performance of specific foot care behaviors were negotiated with patients. Behavioral contracts were subsequently reiterated via a schedule of telephone contact and mailed reminders. Assessments 1 year later indicated that compared to controls, patients who received the intervention had fewer serious foot lesions and other dermatologic abnormalities, and reported more frequent and appropriate foot self-care behavior. A simpler, individualized intervention is described by Lowe and Lutzker.[46] Contingency contracting and a positive reinforcement system improved foot and other self-care behaviors in an adolescent female with poorly controlled type 1 diabetes.

Behavioral interventions have also been used to improve general diabetes regimen adherence. Written cues and positive reinforcement may improve dietary adherence and glucose testing.[46] Hartwell et al.[32] describe a comprehensive behavioral dietary intervention for type 2 patients featuring the identification and alteration of environmental cues associated with eating and health care behaviors, self-monitoring of medication and food intake, self-reinforcement of desired behavior changes using nonfood positive reinforcers, modification and self-defeating cognitions related to the regimen, and an emphasis upon treatment goals that are clear, discrete, verifiable, and realistic.

In the management of diabetic obesity, progress may be slow and inconsistent, and each observable improvement needs to be reinforced. It is advisable to avoid narrow emphasis upon weight loss per se, instead emphasizing the establishment and maintenance of healthy eating patterns. One review of diabetes behavioral weight loss studies[19] concluded that men respond better to individual treatment, whereas women respond better to couples treatment, long-term medical improvement correlates positively with posttreatment weight loss, and the most effective treatments are those that incorporate routine physical exercise and very-low-calorie diets. Finally, maintenance of behavioral improvements differs by regimen area,[72] with improved medication and blood glucose monitoring tending to maintain better than changes in diet and exercise behavior.

Smoking Cessation

Behavioral interventions to reduce or eliminate smoking typically combine several components. The list of empirically supported treatment techniques includes self-monitoring of cigarettes smoked, contracting for behavioral change, positive reinforcement for smoking reduction, programmed delay of smoking, aversive treatment of smoking urges (e.g., sniffing a jar full of used cigarette butts) or smoking behavior (e.g., losing a usual privilege), stimulus control (e.g., smoking only in one setting, or substituting time-contingent for prn smoking), relaxation training, and systematic fading of nicotine intake.[80] Although several nicotine-releasing adhesive skin patches are now Food and Drug Administration (FDA) approved to aid smoking withdrawal, all current patch manufacturers recommend using the patches in conjunction with a behavioral program.[6] Specific relapse prevention techniques are also deemed important. These include developing ways to cope with likely situational relapse triggers, continued positive reinforcement, and teaching strategies to minimize negative emotional reactions to occasional minor relapses.

Treatment of Alcohol Abuse and Dependence

For mild problem drinkers who are not alcohol-dependent, brief counseling interventions delivered by non–mental health personnel are a surprisingly effective way to reduce consumption and prevent progression to alcohol dependence.[7] These entail providing information regarding the risks of excessive consumption, urging responsibility over drinking, recommending decreased consumption and presenting methods to achieve it, and fostering an empathic atmosphere and an optimistic attitude regarding improvement.

For more severe problem drinkers requiring more intensive intervention, a formalized cognitive-behavioral program is effective.[7] Components include self-monitoring of alcohol intake, identification and avoidance of drinking triggers, active modification of the antecedants and consequences of alcohol use, social support, and goal-setting. A "controlled drinking" goal (short of complete abstinence) is usually not advised for those with prior alcohol treatment history, current physical dependence, or alcohol-related liver damage.[7] Alcoholics Anonymous (AA) clearly endorses complete abstinence and emphasizes confrontation, peer support, and spirituality, as well as several elements shared with cognitive-behavioral interventions.[78] Inpatient or residential treatment programs are advised for individuals who are medically frail or have severe additional psychiatric disorders, physiologic withdrawal symptoms, chronic alcoholism, liver disease, or prior treatment failure.[7] Effective pharmacologic approaches include benzodiazepines for acute management of physiologic withdrawal, disulfiram to induce alcohol aversion, and naltrexone to reduce craving.[7]

Management of Depression

Data from controlled studies indicate that depression and anxiety are significantly more prevalent in diabetic patients than in the general U.S. population[25, 26, 61, 67, 83, 87, 88, 91] and at any given time afflict about 25% of patients with type 1 or type 2 diabetes. The risk of psychiatric illness is greater in diabetic patients with versus without complications of the metabolic disorder.[15, 35, 38, 44]

Lustman et al.[49] recently reported a series of placebo-controlled trials of pharmacotherapy in diabetes. These studies showed significant beneficial effects of nortriptyline on depression and of alprazolam on anxiety. In both studies, psychiatric treatment was associated with significant improvements in glycemic control. Alprazolam had a direct hypoglycemic effect that was not dependent upon improvement in anxiety. Nortriptyline had a direct hyperglycemic effect; however, independent of this direct drug effect, depression relief had a significant beneficial effect on glycemic control. A complete remission of depression was associated with a 0.8% to 1.2% improvement in glycated hemoglobin (GHb) over the 8-week study period. Sustained reductions in GHb of this magnitude decrease the rate of retinopathy progression by as much as one third.[60] The significant improvement in glycemic control attributable to depression improvement has stimulated interest in studying more contemporary antidepressants such as the selective serotonin reuptake inhibitors (SSRIs): fluoxetine, paroxetine, and sertraline.

Psychotherapy is generally as effective as medication for relief of anxiety or depression and the treatment is without risk of physical side effects. Findings from a controlled study indicate that cognitive behavioral therapy (CBT), a specific form of psychotherapy, is an effective treatment for depression in diabetes.[55] Patients treated with CBT also realized significant improvements in glycemic control over the 6-month study.

The positive effects of psychiatric management frequently go beyond improved mood. Some of these secondary benefits are listed in Table 35–3 and occur in conjuction with mood improvement.[48, 49] Unfortunately, even after successful treatment, recurrence of anxiety and depression in diabetes is very common. Afflicted diabetic subjects are seldom asymptomatic for an entire year at a time. The physician caring for an anxious or depressed diabetic patient thus can anticipate repeated treatment of the psychiatric illness over the patient's lifetime. The presence of diabetes complications, chronic hyperglycemia, and poor compliance with diabetes treatment have each been associated with diminished response to depression treatment and with recurrence of depression following successful treatment.[51] These findings suggest that optimal relief of emotional disorders in diabetes may require vigorous,

Table 35–3 ■ POTENTIAL BENEFITS OF PSYCHOLOGICAL AND PSYCHIATRIC MANAGEMENT*

Depression relief, anxiolysis
Restoration of normal sleep and eating habits
Behavioral activation†
Pain relief, improved pain tolerance
Improved illness coping and general functioning
Decreased somatic preoccupation
Enhanced sexual functioning
Improved treatment compliance and glycemic control

* Adapted from Lustman PJ, Clouse RE, Alradawi A, et al: Treatment of major depression in adults with diabetes: A primary care perspective. Clin Diabetes 15:122–126, 1997; and Lustman PJ, Clouse RE, Freedland KE: Management of major depression in adults with diabetes: Implications of recent clinical trials. Semin Clin Neuropsychiat 3:102–114, 1998, with permission.
† For example, increased social, occupational, and physical activity.

simultaneous management of the medical and psychiatric conditions.

Social System Interventions

Because diabetic individuals with foot complications may experience a number of difficulties in the areas of general social functioning, individual and group therapies have been widely advocated to facilitate adaptation to diabetes.[66, 75, 81] Indeed, many clinics offer support groups for children with diabetes and their parents, entire families, and general adults with diabetes.[71] Improved type 1 diabetes control in adolescents has been demonstrated following family therapy[59] as well as multifamily group therapy.

Summary and Conclusions

Psychosocial problems are more prevalent in diabetes than in the general U.S. population and are more prevalent in those with diabetes complications than in those without. The difficulties most often encountered in patients with foot complications include depression, social isolation, physical inactivity, and obesity. The etiology of these psychosocial problems is unknown but probably complex, and these problems may contribute to and/or result from diabetes complications. An impressive armamentarium of behavioral and somatic treatments are available to reduce the risk of diabetes complications and combat the problems and symptoms associated with complications. Data regarding the effectiveness of these interventions is scant but promising, and suggests that psychosocial treatment may both restore emotional well-being and improve glycemic control.

REFERENCES

1. Aikens JE, Kiolbasa TK, Sobel RS: Psychological predictors of glycemic change with relaxation training for non-insulin dependent diabetes mellitus (NIDDM). Psychother Psychosom 66:302–306, 1997.
2. Aikens JE, Mayes R: Elevated glycosylated albumin in NIDDM is a function of recent everyday environmental stress. Diabetes Care 20:1111–1113, 1997.
3. Aikens JE, Wagner LI: Diabetes and other endocrinological disorders. In Knight SJ, Camic PM (eds): Clinical Handbook of Health Psychology: A Guide to Practical Interventions. Seattle: Hofgrefe and Huber, 1998.
4. Aikens JE, Wallander JL, Bell DSH, Cole JA: Daily stress variability, learned resourcefulness, regimen adherence, and metabolic control in Type I diabetes mellitus: Evaluation of a path model. J Consult Clin Psychol 60:113–118, 1992.
5. Anderson BJ: Diabetes and adaptation in family systems. In Holmes CS (ed): Neuropsychological and Behavioral Aspects of Diabetes. New York: Springer-Verlag, 1990, pp 85–101.
6. Anonymous: Nicotine patches. Med Lett Drugs Ther 34:1–2, 1992.
7. Anonymous: Ninth Special Report to the US Congress on Alcohol and Health from the Secretary of Health and Human Services. Bethesda, MD: US Department of Health and Human Services, 1997.
8. Bernbaum M, Stewart G, Albert G, Duckro PN: Personal and family stress in individuals with diabetes and vision loss. J Clin Psychol 49:670–677, 1993.
9. Bowker JH, Pfeifer MA (eds): Levin and O'Neal's The Diabetic Foot, 5th ed. St. Louis, Mosby.
10. Bradley C, Moses JL, Gamsu DS, et al: The effects of relaxation on metabolic control of type I diabetes: A matched controlled study. Diabetes 34:S17A, 1985.
11. Bresater LE, Welin L, Romanus B: Foot pathology and risk factors for diabetic foot disease in elderly men. Diabetes Res Clin Pract 32:103–109, 1996.
12. Breuer U: Diabetic patient's compliance with bespoke footwear after healing of neuropathic foot ulcers. Diabetes Metab 20:415–419, 1994.
13. Carney RM, Freedland KE, Lustman PJ, et al: Depression and coronary artery disease in diabetic patients: A 10-year followup. Psychosom Med 56:149, 1994.
14. Carney RM, Freedland KE, Sheline YI, Weiss ES: Depression and coronary heart disease: A review for cardiologists. Clin Cardiol 20:196–200, 1997.
15. Carney RM, Rich MW, Freedland KE, et al: Major depressive disorder predicts cardiac events in patients with coronary artery disease. Psychosom Med 50:627–633, 1988.
16. Carrington AL, Mawdsley SKV, Morley M, et al: Psychological status of diabetic people with or without lower limb disability. Diabetes Res Clin Pract 32:19–25, 1996.
17. Chantelau E, Haage P: An audit of cushioned diabetic footwear: Relation to patient compliance. Diabet Med 11:114–116, 1994.
18. Coleman WC, Brand PW: The diabetic foot. In Porte D, Sherwin RS (eds): Ellenberg & Rifkin's Diabetes Mellitus. New York: McGraw-Hill, 1998, pp 1159–1182.
19. Cox DJ, Gonder-Frederick L: Major developments in behavioral diabetes research. J Consult Clin Psychol 60:628–638, 1992.
20. Davis WK, Hess GE, Hiss RG: Psychosocial correlates of survival in diabetes. Diabetes Care 7:538–545, 1988.
21. DCCT Research Group: Reliability and validity of a diabetes quality-of-life measure for the diabetes control and complications trial (DCCT). Diabetes Care 11:725–732, 1988.
22. deGroot M, Jacobson AM, Samson JA: Psychiatric illness in patients with type I and type II diabetes mellitus [abstract]. Psychosom Med 56:176A, 1994.
23. de Heus-van Putten MA, Schaper NC, Bakker K: The clinical examination of the diabetic foot in daily practice. Diabet Med 13(Suppl 1):S55–S57, 1996.
24. Delameter AM, Kurtz SM, Bubb J, et al: Stress and coping in relation to metabolic control of adolescents with type I diabetes. Dev Behav Pediatr 8:136–140, 1987.
25. Friis R, Nanjundappa G: Diabetes, depression and employment status. Soc Sci Med 23:471–475, 1986.
26. Gavard JA, Lustman PJ, Clouse RE: Prevalence of depression in adults with diabetes: An epidemiological evaluation. Diabetes Care 16:1167–1178, 1993.
27. Gavfels C, Lithner F, Borjeson B: Living with diabetes: Relationship to gender, duration, and complications. A survey in Northern Sweden. Diabetes Educ 10:768–773, 1993.
28. Glasgow RE, Toobert D: Social environment and regimen adherence among type II diabetic patients. Diabetes Care 11:399–412, 1988.
29. Grabowska MJ: The effect of hypnosis and hypnotic suggestion on blood flow in the extremities. Polish Med J 10:1044–1051, 1971.
30. Greenspan K: Biologic feedback and cardiovascular disease. Psychosomatics 19:725–737, 1978.
31. Greenspan K, Lawrence PF, Esposito DB, Vorhees AB: The role of biofeedback and relaxation therapy in arterial occlusive disease. J Surg Res 29:387–394, 1980.
32. Hartwell S, Kaplan R, Wallace J: Comparison of behavioral interventions for control of type II diabetes. Behav Ther 17:447–461, 1986.
33. Hiss HG: Barriers to care in non-insulin-dependent diabetes mellitus. The Michigan experience. Ann Intern Med 124:146–148, 1996.
34. Irvine AA, Cox D, Gonder-Frederick L: Fear of hypoglycemia: Relationship to physical and psychological symptoms in patients with insulin-dependent diabetes mellitus. Health Psychology 11:135–138, 1992.
35. Jacobsen AM, Rand LI, Hauser ST: Psychologic stress and glycemic control: A comparison of patients with and without proliferative diabetic retinopathy. Psychosom Med 47:372–381, 1985.
36. Kavanagh DJ, Gooley S, Wilson PH: Prediction of adherence and control in diabetes. J Behav Med 16:509–522, 1993.
37. Keeling D, Price R, Jones E, Harding KG: Social support for elderly patients with chronic wounds. J Wound Care 6:389–392, 1997.

38. Kovacs M, Mukerji P, Drash A, Iyengar S: Biomedical and psychiatric risk factors for retinopathy among children with IDDM. Diabetes Care 18:1592–1599, 1995.

39. Lammers CA, Naliboff BD, Straatmeyer AJ: The effects of progressive muscle relaxation on stress and diabetic control. Behav Res Ther 22:641–650, 1984.

40. Lane JD, McCaskill CC, Ross SL, et al: Relaxation training for NIDDM: Predicting who may benefit. Diabetes Care 16:1087–1094, 1993.

41. Lerner RK, Esterhai JL, Polomono RC, et al: Psychosocial, functional, and quality of life assessment of patients with posttraumatic fracture nonunion, chronic refractory osteomyelitis, and lower extremity amputation. Arch Phys Med Rehabil 72:122–126, 1991.

42. Littlefield CH, Craven JL, Rodin GM, et al: Relationship of self-efficacy and bingeing to adherence to diabetes regimen among adolescents. Diabetes Care 15:90–94, 1992.

43. Litzelman DK, Slemenda CW, Langefeld CD, et al: Reduction of lower extremity clinical abnormalities in patients with noninsulin dependent diabetes mellitus: A randomized, controlled trial. Ann Intern Med 119:36–41, 1993.

44. Lloyd C, Wilson R, Forrest K: Prior depressive symptoms and the onset of coronary heart disease. Diabetes 46:13A, 1997.

45. Lloyd CE, Matthews KA, Wing RR, Orchard TJ: Psychosocial factors and the complications of insulin-dependent diabetes mellitus: The Pittsburgh epidemiology of diabetes complications study—VI. Diabetes Care 15:166–172, 1992.

46. Lowe K, Lutzker JR: Increasing compliance to a medical regimen with a juvenile diabetic. Behav Ther 10:57–64, 1979.

47. Lustman PJ: Anxiety disorders in adults with diabetes mellitus. Psychiatr Clin North Am 1 :419–432, 1988.

48. Lustman PJ, Clouse RE, Alradawi A, et al: Treatment of major depression in adults with diabetes: A primary care perspective. Clin Diabetes 15:122–126, 1997.

49. Lustman PJ, Clouse RE, Freedland KE: Management of major depression in adults with diabetes: Implications of recent clinical trials. Semin Clin Neuropsychiat 3:102–114, 1998.

50. Lustman PJ, Frank BL, McGill JB: Relationship of personality characteristics to glucose regulation in adults with diabetes. Psychosom Med 53:305–312, 1988.

51. Lustman PJ, Freedland KE, Griffith LS, Clouse RE: Predicting response to cognitive behavior therapy of depression in type 2 diabetes. Gen Hosp Psychiatry 20:302–306, 1998.

52. Lustman PJ, Griffith LS, Clouse RE: Depression in adults with diabetes: Results of a 5-year follow-up study. Diabetes Care 11:605–612, 1988.

53. Lustman PJ, Griffith LS, Clouse RE, et al: Psychiatric illness in diabetes: Relationship to symptoms and glucose control. J Nerv Ment Dis 174:736–742, 1986.

54. Lustman PJ, Griffith LS, Clouse RE, et al: Effects of nortriptyline on depression and glucose regulation in diabetes: Results of a double-blind, placebo-controlled trial. Psychosom Med 59:241–250, 1997.

55. Lustman PJ, Griffith LS, Freedland KE, et al: Cognitive behavior therapy for depression in type 2 diabetes: Results of a randomized controlled clinical trial. Ann Intern Med 129:613–621, 1998.

56. Lustman PJ, Griffith LS, Freedland KE, et al: The course of major depression in diabetes. Gen Hosp Psychiatry 19:138–143, 1997.

57. Lustman PJ, Griffith LS, Gavard JA, et al: Depression in adults with diabetes. Diabetes Care 15:1631–1639, 1992.

58. Mazze RS, Lucido D, Shamoon H: Psychological and social correlates of glycemic control. Diabetes Care 7:360–366, 1984.

59. Minuchin S, Baker L, Rosman BL, et al: A conceptual model of psychosomatic illness in children. Arch Gen Psychiatry 32:1031–1038, 1975.

60. Morisaki N, Watanabe S, Kobayashi J, et al: Diabetic control and progression of retinopathy in elderly patients: Five-year follow-up study. J Am Geriatr Soc 42:142–145, 1994.

61. Murrell SA, Himmelfarb S, Wright K: Prevalence of depression and its correlates in older adults. Am J Epidemiol 117:173–185, 1983.

62. Needham WE, Eldridge LS, Harabedian B, Crawford DG: Blindness, diabetes, and amputation: Alleviation of depression and pain through thermal biofeedback therapy. J Visual Impair Blindness 87:368–371, 1993.

63. Peyrot M, Rubin RR: Structure and correlates of diabetes-specific locus of control. Diabetes Care 17:994–1001, 1994.

64. Peyrot M, Rubin RR: Levels and risks of depression and anxiety symptomatology among diabetic adults. Diabetes Care 20:585–590, 1997.

65. Peidmont RL: Effects of hypnosis and biofeedback upon the regulation of peripheral skin temperature. Percept Mot Skills 53:855–862, 1981.

66. Piersma HL: The family with a chronically ill child. Fam Ther 13:105–116, 1985.

67. Popkin MK, Callies AL, Lentz RD, et al: Prevalence of major depression, simple phobia, and other psychiatric disorders in patients with long-standing type I diabetes mellitus. Arch Gen Psychiatry 45:64–68, 1988.

68. Reiber GE, Pecoraro RE, Koepsell TD: Risk factors for amputation in patients with diabetes mellitus: A case-control study. Ann Intern Med 117:97–105, 1992.

69. Rice BI, Schindler JV: Effect of thermal biofeedback-assisted relaxation training on blood circulation in the lower extremities of a population with diabetes. Diabetes Care 15:853–858, 1992.

70. Robinson N, Fuller H, Edmeades SP: Depression and diabetes. Diabet Med 5:268–274, 1988.

71. Rubin RR, Peyrot M: Psychosocial problems and interventions in diabetes: A review of the literature. Diabetes Care 15:1640–1657, 1992.

72. Rubin RR, Peyrot M, Saudeck CD: Effect of diabetes education on self regulation and lifestyle behaviors. Diabetes Care 14:335–338, 1991.

73. Sachs G, Spiess K, Moser G, et al: Hormonal and blood glucose responsiveness as an indicator of specific emotional arousal in type I diabetics. J Psychosom Res 37:831–841, 1993.

74. Sarafino EP: Health Psychology: Biopsychosocial Interactions. 2nd ed. New York: John Wiley & Sons, 1994.

75. Satin W, LaGreca AM, Zigo MA, Skyler JS: Diabetes in adolescence: Effects of multifamily group interventions and parent simulation of diabetes. J Pediatr Psychol 14:259–275, 1989.

76. Saunders JT, Cox DJ, Teates CD, Pohl SL: Thermal biofeedback in the treatment of intermittant claudication in diabetes. A case study. Biofeedback Self Reg 19:337–345, 1994.

77. Sheline YI, Wang PW, Gado MH, et al: Hippocampal atrophy in recurrent major depression. Proc Natl Acad Sci U S A 93:3906–3913, 1996.

78. Snow MG, Prochaska JO, Rossi, J: Processes of change in Alcoholic's Anonymous: Maintenance factors in long term sobriety. J Stud Alcohol 55:362–371, 1994.

79. Surwit RS, Schneider MS, Feinglos MN: Stress and diabetes mellitus. Diabetes Care 15:1413–1422, 1992.

80. Tarlow G: Clinical Handbook of Adult Behavior Therapy: Adult Psychological Disorders. Cambridge, MA: Brookline Books, 1989.

81. Tatersall RB, McCullough DK, Aveline M: Group therapy in the treatment of diabetes. Diabetes Care 8:180–188, 1985.

82. Thompson CJ, Cummings JF, Chalmers J, et al: How have patients reacted to the implications of the DCCT? Diabetes Care 19:876–879, 1996.

83. Tun PA, Nathan DM, Perlmuter LC: Cognitive and affective disorders in elderly diabetics. Clin Geriatr Med 6:731–746, 1990.

84. Viinamaki H, Niskanen L, Uuusitupa M: Mental well being in people with non-insulin-dependent diabetes. Acta Psychiatr Scand 92:392–397, 1995.

85. Walsh CH: A healed ulcer: What now? Diabet Med 13:S58–S60, 1996.

86. Weiss GN, Gorton TA, Read RC, Neal LA: Outcomes of lower extremity amputations. J Am Geriatr Soc 38:877–883, 1990.

87. Wells KB, Golding JM, Burnam MA: Affective, substance use, and anxiety disorders in persons with arthritis, diabetes, heart disease, high blood pressure, or chronic lung conditions. Gen Hosp Psychiatry 11:320–327, 1989.

88. Weyerer S, Hewer W, Pfeifer-Kurda M, Dilling H: Psychiatric disorders and diabetes: Results from a community study. J Psychosom Res 33:633–640, 1989.

89. Wikblad K, Leksell J, Wibell L: Health-related quality of life in relation to metabolic control and late complications in patients with insulin dependent diabetes mellitus. Qual Life Res 5:123–130, 1996.

90. Wikblad K, Smide B, Bergstrom A, et al: Outcome of clinical foot examination in relation to self-perceived health and glycaemic control in a group of urban Tanzanian diabetic patients. Diabetes Res Clin Pract 37:185–192, 1997.

91. Wing RR, Marcus MD, Blair EH, et al: Depressive symptomatology in obese adults with type II diabetes. Diabetes Care 13:170–172, 1990.

Chapter 36

EMPOWERMENT IN AMPUTATION PREVENTION

■ William J. Wishner and Richard R. Rubin

While there is no universal agreement on how to best effect the behavioral changes needed to decrease amputations, we do know that, currently, the detection of diabetes-related foot problems generally occurs far too late. As a result, throughout the world, the human and economic cost of foot ulcers and amputations remains very high.

In this chapter you will find information and support for empowered detection of loss of protective sensation by both patients and health care professionals using the monofilament. We believe the future adoption of this or similar empowerment approaches, together with the continued use of other available tools, may reduce the number of amputations and the associated human and economic cost.

To accomplish the broader, global task of prevention of foot ulcers and achieve both the St. Vincent Declaration[9] and Healthy People 2000[12] target goals of 50% reduction of amputations, will require a synergy, created by a coalition of government, voluntary health agencies, industry, health care professionals, and patients. Using newer technologies to distribute education about the amputation prevention will enhance the empowerment process.

Foot Ulcers and Amputations Are Preventable

The antecedent events to amputation are well known and have been disseminated both in professional and public arenas for several decades.[17] Pecoraro, Reiber, and Burgess published their seminal work describing the amputation cascade and how intervention in any of the component causes could prevent amputations.[21] Despite this, overall rates of lower extremity amputation in the United States and other countries have not significantly declined.

The cost, both human and economic, associated with foot ulcers and amputations remains high. Economic costs relating to amputations and rehabilitation are likely to grow with improved and expanded application of technology to the treatment of both foot ulcers and limb salvage. Currently, an estimated 54,000 diabetes-related amputations are performed annually in the United States alone leading to hospital and surgical costs estimated at $500 million per year.[23] This cost does not include the inpatient and outpatient costs of foot ulcers not requiring amputation. More importantly, the 5-year survival rate for patients undergoing an amputation remains about 50%.[23] Clearly, these costs, both human and economic, can be far lower when problems are identified and effectively treated earlier rather than at later stages of a first foot ulcer, indolent infection, destructive deformities, gangrene, or amputation.

We know how to screen for the high-risk foot. A previous history of foot ulcer or amputation, foot deformities, absent pedal pulses, and loss of protective sensation defines the high-risk foot.[22, 24] There are effective, inexpensive screening techniques which, when used consistently, will allow early identification. Finding the high-risk foot allows early preventive intervention before the first foot ulcer.[30] When patients are provided with foot screening, education, proper fitting footwear, and routine care for foot problems, ulcers and amputation rates have been reduced.[2, 16] Unfortunately, we have not been able to consistently and universally foster use of these approaches.[32]

If we are to foster the concept of preventive care, the detection process must focus on the earliest identifiable point in the amputation cascade, that is, on the detection of loss of protective sensation.

Use of the Monofilament to Detect Loss of Protective Sensation

Protective sensation is the sensation that allows a person to feel discomfort and take action to avoid injury. Most protective sensation takes place below the threshold of consciousness and corrective action is taken automatically. Loss of this protective sensation in the feet as a result of diabetes prevents recognition of injury or repetitive trauma and sets the stage for the development of injury and foot ulcers.[6] The loss of protective sensation does not imply that there is a total absence of sensation. In fact, most people will still "feel" their feet as well as other types of sensation such as deep pain, heat, or cold. When patients say they have no feeling in their feet, the feet are clearly at risk.

The early identification of loss of protective sensation is a key to reducing the rate of foot ulcers and ultimately of amputations. One can use a nylon monofilament to identify this loss.[15] This tool is most useful when the loss is asymptomatic or subclinical.

The history of the use of these filaments to test for the presence or absence of sensation dates back to before 1900, when horse hairs were first used. In 1960, Josephine Semmes and Sidney Weinstein began to use the current type of monofilament. Their premise was that increasing the diameters of the monofilament would be accompanied by increased force to bend, thus identifying a progressive scale for sensory neurologic testing. There are numerous sizes of the monofilament, but the size that is used to identify loss of protective sensation is, by convention, the 5.07/10-gm monofilament. The 5.07 refers to the monofilament size (the actual diameter is 0.44 mm) and the 10 gm refers to the force necessary to just bend the filament. Application of more than 10 gm of force will not significantly increase the sensation felt by the patient.[34]

While there is no agreement on the exact number of places to test on the foot, a loss of sensation at any point is considered sufficient for the diagnosis. Use of a standardized testing procedure and standardized monofilament generates reproducible results.[34] The loss of protective sensation is correlated with development of foot ulcers. In one study,[25] 20% of a sample of 358 patients with diabetes were found to have loss of protective sensation by monofilament testing. This 20% accounted for 80% of foot ulcers and 100% of amputations during the next 32 months (see Fig. 36–1).

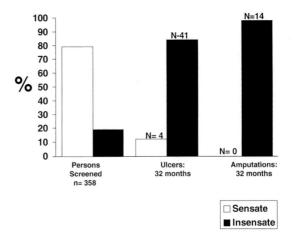

Figure 36–1 ▪ Predictive value of loss of protective sensation detected by the 5.07/10-gm monofilament; 358 persons screened and followed for 32 months. (Adapted from Rith-Najarian SJ, Stolusky T, et al: Diabetes Care 15:1386–1389, 1992, with permission.)

While more and more health care professionals now are becoming aware of the monofilament and the predictive value of this tool, to this point, availability of the monofilament has been limited by cost ($10 to $20) and by limited distribution. In 1996 a new production technique was introduced by the Lower Extremity Amputation Program (LEAP), making it possible to produce the standard 5.07/10-gm monofilament at a cost of only pennies. An industry-sponsored amputation prevention initiative was begun in 1997 to manufacture and distribute these inexpensive monofilaments as well as information on their use in preventive foot care (see Fig. 36–2). Together, these projects have begun to make possible wider distribution of monofilaments, at least in the United States.

Targeting Health Care Professionals to Screen for Feet At Risk

Traditionally, health care professionals have been provided with education focused on encouragement to teach good foot care to patients, examine patients' feet at each visit, and provide early and effective treatments of injuries or superficial ulcerations. Clearly, in the doctor's exam room this has not been a universally successful approach to detection and prevention.[3, 13, 32] The reasons for this lack of success include minimal training to examine feet properly, lack of a standardized tool to diagnose loss of protective sensation, lack of time to do the exam, and finally inadequate information about prevention resources available to the patient. These problems reflect the fact that while the diabetes foot care literature is replete with instructions for foot care, treatment of foot ulcers, and limb salvage, little advice is offered regarding application-specific primary prevention techniques. Frequently, the exam itself is relegated to others in the health care team. Specifically, podiatrists and nurses have taken up this task and have shown much more resolve to identify early problems, but until now, not specifically the detection of loss of protective sensation.

Obviously, the mere act of looking at the feet is important. Relatively unskilled examiners can detect conditions such as poorly trimmed nails, deformities, inadequate footwear, or early infections that are antecedents of future foot ulcers, but it is ultimately the lack of resolve to examine feet at each visit that limits the potential effectiveness of these provider-initiated interventions. Many providers still assume that if patients report that their feet look and feel normal there is no problem. This has ultimately lessened the imperative to examine feet at office visits.

One study[13] found that only 53% of family physicians reported adhering to recommendations for semiannual foot exams for patients with type 2 diabetes. Sixty-seven percent of physicians surveyed said they adhered to the same guidelines for patients with type 1 diabetes. In another study, del Aquila found that while patients with prior foot ulcers were more likely to see a podiatrist and receive outpatient diabetes education and instructions for foot self-care, there was no significant increase in the actual number of visits (podiatry visits or diabetes education) for peripheral neuropathy or peripheral vascular disease; this despite the fact that these conditions had been identified as risk factors for foot ulcers and amputations.[8]

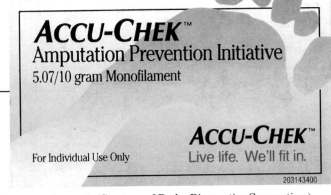

Figure 36–2 ■ 5.07/10-gm monofilament. (Courtesy of Roche Diagnostics Corporation.)

Finally, there has not been a readily available clinical tool to identify loss of protective sensation. In the past, the 128-Hz tuning fork has been shown to correlate well with the loss of protective sensation (when compared to the 5.07/10-gm monofilament).[31] Still, many physicians do not have the required tuning fork (most have a 256-Hz fork) or were never adequately trained in its use or in what constitutes a normal response. Some of the same considerations apply to other testing devices or techniques to test superficial pain or light touch. It is hoped that the use of the monofilament will help in changing this paradigm of testing.

Targeting the Person with Diabetes to Find and Prevent Foot Problems

The patient, in the past, has been consigned the role of following foot care directions from health care providers. These directions include examining feet daily, following good foot care rules, and promptly reporting any possible problems. While it is true that patients who comply with such instructions have fewer ulcers and amputations, such adherence is far from universal.[4] Even when patients receive advice regarding foot care, they frequently do not remember what they are told, and many of those who remember the recommendations do not follow them. One study found that 55.7% of the patients surveyed recalled foot care recommendations they received from their health care providers. Of this group, about two thirds (64.4%) said they followed the recommendations. Among those who did not remember the recommendations they received (44.3%), only about one third said they engaged in foot self-care.[14] Yet many patients say they want information and education concerning foot care. In a VA Medical Center population, 27.5% of the patients said they needed education concerning foot self-exams, 38.6% wanted information about selecting proper shoes, 41.5% wanted to know when to call a provider concerning foot problems, and 39.6% said they needed to know whom to call for an urgent problem.[22]

Unfortunately, most people with diabetes still receive little or no formal diabetes education. In a nationwide sample, 41% of those with type 1 diabetes, 51% of those with insulin-treated type 2 diabetes, and 76% of those with non–insulin-treated type 2 diabetes said they never attended a diabetes education class, course, or education program.[7] No useful data are available concerning the frequency with which people receive foot-related self-care education, but it is probably safe to assume that the rates for this specific type of education are low as well.

If the patient does not perceive a problem or cannot detect it by self-examination, no significant preventive intervention will follow. For instance, patients may view their own calluses and bunions as being normal. Even if they recognize a problem, they may be defeated by the lack of clear directions as to what relief to apply.

There are certain pathophysiologic risk factors for amputations that patients can understand and recognize.[19, 22] These include signs of severe peripheral neuropathy such as total absence of distal sensation (carrying a five-fold increase in risk for amputation), signs of increased propensity to infection, including ulcers becoming infected (ten-fold increase in amputation risk), infected ingrown toenails (seven-fold increase in amputation risk), and infected cuts (three-fold increase in amputation risk).

Diabetes fundamentally remains a self-managed disease, with patients providing the vast majority of their care.[1] It has been shown that patients who are empowered with an awareness of their own diabetes-related problems, the treatment options available, and adequate tools for self-care, make healthier choices in the management of their disease.[5, 18] Thus, facilitating patient empowerment in the area of foot care may be critical to the success of any efforts to reduce amputation rates in people with diabetes.

Patient behavior has been related directly to risk for lower extremity amputations. For example, Reiber found that those who changed their shoes during the day, recognized the importance of diabetes self-care, and who exercised at least 20 minutes three or more times weekly were about half as likely to have an amputation as those who did none of these things.[23]

Effective self-management of blood glucose levels and weight is also associated with reduced amputation rates. Reiber found that amputation rates were elevated for patients whose hemoglobin A_{1C} (HbA_{1c}) and body mass index (BMI) levels were elevated. Those with elevated HbA_{1c} levels had 1.7 times as many amputations as those with lower HbA_{1c} levels, and those with BMI greater than 25 had 1.9 times as many amputations as those with lower BMIs.[23] Both glycemic control and weight are affected by individual behavior.

All this suggests that patient awareness, patient attitudes, and patient involvement in self-care behavior can play a crucial role in reducing the rate of diabetes-related amputations. Unfortunately, for many people with diabetes the importance of preventive foot care and information regarding this care may remain obscure.

Should we then focus efforts to prevent foot problems on the health care professional or the patient, or both? Can both provider and patient be encouraged to focus on the same element of prevention to increase the effectiveness of the prevention process?

Can the Monofilament Be Used by Patients to Detect Loss of Protective Sensation?

The monofilament was originally designed to be used exclusively by health care providers, but there is recent evidence that the monofilament can be used by patients themselves, thus alerting them to potential problems at an early stage. Birke and Rolfsen[5] reported the results of a study of 145 patients who completed self-screening for loss of protective sensation using a monofilament. The results suggest that the test is easy for patients and their families: 68% of the patients were able to use the monofilament as directed without assistance and the rest with assistance from a family member. Almost all study participants said the instructions for the tests were clear (98%) and that the filament was easy to use (97%). More importantly, test results obtained by the patients were highly correlated with those obtained by health care providers, with an 87% agreement on patient/provider findings, indicating that most patients were able to accurately identify loss of protective sensation in their own feet. Finally, and perhaps most striking, among study participants who accurately identified loss of protective sensation, 37% of the total sample, almost half (23 people) discovered sensory loss previously undetected by providers. While directions for self-testing with the monofilament cannot be written to be univer-

sally understood, Figure 36–3 represents one example of such testing directions.

By objectively assessing the presence or absence of sensation, patients are more likely to become empowered to care for their feet. Indeed, using the monofilament gives patients the first real opportunity of detecting this problem in their own homes. This awareness could intensify patient involvement in their own care, including more frequent foot inspections, making sure their shoes fit properly, keeping appointments with their health care professional, and intensifying efforts to manage their blood sugar, weight, and other risk factors. As Levin notes, "the bottom line would be a decrease in the number of amputations."[18]

While the monofilament may seem like the ultimate tool for self-testing, it is not a panacea. Some people with diabetes will continue to deny their disease or feel there is nothing they can do to avoid the catastrophic complications. While these people may never seek empowerment regarding diabetes self-care in general or foot care in particular, some efforts to help patients modify health-related beliefs have proven successful.[27-29] In addition, it should be noted that 75% of the patients that were approached to participate in the Birke and Rolfsen study completed the protocol.[5] Thus, it would appear that there is a general willingness to engage in empowered foot care.

Some patients may have difficulties understanding and following directions for use of the monofilament, but the findings of Birke and Rolfsen suggest that this may be a rare phenomenon.[5] Still other patients may be unable to test on their own due to limited mobility or limited vision. This category accounted for 32% of Birke and Rolfsen's subjects.[5] While age was not a factor in determining whether a person required assistance in using the monofilament, age was found to influence the accuracy of self-testing. This finding is consistent with those of an earlier study which reported that 86% of elderly subjects (age >65 years) where not able to inspect and remove a simulated lesion spot from their foot because of immobility, obesity, or poor vision.[33]

A concern about monofilament testing is the issue of false-positives and false-negatives. While false-positives may create temporary anxiety for the patient, retesting by the health provider will alleviate this concern. The retesting process can also be a

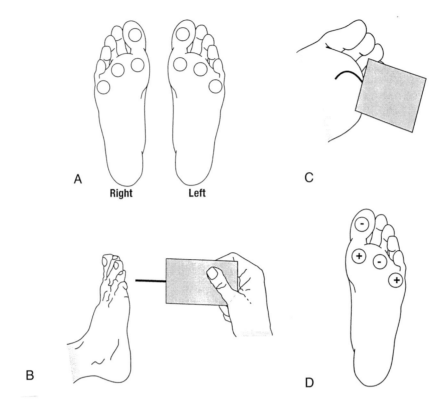

How do I find out if I have normal sensation in my feet?

Use the nylon monofilament and do this simple test.
If you can't reach or see your feet, have a friend
or family member help you with testing.

Test at the spots shown in **A**.
Hold the card so you can touch your foot with the
tip of the monofilament as shown in **B**.
Push just hard enough to just make the monofilament
bend as shown in **C**.

On the report card, place a "+" in sites where
you feel the monofilament. Place a "−" in sites
where you don't feel the monofilament, as shown in **D**.

Figure 36–3 ■ Patient self-testing guidelines for use of the monofilament. Directions for self-testing should be written and adapted to specific education and language levels. (Courtesy of Roche Diagnostics Corporation.)

Illustration continued on opposite page

highly effective "teachable moment." It may provide the opportunity to reinforce the patient's active participation in foot care including the use of the monofilament for future detection. Retesting also provides time to answer any questions the patient may have re-garding foot care. False-negatives can be more problematic, since these results can create a false sense of security and possibly lead to reduced efforts on the part of the patient to protect the feet. This eventuality should be addressed by proper retesting by

Monofilament Test Report Card

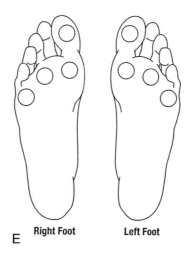

E   **Right Foot**   **Left Foot**

If you cannot feel the monofilament in one
or more spots, you are at high risk for
developing a foot ulcer in the future.

Take this report card **and the monofilament**
to your doctor or nurse to re-test
and confirm your results.

Develop a plan of foot care and protection
to prevent future injury and foot ulcers.

Figure 36–3 *Continued*

the health care provider at the office visit and continuing efforts to improve the patient's self-testing skill.

Awareness of loss of protective sensation will not in and of itself lessen amputation rates. To accomplish this goal, many behaviors related to the amputation cascade pathway must be modified. Critical questions surrounding the empowered use of the monofilaments must be answered: Will discovery of loss of protective sensation lead to an increase in effective preventive behavior on the part of the patient or provider? What type of preventive care is increased? How long are changes in preventive care maintained? How often should monofilament testing be done? Can we measure the effect of monofilament testing directly on the rate of foot ulcers or amputations?

Patient self-testing with the monofilament or any device should be seen as a part of the total prevention process. It may or may not be appropriate for given individuals.

How Can We Better Empower Patient and Provider in the Prevention Process?

The goal of empowerment is generally seen as helping patients make informed decisions concerning their own health care.[26] An equally important goal is that of provider empowerment; that is, helping health care professionals make informed decisions concerning the care they provide their patients. It is apparent that hopes for more effective preventive foot care rest in our ability to empower all key members of the therapeutic team.

The patient empowerment perspective holds that the costs and benefits of diabetes self-care must be seen in the broader personal and social context of a person's life. Patients must be seen as experts in their own lives just as health care providers are experts in the clinical aspects of diabetes. Ninety-nine percent of diabetes care is self-care. The vast majority of clinically relevant decisions are not made three or four times a year in the health care provider's office, but literally countless times each day in the context of the person's normal life. Empowered diabetes care requires that patients have specific self-care information and skills (such as how to test blood sugar, take medications, and deal with hypoglycemia) that are necessary to effectively manage their disease. But empowered diabetes care requires another set of skills as well—those problem-solving skills that allow patients to actually enact specific self-care behaviors in the real context of daily life. For example, it is one thing to know what to eat to maintain good blood sugar levels. It is another thing to eat the right foods and quantities to maintain that blood sugar when one is at a party. The latter requires effective application of problem-solving skills. Behavior change takes place as the health care provider helps the patient make informed decisions about self-care.[11, 29] The provider's efforts to understand the patient's perspective, acknowledge the patients feelings, and offer relevant information to help the patient make informed choices are the cornerstones of the provider's role in facilitating empowerment.[10] People with diabetes have always chosen what to do with the recommendations they receive from their health care providers. Accordingly, the empowerment perspective seeks to clarify the patient's role as an informed, active partner in formulating and maintaining the treatment program. This approach avoids the dilemma in which patients exercise their power to choose by vetoing (usually without expressly stating the veto) recommendations made by the health care provider without effectively utilizing the provider's expertise to develop a more workable plan. This is especially true with regard to the examination of their feet.

Even if health care providers always thoroughly examine patient's feet during appointments, a critical role remains for empowered foot self-care in reducing amputations. This is true for several reasons: First, while the health care provider can identify some serious diabetes-related foot problems by looking at and feeling the patient's feet, some problems may be missed. Looking at the feet allows the provider to identify problems and potential risk factors such as deformities, areas of pressure (calluses), poor nail care, poor footwear, reddened areas, or limited joint movement. Feeling the feet allows the health care provider to identify some additional problems including increased heat and absence or diminution of pulses. Unfortunately, everything may appear normal and the person may still be at increased risk for foot ulcers by virtue of loss of protective sensation. Thus, it is essential that the patient also know how to identify this loss himself, even if the physician for any reason is unable to determine the loss.

If any loss in protective sensation is discovered by patients, they themselves can take action to prevent injury or foot ulcers. Additionally, the patient can inform the health care provider in a timely manner whenever this loss in sensation is observed; the detection process is reinforced for the provider. Finding loss of protective sensation, patients can work on self-care beliefs and behaviors that proximally or distally affect the development of foot ulcers. These include general and diabetes-specific health beliefs, exercise, and other preventative foot care behaviors.

In summary, there are three keys to patient empowerment that may contribute to a reduction in foot ulcers. First, information concerning risk factors for the development of foot ulcers; second, the monofilament necessary for identifying the loss of protective sensation; and third, the skills necessary to take appropriate action when problems have been identified. With regard to the health care professional, these empowerment issues are exactly the same; that is, information concerning risk factors for foot ulcers, the knowledge that loss of protective sensation places the person at great risk, and of course, all of the other well-known signs of potential foot problems. They too need the tools, hopefully the same as patients (the monofilament), to correctly identify the loss of protective sensation, coupling this with other foot examination skills. Lastly, the health care provider needs the skills to actually protect the foot from future ulceration.

In reality, health care providers and patients need virtually the same resources to prevent foot ulcers. The common thread and possible synergy is use of the monofilament by both patient and health care providers.

What Can Providers Do to Facilitate Empowered Patient Foot Care?

Providers can model effective foot care screening behavior by using the monofilament to test for loss of protective sensation and in doing so perform adequate foot examinations. At the same time, they can do any or all of the following: give essential preventive information, teach critical foot care skills, answer questions regarding foot care, and facilitate foot care–related problem solving. Effective health care behavior-related problem solving is critical if patients are to initiate and maintain effective self-care of their feet and of diabetes itself.

Health care providers can facilitate the development of these problem-solving skills. For example, when recommending therapeutic shoes to a patient at risk, the provider might ask the patient if the cost of these shoes is a problem, if the patient will have any difficulty finding a store that sells the shoes, and whether the patient has any reservations about wearing shoes that might be less fashionable than the one he or she currently is wearing. This process will reduce resistance to wearing protective shoes. A similar approach could be taken to helping patients overcome resistance to regular foot self-examination. Identifying common barriers to foot care and helping the patient decide how to deal with any barriers he or she might have can go a long way towards helping patients play an active role in the care of their own feet.

The same approach can also be taken to helping patients become empowered concerning their interactions with health care providers at the office visit. Despite the fact that the majority of diabetes care is self-care, an active coalition between the provider who is an expert in clinical aspects, and the patient who is an expert on the equally critical issue of his or her life, is essential if health and well-being are to be maximized. The physician should point out that the provider's primary role is to help patients make well-informed decisions concerning their health care, which means that the patient must develop skill in asking questions, getting answers, and solving health related problems.

Can the Monofilament Facilitate Synergy and Help Build a Coalition in Amputation Prevention?

Synergy is possible when identical information on the loss of protective sensation is promoted and used by all stakeholders in the amputation prevention process. These stakeholders include physicians, patients, podiatrists, pharmacists, the pharmaceutical industry, footwear companies, diabetes suppliers, governmental agencies, and voluntary diabetes health agencies.[35]

Since the social and economic costs of serious diabetes-related foot problems are borne by society as a whole, success in reducing amputation rates requires a national coalition of stakeholders. Their collective efforts could provide resources for financing, production, and distribution of both information and the monofilament.[35]

The monofilament can be the "calling card" of the amputation prevention process. There have been in the past many other approaches to prevention, but none so far has been universally accepted and understood by both provider and patient.

To create synergy, patients can get the monofilament-prevention message from pharmacists, footwear providers, voluntary and governmental agencies, and from their provider. It can be enclosed with each medication, test strip, or syringe prescription. Increased dissemination of the monofilament and supporting prevention information increases the likelihood that patients will test for loss of protective sensation (and in doing so look at their feet); undertake protective foot care if there is loss of protective sensation (even before they see the provider); discuss foot care with their provider; retest for loss of protective sensation as part of their ongoing self-management; and finally, attempt better control of their diabetes in the process.

To create synergy, providers can get the monofilament-prevention message from the pharmaceutical industry, professional societies, governmental agencies, and patients themselves. With the monofilament and supporting prevention information, the provider will be encouraged to test with the monofilament (in doing so look at the feet); recommend protective footwear and care if there is loss of protective sensation; reinforce the importance of the prevention process; make retesting part of the regular reevaluation process; and finally, encourage better control of diabetes. The end result of the synergy would be a focus on the same preventive message: look at the feet, use the monofilament, detect loss of protective sensation, then protect the feet. It is hoped that the message would be carried to those providers not adequately screening for feet at risk, and to those patients who are unaware of the potential problem and have not yet noted loss of protective sensation or developed their first foot ulcer.

Many stakeholders are already working cooperatively to achieve these goals. The American Diabetes Association (ADA), American Association of Diabetes Educators (AADE), American Podiatric Association, National Institutes of Health (NIH), and the Centers for Disease Control and Prevention (CDC) all have foot care interest groups, and supply information to both providers and patients. The CDC has sponsored foot care initiatives through their state outreach programs. Pharmaceutical industry sponsored programs already distribute foot education materials, practical foot care training guides and, more recently, the monofilament itself. The health care industry has developed a broad, effective distribution system that health care providers, voluntary agencies, and even governments lack. Recently, a monofilament provided by industry was placed in each "Feet Can Last a Lifetime" kit distributed by the National Institute of Diabetes and Digestive and Kidney Disease (NIDDK).

A Model Program: Feet Can Last a Lifetime

In November 1995, the first nationwide campaign to increase awareness that diabetes-related amputations can be prevented was announced. This campaign, called "Feet Can Last A Lifetime," was championed by the NIDDK. The program featured patient workshops on foot care, health care provider workshops on detecting loss of protective sensation, a mass media public information campaign, and dissemination of foot care information kits to both people with diabetes and health care providers.[20]

Materials in the patient/consumer kits were designed to facilitate empowered foot care. In 1995, the first kit was distributed to 100,000 patients. Patients who returned response cards included with their kits indicated they had read the materials. Seventy-eight percent of those responding indicated they would like to see a mirror added to the kit, and 35% requested additional information on topics such as neuropathy, diet, and exercise. Four thousand health care provider kits were also distributed. Health care providers who returned response cards included with their kits said the monofilament provided in the kit was one of the most useful items. Seventy-five percent of the responding providers said they had shared all the information with their patients. A technical assistance kit was also developed for the program, to help partner organizations plan and conduct local workshops and generate media coverage.[20]

An updated version of this program released in 1998 includes reproducible foot screening and patient counseling tip sheets, two publications, "Feet Can Last a Lifetime" (a health care providers guide to preventing diabetic foot problems) and "Taking Care of Your Feet for a Lifetime" (a patient guide for foot care), Medicare guidelines for therapeutic shoe reimbursement, and "high-risk feet" stickers for patient charts. Also in the kit is an industry sponsored 5.07/10-gm monofilament.

A recent article that describes the "Feet Can Last a Lifetime" program[20] includes practical guidelines for holding local foot care workshops pointing out that while mass media strategies can be effective for reaching large, diverse audiences, messages are usually more believable when heard from a trusted source such as a local physician, nurse, or other health care provider.

The Use of Newer Technologies for Facilitating Empowered Foot Care

Traditional approaches to facilitating health-related behavior change depended on face-to-face education and the distribution of printed material. Today and in the future, the Internet may offer a promising alternative, making possible nearly instantaneous interactive communication in which all parties can exchange and share prevention information around the globe. The medium is not without its problems. Not all patients or professionals are currently linked with the Internet. Older and poorer patients are least likely to be on-line. Still, the number of people using the Internet is likely to dramatically increase in the next few years. Before the next edition of this book is published, the number of Internet users is likely to quadruple and access will be available throughout the world. In the meantime, energy should be devoted to developing accurate practical information and services for empowered foot care for placement on the Internet. Information on amputation prevention is currently available on the industry sponsored website: *www.diabetesresource.com*. This represents an example of coalition between the pharmaceutical industry and health care community to promote the common goal of amputation prevention.[20] Web sites from professional organizations, such as the American Podiatric Association and the American Diabetes Association, also contain specific foot care information as well.

Conclusions

Foot ulcers and amputations can be prevented using available examinations and the monofilament. Still, to maximize the benefits of these techniques and all our education efforts, the patient must be seen as an active participant in preventive care and a synergy must be created between patient and health care provider efforts. Thus, empowerment of the patient and health care professional should be one of the primary targets in reducing diabetes-related amputation rates. Effective empowerment requires the building of a national coalition of all stakeholders. Individual communities will need to tailor their coalitions to their own needs.

Wider use of the monofilament will facilitate these efforts. At the same time, all potentially effective tools and techniques for the early detection of foot problems should be explored if we are to successfully prevent foot ulcers and reduce amputation rates. The creation of synergy in the amputation prevention message across all stakeholders may be instrumental in future reduction of amputation rates. The authors of this chapter look forward to hearing readers' comments, and to sharing ideas and successes in the prevention process before the next edition.

REFERENCES

1. Arnold MS, Butler PM, et al: Guidelines for facilitation of a patient empowerment program. Diabetes Educ 21:308–312, 1995.
2. Assal JP, Muhlhauser I, et al: Patient education as the basis for diabetes care in clinical practice. Diabetologia 28:602–613, 1985.
3. Bailey TS, Yu HM, et al: Patterns of foot examination in a diabetes clinic. Am J Med 78:371, 1985.
4. Barth R, Campbell LV, et al: Intensive education improves knowledge, compliance and foot problems in type 2 diabetes. Diabet Med 8:111–117, 1991.
5. Birke JA, Rolfsen RJ: Evaluation of a self-administered sensory testing tool to identify patients at risk of diabetes-related foot problems. Diabetes Care 21:23–25, 1998.
6. Birke JA, Sims DS: Plantar sensory threshold in the ulcerative foot. Lepr Rev 57:261–267, 1986.
7. Clement S: Diabetes self management education. Diabetes Care 18:1204–1214, 1995.
8. Del Aguila MA, Reiber GE, et al: How does provider and patient awareness of high-risk status for lower-extremity influence foot care practice. Diabetes Care 17:1050–1054, 1994.
9. Diabetes care and research in Europe. The Saint Vincent Declaration. Diabetologia 10(Suppl):143–144, 1990.
10. Glasgow RE, Eakin EG: Dealing with diabetes self management. *In* Anderson BJ, Rubin RR (eds): Practical Psychology for Diabetes Clinicians. Alexandria, VA: American Diabetes Association, 1996.
11. Golin CE, DiMatteo MR, et al: The role of patient participation in the doctor visit: Implications for adherence to diabetes care. Diabetes Care 19:1153–1164, 1996.
12. Healthy People 2000: *In* National Health Promotion and Disease Prevention Objectives. U.S. Department of Health and Human Services, DHHS Pub. No. PHS 91-50212, Washington, DC, 1991.
13. Kenny SJ, Smith PJ: Survey of physician practice behaviors related to diabetes mellitus in the U.S. Diabetes Care 16:1507–1510, 1993.
14. Kravitz RL, Hays RD, et al: Recall of recommendations and adherence to advice among patients with chronic medical conditions. Arch Intern Med 153:1869–1878, 1993.
15. Kumar S, Fernado DJ, et al: Semmes-Weinstein monofilaments: A simple, effective and inexpensive screening device for identifying diabetic patients at risk of foot ulceration. Diabetes Res Clin Pract 13:63–67, 1991.
16. Larsson J, Apelqvist, et al: Decreasing the incidence of major amputation in diabetic patients: A consequence of a multidisciplinary foot care team. Diabet Med 12:770–776, 1995.
17. Levin ME: Preventing amputation in the patient with diabetes. Diabetes Care 18:1383–1394, 1995.
18. Levin ME: Diabetes and peripheral neuropathy [editorial]. Diabetes Care 21:1, 1998.
19. Litzelman DK, Marriott DJ: Independent physiological predictors of foot lesions in patients with NIDDM. Diabetes Care 20:1273–1278, 1997.

20. Marchand LH, Campbell W, et al: Lessons from "Feet Can Last a Lifetime": A public health campaign. Diabetes Spectrum 9:214–218, 1996.

21. Pecoraro RE, Reiber GE, et al: Pathways to diabetic limb amputation: Basis for prevention. Diabetes Care 13:513–521, 1990.

22. Reiber GE: Who is at risk of limb loss and what to do about it? J Rehabil Res Dev 31:357–362, 1994.

23. Reiber GE, Boyko, EJ, et al: Lower extremity foot ulcers and amputations in diabetes. In Diabetes in America, 2nd ed. Washington DC: National Institutes of Health, 1995, pp 409–428.

24. Reiber GE, Pecoraro RE, et al: Risk factors for amputation in patients with diabetes mellitus. Ann Intern Med 117:97–105, 1992.

25. Rith-Najarian SJ, Stolusky T, et al: Identifying diabetic patients at high risk for lower extremity amputation in a primary care setting. Diabetes Care 15:1386–1389, 1992.

26. Rubin RR: Behavior change. In Funnell M (ed): Core curriculum for diabetes educators, 3rd ed. Chicago, IL: American Association of Diabetes Educators, (in press).

27. Rubin RR, Peyrot M, et al: Effect of diabetes education on self-care, metabolic control, and emotional well-being. Diabetes Care 12:673–679, 1989.

28. Rubin RR, Peyrot M, et al: Differential effect of diabetes education on self regulation and lifestyle behaviors. Diabetes Care 14:335–338, 1991.

29. Rubin RR, Peyrot M, et al: The effect of a diabetes education program incorporating coping skills training on emotional well-being and diabetes self efficacy. Diabetes Educ 19:210–214, 1993.

30. Sanders LJ: Diabetes mellitus—prevention of amputation. J Am Podiatr Med Assoc 84:322–328, 1994.

31. Sosenko JM, Kato M, et al: Comparison of quantitative sensory threshold measures for their association with foot ulceration in diabetic patients. Diabetes Care 13:1057–1061, 1990.

32. Sussman KE, Reiber GE, et al: The diabetic foot problem—a failed system of health care. Diabetes Res Clin Pract 17:1–8, 1992.

33. Thompson EJ, Masson EA: Can elderly patients cooperate with routine foot care? Age Aging 21:171–174, 1992.

34. Valk GD, de Sonnaville JJ, et al: The assessment of diabetic polyneuropathy in daily clinical practice: Reproducibility and validity of Semmes Weinstein monofilaments examination and clinical neurological examination. Muscle Nerve 20:116–118, 1997.

35. Wishner WJ: Worldwide support to reduce amputations. Pract Diabetes Int 14:52, 1997.

Chapter 37

IMPROVEMENTS IN DIABETIC FOOT CARE WITH CLINICAL INFORMATION SYSTEMS

■ Allan Khoury, Mark Roth, and Patrick Landers

It is clear that diabetic foot care can be improved.[1–3, 5, 6] However, developing systems that allow primary care physicians to do appropriate screening and care interventions, on a regular basis, has been difficult.

Work in several institutions now demonstrates that clinical information systems can help to improve diabetic foot care. This chapter describes the work of three institutions that have been using clinical information systems long enough to improve outcomes in diabetic foot care.

The steps in improving diabetes foot care are as follows. First, physicians need to recognize that a patient being seen in diabetic. This seems obvious, but it is something that can be easily overlooked. For example, if a diabetic comes to see a busy practitioner for an upper respiratory infection, the physician may not remember that the patient is a diabetic.

Once the presence of diabetes is recognized, the proper type of foot examination needs to be done. Performing an appropriate foot exam requires the following elements. First, the physician must be motivated to do the foot exam. Second, the physician needs to be reminded which elements of the foot exam are important.

After the foot exam has been done, the physician needs to apply a stratification grid to the findings, to determine the risk for diabetic amputation. This has been particularly challenging to implement in the typical outpatient setting. Consider the plight of the primary care physician. There are stratification tools not only for diabetes, but for asthma, depression, congestive heart failure, coronary artery disease, hypertension, and other conditions. The ability to track and organize disease severity for a multiplicity of chronic illnesses has proven to be difficult.

Once the stratification tool has been applied, the care intervention should be layered as to level of risk, with the patients at highest risk getting the most intensive care. The rules for this layering are difficult for a busy primary care physician to remember.

If the intervention is appropriately applied, the physician needs to be assured that the patient has complied with it. For example, has the patient seen the podiatrist for further education?

Lastly, an outreach system, to generate mailings, or phone calls, to diabetics who have not had their feet evaluated in a particular time interval, is necessary to treat an entire population of diabetic patients. Again, this sort of intervention is beyond the capabilities of most primary care physician offices.

The systems to be described in this chapter have resolved some, or all of these problems. All use computerized medical records. All, at the moment, are in place in the managed care organizations described, and are used for all diabetic encounters. This chapter will describe these systems, analyze their successes, and evaluate potential obstacles in propagating this approach to care in various settings.

Existing Systems

Group Health Cooperative of Puget Sound

Group Health Cooperative of Puget Sound began to deploy, in 1996, a diabetes "risk registry." Their diabetes risk registry presents, in both paper and electronic form, the status of a diabetic patient and guidelines for diabetic care. The risk registry can be used by practitioners at a patient visit. A paper version of the registry (Fig. 37–1) can be generated, and can be used as a charting form. Alternatively, the same information can be accessed electronically.

The risk registry can also be used for population management. All diabetic patients can be electronically scanned and sorted by various criteria. For example, diabetics who have not had a foot exam in the past year could be identified and notified. Alternatively, all diabetics whose low-density lipoprotein (LDL) cholesterol level is greater than 130, or who have, by the Framingham equation, an increased coronary artery event risk in the upcoming 5 years, could be identified and notified.

The risk registry has led to substantial improvements in the quality of care. Of particular note is the increases in compliance with the foot exam.[7] The percent of diabetic patients with foot exams increased from 26% to 60% in the year after the full system was implemented.

Lovelace Health Systems

Lovelace Health Systems, in Albuquerque, New Mexico, a Division of CIGNA Health

Care, has in place a diabetes information system that has also resulted in improved care in diabetic patients. Again, for each patient, compliance with the organization's diabetes guidelines, which include a periodic foot exam, can be assessed electronically. In addition, practitioners receive batch reports, regarding guideline compliance in their panel of patients, on a quarterly basis. These reports may provide motivation for the practitioners to access the electronic system when diabetic patients are seen.

As in Group Health Cooperative, substantial gains in diabetic care compliance were seen in the 2 years after the implementation of the system, with glycated hemoglobin levels decreasing by approximately 2%. The organization also demonstrated an increase in the number of diabetic foot exam (J. Byrnes, M.D., personal communication).

The Lovelace system is mainframe based and constructed from legacy systems. Electronically accessed information is available on mainframe terminals. Therefore, this system was inexpensive to build.

Kaiser Permanente of Ohio

Kaiser Permanente of Ohio has developed a Medical Automated Record System (MARS) that supports disease management in many areas. The organization has concentrated on improving diabetic foot care for several years. The interventions are as follows.

The practitioner's support staff is required to review the diagnosis list, which is electronically generated, at the time of a visit, and specific to the patient being seen. Diabetic patients are instructed to remove their shoes and shocks before the examination, to facilitate a foot exam by the practitioner. In addition, the organization has stratified the entire diabetic population as to risk for amputation. The stratification grid was taken from the literature.[4] Stratification is accomplished by generating a reminder, at the time of a visit, using the automated medical record system, if the patient is diabetic and has not been stratified as to risk for amputation. The stratification grid is printed, which reminds the practitioner of the stratification mechanism (Fig. 37–2). If the practitioner notes, after the diagnosis of diabetes in the diagnosis column, the risk level for amputation (low, moderate, or high), the grid no longer prints.

Group Health Cooperative of Puget Sound

Patient Summary Sheet

Primary Phone #:   425 123-■■■■
Alternate Phone #:   —

Date: 12-May-1998
Consumer # _____
Patient Name: _____
Patient Age: __50__
Primary Practitioner: _____

Roadmap Populations	*Diabetes & Primary HC*
Date of Diabetes Diagnosis:	
Ketoacidosis Diagnosis Ever?	N
Smoking Status:	N

Vital Signs:	**Last visit**	**Today**
Weight (Lbs):	296	
Height (Inches):	70	
Blood Pressure:	122/80	
Body Mass Idx:	42.6	
Vitals Signs Date:	14-May-1997	

Priority Registry Health Risk Factors	**Working Notes**

1. CAD/CVD Risk Estimate
5 Year CHD Risk %   Risk Cat.
Family history of PREMATURE CAD?
Prior ECG evidence of LVH?
Most Recent Lab Values

Total Chol	195	HDL	33	
TC/HDL	5.9	Date	06-Mar-1997	
LDL	125	Date	07-Mar-1997	
TG	183	Date	06-Mar-1997	

Baseline LDL   Goal (20% Reduction) =
Moderate/High Risk: *Aspirin/day?*   ?

2. Kidney Risks
Albuminuria/Creat. ratio   6   Date   20-Nov-1997
Serum Creatinine   0.9   Date   09-Jun-1997

3. Retinal Screening
Latest Eye Exam: 02-Jun-1997
L. Retin. Sts.   ?   *R. Retin. Sts.*   ?

4. Foot Risk Status   High Risk Foot?   Y
Date of Last Foot Exam: 19-Nov-1997
Patient Foot Care Contract offered?   Y
History of ulcer or amputation?   N
Foot deformity?   Y   Bunion/callus?   Y
Insensate to 5.07 monofilament?   N
Ulcer Present?   N

5. Glycemic Control
HbAlc: 9.5   Date: 21-Nov-1997
Frequency of SMBG:
Shots/day: —   Insulin Dose: —

6. Cardiac/Diabetic Meds filled in last 6 mos
Niacin
BAS/Fibrate
Statin
ACE Inhibitor
Beta Blocker
Diabetic Meds: GLYBURIDE   29-Apr-1998
                 METFORMIN   29-Apr-1998

Changes:

Figure 37–1 ■ Paper GHC registry.

Illustration continued on following page

Patients who are stratified to moderate or high risk are automatically tracked for the organization's intervention, which is a visit to podiatry, in which the patient sees a video on foot care, and receives personalized instruction on foot care. The system has been successful in referring only those at medium and high risk, for the intervention.[8] An analysis of data in 1996, assessing the risk level of diabetics who came to foot surgery, found

Group Health Cooperative of Puget Sound

Patient Summary Sheet

Date: 12-May-1998

Consumer # _____

Patient Name: _____

Patient Age: ___50___

Primary Practitioner: _____

Primary Phone #:   425 123-■■■■

Alternate Phone #:   —

Clinical Roadmap Populations

   Diabetes, Primary Prevention Heart Care

Identified Diabetes-related Risk Factors for this person:

Kidney Risks

Retinal Screening

Foot Risk

   High risk foot, initiate prophylactic intervention program per Diabetic Foot Screening guideline.

Glycemic control

   HbAlc > 8.0%, refer to Glycemic Control Guideline.
   BMI > 27.0

Figure 37–1 *Continued*

that the risk ratio for moderate- and high-risk patients, in patients who required diabetic amputation, was 17.4, a highly significant number. This demonstrated that the stratification tool was an effective one.

The organization is measuring the number of diabetic amputations on its members. This number decreased by approximately 20% between 1995 and 1996, a result that is encouraging, but not yet statistically significant.

Conclusions

Electronic medical record systems can improve diabetic foot care. A successful implementation combines a reporting mechanism, which allows practitioners to compare their performance to their colleagues, and a mechanism to quickly assess, at the point of care, the diabetic patient's compliance with the organization's guidelines. In addition, electronic systems can facilitate the ability to do outreach to diabetic patients whose care is deficient. The importance of each of these components is hard to assess, but in total, they represent a significant breakthrough in the ability to improve diabetic foot care.

Obstacles to Future Progress

The successful examples described occurred in group and staff model managed care orga-nizations. Relevant clinical data was stored in the organization's computers, and, consequently, easily available. To extend this model to managed care organization that rely on networks of private physicians presents some challenges; extending them to fee-for-service physicians presents even greater challenges. A system needs to be developed that brings information regarding a particular diabetic patient to bear at the moment of care. To do this, several functionalities are needed. Patient indexes need to be developed that accurately identify the patient being seen. Electronic systems need to be accessed at each visit to determine if the patient is diabetic, and whether they have had the appropriate intervention. Many organizations have the ability to do this, but have been struggling with ways to send this information without interfering with the doctor's office workflow. To deliver diabetic care, other than foot care, laboratory information needs to be available, and presented to the physician, with the notification that the patient is diabetic. This laboratory information may have been generated by many different lab vendors. Pharmacy information, also from many vendors, needs to be included in the information presented.

These tasks seem daunting, but with the advent of the Internet significant progress is being made for each of them. When they are solved, many more patients should be able

PROV: 00666   KHOURY, ALLAN M.D.
                      INTERNAL MEDICINE
LOC: 60   WILLOUGHBY MED. CENTER
DSK: 2E   MEDICINE 3
APPT DATE: 07-15-1997   APPT TYPE: SD
APPT TIME: 10:30 A   CHK IN TIME: 10:16 A
ENCTR NBR: 000407028198

REMINDER SHEETS

DO NOT SCAN

HOME: WORK: 000-000-0000   RECBASE: 60
DOB: 07-01-1957   SEX: M
GRP/SGRP: BENEFITS NOT AVAILABLE

```
*** REMINDER NOTICE***

DO NOT CHART  **  DO NOT CHART  **  DO NOT CHART

DO NOT WRITE NOTES ON REMINDER—USE PROGRESS SHEET
```

Medical Reminders:

* *

THIS PATIENT HAS BEEN NOTED TO HAVE DIABETES, BUT THERE IS NO DESIGNATION AS TO WHETHER

THE PATIENT IS AT LOW, MEDIUM OR HIGH RISK FOR AMPUTATION. PLEASE COMPLETE THE ENCLOSED

GRID, AND DETERMINE WHETHER THE PATIENT IS AT LOW, MEDIUM OR HIGH RISK FOR AMPUTATION.*

ONCE THE RISK IS DETERMINED, PLEASE WRITE AN EXACT DESIGNATION, SUCH AS "MEDIUM

AMPUTATION RISK", IN THE DIAGNOSIS COLUMN. AFTERWARD, THE QUESTION GRID WILL NO LONGER

PRINT AND AN INTERNAL REFERRAL TO THE PODIATRY DEPARTMENT WILL BE AUTOMATICALLY

GENERATED FOR MEDIUM OR HIGH RISK PATIENTS.

**** QUESTION GRID ****

LOSS OF PROTECTIVE SENSATION	3
HX FOOT ULCER/LOWER EXTREMITY AMPUTATION	3
FOOT DEFORMITY	2
DIABETES GREATER THAN 10 YEARS	2
VASCULAR DISEASE	1
SMOKING OR CORONARY ARTERY DISEASE	1
NEPHROPATHY OR RETINOPATHY	1

Figure 37–2 ■ Diabetes stratification grid.

Illustration continued on following page

1 TO 3 POINTS INDICATES LOW RISK, 4 TO 7 POINTS INDICATES MEDIUM RISK AND 8 TO 13 POINTS

INDICATES HIGH RISK.

* (GAVIN ET AL, WEST. J. MED. 158, 47–55)

* *

* *

THIS PATIENT IS IDENTIFIED AS HAVING DIABETES, AND DOES NOT APPEAR TO HAVE HAD A DILATED

RETINAL EXAM IN THE PAST YEAR. IF THAT IS IN FACT THE CASE, PLEASE REFER THE PATIENT FOR A

DILATED RETINAL EXAM.

* *

Alert Reminders:

Educational Interventions:

Figure 37–2 *Continued*

to benefit from the models developed in the managed care organizations described.

REFERENCES

1. Assai JP, et al: Patient education as the basis for diabetes care in clinical practice and research. Diabetologist 28:602–613, 1985.
2. Bild DE, Selby JV, Sinnock P, et al: Lower extremity amputation in people with diabetes. Diabetes Care 12:24–30, 1989.
3. DHHS publication #91-5021.
4. Gavin LA, Stress RM: Goldstone DJ: Prevention and treatment of foot problems in diabetes mellitus. West J Med 158:47–55, 1993.
5. Litzelman D, et al: Reduction of lower extremity clinical abnormalities in patients with non-insulin dependent diabetes mellitus. Ann Intern Med 119:36–41, 1993.
6. Pinzur MS, et al: Benchmark analysis on diabetics at high risk for lower extremity amputation. Foot Ankle Int 17:695, 1996.
7. McCulloch DK, Price MJ, Hindmarsh M, Wagner EH: A population-based approach to diabetes management in a primary care setting: Early results and lessons learned. Effect Clin Pract 1:12–22, 1998.
8. Khoury A, Landers P, Roth M, et al: Computer supported identification and intervention for diabetic patients at risk for amputation. MD Comput 15:307–310, 1998.

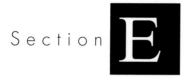

Section **E**

MEDICOLEGAL ASPECTS

Chapter 38

MEDICOLEGAL ASPECTS OF CARE AND TREATMENT OF THE DIABETIC FOOT*

■ John J. Frank and Joseph A. Frank

This chapter discusses the legal implications of the health care provider's care and treatment of the diabetic foot. We believe that this topic can best be addressed by what the personal injury attorney looks for when a client presents himself or herself with a potential malpractice case against a health care provider for the negligent treatment of the diabetic foot.

Plaintiff's Case

A plaintiff in a malpractice suit must overcome five hurdles to satisfy his or her burden of proof:

1. Plaintiff and defendant were in a patient–health care provider relationship.
2. During the course of such relationship plaintiff had condition X.

3. There was a standard of care with regard to the care and treatment of condition X.
4. The defendant's care fell below that standard of care and was thereby negligent.
5. As a direct and proximate result of defendant's negligence, the plaintiff sustained damages.

This chapter discusses each of these five elements as they apply to the care and treatment of the diabetic foot.

Patient–Health Care Provider Relationship

In cases involving the diabetic foot, the patient–health care provider relationship issue can present itself in two ways. First, there is the scenario where the patient comes to the health care provider for care of the diabetic condition. Often the patient will come to the health care provider with a callus or a sore on the foot that will not heal. Second, there is the situation where the patient is under the care of the health care provider for a condition unrelated to the patient's diabetes, or the patient is receiving long-term care

---

* This chapter states general principles of law from a plaintiff's attorney's viewpoint. The information provided in this chapter should not be considered as a substitute for independent research and independent counsel from one's attorney or insurer's attorney. It should also be noted that rules of law may vary from jurisdiction to jurisdiction.

from the health care provider (e.g., the patient is a resident in a nursing home). Depending on which of these two scenarios is presented, the standard of care applicable to the patient will differ. Those differences are discussed later in the chapter.

The patient–health care provider relationship is based on contract. The patient promises that he or she will pay for the services of the health care provider. The health care provider promises that he or she will treat the patient with the best possible skill and care. The contractual relationship is formed when the patient seeks a health care provider to render services, and the health care provider accepts the patient.

Patient with Diabetes

The fact that the patient has diabetes is presupposed by the fact that he or she has come to our office with a potential malpractice claim for the amputation of a diabetic foot. One issue that arises in this area is whether the patient was already diagnosed with diabetes. If the patient had not, the attorney is concerned with whether the physician's failure to diagnose constitutes a breach of the standard of care.

If the patient had been diagnosed with diabetes, the attorney looks to see if adequate preventive and curative steps were taken to prevent the necessity for amputation. These preventive and curative steps are discussed later in the chapter.

Standard of Care

In nearly every medical malpractice action the plaintiff is required to present expert medical testimony as to the standard of care and whether the care provided by the physician was within that standard. Cases involving care and treatment of the diabetic foot are no exception. After the attorney has been hired, he or she orders all of the medical records regarding the care of the client. Once all of the records have been gathered, the file is sent to a medical expert for review. The expert then reports back to the attorney and gives his or her opinion as to whether the client has a case for malpractice.

The first thing that the attorney wants to know is if the care provided to the patient fell below the standard of care. In most states the standard of care is defined as that degree of skill and learning ordinarily used under same or similar circumstances by members of that profession. In addition, in many states specialists are held to the degree of skill and learning ordinarily used under same or similar circumstances by members of the profession who practice within that specialty. If the expert indicates that the care provided by the physician did not fall below the standard of care, the attorney will either withdraw from the case or seek another opinion. On the other hand, if the expert expresses an opinion that the care provided to the patient fell below the standard of care, and that the breach was negligent, the focus will turn to whether the breach of the standard of care caused the patient's injuries. (Causation is discussed more fully later in the chapter.)

Negligence

There are numerous ways in which a health care provider's treatment of a diabetic patient can fall below the standard of care. A discussion of the most common areas follows.

Failure to Diagnose

A health care provider can be subject to liability on a claim for negligence for failing to diagnose the patient's diabetes or for failure to diagnose the patient's foot problem, for example, the existence of neuropathy or vascular disease. The standard that applies here is whether, in light of the circumstances presented by the patient's condition, the physician should have ordered appropriate tests.

Numerous "red flags" should alert the physician to the possibility that the patient has diabetes. Failure to recognize these red flags and conduct the appropriate tests will most probably be characterized as negligent and thus expose the physician to liability for failure to diagnose diabetes. Also, within the realm of negligent failure to diagnose is the situation where the diabetes mellitus is not noticed or is ignored. Again, the standard will vary depending on whether the patient is a diagnosed diabetic. If the patient is a diagnosed diabetic and has a foot problem, a physician will most likely be found negligent for failure to control the diabetes and properly examine the patient. If the patient has not been diagnosed as having diabetes, the standard referred to earlier will be applied to determine whether the physician was negligent.

Failure to Prevent Pressure Ulcers

When a diabetic patient is under the care of a hospital or nursing home, that facility and the patient's attending physician have a duty to take all reasonable measures to prevent the development of pressure ulcers on the patient's feet. This duty may require the physician to order protective apparatuses such as heel protectors and air mattresses. The physician may also be required to order daily examinations of the patient's feet to discover the development of erythema or ulcers. Regular turning and movement of the patient may also be required to prevent the development of ulcers. Regular visits by the attending physician may also be required. When a diabetic patient is admitted for long-term care, a complete physical, neurologic, and vascular examination should be performed to identify the patient's risks of decubitus ulcers.

A diabetic patient admitted for long-term care is at a high risk for development of pressure ulcers. In some situations, even when the highest degree of care is exercised, the patient can develop them. In such cases, the health care provider is not guilty of medical malpractice. A legal cause of action for medical malpractice is not based on a bad result but on bad care. The errors and omissions just described all can be characterized as bad care.

To adequately defend a claim for negligent failure to prevent development of pressure ulcers, the health care provider needs to show adequate documentation of the precautionary procedures. The medical record is the most crucial piece of evidence in cases brought under this theory. The attorney bringing the action and his or her expert will look to the attending physician's orders and the nurses notes to make sure that due care was taken to prevent pressure ulcers. When reasonable preventive measures had been taken and documented, the patient's case is not likely to receive a favorable review from an expert. It must also be kept in mind that the patient's claim for damages must also be "sold" to a jury. A health care provider's best defense is that they did everything in their power to prevent this type of injury to the patient. Without adequate documentation of

the measures taken, this defense is not likely to be believed (see Case Study No. 1).

Failure to Adequately Treat Ulcers

Because the patient has come to an attorney, he or she, in all probability, has already had an amputation. This amputation can be the result of severe peripheral arterial disease. This is not rare in diabetic patients, particularly in those who smoke, and have a large number of vascular risk factors. The most common cause for amputation in the diabetic is a foot ulcer complicated by infection and peripheral arterial disease. Substandard treatment accounts for approximately 50% of these amputations. Since attorneys are also aware of these statistics, when a person who has suffered an amputation comes to an attorney, the attorney will be inclined to gather the medical records from the doctors and hospitals and look for the following information: Was the patient adequately educated in foot care to prevent the development of ulcers? Has the physician routinely examined the patient's foot and done at least yearly neurologic and vascular examinations? If vascular insufficiency has been documented, was adequate consultation obtained? If an ulcer had developed, was it adequately treated? Was proper debridement carried out? Were both aerobic and anaerobic cultures obtained? Was the antibiotic selected a proper one? Because the outcome of infection can relate, at least in part, to the degree of hyperglycemia, were routine serum glucose levels obtained, and were the appropriate changes made in insulin and oral hypoglycemic agents' dosages? Was hospitalization carried out at the proper time? If the lesion was not responding to treatment, did the treating physician have the necessary expertise to adequately treat the patient's condition? If not, were proper consultations obtained (e.g., from an endocrinologist, diabetologist, infectious disease expert, vascular surgeon)?

A serious error of omission in many cases has been lack of proper inspection and prophylactic treatment to prevent pressure ulcers of the heel in diabetics confined to bed. Failure to document orders to use heel protectors or special mattresses and to do daily inspection of the heels can be considered a significant error of omission. It has been shown in many cases that patients who have not been properly managed have developed pressure necrosis of the heels and ultimately have come to amputation. Settlements out of court in these situations have been sizable (see Case Study No. 1).

Another situation resulting in amputations has occurred in patients treated at home for foot infection who have not been carefully instructed to watch for signs and symptoms of worsening infection. It is very important that these patients be instructed in the signs and symptoms of worsening infection (see Chapter 9). Patients who have not been so instructed and who have not been informed to contact the physician at once, should any of these signs or symptoms develop, can make the physician liable for substandard care. Because patients frequently forget what they have been told, the best way for physicians to defend themselves is to carefully document in the chart the instructions that were given. The physician's best chance for a successful defense is adequate documentation in the medical record, careful patient education, and proper use of consultation with experts in the field. The physician's credibility is usually one of the strengths of the defense of a claim. However, that credibility can be seriously diminished by a failure to adequately document the chart.

Because all amputations cannot be prevented, the lay jury, with the help of the defendant's attorney and experts, realize that the serious situation presented by a diabetic patient's limbs cannot always be successfully treated. Thus, the health care provider's best defense is that everything that could be done was done to prevent the tragic results suffered by the patient.

A glaring example of very superficial treatment and lack of follow-up can be noted in Case Study No. 2.

Abandonment

A claim brought under an abandonment theory is based on the patient's assertion that the physician knew or should have known that the patient's condition required continued expert medical attention and that the physician's failure to provide this care, or to at least ensure that such care was rendered by another qualified person, contributed to the patient's tragic result. This theory can be presented in several different situations. The most common situations that give rise

to a claim of abandonment are when the physician unilaterally withdraws from the care of the patient or when the physician has performed a procedure on the patient and fails to follow-up with the patient for postoperative complications.

A physician who has a diabetic patient with an ulcer or a traumatic injury to the lower limbs should not withdraw from the patient's care or leave town and so forth, until such time as that patient has obtained another physician. That physician would not likely get much sympathy from a jury, especially after the patient's attorney argues to the jury that his or her client was in grave danger of developing infection and gangrene and the defendant physician left the patient "out in the cold" with no one to treat the condition (e.g., went on vacation; see Case Study No. 2). When the patient has refused to follow the orders and advice given by the physician, a claim of abandonment may successfully be defended.

Another example of abandonment is failure to treat because of the patient's refusal or inability to pay for services previously rendered. In this era of public dissatisfaction with the health insurance industry, the physician is not likely to succeed if his or her defense is based on the patient's failure to pay the bill. A physician's duty to the patient cannot be excused for nonpayment of the bill. In addition, such an assertion is likely to inflame a jury, resulting in an even higher award against the medical provider.

Once a successful operation or procedure has been performed, the physician has a continuing obligation to the patient. Unless the physician–patient relationship is mutually terminated by the parties, the physician's obligation to the patient continues until ended by the cessation of the necessity that gave rise to the relationship. A physician performing an operation on the lower limbs of a diabetic patient should continue to monitor the patient's surgical wounds until these wounds have completely healed. Otherwise, the patient will have a very strong case of abandonment against the operating physician.

Informed Consent and Surgical Battery

A patient is entitled to full disclosure of the risks involved in a procedure that is to be performed. A physician's failure to so inform may give rise to a claim by the patient that the procedure was performed without his or her informed consent. A related cause of action is that of surgical battery. A claim for surgical battery is based on an assertion by the patient that a procedure was performed on him or her without consent or that the procedure performed exceeded the scope of the consent that he or she gave.

Surgical procedures performed on the lower limbs of a diabetic patient pose great risks of infection and postsurgical complications. It is imperative that all of these risks be explained in detail to the patient. It would be wise to prepare a pamphlet outlining these risks that could be left with the patient for his or her consideration. Finally, the physician should have the patient sign a consent form after the patient has been given sufficient time to review the material and discuss the options with the physician and the patient's family. The form should indicate that the physician has discussed the risks of the procedure with the patient (the physician may also want to enumerate what these risks are) and that the patient has been given time to weigh his or her options and has chosen to proceed with the procedure.

Failure to Educate Patient

A physician may be found negligent for failing to educate a diabetic patient as to proper foot care. The patient should be informed of the serious and possibly tragic consequences of infection in the foot area. A physician should instruct the patient as to the proper footwear (shoes, socks, stockings, etc.). The patient should be instructed to inspect his or her feet regularly for cuts, blisters, calluses, and so forth (see Chapter 9) and to recognize the warning signs of infection. The physician should instruct the patient to seek medical treatment at the first signs of infection.

A common defense of physicians in cases involving amputation of the diabetic foot is the patient's own negligence. Depending on the jurisdiction, a patient's own negligence may reduce the amount of recovery or bar recovery altogether. The defense of contributory fault can be very effective if the patient had been adequately educated regarding foot care. A physician cannot assert that the patient should have sought treatment sooner if the physician had not warned the patient of the serious consequences of infection and had

not instructed the patient as to the warning signs of infection. If the physician has provided the patient with a pamphlet describing the signs of infection, the serious health risks posed by infection, and the need to seek medical treatment at the first signs of infection, that pamphlet will be compelling evidence of the patient's contributory fault.

Contributory fault of the patient may be the physician's best defense to a patient's claim for negligent treatment of the diabetic foot. However, this shield may be used as a sword against the physician if he or she has not adequately educated the patient (see Case Study No. 2).

Causation

Once it has been established that the physician's care of the patient fell below the standard of care and was negligent, the patient's attorney must prove with a reasonable degree of medical certainty that the physician's negligence caused or contributed to cause the injury to the plaintiff. Again, this requires expert testimony on behalf of the patient. In medical malpractice cases involving the care and treatment of the diabetic foot, causation is one of the most difficult elements for the patient to prove. In almost every case involving the care and treatment of the diabetic foot, the physician can raise the defense that the patient would have suffered the same result even if the highest degree of care had been exercised on the patient's behalf. A diabetic patient with an ulcer or a traumatic injury to his or her feet is at great risk of infection and gangrene. Often, no matter what the physician does, the patient will suffer amputation or serious infection. Unless the patient's expert can testify that the negligence of the physician caused or substantially contributed to cause the patient's injury, the patient will not succeed in his or her claim of malpractice.

Defendant Case

Attorneys who represent patients in medical malpractice cases try to anticipate the defenses that the physician will raise before filing the claim. There are several defenses that are raised routinely that the experienced attorney can defeat and even possibly turn against the physician. These common defenses are as follows:

1. Judgment defense
2. General practitioner defense
3. "Patient would have lost his leg anyway" defense
4. Informed consent
5. Comparative fault/contributory negligence
6. "Empty chair" defense

A detailed discussion of the defenses follows.

Judgment Defense

This defense is based on the physician's assertion that several courses of treatment could have been taken, but, in hindsight, another course of action should have been taken. In most states, this is a valid defense. The patient's attorney will try to counter this defense by establishing that there was only one proper course of treatment for the patient and that the physician was negligent for failing to follow that course. What usually results from this defense is a battle of experts and authoritative texts. There is a saying among attorneys who practice in the area of medical malpractice: "Medical books don't treat patients, doctors do." What we mean when we say that is that juries are more impressed by live witnesses than medical texts. Therefore, a credible physician, either as a client or an expert witness, is better than a stack of medical textbooks.

General Practitioner Defense

It has been estimated that approximately 80% of all diabetics are treated by general practitioners as opposed to diabetes specialists. Therefore, it is a common defense in these cases that the treating physician, as a general practitioner, should not be held to the same standard as a diabetes specialist. This defense is rarely effective. The patient's attorney will argue that all physicians have medical training and that even a general practitioner should be able to identify the serious consequences of traumatic injury or pressure ulcers on the diabetic foot. The physician will also be questioned as to why he or she did not refer the patient to a specialist.

"Patient Would Have Lost the Leg Anyway" Defense

The basis of this defense is regardless of whether the physician was negligent or not, the patient was going to require amputation. In cases involving pressure ulcers or traumatic injury to the diabetic foot, this is sometimes true. Because of these patients' poor circulation, there is always a risk of infection or gangrene. However, some states allow a patient to recover for the loss of the chance to save the leg, thus defeating this defense.

Informed Consent

Another common defense raised is that the patient was advised of all of the risks involved in the procedure and signed a consent form indicating that he or she understands the risks and consents to the procedure. The first pitfall to this defense is that the physician is most likely to be perceived as more knowledgeable in the area of medicine than the patient. If the patient testifies that the risks were not explained to him or her or that the risks were explained to him or her but he or she did not understand them, the jury is likely to believe the patient. Also, most consent forms are preprinted forms with the name of the procedure written in. The signed form is not likely to sway the jury to the fact that the patient consented because most jurors can relate to the situation where they are asked to sign something they have not read by a person of authority, and, in reliance on that person, they sign it. For a physician to effectively use a consent form as a defense, the form should enumerate each of the risks involved in the procedure. The physician may also want to have the patient put his or her initials after each paragraph.

Comparative Fault and Contributory Negligence

This defense blames the patient's condition on his or her own acts of negligence. For example, a physician would claim that the patient's foot had to be amputated because the patient did not practice good foot care. In some states the contributory negligence of the patient is not a defense to the negligence of the physician. Other states ask the jury to assess the percentages of fault attributable to the physician and the patient. The damages awarded to the patient are then reduced by the percentage of fault attributed to him or her. This defense is ineffective if the patient had not been adequately educated by the physician. In addition, the patient is not likely to be held to the same standard as the physician because of the physician's training and experience.

"Empty Chair" Defense

Perhaps the most effective defense that can be raised by the physician accused of negligence is that someone else or some other entity caused the patient's injuries. The physician will want to show that he or she ordered the appropriate tests or prescribed the proper care. It is very difficult for the patient's attorney to counter such a defense when the accused party is not in the suit or present at trial. Attorneys who represent patients in response to the increased successful use of this defense have been joining all of the parties involved in the care of the patient and then eliminating the unnecessary parties once they have been cleared of negligence.

The Physician As a Witness

When a physician is sued by a patient it is important that the physician be a credible, effective witness. This is true for depositions as well as trial. At the defendant physician's deposition, the attorney for the patient will be evaluating the physician's effectiveness as a witness as well as discovering facts about the case. It is important that the physician make a good impression at the deposition because the patient's lawyer is the one who controls the litigation. If the patient's lawyer is impressed with the physician as a witness, that lawyer is likely to want to resolve the case before trial. Things that impress an attorney about a physician as a witness are: the physician's grasp of the facts of the case; the physician's knowledge of the medical issues in the case; the physician's demeanor and body language; and the believability of the physician's testimony.

If the patient's attorney is unimpressed with the physician witness, the attorney is more likely to be willing to take the case to trial. If a physician witness is evasive, argumentative, or displays a lack of knowledge of the facts or medicine, a jury is not likely to believe that witness.

In this era of public skepticism about injury claims and claimants, a physician being sued for medical malpractice has an advantage from the start. However, that advantage can be lost if the physician is not a credible witness. Jurors tend to side with the party they perceive as the victim in a lawsuit. Public opinion polls show that a majority of people believe the victim in a lawsuit is the person being sued. A physician can quickly lose the sympathy of the jury if he/she does not appear to be familiar with the facts or medicine of the case, or if the physician is evasive or argumentative in providing answers. Therefore, a prepared physician witness is critical to a successful defense of a medical malpractice claim.

Jury Verdict Statistics

Between 1988 and 1998, 51 verdicts in diabetic foot cases were reported nationwide by LRP Publications. Forty-one of those cases resulted in verdicts for the defendants. The ten cases in which the plaintiffs prevailed had a verdict range between $63,000.00 and $3,523,375.00, with an average award of $851,229.50.[1] These figures do not reflect the cases which were dismissed prior to trial or settled. Eleven settlements were reported during that same time frame with a range between $125,000.00 and $750,000.00, with an average settlement of $421,590.90.[2]

Case Study No. 1

L.B. was a diabetic who had suffered a stroke in June 1988. On July 1, 1988, she was admitted to defendant nursing home on her release from the hospital. L.B. suffered from left side paralysis and was in a leg brace. During her stay at the nursing home, she developed an ulcer on her left heel, which was first noted on October 19. On that day the ulcer was treated with povidone-iodine (Betadine) and whirlpool treatment. The next note in the record is from November 12,

---

[1] LRP Publications, Copyright 1997.
[2] Ibid.

at which point the nurse noted a foul odor. On November 15, L.B.'s temperature spiked at 39.7°C. Her physician performed a culture. The following day, she was admitted to the hospital and her ulcer was described as gangrenous, 5 cm, and stage II. Extensive debridement was performed on November 19. L.B.'s condition worsened and her left leg was amputated above the knee on November 28. In September 1989, L.B.'s right foot and leg were amputated above the knee.

After the amputation of her left leg, L.B. retained an attorney for a potential medical malpractice claim against the nursing home. L.B's attorney ordered all of the medical records and send them to an expert for review. The expert found that the nursing home personnel were negligent in the following respects:

1. The nurses failed to notify L.B.'s physicians about the condition of her foot or heel on any regular basis.
2. There was a lack of daily observation or supervision of L.B.'s feet, heels, and legs.
3. The patient was not provided with heel protectors.
4. The patient was not provided with an air mattress or any other special mattress.
5. Inadequate bandaging of the ulcerated area after the ulcer had developed.

In addition to his findings of negligence on the part of the nursing home, the expert also found negligence on the part of L.B's attending physicians. L.B's attending physicians were, in the expert's opinion, negligent in the following respects:

1. After her admission, L.B. was seen by a physician only three times, and not for the first time until August 22, six weeks after her admission.
2. At no point in the record did it indicate that a physical examination or a neurologic examination was performed, even though L.B. had suffered a stroke.
3. There was no examination recorded of her heart, lungs, or peripheral circulation, nor was there an examination of her skin.
4. There were no notes regarding her brace.
5. No orders were left to the nursing home personnel to examine her lower limbs on a daily basis.
6. The physicians did not order special mattresses, air mattresses, or heel protectors.

7. Once the lesion developed, no culture was taken until the day before admission to determine whether or not it was infected.
8. On November 12, the nurses noted a foul odor, but nothing was done until three days later when L.B.'s temperature spiked at 39.7°C. At that point a culture was done, but it was too late.
9. Once the patient's temperature hit 39.7°C, she should have received intensive antibiotic treatment and should have been hospitalized, but only cefaclor (Ceclor) was given. No white blood cell counts or blood glucose levels were obtained either.
10. The patient's ulcer should have been debrided.

The defendant physicians' defense was that they did everything that they could to prevent the injuries suffered by the patient L.B. and that if there was any negligence, it was on the part of the nursing home staff. The nursing home's defense was similar in that they claimed they did everything they could and that if anyone was negligent, it was the defendant physicians. This case was not tried but was settled out of court for a substantial sum of money.

Case Study No. 2

L.N. was diagnosed as a diabetic in 1960. L.N. remained under the care of the same physician for 20 years until he switched to Dr. Doe for convenience purposes. On Feb. 11, 1985, L.N. fell on a patch of ice and sprained his ankle. The ankle became badly swollen and discolored. Eventually, on March 9, L.N. saw Dr. Doe about his sprained left ankle. On examination of L.N.'s feet, Dr. Doe found an infected callus, he described a draining diabetic ulcer on the ball of L.N.'s left foot. Dr. Doe trimmed the callus and painted it with merthiolate. Dr. Doe told L.N. to soak the foot and to come back if it did not get any better. No other instructions were given to the patient. L.N. told Dr. Doe that he did not think he could walk with his swollen ankle, so Dr. Doe gave him an off-work slip for the next 3 days.

At no time did Dr. Doe instruct L.N. that the condition of his ulcer could deteriorate and quickly turn to gangrene, requiring amputation. Dr. Doe then went on vacation until

April 4. No one answered the telephone at the physician's office while he was gone. During the physician's vacation, L.N. continued to have problems with his foot. On April 4 he returned to Dr. Doe. L.N.'s wife told the physician that she wanted him to put her husband in the hospital. The physician disagreed and made an appointment for L.N. to see a specialist that treated him in 1982.

The specialist diagnosed gangrene of the left foot. Despite efforts to save the foot, the patient's left leg had to be amputated just below the knee. After his recovery, L.N. retained an attorney for a possible malpractice claim against Dr. Doe. L.N.'s attorney ordered the entire medical record and sent it to his expert for review. The expert communicated to the attorney that the care Dr. Doe gave to L.N. fell below the minimum standard of care in the following respects:

1. Dr. Doe did not perform adequate tests to make sure that L.N.'s diabetes was under control.
2. Dr. Doe's use of merthiolate on the ulcer was wholly ineffective.
3. No cultures were taken of the wound to determine the nature and extent of the infection.
4. Dr. Doe did not instruct L.N. to stay off his feet.
5. Antibiotics were not prescribed.
6. Dr. Doe did not adequately instruct L.N. or warn him of the elementary damages inherent to his condition.
7. Insulin was administered improperly.
8. L.N. should have been hospitalized so that the wound could have been cultured, medicated, and brought under control.
9. Dr. Doe did not examine the patient for loss of sensation.
10. No radiographs or bone scans were performed.
11. Merely telling the patient to soak the foot was bad medicine.
12. Dr. Doe should have referred the patient to the specialist immediately.

The plaintiff's expert also testified that if Dr. Doe had met the minimum standards, the patient would have stood an excellent chance of not losing his leg. The expert who testified on behalf of Dr. Doe testified that

L.N.'s own negligence was the cause of his infection, not the negligence of Dr. Doe. L.N.'s expert responded to this claim by pointing out that L.N. was not properly educated with regard to proper foot care, nor was he warned of the seriousness of infection and the need for regular foot inspection. L.N.'s case was never tried before a jury. His case was settled out of court for a substantial amount of money.

Do

- Educate the patient with regard to diabetes and foot care.
- Refer to an expert in the field if you believe you may be getting in over your head.
- Document in the patient's chart all that is done on behalf of the patient.
- Use aggressive treatment for foot ulcers.
- Include regular patient follow-up.

Don't

- Treat if you are in doubt about the patient's condition.
- Treat a diabetic with foot ulcers if that is not within your field.
- Delay in your treatment of the diabetic foot.
- Let the patient go untreated for an extended period.

Conclusion

There have been hundreds of cases brought against health care providers alleging negligent treatment of the diabetic foot. Most of these cases involve amputation of the patient's foot or leg. Because of the very serious injuries involved, settlements and verdicts in these cases are usually quite high.

Almost 80% of all diabetics are treated by general practitioners instead of diabetic specialists. Therefore, the general practitioner should be aware of the potential legal consequences of his or her care of the diabetic foot. Serious injuries to the patient and malpractice suits against the health care provider can be prevented by following the simple legal rules discussed in this chapter.

INDEX

Note: Page numbers in *italics* refer to illustrations; page numbers followed by t refer to tables, and those followed by pl refer to plates.

AAI. See *Ankle-arm index (AAI)*.
AAWM (American Academy of Wound Management), certification programs of, 678, 678t
Abandonment, as legal issue, 760
Abdominal aortic aneurysm(s), computed tomographic angiography of, *377*
Abdominal obesity, and peripheral arterial disease, 226
Abductor digiti minimi muscle flap(s), 578, *581*
Abductor digiti quinti muscle, 488, *489, 492*
Abductor digiti quinti tendon, *495*
Abductor hallucis brevis tendon, *495*
Abductor hallucis muscle, 488, *489–492*
ABI. See *Ankle-brachial index (ABI)*.
Abrasion(s), from total-contact cast, 306
Abscess(es), magnetic resonance imaging of, 350
    plantar, 499, *500*, 509–510, *510*
        drainage of, 613
        management of, 570, *570*
Acarbose, perioperative use of, 520
Acetic acid solution, home preparation of, 661t
Achilles tendon, anatomy of, 488
    lengthening of, 187
    partial excision of, in midtarsal disarticulation, 626, *627*
Achilles tendon reflex, 44–45
Acidic fibroblast growth factor (aFGF), 399
Activated protein C, in thrombosis, 90
Activity, assessment of, 182
    level of, and footwear prescription, 184t
ADA. See *American Diabetes Association (ADA)*.
Adductor hallucis muscle(s), 488, 492
Adductor magnus muscle, division of, in transfemoral amputation, 632, 634
Adhesion molecule(s), and endothelium, 75–76
Advanced glycation end-product(s) (AGE), and low-density lipoprotein, in atherosclerosis, 67–68
    direct removal of, 87–88
    in diabetic neuropathy, 40–41
    receptor for, 84–86
aFGF (acidic fibroblast growth factor), 399
AFO. See *Ankle-foot orthosis (AFO)*.
Africa, foot care in, 268
AGE. See *Advanced glycation end-product(s) (AGE)*.
Age, and incidence of lower limb amputation, *20,* 20t
    and risk of foot ulcers, 14, *15*
    and risk of lower limb amputation, 22, *22*

AirCast brace, 152
Albumin, serum, and stress response, 216
    and wound healing, 610
Alcohol abuse, treatment of, 732
Alcohol use, and risk of diabetic neuropathy, 51
Aldose reductase inhibitors (ARIs), and nerve conduction velocity, 40
Alendronate, for Charcot foot, 462
Algeria, foot care in, 268
Alginate dressing(s), 294t
Alprazolam, 733
Ambulation, after amputation, 611
    energy expenditure from, 636–638, 637t
    gait training and, 648–651
    of rays, 622–623, *623*
    transfemoral, 632, 634
    transmetatarsal, 625
    transtibial, 632
    with assistive devices, 640
    after disarticulation, Lisfranc, 625, *626*
    midtarsal, 626–627
    of toes, 618–619
    Syme ankle, 629, *631*
    with total-contact cast, 313–314
American Academy of Wound Management (AAWM), certification programs of, 678, 678t
American Diabetes Association (ADA), classification system of, 4
    Clinical Practice Recommendations of, 10–11
    diagnostic criteria of, 4
    position statement on foot care by, 682
    recommendations on glycemic control by, 6–7
Aminoglycoside, for foot infections, 476t
Aminoguanidine, and glycoxidation products, 87
Amitriptyline, for paresthesia, 55
Amputation. See also specific level, e.g., *Transtibial amputation*.
    ambulation after, 611. See also *Ambulation*.
    complications of, 187
    cosmetic results of, 610–611
    cost of, 220, 404–405
    dressings after, 639
    emergency, 611–615, *612, 614*
    epidemiology of, 263t
    exercise after, 253
    for Charcot foot, *vs.* reconstruction, 601–602
    gait after, 644–645

766

Amputation (*Continued*)
  goals of, 608
  "guillotine," 614
  historical perspective on, 65–66
  in foot infections, predictors of, 478
  incidence of, 636
    patient education and, 666
  inevitability of, as legal defense, 762
  level of, determination of, 609–610
    geographic variation in, 608
  litigation after, 254–255
  lower limb, and subsequent mortality, 27, 27t
    aspirin and, 24–25
    economic impact of, 29–30, 30t
    epidemiology of, 19–27, *20–22,* 20t–27t
    glycemic control and, 24
    level of, 20, 21t
    prevalence of, 19–20, *20–21,* 20t–21t
    risk factor(s) for, 20–25, *22,* 23t, 221. See also
      Risk determination.
      age as, 22, *22*
      duration of diabetes as, 22, 23t, 24
      education and, 25
      footwear and, 25
      gender as, 22, *22*
      glycosylated hemoglobin as, 23t
      intermittent claudication as, 24
      peripheral neuropathy as, 24
      race as, 22, *22*
      retinopathy as, 23t, 25
      smoking as, 23t
    subsequent, risk of, 25, 26t, 27, 29, 30t
  morbidity from, 220
  mortality after, 636
  open, postoperative management in, 614–615
  partial foot. See also specific type, e.g., *Toe(s),*
    disarticulation of.
    advantages of, 607, 615
    footwear prescription for, 185, 186t
    pedorthic care for, 715–717
    prevention of equinus ankle contracture in, 609
  peripheral neuropathy and, pathogenesis of, 231
  positioning after, 639
  postoperative management in, 611
  prevention of, coalition-building and, 745–746
    feasibility of, 737–738
    health care provider empowerment in, 743–745
    model program for, 746
    patient empowerment in, 743–745
    technological resources for, 746–747
  prognosis in, 220–221
  progression of pathology in, *684*
  psychosocial issues in, 728
  rate of, hyperbaric oxygen therapy and, 414–416,
    415t
  rehabilitation after, 255
    bed mobility and, 639
    bedside management in, 638–639
    metabolic cost of ambulation and, 636–638, 637t
    patient education and, 642, *643*
    physical conditioning and, 647–648
    prosthesis management and, 645–647
    residual limb care and, 640–642
    sound limb management and, 642, 644–645
    transfers and, 639–640
  skin graft for, 608–609, *609*
  soft tissue envelope from, 608
  wound healing after, 611. See also *Wound healing.*
Anaerobic infection(s), of foot, 470

Anemia, and wound healing, 214
Anesthesia, and hypoglycemia, 516
  general, and insulin therapy, 516–519, 517t–518t
  local, and insulin therapy, 520–521
  metabolic response to, and perioperative diabetes
    management, 514–515
Aneurysm(s), abdominal aortic, computed
    tomographic angiography of, *377*
Angiogenesis, in wound healing, 397
  oxygen and, 408, *409*
Angiography, and nephrotoxicity, 532
  computed tomography, 377, *377*
  contrast, 374–376, *375*
  digital subtraction, 375, *375*
  magnetic resonance, 377, *378–379,* 379
    in peripheral arterial disease, 369–370
    indications for, 534
Angioplasty, aortic, *385*
  balloon, for peripheral vascular disease, 536–537
  femoropopliteal, 385, *388–389*
  of bypass grafts, 385, 388, *392*
  peripheral arterial. See *Peripheral arterial*
    angioplasty.
  tibial, 385, *390–391*
Animal oil(s), for diabetic foot care, 59–60
Ankle, controlled motion of, devices for, 705–706,
    706
  deep tendon reflex in, 44–45
  destruction of, in Charcot foot, 454–456, *456*
  diabetic neuropathy in, radiography of, *339–340*
  disarticulation of, Syme, 627–629, *628–631.* See
    also *Syme ankle disarticulation.*
  dorsiflexion of, assessment of, 181
  equinus contracture of, prevention of, in partial foot
    amputation, 609
  fractures of, management of, in prevention of
    Charcot foot, 602, *603–605*
  motion of, after Lisfranc disarticulation, 625, *626*
  neuropathic arthropathy of, *592*
  realignment of, in Charcot foot, *596*
Ankle pressure, in peripheral arterial disease, 223,
    224, 358, *359*
  measurement of, equipment for, *361*
Ankle-arm index (AAI), and risk of amputation, 23t,
    24
  and risk of foot ulcers, 15, 17t
  in peripheral arterial disease, 366, *366*
Ankle-brachial index (ABI), compression stockings
    and, 329, 329t
  in peripheral vascular disease, 528
  indications for, 370
Ankle-foot orthosis (AFO), as alternative to total-
    contact cast, 317, *317,* 323, *323*
  for Charcot foot, 461
    after arthrodesis and realignment, *599–600,*
      600–601
Ankle-toe pressure, in peripheral arterial disease,
    366–367, *366–367*
Antibacterial agent(s), sensitization to, 290
  topical, for wound care, 289–290, 291t
Antibiotic(s), for foot infections, 473–477, 476t–477t
  choice of, 474–475, 476t–477t
  cost of, 475
  duration of, 475, 477
  indications for, 473–474
  route of administration for, 474
  with osteomyelitis, 477
  for foot ulcers, 244
Anticoagulant(s), for peripheral vascular disease, 535

Antidepressant(s), and glycemic control, 733
  tricyclic, for paresthesia, 55
Antiplatelet agent(s), clinical trials of, 9–10
  for peripheral vascular disease, 535
  for prevention of thrombosis, 91–92
Antithrombin III, activity of, glycation and, 84
  in thrombosis, 89–90
Anxiety, treatment of, 732–733, 733t
Aorta, angioplasty of, 385
  calcification of, 530
Aortobifemoral graft(s), for aortoiliac occlusive
    disease, 540, 542, 542t
Aortofemoral reconstruction, limb salvage rate in,
    538–539
Aortoiliac endarterectomy, 540, 540–541, 541t
Aortoiliac occlusive disease, surgical management of,
    538–543, 539–542, 541t–542t
  angioplasty with stenting in, 541–542
  aortobifemoral grafts in, 540, 542, 542t
  aortoiliac reconstruction in, 540–541, 543t
  endarterectomy in, 540, 540, 541t
  extra-anatomic bypass in, 542–543
  results of, with inflow procedure alone, 538–539
Apligraft, 296
Aponeurosis, plantar, 488, 489–491, 495
Arch length, vs. foot length, 704
Arglaes, 290
ARIs (aldose reductase inhibitors), and nerve
    conduction velocity, 40
Arm, deep tendon reflex in, 46–47
Arterial angioplasty, peripheral, 383–388, 385–392
Arterial bypass surgery, imaging of pedal arch before,
    533–534
Arterial occlusion. See also specific site.
  acute, 230–231, 230t
Arterial waveform(s), in peripheral arterial disease,
    363–364, 363–365, 529, 529
Arteriography, before bypass surgery, 534
  transfemoral, 532
Arteriosclerosis, in lower extremities, in diabetics vs.
    nondiabetics, 501
Arteriovenous shunt(s), plantar, in diabetic
    neuropathy, 36, 37–38, 59
Arteritis, septic, 498–499, 498–499
Artery(ies), blood flow in, 109, 109t
  calcification of, in peripheral vascular disease,
    530–531, 530–531
  stiffness of, in diabetes mellitus, 84
  to leg, calcification of, 111
Arthritis, septic, of metatarsophalangeal joint, 280
Arthrodesis, with realignment, for Charcot foot, 591,
    592–601, 600–601
Arthropathy, Charcot. See Charcot foot.
Asia, foot care in, 265–267
Aspirin, and risk of lower limb amputation, 24–25
  clinical trials of, 9–10
  for peripheral vascular disease, 535
  for prevention of thrombosis, 91–92
Assistive device(s), ambulation with, after
    amputation, 640
  with total-contact cast, 318
Atherosclerosis, and thrombosis, 88–91, 88t
  cutaneous manifestations of, 197
  endothelium in, 71–77
    cell adhesion molecules and, 75–76
    endothelin-1 and, 74–75
    nitric oxide and, 71–73
    prostacyclin and, 73–74
    thromboxane and, 74

Atherosclerosis (Continued)
    transport of low-density lipoprotein through,
      67–71, 71
    von Willebrand factor and, 76–77
  glycation in, 80–81
    and lipoprotein metabolism, 81–82
  glycoxidation of vascular structural proteins in,
      84–88, 85
  historical perspective on, 65–66
  in arteries to leg, 110
  in vitro studies of, 92
  lipids and, 77–80
  lipoproteins and, 77–80
  of tibial artery, 525–526
  pathogenesis of, 67–71, 71
    low-density lipoprotein in, 67–71, 71
    oxidation hypothesis in, 73
Athletic shoes, and peak pressure, 168
Australia, foot care in, 267
Austria, foot care in, 265
Autoamputation, 611, 612
Autolytic debridement, 287
Autonomic neuropathy, and blood flow, 112, 112–113
  and risk of foot ulcers, 683–684
  assessment of, 660
  dermatologic manifestations of, 689–690, 690
  in Charcot foot, 444–445
  preoperative assessment of, 516
Avulsion fracture(s), 456–457, 457–458
Axillobifemoral bypass, 543
Aztreonam, for foot infections, 476t

Bacteria, classification of, 469
  killing of, oxygen tension and, 407, 408–409
Bacterial colonization, 468
"Baked potato toe," 686, 686
Balance, assessment of, 181–182
  in total-contact cast, 305
  standing, with amputee prosthesis, 648–649
Balloon angioplasty, for peripheral vascular disease,
    536–537
Bandages, types of, 294t
Basic fibroblast growth factor (bFGF), 399
Battery, surgical, 760–761
Bed mobility, after amputation, 639
Behavioral intervention(s), for noncompliance,
    731–732
  for smoking cessation, 732
Belgium, foot care in, 264
Beraprost sodium, efficacy of, 73–74
Beta-blocker(s), and gangrene of toes, 227
bFGF (basic fibroblast growth factor), 399
Biceps tendon reflex, 46
Biofeedback, 730–731
Biomechanical problem(s), and ulcers, 126t
  clinical approach to, 177–185, 179t, 183, 184t–186t,
      694–695, 695
    activity assessment in, 182
    assessment of foot deformity in, 179–180, 179t
    assessment of sensory loss in, 177–178, 179t
    assessment of soft tissue changes in, 180
    footwear prescription in, 182–185, 183,
      184t–186t. See also Footwear, prescription of.
    gait assessment in, 182
    measurement of plantar pressure in, 178–179.
      See also Plantar pressure, measurement of.
    surgical, 185–188
    with callus, 180–181

Biomechanical problem(s) (*Continued*)
  with imbalance, 181–182
  with limited joint mobility, 181
  with weakness, 181–182
Biopsy, of bone, in osteomyelitis, 472–473
  of foot ulcer, 242–243, 243pl
Biosynthetic dressing(s), 294t
Biothesiometer, *688,* 688–689
Bisphosphonate(s), for Charcot foot, 462
Blister(s), 202, *202*
Blood, as shear thinning fluid, 113–114, *114*
  components of, 107
  relative force of, 107
  transient resistance of, 115t, 116, *117*
  viscoelasticity of, 115t, 116
  viscosity of, and shear thinning, 115
    diet and, 118, 118t
    exercise and, 118, 118t
Blood flow, autonomic neuropathy and, *112,* 112–113
  cessation of, 109
  destabilization of, 115, 115t
  exercise and, in peripheral arterial disease,
    358–360, *359,* 360t
  in arteries, 109, 109t
  in capillaries, 109t, 110
  in leg veins, 111–112
  inertial, *vs.* viscous, 109–110, 109t
  leukocytes and, 113, *114*
  nonnewtonian properties of, 115, 115t
  peripheral, increased, in Charcot foot, 444–445
  pharmacologic agents affecting, 118–121, 119t–120t
  principles of, 107–109
  proteins and, 108
  time-based properties of, 115–116, 115t, *117*
  to leg and foot, 110–111, *111*
Blood pressure, control of, 7–8
Blood vessel(s), in foot, anatomy of, 486
  Reynolds numbers for, 109, 109t
  stiffness of, in diabetes mellitus, 84
Blue toe syndrome, 227
Body image, amputation and, 610–611
Body weight. See *Weight* entries.
Bone, demineralization of, 334–336, *336–338*
  destruction of, in Charcot foot, 448–459, *449–458.*
    See also *Charcot foot, bone and joint*
    destruction in.
  healing of, in Charcot foot, *442,* 443
  resorption of, in Charcot foot, 443
Bone biopsy, 472–473
Bone graft(s), for arthrodesis, in Charcot foot, 591
Bone infection(s), of foot, 471–473. See also
  Osteomyelitis.
Bone mineral density, in Charcot foot, 445
Bone scintigraphy, 344, *346,* 347
  in osteomyelitis, 472
Bone spur(s), calcaneal, 333, *335*
Boot(s). See also *Footwear.*
  fixed-ankle-brace, 434, *435*
Brace(s), for ulcer healing, 152
  patellar tibial, 584, *584*
Brachioradialis tendon reflex, 45–46
Brazil, foot care in, 268
Bridge shoes, 324, *326*
Bruit(s), in peripheral arterial disease, 357
Bullae, diabetic, *202–203,* 202–204. See also *Diabetic*
  bullae.
Bunion(s), 180, *504*
  after disarticulation of second toe, 617, *617*
  footwear for, *428*

Bunion(s) (*Continued*)
  infection of, and plantar space abscess, 509–510,
    510
  tailor's, 506
Burden of proof, in plaintiff's malpractice suit, 757
Burn(s), of foot, *685*
Bypass graft(s), angioplasty of, 385, 388, *392*
  failure of, *554,* 554–555
  patency rates of, 545t, 547

Cadexomer iodine, 290, 291t
Calcaneal artery flap, lateral, *578*
  medial, 578, *579*
Calcaneal nerve, anatomy of, *489*
Calcaneocuboid joint, destruction of, in Charcot foot,
  449, 452–454, *455–456*
Calcaneus, anatomy of, *494*
  destruction of, in Charcot foot, 456–457, *457–458*
  spurs of, 333, *335*
Calcification, arterial, 530–531, *530–531*
  in leg, 111
Calcium alginate(s), 288
Calcium channel blocker(s), for peripheral vascular
  disease, 535
Callus(es), 180–181
  filing of, 254
  formation of, and ulceration, 140
  hemorrhage into, 181
  home surgery on, 233, *234*
  in diabetic neuropathy, 57
  of distal foot, 506, *507*
  pathophysiology of, 690
  plantar, and risk of ulceration, 142–143
  ulceration of, and mal perforans, 510–512, *511*
Calories, expenditure of, 213, 213t
Cancellous screw(s), *597*
Capillary(ies), blood flow in, 109t, 110
Capillary filling time, in peripheral arterial disease,
  230, 230t
Capillary refill time, 357
Capsaicin, for dysesthesia, 53
Carbamazepine, for paresthesia, 55
Carbohydrate(s), and wound healing, 214
Carbonyl(s), reactive, scavenging of, 87
Carbonyl stress, 81
Cardiovascular system, preoperative assessment of,
  515
CARE (Cholesterol and Recurrent Events) Trial, 8–9
Carnitine, for peripheral vascular disease, 535–536
Carotenoderma, 206
Cartilage, decreased growth of, in Charcot foot, 448
Carville splint, 150
Case management, by wound care nurse, 680
Cast(s), plaster, 712–713
  total-contact. See *Total-contact cast (TCC).*
Cast boot(s), 150
  for total-contact cast, 311, *312*
Cast shoe(s), 326–328, *327–328*
  resource list for, 331
Catheter(s), for percutaneous transluminal
  angioplasty, 379, *380*
Causation, as legal issue, 761
"Cayenne pepper spots," 693
β-Cell(s), destruction of, nitric oxide and, 72
Cell adhesion molecule(s), and endothelium, 75–76
Cellulitis, magnetic resonance imaging of, *349*
  vs. osteomyelitis, advanced imaging of, 342
Central America, foot care in, 268

Cephalosporin(s), for foot infections, 476t
Certification program(s), for wound care nurses, 677–678, 678t
Charcot foot, 237, 237–238, 239, 439–462
  bone and joint destruction in, 448–459, 449–458
    in ankle, 454–456, 456
    in calcaneocuboidal joint, 452–454, 455–456
    in calcaneus, 456–457, 457–458
    in forefoot, 448–450, 450–451
    in naviculocuneiform joints, 452–454, 455–456
    in subtalar joint, 454–456, 456
    in talonavicular joint, 452–454, 455–456
    with collapsed medial column, 695
  classification of, Eichenholtz, 587
  clinical features of, 440–441, 441t
  diagnosis of, 457–459
  disorders causing, 440
  foot ulcers in, 565, 566–567, 588
  historical perspective on, 439–440
  in diabetic neuropathy, 57
  management of, 459–462, 460
    algorithm for, 460
    bisphosphonates in, 462
    early recognition in, 460
    footwear in, 461–462
    goals of, 459
    immobilization in, 460–461
    orthotics in, 461–462
    pedorthic care in, 717
    surgical, 462, 587–605
      goals of, 588
      indications for, 587–588
      osteotomy in, 589, 590, 591
      realignment and arthrodesis in, 591, 592–601, 600–601
      results of, 601
      timing of, 588–589
      use of ankle-foot orthosis after, 599–600, 600–601
      vs. amputation, 601–602
    total-contact cast in, 662. See also Total-contact cast (TCC).
  natural history of, 441–443, 442
  pathogenesis of, 443–448, 444, 446
    collagen glycosylation in, 447–448
    decreased cartilage growth in, 448
    equinus deformity in, 447
    fractures in, 446, 446–447
    increased peripheral blood flow in, 444–445
    mechanical stress in, 445–446
    renal transplantation in, 447, 457
  pedorthic care for, case study of, 722–724, 723–724
  plantar stress in, 129, 130
  prevalence of, 440–441
  prevention of, 459–460
    fracture management in, 602, 603–605
  stages of, 442–443
  with heel ulcer, 573
Charcot fracture(s), clinical features of, 180
  surgical treatment of, 185–188
Charcot Restraint Orthotic Walker (CROW), 152, 461
China, foot care in, 266
Cholesterol and Recurrent Events (CARE) Trial, 8–9
Cholesterol embolism, and gangrene of toes, 227, 227pl, 228
Cholesterol ester(s), in atherosclerosis, 69–70
Chopart disarticulation, 626–627, 627
Chopart's joint, 494
Cigarette smoking. See Smoking.

Circulation, in foot ulcers, assessment of, 285
Clamshell ankle-foot orthosis, after Charcot foot surgery, 600
Claudication, and risk of lower limb amputation, 24
  clinical features of, 357, 526, 686
  in peripheral arterial disease, 227–230, 228t, 230, 230t
  management of, biofeedback in, 730–731
    conservative, 534–535
    pharmacologic, 535–536
  pathophysiology of, 356
  progression of, 526
Claustrophobia, during hyperbaric oxygen therapy, 413
Clavus, 505, 505
Claw foot deformity, 57, 58
Claw toe, 179
  and risk of ulceration, 141
  footwear for, 428
Cleanser(s), for wound care, toxicity of, 289, 289t
  types of, 294t
Clindamycin, for foot infections, 476t
Coagulation cascade, 396
Cock-up toe(s), 503
Cognitive ability, and patient education, 668
Cognitive-behavioral therapy, 733
Cold feet, in peripheral arterial disease, 229
Collaboration, interdisciplinary. See Interdisciplinary collaboration.
Collagen, and wound healing, 397
  cross-linking of, 84
  glycosylation of, and Charcot foot, 447–448
  glycoxidation of, and diabetic complications, 86
  production of, 406, 406
Collagen dressing(s), 294t
Colonization, bacterial, 468
Comparative fault, 762–763
Complement cascade, in wound healing, 396
Compliance, wound care nurse and, 680
Composite dressing(s), 294t
Compression bandage(s), 294t
Compression dressing(s), 642
Compression stocking(s), 329, 329t
Computed tomography (CT), 347–348, 348
  of Charcot foot, 458
Computed tomography angiography, 377, 377
Confinement anxiety, during hyperbaric oxygen therapy, 413
Consent, informed, 760–762
Contrast agent(s), interaction of, with metformin, 532
  nephrotoxicity of, 376, 532–533
  toxicity of, 342–343
Contrast angiography, 374–376, 375
Contributory negligence, 762–763
Controlled ankle motion device(s), 705–706, 706
Copper, and wound healing, 214–215
Corn(s), 505, 505
Corticosteroid(s), and Charcot foot, 447
  and wound healing, 215
  for necrobiosis lipoidica diabeticorum, 200
Cortisol, surgery and, 515
Cosmesis, after amputation, 610–611
Counterregulatory hormone(s), surgery and, 515
Cream(s), for diabetic foot care, 59–60
  for wound care, 294t
CROW (Charcot Restraint Orthotic Walker), 152, 461
CT. See Computed tomography (CT).
Cuboid bone, 495

Cuneiform bone, *495*
  osteomyelitis of, magnetic resonance imaging of, *351*
Cushion heel(s), in footwear, 710, *710*
Custom-made footwear, 713–714, *714*
  for Charcot foot, 723–724, *724*
Cutaneous nerve(s), 486, *487*

Damping element(s), and ground-footwear interaction, 159, *160,* 161
DCCT. See *Diabetes Control and Complications Trial (DCCT).*
Debridement, 287–288
  during initial evaluation, 613–614
  efficacy of, *vs.* total-contact cast, *304*
  hemostasis after, 288
  Kritter flow-through irrigation system after, 614, *614–615*
  of foot infections, 473
  of foot ulcers, 244
Deep peroneal nerve, assessment of, in diabetic neuropathy, 47
Deep tendon reflex(es), in diabetic neuropathy, 44–47
Demineralization, radiography of, 334–336, *336–338*
Depression, biochemical basis of, 729
  diabetes mellitus complications and, 729, 729t
  management of, 732–733, 733t
Depth-ischemia classification system, for diabetic wounds, 276–282, 276t, *277–281*
  flow chart for, *278*
  grade 0, 276, *277, 279*
  grade 1, *277, 278, 279*
  grade 2, *277, 279*
  grade 3, 279, *280–281*
  grade A, *277, 279*
  grade B, 280
  grade C, 280
  grade D, 280
  prognosis in, 282
Dermagraft, 249–250, 296
Dermatologic examination, *689–693,* 689–694
  for calluses, 690
  in autonomic neuropathy, 689–690, *690*
Dermatosis, perforating, 205, *205*
Dermopathy, diabetic, 201–202, 201pl, 693
Desensitization, of residual limb, 641–642
Dextran, and shear thinning, 114
  for hemorheologic disorders, 118, 119t
DH Pressure-Relief Walker, 152, 317, *317*
Diabetes Control and Complications Trial (DCCT), 5–6
  on hyperglycemia, 37, 39t
Diabetes mellitus, classification of, 4
  complications of, psychosocial factors in, 728–729, 729t
  cost of, 524
  cutaneous manifestation(s) of, 197–208
    bullae as, *202–203,* 202–204. See also *Diabetic bullae.*
    dermopathy as, 201–202, 201pl, 693
    from vascular changes, 197–198
    granuloma annulare as, 200–201, 200pl, *201*
    necrobiosis lipoidica diabeticorum as, 198–200, *199–200*
    scleroderma diabeticorum as, 204–205
  dermatosis in, 205–208, *205–208*

Diabetes mellitus (*Continued*)
  diagnostic criteria for, 4
  duration of, and onset of Charcot foot, 441, 441t
    and risk of foot ulcers, 14–15, 17t
    and risk of lower limb amputation, 22, 23t, 24
  economic impact of, 3, 404–405
  erythrocyte deformability in, 116–117
  exercise and, 252–253, 253t–254t
  incidence of, 3, 524
  leukocyte deformability in, 117–118
  morbidity from, 3
  mortality from, 3
  pathogenesis of, 72–73
  perioperative management of, 513–522
    for type 1 disease, 516–519, 517t–518t
      vs. type 2 disease, 514
    for type 2 disease, 519–521, 520t
    hyperglycemia and, 514
    interdisciplinary collaboration in, 516
    metabolic response to anesthesia in, 514–515
  plasma lipoproteins in, 77–78
  postoperative management of, 521–522
  preoperative evaluation of, 515–516
  risk determination in. See *Risk determination.*
  treatment of, hemorheology and, 118–121, 118t–120t
  type 2, screening for, 4
  upper extremity complications of, 556–557, *557*
  vascular complications of, 524. See also *Vascular disease.*
Diabetic bullae, *202–203,* 202–204
  blisters in, 202, *202*
  glycemic control and, 204
  limited joint mobility in, 202–204, *203*
  waxy skin syndrome in, 202–204
Diabetic dermopathy, 201–202, 201pl, 693
Diabetic foot clinic(s), 657–664
  acute problems in, management of, 661–662, 661t
  chronic care program of, 662–664
  equipment for, 661–662, 661t
  first-tier program for, 658–661
    intake evaluation in, 658–660
  organization of, 658
  personnel for, 658
  telephone "hotlines" in, 663
Diabetic Foot Study Group, 261
Diabetic nephropathy. See *Nephropathy.*
Diabetic neuropathic osteoarthropathy (DNOAP). See *Charcot foot.*
Diabetic neuropathy, clinical features of, 526–527
  definition of, 33–34
  diagnosis of, 41–50, 44t, *45–49,* 50t
    nerve fiber tests in, 49–50, 50t
    neurologic examination in, 41–49, 44t, *45–49,* 687–689, *687–689*
      limited, 42, 44t, *45–46*
      of balance, 48
      of deep tendon reflexes, 44–47
      of foot shape, 49
      of joint flexibility, 48–49
      of muscle strength, 47
      of muscle tightness, 48
      of proprioception, 47
      of sense of touch, 47–48
      pinprick testing for, 43–44
      two-point discrimination for, 42–43, *45*
      using Harris foot mat, 49, *49*
    Semmes-Weinstein monofilament in. See *Semmes-Weinstein monofilament(s).*

Diabetic neuropathy (*Continued*)
  differential diagnosis of, 687
  diffuse, 35–36, *36–38*
    plantar arteriovenous shunts in, 36, *37–38,* 59
    stocking-and-glove nerve damage in, 35–36, *36*
  epidemiology of, 34
  etiology of, 36–41, *39,* 39t, *42–43*
    abnormal fatty acid metabolism in, 40
    advanced glycosylated end products in, 40–41
    confirmation of, 41, *42–43*
    hyperglycemia in, 36–37, 39t
    myo-inositol in, 40
    nerve growth factor in, 41
    neural tissue antibodies in, 41
    polyol pathway in, *39,* 40, 72
    vasa nervorum in, 37–40, *39*
  focal, 34–35
  in joints, 337, *339–341*
    vs. malignancy, 340
  large fiber, 35
  pathogenesis of, 72
  progression of, *684*
  radiography in, 336–340, *339–341*
  reversible components of, 41, *43*
  risk factors for, 50–51, 50t
  scope of, *687*
  small fiber, 35
  stages of, 34, 34t
  subclinical, 33
  treatment of, 50–61, 50t, *51–59,* 60t–61t
    avoidance of future complications in, 56–61,
      58–59, 60t–61t
      routine office examination in, 57–60, *58–59*
    foot care in, 57–60, *58–59.* See also *Foot care.*
    risk stratification and, 60, 60t
    pain management in, 51–56, *51–57,* 52t, 55t, 58t
      acute *vs.* chronic, 52, 52t
      algorithm for, *51,* 56, *56–57,* 58t
      for dysesthesia, 53, *54,* 54t
      for muscular pain, *54,* 55–56
      for paresthesia, 53, *54,* 55
      nerve function and, 52, *52*
    patient education in, 61, 61t
    risk factor modification in, 50–51, 50t
  types of, 34–36, 35t, *36–38*
Diet. See also *Nutrition.*
  and blood viscosity, 118, 118t
Diffuse idiopathic skeletal hyperostosis (DISH), 333
Digital subtraction angiography, *375*
Digital vascular imaging (DVI), 534
Dilantin. See *Phenytoin.*
Disarticulation(s). See at specific site, e.g., *Toe(s),*
    disarticulation of.
DISH (diffuse idiopathic skeletal hyperostosis), 333
Distal symmetric polyneuropathy, 35–36, *36*
Diuretic(s), for hypertension, 225
DNOAP (diabetic neuropathic osteoarthropathy). See
    Charcot foot.
Documentation, as legal issue, 760
Doppler ultrasonography, of peripheral arterial
    disease, 361–362, 568
Dorsal interossei muscle(s), 492, *492*
Dorsal ulcer(s). See also *Foot ulcer(s).*
  pedorthic care for, case study of, 719, *720*
Dorsalis pedis artery, 486
Dorsalis pedis artery flap, 578, *580*
Double rocker bottom shoes, *708,* 708–709
  plaster, 315, *315–316*
Doxycycline, for foot infections, 476t

Drag, nonnewtonian fluids and, 115, 115t
Dressing(s), 290–293, 292t–295t
  advanced, 292
  after amputation, 639
  after open amputation, 615
  alginate, 294t
  antimicrobial, 294t
  application of, before total-contact cast, 306, *307*
  biosynthetic, 294t
  collagen, 294t
  composite, 294t
  compression, for residual limb, 642
  conventional, 292
  efficacy of, *vs.* total-contact cast, *304*
  film, 295t
  foam, 294t
  for foot ulcers, 152–153, 245
  hydrogel, 295t
  ideal, 292t
  moist, for autolytic debridement, 287
  occlusive *vs.* nonocclusive, 293
  primary, 292–293
  secondary, 292–293
  solutions for, home preparation of, 661t
  sterile *vs.* nonsterile, 293
Dry gangrene, 611, *612*
Dry skin, in diabetic neuropathy, 59
Duplex ultrasonography, of peripheral arterial
    disease, 368–369
DVI (digital vascular imaging), 534
Dysesthesia, in diabetic neuropathy, treatment of, 53,
    54, 54t

Early Treatment Diabetic Retinopathy Study
    (ETDRS), 9
Eastern Europe, foot care in, 265
Edema, as contraindication to total-contact cast,
    304–305
Education, of patient. See *Patient education.*
Educational material(s), for patients, 671
EGF. See *Epidermal growth factor (EGF).*
Eichenholtz classification, of Charcot foot, 587
Elastin, and wound healing, 397
Electrical stimulation, for wound healing, 250,
    296–297
Electronic information system(s). See *Information
    system(s).*
Embolism, and acute arterial occlusion, 230–231,
    230t
EMED peak pressure measurement platform,
    134–135
Emphysema, subcutaneous, 341–342
Empowerment, of patient, and prevention of foot
    ulcers, 740–741, 743–745
"Empty chair" defense, 763
Endarterectomy, aortoiliac, 540, *540–541,* 541t
End-artery disease, progression of, 499–501, *500–501*
Endothelial cell adhesion molecule (ELAM), and
    atherosclerosis, 76
Endothelin-1, activity of, 74–75
Endothelium, in atherosclerosis, 71–77. See also
    Atherosclerosis, endothelium in.
Endovascular procedure(s), for peripheral vascular
    disease, 536–537
Energy expenditure, after transfemoral amputation,
    632, 634
  from ambulation, after amputation, 636–638, 637t
  resting, 213, 213t

Enteral nutrition, postoperative, 218
Entrapment neuropathy, 35
Enzymatic debridement, 288, 294t
Enzyme(s), plasmin-activating, for hemorheologic
    disorders, 118, 119t
Epidermal growth factor (EGF), and wound healing,
    400
Epidural spinal stimulation, for intractable pain, 556
Epinephrine, surgery and, 515
Equinus deformity, and Charcot foot, 447
Erectile dysfunction, endothelin-1 and, 75
Eruptive xanthoma, 207, *207*
Erythrocyte(s), and blood shear thinning, 113–114
    deformability of, in diabetes mellitus, 116–117
    in rouleaux form, 116
Escharotomy, in foot ulcers, 244
ETDRS (Early Treatment Diabetic Retinopathy
    Study), 9
Euglycemic diabetic ketoacidosis, 515
Europe, foot care in, 262–265
European Association for Study of Diabetes, 261
Exercise, after amputation, 647–648
    and blood viscosity, 118, 118t
    for diabetic patient, 252–253, 253t–254t
    for intermittent claudication, 229
    patient education about, 672–673
    vascular response to, in peripheral arterial disease,
        358–360, *359,* 360t
Exercise stress testing, in peripheral arterial disease,
    365, 365–366
Extensor digitorum brevis muscle flap, 578, *580*
Extensor digitorum brevis tendon, *494*
Extensor hallucis brevis tendon, *494*
Extensor hallucis longus tendon, *494*
Extra-anatomic axillobifemoral bypass, 543
Extra-depth footwear, 432, *433*
Extremity(ies). See *Lower extremity(ies); Upper*
    extremity(ies).

FAB (*fixed-ankle-brace) walker, 434, 435*
Failure to diagnose, as legal issue, 758–759
Failure to educate patient, as legal issue, 761
Failure to prevent pressure ulcers, as legal issue, 759
Failure to treat pressure ulcers, as legal issue,
    759–760
Fall(s), risk of, assessment of, 181–182
    ulcer healing devices and, 153
Fasciocutaneous flap, for free tissue transfer, 578,
    582t
Fasting plasma glucose (FPG), and retinopathy
    risk, 4
    and risk of amputation, 23t
Fat(s), and wound healing, 214
    metabolism of, counterregulatory hormones and,
        515
Fatty acid(s), metabolism of, in diabetic
    neuropathy, 40
Fatty streak(s), in atherosclerosis, 67
Fault, comparative, 762–763
"Feet Can Last A Lifetime" program, 746
Felt padding, for total-contact cast, 309
Femoral artery, calcification of, *531*
    occlusion of, waveforms in, *363–364*
        with sparing of aorta and iliac artery, 532, *532*
Femoral distractor, for realignment of valgus
    deformity, *598*
Femoral posterior tibial bypass, *551–552*
Femoral-to-tibial bypass, *363*

Femoroperoneal artery bypass, 549, *549, 551*
Femoropopliteal angioplasty, 385, *388–389*
Femoropopliteal bypass, 543–547, *544,* 545t
    above-knee technique in, *544*
    below-knee technique in, *544*
    patency rates in, 545t, 547
    saphenous vein graft in, 544, 545t
    synthetic grafts for, 543–546, 546t
Femoropopliteal occlusive disease, surgical
    management of, 543–547, *544,* 545t. See also
    Femoropopliteal bypass.
Femoropoplitel artery bypass, *vs.* angioplasty, 385
FGF. See *Fibroblast growth factor (FGF).*
Fibrinogen, and blood flow, 109
    and shear thinning, 114–115
    in thrombosis, 89
    plasma, drugs affecting, 119–121, 120t
Fibrinolysis, low-density lipoprotein and, 82
Fibrinolytic system, in thrombosis, 90–91
Fibrinopeptide A, in thrombosis, 89
Fibroblast(s), proliferation of, hyperbaric oxygen
    therapy and, 407, *407–408*
Fibroblast growth factor (FGF), 399, 406
Fibroplasia, in wound healing, 396–397
Fiji, foot care in, 267
Film dressing(s), 295t
Finite element analysis, 163–164, *164–165*
Fixed-ankle-brace (FAB) walker, 434, *435*
Flap(s), local, 570, 577–578, *577–582*
    abductor digiti minimi muscle, 578, *581*
    extensor digitorum brevis muscle, 578, *580*
    lateral calcaneal artery, *578*
    medial calcaneal artery, 578, *579*
    medial plantar artery, *577*
    toe fillet, 578
    myofasciocutaneous, for knee disarticulation, 632
Flare reaction, 239
Flexor digiti quinti muscle, 488, *489–492*
Flexor digiti quinti tendon, *495*
Flexor digitorum brevis muscle, 488, *490, 492*
Flexor digitorum brevis muscle flap, 578, *582*
Flexor digitorum brevis tendon, *495*
Flexor digitorum longus muscle, *492*
Flexor digitorum longus tendon, 488, *489, 491 495*
Flexor hallucis brevis muscle, 488, *489–492*
Flexor hallucis brevis tendon, *495*
Flexor hallucis longus muscle, 488, *489–491*
Flexor hallucis longus tendon, *495*
Flexor muscle(s), 488
Flexor tendon, 492
Fluid(s), deformation of, *vs.* solids, 107, *108*
    nonnewtonian, 107
    properties of, 115, 115t
Fluoroquinolone(s), for foot infections, 474, 476t
Foam, for foot impressions, 713
    for total-contact orthosis, 713
Foam cell(s), in atherosclerosis, 69
Foam dressing(s), 294t
Focal neuropathy. See *Diabetic neuropathy, focal.*
Foot, and risk of ulceration, 140–142
    and susceptibility to infection, 468
    arterial calcification in, 111
    arteries to, 110–111, *111*
    bones of, 493, *494–495*
    burns of, *685*
    Charcot neuroarthropathy of, 439–462. See also
        Charcot foot.
    deformities of, 501–507, *502–508,* 502t
        and ulcers, 236–238, *236–239*

Foot (*Continued*)
   assessment of, 179–180, 179t, 669
   at heel, 507, *508*
   at midfoot, 506–507
   distal, 506, *507*
   footwear for, 427–428, *428,* 701
   in toes, 503–506, *504–507*
   motor neuropathy and, 395
   prophylactic surgery for, 507–509
   risk factors for, 493, 496
   dorsal, phlegmon of, 510
      skin grafts in, 570, *575–576*
   dorsiflexion of, in diabetic neuropathy, 47
   erythema of, 198
   examination of, 177–178, 179t, 240–242, *241,*
      684–695, *684–695*
      acute *vs.* chronic presentation for, *685*
      at intake evaluation, 658–660
      dermatologic, *689–693,* 689–694. See also *Skin,*
         examination of.
      in peripheral arterial disease, 357
      inspection in, 241, *241*
      musculoskeletal, 694–695, *695*
      neurologic, 687–688, *687–689*
      palpation in, 241
      patient education about, 668–670
      psychological effects of, 731
      sensory, 241–242
      vascular, 685–687, *686*
   forces at, and gait, 127, *130*
   impressions of, for total-contact orthosis, 712
   insensitive, detection of, Semmes-Weinstein
      monofilament in. See *Semmes-Weinstein*
      monofilament(s).
      examination of, 425, 425t
      progression of lesions in, 527
      protection of, 427
   intrinsic minus, 505, *505,* 687, *688*
   length of, *vs.* arch length, *704*
   muscles of, 488, *490–492,* 492
   nerves of, 486, *487*
   plantar flexion of, in diabetic neuropathy, 47
   range of motion in, evaluation of, 694
   regions of, for reconstructive surgery, 570, *573–575*
   shortened, footwear for, 433–435, *435*
   tendons of, 488, 493
Foot care, after ulcer healing, 250–251, *251*
   American Diabetes Association position statement
      on, 682
   by wound care nurses, 679
   complexity of, 283
   epidemiologic studies of, 263t
   exercise in, 252–253, 253t–254t
   in Africa, 268
   in Australia, 267
   in Austria, 265
   in Belgium, 264
   in Central America, 268
   in China, 266
   in diabetic neuropathy, 57–60, *58–59*
      and risk stratification, 00, 60t
   in Eastern Europe, 265
   in Fiji, 267
   in France, 264
   in Germany, 264
   in Greece, 265
   in India, 266
   in Italy, 264
   in Japan, 266

Foot care (*Continued*)
   in Nauru, 267
   in Netherlands, 264
   in New Zealand, 267
   in Philippines, 266
   in Scandinavia, 264–265
   in Singapore, 266
   in South America, 268
   in Spain, 265
   in Switzerland, 265
   in United Kingdom, 262, 264
   information systems for, 749–754. See also
      Information system(s).
   international conferences on, 261–262
   legal issues in, 254–255. See also *Legal issue(s).*
   noncompliance with, psychosocial issues in,
      729–730
   patient education about, 253–254, *254,*
      255t
      effectiveness of, 665–666
   psychosocial issues in, 252
Foot clinic(s). See *Diabetic foot clinic(s).*
Foot infection(s), 244–245, 244t, 467–479
   classification of, 471, 471t–472t
   clinical features of, 470
   complications of, 467
   cultures of, 469–470
   diagnosis of, 470, 470t, 691–692, *692*
   epidemiology of, 467–468
   indications for hospitalization in, 471
   involving bone, 471–473. See also *Osteomyelitis.*
   major, 509–512, *510–511*
   management of, 284–285
      with wet gangrene, 612–613
   of malleolus, *574*
   pathophysiology of, 468, 565, *568*
   progression of, 497–501, *498–501*
      initial lesion in, 497–498
      local, 498
      to end-artery disease, 499–501, *500–501*
      to septic arteritis, 498–499, *498–499*
   treatment of, 473–478, 476t–477t
      adjuvant, 477–478
      antibiotics in, 473–477, 476t–477t
         choice of, 474–475, 476t–477t
         cost of, 475
         duration of, 475, 477
         indications for, 473–474
         route of administration for, 474
         with osteomyelitis, 477
      debridement in, 473
      outcome of, 478
      surgical, 473
Foot pain, nondiabetic causes of, radiography in,
   333–334, *334–335*
Foot soak(s), efficacy of, 288
Foot ulcer(s). See also *Wound(s); Wound care.*
   base of, 691
   biopsy of, 242–243, 243pl
   circulation in, 285
   clinical features of, 242, 242pl
   culture of, 285
   depth of, 691, *692*
   economic impact of, 27, 28t, 29
   epidemiology of, 13–18, 14t–19t, *15–19,* 220, 263t
   exercise and, 252–253, 253t–254t, 673
   foot deformities and, *236–238,* 236–239
   from foreign bodies, 242
   from tight footwear, 429, *429*

Foot ulcer(s) (*Continued*)
  healing of, 146–153, *147–148,* 147t
    exercise after, 673
    impediments to, 248–249, 248t
    load relief and, 146, *147–148,* 147t
    maximum peak pressure for, 153
    non–weight-bearing for, 151
    risk of falls during, 153
    times for, 146, *147–148,* 147t
  history of, and risk of future ulceration, 143
  in Charcot foot, 448, 458, *458*
  incidence of, 13–14, 14t
  ischemic, 692, *692–693*
  margins of, 691, *691*
  morbidity from, 220
  nonhealing, skin equivalents for, 295–296, 295t
    management of, 286–287
  nutrition and, 212–218. See also *Nutrition.*
  osteomyelitis in, incidence of, 511
  pathogenesis of, 139–140, 221–239, *222–238,*
      405
    callus formation in, 140
    Charcot foot in, 565, *566–567.* See also *Charcot
      foot.*
    foot deformities in, *236–238,* 236–239
    infection in, 239
    peripheral arterial disease in, 221–231, *224–230.*
      See also *Peripheral arterial disease.*
    peripheral neuropathy in, 231–236, *232–236.* See
      also *Peripheral neuropathy.*
    tissue ischemia in, 139
  penetrating, *243,* 243–244
  preparation of, for total-contact cast, 306
  prevention of, 565, 567
    failure of, as legal issue, 759
    feasibility of, 737–738
    health care provider empowerment in, 743–745
    patient education in, 426–429, *428,* 663
    patient empowerment in, 740–741, 743–745
    surgical procedures for, 185–188
  psychosocial issues in, 728
  recurrence of, after total-contact cast, 314
    footwear compliance and, 428–429
    risk factors for, 18
  risk factor(s) for, 140–146, 493, 496–497. See also
      Risk determination.
    age as, 14, *15*
    autonomic neuropathy as, 683–684
    body weight as, 144
    component causes in, 18, *18–19*
    duration of diabetes as, 14–15, 17t
    footwear as, 145, 232, *232*
    fractures as, 143
    gait abnormalities as, 144–145
    gender as, 14, *16,* 17t
    glycosylated hemoglobin as, 16, 17t
    history of ulcers as, 143
    insulin resistance syndrome as, 684
    leg weakness as, 143
    limited joint mobility as, 142
    noncompliance as, 496–497, *497*
    peripheral neuropathy as, 15, 17t
    plantar callus as, 142–143
    posture as, 144–145
    race as, 14, *18*
    shear stress as, 143–144
    smoking as, 16, 17t
    structure-function relationships in, 140–142
    tissue-related, 142

Foot ulcer(s) (*Continued*)
  screening for, 738
    targeting health care providers for, 739–740
  site of, 14, 14t–15t
    distribution of, 125, 139, *139*
  size of, documentation of, before total-contact cast,
      306, *306*
  threshold pressure for. See *Threshold pressure.*
  treatment of, 242–249, 242t–248t, *243–248*
    adjunctive, 249–250
    ankle-foot orthosis in, 317, *317,* 323, *327*
    antibiotics in, 244
    braces in, 152
    cast shoe in, 326–328, *327–328*
    Charcot Restraint Orthotic Walker in, 152
    cost of, international comparison of, 261
    custom sandals in, 325
    debridement in, 244
    DH Pressure Relief Walker in, 152, 317, *317*
    dressings in, 152–153, 245. See also *Dressing(s).*
    escharotomy in, 244
    failure of, as legal issue, 759–760
    "half shoes" in, 151
    healing shoes in, 325–326, *327*
    holistic, 679
    hyperbaric oxygen therapy in. See *Hyperbaric
      oxygen therapy.*
    MABAL shoe in, 150–151
    neuropathic walker in, *323,* 323–324
    non–weight-bearing in, 245
    orthopedic scooters in, 151
    orthotic dynamic system splint in, 322, *322*
    pedorthic care in, 714–715
      case study of, 718–719, *718–719*
    posterior splint in, 322–323, *323*
    skin grafts in, *234*
    total-contact cast in, 146–151, 245. See also
      Total-contact cast (TCC).
    weight relief shoes in, 324–325, *325–326*
    whirlpool therapy in, 245, 288
Footwear, 154–177
  acceptance of, 176–177
  accommodative behavior of, 156, *157*
  after transmetatarsal amputation, 625
  after ulcer healing, 250–251, *251*
  and cushioning, static and dynamic phases of, 154,
      155, 156
  and ground plane properties, 159, *160,* 161
  and risk of lower limb amputation, 25
  and risk of ulceration, 145
  and shear stress, 159
  biomechanics of, computer models of, 163–164,
      164–165
  compliance with, and recurrent ulcers, 428–429
  components of, 702, *702*
  cushion heels in, 710, *710*
  customized uppers for, 710, *711*
  custom-made, 713–714, *714*
  distribution of force by, 156–157, *157–158*
  evaluation of, by podiatrist, 695–696
  examination of, 660–661
  extended steel shanks for, *709,* 709–710
  extra-depth, 432, *433*
  fit of, 175–176, *176*
  fitting of, 430, *430–431,* 702–704, *702–704*
    guidelines for, 703–704
    shoe shape and, 702–703, *702–703*
    shoe size and, 703, *704*
  for Charcot foot, 461–462, 717

Footwear (*Continued*)
  for diabetic neuropathy, 60–61
  for dorsal ulcers, 715
  for injury prevention, risk determination in,
      423–425, *424*
  for plantar ulcers, 714
  for shortened feet, 433–435, *435*
  for tarsometatarsal amputations, 716
  for toe and ray amputations, 715–716
  for transmetatarsal amputations, 716
  healing, 704–706, *704–706*
  heel relief, 705, *706*
  in-depth, 706
    with orthotics, 326
  insoles for, biomechanical studies of, 164–170,
      166–170, 166t. See also *Insole(s).*
  Medicare reimbursement for, 423
  negative heel, 705, *705*
  outsoles of, 171–175, *172–173,* 172t–175t
  patient education about, 254, *254,* 671–672
  plantar pressure measurement in, 133, *134*
  poorly fitting, and foot ulcers, 232, *232*
  postoperative, 705, *705*
  prescription of, 182–185, *183,* 184t–186t, 717
    activity level and, 184t
    examination of existing footwear in, 182
    for partial amputation, 185, 186t
    plantar pressure measurement and, 176
    recommendations for, 183–185, 186t
    stepwise approach to, 182–183, *183*
  rocker soles for, 706–709, *707–708*
  stabilization of, 709, *709*
  temporary, 435–436, *436–437*
  tight, ulceration from, 429, *429*
  tissue properties and, 161–163, *162*
  uppers of, and shear strain on plantar tissue,
      175–176, *176*
  wedges for, 710, *710*
Force, distribution of, by footwear, 156–157, *157–158*
  ground reaction, 129, *130*
  harm done by, 127–129, *130*
Force platform(s), 127, *130*
Force-time integral, in plantar pressure
    measurement, 134–135, *135*
Forearm, flexion of, in diabetic neuropathy, 47
Forefoot, bone and joint destruction in, from Charcot
    foot, 448–450, *450–451*
  contour of, after ray amputation, 619, *620*
    after toe disarticulation, 618, *618*
  pronation of, 179
  supination of, 180
Forefoot-relief shoe(s), 324, *325*
Foreign body(ies), in foot, 242
Fosamax. See *Alendronate.*
FPG. See *Fasting plasma glucose (FPG).*
Fracture(s). See also specific site.
  acute management of, for prevention of Charcot
      foot, 602, *603–605*
  and risk of ulceration, 143
  avulsion, 456–457, *457–458*
  in Charcot foot, *446,* 446–447
  in neuroarthropathy, radiography of, 337, 340
  stress, 333–334, *335*
    after tibiotalocalcaneal arthrodesis, 601, *601*
    magnification radiography in, *345*
France, foot care in, 264
Free tissue transfer, case study of, 578, 583, *583*
  fasciocutaneous flap for, 578, 582t
  indications for, 578

Free tissue transfer (*Continued*)
  muscle flap for, 578, 582t
  types of, advantages and disadvantages of, 582t
Freiberg's infraction, 340
Fungal infection(s), from total-contact cast, 306
Fusidic acid, 291t

Gabapentin, for dysesthesia, 53
Gait, 126–129, *128–130*
  abnormalities of, and risk of ulceration, 144–145
  after amputation, 644–645
  assessment of, 182
  forces at foot and, 127, *130*
  in peripheral neuropathy, 235–236
  in rocker shoes, 174
  kinematics and, 127, *128–129*
  pressure and, 127–129, *130*
  rationale for study of, 126–127
  speed of, in measurement of plantar pressure, 131
  with prosthesis, 648–651
    goals of, 651
    horizontal tilt and, 649–650
    lateral shift and, 649
    standing balance and, 648–649
    transverse rotation and, 650–651
    vertical displacement and, 649
Gallium-67 citrate scintigraphy, in osteomyelitis, 347
Ganglioside(s), and diabetic neuropathy, 41
Gangrene, dry, 611, *612*
  factors precipitating, 608
  from mal perforans, *511,* 512
  historical accounts of, 219
  in upper extremities, 556–557, *557*
  of heel, 240, *240,* 507, *508*
  of toes, 227, 227pl, *228*
    from thermal injury, 233, *235*
  progression of, 499, *500–501,* 501
  wet, 611–614, *614*
Gastrocnemius muscle, 488
Gastrointestinal disease, and micronutrient
    deficiency, 215
Gauze, for dressings, 292, 294t–295t
G-CSF (granulocyte colony-stimulating factor), for foot
    infections, 239, 477–478
Gender, and risk of foot ulcers, 14, *16,* 17t
  and risk of lower limb amputation, 22, *22*
General practitioner defense, 762
Germany, foot care in, 264
GLA (γ-linoleic acid), metabolism of, 40
Glucagon, surgery and, 515
Glucagonoma, 207, *208*
Glucophage. See *Metformin.*
Glucose, blood levels of, control of. See *Glycemic
    control.*
    perioperative, 518–519
    postoperative, 521
    stress mediated by, reduction of, 86
Glucose tolerance, impaired, 4
Glucose tolerance test, oral, as screening tool, 4
Glycation, and antithrombin III activity, 84
  and atherosclerosis, 80–81
  of lipoprotein(a), 83
  of lipoproteins, 81–82
  of vascular structural proteins, inhibition of, 86–88
Glycemic control, 4–7
  and diabetic bullae, 204
  and neuropathic pain, 52
  and risk of amputation, 24, 221

Glycemic control (*Continued*)
  and risk of diabetic neuropathy, 50–51
  biofeedback and, 731
  clinical trials of, 5–6
  during nutritional support, 218
  epidemiologic studies of, 4–5
  in wound care, 285
  intensive *vs.* conventional, 5–6
  pharmacologic, 7
  treatment of depression and, 733
Glycosylated hemoglobin (HbA$_{1c}$), and risk of foot
    ulcers, 16, 17t
  and risk of limb amputation, 23t
  and vascular disease, 525
  and wound healing, 610
Glycosylation, and risk of ulceration, 142
  of collagen, and Charcot foot, 447–448
Glycoxidation, and collagen cross-linking, 84
  of collagen, and diabetic complications, 86
  of vascular structural proteins, in atherosclerosis,
    84–88, *85*
  products of, aminoguanidine and, 87
    and renal impairment, 86
    in diabetes mellitus, 80–81
Graft(s), skin. See *Skin graft(s)*.
Granulation tissue, assessment of, 286
Granulocyte colony-stimulating factor (G-CSF), for
    foot infections, 239, 477–478
Granuloma annulare, 200–201, 200pl, *201*
Greece, foot care in, 265
Ground reaction force, 129, *130*
Group Health Cooperative of Puget Sound, 750,
    751–752
Growth factor(s), and wound healing, 295–296, 295t,
    397–401, 556
  in atherosclerosis, 69–70
Guide pin(s), insertion of, *595*
"Guillotine" amputation, 614

"Half shoes," 151
Hallux, disarticulation of, 616, *616–617*
  metatarsophalangeal joint of, septic arthritis of,
    280
  pressure in, measurement of, *361*
  ulcers of, limited metatarsophalangeal joint
    mobility and, 127, *129*
Hallux extensus, *687*
Hallux interphalangeal sesamoid, *695*
Hallux valgus deformity, 333, *334*, 506, *507*
  after disarticulation of second toe, 617, *617*
Hammer toe(s), 503, *504–505*, 505
  and foot ulcers, *236*, 567
Hand, limited joint mobility in, 203, *203*
Haptoglobin, and shear thinning, 114–115
Harris foot mat, 49, *49*
Harris-Benedict equation, 213, 213t
HbA$_{1c}$. See *Glycosylated hemoglobin (HbA$_{1c}$)*.
HDL. See *High-density lipoprotein (HDL)*.
HDS (Hypertension in Diabetes Study), 7
Healing shoes, 704–706, *704–706*
  with orthosis, 325–326, *327*
Health, beliefs about, 667
Health care provider(s), empowerment of, 743–745
  foot ulcer screening by, 739–740
  relationship with patient, legal issues in, 757–761.
    See also *Legal issue(s)*.
Heat-moldable healing shoe(s), 704, 704–705,
    719

Heel, ability to walk on, 48
  deformities of, 507, *508*
  trauma to, 239–240, *240*
Heel pad, preservation of, in Syme ankle
    disarticulation, 629, *629–631*
Heel relief shoe(s), 705, *706*
Heel ulcer(s), progression of, 497, *508*
  treatment of, 245, *246–248*, 248
    total-contact cast for, 150
  with Charcot foot, *573*
Heel-relief shoe(s), 324, *326*
Heel-to-toe rocker bottom shoe(s), 707, *708*
Heloma molle, 505–506, *506*
Hemoglobin (HbA$_{1c}$), glycosylated. See *Glycosylated*
    hemoglobin (HbA$_{1c}$).
Hemorheology, 107–121. See also *Blood; Blood flow*.
  and treatment of diabetes mellitus, 118–121,
    118t–120t
Hemostasis, after debridement, 288
High-density lipoprotein (HDL), decreased levels
    of, 66
  glycation of, 83
  in atherosclerosis, and qualitative abnormalities in
    diabetes, 79
  in diabetes mellitus, 77–78
  in peripheral arterial disease, 225
Hindfoot, neuropathic arthropathy of, *592, 594, 597*
  varus deformity of, *592, 594, 597*
"Home surgery," dangers of, 685, *685*
  trauma from, 233, *234*
Hormone(s), counterregulatory, 515
HOT (Hypertension Optimal Treatment) Study, 7
Hourglass appearance, of phalanges, *450*
Humalog, perioperative use of, 518–519
Human skin equivalent(s), 295–296, 295t
Hydrogel dressing(s), 295t
Hygiene, patient education about, 671
Hyperbaric oxygen therapy, adjunctive use of, 405
  and angiogenesis, 408, *409*, 414
  and fibroblast proliferation, 407, *407–408*
  and leukocyte killing ability, 412
  and neovascularization, 411
  and tissue oxygen tension, 413–414, *413–414*
  and vasoconstriction, 412
  and wound healing, 415, 415t, *416*
  case study of, 417, 417pl
  chambers for, 409, *410–411*
  clinical studies of, 414–416, 415t, *416*
  confinement anxiety during, 413
  cost of, 414–415
  definition of, 408–409
  efficacy of, 556
  for foot infections, 478
  for wound healing, 250
  future trends in, 417
  history of, 405
  mechanism of action for, 411, 412t
  patient selection for, *416*, 416–417
  protocols for, 417
  rationale for, 405–407, *406–409*
  side effects of, 412
  toxicity of, 412–413, *413*
Hyperglycemia, and peripheral arterial disease,
    225
  and postoperative infection, 217
  and wound healing, 216–217
  in diabetic neuropathy, 36–37, 39t
  pathophysiology of, and perioperative diabetes
    management, 514

Hyperinsulinemia, 66–67, 225–226
Hyperlipidemia, 51, 225
  control of, 8–9
Hypertension, 51, 66, 225
  control of, 7–8
Hypertension in Diabetes Study (HDS), 7
Hypertension Optimal Treatment (HOT) Study, 7
Hypoalbuminemia, and stress response, 216
Hypoglycemia, anesthesia and, 516
Hypoglycemic agent(s), perioperative use of, 519–520, 520t
Hysteresis, and ground-footwear interaction, 159, 160, 163

IGF. See Insulin-like growth factor (IGF).
Iliac artery(ies), occlusion of, magnetic resonance angiography in, 378
    thrombolysis of, 384
    waveforms in, 364
Iliofemoral endarterectomy, 540
Imaging study(ies), 333–351. See also under specific type.
  selection of, 350–351
Imipenem-cilastatin, for foot infections, 476t
Imipramine, for paresthesia, 55
Immediate postoperative prosthesis (IPOP), 639
Immobilization, after fracture treatment, 602
  for Charcot foot, 460–461
Immune complex(es), in atherosclerosis, 68–69
Immune function, in diabetes mellitus, 468
  low-density lipoprotein modification and, 83–84
Immunosuppression, and wound healing, 249
Immunosuppressive therapy, and Charcot foot, 447
Impaired glucose tolerance, 4
In-depth shoes, 706
  with orthoses, 326
India, foot care in, 266
Indium-111 white blood cell imaging, 347
  in Charcot foot, 458–459
  in osteomyelitis, 472
Infection(s), and foot ulcers, 239
  of foot, 244–245, 244t. See also Foot infection(s).
  postoperative, hyperglycemia and, 217
  radiography of, 340–342, 342–344
  superficial vs. deep, 468–469
Inflammation, in wound healing, 396
Information system(s), 749–754
  future progress of, 752, 754
  Group Health Cooperative of Puget Sound, 750, 751–752
  Lovelace Health Systems, 750
  of Kaiser Permanente of Ohio, 750–753
  stratification grids in, 753–754
Informed consent, 760–762
Infrainguinal arterial occlusive disease, 537–538, 537–539
Infrapopliteal vascular occlusive disease, surgical management of, 547–550, 548–552
  choice of site for, 547
  femoral posterior tibial bypass in, 551–552
  femoroperoneal artery bypass in, 549, 549, 551
  patency rates in, 549
  popliteal to dorsalis pedis bypass in, 551, 553
  PTFE grafts in, 548–549

Infrapopliteal vascular occlusive disease (Continued)
    results of, in diabetic vs. nondiabetic patients, 547–548, 548t
    saphenous vein graft in, 547, 550, 550
Infrared thermometry, in Charcot foot, 460
  in diagnosis of infected foot ulcers, 285
  in diagnosis of inflammation, 427
Ingrown toenail(s), 503–504
Injury. See Trauma.
Insole(s), biomechanical studies of, compression tests in, 165–166, 166, 166t
    pressure reduction properties in, 165–166
    redistribution of load in, 168–170, 169–170
    stress-strain curves in, 164, 166
    thickness in, 167
    using "plugs," 167, 168
    with metatarsal pads, 166–167
  evaluation of, 433
  for control of pronation, 431
  for diabetic neuropathy, 60
  materials for, 156–157, 158, 431–432, 432
Insulin, and endothelin production, 75
  and platelet function, 91
Insulin resistance syndrome, and risk of foot ulcers, 684
Insulin therapy, during nutritional support, 218
  for type 1 diabetes mellitus, 516–519, 517t–518t
  for type 2 diabetes mellitus, 519–521
  intensive vs. conventional, 6
  postoperative, 521
Insulin-like growth factor (IGF), and cartilage formation, in Charcot foot, 448
  and wound healing, 400–401
Interdisciplinary collaboration, in foot care, 251–252, 252t
  in interventional radiology, 375
  in management of foot ulcers, 251–252, 252t
  in perioperative diabetes management, 516
  in wound care, 284
Interleukin-1 (IL-1), 69
Intermittent claudication. See Claudication.
Internal vascular belt, anatomy of, 486
International Consensus Group on the Diabetic Foot, 261–262
Internet, for prevention programs, 746–747
Interossei muscle(s), anatomy of, 492, 492
Interphalangeal joint(s), destruction of, in Charcot foot, 449
Interventional radiology, 374–388
  in peripheral vascular disease, 536–537
  interdisciplinary collaboration in, 375
  new techniques in, 376–379, 376–379
  percutaneous transluminal angioplasty in, 379–383, 380–384
  peripheral arterial angioplasty in, 383–388, 385–392. See also Peripheral arterial angioplasty.
Intravascular ultrasonography (IVUS), 376, 376
Intrinsic minus foot, 505, 505, 687, 688
Iodine, cadexomer, 290, 291t
IPOP (immediate postoperative prosthesis), 639
Iron, and wound healing, 214
Irrigation, Kritter flow-through, 614, 614–615
  of wounds, 289
Ischemic neuritis, in peripheral arterial disease, 229
Italy, foot care in, 264
IVUS (intravascular ultrasonography), 376, 376

Japan, foot care in, 266
Joint(s). See also named joint, e.g., *Ankle.*
    destruction of, in Charcot foot, 448–459, *449–458.*
        See also *Charcot foot, bone and joint
        destruction in.*
    diabetic neuropathy of, 337, *339–341*
        vs. malignancy, 340
    flexibility of, 48–49
    mobility of, assessment of, 694–695
        limited, and risk of ulceration, 142
            as goal of pedorthist, 701
            clinical approach to, 181
            in diabetic bullae, 202–204, *203*
    pain in, after amputation of contralateral limb,
        644–645
Judgment defense, 762
Jury(ies), verdicts of, statistics on, 763–765

Kaiser Permanente of Ohio, information system of,
        750–753
Kaposi's sarcoma, 207
Keratinocyte growth factor (KGF), 399
Keratosis, in perforating dermatosis, 205, *205*
Ketoacidosis, euglycemic, 515
Ketonuria, 521
KGF (keratinocyte growth factor), 399
Kidney. See *Renal* entries.
Kinematic viscosity, 109
Kinematics, 127, *128–129*
"Kissing" balloon technique, in peripheral arterial
        angioplasty, 383, *386*
Knee, deep tendon reflex in, 45
    disarticulation of, 632
        energy expenditure from ambulation after,
            636–637
    leg flexion/extension at, 47
    preservation of, in transtibial amputation, 630–632
Kritter flow-through irrigation system, 614, *614–615*
Kyrle's disease, 205, *205*

Lanolin, for diabetic foot care, 60
Larval therapy, for foot infections, 478
Laser Doppler velocimetry (LDV), 368, 530
Last(s), for footwear, 702
Laws of motion, and behavior of fluids, 107
Lawsuit(s), malpractice. See Legal issue(s);
        Malpractice suit(s).
LDL. See *Low-density lipoprotein (LDL).*
LDV (laser Doppler velocimetry), 368, 530
Learning, by adults, 666–667
Leg ulcer(s), treatment of, 401–402
Leg vein(s), blood flow in, 111–112
Legal issue(s), 757–765
    abandonment as, 760
    case studies of, 763–765
    causation as, 761
    comparative fault as, 762–763
    contributory negligence as, 762–763
    defendant's case and, 761–763
    "do's and don't" pertaining to, 765
    "empty chair" defense as, 763
    failure to diagnose as, 758–759
    failure to educate patient patient as, 761
    failure to prevent pressure ulcers as, 759
    foot care and, 254–255

Legal issue(s) (*Continued*)
    informed consent as, 760–761
    negligence as, 758
    plaintiff's case and, 757–761
    standards of care as, 758
    surgical battery as, 760–761
Lente insulin, perioperative use of, 519
Leriche's syndrome, 228, 357
Leukocyte(s), and blood flow, 113, *114*
    deformability of, in diabetes mellitus, 117–118
    imaging of. See *White blood cell imaging.*
    killing ability of, hyperbaric oxygen therapy and,
        412
Lichen planus, 206
Ligament(s), weakening of, in Charcot foot, 442
Limb salvage, algorithm for, *585*
    principles of, 584, *585,* 586
    rates of, hyperbaric oxygen therapy and, 414–416,
        415t
    with tissue transfer, in peripheral vascular disease,
        550–552, *553*
Limb-threatening emergency(ies), management of,
        611–615, *612, 614*
    with dry gangrene, 611, *612*
    with wet gangrene, 611–614, *614*
γ-Linoleic acid (GLA), metabolism of, 40
Lipid(s), and atherosclerosis, 77–80
    qualitative abnormalities in diabetes and, 78
    control of, 8–9
    stress mediated by, reduction of, 86–87
α-Lipoic acid, for paresthesia, 55
Lipoprotein(s), 77–80. See also *High-density
        lipoprotein (HDL); Low-density lipoprotein
        (LDL); Very low-density lipoprotein (VLDL).*
Lipoprotein(a), glycation of, 83
Lipoprotein(s), glycation of, 81–82
    oxidation of, 73
    plasma, in diabetes, 77–78
Lipoprotein-deficient serum, in diabetes mellitus, 80
Lisfranc disarticulation, 625, *626*
Lisfranc's joint. See *Tarsometatarsal joint(s).*
Lisinopril, and nerve conduction velocity, in diabetic
        neuropathy, 37–38
Literacy, and patient education, 668
"Livingston's vicious cycle," 55
LLADM (lower limb arterial duplex mapping), 369
Load, redistribution of, by insoles, 168–170, *169–170*
Loading analysis, in plantar pressure measurement,
        133–135, *135*
Local flap(s), 570, 577–578, *577–582.* See also *Flap(s),
        local.*
Lotion(s), for diabetic foot care, 59–60
Lovelace Health Systems, 750
Low-density lipoprotein (LDL), and peripheral
        arterial disease, 225
    glycation of, 81–82
    in atherosclerosis, 79
    modification of, 83–84
    oxidation of, dietary monounsaturated fats and, 77
    in atherosclerosis, 67–71, *71*
Lower extremity(ies). See also specific part, e.g., *Foot.*
    amputation of. See *Amputation, lower limb.*
    arteriosclerosis in, in diabetics *vs.* nondiabetics, 501
    artificial calcification in, 111
    biomechanics of, and design of total-contact
        orthosis, 711–712
    flexion-extension of, at knee, 47
    peripheral arterial disease in. See *Peripheral
        arterial disease, in lower extremities.*

Lower extremity(ies) (*Continued*)
  physical examination of, 527
  surgery on, diabetic management during, 513–522.
    See also *Diabetes mellitus, perioperative management of.*
  weakness in, risk of ulceration and, 143
Lower Extremity Amputation (LEA) Group, 261
Lower limb arterial duplex mapping (LLADM), 369
Lumbar sympathectomy, 552
Lumbrical muscle(s), 488
Lysine, hydroxylation of, *406,* 406–407

MABAL shoe, 150–151
Macronutrient(s), and wound healing, 214
Macrophage(s), activation of, in atherosclerosis, 69
  and wound healing, 396
Maggot therapy, for foot infections, 478
Magnetic resonance angiography (MRA), 377,
  378–379, 379
  indications for, 534
  of peripheral arterial disease, 369–370
Magnetic resonance flowmetry, of peripheral arterial
  disease, 369–370
Magnetic resonance imaging (MRI), 348–350,
  349–351
  of Charcot foot, 458
  of osteomyelitis, 472
Magnetoresistive device(s), 144
Mal perforans, 510–512, *511*
Malignancy, in joints, *vs.* neuropathy, 340
Malleolus, wound infection of, *574*
Malpractice suit(s), plaintiff's case in, burden of proof
  and, 757
Managed care, and wound healing, 249
Mask(s), for plantar pressure measurement, 132–133,
  132–133
Mechanical stress, and Charcot foot, 445–446
Median nerve, assessment of, in diabetic neuropathy,
  47
Medical record(s), electronic. See *Information system(s).*
Medicare, reimbursement for footwear by, 423
Medicolegal issue(s). See *Legal issue(s).*
Meggitt classification system, for diabetic wounds,
  274–275
Metacarpophalangeal joint(s), osteomyelitis of, *346*
Metatarsal(s), *494*
Metatarsal bar(s), *433*
Metatarsal "cookies," 430
Metatarsal fracture(s), in Charcot foot, 451, *452*
Metatarsal head(s), cupping of, in Charcot foot, 450,
  450
  mal perforans of, 510–512, *511*
  osteomyelitis of, 341, *343*
    computed tomography of, *348*
    management of, *571–572*
  resection of, for recurrent ulcers, 186, 186pl
  resorptive changes in, 334, 336
  soft tissue thickness under, 180
  ulcers of, *573*
    magnification radiography of, *345*
Metatarsal ligament, *491*
Metatarsal pad(s), biomechanical studies of, 166–167
Metatarsal shaft, shortening of, in ray amputation,
  619, *619*
Metatarsophalangeal joint(s), destruction of, in
  Charcot foot, 448, *449, 451*
  disarticulation of toes at, 616–617, *617*

Metatarsophalangeal joint(s) (*Continued*)
  excision of, 622–623, *623*
  kinematics of, 127, *128–129*
  of hallux, septic arthritis of, *280*
  pencil-cup deformity of, *344*
Metaxalone, for paresthesia, 56
Metformin, interaction of, with contrast agents,
  342–343, 376, 532
  perioperative use of, 520, 520t
  vs. conventional therapy, 6
Methicillin-resistant *Staphylococcus aureus* (MRSA),
  290, 470
Metronidazole, for foot infections, 476t
  for wound care, 291t
Mexiletine, for paresthesia, 55
Microangiopathy, in peripheral arterial disease, 223
  obliterative, 498–499, *499*
Micronutrient(s), and wound healing, 214–215
  deficiency of, comorbid conditions and, 215
Microvascular disease, history of, and risk of foot
  lesions, 683
Midtarsal amputation, pedorthic care for, 716
  case study of, 722, *722*
Midtarsal disarticulation, 626–627, *627*
Mild rocker bottom shoes, 707, *708*
Mineral(s), and wound healing, 214–215
Mobility, after amputation, 639–640
Moist dressing(s), 287
Moisturizer(s), for diabetic foot care, 59–60
Monofilament(s), Semmes-Weinstein. See *Semmes-Weinstein monofilament(s).*
Monounsaturated fat(s), dietary, and low-density
  lipoprotein oxidation, 77
Morocco, foot care in, 268
Motor neuropathy, and foot deformity, 395
  assessment of, 660
  complications of, 687, *688*
MRA. See *Magnetic resonance angiography (MRA).*
MRI. See *Magnetic resonance imaging (MRI).*
MRSA (methicillin-resistant *Staphylococcus aureus*),
  290, 470
Mupirocin polyethylene glycol ointment, 290, 291t
Muscle(s). See also named muscle.
  tightness of, in diabetic neuropathy, 48
Muscle flap(s), for free tissue transfer, 578, 582t
Muscle strength testing, in diabetic neuropathy, 47
Muscular pain, in diabetic neuropathy, *54,* 55–56
Myofasciocutaneous flap, for knee disarticulation,
  632
Myo-inositol, in diabetic neuropathy, 40

Naftidrofuryl, for peripheral vascular disease,
  535–536
Nail(s). See *Toenail(s).*
National Pressure Ulcer Advisory Panel/Agency for
  Health Care Policy and Research (NPUAP/
  AHCPR) staging system, 286
Nauru, foot care in, 267
Navicular bone, anatomy of, *494–495*
  displacement of, in Charcot foot, *454*
  osteomyelitis of, magnetic resonance imaging of,
  351
Naviculocuneiform joint, destruction of, in Charcot
  foot, *449,* 452–454, *455–456*
NCV. See *Nerve conduction velocity (NCV).*
Necrobiosis lipoidica diabeticorum, 198–200, *199–200*
Negative heel shoes, 705, *705*
  rocker bottom, 707–708, *708*

Negligence, 758
    case study of, 763–764
    contributory, 762–763
Neovascularization, hyperbaric oxygen therapy and,
        411
Nephropathy, pathogenesis of, nitric oxide in, 72
    proteinuria and, 516
Nephrotoxicity, contrast agents and, 376, 532–533
Nerve(s), of foot, 486, *487*. See also specific nerve.
Nerve conduction velocity (NCV), aldose reductase
        inhibitors and, 40
    in diabetic neuropathy, deterioration of, 41, *42*
        lisinopril and, 37–38
Nerve fiber test(s), in diabetic neuropathy, 49–50, 50t
Nerve function, and neuropathic pain, 52, *52*
Nerve growth factor, and diabetic neuropathy, 41
Netherlands, foot care in, 264
Neural tissue, antibodies to, in diabetic
        neuropathy, 41
Neuritis, ischemic, in peripheral arterial disease,
        229
Neuroarthropathy, Charcot. See *Charcot foot.*
    fractures in, radiography of, 337, 340
Neurologic examination, in diabetic neuropathy,
        41–49, 44t, *45–49.* See also *Diabetic
        neuropathy, diagnosis of, neurologic
        examination in.*
Neurontin. See *Gabapentin.*
Neuropathic arthropathy. See *Charcot foot.*
Neuropathic osteoarthropathy. See *Charcot foot.*
Neuropathic walker(s), *323,* 323–324
Neuropathy, autonomic. See *Autonomic neuropathy.*
    diabetic. See *Diabetic neuropathy.*
    entrapment, 35
    motor. See *Motor neuropathy.*
    peripheral. See *Peripheral neuropathy.*
New Zealand, foot care in, 267
Newton, Sir Isaac, study of fluids by, 107
Nitric oxide, 71–73
Noncompliance, and risk of foot ulcers, 496–497, *497*
    behavioral interventions for, 731–732
    factors in, 729–730
Nonenzymatic glycosylation, 142
Nonnewtonian fluid(s), 107
    properties of, 115, 115t
Non–weight-bearing, for ulcer healing, 151, 245
    patellar tibial brace for, 584, *584*
NPH insulin, perioperative use of, 519
    postoperative use of, 521
Nursing education program(s), wound care component
        of, 676–677
Nutrition, and foot ulcer(s), 212–218
    and wound healing, 212–213, 248–249, 610
    assessment of, 213–216, 213t
        biochemical, 216
        caloric expenditure in, 213–214, 213t
        evaluation of comorbid conditions in, 215
        evaluation of pharmacotherapy in, 215
        macronutrients in, 214
        psychosocial factors in, 215–216
        weight loss in, 213–214
Nutritional support, postoperative, 218
Nutritional therapy, compliance with, 217
    hyperglycemia and, 216–217
    perioperative, 216t, 217–218

Obesity, behavioral interventions for, 732
    truncal, and peripheral arterial disease, 226

Obliterative microangiopathy, 498–499, *499*
Occlusive dressings, *vs.* nonocclusive dressings,
        293
ODS (orthotic dynamic system) splint(s), 322, *322*
Off-loading, 695–697, *696–697*
Oil(s), for wound care, 294t
Onychauxis, 502t
Onychia, 502t
Onychoatrophy, 502t
Onychodystrophy, 502t
Onychogryposis, *503*
Onycholysis, 502t
Onychomadesis, 502t
Onychomalacia, 502t
Onychomycosis, *502,* 502t, *689,* 694
Onychophosis, 502t
Onychophyma, 502t
Onychoschizia, 502t
Oral glucose tolerance test, 4
Orthopedic scooter, 151
Orthosis(es). See also *Insole(s).*
    for Charcot foot, 461–462
    healing shoes with, 325–326, *327*
    in-depth shoes with, 326
    materials for, 329
    resource list for, 331
    total-contact. See *Total-contact orthosis (TCO).*
Orthotic dynamic system (ODS) splint(s), 322, *322*
Osteoarthritis, in contralateral limb, after
        amputation, 644–645
Osteoarthropathy, neuropathic. See *Charcot foot.*
Osteolysis, focal, 334–336, *337–338*
    in Charcot foot, 443
Osteomyelitis, 239, 471–473
    classification of, 472
    diagnosis of, 472
        computed tomography in, 347–348, *348*
        magnetic resonance imaging in, 348, 350,
            350
        radiography in, 340–342, *342–344*
        scintigraphy in, 344, *346,* 347
    in foot ulcers, incidence of, 511
    in grade 3 infection, *280*
    management of, 570, *571–572*
    treatment of, antibiotics in, 477
        before surgery for Charcot foot, 589
    vs. cellulitis, advanced imaging in, 342
    vs. osteoarthropathy, in Charcot foot, 443
Osteotomy, for Charcot foot, 589, *590,* 591
Outsole(s), 171–175, *172–173,* 172t–175t
    modifications to, 433, *433–434*
Oxidation, lipoprotein glycation and, 82
    stress from, reduction of, 87
Oxidation hypothesis, in atherosclerosis, 73
Oxygen, and angiogenesis, 408, *409,* 414
    in collagen production, 406, *406*
    topical, for wound care, 297
Oxygen pressure, inspired, and tissue oxygen tension,
        411, 412t
Oxygen tension, and killing of bacteria, 407,
        408–409
    in tissue, hyperbaric oxygen therapy and, 413–414,
        413–414
        inspired oxygen pressure and, 411, 412t
    transcutaneous. See *Transcutaneous oxygen tension
        (TcPO$_2$).*
Oxygen therapy, hyperbaric. See *Hyperbaric oxygen
        therapy.*
    topical, 409, 411

PAI (plasminogen activator inhibitor), 90–91
Pain, after amputation, in residual limb, 640–641
  from foot ulcers, grading of, 286
  in Charcot foot, 460
  in diabetic neuropathy, 526–527
  in intermittent claudication, 226–230
  in joints, after amputation of contralateral limb,
      644–645
  insensitivity to. See Foot, insensitive.
  intractable, management of, 556
Pain management, in diabetic neuropathy, 51–56,
      51–57, 52t, 55t, 58t
Palmaz stent(s), for percutaneous transluminal
      angioplasty, 381, 382
Palpation, in foot examination, 241
Pamidronate, for Charcot foot, 462
Paresthesia, 53, 54, 55
Paronychia, 693–694
Partial weight-bearing, with total-contact cast, 318
Partial-foot sock(s), 329
Patellar deep tendon reflex, 45
Patellar tibial brace, 584, 584
Patient education, 665–670
  about diabetic neuropathy, 61, 61t
  about exercise, 672–673
  about foot care, 253–254, 254, 255t
  about total-contact cast, 312–314, 313t
  after amputation, 642, 643
  failure of, as legal issue, 761
  for prevention of foot ulcers, 426–429, 428, 740–741
  goal-setting in, 670
  in diabetic foot clinic, 662–664
  role of pedorthist in, 700
  teaching methodology in, 670–672
Patient–health care provider relationship, legal issues
      in, 757–761. See also Legal issue(s).
PDGF. See Platelet-derived growth factor (PDGF).
PDWHF(s) (platelet-derived wound-healing factors),
      556
Peak pressure, athletic shoes and, 168
  in plantar pressure measurement, expected values
      for, 135–136, 136
    plot of, 131–132, 132pl
  maximum, for foot ulcer healing, 153
  with use of total-contact cast, 148–149
Pedal arch, imaging of, before bypass surgery,
      533–534
Pedorthic care, for Charcot foot, 717
  case study of, 722–724, 723–724
  for dorsal ulcers, case study of, 719, 720
  for midtarsal amputation, case study of, 722, 722
  for partial foot amputations, 715–717
  for plantar ulcers, case study of, 718–719, 718–719
  for ray amputation, case study of, 719–720, 721
  for transmetatarsal amputation, case study of,
      720–721, 721
  for ulcers, 714–715
Pedorthist(s), objectives of, 701–702
  role of, 700–701
Pelite, for insoles, 432
  mechanical properties of, 158, 162
Pelvis, motion of, and gait training after amputation,
      648–651
Pencil-cup deformity, of metatarsophalangeal joint,
      344
Penciling, in diabetic osteolysis, 337–338
Penicillin, for foot infections, 476t
Pentoxyfylline, for peripheral vascular disease,
      535–536

Peppermint stick sign, in Charcot foot, 237, 237, 450,
      451
Percutaneous transluminal angioplasty (PTA),
      379–383, 380–384
  advantages of, 379, 388, 393
  catheters for, 379, 380
  in bypass grafts, 385, 388, 392
  mechanism of action in, 380–381, 381
  technique of, 379–380, 380
  with stent, 381, 382–383
    for aortoiliac occlusive disease, 541–542
  with thrombolytic therapy, 381–383, 384
Perforating dermatosis, 205, 205
Perioperative period, diabetes management during,
      513–522. See also Diabetes mellitus,
      perioperative management of.
  nutritional therapy during, 216t, 217–218
Peripheral arterial angioplasty, 383–388, 385–392
  distal abdominal aortic view in, 383, 385
  "kissing" balloon technique in, 383, 386
  patient preparation for, 383
  stents for, 383, 385, 387
Peripheral arterial disease, 221–231, 223t–230t,
      224–230
  acute occlusion in, 230–231, 230t
  ankle pressure in, 223, 224, 358, 359
  capillary filling time in, 230, 230t
  gangrene of toes in, 227, 227pl, 228
  in diabetic vs. nondiabetic patients, 221, 223, 223t
  in lower extremities, clinical diagnosis of, physical
      examination in, 356–357
    morbidity from, 355
    noninvasive studies of, ankle-toe pressure in,
        366–367, 366–367
      choice of, 371
      Doppler ultrasonography in, 361–362, 568
      duplex ultrasonography in, 368–369
      exercise stress testing in, 365, 365–366
      history of, 360
      indications for, 360–361, 370–371
      induction of reactive hyperemia in, 365
      magnetic resonance flowmetry in, 369–370
      photoplethysmography in, 361, 361
      prognostic value of, 356
      radioisotope imaging in, 529
      regional tissue perfusion measurements in,
          367–368
      segmental pressure in, 362, 528, 528
      toe pressure in, 223, 224, 362–363
      waveform evaluation in, 363–364, 363–365,
          529, 529
    pathophysiology of, 357–360, 358–359, 360t
      degree of stenosis in, 358, 358
      segmental pressure in, 358, 359
      vascular response to exercise in, 358–360, 359,
          360t
  microangiopathy in, 223
  pathogenesis of, hyperglycemia in, 225
    hyperinsulinemia in, 225–226
    hyperlipidemia in, 225
    hypertension in, 225
    obesity in, 226–227
    smoking in, 223–225, 224t, 226
  signs and symptoms of, 227–230, 228t, 230, 230t
  skin lesions in, 230, 230
Peripheral neuropathy, 231–236, 232–236
  and amputation, pathogenesis of, 231
  and risk of foot ulcers, 15, 17t
  clinical features of, 231

Peripheral neuropathy (*Continued*)
  etiology of, nondiabetic, 231
  gait in, 235–236
  monofilament testing in, 236, *236*
  painless trauma in, 231–233, *232–235*
Peripheral vascular disease, clinical features of,
    526–527
  diagnosis of, 527–534, *528–533*
    history in, 526
  historical perspective on, 65–66
  in upper extremities, 556–557, *557*
  intractable pain in, management of, 556
  management of, 534–558
    conservative, 534–535
    interventional radiology in, 536–537
    pharmacologic, 535–536
    surgical, *537–554,* 537–555, 541t–546t. See also
      specific disease site, e.g., *Aortoiliac occlusive
      disease.*
      follow-up after, 552–555, *554*
      limb salvage with tissue transfer in, 550–552,
        553
      lumbar sympathectomy in, 552
    nonreconstructible, management of, 555–556
  pathogenesis of, 525–526
  progression of, epidemiology of, 66
  risk factors for, 66–67
  smoking and, 10
Periungual telangiectasia, 197–198
Peroneal artery, 110, *111*
  occlusion of, waveforms in, *364*
Peroneal artery bypass, for infrapopliteal vascular
    occlusive disease, 549, *549, 551*
Peroneal nerve, 486, *487*
  deep, assessment of, in diabetic neuropathy, 47
Peroneus brevis tendon, preservation of, in ray
    amputation, 619, *620*
Peroneus longus muscle, 492, *492*
Peroneus longus tendon, 493, *495*
Pexiganin acetate, for foot infections, 474
PGI₂. See *Prostaglandin I₂.*
Phalanges, hourglass appearance of, in Charcot foot,
    450
  osteomyelitis of, 341, *342*
  resorption of, 336, *338*
    in Charcot foot, *450*
Phantom limb sensation, 640–641
Phenytoin, for paresthesia, 55
Philippines, foot care in, 266
Phlegmon, of dorsal foot, 510
Photoplethysmographically derived digital pressures
    (PPDPs), in peripheral arterial disease,
    366–367, *367*
Photoplethysmography, in peripheral arterial disease,
    361, *361*
Physical conditioning, after amputation, 647–648
Physician, as witness, 763
Physicians' Health Study, 9
Pinprick testing, in diabetic neuropathy,
    43–44
Plantar abscess(es), 499, *500,* 509–510, *510*
  drainage of, 613
  management of, 570, *570*
Plantar aponeurosis, 488, *489–491, 495*
Plantar arteriovenous shunt(s), in diabetic
    neuropathy, diffuse, 36, *37–38,* 59
Plantar artery(ies), 486, *491*
Plantar artery flap, medial, *577*
Plantar callus, and risk of ulceration, 142–143

Plantar fascia, 488, *489*
Plantar flap, for transmetatarsal amputation, 623,
    624
Plantar interossei muscle(s), 492, *492*
Plantar muscle(s), 488, *490–492*
Plantar nerve(s), *487, 490–491*
Plantar pressure, activity level and, footwear
    prescription for, 184t
  areas of, and total-contact orthosis design, 712
  finite element analysis of, 163–164, *164–165*
  high, causes of, 140–146. See also *Foot ulcer(s), risk
    factors for.*
  in rocker bottom foot, 129, *130, 237, 238*
  in rocker *vs.* roller shoes, 172t, *173,* 173–174,
    174t–175t
  measurement of, 129–136, *132–136,* 178–179
    and footwear prescription, 176
    barefoot, 131, 131pl
    data collection in, 131
    devices used in, 129–131
    force-time integral in, 134–135, *135*
    indications for, 138
    in-shoe, 133, *134*
    loading analysis in, 133–135, *135*
    peak pressure in, 131–132, 132pl, 135–136, *136*
    regional analysis in, 132–133, *132–133*
  redistribution of, insoles for, 430–431
  relief of, 701
  threshold for injury from, 136–139, 138pl
  total-contact cast and, 302
Plantar skin, 483
Plantar tissue, shear strain on, shoe uppers and,
    175–176, *176*
Plantar ulcer(s). See *Foot ulcer(s).*
Plantaris muscle, 488
Plantaris tendon, 488
Plaque(s), in necrobiosis lipoidica diabeticorum,
    198–199, *199*
"Plaque cracker" technique, in aortoiliac
    endarterectomy, *541*
Plasma, constituents of, covalent binding of,
    84, *85*
Plasma protein(s), and shear thinning, 114–115
Plasmapheresis, 118, 119t
Plasmin-activating enzyme(s), 118, 119t
Plasminogen activator inhibitor (PAI), 90–91
Plastazote, for insoles, *432*
  for sandals, 325, 435, *435–436*
  for temporary footwear, 435–436, *436*
  mechanical properties of, 157, *158,* 162
Plaster cast(s), for design of total-contact orthosis,
    712–713
Plaster shoe, double-rocker, 315, *315–316*
Plastic surgery. See *Reconstructive surgery.*
Platelet(s), and thrombosis, in diabetes mellitus,
    88–89, 88t
  function of, insulin and, 91
    lipoprotein glycation and, 82
  in atherosclerosis, 70
Platelet releasate(s), for wound healing, 401–402
Platelet-derived growth factor (PDGF), biochemical
    properties of, 398
  for wound healing, 249, 397–399, 556
  in atherosclerosis, 69–70
  receptors for, 398
Platelet-derived wound-healing factor (PDWHFs),
    556
"Plug(s)", for insoles, 167, *168*
Pneumothorax, from hyperbaric oxygen therapy, 412

Podiatrist(s), evaluation by, history in, 683–684
    foot examination by, 684–695, *684–695*. See also
        Foot, examination of.
    frequency of care by, *683*
    off-loading by, 695–697, *696–697*
    role of, 252
Podotrack, 129
Polymyxin B sulfate–bacitracin zinc–neomycin, 291t
Polyneuropathy, distal symmetric, 35–36, *36*
Polyol pathway, in diabetic neuropathy, *39,* 40, 72
Polytetrafluoroethylene (PTFE) graft, for
        femoropopliteal bypass, 543–546, 546t
    for infrapopliteal bypass, 548–549
Popliteal artery, 110, *111,* 486
    calcification of, *531*
    occlusion of, waveforms in, *364*
        with sparing of aorta and iliac artery, 532, *532*
Popliteal to dorsalis pedis bypass, *551, 553*
Positioning, after amputation, 639
Posterior splint(s), for foot ulcers, 322–323, *323*
Postoperative shoe(s), 705, *705*
Posture, and risk of ulceration, 144–145
PPDP(s) (photoplethysmographically derived digital
        pressures), in peripheral arterial disease,
        366–367, *367*
Prandin. See *Repaglinide.*
Pravastatin, clinical trials of, 9
Precose. See *Acarbose.*
Pressure, and gait, 127–129, *130*
Pressure necrosis, of heel, 240, *240*
Pressure ulcer(s). See *Foot ulcer(s).*
Pressure-sensitive socks, 430, *430–431*
Pressure-time integral, in plantar pressure
        measurement, 134
Preulcer(s), 181
Proline, hydroxylation of, and collagen production,
        406, 406–407
Prolyl hydroxylase, kinetics of, *406*
Pronation, control of, insoles for, 431
Proprioception, in diabetic neuropathy, 47
Prostacyclin, and endothelium, 73–74
Prostacyclin stimulating factor (PSF), in
        atherosclerosis, 73
Prostaglandin I$_2$ (PGI$_2$), decreased synthesis of, in
        diabetes mellitus, 73
    for peripheral vascular disease, 535
Prosthesis, ambulation with, metabolic cost of,
        637–638
    fitting of, after transtibial amputation, 630–631, *631*
    for amputees, 645–647
        advances in, 645
        skin care and, 646
        socks for, 646–647
        suspension sleeve for, 646–647
    gait training with, 648–651
        goals of, 651
        horizontal tilt and, 649–650
        lateral shift and, 649
        standing balance and, 648–649
        transverse rotation and, 650–651
        vertical displacement and, 649
    immmediate postoperative, 639
    temporary, for Syme ankle disarticulation, 629, *630*
Protective sensation, loss of. See *Foot, insensitive.*
Protein(s), 108, 214
    plasma, 114–115
    vascular, glycation of, inhibition of, 86–88
        glycoxidation of, 84–88, *85*
    visceral, 216

Protein C, activated, in thrombosis, 90
Protein kinase C, in diabetic neuropathy, 38–39
Proteinuria, 516
Prothrombin fragment, in thrombosis, 89
Pruritus, in diabetes mellitus, 208
Pseudoclaudication, 228
Pseudomonas infection(s), 469–470
PSF. See *Prostacyclin stimulating factor (PSF).*
Psychosocial issue(s), 727–728
    depression as, 732–733, 733t
    diabetic complications as, 728–729, 729t
    in amputation, 728
    in foot care, 252
    in foot ulcers, 728
    in nutrition, 215–216
    interventions for, 730–733, 730t, 733t
    noncompliance as, 729–730
    support groups for, 733
PTA. See *Percutaneous transluminal angioplasty
        (PTA).*
PTB (patellar tendon-bearing) orthosis, for Charcot
        foot, 461
PTFE (polytetrafluoroethylene) graft, for
        femoropopliteal bypass, 543–546, 546t
    for infrapopliteal bypass, 548–549
Pulmonary overpressure accident(s), from hyperbaric
        oxygen therapy, 412, *413*
Pulse, in peripheral arterial disease, 357
Puncture wound(s), 239

Quadratus plantae muscle, 488, *491*
Quality of life, 287

Race, amputation and, 22, *22,* 221
    foot ulcers and, 14, *18*
Radial nerve, 47
Radiography, 333–342, *334–344*
    of bone demineralization, 334–336, *336–338*
    of Charcot foot, 458
    of diabetic neuropathy, 336–340, *339–341*
    of infections, 340–342, *342–344*
    of osteomyelitis, 472
    of skeletal changes, not due to diabetes mellitus,
        333–334, *334–335*
    of vascular disease, *530–533,* 530–534
    magnification, 343–344, *345*
Radiology, interventional. See *Interventional
        radiology.*
Radionuclide imaging, 344, *346, 347,* 472
RAI (resting ankle index), 366
Rancho Los Amigos classification system, for diabetic
        wounds, 274–275
Range of motion, after amputation, 647
    in foot, 694
Ray(s), amputation of, 619, *619–623,* 622–623
    method of, 619, *619–622,* 622
    multiple, 619, *621–622*
    pedorthic care for, 715–716
        case study of, 719–720, *721*
Reactive hyperemia, induction of, 365
Receptors, for advanced glycosylated end products,
        84–86
Reconstructive surgery, clinical assessment in, 568,
        568t
    components of, 567, 568t

Reconstructive surgery (*Continued*)
 free tissue transfer in, 578, 580t, 583, *583*. See also
  Free tissue transfer.
 goals of, 568
 local flaps in, 570, 577–578, *577–582*
 soft tissue, 570, *573–576*
 wound care in, 569–570, *570–572*
  and success of revascularization, 568–569, *569*
Rectus abdominis muscle flap, 583, *583*
Red blood cell(s). See *Erythrocyte(s).*
Regional perfusion index (RPI), 368
Rehabilitation, after amputation. See *Amputation,*
 rehabilitation after.
Relaxation training, 731
Renal failure, and wound healing, 249
 from contrast agents, 343
Renal function, preoperative assessment of, 516
Renal impairment, glycoxidation products and, 86
Renal transplantation, and Charcot foot, 447, 457
Repaglinide, perioperative use of, 520, 520t
Residual limb, care of, 640–642
 compression dressings for, 642
 exercises for, 647–648
Rest pain, in peripheral arterial disease, 229, 357,
 526
Resting ankle index (RAI), 366
Retinopathy, and risk of limb amputation, 23t, 25
 nitric oxide and, 71–72
 pathogenesis of, von Willebrand factor in, 77
 risk of, fasting plasma glucose and, 4
Retrograde venous perfusion, of antibiotics, 474
Revascularization, for foot infections, 478
 success of, wound care and, 568–569, *569*
Reynolds number(s), 109, 109t
Rifampin, for foot infections, 476t
Risk determination, 423–425, *424*
 and patient management, 426–429, *428,* 696–697,
  696–697
  for category 0 patient, 426
  for category 1 patient, 426–427
  for category 2 patient, 427–428, *428*
  for category 3 patient, 428–429
 categorization in, 425–426, 425t
 education and, 16
 information systems for, 749–754. See also
  Information system(s).
 patient education and, 668
 sensory examination in, 423–424, *424*
 vascular examination in, 424–425
Risk stratification grid(s), *753–754*
Rochester Diabetic Neuropathy Study, 34
Rochester Trial, 555
Rocker bottom foot, osteotomy for, *591*
 plantar pressure in, 129, *130,* 237, *238*
Rocker bottom shoe(s), 171–175, *172–173,* 433, *434,*
 706–709, *707–708*
 double, *708,* 708–709
 heel-to-toe, 707, *708*
 mild, 707, *708*
 negative heel, 707–708, *708*
 prescription of, 183–185, 185t
 severe angle, 707, *708*
 toe-only, 707, *708*
Roller bottom shoe(s), 171–175, *172–173,* 172t–175t,
 433, *434*
 prescription of, 183–185, 185t
RPI (regional perfusion index), 368
Rubor, 527
Russia, foot care in, 265

Saline solution, home preparation of, 661t
Sandal(s), custom-made, 325, 714, *714*
 temporary, 435, *435–436*
Saphenous nerve, 486, *487*
Saphenous vein graft, angioplasty of, 388, *392*
 for femoropopliteal bypass, 544, 545t
 for infrapopliteal vascular occlusive disease, 547,
  550, *550*
Scandinavia, foot care in, 264–265
Scandinavian Simvastatin Survival Study, 8
Sciatic nerve, 486, *487*
 assessment of, in diabetic neuropathy, 47
Scintigraphy, 344, *346,* 347, 472
Scleroderma diabeticorum, 204–205
Scooter(s), orthopedic, 151
Seizure(s), from hyperbaric oxygen therapy, 412
Self-care, behavioral interventions for, 731–732
Semmes-Weinstein monofilament(s), 177–178, *236,*
 242
 availability of, 739
 for risk determination, 423–424, *424*
 history of, 738
 in detection of sensation loss, 738–739, *738–739*
 in diabetic neuropathy, 58–59, *59*
 in peripheral neuropathy, 236, *236*
 patient use of, 741–743, *742–743*
 prevention efforts facilitation with, 745–746
Sensation, loss of. See *Foot, insensitive.*
Sensory loss, in foot, 177–178
Sensory neuropathy, 660
Septic arteritis, 498–499, *498–499*
Septic arthritis, of metatarsophalangeal joint, *280*
Sesamoid(s), *492*
Severe angle rocker bottom shoe(s), 707, *708*
Shank(s), steel, for footwear, *709,* 709–710
Sharp-dull test, 688
Shear, reduction of, 701
Shear strain, on plantar tissue, shoe upper and,
 175–176, *176*
Shear stress, 127, 129, *130*
 and risk of ulceration, 143–144
 footwear and, 159
 measurement of, 144
Shock, reduction of, 701
Shoe(s). See also *Footwear.*
 cast, 326–328, *327–328*
  resource list for, 331
 healing, 704–706, *704–706*
  with orthosis, 325–326, *327*
 heel relief, 705, *706*
 in-depth, 706
 negative heel, 705, *705*
 plaster, double-rocker, 315, *315–316*
 postoperative, 705, *705*
 weight relief, 324–325, *325–326*
 wound, *328*
Shoe insert(s). See *Insole(s).*
Short-tau inversion recovery (STIR) imaging, 348, *350*
Shrinker sock(s), 642
Silicon, injection of, 180
Silver, for wound care, 291t
Simvastatin, clinical trials of, 8
Singapore, foot care in, 266
Skin, blood flow to, standing and, 112, *112*
 dry, in diabetic neuropathy, 59
 examination of, *689–693,* 689–694
  for calluses, 690
  for ulcers, 690–692, *690–692*
  in autonomic neuropathy, 689–690, *690*

Skin (*Continued*)
    fragile, as contraindication to total-contact cast, 304
    hypersensitivity of, after amputation, 641–642
    of foot, 483
    xerosis of, *687*
Skin abrasion from total-contact cast, 306
Skin care, with amputee prosthesis, 646
Skin cleanser(s), toxicity of, 289, 289t
    types of, 294t
Skin graft(s), 295–296, 570, *575–576*
    for amputation, 608–609, *609*
    for foot ulcers, *234*
    split-thickness, after osteomyelitis, *572*
        with medial plantar artery flap, *577*
Skin lesion(s), 669–670
    in peripheral arterial disease, 230, *230*
Skin sealant(s), 295t
Skin substitute(s), 295–296, 295t
Small fiber neuropathy, 35
Small fiber test(s), 50, 50t
Smoking, and peripheral vascular disease, 10,
        223–225, 224t, *226*
    and risk of foot ulcers, 16, 17t
    and risk of limb amputation, 23t
    and wound healing, 610
    cessation of, 732
Sock(s), *328,* 328–329, 329t
    biomechanical properties of, 170–171
    for amputee prosthesis, 646–647
    pressure-sensitive, 430, *430–431*
    resource list for, 331
    shrinker, 642
Soft tissue, examination of, 180
    in Charcot foot, 442
    infection of, 341, *343–344*
    reconstructive surgery of, 570, *573–576*
    thickness of, and risk of ulceration, 141
        under metatarsal heads, 180
Soft tissue envelope, from amputation, 608
Soleus muscle, 488
Solid(s), deformation of, *vs.* fluids, 107, *108*
Somatomedin. See *Insulin-like growth factor (IGF).*
South Africa, foot care in, 268
South America, foot care in, 268
Spain, foot care in, 265
Spinal stimulation, epidural, for intractable pain, 556
Splint(s), orthotic dynamic system of, 322, *322*
    plaster, 309, *310*
    posterior, 322–323, *323*
    resource list for, 331
    walking, 150, 316–317
Spring(s), and distribution of force by footwear,
        156–161, *157–158, 160*
    tissue properties and, 162
Stabilizer(s), for footwear, 709, *709*
Standards of care, as legal issue, 758
    case study of, 764–765
Standing, vasoconstrictive response to, 112, *112*
Standing balance, with amputee prosthesis, 648–649
Staphylococcus aureus, and foot infections, 469
Steel shank(s), for footwear, *709,* 709–710
Steinmann pin(s), for arthrodesis, in Charcot foot,
        593, 597, 602, *604–605*
Stent(s), for percutaneous transluminal angioplasty,
        381, *382–383*
    for peripheral arterial angioplasty, 383, 385, *387*
STILE (Surgery Versus Thrombolysis for Lower
        Extremity Ischemia) trial, 555
STIR (short-tau inversion recovery) imaging, 348, *350*

Stockinette, application of, before total-contact cast,
        307–308, *308*
Stocking(s), compression, 329, 329t
Stocking-and-glove nerve damage, in distal symmetric
        polyneuropathy, 35–36, *36*
Stratification grid(s), *753–754*
Stress fracture(s), 333–334, *335, 345*
    after tibiotalocalcaneal arthrodesis, 601, *601*
Stress response, 216
Stress-diathesis model, of depression, 729
Stress-strain relationship, 161–163, *162*
Subchondral bone, microfractures of, 446
Subcutaneous emphysema, 341–342
Suborthelene, for insoles, *432*
Subtalar joint, destruction of, 454–456, *456*
    neuropathy in, 337, *341*
Subungual exostosis, 333, *334*
"Sucked candy" sign, in Charcot foot, 237, *237,* 450,
        451
Sulfonylurea(s), perioperative use of, 519–520, 520t
Support group(s), 733
Sural nerve, 486, *487*
Surgery, metabolic response to, 514–515
Surgery Versus Thrombolysis for Lower Extremity
        Ischemia (STILE) trial, 555
Surgical battery, 760–761
Suspension sleeve, for amputee prosthesis, 646–647
Switzerland, foot care in, 265
Syme ankle disarticulation, 627–629, *628–631*
    ambulation after, 637
    contraindications to, 627, 629
    functional outcome of, 629, *631*
    indications for, 627, *628*
    method of, 627, *629–630*
    postoperative management in, 629, *630*
Sympathetic nervous system, dysfunction of, in
        Charcot foot, 444–445
Syndrome X, 226
Systolic Hypertension in Europe (Syst-Eur) Trial, 7–8

Tabes dorsalis. See *Charcot foot.*
Tailor's bunion, 506
TAL (tendo Achilles lengthening), 187. See also
        Achilles tendon.
Talonavicular joint, destruction of, *449,* 452–454,
        455–456
Tarsal tunnel syndrome, 35, 231
Tarsometatarsal amputation, pedorthic care for, 716
Tarsometatarsal disarticulation, 625, *626*
Tarsometatarsal joint(s), *452*
    arthrodesis of, *598–599*
    destruction of, *449,* 450–452, *452–453*
TBI. See *Toe-brachial index (TBI).*
TCC. See *Total-contact cast (TCC).*
TCO. See *Total-contact orthosis (TCO).*
TcPO$_2$. See *Transcutaneous oxygen tension (TcPO$_2$).*
Technetium-99m scintigraphy, 344, *346,* 347
Tegretol. See *Carbamazepine.*
Telangiectasia, periungual, 197–198
Telephone "hotlines," in diabetic foot clinic(s), 663
Temperature biofeedback, 730–731
Temperature sensation, in foot, assessment of, 242
Tendo Achilles lengthening (TAL), 187. See also
        Achilles tendon.
Tendon. See named tendon.
TGF. See *Transforming growth factor (TGF).*
Thermal injury, 233, 235, *235,* 235pl
Thermal sensitivity, in foot, 242

Thermometry, infrared, in Charcot foot, 460
    in infected foot ulcers, 285
    in inflammation, 427
Thiazolidinedione(s), perioperative use of, 520,
    520t
Thixotropy, 116
Threshold pressure, 136–139
    abnormal values in, definition of, 137
    case study of, 138, 138pl
    factors affecting, 136–137
Throat, on footwear, 702–703, *702–703*
Thrombolysis or Peripheral Arterial Surgery (TOPAS)
    trial, 555
Thrombolytic therapy, for occluded bypass grafts,
    554–555
    with percutaneous transluminal angioplasty,
    381–383, *384*
Thrombosis, activated protein C in, 90
    antithrombin III in, 89–90
    clinical studies of, 91–92
    coagulation in, 89
    fibrinogen in, 89
    fibrinolytic system in, 90–91
    fibrinopeptide A in, 89
    mechanisms of, 88
    platelets in, 88–89, 88t
    prevention of, 91–92
    prothrombin fragment F1+2 in, 89
Thromboxane, and endothelium, 74
Tibia, osteotomy of, for Charcot foot, *595*
Tibial angioplasty, 385, *390–391*
Tibial artery, 110, *111,* 486
    atherosclerosis of, 525–526
    occlusion of, *538*
        digital subtraction angiography in, *375*
        waveforms in, *363–364*
Tibial nerve, 486, *487*
    in diabetic neuropathy, 47
Tibialis anterior tendon, insertion of, *495*
    reattachment of, after midtarsal disarticulation,
    626
Tibialis posterior tendon, *492,* 492–493
Tibiocalcaneal arthrodesis, for Charcot foot,
    593
Tibiotalar joint, fracture-dislocation of, *594–595*
Tibiotalocalcaneal arthrodesis, stress fracture after,
    601, *601*
Ticlopidine, for peripheral vascular disease, 535
Tip-top-toe ulcer syndrome, 236, *236*
Tissue graft(s), for wound healing, 249–250
Tissue ischemia, in foot ulceration, 139
Tissue necrosis, progression of, 498–499, *498–499*
Tissue oxygen tension. See *Oxygen tension, in
    tissue.*
Tissue perfusion, regional, in peripheral arterial
    disease, 367–368
Tissue plasminogen activator (t-PA), 90
Tissue transfer, with limb salvage, in peripheral
    vascular disease, 550–552, *553*
Toe(s), "baked potato," 686, *686*
    claw. See *Claw toe.*
    deformities of, 503–506, *504–507*
    disarticulation of, *616–618,* 616–619
        functional outcome in, 618–619
        pedorthic care for, 715–716
        technique for, 616–618, *616–618*
    gangrene of, 227, 227pl, *228*
        from theraml injury, 233, *235*
    web infections of, 505

Toe fillet flap, 578
Toe pressure, in peripheral arterial disease, 223, *224,*
    362–363
Toe sock(s), 328, *328*
Toe spring, from rocker *vs.* roller shoes, *172,* 172–173,
    183
Toe-brachial index (TBI), 528–529
Toenail(s), anatomy of, 484, *485*
    care of, patient education about, 671
    deformities of, 501–503, *502–504,* 502t
    examination of, 689, *689*
    ingrown, *503–504*
    terminology related to, 502t
    yellow, 206
Toe-only rocker bottom shoe(s), 707, *708*
TOPAS (Thrombolysis or Peripheral Arterial Surgery)
    trial, 555
Topical oxygen therapy, 409, 411
    for wound care, 297
Total-contact cast (TCC), 146–151, 245, 301–319,
    321–322, *322*
    advantages of, 305, 305t
    ambulation with, 313–314
    and plantar pressure, 302
    application of, *306–312,* 306–314, 313t
        cast boot for, 311, *312*
        documentation of ulcer size before, 306, *306*
        donning of stockinette before, 307–308, *308*
        felt padding in, 309
        foam layer in, 308, *308*
        patient positioning for, 307, *307*
        patient preparation for, 306–311, *306–311*
        plaster for, 309, *309–310*
        precautions for, 315
        protective board for, 309, *311*
        use of dressings before, 306, *307*
        walking heel for, 309–311, *311*
    bivalved, 150
    case study of, 318, *319*
    changing of, 314, *314*
    clinical trials of, 149–150
    compliance with, 317–318
    complications of, 150
    contraindications to, 304–305, 304t
    development of, 146, 148
    disadvantages of, 305–306, 305t
    efficacy of, 302–303, *303–304*
    follow-up with, 314
    for Charcot foot, 461, 662
    for heel ulcers, 150
    healing curves for, *147*
    history of, 301–302
    indications for, 303, 304t
    load relief from, 148
    modifications of, 315–317, *315–317*
    partial weight-bearing with, 318
    patient education about, 312–314, 313t
    peak pressure with, 148–149
    principles of, 301–302
    removal of, 314, *314*
    ulcer recurrence rate after, 314
    with assistive devices, 318
Total-contact orthosis (TCO), 710–713, *712*
    design of, evaluation of lower limb biomechanics
        and, 711–712
        foot impression techniques for, 712
        identification of plantar pressure areas and,
        712
        plaster casts for, 712–713

Total-contact orthosis (TCO) (*Continued*)
  for Charcot foot, 717, 722–723, *723*
  for foot ulcers, 714–715
  for plantar ulcers, 714–715
  for tarsometatarsal amputation, 716–717
  for toe and ray amputations, 716
  for transmetatarsal amputations, 716
  materials for, 713
Touch, sense of, in diabetic neuropathy, 47–48
t-PA. See *Tissue plasminogen activator (t-PA)*.
Tramadol, for paresthesia, 55
Transcutaneous oxygen tension (TcPO₂), and
      indication for hyperbaric oxygen therapy, 416,
      416
  and risk of amputation, 23t
  and risk of foot ulcers, 15, 17t
  in peripheral arterial disease, 368, 529–530,
      568
  stage of neuropathy and, *38*
Transfemoral amputation, 632, 634
  ambulation after, energy expenditure from,
      637
  gait after, 644–645
Transfemoral arteriography, 532
Transfer(s), after amputation, 639–640
Transforming growth factor (TGF), 399–400
Transmetatarsal amputation, 623–625, *624*
  complications of, 188
  footwear prescription for, 185, 186t
  pedorthic care for, 716
    case study of, 720–721, *721*
Transplantation, renal, and Charcot foot, 447,
      457
Transtibial amputation, 630–632, *631, 633*
  ambulation after, energy expenditure from,
      637
  contour of, for prosthesis fitting, 630–631,
      631
  functional outcome of, 632
  gait after, 644–645
  method of, 630–632, *631, 633*
  preservation of knee in, 630–632
  wound closure after, 632, *633*
Trauma, and Charcot foot, 565, *566–567*
  and development of foot lesion, 497
  and diabetic dermopathy, 202
  and peripheral vascular disease, 525
  from home surgery, 233, *234*
  mechanical, and Charcot foot, 445–446
  painless, in peripheral neuropathy, 231–233,
      232–235
  to heel, 239–240, *240*
Treadmill exercise stress testing, in peripheral
      arterial disease, *365*, 365–366
Triamcinolone acetonide, for necrobiosis lipoidica
      diabeticorum, 200
Triceps tendon reflex, 46–47
Trichophyton rubrum infection(s), from total-contact
      cast, 306
Tricyclic antidepressant(s), for paresthesia, 55
Triglyceride(s), and risk of peripheral vascular
      disease, 66
Trimethoprim-sulfamethoxazole, for foot infections,
      476t
Trovafloxacin, for foot infections, 475
Truncal obesity, and peripheral arterial disease,
      226
Tumor necrosis factor-α (TNF-α), in
      atherosclerosis, 69

Tuning fork, for foot examination, 241
  training in use of, 740
Two-point discrimination, in diabetic neuropathy,
      42–43, *45–46*

UKPDS. See *United Kingdom Prospective Diabetes
      Study (UKPDS)*.
Ulcer(s), biomechanical problems and, 126t
  foot. See *Foot ulcer(s)*.
  heel. See *Heel ulcer(s)*.
  in necrobiosis lipoidica diabeticorum, *200*
  venous stasis, 557–558
Ultralente insulin, perioperative use of, 519
  postoperative use of, 521
Ultram. See *Tramadol*.
Ultrasonography, Doppler, 361–362, 568
  duplex, 368–369
  for wound healing, 250, 297
  intravascular, 376, *376*
Ungius incarnatus, 502t, *503–504*
United Kingdom, foot care in, 262, 264
United Kingdom Prospective Diabetes Study
      (UKPDS), 6
  on hyperglycemia, 37, 39t
University of Texas Diabetic Foot Classification
      System, 696–697, *696–697*
University of Texas Wound Classification System,
      691, *692*
Upper extremity(ies), vascular disease in, 556–557,
      557

Vacuum-assisted closure, for wound care, 297,
      583–584
Valgus deformity, realignment and arthrodesis for,
      598–599
Vancomycin, for foot infections, 476t
Varus deformity, in Charcot foot, *592, 594, 597*
  of toes, 505
Vasa nervorum, in diabetic neuropathy, 37–40, *39*
Vascular belt, internal, 486
Vascular cell adhesion molecule (VCAM), and
      atherosclerosis, 75–76
Vascular disease, diagnosis of, 527–534, *528–533*
    noninvasive imaging in, 527–530, *528–529*
    physical examination in, 527, 685–687, *686*
    radiography in, *530–533*, 530–534
  incidence of, 524–525
  pathogenesis of, 525–526
  peripheral. See *Peripheral vascular disease*.
Vascular endothelial growth factor (VEGF), and
      wound healing, 397
  oxygen and, 408
Vascular occlusive disease, infrapopliteal. See
      Infrapopliteal vascular occlusive disease.
Vasoconstriction, hyperbaric oxygen therapy and, 412
  in wound healing, 396
  standing and, 112, *112*
Vasodilatation, in wound healing, 396
Vasodilator(s), 535
Vasopressor(s), 227
VCAM. See *Vascular cell adhesion molecule (VCAM)*.
VEGF. See *Vascular endothelial growth factor
      (VEGF)*.
Vein graft(s), angioplasty of, 385, 388, *392*
Venous filling time, 669

Venous insufficiency, management of, 557–558
Venous refill time, 357
Venous stasis ulcer(s), 557–558
Verapamil, for claudication, 535
Very low-density lipoprotein (VLDL), and risk of
    peripheral vascular disease, 66
  glycation of, 83
  in diabetes mellitus, 77–78
Veterans Administration Cooperative Study on
    Antiplatelet Agents in Diabetic Patients After
    Amputation for Gangrene, 9–10
Vibration perception threshold (VPT), and risk of
    amputation, 23t
  and risk of foot ulcers, 15, 17t
  measurement of, *688*, 688–689
Visceral protein, in nutritional assessment,
    216
Viscoelasticity, of blood, 115t, 116
Viscosity, and blood flow, 109–110
  kinematic, 109
Visual analog scale, for pain assessment, 286
Vitamin(s), and wound healing, 214–215
Vitiligo, 206, 206pl
VLDL. See *Very low-density lipoprotein (VLDL)*.
von Willebrand factor, and endothelium, in
    atherosclerosis, 75–77
VPT. See *Vibration perception threshold (VPT)*.

Wagner classification system, for diabetic wounds,
    274–275
  for risk categorization, 425–426, 425t
Walker(s), neuropathic, *323*, 323–324
  prefabricated, 324, *324*
Walking heel, for total-contact cast, 309–311,
    311
Walking splint(s), 150, 316–317
Wallstent, for percutaneous transluminal angioplasty,
    381, *383*
Warmth therapy, for wound care, 297
Wartenberg pinwheel, use of, 43
Waveform(s), in peripheral arterial disease, *363–364,*
    363–365, 529, *529*
Wax, for foot impressions, 713
Waxy skin syndrome, 202–204
Weakness, 181–182
  and risk of ulceration, 143
Web infection(s), 505
Wedge(s), for footwear, 710, *710*
"Wedge effect," 691
Weight, body, and risk of ulceration, 144
Weight loss, assessment of, 213–214
  behavioral interventions for, 732
Weight relief shoe(s), 324–325, *325–326*
Weight-bearing, concentrated, and development of
    foot lesions, 497, *505*
  partial, with total-contact cast, 318
Werner's syndrome, 207–208
WESDR (Wisconsin Epidemiologic Study of Diabetic
    Retinopathy), 5
Wet gangrene, 611–614, *614*
Wheelchair mobility, 640
Whirlpool therapy, for foot ulcers, 245, 288
White blood cell(s). See *Leukocyte(s)*.
White blood cell imaging, indium-111, 347
  in Charcot foot, 458–459
  in osteomyelitis, 472
Wisconsin Epidemiologic Study of Diabetic
    Retinopathy (WESDR), 5

Witness(es), physicians as, 763
World Health Organization (WHO), St. Vincent
    Declaration of, 262
Wound(s), classification systems for, by etiology,
    274
  depth-ischemia, 276–282, 276t, *277–281*
    flow chart for, *278*
    grade 0, 276, *277, 279*
    grade 1, *277, 278, 279*
    grade 2, *277, 279*
    grade 3, 279, *280–281*
    grade A, *277, 279*
    grade B, 280
    grade C, 280
    grade D, 280
    prognosis in, 282
    purpose of, 276
  history of, 273–274
  ideal characteristics of, 273
  of Lavery, Armstrong, and Harkless, 274
  of Pecoraro and Reiber, 274
  University of Texas, 691, *692*
  Wagner, 274–275
  cleansing of, 288–289, 289t
  cultures of, 285, 469–470
  debridement of, 287–288
  description of, documentation of, 285–286
  irrigation of, 289
    Kritter flow-through system for, 614,
      614–615
  puncture, and infection, 239
Wound care, adjunctive therapy for, 296–297
  algorithm for, *298, 585*
  ancient, 242t
  and success of revascularization, 568–569, *569*
  antibacterial agents for, topical, 289–290,
    291t
  complexity of, 283–284
  dressings for, 290–293, 292t–295t. See also
    Dressing(s).
  glycemic control in, 285
  goals of, 286–287
  holistic approach to, 297–299, *298*
  in diabetic foot clinic, 661–662, 661t
  in reconstructive surgery, 569–570, *570–572*
  initial assessment in, 284–286
  interdisciplinary collaboration in, 284
  products for, 294t–295t
  sterile *vs.* nonsterile, 293
Wound care nurse(s), benefits provided by, 680
  qualifications of, 676–678, 678t
  role of, 680
  services provided by, 678–679
Wound filler(s), 295t
Wound healing, adjunctive therapy for, 249–250
  after amputation, 611
  complexity of, 283–284
  drugs affecting, 215
  factors affecting, 610
  fibroplasia in, 396–397
  growth factors and, 295t, 397–401, 556
  hyperbaric oxygen therapy and, 404–417, 415, 415t,
    416. See also *Hyperbaric oxygen therapy*.
  hyperglycemia and, 216–217, 514
  immunosuppression and, 249
  impediments to, 248–249, 248t
  inflammation in, 396
  macronutrients and, 214
  macrophages and, 396

Wound healing (*Continued*)
  micronutrients and, 214–215
  nutrition and, 212–213, 248–249, 610
  phases of, 396–397
  platelet releasates for, 401–402
  smoking and, 610
Wound margin(s), assessment of, 286
Wound Ostomy Continence Nurses Society, programs
    of, 676–677, 678t
Wound pouch(es), 295t
"Wound score," 274
Wound shoe(s), *328*
Wrist, deep tendon reflex in, 45–46
  extension of, 47
  flexion of, 47

Xanthoma, eruptive, 207, *207*
Xenon-133, clearance of, in peripheral vascular
    disease, 529
Xerosis, *687*

Yellow nail(s), 206
Yellow skin, 206

Zinc, and wound healing, 214–215

ISBN 1-55664-471-X